Dukes' Physiology of Domestic Animals

This book is dedicated to my wife Shirley Ann Bruckner Reece, born 12/03/1932, died 09/29/1999.

Thanks to God for the gift of Shirley for the 46 years of our marriage and for the seven children (Mary Kay, Kathy Ann, Barbara Jean, Sara Lucinda, Anna Marie, Susan Theresa, and William Omar II) we were privileged to bring forth. Shirley was raised in Chicago, and received her BS in Foods and Nutrition at Iowa State University. We were united in marriage prior to receiving our degrees in 1954.

Shirley was a model wife and mother. At every age, she had wisdom beyond her years and was admired by all who knew her. She personified joy, received by grace through God, enjoyed life and loved Ames. Because of her example, support for my vocation, and enthusiasm for family, church, community, and the veterinary profession, I have been encouraged to continue with *Dukes' Physiology of Domestic Animals* and thereby give honor for her presence throughout much of my life.

W.O.R.

Dukes' Physiology of Domestic Animals

Thirteenth Edition

Editor

William O. Reece DVM, PhD

University Professor Emeritus
Department of Biomedical Sciences
College of Veterinary Medicine
Iowa State University, Ames, Iowa
USA

Associate Editors

Howard H. Erickson DVM, PhD

Professor Emeritus of Physiology
Department of Anatomy and Physiology
College of Veterinary Medicine
Kansas State University, Manhattan, Kansas
USA

Jesse P. Goff DVM, PhD

Professor and Anderson Chair
Department of Biomedical Sciences
College of Veterinary Medicine
Iowa State University, Ames, Iowa
USA

Etsuro E. Uemura DVM, MS, PhD

Professor
Department of Biomedical Sciences
College of Veterinary Medicine
Iowa State University, Ames, Iowa
USA

WILEY Blackwell

The first through twelfth editions of this volume were published by Comstock Publishing Associates, an imprint of Cornell University Press. Publication of the 13th edition has been made possible by arrangement with Cornell University Press.

Editorial Offices
1606 Golden Aspen Drive, Suites 103 and 104, Ames, Iowa 50010, USA
The Atrium, Southern Gate, Chichester, West Sussex, PO19 8SQ, UK
9600 Garsington Road, Oxford, OX4 2DQ, UK

For details of our global editorial offices, for customer services and for information about how to apply for permission to reuse the copyright material in this book please see our website at www.wiley.com/wiley-blackwell.

Authorization to photocopy items for internal or personal use, or the internal or personal use of specific clients, is granted by Blackwell Publishing, provided that the base fee is paid directly to the Copyright Clearance Center, 222 Rosewood Drive, Danvers, MA 01923. For those organizations that have been granted a photocopy license by CCC, a separate system of payments has been arranged. The fee codes for users of the Transactional Reporting Service are ISBN-13: 978-0-1185-0139-9/2015.

Library of Congress Cataloging-in-Publication Data
Dukes' physiology of domestic animals. – 13th edition / editor, William O. Reece ; associate editors, Howard H. Erickson, Jesse P. Goff, Etsuro E. Uemura.
　　p. ;　cm.
　　Physiology of domestic animals
　　Preceded by Dukes' physiology of domestic animals. 12th ed. / edited by William O. Reece. Ithaca, N.Y. : Comstock Pub./Cornell University Press, 2004.
　　Includes bibliographical references and index.
　　ISBN 978-1-118-50139-9 (cloth)
　I. Reece, William O., editor.　II. Erickson, Howard H., 1936- , editor.　III. Goff, Jesse P., editor.　IV. Uemura, Etsuro E., editor.
　V. Title: Physiology of domestic animals.
　[DNLM: 1. Animals, Domestic–physiology. 2. Physiology, Comparative. SF 768]
　SF768
　636.089′2–dc23
　　　　　　　　　　　　　　　　　2014050190
A catalogue record for this book is available from the British Library.

Contents

List of Contributors

Michele Borgarelli DMV, PhD
Diplomate
European College of Veterinary Internal Medicine (Cardiology)
Associate Professor of Cardiology
Virginia-Maryland Regional College of Veterinary Medicine
Blacksburg, VA
USA
(Senior author of Chapter 39)

Scott A. Brown VMD, PhD
Diplomate
American College of Veterinary Internal Medicine
Edward H. Gunst Professor of Small Animal Studies and Josiah Meigs
Distinguished Teaching Professor
Departments of Physiology and Pharmacology and Small Animal Medicine
and Surgery
College of Veterinary Medicine
University of Georgia
Athens, GA
USA
(Author of Chapter 40)

Richard L. Engen MS, PhD
Professor Emeritus
Department of Biomedical Sciences
College of Veterinary Medicine
Iowa State University
Ames, IA
USA
(Coauthor of Chapter 30)

Howard H. Erickson DVM, PhD
Emeritus Professor
Department of Anatomy and Physiology
College of Veterinary Medicine
Kansas State University
Manhattan, KS
USA
(Coauthor of Chapters 37 and 41; Editor of Section VI; volume Associate
Editor)

Robert F. Gilmour, Jr PhD
Vice President, Research and Graduate Studies
Professor of Biomedical Sciences
University of Prince Edward Island
Charlottetown, PE
Canada
(Senior author of Chapters 31 and 32)

Jesse P. Goff DVM, PhD
Professor and Anderson Chair
Department of Biomedical Sciences
College of Veterinary Medicine
Iowa State University
Ames, IA
USA
(Author of Chapters 42–45, 47–50, and 51; Editor of Sections VII, VIII, and IX;
volume Associate Editor)

Patrick J. Gorden DVM
Director
Food Supply Veterinary Medicine
Veterinary Diagnostic and Production Animal Medicine
College of Veterinary Medicine
Iowa State University
Ames, IA
USA
(Senior author of Chapter 54)

Jens Häggström DVM, PhD
Diplomate
European College of Veterinary Internal Medicine (Cardiology)
Department of Clinical Sciences
Faculty of Veterinary Medicine and Animal Science
Swedish University of Agricultural Sciences
Uppsala
Sweden
(Coauthor of Chapter 39)

Eileen M. Hasser PhD
Professor
Department of Biomedical Sciences, College of Veterinary Medicine
Department of Medical Pharmacology and Physiology
Resident Investigator, Dalton Cardiovascular Research Center
University of Missouri
Columbia, MO
USA
(Coauthor of Chapters 34 and 35; Senior author of Chapter 38)

Cheryl M. Heesch PhD
Professor
Department of Biomedical Sciences, College of Veterinary Medicine
Resident Investigator, Dalton Cardiovascular Research Center
University of Missouri
Columbia, MO
USA
(Senior author of Chapter 35; Coauthor of Chapters 34 and 38)

Patricia A. Johnson PhD
Professor and Chair
Department of Animal Science
College of Agriculture and Life Sciences
Cornell University
Ithaca, NY
USA
(Author of Chapter 55)

David D. Kline PhD
Associate Professor
Department of Biomedical Sciences, College of Veterinary Medicine
Resident Investigator, Dalton Cardiovascular Research Center
University of Missouri
Columbia, MO
USA
(Senior author of Chapter 34; Coauthor of Chapters 35 and 38)

M. Harold Laughlin PhD
Curators' Professor and Chair
Department of Biomedical Sciences, College of Veterinary Medicine
Professor
Department of Medical Pharmacology and Physiology
Investigator, Dalton Cardiovascular Research Center
University of Missouri
Columbia, MO
USA
(Coauthor of Chapters 36 and 38)

John W. Ludders DVM
Diplomate
American College of Veterinary Anesthesia and Analgesia
Professor Emeritus
Department of Clinical Sciences
College of Veterinary Medicine
Cornell University
Ithaca, NY
USA
(Author of Chapter 26)

Luis A. Martinez-Lemus DVM, PhD
Associate Professor
Department of Medical Pharmacology and Physiology and Dalton Cardiovascular Research Center
University of Missouri
Columbia, MO
USA
(Senior author of Chapter 36)

N. Sydney Moïse DVM, MS
Diplomate
American College of Veterinary Internal Medicine
Professor of Medicine
Department of Clinical Sciences
College of Veterinary Medicine
Cornell University
Ithaca, NY
USA
(Coauthor of Chapter 32)

David C. Poole PhD, DSc
Fellow, American College of Sports Medicine
Professor
Departments of Kinesiology, Anatomy and Physiology
Kansas State University
Manhattan, KS
USA
(Senior author of Chapters 37 and 41)

William O. Reece DVM, PhD
University Professor Emeritus
Department of Biomedical Sciences
College of Veterinary Medicine
Iowa State University
Ames, IA
USA
(Author of Chapters 11–25, 27–29, 52, and 53; Senior author of Chapter 46; Editor of Sections II, III, IV, and V; volume Editor)

Dean H. Riedesel DVM, PhD
Diplomate
American College of Veterinary Anesthesia and Analgesia
Professor
Department of Veterinary Clinical Sciences
College of Veterinary Medicine
Iowa State University
Ames, IA
USA
(Author of Chapter 33; Senior author of Chapter 30)

Leo L. Timms PhD
Morrill Professor
Departments of Animal Science and Veterinary Diagnostics and Production Animal Medicine
Colleges of Agriculture and Veterinary Medicine
Iowa State University
Ames, IA
USA
(Coauthor of Chapter 54)

Darrell W. Trampel DVM, PhD (Deceased)
Professor
Poultry Extension Veterinarian
Department of Veterinary Diagnostic and Production Animal Medicine
College of Veterinary Medicine
Iowa State University
Ames, IA
USA
(Coauthor of Chapter 46)

Etsuro E. Uemura DVM, PhD
Professor
Department of Biomedical Sciences
College of Veterinary Medicine
Iowa State University
Ames, IA
USA
(Author of Chapters 1–10; Editor of Section I; volume Associate Editor)

Preface

We are pleased to continue the legacy established in 1933 by Dr H. Hugh Dukes when the lithoprinted first edition of *The Physiology of Domestic Animals* was published by Edwards Brothers, Inc., Ann Arbor, Michigan. The preface by H.H. Dukes included the following opening statement:

> This book was written mainly at Iowa State College; it was completed at Cornell University. Based on nearly fifteen years of experience in the field of animal physiology, it represents an attempt to provide students of veterinary medicine with a suitable textbook for their course in physiology. I believe also, on the basis of experience, that much of the book will be useful to students of animal husbandry. Furthermore, I venture the opinion that practitioners of veterinary medicine who wish to keep up with the trend in physiology will find the book helpful.

The first two lithoprinted editions were followed by the third revised edition in 1935 with an improved format, printed from type, by Comstock Publishing Company, Inc., Ithaca and New York. The seventh edition, the last edition authored by Dr Dukes, was published in 1955. It was the first to be published by Comstock Publishing Associates, a Division of Cornell University Press, Ithaca and London, who continued as publishers for the 8th, 9th, 10th, 11th, and 12th editions, which published in 2004.

The 8th edition was the first to be multiauthored and was begun by Dr Melvin J. Swenson as editor. Dr Swenson continued as editor for the 9th and 10th editions and coedited with Dr William O. Reece for the 11th edition. Dr Reece edited the 12th edition, the last one to be published by Cornell University Press. Publishing rights were licensed by Cornell University Press to John Wiley & Sons, Inc. for the 13th multiauthored book with William O. Reece, Editor, and Howard H. Erickson, Jesse P. Goff, and Etsuro E. Uemura, Associate Editors.

The vision of Dr Dukes for his textbook *The Physiology of Domestic Animals*, which was to provide students of veterinary medicine with a suitable textbook for their courses in physiology, and to be useful to students in animal husbandry and practitioners of veterinary medicine, has been a goal throughout all the years since the first edition and is being continued with the 13th edition.

Many features of the previous edition will be continued that include the following for each chapter.

1 The text content is preceded by an outline listing the first- and second-order headings.
2 A brief introduction.
3 A list of questions that precede each first-order heading that alert students to important information that follows. Answers to the questions will be found in the text that follows.
4 Key words are in bold color on first use.
5 Meaningful self-evaluation exercises are provided at the end of each chapter that feature important facts or concepts.
6 Answers, explanations, or solutions are provided for each self-evaluation exercise.

Conscientious use of the above features provide not only an organized study when first used, but also a quick review when needed for future use.

Our effort to identify the 13th edition as an all-new work is apparent in many ways. The chapters within several sections have a single author and their number reduced in other sections. This permits greater consistency of presentation and content overlap is minimized.

An important change was made for the renal and respiratory chapters. Previously the entire topic of each was presented in a single chapter. Now, the one single chapter has been divided into several chapters where emphasis can be focused on a single concept. This will facilitate lecture organization and selective referral.

A notable addition to this edition is the provision of full color throughout. The use of color not only enhances the attractiveness but also provides a means for contrast within the text and figures.

Other features include a downloaded version of the 13th edition available online. All figures and tables will be on PowerPoint to facilitate lecture presentations. An effort has been made to reduce pagination of the volume while at the same time providing increasing font size and space for figures and tables. Overall, the 13th edition of *Dukes' Physiology of Domestic Animals* will continue with its classic stature as a comprehensive resource, not only stressing basic physiology with application to animals, but also with updated features to assist teaching effectiveness.

William O. Reece

Acknowledgments

We are grateful for the efforts of Erica Judisch, Commissioning Editor, Veterinary Medicine, Wiley Blackwell, Heidi Lovette, Science Editor, Cornell University Press, and Tonya Cook, Rights Manager, Cornell University Press, for successfully negotiating the transfer of rights from Cornell University Press to Wiley Blackwell. Their professionalism and patience throughout a complex process is appreciated.

Cornell University Press has been as important to the success of the book as the legacy of *The Physiology of Domestic Animals*, that began with Dr Dukes, whose publishing career was spanned at Ithaca. The continued integrity and cooperation of Cornell University Press as publisher during my tenure was always apparent. My appreciation and thanks are extended to all directors, science editors and staff throughout the years for their efforts.

A project of this complexity requires participation by many individuals. My indebtedness and thanks are extended to these very nice people.

The authors and section editors, in addition to their teaching, research, service, and administrative duties, devoted their talents to this project.

Much of my time during the preliminary phases and preparation of manuscripts involved the Veterinary Medical Library, Iowa State University. Kristi Schaaf, Director, was a friendly, knowledgeable resource for location of reference material and other information as needed. Also helpful was Lana Greve, Library Assistant.

Dr Anumantha Kanthasamy, Professor and Chair, Department of Biomedical Sciences, College of Veterinary Medicine, Iowa State University, provided office resources and services, assisted by Linda Erickson, Administrative Specialist, William Robertson, Laboratory Supervisor, and Kim Adams. Paige Behrens, Office Assistant and Iowa State University student in Graphic Design, assisted by Megan Demoss, transformed my manuscripts and all other essential items to computer documents.

Drs Howard Erickson, Jesse Goff, and Etsuro Uemura, Associate Editors for this volume, helped in the planning and its execution. Their advice, enthusiasm, and hard work have never wavered, and their innovations have provided a new freshness. In addition, Dr Howard Erickson provided faithful support and planning for the 12th edition.

Mal Rooks Hoover, Certified Medical Illustrator, College of Veterinary Medicine, Kansas State University, generously provided her expertise to enhance the effectiveness, for many of the figures, including color, that appear in the chapters authored by Dr Reece, Dr Erickson, and several other authors in the cardiovascular section. We are grateful for her effort on our behalf.

Dr Darrell Trampel sadly passed away during the production of this book. He will be greatly missed by colleagues and friends.

Nancy Turner, Senior Development Editor, Wiley Blackwell, provided timely information and guidance from the very beginning of the project. Her knowledge, experience, professionalism, and assistance in all phases were extremely helpful. This effort was continued by the expertise of Catriona Cooper, Senior Project Editor, Wiley Blackwell, in finalizing the manuscript and the associated details required for submission to the copy editor. Our thanks are extended to Nancy and Catriona on behalf of all the authors, for their patient and friendly assistance and attention to details. Extended thanks to Kathy Syplywczak, Project Manager, and Jolyon Philips, copy editor, for their expertise and attention to detail that was needed in making this edition a volume for which we can all be proud.

Above all, I thank God for this community of people and for His answer to my many prayers for this project.

William O. Reece

Tributes to Drs H. Hugh Dukes and Melvin J. Swenson

Veterinary educators, researchers, authors, and administrators

Dr H. Hugh Dukes (1895–1987)

Dr Melvin J. Swenson (1917–2005)

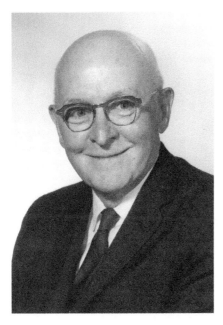

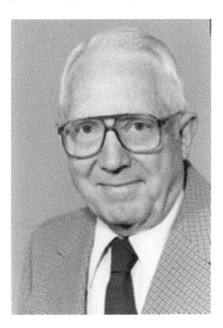

BS, Clemson College, 1915; DVM, Iowa State College, 1918; United States Army, 1918–1920; MS, 1923, Iowa State College; Assistant Professor, Veterinary Physiology and Physiology Research, Division of Veterinary Medicine, Iowa State College, 1921–1932; Professor and Head, Department of Veterinary Physiology, New York State Veterinary College at Cornell University, 1932–1960. Author, *The Physiology of Domestic Animals*, Editions 1–7, 1933–1955.

DVM, 1943, College of Veterinary Medicine, Kansas State University; United States Army Veterinary Corps, 1943–1946; MS, 1947, PhD, 1950, College of Veterinary Medicine, Iowa State University; Professor and Head, Veterinary Physiology and Pharmacology, College of Veterinary Medicine, Iowa State University, 1957–1973; Professor of Veterinary Anatomy, Physiology, and Pharmacology, College of Veterinary Medicine, Iowa State University, 1973–1987; Editor, *Dukes' Physiology of Domestic Animals*, Editions 8–11, 1970–1993.

About the companion website

This book is accompanied by a companion website:

www.wiley.com/go/reece/physiology

The website includes:

- Review questions and self-evaluation exercises from the book
- Powerpoints of all figures from the book for downloading
- PDFs of all tables from the book for downloading

Neurophysiology

Section Editor: Etsuro E. Uemura

1 Nervous Tissue

Etsuro E. Uemura

Iowa State University, Ames, IA, USA

The nervous system has two categories of cells, neurons (Greek *neuron*, nerve) and neuroglia (Greek *glia*, glue). Their names reflect the fact that neurons give rise to nerves, while neuroglia are thought of as cells simply holding neurons together. Neurons and neuroglia are far more complex in their shape than cells in any other tissue. Their morphological heterogeneity reflects the functional complexity of the nervous system. Neurons and neuroglia play different roles in the nervous tissue. Neurons are specialized in information processing. Specialized contact areas called synapses mediate signals from one neuron to others. Synapses are the basis of complex neuronal networks designed for information processing. Neurons stop dividing within a few months after birth. Therefore, if nerve damage involves cell bodies in the adult animal, resulting neuronal death will permanently change the structure and functions of the affected areas. Unlike neurons, neuroglia continue to divide. This glial capacity to divide is essential for their structural and functional support of neurons. Neurons and glial cells require a chemically stable environment. Endothelial cells of the central nervous system and the choroid plexus help maintain such an environment by regulating molecules secreted into the interstitial fluid and cerebrospinal fluid (CSF).

system. All nervous tissue other than the cerebrum, brainstem, cerebellum, and spinal cord is referred to as the **peripheral nervous system (PNS)**. The PNS comprises the nerves, ganglia (spinal, cranial, sympathetic trunk, collateral, terminal), and sensory receptors. The PNS conveys (i) sensory signals about the external and internal environment of the body to the CNS and (ii) motor signals from the CNS to the peripheral effectors (skeletal muscle, cardiac muscle, smooth muscle, secretory glands). Certain neural components of the CNS and PNS regulate the visceral organs, smooth muscles (e.g., vascular, pupillary dilator, pupillary sphincter, ciliary, orbital, arrector pili), and glands (salivary, lacrimal, nasal, adrenal). These neural components of the CNS and PNS are collectively referred to as the **autonomic nervous system (ANS)**. The ANS is, in general, not under voluntary control, but rather its action is controlled by the hypothalamus. The ANS consists of many specialized neural components (e.g., nuclei, ganglia, nerves, tracts and visceral plexus). For example, the increased heart rate in the "fight or flight" response involves the hypothalamus (i.e., CNS), intermediolateral nucleus in the spinal cord (i.e., CNS), ganglia (i.e., PNS) and peripheral nerves (i.e., PNS).

Division of the nervous system

> 1 Differentiate between the central nervous system and the peripheral nervous system.
> 2 What is the relationship between the autonomic and the central nervous systems?

The nervous system can be classified into three systems: the central nervous system, peripheral nervous system and autonomic nervous system. The **central nervous system (CNS)** is composed of the cerebrum, cerebellum, brainstem, and spinal cord. It is the central processing unit of the entire nervous

Cells of the nervous system

> 1 What are three different types of neurons?
> 2 What are the functions of an axon and a dendrite?
> 3 What is the axon hillock? What is its functional significance?
> 4 What are the structural and functional differences between myelinated and nonmyelinated axons?
> 5 Name the neuroglia of the CNS and PNS, and explain their functions.
> 6 How do Schwann cells differ from oligodendrocytes?
> 7 What are the bases of classifying peripheral nerve fibers?

Dukes' Physiology of Domestic Animals, Thirteenth Edition. Edited by William O. Reece, Howard H. Erickson, Jesse P. Goff and Etsuro E. Uemura.

© 2015 John Wiley & Sons, Inc. Published 2015 by John Wiley & Sons, Inc.

Companion website: www.wiley.com/go/reece/physiology

Neurons and neuroglia are the two categories of cells of the nervous system. **Neurons** share certain universal cellular features with all other cells in the body; however, neurons have certain unique features that separate them from other cells. For example, they have distinctive cell shapes with a membrane capable of generating electrical impulses. They transfer impulses from one neuron to the next via synapses (Greek *synapsis*, a connection), the specialized contact areas between two neurons. Although transmission of impulses is a basic biological function performed by all neurons, their electrical property alone does not explain the diverse roles they play in a complex neural network. **Neuroglia** are the most abundant cells in nervous tissue (over 90%), filling essentially all the space in the nervous system not occupied by neurons and blood vessels. They provide structural, metabolic, and protective support for neurons.

Neurons

The most obvious difference between neurons and other cells in the body lies in their great variety of shapes and sizes. Neurons have highly irregular shapes with one or more cellular processes extending from the cell body (Figure 1.1). The **neuronal cell body** (also referred to as the **soma** or **perikaryon**) contains the same organelles found in other cells. However, the rough endoplasmic reticulum and polysomes (collectively referred to as **Nissl substance**) are especially abundant in perikarya. Each neuron has a single axon. The area of the cell body where an axon originates is the **axon hillock**. The axon hillock is also referred to as the trigger zone, as action potentials are generated here. Just distal to the axon hillock is the **initial segment** of the axon.

Axons frequently branch at a distance from the cell body, forming synapses with other neurons, muscle cells, or glands. The remaining neuronal processes are **dendrites** (Greek *dendron*, tree) that resemble trees (Figure 1.1). Dendrites and perikarya are the primary receptive sites of impulses from other neurons. The number of dendrites varies depending on the type of neuron (Figure 1.2). Action potentials are generated at the axon hillock. An action potential travels along the axon at a speed that varies from 0.5 to 120 m/s. Larger axons, over 1 μm in diameter, are myelinated in both the CNS and PNS, while axons less than 1 μm in diameter are not myelinated. Myelinated axons conduct impulses much faster than nonmyelinated axons. There is a constant relationship between axon diameter, internodal length (i.e., length of each myelin sheath), and conduction velocity. Larger axons have longer internodes and faster conduction velocities. Neurons are contiguous not continuous and they communicate with each other via synapses. If a neuron is linked to more than one recipient neuron, its axon branches to make synaptic connections with all the recipient neurons. Neurons, like muscle cells, do not divide once they reach maturity. Therefore, any physical injury that leads to neuronal death will permanently change the structure and functions of the affected areas.

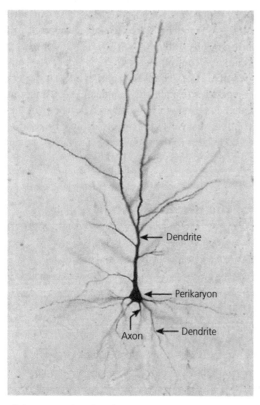

Figure 1.1 A cortical multipolar neuron stained with the Golgi silver impregnation method showing the perikaryon, axon, and dendrites. Only one axon emerges from the perikaryon. All other neuronal processes are dendrites.

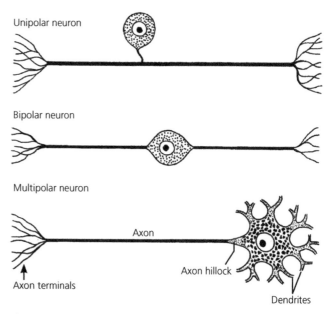

Figure 1.2 The classification of neurons is based on the number of cell processes emerging from the cell body. Cell bodies of unipolar neurons are present in the spinal and cranial ganglia. Cell bodies of bipolar neurons are present in the retina of the eye, spiral ganglia of the auditory nerve, vestibular ganglia of the vestibular nerve, and olfactory epithelium. The majority of neurons are multipolar neurons.

The color of fresh nervous tissue reflects neuronal cell bodies and axons. Areas with a high population of perikarya (e.g., cerebral cortex) appear gray and are referred to as the **gray matter**. In contrast, areas mainly made of myelinated axons appear white because of the presence of lipid in myelin. The name **white matter** is used to indicate such areas.

Classification of neurons

Neurons are classified into three types (unipolar, bipolar, and multipolar) based on the number of cellular processes extending from the cell body (Figure 1.2). **Unipolar neurons** have a single stem process that bifurcates to form two processes, the peripheral and central. Unipolar neurons innervate peripheral tissues, bringing somatic and visceral sensory information to the CNS. Thus they are also referred to as primary sensory neurons. **Bipolar neurons** have two processes. Bipolar neurons are located in the retina of the eye (see Figure 7.4), spiral ganglion of the cochlea (see Figure 6.2B), vestibular ganglion of the vestibular organ (see Figure 9.1), and olfactory epithelium (see Figure 5.2). Bipolar neurons are sensory neurons. Their peripheral processes innervate sensory receptors, bringing sensory signals to the CNS. An exception to this rule is the olfactory cells. A terminal branch of the olfactory cell forms a dendritic bulb and its cilia act as receptors detecting the chemical environment in nasal air. **Multipolar neurons** are the most prevalent type. As the name "multipolar" suggests, each neuron has numerous cell processes (one axon and many dendrites). The length and arrangement of neuronal processes vary considerably.

Neuroglia

Neuroglia are generally small in size and outnumber neurons by as much as 10 : 1 to 50 : 1. Their small size is such that only their nuclei are clearly seen in routine histological preparations. The nuclei range in diameter from 3 to 10 μm, which is about the size of the smallest neurons. Unlike neurons, neuroglia have the capacity to divide. Schwann cells are the only neuroglia of the PNS. Neuroglia of the CNS are oligodendrocytes, ependymal cells, microglia, and astrocytes.

Schwann cells (also referred to as neurolemmocytes) support axons of the PNS, depending on the size of the axon, in two ways. Schwann cells associated with most axons over 1 μm in diameter form myelin sheaths by concentrically wrapping their plasma membrane around the axon (up to 50 or more layers) (Figure 1.3C). Schwann cells are arranged side by side along the axon. Each Schwann cell forms an **internode** of the myelin sheath of various lengths (25–1000 μm). The larger axons have longer internodes and faster conduction speed. The junction between each internode is the **node of Ranvier** (Figure 1.3B). Schwann cells are also associated with most axons less than 1 μm in diameter. Schwann cells associated with smaller axons do not form a myelin sheath, but they hold many smaller axons in their processes. **Oligodendrocytes** (Greek *oligos*, little; *dendron*, dendrite) are small neuroglia of the CNS. They are present

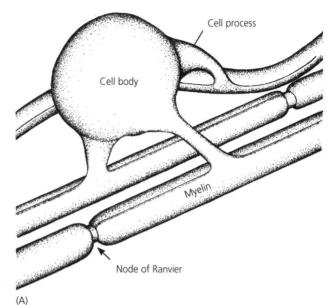

(A)

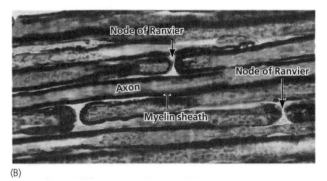

(B)

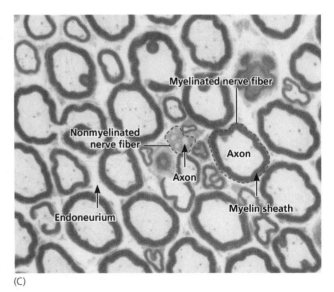

(C)

Figure 1.3 (A) Oligodendrocytes myelinate most axons about 1 μm and over in diameter. Each oligodendrocyte contributes segments of myelin sheath (i.e., internodes) for many axons. (B) Longitudinal section of a peripheral nerve showing axons and their darkly stained myelin sheath, and nodes of Ranvier. (C) Electron micrograph of nonmyelinated and myelinated axons. Nonmyelinated axons are much smaller in size than myelinated ones. Each axon is surrounded by endoneurium.

in both the white and gray matter. Oligodendrocytes have numerous cell processes that extend to adjacent axons to form myelin sheaths (Figure 1.3A). Generally, oligodendrocytes myelinate most axons over 1 μm in diameter to speed conduction velocity (Tables 1.1 and 1.2).

Table 1.1 Classification of peripheral nerve fibers by the letter system.

Type	Diameter (μm)	Conduction velocity (m/s)	Function
Aα	12–22	70–120	Somatic motor, proprioception
Aβ	5–12	30–70	Touch, pressure
Aγ	3–8	15–30	Motor to muscle spindle
Aδ	1–5	12–30	Fast pain and temperature
B	1–3	3–15	Visceral motor (preganglionic)
C	0.3–1.5	0.3–1.5	Visceral motor (postganglionic), slow pain and temperature

Table 1.2 Classification of peripheral sensory nerve fibers by the numerical system.

Type	Letter equivalent	Diameter (μm)	Origin
Ia	Aα	12–22	Muscle spindle (primary)
Ib	Aα	10–15	Golgi tendon organ
II	Aβ, Aγ	5–12	Muscle spindle (secondary), touch, pressure
III	Aδ	1–5	Fast pain and temperature
IV	C	0.3–1.5	Slow pain and temperature

An axon and myelin sheath (if present) together form a **nerve fiber**. Peripheral nerve fibers vary in diameter, ranging from 0.3 to 22 μm. Nerve fibers are classified according to their fiber diameter, speed of conduction, and functions. The largest nerve fibers are classified as Aα and the smallest ones as C (Table 1.1). Since the conduction velocity reflects myelination and the axonal diameter, Aα nerve fibers that innervate the skeletal muscle are heavily myelinated and have the fastest conduction velocity. Other type A (β, γ, δ) and B nerve fibers are progressively smaller and poorly myelinated. Most nerve fibers classified as C are not myelinated and have a slow conduction velocity. A numerical system (I, II, III, IV) is used to classify sensory nerve fibers (Table 1.2). The largest sensory fibers are classified as Ia and the smallest ones as IV. Type IV sensory fibers are mostly nonmyelinated.

Microglia comprise 10–20% of all neuroglia. Microglia are the macrophages of the CNS and act as the first line of defense against tissue injury or infection. Once activated, microglia proliferate and assume a phagocytic role by developing into round, often large cells. They clear debris from the injured area. However, phagocytosis is not the only means of destroying foreign invaders. For example, microglia are also known to release nitric oxide, which prevents viral replication.

Astrocytes (Greek *astron*, star) are star-shaped cells with numerous long cell processes (Figure 1.4). However, they appear as cells with pale ovoid nuclei with routine staining. Astrocytes represent approximately 50% of the glial cell population in the CNS. They provide structural and metabolic support for neurons. For example, astrocytes seal the outer and inner surfaces of the CNS by forming the outer and

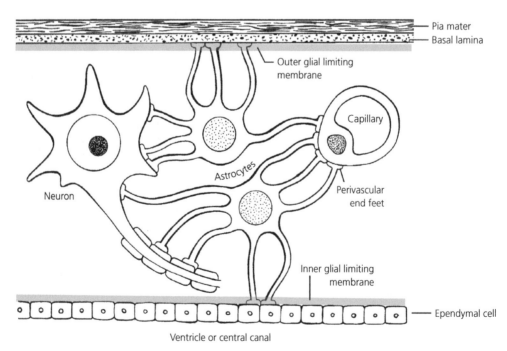

Figure 1.4 Relationship of astrocytes to other cellular and structural components of the central nervous system. Astrocytic processes surround neurons, individual or groups of synapses, capillaries and internodal areas between myelin sheaths. They also form a plexus beneath the pia mater (outer glial limiting membrane) and ependyma (inner glial limiting membrane).

inner glial limiting membranes, respectively. Astrocytes release **neurotrophic factors** (e.g., nerve growth factor), which are important for neuronal survival. Elongation of axons and dendrites requires not only the physical presence of astrocytes, but also **extracellular adhesion molecules** (e.g., laminin, fibronectin) released from astrocytes. Astrocytic processes cover the greater part of neurons, synaptic sites, internodal areas, and capillaries. Astrocytic covering of synaptic sites and internodal areas may prevent signal interference from nearby synapses and axons.

The astrocytic processes that cover capillaries are the **perivascular end feet**. Experimental studies suggest that such close contact between astrocytes and the capillary endothelium is important for glucose transport, regulation of extracellular environment (pH, ion concentration, osmolarity), glutamate metabolism, and maintenance of the endothelial blood–brain barrier. Astrocytes maintain the optimal extracellular environment for neurons and neuroglia. For example, astrocytes are equipped with ionic channels for potassium (K^+), sodium (Na^+), chloride (Cl^-), bicarbonate (HCO_3^-) and calcium (Ca^{2+}). Therefore, they are capable of exchanging these ions with neighboring cells, including neurons. Excitation of neurons accompanies a marked flux of K^+ into the extracellular space. However, an increase in K^+ concentration is prevented by astrocytes, which take up K^+ and relocate it to areas with low neuronal activities or release it to the blood and CSF. Astrocytes also prevent the build-up of potentially neurotoxic substances. Glutamate, for example, is a neurotransmitter that excites postsynaptic neurons (see Figure 3.2B). It is also neurotoxic if accumulated beyond a certain concentration. Astrocytes prevent excess accumulation of extracellular glutamate by metabolizing glutamate into glutamine. Glutamine from astrocytes is used by neurons for synthesis of new glutamate, which is repackaged into synaptic vesicles to be used as a neurotransmitter.

Astrocytes participate in the repair process following tissue injury. Under slowly degenerative conditions, astrocytes retain their small size. Thus only special stains can observe their reactive cytoplasm and cell processes. However, typical astrocytic reactions to pathological conditions are cellular swelling and hyperplasia (Greek *hyper*, above; *plasis*, formation; a condition characterized by an increase in the number of cells). Astrocytic swelling is often induced by injuries from hypoxia (a condition where oxygen levels are below normal), trauma, and hypoglycemia (Greek *hypo*, under; *glykys*, sweet; *haima*, blood; the presence of low sugar levels in the blood). Swelling usually reflects changes in extracellular ionic concentrations (e.g., increase in K^+, decrease in Na^+ and Cl^-, accumulation of glutamate). Destructive lesions of the CNS, especially those caused by trauma, promote astrocytic hyperplasia. In a cerebral infarct, i.e., an area of necrosis (Greek *nekrosis*, deadness; death of tissue) resulting from insufficient blood supply, astrocytes proliferate along the edge of the necrotic area, often sealing off the lesioned area.

Ependymal cells (Greek *ependyma*, upper garment) cover the ventricles and central canal of the CNS (Figure 1.5). They

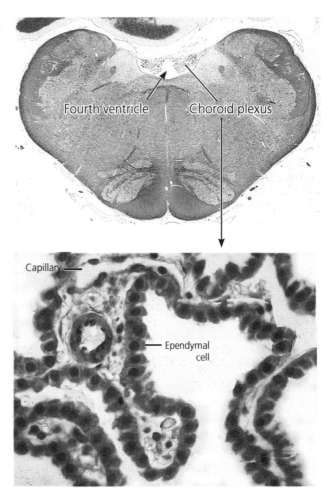

Figure 1.5 The choroid plexus in the fourth ventricle of the medulla oblongata. The choroid plexus is composed of vascular connective tissue lined with ependymal cells on the ventricular surface.

Table 1.3 Normal CSF values.

Color: clear
Cells: <5/mm³
Protein: <25 mg/dL
Glucose: 2.7–4.2 mmol/L
Pressure: <170 mmH₂O

also line the choroid plexus. The ependymal cells of the ventricles and central canal form a selective barrier between the nervous tissue and **CSF**. Junctional complexes are present between adjacent ependymal cells, enabling them to modify the CSF by secretory or absorptive processes. The choroid plexus secretes CSF (Table 1.3). However, it is not the only source of CSF. CSF is also released from the brain through (i) the ependymal lining of the ventricles and central canal and (ii) the pia–outer glial limiting membrane that covers the external surface of the CNS.

The CSF leaves the ventricular system via a small opening, the lateral aperture of the fourth ventricle, to enter the subarachnoid space. It also enters the central canal of the caudal medulla oblongata and spinal cord. The CSF in the subarachnoid space is drained into the dorsal sagittal sinus, which also receives numerous tributary veins from the cerebral hemispheres and passes blood to the maxillary, internal jugular and vertebral veins and to the vertebral venous plexuses. The CSF in the subarachnoid space of the meninges not only protects the brain and spinal cord from trauma, but also reduces the effective weight of the brain significantly by providing a buoyancy effect.

Extracellular environment of the CNS

1 What are the blood–CSF and blood–brain barriers? Where are they located?

2 What transport mechanisms are involved in production of the CSF by the choroid plexus?

3 Explain the formation, circulation, and function of the CSF.

4 What structure represents the blood–brain barrier?

5 What transport mechanisms are involved in the blood–brain barrier?

6 List the areas of the brain where the blood–brain barrier is absent and explain the reason.

Neurons and neuroglia require a chemically stable environment. Thus, the brain receives only the essential materials from the blood and CSF. Two structures acting as gatekeepers to the brain's interior are (i) the **choroid epithelium** of the choroid plexus that acts as the blood–CSF barrier and (ii) the **capillaries** of the nervous tissue that act as the blood–brain barrier.

Blood–CSF barrier

The choroid plexus is present in the lateral, third and fourth ventricles (Figure 1.6). It is formed by invagination of the pia mater covered with choroid epithelial cells on the surface facing the ventricle. Vasculature of the pia mater follows the choroid plexus, providing rich capillary networks. The choroid epithelial cells are modified ependymal cells (they have microvilli instead of cilia on the apical surface). The capillary endothelium of the choroid plexus has many fenestrations in its wall, allowing passage of many small molecules. In contrast, choroid epithelial cells are sealed together by a tight junction that prevents the passage of water-soluble molecules into the CSF. Tight junctions are the anatomical basis of the **blood–CSF barrier** (Figure 1.7) Thus, **choroid epithelial cells** play a key role in regulating what can enter and leave the CNS tissue, maintaining an optimal environment for neurons and neuroglia. The choroid plexus relies on carrier proteins to transport essential molecules. Carrier proteins are located on the basal surface of the choroid epithelial cells. Essential molecules are released into the ventricle through the apical surface of the choroid epithelial cells, probably by facilitated diffusion. The CSF is also important for removing waste products from the CNS. Waste products removed from the CNS are drained into the dorsal sagittal sinus via the arachnoid villi.

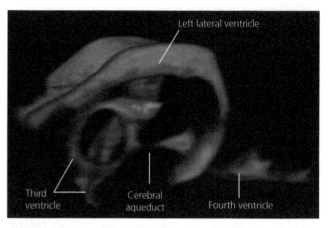

Figure 1.6 MRI reconstruction of the ventricles of a dog showing the lateral ventricles, third ventricle, cerebral aqueduct, and fourth ventricle. Dr A. Zur Linden, Iowa State University College of Veterinary Medicine. Reproduced with permission from Dr A. Zur Linden.

Clinical correlations

Certain antibiotics (e.g., penicillin and most cephalosporin antibiotics) are actively removed from the CSF. Thus, the concentration of penicillin in CSF is about 1% of that in the blood. Interestingly, the choroid plexus under inflammatory conditions (e.g., meningitis) becomes leaky, resulting in a partial breakdown of the blood–CSF barrier. Consequently, the concentration of penicillin in CSF increases to 20% or more of that in the blood, preventing further bacterial growth or even killing bacteria. As inflammation subsides, the choroid plexus regains the function of the blood–CSF barrier and resumes removal of penicillin from CSF, allowing the possibility of a relapse of bacterial growth. Therefore, use of antibiotics that are not actively removed from the CSF (e.g., ceftriaxone with broad-spectrum activity against Gram-positive and Gram-negative bacteria) must be considered for treating many types of meningitis.

Cerebrospinal fluid is 99% water, which the choroid plexus secretes into the ventricles by creating ion gradients on both apical and basal surfaces of choroid epithelial cells (Figure 1.7). Water in the choroid epithelial cells dissociates into hydrogen (H^+) and hydroxyl (OH^-) ions. OH^- combines with intracellular CO_2 produced by cell metabolism to form bicarbonate ions (HCO_3^-). At the basal surface of the cells, H^+ is exchanged for extracellular sodium ions (Na^+) from the blood. Na^+ is pumped out through the apical surface into the ventricles. The flux of Na^+ results in an excess positive charge in the ventricles. To neutralize this excess positive charge, chloride ions (Cl^-) and HCO_3^- move into the ventricles. Water also diffuses into the ventricles to maintain osmotic balance. These processes maintain water and concentration of ions in the CSF appropriate for the brain and spinal cord. Water and ions are not the only substances that the CNS must obtain from the blood. The majority of micronutrients

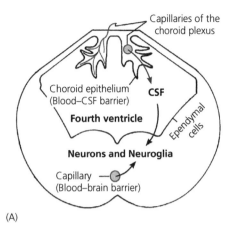

(A)

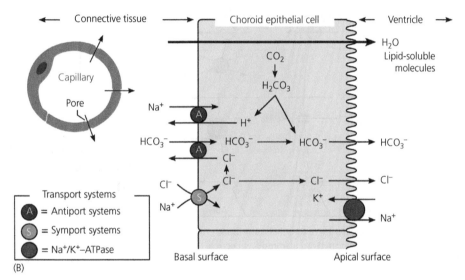

(B)

Figure 1.7 (A) Neurons and neuroglial cells receive essential materials via two routes. Capillaries in the choroid plexus provide micronutrients, whereas interstitial capillaries provide oxygen and substances that the CNS consumes rapidly and in large amounts. The fourth ventricle is exaggerated here and not proportional to the size of the medulla oblongata. (B) The capillaries in the choroid plexus do not act as the blood–CSF barrier, as they are fenestrated (i.e., many pores) and intercellular gaps between endothelial cells are not tight as those found in capillaries of the CNS. As a result, molecules easily cross the capillary endothelial cell of the choroid plexus. The blood–CSF barrier is provided by the choroid epithelial cells, which are joined together by tight junctions. Microvilli of the choroid epithelial cells are present on the ventricular side of the epithelium. The choroid plexus produces CSF by diffusion, facilitated diffusion, and active transport systems. The choroid plexus epithelium also transports metabolites from CSF to blood (not shown).

(substances that are essential to the brain but only needed in relatively small amounts) come from the CSF. Micronutrients include vitamin B_6 (pyridoxine), folates (members of vitamin B-complex class) and vitamin C. In contrast, nutrients (glucose, amino acids, lactate) that the CNS requires in large amounts are delivered directly into the interstitial fluid by the capillary endothelium. This process depends on a facilitated-diffusion system.

Blood–brain barrier

It is known that a dye such as trypan blue, injected intravenously, stains all tissues of the body except the brain and spinal cord. Animals do not show any adverse effects from this procedure. However, when the dye is injected into the ventricle, the whole brain is diffusely stained and animals suffer from neurological problems. Clearly, the central nervous tissue has some barrier against the passage of a circulating dye, and this barrier is referred to as the blood–brain barrier (Figure 1.8). The site of the blood–brain barrier was shown by use of a tracer, horseradish peroxidase (HRP). HRP injected into the ventricle easily enters the extracellular spaces of the brain by crossing the ependymal cells. Although HRP in the brain passes through the capillary basement membrane, it is prevented from crossing the capillary wall into the lumen. However, there are a few specialized areas in the brain that allow entry of dyes or HRP. These nonbarrier regions include the choroid plexus, hypophysis,

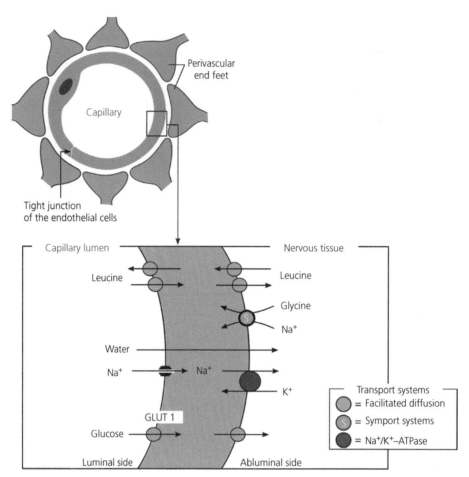

Figure 1.8 Transport of molecules across capillaries of the CNS. Continuous tight junctions of endothelial cells restrict the diffusion of large and small solutes across the endothelial cells. The perivascular end feet encircle the capillary. Transport carriers for essential amino acids and glucose facilitate their movement into the CNS. Active transport systems moves small nonessential amino acids from brain to blood. Na^+ is transported from blood to the CNS by Na^+ transporters on the luminal membrane and Na^+/K^+-ATPase on the abluminal membrane. This Na^+ movement drives transport of water into the CNS.

median eminence, pineal gland, and area postrema. Capillaries in these areas are fenestrated, which is essential for these areas to carry out their function (e.g., release of hormones into the circulation, monitoring circulating molecules). Thus, capillaries are the factor that restricts what can enter the brain from the blood.

The morphological basis of the blood–brain barrier is established by the electron microscope. Capillaries of the CNS are associated with three unique features: (i) continuous **tight junctions** that seal neighboring endothelial cells, (ii) absence of **fenestrations** and (iii) only a small number of **pinocytotic vesicles**. Although capillary endothelium is the structural basis of the blood–brain barrier, such a property appears to be maintained by astrocytes that form perivascular end feet around the entire outer surface of the capillary endothelium (Figure 1.8). This association suggests that the interaction between astrocytes and endothelial cells is important for the maintenance of

the blood–brain barrier. Thus, it is not surprising to see the absence of normal astrocyte–endothelial cell relationships in the nonbarrier regions of the brain mentioned above and in brain tumors. The transcellular transport is the only way for any substance in the blood to enter the CNS. The plasma membrane is made of a lipid bilayer. It is not permeable to charged molecules and most polar molecules such as sugars and amino acids. Anions in water are attracted electrostatically to the hydrogen atom of water, whereas cations are attracted to the oxygen atom of water. Such attraction of ions to water molecules imposes a barrier for ions to pass through the hydrophobic lipid bilayer of membrane. Thus, lipophilic substances (e.g., nicotine and ethanol) are very permeable and their transport through the endothelial cells is only limited by blood flow. Gases (e.g., CO_2, O_2, N_2O) diffuse rapidly into brain. Water also crosses freely in either direction through the membrane by diffusion as the osmolality of the plasma changes.

The brain needs certain water-soluble nutrients, such as glucose or certain essential amino acids. However, water-soluble compounds are restricted from passing through the blood–brain barrier into the brain. Glucose is a vital source of energy in the brain and its transport depends on a specific glucose carrier (GLUT 1) in the capillary endothelial cells. GLUT 1 is a facilitative transporter located at both the luminal and the abluminal side of the endothelial membrane. Facilitated diffusion carried out by the carriers does not consume energy. Facilitated diffusion moves molecules in both directions across the membrane, but the net flow is from the side of higher concentration to that of lower concentration. Since glucose is rapidly consumed in the CNS, the glucose concentration in interstitial fluid is normally lower than in blood plasma. As a result, the net flow of glucose across the blood–brain barrier is from blood to interstitial fluid. Specific carriers have substrate specificity. Thus, the carriers that transport D-glucose do not transport the L-enantiomer.

Large neutral amino acids (e.g., phenylalanine, leucine, tyrosine, isoleucine, valine, tryptophan, methionine histidine, and L-dopa) are transported by facilitated diffusion both on the luminal and abluminal sides of the endothelial cells. Some of them, for example tryptophan, are precursors for neurotransmitters (serotonin, melatonin) synthesized in the CNS. Serotonin is involved in mood and sleep and melatonin regulates the sleep–wake cycle (circadian rhythm). Smaller neutral amino acids such as glycine, alanine, serine, cysteine, proline, and γ-aminobutyric acid (GABA) are synthesized in the CNS. These amino acids are also transported primarily from the brain to the circulation. Their transport requires an energy-dependent and Na^+-dependent symport carrier located at the abluminal side of the endothelial cell membrane. Na^+/K^+-ATPase located on the abluminal endothelial membrane provides the energy to drive the Na^+ and amino acid symport carrier by maintaining high extracellular Na^+ concentration in the CNS. Ion channels are also present in the luminal endothelial membrane. These ion channels and Na^+/K^+-ATPase work together to remove K^+ from the interstitial fluid of the CNS in order to maintain a constant K^+ concentration.

It appears that essential amino acids which are precursors for catecholamines (epinephrine and norepinephrine synthesized from tryosine) and indolamine (e.g., serotonin and melatonin synthesized from tryptophan) are transported into the CNS. On the other hand, amino acids that are synthesized in the CNS and which function as neurotransmitters are not just restricted from crossing the blood–brain barrier into the CNS, but are transported out of the CNS. This lopsided transport across the blood–brain barrier may ensure that neurotransmitters will not accumulate in the brain, preventing the potential neurotoxic glutamate effect and unwanted inhibition of neurons by glycine and GABA.

Clinical correlations

Water crosses the membrane freely in either direction by diffusion. This property of water across the membrane can be clinically useful in osmotherapy. For example, mannitol, $C_6H_8(OH)_6$, is poorly permeable and intravenous administration of mannitol osmotically dehydrates the brain. Thus, mannitol can be used to reduce dangerously elevated intracranial pressure (e.g., after head trauma). Mannitol is also used experimentally to deliver drugs to the CNS by temporarily opening the blood–brain barrier. This osmotic disruption approach uses a concentrated dose of mannitol to remove fluid from the brain's endothelial cells, which causes endothelial cells to shrink and the tight junctions to open. However, the temporary opening of the blood–brain barrier is only applicable in disorders that do not require long-term treatment.

The blood–brain barrier is essential for maintaining stable functions of the CNS. The barrier imposed by the capillary endothelium ensures that any changes in nutrients, ions, and hormones do not directly influence synaptic functions. Unfortunately, the strict criteria set by the barrier applies equally to therapeutic drugs. The lipophilic antibiotic chloramphenicol crosses the blood–brain barrier without problems, but the highly hydrophilic penicillin is prevented from crossing the barrier. A high proportion (over 95%) of large-molecule drugs do not cross the blood–brain barrier, which includes all the products of biotechnology, recombinant proteins, and monoclonal antibodies. Thus, most drugs that are effective in the treatment of systemic diseases are not effective for treating CNS diseases. It is highly desirable that drugs are developed which can either directly or indirectly bypass the blood–brain barrier. Fortunately, inflammation associated with certain diseases affects the blood–brain barrier by increasing the permeability of endothelial membranes to certain antibiotics, allowing drugs to enter the CNS. As the inflammation decreases, entrance of the antibiotic also decreases, lowering the effectiveness of treatment.

Self-evaluation

Answers can be found at the end of the chapter.

1 Dendrites of neurons receive signals from other neurons.
   A True
   B False

2 Neurons that have one axon and numerous dendrites are classified as:
   A Bipolar neuron
   B Multipolar neuron
   C Unipolar neuron

3 Axon hillock is a site that generates action potentials.
   A True
   B False

4 Neuroglia that is part of the choroid plexus comprises:
   A Astrocytes
   B Ependymal cells
   C Microglia
   D Oligodendrocytes

5 Which statement about astrocytes are not correct?
   A Astrocytes form the choroid plexus
   B Astrocytes transport glucose from capillaries to neurons
   C Astrocytes form perivascular end feet
   D Astrocytes continue dividing after birth
   E Astrocytes prevent intercellular accumulation of the neurotransmitter glutamate

6 The myelin sheath:
   A Is made by oligodendrocytes in the PNS
   B Is made by Schwann cells in the CNS
   C Slows the nerve impulse traveling along axons
   D Enables faster conduction velocity

7 A nerve fiber is made of:
   A An axon only
   B An axon and Schwann cells.
   C An axon and endoneurium
   D An axon and epineurium

8 Leucine is transported by facilitated diffusion at the blood–brain barrier.
   A True
   B False

9 What structure represents the blood–brain barrier?
   A Choroid plexus
   B Microglia
   C Endothelial cells
   D Astrocytes
   E Meninges

10 Nerve fibers classified as Aα are larger in diameter and faster in conduction than those fibers classified as C fibers.
   A True
   B False

11 Axons in the CNS are myelinated by:
   A Astrocytes
   B Schwann cells
   C Ependymal cells
   D Oligodendrocytes

12 Na^+/K^+-ATPase is located on which membrane of endothelial cells?
   A Luminal
   B Abluminal

13 Glucose in the CNS is transported by:
   A Simple diffusion
   B GLUT 1
   C Facilitated diffusion
   D Na^+-dependent symport carrier
   E Na^+/K^+-ATPase

14 The choroid plexus produces the CSF.
   A True
   B False

15 The CSF in the third ventricle enters the fourth ventricles via cerebral aqueduct.
   A True
   B False

16 What represents the blood–CSF barrier?
   A Meninges
   B Capillary endothelium of the choroid plexus
   C Perivascular end feet
   D Choroid epithelium
   E Astrocytes

17 The blood–brain barrier is absent in the:
   A Spinal cord
   B Cerebellum
   C Choroid plexus
   D Area postrema
   E Two of the above

Suggested reading

Abbott, N.J. (2002) Astrocyte–endothelial interactions and blood–brain barrier permeability. *Journal of Anatomy* 200:629–638.

Cserr, H.F. (1971) Physiology of the choroid plexus. *Physiological Reviews* 51:273–311.

De Terlizzi, R. and Platt, S.R. (2006) The function, composition and analysis of cerebrospinal fluid in companion animals. Part I. Function and composition. *Veterinary Journal* 172:422–431.

Eurell, J.A. and Frappier, B.L. (2006) *Dellmann's Textbook of Veterinary Histology*, 6th edn. Wiley-Blackwell, Hoboken, NJ.

Fitzgerald, T.C. (1961) Anatomy of the cerebral ventricles of domestic animals. *Veterinary Medicine* 56:38–45.

Goldstein, G.W. and Betz, A.L. (1986) The blood–brain barrier. *Scientific American* 255(3):74–83.

Gomez, D.G. and Potts, D.G. (1981) The lateral, third and fourth ventricle choroid plexus of the dog: a structural and ultrastructural study. *Annals of Neurology* 10:333–340.

Janzer, R.C. and Raff, M.C. (1987) Astrocytes induce blood–brain barrier properties in endothelial cells. *Nature* 325:253–257.

Masuzawa, T., Ohta, T., Kawakami, K. and Sato, F. (1985) Immunocytochemical localization of Na^+, K^+-ATPase in the canine choroid plexus. *Brain* 108:625–646.

Segal, M.B. and Pollay, M. (1977) The secretion of cerebrospinal fluid. *Experimental Eye Research* 25(Suppl.):127–148.

Spector, R. and Johanson, C.E. (1989) The mammalian choroid plexus. *Scientific American* 261(5):68–74.

Answers

1 A	10 A
2 B	11 D
3 A	12 B
4 B	13 B
5 A	14 A
6 D	15 A
7 B	16 D
8 A	17 E
9 C	

2 Electrochemical Basis of Neuronal Function

Etsuro E. Uemura
Iowa State University, Ames, IA, USA

Neurons function by establishing communication mediated by electrical and chemical means. Thus the excitability of neurons and their ability to propagate electrical signals are one of the most prominent features of the nervous system. The relatively static membrane potential of inactive cells is the **resting membrane potential**. It reflects selective ionic permeability of the plasma membrane, maintained at the expense of continuous basal metabolism. The resting membrane potential plays a central role in the excitability of nerves. When a neuron receives excitatory or inhibitory signals, the neuronal membrane generates excitatory or inhibitory graded membrane potentials (i.e., transient changes in the resting membrane potential). Once the electrical stimulus fulfills specific criteria, the neuronal membrane undergoes dynamic reversal of membrane potential, known as an action potential. In this chapter, four basic physiologic properties of neurons (resting membrane potential, graded potential, action potential, and propagation of action potential) are discussed for a better understanding of neuronal functions.

Distribution of intracellular and extracellular ions

1 Name five major intracellular and extracellular ions and indicate which ions are more highly concentrated inside neurons relative to outside.

2 What two energy gradients drive the movement of ions across the membrane?

3 What is the equilibrium potential?

4 What happens to the membrane potential if an ion is allowed to selectively cross the membrane?

5 What are the properties and functions of Na⁺/K⁺-ATPase?

The neuronal membrane, like other cell membranes, is made of a lipid bilayer. It is not permeable to charged molecules and most polar molecules such as sugars and amino acids. Anions in water are attracted electrostatically to the hydrogen atom of water and cations to the oxygen atom. Attraction of ions to water molecules acts as a barrier for passage of ions across the hydrophobic lipid bilayer of the membrane. This property is the basis for the unique distribution of inorganic ions (e.g., Na^+, K^+, Cl^-) across the neuronal membrane. The proteins present in the membrane are receptors, transporters, and enzymes. The selective permeability of the neuronal membrane reflects the presence of ion channels. These ion channels allow some ions to pass through the membrane in the direction of their concentration and electrostatic gradients. The neuron has four main types of selective ion channels: Na^+, K^+, Ca^{2+}, and Cl^- channels. These ion channels are either in an open state (also referred to as nongated or leak channels) or have gates that may open or close in response to specific stimuli (e.g., voltage or chemicals). Nongated channels play a role in maintaining the intracellular and extracellular ion concentrations. Voltage-gated ion channels are important for generation of action potentials and their propagation along axons. Chemically gated ion channels play a role in synaptic transmission by opening ion channels when they bind with a variety of ligands, such as a neurotransmitter or intracellular signaling molecules. Channel proteins mediate **passive transport** of molecules across the membrane and metabolic energy is not necessary. Uncharged molecules are passively transported across the membrane according to the concentration gradient of the solute. Uncharged molecules diffuse through the membrane from the side of higher concentration to the side of lower concentration. Charged molecules cross the membrane according to the electrochemical gradient (i.e., the combination of the concentration and electrical

Dukes' Physiology of Domestic Animals, Thirteenth Edition. Edited by William O. Reece, Howard H. Erickson, Jesse P. Goff and Etsuro E. Uemura.

© 2015 John Wiley & Sons, Inc. Published 2015 by John Wiley & Sons, Inc.

Companion website: www.wiley.com/go/reece/physiology

gradients). **Active transport** requires specific carrier proteins and metabolic energy, such as hydrolysis of ATP.

In the resting state of neurons, the electrolyte content differs greatly from that of the extracellular fluid (Table 2.1). The concentration of Na^+ ions is approximately 10 times greater in the extracellular fluid (150 mmol/L) than in the intracellular fluid (15 mmol/L). Similarly, the concentration of Cl^- ions is much greater in the extracellular fluid (150 mmol/L) than in the intracellular fluid (13 mmol/L). In contrast, the concentration of intracellular K^+ (100 mmol/L) is approximately 20 times higher

Table 2.1 Intracellular and extracellular distribution of ions across the neuronal membrane.

Ion	Extracellular concentration (mmol/L)	Intracellular concentration (mmol/L)
Na^+	150	15
K^+	5	100
Ca^{2+}	2	0.0002
Cl^-	150	13
Fixed anions	—	385

than in the extracellular fluid (5 mmol/L). There are many negatively charged intracellular organic molecules (e.g., proteins, nucleic acids, carboxylic groups, and metabolites carrying phosphate). Since the organic anions are too large to pass through the membrane, they are called **fixed anions**. They drive the electrical charge of cytoplasm facing the plasma membrane towards negative relative to the outside of the membrane.

The selective permeability of the membrane is key for maintaining the separation of charges across the membrane (Figure 2.1). If the neuronal membrane is selectively permeable only to K^+, the high **concentration gradient** of K^+ should drive them from inside the cell to outside through K^+ nongated channels. However, intracellular fixed anions prevent an efflux of K^+ ions. At the same time, extracellular positive charges drive K^+ into the neuron due to **electrostatic forces**. However, the distribution of K^+ remains stable as the movement of ions in one direction under the influence of the concentration gradient is precisely balanced by the movement of ions in the opposite direction due to the **electrochemical gradient**. When the two opposing forces (concentration gradient, electrostatic forces) are equal, intracellular and extracellular K^+ concentrations are in equilibrium. The membrane potential derived at the equilibrium of K^+ is called the K^+ equilibrium potential (approxi-

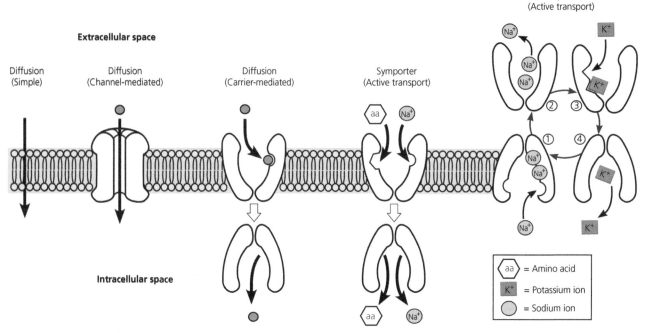

Figure 2.1 Transport of solute across the neuronal membrane. *Simple diffusion*: the molecules move according to their concentration gradient. Simple diffusion does not require input of energy and net movement of the molecules stops after reaching equilibrium. *Channel-mediated diffusion*: when the channel is in the open state, certain charged ions (e.g., Na^+ and K^+) are able to pass through the pore to reach the other side of the plasma membrane. *Carrier-mediated diffusion*: movement of substances across cell membranes with the aid of a carrier protein (e.g., GLUT transporter that move hexoses such as glucose, galactose, mannose, and fructose). *Symporter*: a carrier protein cotransports two or more molecules in the same direction across the cell membrane. Examples include Na^+–glucose, Na^+–amino acid, Na^+–neurotransmitter uptake. *Antiporter*: exchange of molecules takes place in opposite directions, i.e., one enters the cell as the other exits the cell. An example is Na^+/K^+-ATPase that maintains the concentration gradients of Na^+ and K^+ across the cell membrane. The following steps are involved in moving molecules against their concentration gradient. (1) An ATP molecule binds to the ATPase. This step creates binding sites for three Na^+ ions on the intracellular side of the carrier. (2) The energy released by hydrolysis of the high-energy bond changes the conformation of the carrier protein so that the channel opens to the extracellular side. At the same time, the binding affinity for Na^+ decreases and the Na^+ ions are released into the extracellular side. (3) After the loss of Na^+, the phosphate group detaches, creating high-affinity binding sites for K^+ on the extracellular side of the carrier channel. Two K^+ ions from the extracellular fluid attach to the carrier protein. (4) A new ATP molecule binds to the ATPase, changing the conformation. Subsequent opening of the channel to the cytoplasmic side releases K^+ into the cytoplasm.

Table 2.2 Nernst equation to determine equilibrium potential of ions.

The Nernst equation for calculating the equilibrium potential of an ion present on both sides of the cell membrane is as follows:

$$E_{ion} = 2.303 \frac{RT}{zF} \log \frac{[ion]_o}{[ion]_i}$$

where:
E_{ion} = ionic equilibrium potential
R = gas constant (8.314 J mol^{-1} K^{-1})
T = temperature of Kelvin scale (273.15 + temperature in °C)
z = valence of the ion
F = Faraday constant (96 485 C mol^{-1})
$[ion]_o$ = ionic concentration outside the cell
$[ion]_i$ = ionic concentration inside the cell

The equilibrium potential calculated by the Nernst equation:
E_K = 61.5 mV log 5/100 = −80 mV
E_{Na} = 61.5 mV log 150/15 = +62 mV
E_{Cl} = 61.5 mV log 150/13 = −65 mV

mately −80 mV) (Table 2.2). Similarly, if the membrane is selectively permeable only to Na$^+$, the electrochemical gradient drives Na$^+$ into the neuron to establish the equilibrium. The membrane potential derived from the equilibrium of Na$^+$ is the Na$^+$ equilibrium potential (approximately +62 mV). The Cl$^-$ equilibrium potential is very similar to the K$^+$ equilibrium potential.

Resting membrane potential

1 Explain the ionic mechanisms contributing to the resting membrane potential and approximate voltage in most mammalian neurons.

2 What is the relationship between ionic driving forces, ion channels, and the membrane potential?

3 What role does the Na$^+$/K$^+$-ATPase play in maintaining the resting membrane potential?

The potential difference across the membrane of resting neurons is referred to as the resting membrane potential. It is about −65 mV (i.e., the inside of the neuron is about 65 mV less than the outside). The resting membrane potential reflects asymmetric distribution of certain ions (K$^+$, Na$^+$, Cl$^-$, fixed anions) across the neuronal membrane. The resting membrane potential of a neuron is far from the equilibrium potential for K$^+$ (−80 mV) or Na$^+$ (+62 mV). This is because the membrane of resting neurons is selectively permeable to K$^+$ due to the presence of high numbers of nongated K$^+$ channels. Na$^+$ ions are driven inwards across the membrane by the electrochemical gradient. However, the Na$^+$ conductance is extremely small due to limited Na$^+$ nongated channels available. This significantly limits Na$^+$ influx despite their large electrochemical gradient. Thus the resting potential reflects the unequal distribution of ions across the neuronal membrane.

The asymmetric distribution of K$^+$ and Na$^+$ across the membrane is maintained by the Na$^+$/K$^+$-ATPase (Na$^+$/K$^+$ pump) in the membrane (Figure 2.1). The Na$^+$/K$^+$-ATPase moves Na$^+$ and K$^+$ against their electrochemical gradient, removing Na$^+$ and bringing

K$^+$ into the neuron. The pumping of Na$^+$ and K$^+$ can be turned off reversibly by the use of metabolic inhibitors (e.g., dinitrophenol, azide, cyanide), while intracellular injection of ATP can reverse such an inhibitory effect. The Na$^+$/K$^+$ pump works continuously, regardless of the state of electrical activity of a neuron, maintaining the large ionic concentration gradients across the membrane.

Graded potential

1 What are the two types of postsynaptic potentials and how do they generate membrane depolarization or hyperpolarization?

2 Where is the axon hillock located in a neuron and what role does it play in postsynaptic membrane potentials?

3 What are the two mechanisms that modify membrane potentials at the axon hillock?

A neuron receives hundreds of inputs from other neurons primarily via axodendritic and axosomatic synapses. In response to neurotransmitters from presynaptic neurons, brief local changes in postsynaptic membranes are generated at each synaptic site. These local membrane potentials are referred to as **graded potentials**, as their amplitude is directly proportional to the intensity of the stimulus applied at synaptic sites. Each synaptic site generates graded potentials, so that thousands of graded potentials occur at cell bodies and dendrites. Graded potentials generated by synaptic sites at dendrites and cell bodies travel to reach the axon hillock (also referred to as the **trigger zone**) of a neuron (see Figure 1.2). The axon hillock is where graded potentials are integrated to generate action potentials. In unipolar and bipolar neurons, the trigger zone is at a terminal area of a neuronal process that is equivalent to a dendrite. The trigger zone is most sensitive to the depolarizing action of the local currents and is a crucial region of neurons that generates action potentials in response to incoming graded potentials. Graded potentials reaching the trigger zone must be strong enough to depolarize the membrane to the level known as the **threshold potential** (or voltage), about −55 mV. Once the sum of graded potentials exceeds the threshold, the trigger zone triggers action potentials that propagate along the axon. If the depolarization does not reach the threshold, an action potential is not generated and the graded potentials decay.

Excitatory and inhibitory postsynaptic potentials

Graded potentials modulate the postsynaptic neuron by shifting the resting membrane potential toward or away from the threshold potential. Shifting the membrane potential toward more positive is called **depolarization** (Figure 2.2) and a depolarizing graded potential is referred to as an **excitatory postsynaptic potential (EPSP)** (Figure 2.3A). For example, acetylcholine and glutamate induce depolarizing graded potentials by opening ligand-gated Na$^+$ channels, triggering an influx of Na$^+$. Synapses that induce EPSPs are called **excitatory synapses**, as they drive the postsynaptic membrane potential toward the threshold. In contrast, neurotransmitters such as γ-aminobutyric acid (GABA) and glycine bind to ligand-gated Cl$^-$ channels

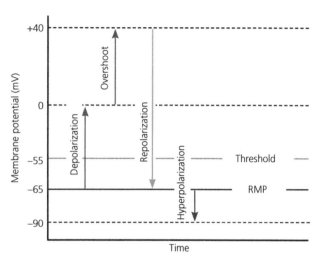

Figure 2.2 Terminology related to membrane potential of neurons. *Depolarization*: decrease in the potential difference across the plasma membrane, going to more positive. *Overshoot*: a portion of depolarization that causes the inside of the cell to be positively charged with respect to the outside. *Repolarization*: change in potential that returns the membrane potential to a negative value after the depolarization phase of an action potential. Repolarization returns the membrane potential to the resting membrane potential (RMP) (–65 mV). *Hyperpolarization*: increase in the potential difference across the membrane to more negative, away from the RMP. *Threshold*: critical membrane voltage (–55 mV) to which the membrane potential must be depolarized in order to generate an action potential. When the graded potential reaches the threshold potential, there is about a 50% chance of generating an action potential. The membrane potential must exceed the threshold to generate an action potential.

that trigger influx of Cl⁻. Subsequent shifting of the membrane potential toward more negative is called **hyperpolarization** (Figure 2.2). A hyperpolarizing graded potential is called an **inhibitory postsynaptic potential (IPSP)** and synapses that induce IPSPs are called **inhibitory synapses** (Figure 2.3B). Thus, the postsynaptic membrane can be stimulated or inhibited, depending on the transmitter involved and the subsequent change in ion permeability that alters membrane excitability.

Summation of graded potentials

Numerous presynaptic axons converge on a postsynaptic neuron, generating thousands of EPSPs and IPSPs. The axon hillock is able to process all graded potentials by algebraic processing, i.e., adding or subtracting potential changes. The axon hillock continues to process graded potentials as long as (i) the sum of all graded potentials stays under the threshold potential and (ii) the presynaptic changes occur faster than the decay rate of the graded potential in the postsynaptic neuron. Thus, when a synapse triggers a small depolarization (EPSP), a simultaneous depolarization at another synapse located at a different site on the same cell body or dendrites is summated to induce a larger depolarization. However, simultaneous hyperpolarization (IPSP) at another synapse located elsewhere on the same cell body or dendrites results in a smaller membrane depolarization.

There are two modes of summation, spatial and temporal (Figure 2.4). In **spatial summation**, graded potentials induced by

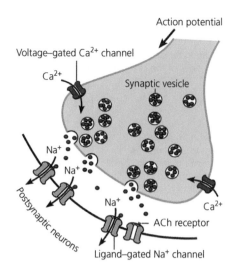

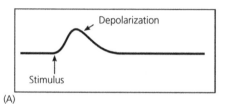

(A)

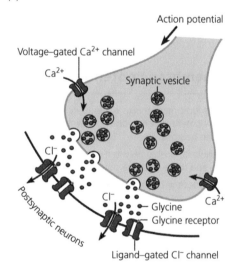

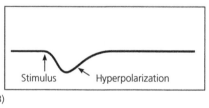

(B)

Figure 2.3 Postsynaptic potentials generated at the postsynaptic cell body and dendrites. (A) Neurotransmitters, for example acetylcholine (ACh) and glutamate, induce excitatory postsynaptic potentials (EPSPs) by opening ligand-gated Na⁺ channels, triggering an influx of Na⁺. EPSPs drive the membrane potential toward threshold voltage. (B) The neurotransmitters glycine and GABA induce inhibitory postsynaptic potentials (IPSPs) by binding to ligand-gated Cl⁻ channels that trigger an influx of Cl⁻ ions. IPSPs drive the membrane potential away from threshold voltage.

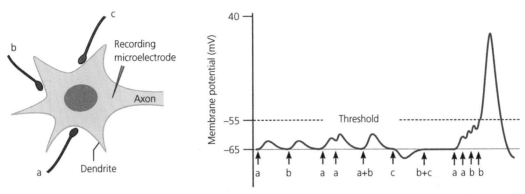

Figure 2.4 Summation of EPSPs and IPSPs at the postsynaptic neuron. Three presynaptic neurons (a, b, c) were stimulated at times indicated by the arrows on the graph, and the membrane potential was recorded in the postsynaptic neuron. An action potential is generated when the EPSP is large enough to exceed the threshold voltage (–55 mV). Axons a and b are excitatory, and axon c is inhibitory to the postsynaptic neuron.

different synapses summate in the postsynaptic dendrites and cell body. In **temporal summation**, graded potentials induced by the successive action of presynaptic terminals summate in the postsynaptic neuron. When EPSPs and IPSPs occur simultaneously in the same cell, their relative strengths determine the response of the postsynaptic neuron. Thus, the axon hillock of postsynaptic neurons summates every local graded potential generated by incoming afferent axons and triggers action potentials once the sum of all graded potentials exceeds the threshold. This summation of graded potentials processed at the subthreshold membrane potential is a key step in integration of electrical signals occurring at neuronal levels. A graded potential surpassing the threshold potential at the trigger zone generates a burst of action potentials, not just one action potential. Furthermore, the intensity of the graded potential is proportional to the frequency of action potentials generated at the trigger zone.

Action potential

1 Explain an action potential and graded potential with respect to:
   (a) Location on the neuron in which they occur
   (b) Ion channels involved in generating these potentials.
2 What is 'threshold potential' with respect to an action potential?
3 What are the ionic mechanisms responsible for generating an action potential?
4 Illustrate an action potential with labels, including:
   (a) Depolarization, overshoot, repolarization and hyperpolarization
   (b) Approximate peak voltage and duration.
5 Describe three stages of voltage-gated Na⁺ channels and explain how each of these stages relates to action potentials.
6 What are the two phases of refractory period of an action potential and why are they important?
7 What is responsible for maintaining ionic concentration gradients across the membrane despite continued generation of action potentials?
8 How do local anesthetics block sensory signals from reaching their destinations?

An action potential is a brief reversal in membrane potential when membrane permeability of Na⁺ and K⁺ increases subsequent to activation of voltage-gated Na⁺ and K⁺ channels (Figure 2.5B). The membrane potential at which a sufficient number of voltage-gated Na⁺ channels open for generating an action potential is called the **threshold potential** (about –55 mV). To generate an action potential, the EPSPs generated at the cell body and its dendrites must be large enough to depolarize the trigger zone beyond the threshold (Figure 2.5A). Action potentials represent identical membrane depolarizations of about 100 mV in amplitude. The strength of the EPSP that initiates an action potential has no influence on its amplitude. It is important to note that not all voltage-gated Na⁺ channels open simultaneously at the threshold potential. Some voltage-gated Na⁺ channels start to open as the membrane starts to depolarize. When the graded potential reaches the threshold potential, more voltage-gated Na⁺ channels open, and there is about a 50% chance of generating an action potential. Only when membrane depolarization exceeds the threshold potential do sufficient numbers of voltage-gated Na⁺ channels open, ensuring the generation of an action potential. Since the generation of an action potential hinges on the threshold potential (i.e., the membrane voltage must reach the threshold to generate an action potential and nothing happens below the threshold), an action potential is often referred to as an **all-or none** phenomenon. The entire duration of an action potential in a neuron is about 2 ms.

Voltage-gated Na⁺ channels

Action potentials have two phases, the rising phase and falling phase. Key to understanding an action potential are the voltage-gated Na⁺ channels. This channel has activation and inactivation gates. Depending on which gate is open or closed, Na⁺ channels undergo the three states (resting, activated, or inactivated) during an action potential (Figure 2.6). The **resting state** of voltage-gated Na⁺ channels is maintained when a neuron is under the resting membrane potential. During the resting state, the activation gate closes the channel pore, while the inactivation gate is open (Figure 2.6A). As the activation gate closes, Na⁺ cannot flow into the neuron. Na⁺ channels in the resting state

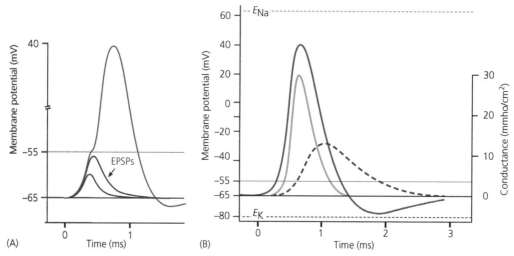

Figure 2.5 (A) Subthreshold excitatory postsynaptic potentials (EPSPs) do not trigger an action potential. When the EPSP is large enough to elevate the membrane potential at the trigger zone (i.e., axon hillock) so that it exceeds the threshold, then the trigger zone generates an action potential that propagates along the axon. (B) Time-course of changes in membrane potential and membrane permeability during one cycle of activity. Inward and outward current flows are due to the influx of Na^+ and efflux of K^+ during the rising and falling phases of the action potential, respectively. The peak of the sodium conductance occurs near the time when the membrane potential crosses the zero line. The decay in sodium conductance is accompanied by an increase in K^+ conductance. The combined effect is membrane repolarization, then hyperpolarization, before return to the resting membrane potential. The horizontal dashed lines represent the equilibrium potential as calculated from the Nernst equation for K^+ (E_K) and Na^+ (E_{Na}).

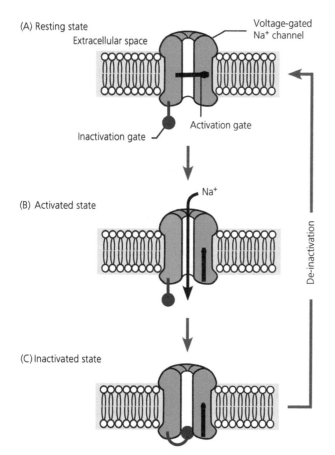

Figure 2.6 Three states of voltage-gated Na^+ channel: (A) resting state, (B) activated state, and (C) inactivated state.

change to the activated state during the rising phase of the action potential. During the **activated state**, both activation and inactivation gates of the Na^+ channel are open, and Na^+ ions flow into the neuron (Figure 2.6B). The inactivated state immediately follows the activated state. During the **inactivated state**, the inactivation gate closes the channel, preventing Na^+ from entering the neuron, but the activation gate is still open (Figure 2.6C). The inactivated state reverts to the resting state (i.e., the inactivation gate opens and the activation gate closes) to repeat the cycle of activation and inactivation of the Na^+ channels. The process of changing the inactivated state to the resting state is called **de-inactivation** and this process occurs only when the repolarizing membrane potential is sufficiently negative (i.e., below the threshold voltage). An action potential cannot be generated without reverting the inactivated state of the Na^+ channels back to the resting state. Thus, sufficient membrane repolarization and hyperpolarization are critical requirements for voltage-gated Na^+ channels to become de-inactivated.

Two phases of the action potential

Na^+ and K^+ permeabilities do not increase simultaneously during the action potential. The voltage-gated Na^+ channels open first, followed by K^+. Subsequently, there are two phases of the action potential, the rising and falling phases. During the **rising phase**, the neuronal membrane rapidly depolarizes subsequent to the opening of voltage-gated Na^+ channels and the increase in membrane permeability to Na^+ (Figure 2.5B). As the channels for Na^+ open, an influx of Na^+ drives the membrane potential toward the

Na⁺ equilibrium potential (+62 mV). This portion of the action potential, where the inside of the neuron is positive relative to the outside, is referred to as the **overshoot** (Figure 2.2). Voltage-gated Na⁺ channels do not stay open long. They are quickly inactivated and the influx of Na⁺ through these channels is terminated.

The **falling phase** of the action potential reflects Na⁺ channel inactivation and opening of voltage-gated K⁺ channels, which open after a delay of about 1 ms after membrane depolarization. The neuron is repolarized by a quick efflux of K⁺. At the end of the falling phase, the membrane potential is far more negative than the resting potential. This reflects the increased K⁺ permeability following the opening of K⁺ channels. Since little Na⁺ permeability exists during this phase, K⁺ outflow drives the membrane potential far below the resting membrane potential –65 mV) and toward the K⁺ equilibrium potential (–80 mV). This portion of the action potential below the resting membrane potential is referred to as **hyperpolarization** (or undershoot) (Figure 2.2). As the voltage-gated K⁺ channels start to close, the resting membrane potential is restored gradually before establishing the K⁺ equilibrium potential.

Na⁺/K⁺-ATPase and action potentials

The Na⁺/K⁺-ATPase plays no direct role in generation of the action potential but simply works all the time, regardless of the state of the membrane potential. Thus, the pump brings in (i) K⁺ that leaks out through the resting membrane, (ii) K⁺ that rushed out during action potentials, and (iii) Na⁺ that rushes in during an action potential. Although, Na⁺/K⁺-ATPase is essential for restoring Na⁺ and K⁺ across the membrane, stopping the pump by use of metabolic inhibitors does not immediately affect membrane excitability. This is because an action potential moves only a small fraction of ions across the membrane and a large reservoir of intracellular K⁺ is sufficient for generating action potentials for a brief period.

Refractory period

The refractory period is the period of time it takes for an excitable membrane to be ready for a second stimulus once it returns to its resting state following excitation. In other words, the refractory period represents the time needed for the voltage-gated Na⁺ channels to revert from the inactivated state to the resting state. When an action potential is initiated, a second action potential cannot be triggered for about 1 ms, regardless of how large a stimulus is applied to a neuron. This period, called the **absolute refractory period**, ensures that a second action potential will not be initiated before the completion of the first action potential, preventing overlap of action potentials. The absolute refractory period corresponds to nearly the entire duration of the action potential (Figure 2.7). It is initiated by the inactivation of the Na⁺ channels that originally opened to depolarize the membrane. The stage that follows the absolute refractory period is known as the **relative refractory period**. This starts when the membrane potential undergoes repolarization and approaches the threshold membrane voltage. It lasts

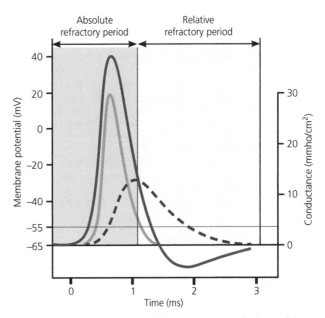

Figure 2.7 The refractory period limits the rate at which signals can be transmitted along a neuron. The absolute refractory period also assures one-way travel of an action potential from cell body to axon terminal by preventing backward conduction of the action potential.

until the time when voltage-gated K⁺ channels are closed. During the relative refractory period, initiation of a second action potential is inhibited, but not impossible, as much stronger depolarizing current that shifts the membrane potential to the threshold can generate an action potential.

There are two reasons for the difficulty in generating action potentials.

1 The voltage-gated Na⁺ channels must be de-inactivated before returning to the resting state to generate an action potential and this process requires membrane repolarization that approaches the threshold membrane voltage. Not all inactivated Na⁺ channels undergo de-inactivation simultaneously and generating an action potential requires a much stronger depolarizing potential to recruit a sufficient number of de-inactivated Na⁺ channels.

2 The membrane potential undergoes hyperpolarization as the voltage-gated K⁺ channels start to open, and a much stronger depolarizing current is required to shift the membrane potential to the threshold.

Clinical correlations

Changes in extracellular ion concentrations result in abnormal electrical activity of neurons. For example, **hyperkalemia** shifts the resting membrane potential closer to the threshold. Sustained, chronic hyperkalemia is almost always associated with some impairment in urinary excretion of potassium. An increase in extracellular potassium levels leads to depolarization of the membrane potential of excitable cells (neuron, muscle). The slowly rising depolarization starts to activate some voltage-gated Na+ channels, but their numbers are insufficient to trigger action potentials. These activated Na+ channels immediately undergo the inactivation process and stay inactivated. They cannot be activated again without de-inactivation (Figure 2.6). Furthermore, depolarization also drives opening and closing of voltage-gated K+ channels and cells become refractory. Since no action potentials can be generated under such a condition, widespread impairment of excitable cells is inevitable. The condition of low levels of circulating K+ (i.e., **hypokalemia**) leads to membrane hyperpolarization, shifting the membrane potential away from the threshold. As a result, stronger EPSPs are needed to generate action potentials. Animals with hypokalemia may show muscle weakness, as motor neurons are not properly generating action potentials.

A variety of chemicals affect the conduction of action potentials by binding to ion channels in the membrane. For example, the local anesthetic **lidocaine** (or xylocaine) blocks signal conduction by blocking voltage-gated Na+ channels. As a result, neurons fail to generate an action potential, preventing the initiation of pain signals by sensory neurons. **Tetrodotoxin** (TTX) isolated from puffer fish also binds to voltage-gated Na+ channels. This prevents affected nerve cells from firing action potentials. TTX poisoning is often fatal due to respiratory failure.

Propagation of action potentials

> **1** Explain the sequence of events involved in the movement of the action potential along the axon.
>
> **2** Why is the movement of the action potential along the axon normally unidirectional?
>
> **3** What two factors influence the conduction velocity of action potentials?
>
> **4** Why is the term "saltatory conduction" applied only to myelinated axons, but not to nonmyelinated axons?

All action potentials generated at the **trigger zone** are identical and they propagate along the axons without losing their strength. This unique propagation (also referred to as conduction) property of an action potential enables it to travel a long distance. The propagation of an action potential involves the passive spread of current, by movement of electrons along the axon. This local current opens nearby voltage-gated Na+ channels and generates a new action potential (Figure 2.8A). This cycle continues along an axon. Thus the passive spread of current along an axon is responsible for the active regeneration of an action potential that continues until it reaches the terminal end of an axon. The action potential reaching the terminal end is identical to the initial action potential generated at the trigger zone. This passive spread of current involving an active regeneration process is somewhat similar to the falling movement of a series of dominos laid down to form a line. When the first domino falls, it hits the next domino, passing on its kinetic energy. The second domino falls and it transfers identical kinetic energy to the third domino. This process continues until the last domino falls.

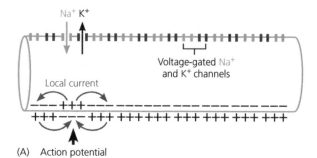

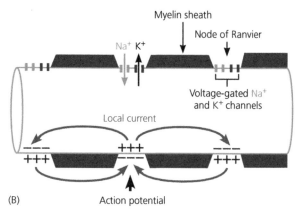

Figure 2.8 Current paths during the propagation of the action potential in myelinated (A) and nonmyelinated (B) axons. In both axons, the top portion of the membrane illustrates the distribution of voltage-gated Na+ and K+ channels. The bottom portion of the axon shows the reversal of membrane polarity triggered by local depolarization. The local currents generated by an action potential flow to adjacent areas of the axonal membrane to depolarize and generate further action potentials. Myelinated axons have Na+ and K+ channels at the node of Ranvier and action potentials jump from one node of Ranvier to the next. This process is referred to as saltatory conduction.

Conduction speed

The **propagation** of action potentials along the axon depends on two principles of cable properties: the diameter of the axon and the resistance of the axonal membrane to current that leaks out (Figure 2.9). Current passing inside an axon is similar to water flowing in a pipe: it faces resistance from the membrane. Since the speed of the passive current depends on the longitudinal conductance of the axoplasm, increasing the axonal size helps increase the conduction velocity of an axon. Another way to help conduction speed is by myelinating axons, which prevents current leakage through the axonal membrane and effectively insulates them.

The myelinated portion of an axon (i.e., internode) has no voltage-gated Na+ and K+ channels. These channels are located at the node of Ranvier. As a result, passive current generated by an action potential must reach the adjacent node of Ranvier to generate a new action potential (Figure 2.8B). Myelination of axons makes this possible. As the passive current generated by an action potential at one node is strong enough to reach the adjacent node, it activates voltage-gated Na+ and K+ channels

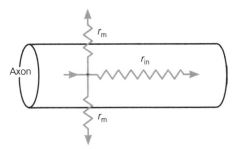

Figure 2.9 An axon is similar to an electrical cable. Local currents that leak across the membrane resistance (r_m) are lost from the axon, whereas those currents that travel through the axoplasm, i.e., longitudinal resistance (r_{in}), carry the electrical signal along the axon. Thus, signal transmission along the axon is more efficient by increasing the ratio of r_m/r_{in}.

and generates a new action potential. At the same time, Na^+ channels at the preceding node of Ranvier are inactivated, K^+ channels open, and repolarization occurs. This cycle continues to the end of the axon. Thus the myelin sheath around an axon makes it possible for current to jump from one node to the adjacent node, instead of traveling along the axon micron by micron. Conduction of the action potential jumping from node to node is called **saltatory conduction** (Latin *saltare*, leap). Myelination increases conduction speed without increasing the axonal diameter. For example, a nonmyelinated axon of 10 μm diameter conducts action potentials at 0.5 m/s as compared with 50 m/s by a myelinated axon of similar diameter. Thus, larger diameter and myelination of axons effectively increase the conduction speed.

A neuron generates action potentials whose amplitude and duration of rising and falling phases are all identical. Postsynaptic neurons determine the stimulus intensity applied to presynaptic neurons by monitoring the frequency of incoming action potentials. It is important to remember that a graded potential exceeding the

threshold at the trigger zone generates a burst of action potentials, not just one action potential. Furthermore, the intensity of the graded potential is proportional to the frequency of action potentials generated at the trigger zone. The quantity of neurotransmitter released at the presynaptic terminal is also proportional to the frequency of action potentials reaching the presynaptic site.

Self-evaluation

Answers can be found at the end of the chapter.

1 Which of the following best describes a neuron at the resting state?
  A Na^+/K^+-ATPase pumps are not active
  B The resting membrane potential is about +65 mV
  C K^+ ions leak out of a neuron via nongated K^+ channels
  D Voltage-gated K^+ channels are open
  E The resting state represents the relative refractory period

2 A local anesthetic, such as lidocaine, prevents generation of action potential by inactivating:
  A Receptors for GABA
  B Nongated Na^+ channels
  C Voltage-gated Ca^{2+} channels
  D Voltage-gated Na^+ channels
  E Release of the neurotransmitter acetylcholine

3 The rising phase of an action potential is triggered by:
  A Inhibitory postsynaptic potentials (IPSP)
  B Na^+/K^+-ATPase pumps
  C Opening of voltage-gated K^+ channels
  D Inactivation of voltage-gated Na^+ channels
  E Activation of voltage-gated Na^+ channels

4 Graded potentials occur at:
  A Presynaptic sites
  B Postsynaptic sites

5 Action potentials follow the all-or-none principle.
  A True
  B False

6 Which of the following is a characteristic of a graded potential?
  A Adheres to the all-or-none principle of the stimulus applied at synaptic sites
  B Depolarizes or hyperpolarizes postsynaptic membrane
  C Opens voltage-gated Na^+ channels
  D Propagates along axons

7 The membrane of resting neurons is selectively permeable to K^+ due to the presence of high numbers of nongated K^+ channels.
  A True
  B False

8 An EPSP is a local hyperpolarization of the membrane.
  A True
  B False

Clinical correlations

Demyelination can result from certain diseases, such as degenerative myelopathy and canine distemper in animals and multiple sclerosis in humans. **Canine degenerative myelopathy** is an incurable, slowly progressive disease of the spinal cord. This degenerative disease is similar to amyotrophic lateral sclerosis in humans. In **canine distemper**, the virus targets glial cells leading to demyelination of axons. Clinical signs associated with demyelination depend on whether the damage involves motor or sensory fibers. The loss of myelin can have devastating effects on neuronal signaling. The strength of current generated by action potentials decreases when current leaks out of the demyelinated areas of axons. As a result, current is no longer able to travel far to reach the adjacent node of Ranvier, where voltage-gated Na^+ and K^+ channels are located, and current simply disappears. After demyelination, therefore, axons fail to conduct action potentials.

9 An IPSP is a local depolarization of the membrane.
   A True
   B False

10 For inhibitory graded potentials (IPSPs) to occur during synaptic transmission, an inhibitory neurotransmitter must bind to the:
   A Ligand-gated receptors to trigger influx of Cl⁻
   B Ligand-gated receptors to trigger influx of Na⁺
   C Voltage-gated Na⁺ channels to trigger influx of Na⁺
   D Voltage-gated K⁺ channels to trigger influx of K⁺

11 What is the result in the postsynaptic neuron when EPSPs increase but IPSPs stay the same?
   A The likelihood of an action potential increases
   B The likelihood of an action potential decreases
   C The likelihood of an action potential stays the same
   D EPSPs and IPSPs do not affect the postsynaptic neuron

12 What triggers depolarization phase of an action potential?
   A Na⁺ moves into the cell.
   B Na⁺ moves out of the cell
   C Increased permeability to K⁺ ions
   D K⁺ moves into the cell

13 Hypokalemia induces _____ of the neuronal membrane and makes neurons _____ _____.
   A Hyperpolarization, more excitable
   B Hyperpolarization, less excitable
   C Depolarization, more excitable
   D Depolarization, less excitable

14 During the absolute refractory period, which gate on the voltage-gated Na⁺ channel is closed?
   A Activation
   B Inactivation
   C Both activation and inactivation
   D Neither activation nor inactivation

15 Which neurotransmitter generates EPSPs that depolarize the post-synaptic membrane during synaptic transmission?
   A Glycine
   B Acetylcholine
   C GABA
   D All of the above

16 The conduction of an action potential from one node of Ranvier to the next node is referred to as:
   A EPSP
   B Saltatory conduction
   C Ionic conduction

17 Depolarization during an action potential is caused by opening of which gate on the voltage-gated Na⁺ channels?
   A Activation
   B Inactivation
   C Both activation and inactivation

18 When two action potentials arrive from two separate presynaptic neurons to the same postsynaptic neurons simultaneously, summation of postsynaptic graded potentials is called:
   A Spatial summation
   B Temporal summation

Suggested reading

Aidley, D.J. (1998) *The Physiology of Excitable Cells*, 4th edn. Cambridge University Press, Cambridge, UK.

Berne, R.M., Levy, M.N., Koeppen, B.M. and Stanton, B.A. (2008) *Physiology*, 6th edn. Mosby Elsevier, Philadelphia.

Dwyer, T.M. (2006) The electrochemical basis of nerve function. In: *Fundamental Neuroscience for Basic and Clinical Applications*, 3rd edn (ed. D.E. Haines), pp. 35–68. Elsevier, Philadelphia.

Kandel, E.R., Schwartz, J.H. and Jessell, T.M. (eds) (2000) *Principles of Neural Science*, 4th edn. McGraw-Hill, New York.

Magee, J.C. and Johnston, D. (1995) Synaptic activation of voltage-gated channels in the dendrites of hippocampal pyramidal neurons. *Science* 268:301–304.

Narahashi, T., Moore, J.W. and Scott, W.R. (1964) Tetrodotoxin blockage of sodium conductance increase in lobster giant axons. *Journal of General Physiology* 47:965–974.

Poo, M. (1985) Mobility and locations of proteins in excitable membranes. *Annual Review of Neuroscience* 8:369–406.

Siegel, A. and Sapru, H.N. (2006) *Essential Neuroscience*, revised 1st edn. Lippincott, Williams & Wilkins, Baltimore.

Stein, W.H. (1990) *Channels, Carriers, and Pumps: An Introduction to Membrane Transport*. Academic Press, San Diego, CA.

Answers

1	C	10	A
2	D	11	A
3	E	12	A
4	B	13	B
5	A	14	B
6	B	15	B
7	A	16	B
8	B	17	C
9	B	18	A

3 Synaptic Transmission

Etsuro E. Uemura
Iowa State University, Ames, IA, USA

A synapse is a special site of contact, where one neuron communicates with others. Transfer of signals from one neuron to another via synapses is called synaptic transmission. Synaptic transmission also occurs between motor neurons (somatic, visceral) and their target tissues (skeletal muscle, cardiac muscle, smooth muscle, glands). There are two distinct classes of synapses, electrical and chemical, but the majority of synapses present in the mammalian nervous system are chemical synapses. In an **electrical synapse**, ion channels connect the cytoplasm of the presynaptic and postsynaptic cells at a gap junction, allowing ionic current to flow passively through the gap junction pores from one neuron to another. Electrical synapses occur, for example, in the hypothalamus, neocortex, hippocampus, and thalamus. In the hypothalamus, electrical synapses enable groups of connected neurons to fire and secrete hormones almost simultaneously into the circulation. In contrast, a **chemical synapse** has no gap junctions. Instead, there is a narrow space, called the synaptic cleft, between the presynaptic and postsynaptic membrane. The presynaptic terminal contains numerous synaptic vesicles filled with a neurotransmitter and the postsynaptic membrane is equipped with receptors for that specific neurotransmitter. Synaptic transmission involves the release of a neurotransmitter from presynaptic terminals and then the binding of the neurotransmitter to postsynaptic receptors. The receptors, in response, open specific ion channels that lead to changes in postsynaptic membrane potential.

Neurotransmitters

1 What are the major neurotransmitters of the CNS and PNS?
2 What are examples of amine, amino acid and peptide neurotransmitters?

3 Explain the synthesis and recycling of the excitatory neurotransmitters acetylcholine and glutamate.
4 Explain how nerve impulses are transmitted from one neuron to others.

An action potential depolarizes the presynaptic terminal. This leads to opening of voltage-gated Ca^{2+} channels in the presynaptic membrane (Figure 3.1). Calcium is highly concentrated outside the cell (2 mmol/L) compared with inside the cell (0.0002 mmol/L). Ca^{2+} enters the neurons due to the electrochemical gradient. Calcium entry triggers the sequence of events that lead to fusion of synaptic vesicles with presynaptic membrane and release of the neurotransmitter into the synaptic cleft by the process of exocytosis. Neurotransmitters are released in packets of discrete numbers of molecules from synaptic vesicles of approximately 50 nm in diameter. Neurotransmitters in the synaptic cleft then bind with their specific postsynaptic receptors. This action causes the ligand-gated channels to open. The type of neurotransmitter and its specific ligand-gated receptors determine what ions enter or leave.

Neurotransmitters of the PNS and CNS

Neurotransmitters present in the peripheral nervous system (PNS) are acetylcholine (ACh), norepinephrine, and epinephrine. In the central nervous system (CNS), a variety of chemicals act as neurotransmitters, including ACh, amines, serotonin, dopamine, norepinephrine, epinephrine, glutamate, aspartate, glycine, γ-aminobutyric acid (GABA), peptides, and nitric oxide (Table 3.1). **Acetylcholine** is synthesized from choline and acetyl coenzyme A (acetyl-CoA) in the axon terminal (Figure 3.2A). Neurons that release ACh are

Dukes' Physiology of Domestic Animals, Thirteenth Edition. Edited by William O. Reece, Howard H. Erickson, Jesse P. Goff and Etsuro E. Uemura.
© 2015 John Wiley & Sons, Inc. Published 2015 by John Wiley & Sons, Inc.
Companion website: www.wiley.com/go/reece/physiology

Table 3.1 Major neurotransmitters of the central nervous system.

Acetylcholine
Amino acids
  Glutamate
  Aspartate
  Glycine
  γ-Aminobutyric acid (GABA)
Amines
  Dopamine
  Norepinephrine
  Epinephrine
  Serotonin
  Histamine
Peptides
  Endorphins
  Enkephalins
  Substance P
Purines
  ATP
Gases
  Nitric oxide

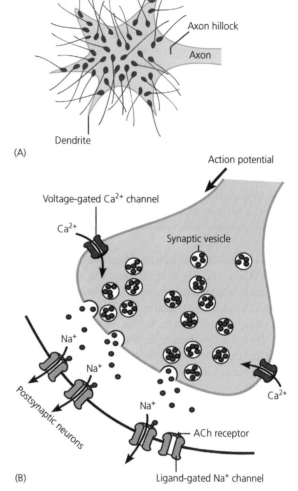

(A)

(B)

Figure 3.1 Synapse in the central and peripheral nervous systems. (A) Postsynaptic neuron receives numerous excitatory and inhibitory axons. (B) Presynaptic membrane contains voltage-gated Ca^{2+} channels. Numerous synaptic vesicles are also present in presynaptic terminals. When an action potential reaches the terminal end, voltage-gated Ca^{2+} channels open, resulting in influx of Ca^{2+} into the terminal end. Ca^{2+} triggers the sequence of events that lead to fusion of synaptic vesicles with presynaptic membrane, and release of the neurotransmitter into the synaptic cleft by exocytosis. Binding of neurotransmitters with a ligand-gated postsynaptic receptor induces a specific postsynaptic response. The neurotransmitters are then eliminated from the synaptic cleft by enzymatic degradation or reuptake by neurons.

called cholinergic neurons. The **amine** neurotransmitters (e.g., dopamine, norepinephrine, epinephrine, serotonin, histamine, tyrosine) are derived from amino acids. Dopamine, norepinephrine, and epinephrine are synthesized from tyrosine. Neurons that release norepinephrine or epinephrine are called adrenergic neurons. Serotonin (or 5-hydroxytryptamine or 5-HT) is derived from the amino acid tryptophan and histamine from histidine. **Glutamate** and **aspartate** are the excitatory neurotransmitters of the CNS. The primary inhibitory neurotransmitters in the CNS are **GABA** and **glycine**. Peptides that act as neurotransmitters include substance P and opioid peptides such as enkephalins and endorphins. Substance P is involved in pain pathways and enkephalins and endorphins mediate analgesia. An unusual neurotransmitter, **nitric oxide (NO)**, diffuses freely into the target neuron to bind to intracellular proteins. Nitric oxide is synthesized from oxygen and the amino acid arginine.

Neurotransmitters are removed quickly from the synaptic cleft after detaching from their receptors. This involves at least two processes: (i) enzymatic inactivation in the synaptic cleft and (ii) diffusion away from the synaptic cleft. **Enzymatic inactivation** in the synaptic cleft is followed by subsequent uptake of constituents by the presynaptic terminal for resynthesis of neurotransmitter. For example, ACh released into the synaptic cleft attaches to postsynaptic receptors and quickly detaches before being broken down to choline and acetate by acetylcholinesterase (AChE) present on the postsynaptic membrane (Figure 3.2A). Choline is actively transported back into the presynaptic terminal for resynthesis of more ACh neurotransmitter. The other process for removing neurotransmitters from the synaptic cleft is **diffusion**. This allows neurotransmitters to enter the circulation or be transported back into the

neuron or into astrocytes. For example, glutamate is transported back into the presynaptic terminal or astrocytes (Figure 3.2B). In the presynaptic terminal, glutamate is repackaged into synaptic vesicles. In the astrocytes, glutamate is converted to glutamine by glutamine synthetase. Glutamine is then transported to the presynaptic terminal by glutamine transporters, and it is repackaged into synaptic vesicles to be used as neurotransmitter.

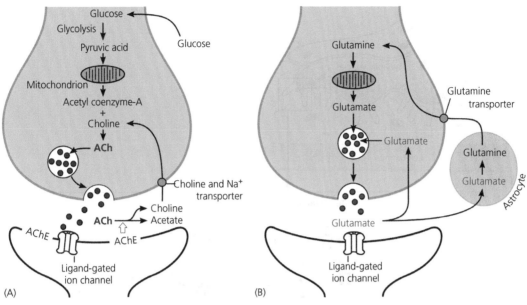

Figure 3.2 Synthesis and recycling of the excitatory neurotransmitters acetylcholine (ACh) and glutamate. (A) ACh released into the synaptic cleft attaches to ACh receptors, then quickly detaches from the receptors. Acetylcholinesterase (AChE) breaks down ACh in the synaptic cleft to choline and acetate. Choline is actively transported back into the presynaptic terminal for synthesis of new ACh. (B) Glutamate released into the synaptic cleft is transported back into the presynaptic terminal or into astrocytes. In the presynaptic terminal, glutamate is repackaged into synaptic vesicles. Astrocytes convert glutamate into glutamine, which is used to synthesize glutamate in neurons.

Receptors for neurotransmitters

> 1 Define an ionotropic and a metabotropic receptor.
>
> 2 Describe the spatial relationship between the receptor and effector cell.
>
> 3 What are the subtypes of cholinergic and adrenergic receptors and where are they located in the body?

Neurotransmitters released from presynaptic sites bind with receptors on the postsynaptic membrane. Postsynaptic receptors are special signal recognition proteins. Their binding with a neurotransmitter changes the permeability to selected ions through their ion channels. This enables ions to distribute across the neuronal membrane according to their electrochemical gradient. The ion channels are gated either directly or indirectly by activating a second-messenger system of the postsynaptic neuron. In **directly gated ion channels**, the binding site for the neurotransmitter is part of the ion channel and neurotransmitter binding results in a conformational change that leads to opening of the ion channel. A receptor with directly gated ion channels is referred to as an **ionotropic receptor**. This quick synaptic response occurs in just a few milliseconds. Neurotransmitters that bind to ionotropic receptors include ACh, glutamate, glycine, and GABA. **Indirectly gated channels**, in contrast, are separated from the binding site of the neurotransmitter. Such receptors are called **metabotropic receptors**. Binding of neurotransmitters to metabotropic receptors activates a guanosine 5′-triphosphate (GTP)-binding protein (G-protein). G-protein, in turn, activates a second messenger system that either (i) opens the ion channel by directly acting on it or (ii) activates an enzyme that opens the channel by phosphorylating the channel protein. Closure of the ion channels is induced by their dephosphorylation. Activation of metabotropic receptors leads to slow and long-lasting synaptic action. Neurotransmitters in the CNS and PNS, with the exception of nitric oxide, bind to several different receptor types. Each receptor type may have numbers of subtypes, which trigger different effects on binding with a given neurotransmitter.

Cholinergic receptors

There are two subtypes of **cholinergic receptors** (i.e., receptors that bind ACh), nicotinic and muscarinic. The name simply indicates that nicotine is an agonist of the nicotinic receptor and muscarine, found in some fungi, is an agonist of the muscarinic receptor. **Nicotinic acetylcholine receptors (nAChRs)** are present in the skeletal muscle as well as the central and autonomic nervous systems (Figure 3.3, see also Figure 10.7). Ion channels of nicotinic receptors allow passage of both Na^+ and K^+ based on the electrochemical gradient. However, Na^+ inflow far exceeds the small K^+ outflow. Activation of nicotinic receptors leads to generation of excitatory postsynaptic potentials (EPSPs).

Muscarinic acetylcholine receptors (mAChRs) are present in the CNS and parasympathetic division of the autonomic nervous system (Figure 3.4, see also Figure 10.7). There are several subtypes of muscarinic receptors (M_1, M_2, M_3, etc.) and

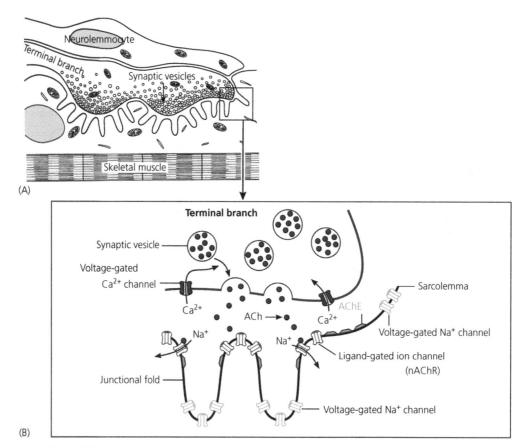

Figure 3.3 (A) Lateral view of the neuromuscular synapse, which comprises a terminal branch of the motor end plate and junctional folds of sarcolemma. A terminal branch of the motor end plate contains numerous synaptic vesicles with acetylcholine. (B) Synaptic transmission at the neuromuscular synapse involves (1) depolarization of the terminal branch that opens the voltage-gated Ca^{2+} channel and subsequent influx of Ca^{2+} into the terminal branch, resulting in the release of ACh into the synaptic cleft by exocytosis; and (2) ACh binding with nicotinic ACh receptors (nAChR) on the sarcolemma and subsequent net influx of Na^+ that results in generation of an EPP. Voltage-gated Na^+ channels are present in the depths of postsynaptic junctional folds and in the perijunctional area. If the EPP reaches the threshold voltage (–50 mV), voltage-gated Na^+ channels open to generate an action potential.

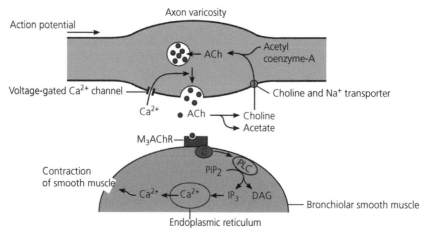

Figure 3.4 Terminal axons of parasympathetic postsynaptic neurons have bead-like swellings known as boutons en passage. These varicosities contain neurotransmitter ACh. Released ACh binds to postsynaptic G protein-coupled muscarinic (M_3) acetylcholine receptors that activate phospholipase C (PLC). PLC converts membrane lipids into inositol trisphosphate (IP_3) and diacylglycerol (DAG). IP_3 releases Ca^{2+} stored in the endoplasmic reticulum, increasing cytoplasmic Ca^{2+}. This leads to smooth muscle contraction (bronchoconstriction).

all are coupled to G proteins, which are linked to second messenger systems. The action of ACh differs depending on the muscarinic receptor subtypes present in the tissue. Binding of neurotransmitters to their receptors leads to generation of either excitatory or inhibitory postsynaptic graded potentials. The receptor subtypes activated by neurotransmitters and subsequent opening of ligand-gated channels for specific ions determine such a change in postsynaptic membrane potential. For example, ACh contracts bronchiolar smooth muscle by binding to the cholinergic M_3 receptor. In contrast, ACh induces a decrease in heart rate by binding to the cholinergic M_2 receptor present in the heart.

Adrenergic receptors

There are two subtypes of **adrenergic receptors** (i.e., receptors that bind epinephrine and norepinephrine), the α and β. Adrenergic receptors, like cholinergic muscarinic receptors, are linked to G proteins and initiate second messenger cascades (Figure 3.5). However, α- and β-adrenergic receptors initiate different second messenger pathways.

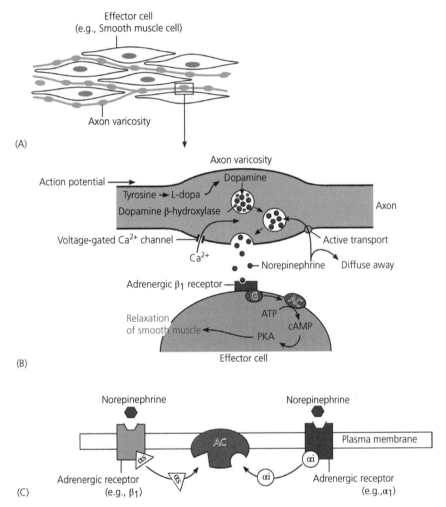

Figure 3.5 (A) Terminal axons of autonomic postsynaptic neurons have bead-like swellings known as boutons en passage. These axon varicosities contain neurotransmitters. They stay close to the surface of the effector cells, but structures similar to the neuromuscular synapse are generally not present. (B) Norepinephrine is released at a varicosity of a sympathetic axon. An action potential opens voltage-gated Ca^{2+} channels, triggering the fusion of synaptic vesicles with the membrane of a varicosity and the release of norepinephrine. Norepinephrine in the synaptic cleft binds to adrenergic receptors, diffuses away from the synapse, or returns to the axon. In the axon, norepinephrine can be metabolized by monoamine oxidase or taken up into synaptic vesicles for release. Adrenergic β receptors, for example, are coupled to G protein, which stimulates adenylyl cyclase (AC). It has been suggested that cAMP-dependent protein kinase A (PKA) increases Ca^{2+} uptake by internal stores, inactivates myosin light chain kinase, and activates cell membrane ion channels, and transporters such as K^+ channels and Na^+/K^+-ATPase. These effects of PKA reduce intracellular Ca^{2+} concentration and increase contractile protein phosphorylation that leads to relaxation of smooth muscle. (C) Adenylyl cyclase (AC) can be stimulated or inhibited via signal transduction pathways. Receptors for agonists that stimulate AC activate G_s, whose α_s subunit dissociates from the $\beta\gamma$ subunits and then interacts with AC to stimulate it. Receptors for agonists that inhibit AC activate G_i, whose α_i subunit inhibits AC.

Glutamate receptors

The main excitatory neurotransmitter in the CNS is glutamate. The response of postsynaptic neurons to glutamate varies depending on the glutamate receptor subtypes present in the tissue. There are two subtypes of glutamate receptors, **NMDA** (*N*-methyl-D-aspartate) and **AMPA** (α-amino-3-hydroxy-5-methyl-4-isoxazole propionic acid). The name reflects that *N*-methyl-D-aspartate is an agonist of the NMDA receptor and α-amino-3-hydroxy-5-methyl-4-isoxazole propionic acid is an agonist of the AMPA receptor. NMDA receptors represent ligand-gated channels that allow passage of Na^+, K^+, and Ca^{2+}. AMPA receptors are also ligand-gated cation channels. Their binding with glutamate opens the channels for Na^+ influx, generating EPSPs.

Neuromuscular synapse

> **1** What are the morphological differences between a neuromuscular synapse and a synapse in the CNS?
>
> **2** What is the neurotransmitter of the neuromuscular synapse?
>
> **3** Define excitatory postsynaptic potential (EPSP) and end-plate potential (EPP).
>
> **4** Explain the major steps involved in synaptic transmission at the neuromuscular synapse.

One motor neuron innervates a group of skeletal muscle fibers. To do so, axons of motor neurons branch at their termini to innervate muscle fibers, all of which contract together as a unit. This unit comprising a motor neuron and the muscle fibers it innervates is known as a **motor unit**. Muscle fibers that belong to one motor unit do not make synaptic contact with any other motor neurons. Nerve impulses to skeletal muscle fibers are mediated by a neuromuscular synapse (also referred to as **neuromuscular junction**). It is composed of a group of several terminal branches and skeletal muscle fibers.

Neuromuscular synapses commonly occur at the midpoint of muscle fibers. At this site, an axon terminates on a muscle fiber as a motor end plate, about $40 \times 60\,\mu m$ in diameter. Many short terminal branches of an axon form a motor end plate. At the light microscopic level, these structures appear as oblong disk-like structures on skeletal muscle fibers. In the terminal branches of the motor end plate are synaptic vesicles containing ACh (Figure 3.3A), where docking proteins are present in close approximation to voltage-gated Ca^{2+} channels. This arrangement allows efficient execution of events associated with synaptic transmission, including opening of voltage-gated Ca^{2+} channels and Ca^{2+} influx into terminal branches, followed by calcium-dependent attachment of synaptic vesicles to presynaptic membranes and release of ACh into the synaptic cleft by exocytosis (Figure 3.3B).

Excitatory neurotransmitters Terminal branches of the motor end plate lie in a primary synaptic cleft of the sarcolemma. The postsynaptic area is increased by junctional folds extending from the primary synaptic cleft. Present on top of the folds are nAChRs (Figure 3.3B). The basement membrane of the postsynaptic sarcolemma contains a high concentration of the enzyme AChE that hydrolyzes the transmitter into choline and acetate. AChE is synthesized in the presynaptic perikarya and transported to the synaptic site.

Synaptic transmission at the neuromuscular synapse

Action potentials reach the terminal branch of an axon and depolarize the presynaptic membrane. Subsequent ionic events that occur at the neuromuscular synapse are similar to the events that occur at synapses between neurons. Depolarization of the terminal branch opens the voltage-gated Ca^{2+} channels. Influx of Ca^{2+} triggers a series of steps that promote fusion of the synaptic vesicle with the terminal membrane and release of ACh into the synaptic cleft by exocytosis. ACh binds to nAChRs on the junctional folds of the sarcolemma. This opens ligand-gated ionic channels that are permeable to both Na^+ and K^+. In skeletal muscle cells at the resting potential ($-90\,mV$), the driving force for Na^+ to enter the cell far exceeds that for K^+ to leave the cell. In fact, K^+ outflow is so small, some textbooks simply indicate that ligand-gated ionic channels only mediate Na^+ influx. A net inflow of Na^+ results in generation of an EPSP, moving the membrane potential from $-90\,mV$ toward zero. In the muscle cells, an EPSP is referred to as an **end-plate potential (EPP)**. Although the postsynaptic sarcolemma is depolarized and generates an EPP, it is not electrically excitable and does not itself generate action potentials.

Voltage-gated Na^+ channels are concentrated in the depths of junctional folds and in the perijunctional area (Figure 3.3B). If the EPP is sufficiently large at the neuromuscular synapse (around $-50\,mV$), voltage-gated Na^+ channels start to open and generate an action potential. Action potentials propagate along the muscle fiber and initiate the series of events that lead to contraction of skeletal muscle. The electrochemical events governing the neuromuscular synapse and the synapse between neurons are similar; however, the neuromuscular synapse is somewhat unique in the following respects.

1 One motor neuron innervates a variable number of muscle fibers, forming a motor unit (whereas synapses between neurons are made by numerous other motor neurons, sensory neurons, and interneurons).

2 Action potentials generate only EPPs (whereas synapses between neurons generate both EPSPs and IPSPs).

3 ACh is the only neurotransmitter (whereas synapses between neurons involves many other neurotransmitters, e.g., ACh, glutamate, aspartate, GABA, glycine, 5-HT, substance P).

4 nAChR is the only receptor type (whereas synapses between neurons utilize many other receptors (e.g., muscarinic, NMDA, AMPA).

Clinical correlations

Impaired synaptic transmission at neuromuscular synapses results in a loss of motor control of skeletal muscle. **Curare**, for example, is a non-depolarizing muscle relaxant that blocks nAChRs at the neuromuscular synapse. The main toxin of curare, D-tubocurarine, binds to the same position on the nAChR as ACh with an equal or greater affinity, making it a competitive antagonist. Thus curare blocks the EPP that normally leads to the initiation of the muscle action potential. South American indigenous people used curare as a paralyzing poison. The prey was shot by arrows or blowgun darts dipped in curare, resulting in asphyxiation due to blocked neuromuscular transmission at respiratory muscles. The antidote for curare poisoning is an anti-AChE that inhibits acetylcholinesterase. Anti-AChE increases the available ACh in the neuromuscular synapse. Since curare is a competitive ACh antagonist, increased levels of ACh activate the AChRs not blocked by toxin at a higher rate.

When synaptic transmission at a presynaptic site is impaired, clinical signs similar to those induced by lesion of a motor neuron occur. For example, tick paralysis and botulism are caused by toxins that act on a presynaptic site of neuromuscular synapses, interfering with the release of ACh. **Tick paralysis** is induced by a neurotoxin secreted by feeding female ticks (*Dermacentor andersoni*, *Dermacentor variabilis*). Clinical signs appear 7–9 days after the attachment of ticks and rapidly progress to hypotonia, areflexia, and paralysis. The prognosis is good if the ticks are removed promptly, with recovery taking place quickly in most instances. **Botulism** is induced by toxins produced by *Clostridium botulinum*. Type C toxin most often affects dogs. Ingestion of contaminated foods is the primary route of exposure to the toxin. The animal will develop acute, progressive quadriplegia with hypotonia and a markedly reduced myotatic reflex. Cranial nerves may be affected, resulting in facial weakness. Since the toxin affects only the neuromuscular synapse, sensory fibers are intact and the dog feels pain.

Loss of the postsynaptic AChR at neuromuscular synapses also leads to loss of muscle strength. For example, **myasthenia gravis** induces clinical signs similar to those of motor neuron disease. It is characterized by progressive muscle weakness and fatigability. Typically, affected dogs suffer exercise-induced weakness that improves following rest. The muscular weakness and fatigability associated with acquired myasthenia gravis are caused by an autoimmune attack on the AChR. The myasthenic antibodies against AChR have been shown to affect neuromuscular transmission by (i) binding to the AChR and altering function; (ii) triggering cross-linking between the receptors, followed by their incorporation into muscle cells by the process of endocytosis, effectively decreasing the number of AChRs available to incoming ACh; and (iii) activating complement leading to destruction of the postsynaptic surface.

Boutons en passage

> 1 What are the morphological differences between neuromuscular synapse and boutons en passage?
>
> 2 Name examples of second messengers at terminal axons of autonomic postsynaptic neurons and explain their pathways associated with G protein-coupled receptors.

The autonomic nervous system innervates smooth muscle cells, cardiac muscle cells, and myoepithelial cells of glands. Autonomic nerve fibers are highly branched and form extensive plexuses. Their terminal axons have bead-like swellings (varicosities) along their length. The varicosities are referred to as boutons en passage (Figure 3.5A). They contain adrenergic neurotransmitters in sympathetic nerve fibers and cholinergic neurotransmitters in parasympathetic nerve fibers. Boutons en passage stay close to the plasma membrane of the effector cells, but structures similar to the neuromuscular synapse are not present.

Sympathetic signal transduction

Neurotransmitters of the **sympathetic division** include norepinephrine and epinephrine. Stimulatory or inhibitory action of these neurotransmitters depends on the receptor. Adrenergic receptors are classified into two categories, α- and β-adrenergic receptors. Each category of adrenergic receptor is further separated into several receptor subtypes (e.g., α_1, α_2, β_1, β_2, β_3). Adrenergic receptors are coupled to G proteins. Those G proteins that are coupled to β-adrenergic subtypes are referred to as G_s. Norepinephrine activates these heterotrimeric G_s-type G proteins, causing the α_s subunit ("s" indicates stimulatory) to dissociate from the βγ subunits and activate adenylyl cyclase. This results in an increase in intracellular cyclic adenosine monophosphate (cAMP), which activates protein kinase A (PKA). The mechanism by which cAMP causes relaxation of smooth muscle is not well understood. However, some studies suggest that cAMP-dependent PKA increases Ca^{2+} uptake by internal stores, inactivates myosin light chain kinase, and activates cell membrane ion channels and transporters such as K^+ channels and Na^+/K^+-ATPase. These effects of PKA lead to reduction of intracellular Ca^{2+} concentration and increased contractile protein phosphorylation, and subsequent relaxation of smooth muscle. In contrast, the G proteins coupled to α-adrenergic receptor subtypes are referred to as G_i. Norepinephrine also activates heterotrimeric G_i-type G proteins, causing dissociation of the α_i subunit ("i" indicates inhibitory) from the βγ subunits of G protein. Subunit α_i inhibits adenylyl cyclase and causes a subsequent decrease in intracellular cAMP, leading to contraction of smooth muscle. Therefore, adenylyl cyclase can be either stimulated or inhibited by G protein.

Parasympathetic signal transduction

There are two subtypes of cholinergic receptors, nicotinic and muscarinic. nAChRs in the autonomic nervous system are found in the presynaptic ganglia of both sympathetic and parasympathetic divisions. Ion channels of nicotinic receptors allow passage of both Na^+ and K^+ based on the electrochemical gradient. Neurons are depolarized, since the driving force for Na^+ to enter the cell far exceeds that for K^+ to leave the cell. mAChRs are present in the postganglionic neurons. They are also present in sweat gland cells. There are several subtypes of muscarinic receptors (M_1, M_2, M_3, etc.) and all are coupled to G proteins. The action of ACh reflects the muscarinic receptor subtypes present in the tissue. For example, ACh contracts the bronchiolar smooth muscle by binding to M_3 receptors (Figure 3.4). The steps involved in the contraction of bronchiolar smooth muscle are as follows: ACh binds to muscarinic receptor M_3. This leads to activation of G protein, followed by stimulation of phospholipase C (PLC). The activation of PLC generates two intracellular second messengers, inositol trisphosphate (IP_3) and diacylglycerol (DAG), from the hydrolysis of phosphatidylinositol 4,5-bisphosphate (PIP_2). IP_3 binds to a calcium channel on the endoplasmic reticulum. This IP_3 binding opens the Ca^{2+} channel, allowing Ca^{2+} to diffuse out of the endoplasmic reticulum into the cytosol. An increase in intracellular Ca^{2+} leads to smooth muscle contraction (bronchoconstriction).

G proteins also modulate certain ion channels without mediation by a second messenger. For example, cholinergic M_2 receptors in the heart activate a specific class of K^+ channels. In response to ACh, M_2 receptors activate G_i-type G proteins, with dissociation of the α_i subunit from the $\beta\gamma$ subunit. The $\beta\gamma$ subunit directly activates a particular class of K^+ channels and hyperpolarizes the cardiac and pacemaker cells. Thus, binding of ACh to M_2 receptors in the heart results in increased K^+ conductance to slow the heart rate.

Self-evaluation

Answers can be found at the end of the chapter.

1 What neurotransmitter is released at the neuromuscular synapse?
   A Norepinephrine
   B Acetylcholine
   C Glutamate

2 Acetylcholinesterase (AChE) present at the postsynaptic membrane breaks up ACh in the synaptic cleft to choline and acetate.
   A True
   B False

3 Choline is actively transported back into the presynaptic terminal for synthesis of new ACh.
   A True
   B False

4 The ion most directly responsible for neurotransmitter release is calcium.
   A True
   B False

5 Which neurotransmitter generates a graded potential that depolarizes the postsynaptic membrane during synaptic transmission?
   A Glycine
   B Acetylcholine
   C GABA
   D All of the above

6 Which of the following is an excitatory neurotransmitter?
   A Glycine
   B Acetylcholine
   C GABA

7 Which of the following is an ionotropic receptor?
   A Acetylcholine
   B Norepinephrine
   C Epinephrine

8 Which statement is true about the neuromuscular synapse?
   A Presynaptic membrane has voltage-gated Na^+ channels
   B Axons of the motor end plate have their cell bodies in the dorsal horn
   C Sarcolemma forms junctional folds
   D Presynaptic membrane has ligand-gated ion channels

9 Enzymatic action is one of the means to clear a neurotransmitter at a synapse.
   A True
   B False

10 Adrenergic β receptors are coupled to G protein, which directly stimulates adenylyl cyclase.
   A True
   B False

11 One of the binding sites of norepinephrine is:
   A Muscarinic receptor subtype M_1
   B Muscarinic receptor subtype M_2
   C Nicotinic receptors
   D β_1 Adrenergic receptor

12 Postganglionic parasympathetic neurons have _____ receptors that bind to neurotransmitter _____.
   A Nicotinic, norepinephrine
   B Adrenergic β_1, norepinephrine
   C Muscarinic, acetylcholine
   D Adrenergic α_1, acetylcholine

13 Which of the followings is affected in a dog with tic paralysis?
   A Sensory neurons in the dorsal horn
   B Postsynaptic acetylcholine receptors
   C Release of acetylcholine at the neuromuscular synapse
   D Release of glycine from the presynaptic sites
   E Motor neurons in the ventral horn

14 Which of the following is affected by myasthenia gravis?
   A Acetylcholinesterase in synaptic cleft
   B Acetylcholine receptors
   C Release of acetylcholine
   D Release of GABA

15 Demyelination of axons is likely to result in:
   A Increased conduction velocity of axons
   B No apparent change in conduction speed as voltage-gated Na^+ and K^+ channels remain available in the demyelinated area
   C Significant loss of conduction of action potential
   D Increased conduction velocity due to loss of resistance imposed by myelin sheath

Suggested reading

Augustine, G.J., Charlton, M.P. and Smith, S.J. (1987) Calcium action in synaptic transmitter release. *Annual Review of Neuroscience* 10:633–693.

Caldwell, J.H. (2000) Clustering of sodium channels at the neuromuscular junction. *Microscopy Research and Technique* 49:84–89.

Cowan, W.M., Sudhof, T.C. and Stevens, C.F. (2001) *Synapses.* Johns Hopkins University Press, Baltimore.

Creese, I., Sibley, D.R., Hamblin, M.W. and Leff, S.E. (1983) The classification of dopamine receptors. *Annual Review of Neuroscience* 6:43–71.

Daw, N.W., Stein, P.S.G. and Fox, K. (1993) The role of NMDA receptors in information processing. *Annual Review of Neuroscience* 16:207–222.

Jahn, R. and Studhof, T.C. (1994) Synaptic vesicles and exocytosis. *Annual Review of Neuroscience* 17:219–246.

Kandel, E.R., Schwartz, J.H. and Jessell, T.M. (eds) (2000) *Principles of Neural Science*, 4th edn. McGraw-Hill, New York.

Moore, R.Y. and Bloom, F.E. (1979) Central catecholamine neuron systems: anatomy and physiology of the norepinephrine and epinephrine systems. *Annual Review of Neuroscience* 2:113–168.

O'Dowd, B.F., Lefkowitz, R.J. and Caron, M.G. (1989) Structure of the adrenergic and related receptors. *Annual Review of Neuroscience* 12:67–83.

Schuman, E.M. and Madison, D.V. (1994) Nitric oxide and synaptic function. *Annual Review of Neuroscience* 17:153–184.

Answers

1	A	9	A
2	A	10	A
3	A	11	D
4	A	12	C
5	B	13	C
6	B	14	B
7	A	15	C
8	C		

4 Somatic and Visceral Senses

Etsuro E. Uemura

Iowa State University, Ames, IA, USA

The nervous system monitors somatic and visceral environments to maintain proper functions of the body. Sensory information is acquired at the terminal end of spinal and cranial sensory nerve fibers and is conveyed to the central nervous system (CNS) for further processing. Some sensory information is consciously detectable, enabling animals to feel pain, touch, temperature, and a full bladder for example. Other information such as blood pressure and the levels of oxygen and carbon dioxide in the blood does not reach conscious levels. Each physical stimulus is recognized by a specific somatosensory or viscerosensory receptor. **Somatosensory** signals originate from the cutaneous areas, muscles, and joints. They respond to mechanical, chemical or thermal stimuli, producing sensations of touch, pressure, vibration, pain, and warm or cold. **Viscerosensory** signals originate from the internal structures of the body. Some viscerosensory signals, such as stretching of the stomach and urinary bladder, are consciously detectable. The sensory signals are carried by various ascending tracts to the thalamus, which then projects to the somatosensory cortex.

Properties of sensory receptors

1 What is the basis of classifying sensory receptors?

2 What are the structural and functional differences between free nerve endings and encapsulated nerve endings?

3 What is the basis of classifying sensory receptors?

4 Describe the receptors associated with the senses of touch, pressure, temperature, pain, or position.

5 What sensory receptors are present in the skeletal muscle? What are their functions?

6 Describe the function of a nociceptor.

7 What ascending tract carries signals for pain? Where in the spinal cord is this tract located?

8 Define thermoreceptors and mechanoreceptors and explain the stimuli that activate them.

9 What are proprioceptors and where are they located?

10 Define physiologic receptors and list examples.

11 What is the main receptor for visceral pain? What causes visceral pain?

Sensory receptors are present in every tissue of the body except the nervous system itself. Most of them are axon terminals of primary sensory neurons. They are classified into two categories based on their terminal morphology. Those receptors with no special modifications are referred to as **free nerve endings** (Figure 4.1). The terminal end of free nerve endings form numerous branches in target tissues. They are not myelinated and ensheathed only by Schwann cells. Free nerve endings are the most widely distributed receptor type in the body. Free nerve endings are receptors for somatic and visceral sense of pain and temperature (warm, cold) and are classified as **nociceptors** and **thermoreceptors**, respectively. There is one sensory receptor that involves specialized cells to detect sensory stimuli. This receptor, known as **Merkel's corpuscle**, is composed of an axon terminal synapsing with a specialized epidermal Merkel cell. Merkel's corpuscles detect pressure: they are **mechanoreceptors** that respond to mechanical deformation of the surrounding tissue and transduce the mechanical force into an electrical potential.

In contrast to free nerve endings, some sensory terminals are ensheathed by a connective tissue capsule. They are classified as **encapsulated nerve endings**. Encapsulated portions of axons are not myelinated. Encapsulated nerve endings are

Dukes' Physiology of Domestic Animals, Thirteenth Edition. Edited by William O. Reece, Howard H. Erickson, Jesse P. Goff and Etsuro E. Uemura.
© 2015 John Wiley & Sons, Inc. Published 2015 by John Wiley & Sons, Inc.
Companion website: www.wiley.com/go/reece/physiology

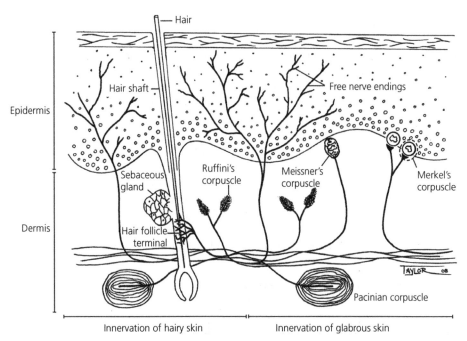

Figure 4.1 Nerve fibers enter the epidermis as free nerve endings. Free nerve endings in the skin are sensitive to pain or temperature. The hair follicle terminal is a nonmyelinated terminal portion of the myelinated nerve fiber. It wraps around the hair follicle below the sebaceous gland. The hair follicle terminals are sensitive to touch. Merkel's corpuscle is composed of epidermal Merkel cells and the terminal ends of sensory fibers innervating them. This receptor is sensitive to touch and pressure. The dermis contains various encapsulated sensory receptors. Ruffini's corpuscle is composed of fine branches of a nonmyelinated axon encapsulated by perineural cells. It is sensitive to stretching of the skin. Those in a joint capsule are proprioceptors. Pacinian corpuscles consist of an axon terminal encapsulated by numerous concentric layers of epineural cells. They are sensitive to high-frequency vibration. Pacinian corpuscles in a joint capsule also serve as proprioceptors.

found mainly in the inner dermis, fasciae, mesenteries, skeletal muscles, and some viscera, and comprise Pacinian corpuscles, Meissner's corpuscles, and Ruffini's corpuscles. All encapsulated endings are **mechanoreceptors**. There are also special mechanoreceptors essential for awareness of kinesthesia (i.e., joint position direction and velocity of joint movements). These receptors, known as Golgi-tendon organs, are located in the tendons and muscle spindles (also called neuromuscular spindles) of the skeletal muscles. They are called **proprioceptors**.

Somatosensory receptors

The sensations detected by the peripheral receptors include pain, temperature, touch, and position of the body (Table 4.1). Each type of sensation to which an animal responds is called modality of sensation. For each modality, specialized sensory receptors respond selectively to the stimulus for that modality and transduce the stimulus into nerve impulses.

In the epidermis, **free nerve endings** detect **pain** and **temperature**. However, hair follicle terminals (i.e., free nerve endings that surround hair follicles immediately below the sebaceous glands) respond to a hair bending. Hair follicle terminals are rapidly adapting receptors: they give a brief initial burst of impulses when the hair is bent and then remain silent until the hair is released, which triggers a second burst of impulses. Hair follicle terminals respond to the sensation of flutter (i.e.,

Table 4.1 Sensory receptors and their function.

Receptor type	Function	Threshold	Adaptation
Nociceptor and thermoreceptor			
Free nerve endings	Pain or temperature (warm, cold)	High	Depends on information
Mechanoreceptor			
Meissner's corpuscle	Touch, vibration (<100 Hz)	Low	Rapid
Merkel's corpuscle	Pressure	Low	Slow
Pacinian corpuscle	High-frequency vibration (100–400 Hz)	Low	Rapid
Hair follicle	Touch		Rapid
Ruffini's corpuscle	Stretch (direction, magnitude)	Low	Slow
	Joint pressure and angle	Low	Slow
Muscle spindles	Proprioception	Low	Rapid initial transient and slow sustained
Golgi tendon organ	Proprioception	Low	Slow
	Muscle tension	Low	Slow

movement with a light irregular motion). Merkel's corpuscles are sensitive to **touch** and **pressure** stimuli and they signal both the displacement and velocity of a stimulus. Merkel's corpuscles are slowly adapting (i.e., they are active as long as the stimulus is present). They are present in the dermal papillary ridges. **Meissner's corpuscles** are low-threshold, rapidly adapting receptors sensitive to touch and **vibration** (<100 Hz) (Figure 4.2).

Pacinian corpuscles (also called lamellar corpuscles) are sensitive to pressure and vibration. They are composed of an axon terminal surrounded by numerous concentric layers of perineural epithelioid cells. Pacinian corpuscles are primarily found in subcutaneous tissues below both hairy and glabrous skin and are especially numerous just beneath the dermis of the digits. They are also present in joint capsules and act as proprioceptors (i.e., sensory receptors that detect a sense of movement and position of the body). Pacinian corpuscles are rapidly adapting mechanoreceptors sensitive to high-frequency vibration (100–400 Hz). Thus they respond to both initial application and removal of a stimulus, but do not respond during maintained stimulation (Figure 4.2). Pacinian corpuscles in the joint capsules are proprioceptors and provide awareness of kinesthesia. **Ruffini's corpuscles** are present in the dermis of the skin and joint capsule. They are sensitive to magnitude and direction of stretch of the skin, but those in the joint capsule are proprioceptors and respond to joint movements. Ruffini's corpuscles are composed of myelinated axon terminals interspersed with collagen fibers and surrounded by several layers of perineural cells. They are slowly adapting mechanoreceptors and have large receptive fields.

Golgi-tendon organs are high-threshold stretch receptors and proprioceptors. They are present in the tendon, where collagen fascicles join the skeletal muscle fibers (Figure 4.3). Golgi-tendon organs are sensitive to increase in muscle tension induced by muscle contraction, but they do not respond to

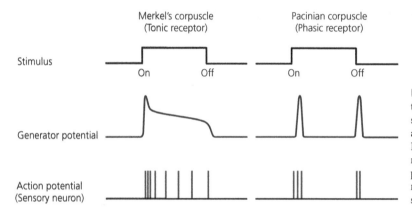

Figure 4.2 Two classes of sensory receptors and their response to a stimulus. Tonic receptors are slowly adapting receptors that continue to discharge at a constant rate as long as the stimulus is maintained. In contrast, phasic receptors are rapidly adapting receptors. They respond with a burst of action potentials when a stimulus is applied, then they rapidly adapt to a constant stimulus. When the stimulus turns off, these receptors are activated again.

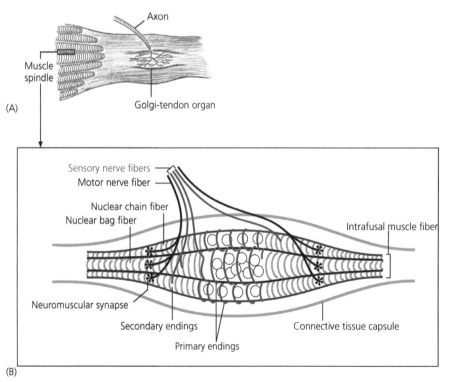

Figure 4.3 (A) Buried among the extrafusal fibers of the muscle are small elongated muscle spindles. They are scattered among and arranged parallel to the extrafusal muscle fibers. Each muscle spindle is made of a connective sheath capsule that encloses a group of intrafusal muscle fibers. Only one of many muscle spindles is illustrated. The Golgi-tendon organ monitors tension applied to tendons during muscular contraction as well as movement and position of the body. (B) Three intrafusal muscle fibers are illustrated. The primary endings (also known as annulospiral endings) wrap around the equatorial regions of intrafusal muscle fibers. Secondary sensory fibers (also known as flower spray endings) are located on each end of the primary endings (shown only on one side of each intrafusal muscle fiber).

passive stretch that occurs when the entire muscle is passively lengthened, for example by striking a tendon with a patellar hammer. **Muscle spindles** are highly specialized stretch receptors and proprioceptors distributed throughout skeletal muscle. These spindle-shaped receptors are composed of several small skeletal muscle fibers and are often referred to as intrafusal muscle fibers (Figure 4.3). Two types of intrafusal muscle fibers are present. The nuclear bag fiber has an enlarged central area where a cluster of nuclei is present. The nuclear chain fiber has a single row of nuclei in a central area of each fiber. A connective tissue capsule encloses intrafusal muscle fibers and nerve fibers.

Terminal portions of sensory fibers wrap around the equatorial region of each muscle fiber. There are two types of sensory receptors associated with intrafusal muscle fibers, primary and secondary. The **primary endings** (also referred to as annulospiral endings) are associated with the central part of the nuclear bag and nuclear chain fibers. They are activated by brief stretching of the intrafusal muscle fibers, detecting muscle length and rate of change. The **secondary endings** (also referred to as flower-spray endings) are located on each end of the primary endings that wrap around the nuclear bag and nuclear chain fibers. The secondary endings respond to sustained stretch of the muscle, detecting muscle length and tension. Equatorial stretching is passive or active. Passive stretch occurs when the entire muscle is passively lengthened, for example by striking a tendon with a patellar hammer. The structural basis for passively stretching the intrafusal muscle includes (i) the connective tissue capsule that is continuous with the perimysium of the extrafusal muscle fibers and (ii) the muscle spindles that are arranged in parallel with the extrafusal muscle fibers. Active equatorial stretching occurs when the intrafusal muscle contracts in response to stimulation of the gamma motor neurons (see Figure 8.7).

Viscerosensory receptors

Sensory receptors of the viscera (or viscerosensory receptors) are composed primarily of free nerve endings. Free nerve endings of the viscera are either nociceptors or physiologic receptors. **Nociceptors** detect changes in visceral structures caused by abnormal physical conditions (e.g., gastrointestinal bloating or cramping) or pathological conditions (e.g., peritonitis, pericarditis). Visceral organs are not sensitive to cutting, heat or cold, but they respond to stretching, distension, spasm, inflammation, or ischemia (Greek *ischein*, to suppress; *haima*, blood; i.e., loss of blood supply). Visceral pain is poorly localized. Receptors that respond to innocuous stimuli are called **physiologic receptors**. For example, the baroreceptors located in the carotid sinus and aortic arch respond to changes in blood pressure. In contrast, the chemoreceptor in the carotid body is sensitive to changes in arterial tension of oxygen (Pao_2) and carbon dioxide ($Paco_2$). These sensory receptors trigger normal visceral reflexes to regulate heart rate and respiration. Some free nerve endings in the respiratory epithelium are sensitive to inhaled particles in the respiratory airways. The coughing reflex, for example, is triggered by these receptors. Other physiologic receptors are located in the smooth muscle layer of the viscera. They respond to stretch or tension. Their sensory signals are important for a sense of fullness in certain organs (e.g., stomach, large intestine, urinary bladder), gastrointestinal motility, micturition and defecation.

Transduction of receptor stimulus

1 What are the tonic and phasic receptors? What receptors belong to these categories?
2 Explain the relationship between stimulus intensity and receptor response.
3 Define receptor adaptation and explain its importance.
4 How do animals detect the location of a sensory stimulus applied to the body?
5 What is the significance of a dermatome?
6 What determines the intensity and duration of sensory stimulus?

For the CNS to recognize sensory stimuli, sensory receptors must convert a stimulus into neural activity (Figure 4.4). This involves a process called **stimulus transduction**. A stimulus applied to a sensory receptor produces a local depolarizing potential in the axonal membrane. The stimulus causes an increase in the permeability of the neuron to Na^+ and the resulting Na^+ influx depolarizes the neuron. If this depolarization, called a **receptor potential**, reaches the threshold membrane potential, an action potential is generated. However, some terminal ends of sensory neurons make synaptic contact with specialized epidermal cells. For example, sensory stimulus to a Merkel cell results in the release of neurotransmitter. When the released transmitters are sufficient to depolarize the terminal axon innervating them, action potentials are generated. **Adaptation** is a unique feature of sensory receptors (Figure 4.2). As the duration of the stimulus increases, the amplitude of the receptor potential decreases. As a result, intensity of the sensation decreases with time as duration of the stimulus increases. Some sensory receptors even turn off and no longer respond to a continuous stimulus. Based on how they respond to continuous stimuli, sensory receptors are classified into two categories, phasic and tonic. Phasic receptors (e.g., Pacinian and Meissner's corpuscles) are rapidly adapting receptors. They fire as they first receive a stimulus, but stop firing if the stimulus magnitude stays unchanged. Tonic receptors are slowly adapting receptors, like Merkel's corpuscles, Ruffini's corpuscles, and baroreceptors. They continue to fire action potentials for the duration of stimulation.

The sensory systems encode four elementary features of stimuli: modality, intensity, duration, and location. Various types of sensory receptors are specialized for detecting particular stimuli, such as pain, temperature (cold, heat), touch, pressure, vibration, and proprioception (Table 4.1). Each type of sensation to which an animal responds is called a **modality** of sensation. For each modality, specialized sensory receptors respond selectively

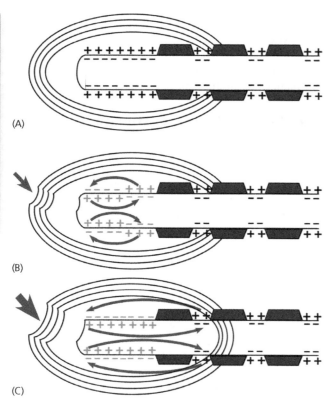

(A)

(B)

(C)

Figure 4.4 Receptor potential and generation of action potential of the Pacinian corpuscle. (A) The resting Pacinian corpuscle. (B) A light mechanical displacement applied to the Pacinian corpuscle changes ionic conduction in the axon within the corpuscle, depolarizing its membrane and inducing a small receptor potential. The receptor potential generates a small current, which travels a short distance down the axon. (C) As the strength of the applied stimulus is increased, the size of the receptor potential and subsequent local current also increases. When the receptor potential exceeds the threshold potential, an action potential is generated at the first node of Ranvier. Action potentials are not generated at the same area of the receptor that induces the receptor potential. The first node continues to generate action potentials so long as the membrane of the first node remains above the excitation threshold.

to stimuli for that modality and transduce the stimulus into nerve impulses. The initial detection of a specific stimulus requires transduction and adaptation. Transduction is the conversion of a stimulus into neural activity that specifies its kind and intensity. Adaptation is a change over time in the responsiveness of the sensory receptor to a constant stimulus. The **intensity** of stimulation is signaled by the firing rates of a receptor, and the **duration** of stimulation is signaled by the time course of firing. The **location** of a stimulus is determined by peripheral and central organization of somesthetic pathways, as well as thalamic and cortical representation of the body surface.

Modality of stimulus

The **somatosensory system** processes signals for specific modalities (i.e., pain, temperature, touch, proprioception). Each of these modalities depends on neurons that are modality

specific. Thus, neurons that respond to "cold" skin do not respond to "warm" skin or to other stimuli (e.g., touch, vibration). Thus, sensory neurons are modality specific and they form ascending somatosensory tracts that carry specific modality signals to the specific areas of the thalamus, which then projects to the specific area of the somatosensory cerebral cortex. The **viscerosensory system** processes sensory signals from viscera. Viscerosensory signals are essential for respiration, heart rate, blood pressure, and micturition. Body sensation is determined by the quality and intensity of the stimulus. The quality of sensation is the subjective interpretation of such stimuli as pain, touch, vibration, cold, warmth, or motion. To generate a sensation, the intensity of the stimulus must reach a subjective threshold. However, any further increase in the intensity of the stimulus alters the quality of sensation and is perceived as unpleasant and painful.

Intensity and duration of stimulus

As mentioned, specialized sensory receptors respond selectively to stimuli and generate signals for a specific modality. However, the process of transduction by sensory receptors is always the same irrespective of the type of receptor. They convert physical changes into an electrical event, i.e., generation of action potentials. The receptor potential induced by stimulation of a sensory receptor mimics the graded potential of postsynaptic neurons. When the receptor potential reaches and then exceeds the threshold membrane potential, an axon of a sensory neuron generates an action potential. Receptor potential is converted into neural code that specifies the pattern of action potentials. For example, an increase in stimulus intensity generates a greater receptor potential (Figure 4.5A), which induces an increased rate of action potentials (Figure 4.5B). Thus, the intensity of sensation reflects the strength of the stimulus applied to sensory receptors. The duration of a stimulus applied to a sensory axon is coded by the duration of action potentials generated by the sensory neuron. The longer a stimulus persists, the longer a series of action potentials are generated in the sensory neuron.

Stimulus location

Animals are able to detect different modalities and know the location of a stimulus applied to the body. As already mentioned, sensory receptors are modality specific and the sensations detected by the peripheral receptors include pain, temperature, touch, and position of the body. The location of a sensory stimulus is determined by (i) the peripheral and central organization of somesthetic pathways (Greek *soma*, body; *aisthesis*, sensation; i.e., pathways that mediate signals from somatosensory receptors) and (ii) thalamic and cortical representation of the body surface.

Dermatome

Each segment of the spinal cord innervates a specific receptive field of the body. The trigeminal nerve fibers also have specific receptive fields in the face. The area of skin innervated by

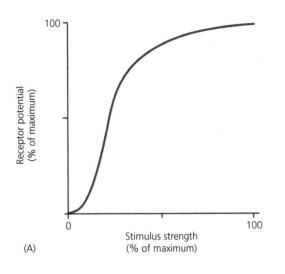

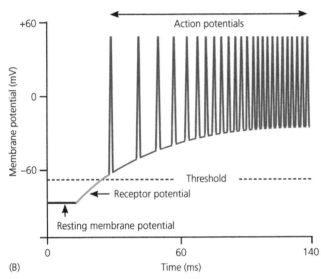

Figure 4.5 (A) The receptor potential increases as a function of stimulus strength. The graph is based on a Pacinian corpuscle and does not apply for other types of sensory receptor. (B) Action potential frequency as a function of receptor potential. Discharge frequency of an axon represents stimulus amplitude (i.e., membrane potential), but the relationship is not linear. Adapted from Hall, J.E. (2011) *Guyton and Hall Textbook of Medical Physiology*, 12th edn. Saunders Elsevier, Philadelphia.

cutaneous branches from a single spinal nerve is termed a **dermatome** (Figure 4.6A). The dermatomes supplied by adjacent spinal nerves overlap (Figure 4.6B). For example, a portion of the C7 area is also supplied by C6 and C8. There is therefore little sensory loss, if any, following interruption of a single dorsal root of a spinal nerve. However, if a peripheral nerve is damaged, there is sensory loss in the area supplied by that nerve. The **receptive field** of a sensory neuron is an area in which a stimulus will alter the firing of that neuron. The size of the receptive field not only varies, but also overlaps to some degree (Figure 4.7). Sensory neurons innervating a given receptor field converge to a smaller number of postsynaptic

neurons. Thus a receptive field covered by a central neuron reflects a combined area monitored by various numbers of primary sensory neurons. The size of a receptive field determines the precise location of stimulus applied to the area. Large receptive fields allow the sensory neuron to detect stimuli applied to a wider area, but results in less precise perception than small ones.

Ascending sensory pathways

> **1** Define a primary afferent fiber, a first-order neuron, and a second-order neuron.
>
> **2** What is the spinothalamic tract? Where does it ascend in the spinal cord? Where does it terminate?
>
> **3** What is the difference in the course of primary sensory fibers from viscera and those from the skin?
>
> **4** Where in the cerebrum are the primary somatosensory, auditory, and visual areas located?
>
> **5** Explain how the CNS detects the specific location of a stimulus applied to the body.

Sensory pathways are organized on a general plan (Figure 4.8). Cell bodies of the primary sensory neurons (also referred to as first-order neurons) are located in the dorsal root ganglia of spinal nerves and ganglia of the cranial nerves. **Peripheral processes** of the primary sensory neurons innervate sensory receptors or terminate as sensory receptors. Peripheral processes pass outward either in the spinal nerves to innervate the skin and deep tissues (e.g., muscles, tendons, joints) or in the rami communicantes and sympathetic trunk to innervate visceral organs. The **central processes** of the primary sensory neurons enter the dorsal spinal cord. Some axons synapse with second-order neurons (i.e., the second neurons to carry information) in the dorsal horn of the spinal cord and some others ascend the spinal cord without synapsing at the cord segments they enter. For example, pain signals carried by the central processes of primary neurons reach the second-order neurons in the dorsal horn of the spinal cord. Axons of the second-order neurons cross the midline to the contralateral white matter and ascend as the **spinothalamic tract** and reach the thalamus (Figure 4.9). The thalamic neurons mediate signals to the ipsilateral primary somatosensory cortex. Signals for proprioception take a different route to the cerebral cortex. Signals from the proprioceptors (e.g., muscle spindles) of the pelvic limbs are carried by the primary sensory neurons in the dorsal root ganglia to the spinal cord. Unlike those axons carrying signals for pain, axons mediating signals for proprioception synapse with neurons of the nucleus thoracicus located in the thoracic and cranial lumbar spinal cord. Their axons enter the lateral funiculus and ascend as the spinomedullary tract to the thalamus. Thus each modality in a given receptive field has its own neural pathways in the spinal cord and the brainstem.

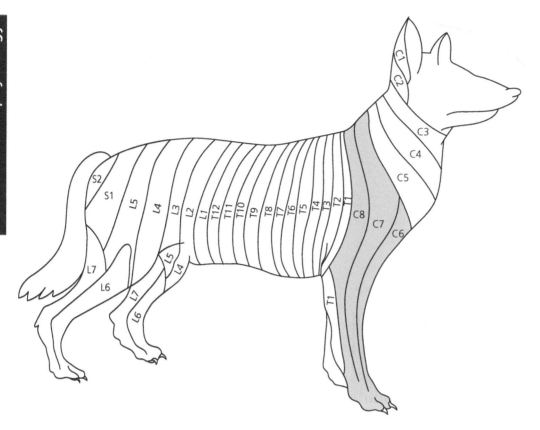

(A)

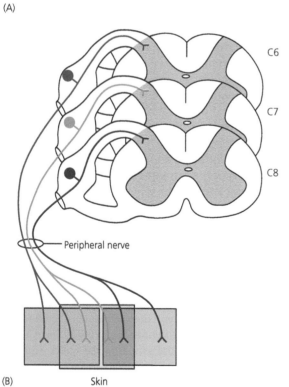

(B)   Skin

Figure 4.6 (A) Dermatomes of the dog. This illustration is a hypothetical composite of several studies (Fletcher and Kitchell, 1966; Hekmatpanah, 1961; Kitchell *et al.*, 1980; Bailey *et al.*, 1982). Spinal cord segments C6, C7 and C8 supply the shaded area. Since cutaneous areas supplied by adjacent spinal nerves overlap, a portion of the C7 area, for example, is also supplied by C6 and C8. (B) Relationship between the area of skin innervated by the peripheral nerve and the dorsal roots. Damage to a peripheral nerve induces a complete loss of sensory information in the area innervated by that nerve. The difference in the skin sizes and shapes highlights the pattern of overlapping areas, but does not suggest an actual size difference in the area of innervation by cord segments.

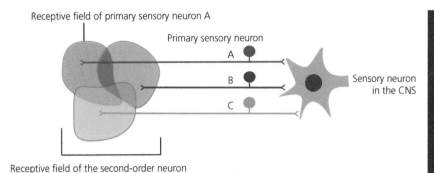

Figure 4.7 Receptive field of primary sensory neurons. Several unipolar neurons, for example A, B, and C, synapse with a second-order neuron in the spinal cord or the brainstem. The receptive field of the second-order sensory neurons is the combined receptive field of primary sensory neurons A, B, and C.

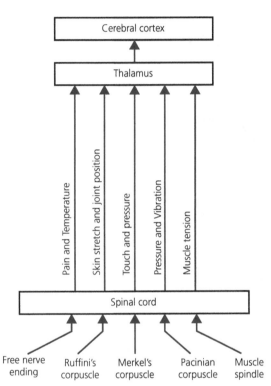

Figure 4.8 Ascending tracts from the spinal cord reach the cerebral cortex via the thalamus. Each tract mediates signals for specific modalities.

Viscerosensory fibers are carried by sympathetic and parasympathetic nerves. Viscerosensory fibers of parasympathetic nerves mediate signals primarily from physiologic receptors, while viscerosensory fibers of sympathetic nerves mediate signals from nociceptors. Although viscerosensory fibers are a structural component of both sympathetic and parasympathetic nerves, they are not considered part of the autonomic nervous system. Visceral sensory signals are carried by viscerosensory fibers that enter the dorsal horn via sympathetic trunk and rami communicantes and synapse with second-order neurons in the dorsal horn. Their axons join the spinothalamic tract and terminate in the thalamus (Figure 4.9). Thus, the cerebral cortex can perceive visceral sensation, such as pain or fullness, of the stomach and urinary bladder.

Receptive field of the body and the cerebral cortex

Sensory receptors are modality specific and their signals are carried to the thalamus by the modality-specific ascending sensory tracts, such as the spinothalamic tract (pain, temperature) and spinomedullary tract (proprioception of the pelvic limbs) (Figure 4.9A). The thalamus sends information topographically to specific areas of the cerebral cortex (Figure 4.9B). Thus the role of the thalamus is to relay specific sensory information to specific somesthetic areas of the cerebral cortex. The somesthetic area of the cerebral cortex consists of the postcruciate, rostral suprasylvian and rostral ectosylvian gyri. The area also extends about 4 mm onto the medial wall of the hemisphere, caudal to the cruciate sulcus. The receptive surfaces of the body are mapped on the cerebral cortex (Figure 4.9B). In humans, this cerebral representation of the primary somesthetic area resembles a little man, hence the name **homunculus** (Latin *homunculus*, a little man) is given to this cerebral map. The cerebral representation is in proportion to their importance in sensory analysis, not their physical size. For example, certain body parts such as the limbs and torso occupy limited areas on the somesthetic cortex. In contrast, the major sensory exploratory surfaces of digits, face, tongue, and lips are greatly magnified. These distortions in the representation of certain body parts reflect the degree to which the cerebral cortex analyzes features of somatic events.

In a dog, two areas of the frontal and temporal lobes represent the body surface. The somesthetic area SI represents a dog that appears to be lying with tail and postaxial thigh on the medial wall of the hemisphere and the preaxial thigh on the dorsal surface. The back of the animal and the occipital aspect of the head fall along the caudal margin of the somesthetic area, toward the parietal lobe. The ventral surface of the trunk, the apices of the limbs and the snout are directed rostrally. The area is activated by stimulation of the contralateral half of the body. The somesthetic area SII shows the back of the dog facing ventrally, along the dorsal border of the rostral ectosylvian sulcus, while the limbs and face extend upward over the rostral suprasylvian gyrus toward SI, with the snout most rostral and the foot most caudal. The area SI can be activated by stimulation of both sides of the body.

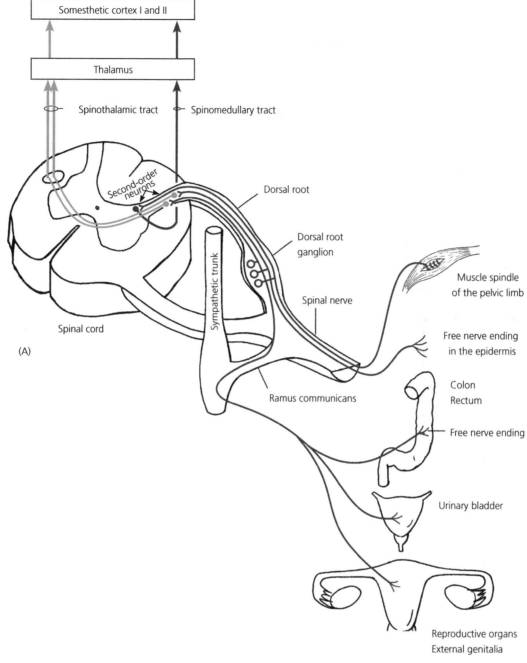

(A)

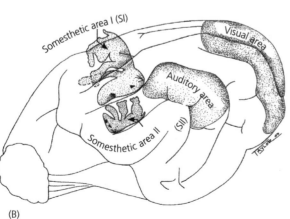

(B)

Figure 4.9 (A) Somatosensory fibers innervating the dermis and muscle spindle of the pelvic limb and viscerosensory fibers from the pelvic viscera. Somatosensory fibers reach the spinal cord via spinal nerves. Sensory fibers carrying signals for epidermal pain or proprioception from the muscle spindle enter the spinal cord. They synapse with the second-order neurons in the dorsal horn that mediate signals for specific modality. The second-order neurons give rise to the ascending tracts, the spinothalamic tract for pain and the spinomedullary tract for proprioception from the pelvic limbs. They reach the thalamus, which projects to the somesthetic cerebral cortex. Viscerosensory fibers pass through the splanchnic nerve and the ramus communicans before reaching the spinal cord and synapse with the second-order neurons in the dorsal horn. Axons of the second-order neurons join the spinothalamic tract. (B) Lateral view of the cerebral hemisphere indicating the somesthetic areas SI and SII.

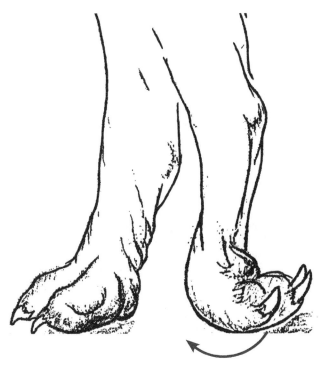

Figure 4.10 Proprioceptive positioning test. When the dorsal surface of the foot is placed on the floor, the animal immediately returns it to the normal position.

Clinical correlations

Unilateral destruction of the somatosensory cortex may cause a transient deficit in the contralateral side of the body. Bilateral destruction of the somatosensory area may result in more pronounced, yet transient deficits. Therefore, it is likely that a small lesion of the somesthetic area will not produce detectable clinical signs. Unilateral lesions of the somesthetic cortex or thalamus may cause a mild hypalgesia (i.e., a decreased sensitivity to painful stimuli). Conscious proprioception from the thoracic and pelvic limbs can be tested by observing the ability of the animal to recognize the location of its limbs without seeing them. For example, when the dorsal surface of the foot is placed on the floor, the animal should immediately adjust it to the normal position (Figure 4.10). This test is referred to as the **proprioceptive positioning test**. The tract involved in proprioceptive positioning of the thoracic limb is the fasciculus cuneatus that occupies the dorsal funiculus of the cervical and cranial thoracic spinal cord segments. Proprioceptive positioning of the pelvic limb requires the spinomedullary tract. This tract occupies the lateral funiculus of the spinal cord.

Self-evaluation

Answers can be found at the end of the chapter.

1 Pacinian corpuscles have rapid adaptation, whereas Merkel's corpuscles have slow adaptation.
   A True
   B False

2 Pain is detected by the:
   A Free nerve endings
   B Pacinian corpuscles
   C Muscle spindle
   D Merkel's corpuscles
   E None of the above

3 Which statement is correct about the system that mediates signals for pain sensation?
   A Ventral roots carry pain signals to the spinal cord
   B Perikarya of the primary sensory neurons is located in the dorsal root ganglion
   C Second-order neurons are located in the ventral horn
   D The spinothalamic tract ascends in the dorsal horn to reach the thalamus

4 Dorsal root ganglion cells are classified as:
   A Multipolar neurons
   B Unipolar neuron
   C Bipolar neurons
   D Neuroglia

5 The dorsal root ganglion cells mediate:
   A Motor signals only
   B Sensory signals only
   C Both motor and sensory signals

6 Which statement is correct for muscle spindles?
   A They are composed of extrafusal muscle fibers surrounded by a connective tissue capsule
   B They are composed of extrafusal muscle fibers with no connective tissue capsule
   C They are composed of intrafusal muscle fibers with no connective tissue capsule
   D They are composed of intrafusal muscle fibers surrounded by a connective tissue capsule
   E They are composed of smooth muscle fibers surrounded by a connective tissue capsule

7 Muscle spindles are innervated by both sensory and motor nerve fibers.
   A True
   B False

8 Receptor potential increases as a function of stimulus strength.
   A True
   B False

9 Frequency of action potentials represents stimulus strength, but the relationship is not linear.
   A True
   B False

10 Receptive fields of primary sensory neurons are circular and identical in size.
   A True
   B False

11 What structure directly projects sensory signals to the cerebral cortex?
   A Dorsal root ganglia
   B Thalamus

   C Primary sensory neurons in the dorsal horn
   D Second-order neurons in the dorsal horn

12 Muscle spindles are:
   A Nonencapsulated receptors
   B Present in the tendon
   C Proprioceptors
   D Synonymous with motor end plates
   E Synonymous with Golgi-tendon organ

13 Conscious proprioception can be evaluated by the proprioceptive positioning test:
   A True
   B False

Suggested reading

Bailey, C.S., Kitchell, R.L. and Johnson, R.D. (1982) Spinal nerve root origins of the cutaneous nerves arising from the canine brachial plexus. *American Journal of Veterinary Research* 43:820–825.

Bell, J., Bolanowski, S. and Holmes, M.H. (1994) The structures and function of Pacinian corpuscles: a review. *Progress in Neurobiology* 42:79–128.

Bennett, G.J., Selzer, Z., Lu, W., Hishidawa, N. Bessen, J.M. and Chaouch, A. (1987) Peripheral and spinal mechanisms of nociception. *Physiological Reviews* 67:67–186.

Boyd, I.A. (1954) The histological structure of the receptors in the knee-joint of the cat correlated with their physiological response. *Journal of Physiology* 124:476–488.

Brown, A.G., Brown, P.B., Fyffe, W. and Pubols, L.M. (1969) Receptive field organization and response properties of spinal neurons with axons ascending the dorsal column in the cat. *Journal of Physiology* 337:231–249.

Brown, A.G. and Fyffe, W. (1981) Form and function of dorsal horn neurones with axons ascending the dorsal columns in cats. *Journal of Physiology* 321:31–47.

Dilly, P.N., Wall, P.D. and Webster, D.E. (1968) Cells of origin of the spinothalamic tract in the cat and rat. *Experimental Neurology* 21:550–562.

Eurell, J.A. and Frappier, B.L. (2006) *Dellmann's Textbook of Veterinary Histology*, 6th edn. Wiley-Blackwell, Hoboken, NJ.

Fletcher, T.F. and Kitchell, R.L. (1966) The lumbar, sacral and coccygeal tactile dermatomes of the dog. *Journal of Comparative Neurology* 128:171–180.

Hall, J.E. (2011) *Guyton and Hall Textbook of Medical Physiology*, 12th edn. Saunders Elsevier, Philadelphia.

Hekmatpanah, J. (1961) Organization of tactile dermatomes, C1 through L4 in cat. *Journal of Physiology* 24:129–140.

Kitchell, R.I., Whalen, L.R., Bailey, C.S. and Lohse, C.L. (1980) Electrophysiologic studies of cutaneous nerves of the thoracic limb of the dog. *American Journal of Veterinary Research* 41:61–76.

Siegel, A. and Sapru, H.N. (2006) *Essential Neuroscience.* Lippincott Williams & Wilkins, Philadelphia.

Willis, W.D. and Coggeshall, R.E. (1978) *Sensory Mechanisms of the Spinal Cord.* Plenum, New York.

Answers

1	A	8	A
2	A	9	A
3	B	10	B
4	B	11	B
5	B	12	C
6	D	13	A
7	A		

5 Olfaction and Gustation

Etsuro E. Uemura
Iowa State University, Ames, IA, USA

Olfactory and taste systems, like other sensory systems, gather information about the external environment. Sensory receptors of these systems respond to chemical molecules mixed in the air or saliva, and the two systems complement each other for better interpretation of what animals eat and smell. **Olfaction** (smell) is an animal's primary special sense and their sense of smell is far more sensitive than that of humans. A dog, for example, has more than 220 million olfactory receptors in its nose, while humans have only 5 million. No wonder they can detect even a trace amount of chemical substances and follow trails of scent of almost any kind. **Gustation** (taste) is the sensation induced by binding of chemical molecules with receptors. Sensory cells of the taste buds are able to differentiate between different tastes by detecting interaction with different molecules or ions. Most importantly, taste and smell determine flavors, the sensory impressions of food or other substances.

Olfaction

1 List the neural structures of the olfactory system.
2 Explain transduction of olfactory stimulus.
3 Describe the central neural pathways for olfaction.

The olfactory system consists of the olfactory bulb, olfactory tract, lateral olfactory gyrus, and piriform lobe (Figure 5.1). Olfaction is essential for the localization of food, reflex-stimulated secretion of digestive enzymes, and detection of danger. The olfactory cells are part of the specialized olfactory epithelium found on the ethmo-turbinate bones of the nasal cavity (Figure 5.2). The olfactory mucosa occupies a relatively large area in dogs (100 cm²) compared with that in humans (about 5 cm²). The olfactory cells give rise to the olfactory nerve fibers that terminate in the olfactory bulb.

Receptors for odorants

Odorant molecules that enter the nasal cavity are dissolved in fluid secreted by the olfactory glands located in the olfactory mucosa. Odorant molecules stimulate olfactory receptors, but it appears that a protein called **olfactory-binding protein** in the mucus is required for this process. The olfactory glands of the nasal mucosa secrete olfactory-binding protein. This protein is thought to carry and/or concentrate the odorant molecules. The olfactory cells are able to distinguish a variety of odors at extremely low concentrations. Sensory neurons in the olfactory mucosa are bipolar neurons. Their cell bodies are present in the olfactory mucosa of the nasal cavity just below a thin sheet of bone, the cribriform plate, of the ethmoid bone (Figure 5.2). A sensory neuron has a single dendrite on one end. It terminates in the surface of the olfactory mucosa as an expanded **olfactory knob**. Each olfactory knob gives rise to about 10–20 cilia, which spread over the surface of the olfactory mucosa. These cilia are covered with mucus. Odor molecules must enter this layer before they can bind to olfactory-binding proteins. The cilia have sensory receptors essential for transduction of the olfactory stimulus. There are groups of sensory neurons expressing olfactory receptors that bind the same set of odors, but not others. However, their affinity for odorant molecules varies widely and such a difference in affinity generates a unique activation pattern of the sensory receptors and subsequently a unique sense of odor.

A single nonmyelinated axon emerges at the opposite end of the sensory neuron. These axons, unlike other cranial nerves, do not form a single nerve, but they come together and form many small fascicles of axons called the **fila olfactoria**. These fascicles pass through foramina in the cribriform plate of the

Dukes' Physiology of Domestic Animals, Thirteenth Edition. Edited by William O. Reece, Howard H. Erickson, Jesse P. Goff and Etsuro E. Uemura.
© 2015 John Wiley & Sons, Inc. Published 2015 by John Wiley & Sons, Inc.
Companion website: www.wiley.com/go/reece/physiology

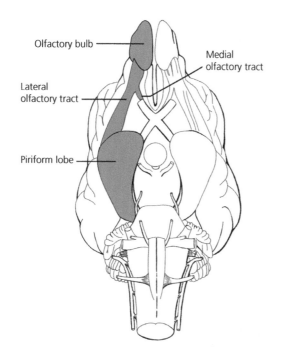

Figure 5.1 Ventral view of the dog brain. The olfactory bulb and its tract mediate olfactory signals originating from the olfactory epithelium in the nasal cavity.

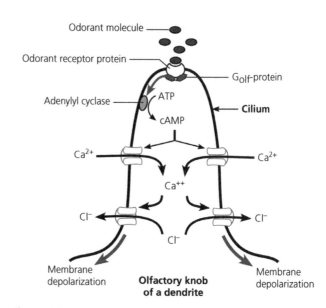

Figure 5.3 Sensory transduction of olfactory signals. The olfactory-binding protein carries odorant molecules to the cilia of the olfactory sensory neurons. A receptor–odorant complex activates a G protein, which leads to activation of a second messenger system and subsequent opening of Ca^{2+} channels and depolarization of the olfactory cells.

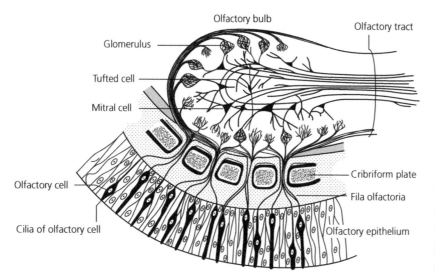

Figure 5.2 Lateral view of the olfactory neurons, fila olfactoria of the olfactory nerve, olfactory bulb and olfactory tract. Dendrites of olfactory bipolar neurons bear 10–20 short cilia. Axons of the olfactory neurons form olfactory fibers, which terminate in the olfactory bulb to synapse with tufted and mitral cells.

ethmoid bone and enter the **olfactory bulb**, where they synapse with tufted and mitral cells.

Transduction of olfactory stimulus

The membrane of cilia is covered with G protein-coupled olfactory receptors (Figure 5.3). Binding of an **odorant** molecule to the receptor on the cilia activates a G protein (G_{olf}), which unites with guanosine triphosphate (GTP). Two second-messenger systems, inositol trisphosphate (IP_3) and cyclic adenosine monophosphate (cAMP), are involved in the transduction of olfactory signals (Figure 5.3). The GTP–G_{olf} complex activates (i) phospholipase C, generating **IP_3** that opens Ca^{2+}

channels and (ii) adenylyl cyclase that produces **cAMP** that opens Na^+ and Ca^{2+} channels in the membrane, permitting Na^+ and Ca^{2+} entry (mostly Ca^{2+}) and subsequent depolarization of olfactory cells. Thus, the GTP–G_{olf} complex leads to a series of events (i.e., increase in intracellular Ca^{2+} concentration, opening of Ca^{2+}-gated Cl^- channels, and efflux of Cl^-) that generate excitatory postsynaptic graded potentials (EPSPs) of the cilia. Ciliary EPSPs travel from cilia to the trigger zone (i.e., axon hillock) of the olfactory cell. When **EPSPs** reaching the axon hillock are strong enough to exceed the threshold potential, action potentials are generated and they propagate along the axons of the olfactory cells to the olfactory bulb. Impulses are then dispersed to wide areas of the central nervous system, including the piriform lobe for perception of smell. A unique feature of olfactory transmission is its rapid adaptation to stimulus. Thus, initial discharge of axons in response to stimulation is followed by quick decline to a steady-state discharge of lower amplitude.

Central pathway for olfaction

Olfactory nerve fibers (i.e., fila olfactoria) terminate in the ipsilateral olfactory bulb. Cells present in the olfactory bulb are tufted cells and mitral cells (Figure 5.2). Dendrites of tufted and mitral cells make synapses with the terminal ends of the olfactory nerve fibers, forming the glomeruli of the olfactory bulb. Neurotransmitters (most likely peptides) released from the terminal end of olfactory axons excite the mitral and tufted cells and the activities of these cells are modulated by inhibitory periglomerular interneurons.

Axons of mitral and tufted cells leave the **olfactory bulb** to reach the various central structures for further processing. These axons form a large lateral olfactory tract (Figures 5.1 and 5.4). The central structures that receive olfactory signals include the amygdala and entorhinal cortex. These areas also send olfactory signals to the hippocampus and frontal cortex. Thus olfactory signals, unlike other sensory systems, do not directly project to the thalamus. The mitral and tufted cells also send their axons to the ipsilateral septal nucleus. Efferents of the tufted and mitral cells reach the contralateral olfactory bulb via the medial olfactory tract and the anterior commissure. The projection of olfactory signals suggests that emotional reaction to olfaction is carried out by the entorhinal cortex, hippocampal

formation, septal nuclei, and amygdala of the **limbic system**. Furthermore, autonomic response to olfaction is carried out by the hypothalamus and periaqueductal gray of the midbrain, as these two areas are a critical part of the autonomic nervous system and intimately associated with the limbic system. Thus, odor signals are not just for olfaction. Processing of odor signals by the limbic system is the basis for forming olfactory memories and olfaction can evoke strong emotional reactions.

Clinical correlations

Anosmia (*an*, negative + Greek *osme*, smell + *ia*, loss of) and hyposmia (reduced ability to smell) are not common clinical problems and the underlying cause of anosmia and hyposmia is not always clear. Anosmia often results from severe inflammation of the olfactory mucosa or bilateral lesions of the olfactory nerve or olfactory bulbs. Anosmia or hyposmia may also result from damage to the olfactory mucosa due to viral infections (e.g., distemper and parainfluenza). In some cases of head trauma, the olfactory bulb moves with respect to the cribriform plate, damaging axons of fila olfactoria passing through the cribriform plate on the way to the olfactory bulb. This results in loss or reduction of the olfactory sense. Deficiencies in the sense of smell can be assessed by observing an animal's response to smell (e.g., turning the head away, contraction of the facial muscles, sniffing). When assessing the sense of smell, irritating substances should be avoided. Any such substances are likely to trigger an animal's response not because of an intact olfactory system, but due to stimulation of sensory nerve endings of the trigeminal nerve in the nasal mucosa.

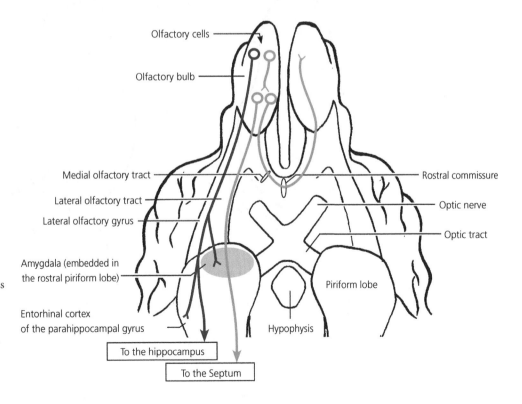

Figure 5.4 Efferent fibers of the olfactory bulb form the lateral and medial olfactory tracts. The lateral olfactory tract reaches the ipsilateral olfactory area (piriform lobe) as well as nonolfactory portions that are part of the limbic system (amygdala, entorhinal cortex of the parahippocampal gyrus, hippocampus of the hippocampal formation, and septum).

Gustation

1 Describe the innervation of the taste buds.
2 Explain transduction of stimulus for salty and sweet taste.
3 Describe the central neural pathway for taste.

Taste buds contain taste receptor cells. In dogs, they are located in various types of papillae (fungiform, vallate, and foliate), which are protrusions on the dorsal and lateral surface of the tongue. The fungiform papillae are distributed throughout the dorsal surface of the rostral two-thirds of the tongue, especially along the lateral margins and the tip. The vallate papillae occupy the caudal portion of the dorsal tongue. The foliate papillae are present on the dorsolateral part of the caudal part of the tongue. The taste receptors of dogs respond to the same chemicals that give the sense of taste in humans. Dogs seem to have sense of taste for sweet, salt, sour and bitter. However, they do not have highly sensitive salt receptors and do not have the strong craving for salt. This may reflect the fact that wild ancestors of dogs, as carnivores, obtained sufficient salt from the diet and there was no need for developing highly sensitive receptors for salt.

Taste buds

Dogs have about 1700 taste buds, while humans have about 9000. Dogs have considerably more taste buds than cats, which average only about 470. The tongue has a unique distribution of the taste buds for the basic flavors (meat, salt, sweet, sour, bitter).

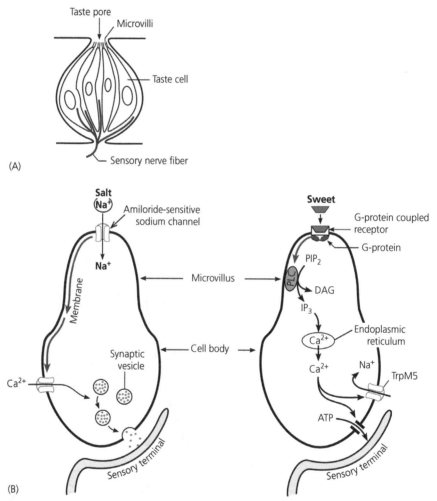

Figure 5.5 (A) The taste bud is composed of a cluster of spindle-shaped cells that extend to a small opening, the taste pore, at the epithelial surface of the tongue. Taste cells have many apical microvilli that project in the taste pore. A taste cell is illustrated with only two microvilli. Receptor cells for sense of sweet or salty taste do not form ultrastructurally identifiable synapses. Instead, axons are closely apposed to these cells. (B) Signal transduction involved in sense of sweet or salty taste. Salty taste of Na$^+$ is detected by influx of Na$^+$ through membrane ion channels, including ENaC, to depolarize the membrane. It is speculated that the transduction of salty taste involves voltage-gated Ca^{2+} channels activated by membrane depolarization subsequent to influx of Na$^+$. Sweet ligand binds to G protein-coupled receptors that activate phospholipase C (PLC), which converts membrane lipids into inositol trisphosphate (IP$_3$) and diacylglycerol (DAG). IP$_3$ releases intracellular Ca^{2+} stored in the endoplasmic reticulum, elevating cytoplasmic Ca^{2+}. The intracellular Ca^{2+} activates taste-selective cation channels (TrpM5) and gap junction hemichannels in the plasma membrane. Influx of Na$^+$ through TrpM5 depolarizes the receptor membrane. The combined action of elevated intracellular Ca^{2+} and membrane depolarization opens the large pores of gap junctions, resulting in ATP release.

The taste buds for meaty tastes are primarily located in the rostral two-thirds of the dorsal surface of the tongue. The rostral and lateral portions of the tongue are sensitive to sweet taste. Salty and sour taste buds are most sensitive on the lateral sides, but more caudal to the area occupied by sweet taste buds. However, the taste buds for salt occupy only a small area. The caudal portion of the tongue is most sensitive to bitter tastes.

Chemical molecules that trigger the sense of taste are dissolved by the saliva. They enter the taste bud through a pore (Figure 5.5A). Taste buds are composed of groups of between 50 and 150 columnar taste receptor cells, bundled together like a cluster of bananas. The taste receptor cells within a bud are arranged such that their tips form a small taste pore, and through this pore extend microvilli. The **taste receptor cells** live for about 10 days and have to be replaced. There are a relatively small number of taste cells compared with the large number of molecules that trigger taste sensations. It also seems that each taste cell has receptors for only one type of flavor. Thus each cell in a taste bud detects either sweet, sour, bitter, or salt. These observations are based on behavioral studies of transgenic mice with absence of one or more taste receptors.

Transduction of gustatory stimulus

Chemical substances dissolved in the saliva enter the taste buds through the pore at the top and bind to the receptors located in the membrane of the microvilli of the taste cells. The binding of molecules with receptors depolarizes the membrane of the taste cells. The mechanisms that generate membrane depolarization depend on the taste molecules that bind to their specific receptors. For example, the transduction of **salty taste** is mediated by Na^+ influx through the amiloride-sensitive Na^+ channel (ENaC) (Figure 5.5B). This induces membrane depolarization. The transduction pathways for salty taste are not well understood. It is speculated that the transduction of salty taste involves opening of voltage-gated Ca^{2+} channels and subsequent influx of Ca^{2+} that leads to the release of neurotransmitters. Taste cells that detect salty taste do not have well-differentiated synapses and their neurotransmitter is not known.

The transduction of **sweet taste** is mediated by G protein-coupled receptors that activate phospholipase C (PLC) (Figure 5.5B). The activation of PLC generates two intracellular second messengers, inositol trisphosphate (IP_3) and diacylglycerol (DAG), from the hydrolysis of phosphatidylinositol 4,5-bisphosphate (PIP_2). IP_3 binds to a calcium channel on the endoplasmic reticulum. This IP_3 binding opens the Ca^{2+} channel, allowing Ca^{2+} to diffuse out of the endoplasmic reticulum into the cytosol. It is speculated that taste-selective cation channels (TrpM5) are calcium sensitive, and IP_3 plays a key role in activating TrpM5. Subsequent Na^+ influx mediated by TrpM5 leads to the generation of a depolarizing receptor potential of the receptor cells. Intracellular elevation of Ca^{2+} combined with membrane depolarization results in ATP release via gap junction channels in the plasma membrane. Transmitter ATP acts on sensory nerve endings, inducing generator potentials. Action potentials follow if generator potentials reach the threshold potential. Taste cells that detect sweet taste do not have well-differentiated synapses.

Central pathway for gustation

The taste cells on the tongue are innervated by bipolar neurons that contribute axons to two cranial nerves, the facial (VII) and glossopharyngeal (IX) (Figure 5.6). Cell bodies of the bipolar neurons are located in the geniculate ganglion of the facial nerve and the distal ganglion of the glossopharyngeal nerve. Peripheral axons from the geniculate ganglion (VII) leave the facial nerve after they leave the cranium to form the chorda tympani nerve and run through the middle ear cavity. The chorda tympani join the lingual nerve, and innervate the taste buds on the rostral two-thirds of the tongue. Central axons from the distal ganglion (IX) reach the tongue via the lingual nerve. It enters the base of the tongue and provides sensory fibers to the taste buds in the caudal portion of the tongue.

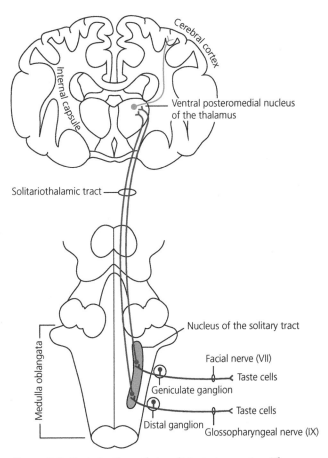

Figure 5.6 Central pathway that mediates taste sensation. The unipolar neurons mediating the sensation of taste via the facial and glossopharyngeal nerves are located in the geniculate and distal ganglia, respectively. Central processes of these ganglia synapse with neurons of the nucleus of the solitary tract in the medulla oblongata. The solitary nucleus gives rise to the solitariothalamic tract and terminates in the ventral posteromedial nucleus of the thalamus, which projects to the cerebral cortex.

The central processes of bipolar neurons in the geniculate and distal ganglia enter the nucleus of the solitary tract in the medulla oblongata. Efferent fibers from the nucleus of the solitary tract ascend as the solitariothalamic tract and terminate in the ventral posteromedial nucleus of the thalamus. The thalamic neurons project to the ipsilateral cerebral cortex. The nucleus of the solitary tract also projects to the amygdala of the limbic system.

Self-evaluation

Answers can be found at the end of the chapter.

1 The olfactory nerve fibers terminate in the:
   A Piriform lobe
   B Thalamus
   C Olfactory bulb
   D Olfactory tract

2 Odorants bind to receptors on the:
   A Cilia of olfactory cells
   B Perikarya of olfactory cells
   C Neurons in the olfactory bulb
   D Axons of olfactory cells

3 Odorant receptor protein is coupled to G protein.
   A True
   B False

4 Membrane depolarization of olfactory cells is triggered by:
   A Voltage-gated Na^+ channels
   B Voltage-gated K^+ channels
   C Ca^{2+}-gated Cl^- channels
   D All of the above

5 Taste molecules bind to receptors on the:
   A Microvilli of receptor cells
   B Perikarya of receptor cells
   C Cranial nerves that mediate signals for taste
   D Axon terminals innervating taste cells

6 The cranial nerves that mediate signals for taste are the facial and glossopharyngeal nerves.
   A True
   B False

7 Which statement is correct about detection of salty taste?
   A Ligand binds to G protein-coupled receptor
   B Amiloride-sensitive sodium channels triggers influx of Na^+, depolarizing receptor cells
   C ATP is the most likely transmitter that depolarizes sensory terminals
   D PLC is involved in signal transduction

8 The primary afferent fibers that mediate taste signals terminate in the:
   A Primary somesthetic cortex
   B Thalamus
   C Nucleus of the solitary tract
   D Ganglia of the glossopharyngeal and vagus nerves

Suggested reading

Bieri, S., Monastyrskaria, K. and Schilling, B. (2004) Olfactory receptor neuron profiling using sandalwood odorants. *Chemical Senses* 29:483–487.

Breer, H., Krieger, J., Meinken, C., Kiefer, H. and Strotman, J. (1998) Expression and functional analysis of olfactory receptors. *Annals of the New York Academy of Sciences* 855:175–181.

Chaudhari, N. and Roper, S.D. (2010) The cell biology of taste. *Journal of Cell Biology* 190:285–296.

Pevsner, J., Sklar, P.B. and Snyser, S.H. (1986) Odorant-binding protein: localization to nasal glands and secretions. *Proceedings of the National Academy of Sciences USA* 83:4942–4946.

Vogt, R.G., Prestwich, G.D. and Lemer, M.R. (1991) Odorant-binding-protein subfamilies associate with distinct classes of olfactory receptor neurons in insects. *Developmental Neurobiology* 22:78–84.

Answers

1 C	5 A
2 A	6 A
3 A	7 B
4 C	8 C

6 Auditory System

Etsuro E. Uemura
Iowa State University, Ames, IA, USA

The auditory system is designed to detect and analyze sound in the environment and much of animal communication relies on this system. Sounds are pressure waves in the air with given frequencies and amplitudes. The auditory system perceives the frequency of sounds as pitch and their amplitude as loudness. Hearing requires at least one ear; however, localization of sound requires two ears as the auditory system must detect the difference in time of arrival or intensity of sound impinging on the two ears. Animals' sense of hearing is also enhanced by their ability to move their ears around to scan the environment for different sounds and locate where the sound is coming from. Hearing is a function of the cerebral cortex, whereas the auditory reflex, such as turning the head in response to sound, is mediated by the brainstem. Hearing involves the external ear, middle ear, and inner ear where the sensory receptor (i.e., the organ of Corti) is located. The cochlear nerve innervates the organ of Corti in the inner ear and relays auditory impulses to the cochlear nuclei in the medulla oblongata. Axons from the organ of Corti ascend the brainstem, synapsing with various relay nuclei before reaching the medial geniculate nucleus of the thalamus, which in turn projects to the auditory cerebral cortex.

External and middle ears

> **1** Describe the structural organization of the external, middle, and inner ears.
>
> **2** What is the function of the middle ear ossicles in transmission of sound?

The **external ear** directs sound waves into the ear canal. Sound waves induce vibration of the tympanic membrane that separates the external ear from the middle ear (Figure 6.1).

The **middle ear** is an air-filled tympanic cavity, separated from the external ear by the tympanic membrane and from the inner ear by the vestibular window and cochlear window. The middle ear communicates with the nasopharynx via the auditory tube, which functions to equalize the pressure in the tympanic cavity with the pressure in the external auditory canal. The middle ear contains a chain of three auditory ossicles, the malleus, incus, and stapes. The **malleus** is attached to the tympanic membrane, whereas the foot plate of the **stapes** fits into the vestibular window in the bony wall between the middle and inner ear. The rim of the base is attached to the margin of the vestibular window by elastic connective tissue. The base of the stapes is in contact with perilymph that fills the inner ear. In dogs, the tympanic membrane and middle ear ossicles have a wide efficiency range and can detect sound between 30 and 35,000 Hz. In contrast, the human ear has greater efficiency within the range 1000–4000 Hz; as the frequency moves beyond this range, efficiency drops off sharply. The ossicles provide a mechanical linkage between the tympanic membrane and the vestibular window. Thus, vibration of the tympanic membrane reaches the inner ear, where the sensory receptor for hearing is located.

Two of the middle ear ossicles, the malleus and incus, constitute a bent lever, with the longer arm of the malleus attaching to the tympanic membrane and the shorter arm of the incus attaching to the stapes. In humans, for example, the handle of the malleus is 1.3 times longer than the long process of the incus. This design, along with the relative size difference between the tympanic membrane and stapes, serves two purposes: (i) it magnifies the vibratory pressure of the tympanic membrane transmitted to the stapes, but (ii) decreases the amplitude of sound waves at the vestibular window. The increase in vibratory pressure is essential as the sound waves are transferred

Dukes' Physiology of Domestic Animals, Thirteenth Edition. Edited by William O. Reece, Howard H. Erickson, Jesse P. Goff and Etsuro E. Uemura.
© 2015 John Wiley & Sons, Inc. Published 2015 by John Wiley & Sons, Inc.

Companion website: www.wiley.com/go/reece/physiology

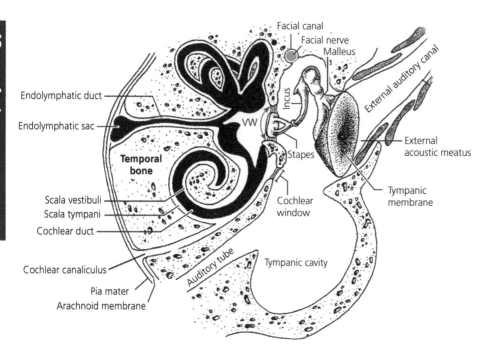

Figure 6.1 The structural components of the external, middle, and inner ear. The tympanic membrane separates the external ear from the middle ear. The middle ear contains three small bones (malleus, incus, stapes) that transmit sound from the tympanic membrane to the inner ear. The stapes fits into a bony opening, the vestibular window (VW). The inner ear is located in the petrous portion of the temporal bone. The sensory receptor for hearing is located in the cochlear duct that lies between the scala vestibuli and scala tympani. The cochlea is simplified in this illustration and does not show its three and one-quarter turns.

from air to a fluid medium (called perilymph) in the inner ear. The decrease in amplitude of sound waves transferred to the perilymph protects the sensitive sensory cells of the organ of Corti.

Inner ear

> 1 What are the three chambers of the cochlea? Which chamber is filled with endolymph?
>
> 2 What cranial nerve innervates the auditory receptors?
>
> 3 Explain how the morphological polarization of sensory cells relates to generation of receptor potentials.
>
> 4 What are the structural and functional differences between the vestibular and cochlear windows?
>
> 5 Explain the structural arrangement of the organ of Corti and explain the functional significance of such an arrangement.
>
> 6 How does the organ of Corti detect different frequencies of sound?

The inner ear contains the sensory organs for both the auditory and vestibular systems. The spiral-shaped cochlea contains three and one-quarter turns. The cochlea is composed of three tubular chambers (Figure 6.2), the vestibular duct (scala vestibuli), cochlear duct, and tympanic duct (scala tympani). A narrow channel called the helicotrema connects the scala vestibuli and scala tympani. They are filled with fluid called **perilymph**, which has a high concentration of Na^+ ions. The scala vestibuli at the basal end faces the vestibular window, whereas the scala tympani faces the cochlear window (Figure 6.1). Thus, pressure on the vestibular window from

movement of the stapes is equalized by fluctuation of the connective tissue sheath that covers the cochlear window. The cochlear duct lies between the scala vestibuli and scala tympani. The cochlear duct is filled with **endolymph**, which has a high concentration of K^+ ions compared with perilymph, maintaining an endolymphatic potential of $+80\,mV$.

Auditory sensory organ

The inner ear contains the sensory organ for the auditory system, the **organ of Corti**. It lies within the cochlea, separating the cochlea into two chambers, the scala vestibuli and the scala tympani (Figure 6.2A,B). The cochlear duct is separated from the scala vestibuli by the vestibular membrane and from the scala tympani by the basilar membrane. The organ of Corti occupies the full extent of the basilar membrane from base to apex (Figure 6.2B). Its structural components include **sensory cells**, supporting cells, and the tectorial membrane (Figure 6.2C). Sensory cells are also referred to as **sensory hair cells** because of their **stereocilia** at the apical surface. Sensory hair cells have 50–100 stereocilia on their apical surface. Stereocilia are connected by tip links at their tips (Figure 6.3B). The tip link is composed of filamentous material, where one end is attached to the side of the stereocilium and the other end to the distal end of the adjacent shorter stereocilium. It is speculated that the tip link is attached to a K^+ channel. This arrangement enables K^+ channels to open when bending of the stereocilia pulls the tip links apart. Stereocilia, once damaged, do not regenerate. It is not known how many of the sensory hair cells must be damaged (due to injury, disease, loud sounds, or aging) before hearing loss becomes obvious. The **tectorial membrane** (Latin *tectum*, roof), a gelatinous structure composed primarily of glycoproteins, overlies the sensory cells, embedding the tips of

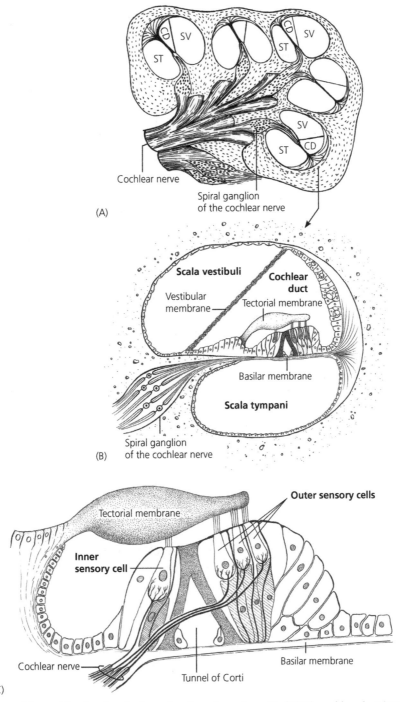

(A)

(B)

(C)

Figure 6.2 (A) Cross-section of the cochlea showing the three chambers, the scala vestibuli (SV), cochlear duct (CD), and scala tympani (ST). (B) The organ of Corti covers the basilar membrane on the side of the cochlear duct. The tectorial membrane overlies the organ of Corti. (C) The organ of Corti is composed of sensory cells and supporting cells. The peripheral processes of bipolar ganglion cells synapse on inner sensory hair cells or travel across the tunnel of Corti to synapse on outer sensory hair cells.

the longest stereocilia of sensory hair cells. Because of this structural arrangement, vibratory movement of the basilar membrane causes stereocilia of the sensory hair cells to bend (Figure 6.3A). The hair cells translate this mechanical bending of stereocilia into voltage changes of the cell membrane.

Transduction of auditory stimulus

Sensory hair cells have a resting intracellular potential of about −70 mV. Endolymph, like extracellular fluid, has a high concentration of K^+, but perilymph has a low concentration of K^+. When the basilar membrane moves upward in response

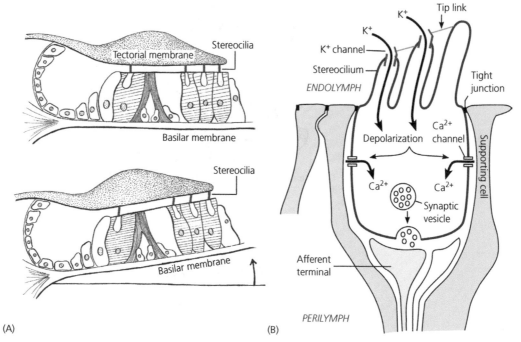

(A)   (B)

Figure 6.3 (A) Deflection of the basilar membrane bends stereocilia of the sensory hair cells. When the basilar membrane makes an upward movement, it creates a shearing force, bending stereocilia toward taller stereocilia. In contrast, downward displacement of the basilar membrane (not shown) causes bending of stereocilia away from taller stereocilia. Such events alter the potential of sensory hair cells, resulting in depolarization or hyperpolarization of the cochlear nerve. (B) Outer sensory hair cell with processes of the supporting cells. They form tight junctions, sealing the soma of the sensory cells from the endolymph in the cochlear duct. Bending the stereocilia toward taller stereocilia opens K^+ channels, resulting in an influx of K^+ into the cell. This depolarizes the sensory hair cell, opening voltage-gated calcium channels. The calcium influx leads to the release of transmitter from the sensory hair cell into the synaptic cleft between the sensory cells and cochlear sensory nerve fibers.

to movement of perilymph in the osseous cochlea, outer rows of the taller stereocilia are displaced against the tectorial membrane, bending all the stereocilia laterally (i.e., toward the taller stereocilia) (Figure 6.3A). This induces (i) ion channels at the tip of the stereocilia to open due to increased tension on the tip link, triggering K^+ influx along the electrical gradient and depolarizing the sensory hair cell (see Figure 9.3B$_2$), (ii) opening of voltage-gated Ca^{2+} channels at the base of the cell and subsequent influx of Ca^{2+}, and (iii) release of a neurotransmitter into the synaptic cleft between sensory hair cells and terminal ends of the cochlear nerve. When the basilar membrane moves downward, stereocilia bend medially, i.e., away from the tallest stereocilium (see Figure 9.3B$_3$). This causes hyperpolarization of the sensory hair cells, possibly involving opening of K^+ channels at the basolateral portion of the cells and an efflux of K^+. Thus, auditory stimuli cause vibration-induced voltage changes, setting up a receptor potential that stimulates terminal ends of the cochlear nerve. An action potential will result if the receptor potential reaches threshold. The cochlear nerve fibers innervate the inner and outer hair cells, mediating auditory signals to the cochlear nuclei in the medulla oblongata. The sensory hair cells also play a role in distinguishing the intensity of sound. There appear to be many sensory hair cells which have progressively

higher thresholds for activation. These cells provide information on loudness by responding only to loud sound.

Detection of the frequency of the tone

When endolymph in the cochlear duct and perilymph in the scala tympani vibrate in resonance, the basilar membrane also vibrates (Figure 6.4A). The **basilar membrane** has a unique physical structure. It is narrow and taut near the base, and wider and more floppy near the apex of the cochlea (Figure 6.4B). Because of its graded stiffness and width, the location of maximum displacement of the basilar membrane is related to the frequency of the tone (Figure 6.5). High-frequency tones selectively distort the basilar membrane close to the base of the cochlea (i.e., close to the vestibular window), intermediate tones distort the basilar membrane from the base to an intermediate region, and low-frequency tones tend to distort the entire basilar membrane with maximum displacement of the membrane occurring near the apex of the cochlear duct. Thus the frequency spectrum of the organ of Corti is precisely laid out on the basilar membrane from base to treble. This orderly arrangement is called tonotopic organization or tonotopy. The tonotopic organization of the organ of Corti is more or less preserved throughout the auditory system.

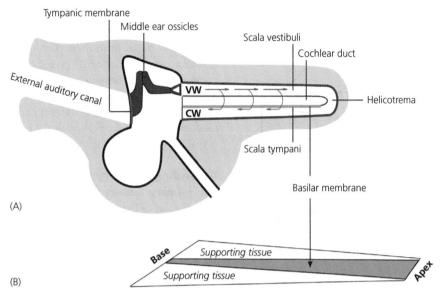

Figure 6.4 (A) The coiled cochlea is depicted as straight to give a clear view of structural relationships. Arrows indicate the manner in which sound waves in the perilymph and endolymph induce vibration of the basilar membrane. Vibration of the stapes causes corresponding waves of perilymph in the scala vestibuli. The basilar membrane vibrates in response to waves of endolymph in the cochlear duct induced by waves transmitted from the scala vestibuli to the scala tympani. The membranous sheath of the cochlear window dampens pressure waves in the cochlea. vw, vestibular window; cw, cochlear window. (B) The basilar membrane and its supporting tissue are shown as if they were uncoiled and stretched out flat. The width of the basilar membrane increases from base to apex.

Clinical correlations

Numerous compounds have been identified as ototoxic and many cause permanent damage to the organ of Corti. A good example of antibiotics known to cause ototoxicity are the aminoglycosides, such as gentamicin and streptomycin. Certain disinfectants, such as chlorhexidine, are also known for their ototoxic effect and potential problems associated with the use of such disinfectants for ear surgery should not be underestimated. Similarly, animals should be examined for otitis externa (i.e., infection of the external ear canal) before the use of chlorhexidine for ear cleaning and flushing. Ototoxic agents must reach the inner ear to induce their toxic effect. For example, chlorhexidine solution may enter the middle ear in an animal with otitis externa and otitis media (infection of the middle ear) via a ruptured tympanum. The round window is a portal for passage of many outside elements (bacteria, toxins, drugs, etc.) into the inner ear and chlorhexidine is no exception. Chlorhexidine in the inner ear ends up in the fluid in the cochlea and once it reaches the organ of Corti and vestibular organ, it causes degeneration of their sensory cells. On recovery from anesthesia after an ear cleaning, the dog becomes deaf in the affected ear and displays abnormal vestibular signs such as ataxia (uncoordinated movement) and nystagmus (oscillation of the eyes).

Ear infection

Otitis media is primarily due to extension of otitis externa. Otitis media often leads to otitis interna (i.e., infection of the inner ear) if not treated properly. Otitis externa and otitis media are usually characterized by inflammation of the ear canal and discharge from the ear. Proper use of antibiotics is essential for treatment of these conditions. **Aminoglycoside antibiotics** (e.g., amikacin, kanamycin, tobramycin, and neomycin) have potential ototoxic effects and they may induce degeneration of the sensory hair cells of the organ of Corti. Otitis media may involve the facial nerve that traverses the facial canal in the petrosal bone. A small portion of the facial canal has no bony wall that separates it from the tympanic bulla (Figure 6.1). At this portion of the canal, the facial nerve is separated from the tympanic cavity only by loose connective tissue lined by simple squamous epithelium. Infection of the facial nerve may further involve the vestibulocochlear nerve, as it accompanies the facial nerve in the inner ear. Thus facial palsy is often associated with vestibular signs. Otitis media may also cause **Horner's syndrome** when infection involves the postganglionic axons that run through the middle ear. In **otitis media interna**, both the facial and vestibulocochlear nerves are often affected because of their location in the inner ear.

Central pathways for hearing

1 Describe the central neural pathway for hearing and explain why an auditory deficit in one ear is only detectable with a lesion of the organ of Corti, cochlear nerve or cochlear nuclei.

2 Describe the central neural pathway that mediates the auditory reflex.

3 How does the auditory system localize sound?

4 How does the auditory system protect sensory hair cells from exceedingly sharp and intense sound?

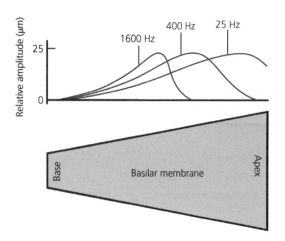

Figure 6.5 The location of the maximum displacement of the basilar membrane is shown in relation to different frequencies of sound.

The auditory system has complex ascending pathways. Auditory signals from the organ of Corti ascend through the cochlea and several relay nuclei in the brainstem to reach the thalamus and auditory cortex (Figure 6.6). There are many ascending auditory pathways in the brainstem and numerous relay neurons along the pathways. They most likely play a role in integrating and processing information. The auditory cortex does not receive signals from every sensory cell, rather it deals with signals preprocessed by multitudes of neurons in the brainstem and thalamus.

Ascending auditory pathways

The **primary sensory neurons** are bipolar cells. Their cell bodies make up the spiral ganglion in the bony cochlea. Central processes of bipolar cells form the cochlear nerve as they leave the cochlea. The **cochlear nerve** carries auditory signals to the cochlear nuclei in the medulla oblongata. In the **cochlear nuclei**,

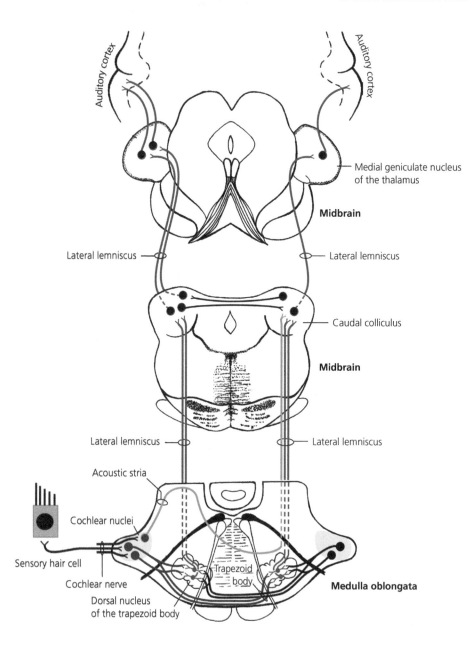

Figure 6.6 Numerous nuclei and ascending pathways are involved in the auditory system. Auditory signals reach the caudal colliculus and the medial geniculate nucleus of the thalamus. The auditory pathway is bilateral, i.e., each ear projects to both sides of the auditory cortex.

the peripheral tonotopic localization is retained. The base of the cochlea is represented dorsally and the apex ventrally, and individual cells respond only over a narrow frequency range. All the cochlear nerve fibers terminate in the dorsal and ventral cochlear nuclei. Fibers from the dorsal nucleus of the trapezoid body form the **acoustic stria**. These fibers decussate to join the lateral lemniscus. Fibers from the ventral cochlear nucleus proceed ventrally to form the **trapezoid body** at the ventral surface of the medulla oblongata. Efferent fibers of the cochlear nuclei either terminate in the ipsilateral or contralateral dorsal motor nucleus. Some fibers ascend, as part of the lateral lemniscus, without terminating in the dorsal nucleus of the trapezoid body. Fibers of the trapezoid body pass ventral to the dorsal nucleus of the trapezoid body. Beyond the cochlear nuclei, the auditory system has many relay nuclei. However, not all the auditory fibers synapse at every relay nuclei. Some fibers bypass certain nuclei and proceed to their next synaptic sites.

The **dorsal nucleus of the trapezoid body** is located in the rostral medulla oblongata, dorsal to the trapezoid body. The dorsal nucleus of the trapezoid body receives bilateral excitatory input from the cochlear nuclei. This binaural input is critical for accurate sound localization. A difference in the time of sound arrival at the two ears results in a delay between the production of impulses. The length of the ipsilateral and contralateral paths determines the arrival of signals at the dorsal nucleus of the trapezoid body via the cochlear nuclei. Almost all ascending auditory fibers terminate in the **caudal colliculus** of the midbrain. Many collicular cells respond to auditory signals from either ear. The caudal colliculus serves as an auditory reflex center (e.g., turning the head in response to a sudden loud sound). Many neurons in the caudal colliculus, like those of the dorsal nucleus of the trapezoid body, are sensitive to the difference in time of sound arrival at the two ears. Therefore, it is important for sound localization. Sound information is processed by the **medial geniculate nucleus** of the thalamus (Figure 6.6) before reaching the auditory cortex of the temporal lobe.

Auditory cortex

The primary auditory cortex is represented primarily by the middle ectosylvian gyrus of the temporal lobe. Each cochlea is mapped bilaterally in the auditory cortex. The auditory cortex is necessary for decoding and feature extraction of complex auditory information. The association cortical areas surrounding the primary auditory cortex integrate various sensory stimuli, and are thus critical to understanding the surrounding environment.

Auditory reflex

1 How are sensory hair cells protected from loud sound?
2 What is the pathway that mediates the middle ear reflex?

Hearing loss occurs when the inner ear suffers an acoustic battering that destroys stereocilia by moving them excessively. The **middle ear reflex** (also referred to as the **acoustic stapedius**

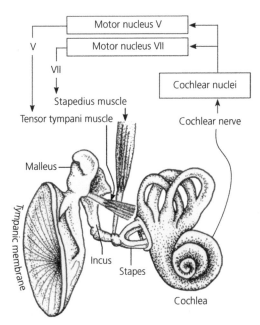

Figure 6.7 The tensor tympani muscle in the middle ear is innervated by the motor nucleus of the trigeminal nerve. The tensor tympani muscle is attached to the muscular process of the malleus. It reflexively contracts in response to loud sound, limiting the movement of the malleus and the tympanic membrane. This action reduces the force and amplitude of sound applied to the organ of Corti in the inner ear. A similar role is also played by the stapedius muscle innervated by the facial nerve. The stapedius muscle attaches to the muscular process of the stapes. Contraction of this muscle pulls the stapes caudally, limiting its movement.

reflex) protects the sensory cells by reflexively contracting the tensor tympani and stapedius muscles in response to loud sound (Figure 6.7). Contraction of these muscles limits the movement of the tympanic membrane and stapes, reducing the force and amplitude of sound applied to the organ of Corti. The reflex involves the motor nuclei of the trigeminal and facial nerves. Efferent fibers of the cochlear nuclei reach the motor nuclei of the trigeminal and facial nerves. The motor nucleus of the trigeminal nerve innervates the **tensor tympani muscle** and the motor nucleus of the facial nerve innervates the **stapedius muscle**. The middle ear reflex is bilateral: loud sound to one ear also triggers the reflex in the opposite ear. This is done by sending signals from the cochlear nuclei to the contralateral dorsal nucleus of the trapezoid body.

Since sensory cells in the organ of Corti can be damaged by excessive movement of endolymph in the inner ear, the reflex contraction of the tensor tympani and stapedius muscles is essential for protection of these sensory cells from sustained loud sounds that might otherwise cause hearing loss. The protection offered against loud sound is only partial, as it takes time for these muscles to contract fully. In a rabbit, for example, the maximum tension can be attained only after 63 ms for the stapedius and 132 ms for the tensor tympani, and in this time the sensory cells can suffer severe damage from the initial waves of sharp and intense sound. Thus, the stapedius and tensor tympani can attenuate loud abrupt sounds only if they come in quick succession.

Self-evaluation

Answers can be found at the end of the chapter.

1 The cochlear duct is filled with:
   A Perilymph
   B Endolymph

2 Which of the following is not a component of the cochlea?
   A Basilar membrane
   B Tectorial membrane
   C Crista ampullaris
   D Spiral ganglion
   E Scala tympani

3 The stapes fits into the vestibular window in the bony wall between the middle and inner ear.
   A True
   B False

4 Tensor tympani muscle is innervated by the facial nerve.
   A True
   B False

5 Which chamber is filled with endolymph?
   A Scala tympani
   B Scala vestibuli
   C Cochlear duct
   D Tympanic cavity

6 Bending the stereocilia toward taller stereocilia opens K^+ channels, resulting in an _____ of K^+ and _____ of sensory hair cells.
   A Outflow, hyperpolarization
   B Outflow, depolarization
   C Influx, hyperpolarization
   D Influx, depolarization

7 High-frequency tones selectively distort the basilar membrane close to the base of the cochlea (i.e., close to the vestibular window), but low-frequency tones tend to distort the entire basilar membrane with maximum displacement of the membrane occurring near the apex of the cochlear duct.
   A True
   B False

8 One of the nuclei of the auditory system that plays a key role in localizing the source of sound is the:
   A Medial geniculate nucleus
   B Cochlear nuclei
   C Dorsal nucleus of the trapezoid body
   D Spiral ganglion

9 The medial geniculate nucleus projects auditory signals to the:
   A Frontal lobe of the cerebrum
   B Parietal lobe of the cerebrum
   C Occipital lobe of the cerebrum
   D Temporal lobe of the cerebrum

10 The acoustic stapedius reflex is mediated by the:
   A Trigeminal and facial nerves
   B Facial nerve only
   C Trigeminal nerve only
   D Vagus nerve

11 Which of the following lesions would best explain complete loss of hearing in the left ear of a dog?
   A Lesion of the left acoustic stria
   B Lesion of the left cochlear nuclei
   C Lesion of the right lateral lemniscus
   D Lesion of the right occipital lobe

12 Which of the following is not part of the auditory pathway?
   A Medial geniculate nucleus
   B Caudal colliculus
   C Cochlear nucleus
   D Nucleus of the solitary tract
   E Temporal lobe

13 The middle ear reflex protects the stereocilia of the sensory hair cells in the organ of Corti.
   A True
   B False

Suggested reading

Borg, E. and Counter, S.A. (1989) The middle-ear muscles. *Scientific American* 261:74–80.

Fettiplace, R. (1999) Mechanisms of hair cell tuning. *Annual Review of Physiology* 61:809–834.

Freeman, D.M. and Weiss, T.F. (1988) The role of fluid inertia in mechanical stimulation of hair cells. *Hearing Research* 35:201–207.

Getty, R.H., Foust, L., Presley, E.T. and Miller, M.E. (1956) Macroscopic anatomy of the ear of the dog. *American Journal of Veterinary Research* 17:364–375.

Gummer, A.W., Hemmert, W. and Zenner, H.P. (1996) Resonant tectorial membrane motion in the inner ear: its crucial role in frequency tuning. *Proceedings of the National Academy of Sciences USA* 93:8727–8732.

Harrison, J.M. and Krving, R. (1964) Nucleus of the trapezoid body: dural afferent innervation. *Science* 143:473–474.

Heine, P.A. (2004) Anatomy of the ear. *Veterinary Clinics of North America: Small Animal Practice* 34:379–395.

Kosmal, A. (2000) Organization of connections underlying the processing of auditory information in the dog. *Progress in Neuropsychopharmacology and Biological Psychiatry* 24:825–854.

Nadol, J.B. Jr (1988) Comparative anatomy of the cochlea and auditory nerve in mammals. *Hearing Research* 34:253–266.

Pickles, J.O. and Corey, D.P. (1992) Mechanoelectrical transduction by hair cells. *Trends in Neurosciences* 15:254–259.

Answers

1 B	8 C
2 C	9 D
3 A	10 A
4 B	11 B
5 C	12 D
6 D	13 A
7 A	

7 Visual System

Etsuro E. Uemura
Iowa State University, Ames, IA, USA

Vision is such an integral part of neural function that even simple tasks, such as standing and walking, are not easy with the eyes closed. Two eyes are necessary for wider peripheral vision and depth perception. Animals have wider peripheral vision than humans because the visual fields of each eye do not completely overlap. In the dog, there is about 50% overlap of the visual fields so that both eyes perceive the middle half of the field of vision. This area of visual overlap provides binocular vision for judgment of distances. The field of vision outside the binocular zone is the monocular zone. Binocular vision varies greatly in different animals, reflecting the position of the eyes in the front of the head. To maintain clear binocular vision, both eyes move as a unit. The eye is equipped with a pupil that adjusts aperture diameter and a lens that focuses light on the retina, where photoreceptor cells receive images. However, the retina is not just converting the image into nerve impulses, it also facilitates feature analysis of the captured image. Feature analysis and visual information processing take place progressively as visual signals are passed to the thalamus, rostral colliculus of the midbrain, and visual cortex.

Structure of the eye

1 What are the three layers of the eye? What functional role does each layer play?
2 Where is the tapetum lucidum located? What is its function?
3 Why does the inner surface of the eye appear black?
4 What structures of the eye does light pass through before reaching the retina?
5 Explain how the eye responds to changes in intensity of ambient light?
6 What is accommodation? What are the structures and the nerve that play a role in accommodation?

The wall of the eye consists of three concentric layers. These layers, proceeding from the outer surface of the eye inward, are the fibrous tunic, vascular tunic, and neuroepithelial (or inner) tunic (Figure 7.1A). The vitreous body and aqueous humor maintain pressure within the eyeball, thus preventing the eyeball from collapsing. The fibrous tunic consists of the **sclera** and **cornea**. It provides mechanical support and protection of the eye. The vascular tunic consists of three major structures: the iris, ciliary body, and choroid. These structures are highly pigmented and vascularized. The retina is the innermost tunic of the eye.

The **iris** contains dilator and sphincter muscles (Figure 7.1B). The dilator muscle opposes the action of the sphincter muscle. The **pupillary sphincter muscle** is circularly arranged in the iris near the pupillary margin (Figure 7.2). It is innervated by the ciliary nerve (postganglionic parasympathetic fibers) from the ciliary ganglion. Contraction of the sphincter muscle results in a decrease in pupillary size (miosis). The **pupillary dilator muscle** is part of the pigmented anterior epithelial cells of the iris. The anterior portion of these cells have cellular extensions that have structural characteristics of smooth muscle cells. Thus, most pigmented anterior epithelial cells are myoepithelial in nature and their cellular extensions represent the dilator muscle. They are radially arranged. This muscle is innervated by the sympathetic postganglionic neurons located in the cranial cervical ganglion. The postganglionic fibers run with the ciliary branch of the ophthalmic nerve to reach the dilator muscle. Contraction of the dilator muscle results in pupillary dilation (mydriasis). Pupillary dilation reflects the general state of sympathetic tone, and certain emotions such as pain, fear, and anger will induce pupillary dilation.

The **ciliary muscle** is the smooth muscle located in the ciliary body (Figure 7.1B). This muscle is innervated by the ciliary

Dukes' Physiology of Domestic Animals, Thirteenth Edition. Edited by William O. Reece, Howard H. Erickson, Jesse P. Goff and Etsuro E. Uemura.
© 2015 John Wiley & Sons, Inc. Published 2015 by John Wiley & Sons, Inc.
Companion website: www.wiley.com/go/reece/physiology

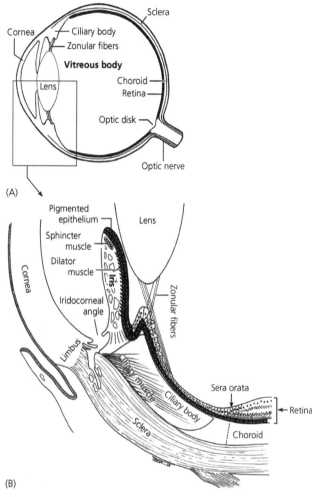

(A)

(B)

Figure 7.1 (A) Midsagittal section of the eye showing its structural components. The iris admits the proper amount of light, which is focused on the retina. A sharp image on the retina is the result of four structural elements: the cornea, aqueous humor, lens, and vitreous body. (B) A portion of the eye is enlarged to show topography of the cornea, iris, ciliary body, and sclera.

nerve (parasympathetic fibers), which contracts the muscle. The ciliary muscle is primarily oriented meridionally in the dog. The meridional fibers originate in the inner surface of the sclera posterior to the iridocorneal angle. They insert in the stroma of the ciliary body. The ciliary muscle contracts in response to parasympapthetic stimulation and decreases tension on the zonular fibers supporting the lens. As a result, the lens becomes more spherical due to its intrinsic viscoelastic properties (Figure 7.3). Focusing on a near object requires a more convex lens that has a shorter focal distance. Consequently, when the gaze is directed at a near object, the ciliary muscle contracts, decreasing the distance between the edges of the ciliary body and relaxing the zonular fibers supporting the lens. This results in a more convex shape of the lens (i.e., more spherical and increased focal power) because of the inherent elasticity of the lens. This process, by which the curvature of the lens changes to

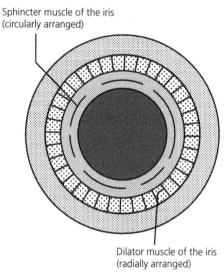

Figure 7.2 Frontal view of the iris and pupil. The radial and circumferential lines in the iris represent the dilator and sphincter muscles, respectively. Pupillary dilation under dim light is caused by constriction of the dilator muscle. This muscle is innervated by sympathetic fibers. Pupillary constriction under bright light is induced by the sphincter muscle, which is innervated by parasympathetic fibers of the ciliary nerve.

focus on a near or far object, is called **accommodation**. When looking at a distant object, the ciliary muscle relaxes and pulls the zonular fibers away from the lens, making the lens less convex with a longer focal distance. This change is necessary for focusing on far objects.

The **choroid** consists of loose connective tissue with numerous vasculature and melanocytes. It serves a nutritive function for ocular tissue. Melanocytes prevent light that escapes past the retina from being reflected back into the retina where it would blur the image. The "eye-shine" that occurs at night when light enters the eye is caused by the **tapetum lucidum** (Latin *tapetum*, carpet; *lucidum*, bright) in the choroid. Although this light-reflective surface enhances dark-adapted vision under dim light, it scatters light in the retina, affecting sharpness of an image. The **retina** is the innermost tunic of the eye and is responsible for detection of light.

Photoreceptor cells

1 What are the structural and functional differences between rod and cone cells of the retina?

2 Explain why dogs are dichromatic and detect only wavelengths within the blue and yellow portion of the light spectrum.

3 List the 10 layers of the retina and explain structural component(s) of each layer.

4 What is the area centralis? How does this area differ from the rest of the retina?

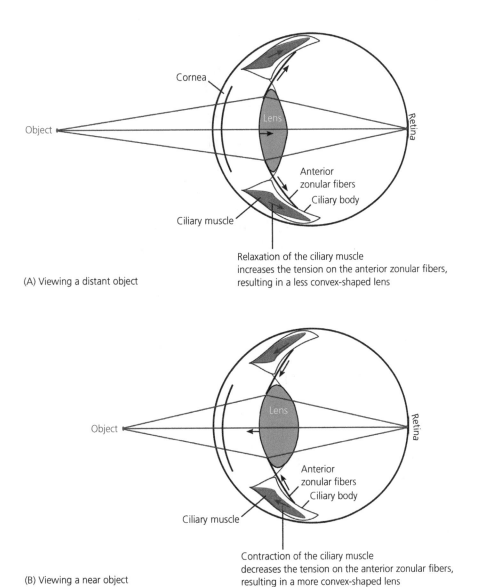

Cornea

Lens

Object

Retina

Anterior
zonular fibers

Ciliary body

Ciliary muscle

Relaxation of the ciliary muscle
increases the tension on the anterior zonular fibers,
resulting in a less convex-shaped lens

(A) Viewing a distant object

Lens

Object

Retina

Anterior
zonular fibers

Ciliary body

Ciliary muscle

Contraction of the ciliary muscle
decreases the tension on the anterior zonular fibers,
resulting in a more convex-shaped lens

(B) Viewing a near object

Figure 7.3 Action of the ciliary muscle on the lens curvature in response to viewing a near or distant object. This process of adjusting the shape of the lens so that the external image falls exactly on the retina is called accommodation. The ciliary muscle in the dog originates in the inner surface of the sclera posterior to the iridocorneal angle and inserts in the stroma of the ciliary body. (A) Relaxation of the ciliary muscle, as shown by the arrow in the ciliary body, increases the tension on the anterior zonular fibers that run between the anterior periphery of the lens to the ciliary body. This results in a less convex-shaped lens. This change is necessary for focusing on far objects. (B) Contraction of the ciliary muscle relaxes the zonular fibers. This results in a more convex-shaped lens (i.e., more spherical with increased focal power) because of the inherent elasticity of the lens. This accommodation is necessary for focusing on near objects.

The key retinal cells include photoreceptor cells, bipolar cells, ganglion cells, horizontal cells, amacrine cells, and pigment epithelial cells (Figure 7.4). There are two types of photoreceptor, rod cells and cone cells, so named because of their shapes (Figure 7.5). Photoreceptor cells consist of two portions, the outer and inner segments. The outer segment is the photosensitive region. In **cone cells**, the outer segment is composed mainly of membranous invaginations. In **rod cells**, the outer segment contains numerous flattened membranous sacs arranged like a stack of coins. The membrane of these invaginations and sacs contains **photopigments**, which convert a light stimulus to a receptor potential. The outer segment of the photoreceptor cells forms the layer of rods and cones of the retina. The inner segment of photoreceptors represents the metabolic region of the photoreceptor cell. The inner segment of the photoreceptor cells forms the outer nuclear layer of the retina. Some 130 million rod and cone cells are present in the retina. The majority (95%) of the photoreceptor cells are rod cells. The photochemical in the rod cells is **rhodopsin**, which is responsible for perception of shades of gray. Rhodopsin has a low threshold of excitability and is easily stimulated by low-intensity light. In fact, rod cells are about 300 times more sensitive to light than are cone cells.

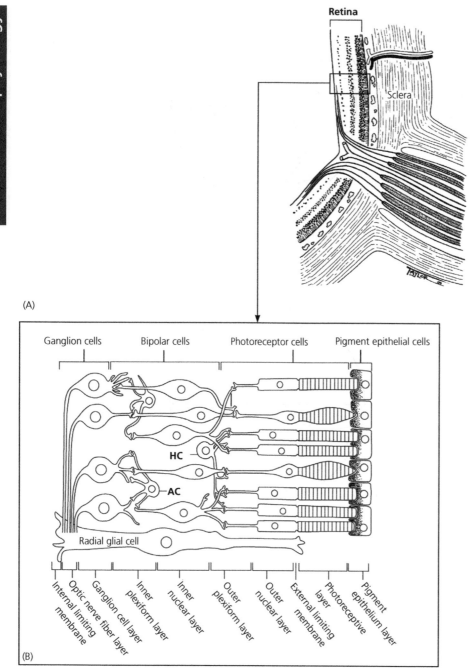

(A)

(B)

Figure 7.4 The retina is the innermost layer of the eye. Its inner surface faces the vitreous body and the outer layer faces the choroid. (A) Illustration of the caudal eye showing the retinal areas shown in (B). (B) Schematic illustration of the retinal layer. The photoreceptor cells form the inner nuclear layer and the photoreceptive layer. The outer and inner plexiform layers are the synaptic sites of two adjacent cell layers. The radial cells extend between the two limiting membranes. The ganglion cells form the optic nerve fiber layer and the pigment epithelium is the outermost cell layer of the retina. Axons of ganglion cells form the inner surface of the retina. They proceed to the optic disk where they exit the eye as the optic nerve. Light must pass through the entire thickness of the retina to reach the photoreceptor cells. HC, horizontal cells; AC, amacrine cells.

Furthermore, hundreds of rod cells feed signals to each ganglion cell, amplifying their stimulating effect on ganglion cells. Thus, rod cells are essential for night vision.

Cone cells have a higher threshold of excitability than rod cells, because the photochemical **iodopsin** requires relatively high-intensity light to be stimulated. Thus, cone cells are less sensitive to light than rod cells. However, cone cells provide color. In primates each cone cell has one of three opsins: a pigment primarily sensitive to blue, green, or red colors with maximum absorptions at 445, 535 or 570 nm, respectively. The

visual system is able to mix and contrast the effect of each cone cell. Thus color is the brain's interpretation of differences in the wavelengths of light. When the light intensity decreases to a point where it is too weak to stimulate cone cells, color vision disappears. This is why night and twilight scenes appear gray. In the dog, each cone has one of two opsins: a pigment sensitive to light with a wavelength of either violet (429–435 nm) or yellow–green (555 nm). Thus, color vision of dogs appears to be dichromatic (Figure 7.6) and they are unable to differentiate between (i) yellow, orange, green, yellow–green, or red, and (ii) gray and greenish-blue. If such is the case, a guide dog at a stop-light may use such clues as the position of light signals and their relative brightness rather than the color of the signals.

The distribution of cone and rod cells also differs. Most cone cells are present in the **area centralis**, the spot where the eye obtains its sharpest images. However, unlike the fovea of the

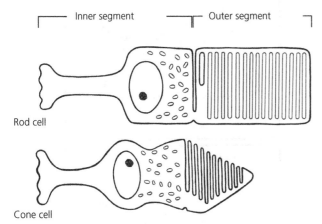

Figure 7.5 The photoreceptor cells (rod and cone cells) are located in the retina. Rod and cone cells have inner and outer segments. The inner segment contains the nucleus and organelles. It is directed toward the center of the eye, while the outer segments are directed toward the choroid. The outer segment of cone cells is composed of numerous membranous invaginations, whereas rod cells have numerous flattened membranous sacs. These membrane invaginations and sacs contain photopigments, which convert a light stimulus to a receptor potential. Rod cells are responsible for perception of shades of gray. Cone cells provide color. In the dog, each cone has one of two photopigments (i.e., opsins): a pigment sensitive to violet or a pigment sensitive to yellow–green. Thus, color vision of dogs appears to be dichromatic.

human eye (equivalent to the area centralis in the dog) where almost all photoreceptors are cone cells, in the dog approximately 5% of photoreceptor cells in the area centralis are cone cells. The area centralis lies dorsolateral to the optic disk. This oval-shaped area centralis is also referred to as the visual streak because of its longer horizontal extension. The visual streak varies greatly among breeds. Since the fovea of the primate contains exclusively cone cells, objects focused on the fovea disappear in darkness. To prevent this loss of image, the eyes of the primate adjust by focusing on the retina outside the fovea. In the dog, this may not be the case as rod cells are the main photoreceptors in the area centralis.

Transduction of visual signals

> **1** Explain the ionic basis for generating receptor potentials in rod and cone cells.
>
> **2** Explain phototransduction of rod cells in the absence or presence of light.
>
> **3** What is the dark current of photoreceptors?

Photoreceptor cells (rods and cones) convert the physical energy of light signals into electrical impulses. This signal transduction process requires opsins present in the rhodopsin of the rod cells and the iodopsin (also known as cone opsin) of the cone cells. Rhodopsin and iodopsin are embedded in the disk membrane of the outer segment. Transduction of visual signals occurs via opsins, which represent the G protein-coupled receptor. Opsins contain the chromophore 11-*cis*-retinal, which is covalently linked to the opsin receptor. When struck by a photon, 11-*cis*-retinal undergoes photoisomerization to all-*trans*-retinal.

Figure 7.6 (A) Humans have full color range because of the presence of numerous cone cells in the retina and because the macula is composed exclusively of cone cells. (B) Dogs are dichromatic: they are able to detect wavelengths within the blue and yellow portion of the light spectrum, but are unable to distinguish reds and oranges. As the photo of the girl shows, her dog is red–green color-blind.

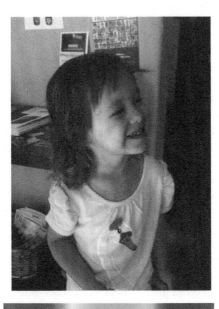

(A)　　　　Human's view

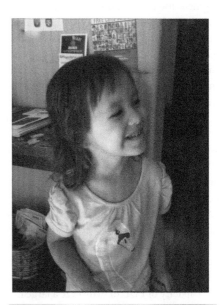

(B)　　　　Dog's view

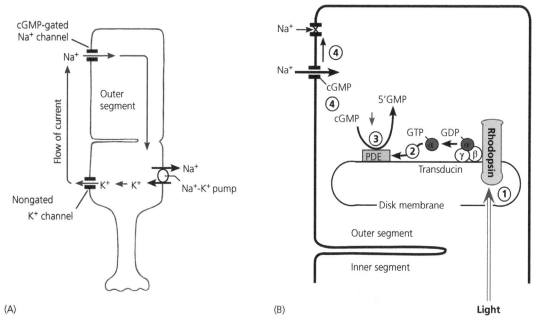

Figure 7.7 Phototransduction of photoreceptors. (A) Phototransduction in a rod cell in darkness. The photoreceptors have cGMP-gated Na⁺ channels in the outer segment membrane, whereas nongated K⁺ channels are present in the inner segment membrane. cGMP binds to the Na⁺ channels and opens the channels, triggering Na⁺ influx. Photoreceptors have high cGMP levels during darkness. This causes Na⁺ channels to open and cause an influx of Na⁺ into photoreceptors, generating inward current. Thus photoreceptors are depolarized during darkness. K⁺ leaks out through nongated K⁺ channels. Na⁺–K⁺ pumps maintain intracellular concentrations of Na⁺ and K⁺. (B) Phototransduction in rod cells under light. The sequence of phototransduction is as follows: (1) light stimulates rhodopsin causing activation of transducin (G protein); (2) transducin stimulates cGMP phosphodiesterase (PDE); (3) cGMP is hydrolyzed by activated PDE, reducing intracellular levels of cGMP; (4) reduction in cGMP leads to closure of cGMP-gated Na⁺ channels, preventing Na⁺ influx and subsequent hyperpolarization of rod cells.

This changes the conformation of the opsin and triggers a signal transduction cascade that decreases the amount of cyclic guanosine monophosphate (cGMP) in photoreceptor cells. The rod and cone cells have cGMP-gated Na⁺ channels in the outer segment membrane and nongated K⁺ channels in the inner segment membrane (Figure 7.7A). The cGMP-gated Na⁺ channels open in the absence of light or close in the presence of light. K⁺ leaks out of the inner segment through nongated K⁺ channels, maintaining proper K⁺ levels. Na⁺/K⁺-ATPases are present in the inner segments of the photoreceptor. These Na⁺–K⁺ pumps maintain intracellular concentrations of Na⁺ and K⁺.

Light absorption by rod cells changes the conformation of rhodopsin (Figure 7.7B). This event stimulates a G protein, which activates cGMP phosphodiesterase (PDE). Activated PDE hydrolyzes cGMP, lowering the concentration of cGMP and subsequent closure of the cGMP-gated Na⁺ channels. This condition prevents Na⁺ influx, causing hyperpolarization of rod cells. Thus, in the presence of light, rod cells are hyperpolarized. Rod cells have a remarkable sensitivity for detecting photons. This sensitivity reflects (i) the large amount of photopigment present in the outer segment and (ii) the ability of rhodopsin to activate hundreds of transduction molecules and the capacity of PDE to hydrolyze a large number of cGMP molecules very quickly. Cone cells have similar phototransduction mechanisms to generate membrane hyperpolarization. The transduction of visual signals is thus not the same as that of

other sensory signals in which sensory receptors are depolarized in response to stimuli.

In **darkness**, photoreceptors are depolarized because of increased levels of cGMP present in photoreceptors. The cGMP binds to the cGMP-gated Na⁺ channels located at the outer segment of the photoreceptors. This triggers the opening of cGMP-gated Na⁺ channels and Na⁺ influx into the outer segment, generating an inward current called the **dark current**. This Na⁺ influx drives the membrane potential toward the Na⁺ equilibrium potential, depolarizing the rod cells. Rod cells in the dark are therefore depolarized and release the neurotransmitter glutamate at synaptic sites on bipolar and horizontal cells of the retina. Thus rod and cone cells only generate receptor potentials, not action potentials.

Visual acuity

> **1** What determines the acuity of visual images?

Each ganglion cell has a small, defined area of retina to which it is linked. These areas are known as receptive fields. The visual field determines acuity of visual images that reflect several factors: population of retinal cells, the ratio of rod to cone photoreceptor cells, and the ratio of photoreceptor cells to ganglion cells. The highest acuity will be achieved if each optic nerve

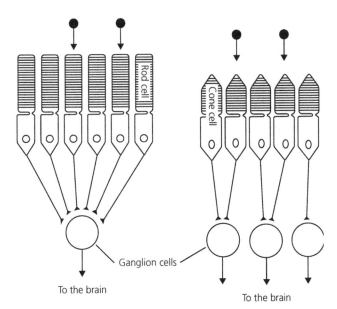

Figure 7.8 Difference in visual acuity of the rod and cone cells reflects their ratio to ganglion cells. Since many neighboring rod cells feed signals via bipolar cells (not shown) to one ganglion cell, two adjacent dots projected to the rod cells are perceived as one dot. In contrast, only one or two cone cells feed information to one ganglion cell, so the same two dots projected on cone cells are seen as two separate dots.

fiber carries signals from a single photoreceptor cell. For example, if an image of two adjacent, but separate, small dots on the retina is carried by two ganglion cells, the visual cortex can perceive them as two dots; however, if two adjacent small dots are fed to a single ganglion cell, the visual cortex fails to recognize them as two separate points. Therefore, an increase in acuity (i.e., increase in visual clarity and sharpness) can be achieved by increasing the number of ganglion cells with fewer photoreceptor cells feeding information to a single ganglion cell. Cone cells provide better acuity than rod cells. This is because hundreds of rod cells feed signals, via bipolar cells, to a single ganglion cell, whereas only a few cone cells feed signals to a single ganglion cell (Figure 7.8). The ratio of cone cells to ganglion cells in dogs is not known. In cats, it is 4 : 1 in the area centralis but 20 : 1 in the periphery. Since the area centralis has some cone cells (about 5% of photoreceptor cells), these areas provide the highest visual acuity in the retina. A high visual acuity in the human is also evident from the approximately 1.2 million optic nerve fibers present in the optic nerve compared with a mere 167,000 optic nerve fibers estimated in the dog.

Pathways of visual signals

> **1** How does the visual field of each eye project to the visual cortex of both cerebral hemispheres?
>
> **2** Describe the visual pathways.
>
> **3** Describe the pathways for pupillary constriction and dilation.

Ganglion cells in the retina give rise to axons of the optic nerve (Figure 7.4), which leaves the eyeball at the optic disk. The optic disk is located ventrolateral to the posterior pole of the eyeball. This small area of the retina, about 1–2 mm in diameter, has no photoreceptor cells and represents the **blind spot** of the eye. Axons of the retinal ganglion cells become myelinated as they leave the eye as the optic nerve. Optic nerve fibers from the medial (i.e., nasal) portion of the retina cross at the optic chiasm, while those from the lateral (i.e., temporal) retina stay on the same side (Figure 7.9A). As a result of the crossover at the optic chiasm, the visual cortex of each occipital lobe is able to analyze the opposite half of the entire visual field. Optic nerve fibers terminate in three nuclei: (i) the **lateral geniculate nucleus** of the thalamus that projects fibers to the visual cortex (Figure 7.9B); (ii) the **rostral colliculus**, which mediates such visual reflexes as turning the head in response to sudden visual stimulus or pupillary dilation (Figure 7.9B); and (iii) the **pretectal nucleus**, which is responsible for pupillary constriction (Figure 7.10).

Visual field

The visual field of each eye is divided into two unequal parts by a plane passing vertically through the fixation point, a larger lateral and a smaller medial (Figure 7.9A), while a plane passing horizontally through the point of fixation divides the visual field into upper and lower parts. The retinal area is also divided into lateral and medial portions by a sagittal plane passing through a line connecting the center of the pupil and the area centralis. A horizontal plane through the middle of the eyeball, at right angles to the sagittal plane, further subdivides the lateral and medial retinal areas into upper and lower quadrants. Light rays from the lateral visual field project to the medial retina, while light rays from medial visual field project to the lateral retina. Thus, each retinal quadrant receives only a portion of the entire scene. In dogs, optic nerve fibers from the lateral 25% of the retina remain ipsilateral, but those from the medial 75% of the retina cross to join the contralateral optic tract. The occipital lobe receives visual information from the contralateral half of the entire visual field. The visual field of each retinal quadrant is precisely mapped in the optic nerve, lateral geniculate nucleus, and visual cortex.

Pupillary light reflex

When bright light shines directly into the eye, the pupil constricts due to contraction of circumferentially arranged smooth muscles of the iris (Figure 7.2). The pupillary light reflex (PLR) requires the retina, optic nerve, two central nuclei (pretectal nucleus and parasympathetic nucleus of the oculomotor nerve), the oculomotor nerve, ciliary ganglion, and ciliary nerve to function normally (Figure 7.10). The pretectal nucleus lies at the junction of the rostral colliculus and the thalamus. The pupillary response to light is consensual: even though only one eye may have been illuminated, the pupillary response occurs in both eyes. The pupillary response that occurs in the illuminated eye is

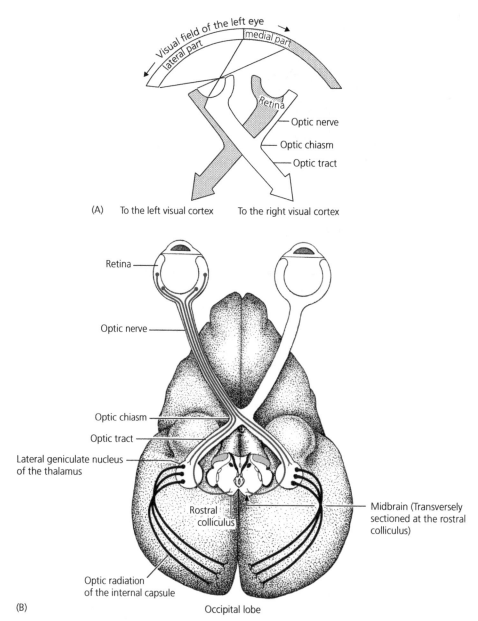

Figure 7.9 (A) The visual field of the left eye in dogs. The medial 75% of the retina receives the entire ipsilateral visual field (i.e., lateral visual field of the left eye) and projects optic nerve fibers to the contralateral visual cortex. In contrast, the lateral 25% of the retina receives the remaining 25% of the visual field (i.e., medial visual field of the left eye). This small portion of the retina projects optic nerve fibers to the ipsilateral visual cortex. Thus, the majority (75%) of the optic nerve fibers in each optic tract originates from the contralateral eye and the remaining fibers (25%) originate in the ipsilateral eye. (B) Ventral view of the brain, showing the visual projection to the lateral geniculate nucleus of the thalamus and rostral colliculus of the midbrain. The lateral geniculate nucleus of the thalamus relays visual information to the visual cortex. The rostral colliculus is the center for the visual reflexes.

the **direct response**, whereas the pupillary response in the eye not directly illuminated is called the **consensual (or indirect) response**. The direct response is much more prominent than the consensual response. There are three reasons for the prominent direct response (Figure 7.11): (i) the pretectal nucleus receives retinal fibers from both eyes, but the majority of fibers come from the contralateral eye; (ii) the right and left pretectal nuclei

exchange fibers; and (iii) the bilateral distribution of pretectal efferent fibers to the parasympathetic nucleus of the oculomotor nerve; however, the majority of pretectal efferent fibers cross to the opposite side to terminate in the contralateral parasympathetic nucleus of the oculomotor nerve. As a result, signals reaching the ipsilateral eye predominate and induce a stronger pupillary response. Instant pupillary response to light is an essential

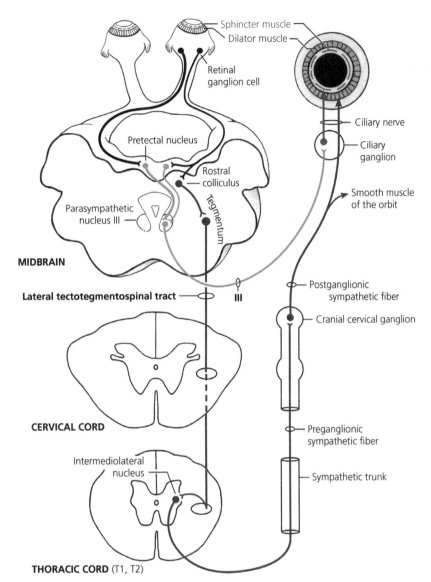

Figure 7.10 Pupillary dilation is mediated by the midbrain tectum, tectotegmentospinal tract and sympathetic system. The lateral tectotegmentospinal tract may send fibers to and receive fibers from the tegmentum. This system also innervates periorbital smooth muscles. Horner's syndrome may result from lesions affecting any portion of the descending central pathway or the sympathetic innervation to the eye. Pupillary constriction in response to light requires the pretectal nucleus, parasympathetic nucleus of the oculomotor nerve, oculomotor nerve, ciliary ganglion, ciliary nerve, and pupillary sphincter muscle. The pupils of both eyes respond to light even though only one eye is exposed. However, the direct response is much more prominent than the consensual response. This difference in pupillary response reflects the major crossing of optic nerve fibers at the optic chiasm and crossing back of pretectal efferent fibers to the parasympathetic nucleus of the oculomotor nerve.

regulatory and safety feature of the visual system. It is also of important diagnostic value. The PLR does not test for vision, but only tests autonomic pupillary control. This is because the PLR is present even with extensive damage to the retina or optic nerve, provided that there are sufficient intact optic nerve fibers to carry light signals to the reflex center.

The optic nerve fibers to the pretectal nucleus are largely from the contralateral eye (Figure 7.11). The pretectal nucleus on each side of the brainstem has reciprocal innervation. The

pretectal neurons also project to the parasympathetic nucleus of the oculomotor nerve in the midbrain, but most (80%) project to the contralateral parasympathetic nucleus of the oculomotor nerve. The preganglionic fibers from the parasympathetic nucleus of the oculomotor nerve reach the ciliary ganglion via the oculomotor nerve. The ciliary ganglion gives rise to the ciliary nerve. This nerve carries postganglionic fibers to the pupillary sphincter muscle of the iris and the ciliary muscle.

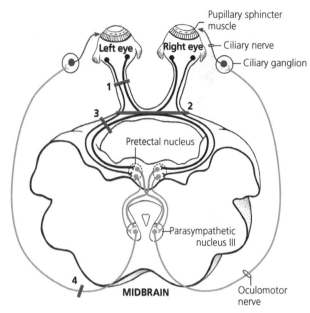

Figure 7.11 Numbers 1–4 indicate the locations of hypothetical lesions. The pupillary light reflex (PLR) is present even with damage to the retina or optic nerve provided there are sufficient intact nerve fibers to carry light signals to the reflex center. Lesion 1: a lesion of the left optic nerve induces blindness of the left eye. Shining a light in the left eye does not induce the PLR in either eye, whereas shining a light in the right eye induces both direct and consensual responses. Lesion 2: blindness of both eyes results from a lesion of the optic chiasm. There is no PLR in either eye. Lesion 3: a lesion that involves one optic tract partially impairs vision, but does not affect the pupillary response of either eye. Lesion 4: a lesion of the oculomotor nerve induces lateral strabismus, ptosis (i.e., narrowed palpebral fissure), and pupillary dilation. There is no PLR in the left eye.

Clinical correlations

Miosis (Greek *meiosis*, diminution) is a condition of excessive constriction of the pupil. It occurs when loss of pupillary dilator tone offsets the tone of pupillary constrictors. Miosis suggests injury to the sympathetic innervation of the eye. Three possible lesions disrupt the sympathetic pathway to the eye: (i) interruption of the lateral tectotegmentospinal tract by a lesion of the lateral funiculus; (ii) interruption of the vagosympathetic trunk in the cervical region due to avulsions or direct injury; and (iii) interruption of postganglionic fibers in the middle ear due to otitis media. Absence of the PLR accompanied by fixed pupillary dilation suggests a lesion of the midbrain or ipsilateral oculomotor nerve. The PLR examines autonomic pupillary control, not vision. Under normal conditions, light directed into one eye will induce pupillary constriction in both eyes. The PLR varies according to the site of the lesion affecting the PLR pathway. If the left optic nerve is damaged, light directed into the left eye will not elicit pupillary constriction in either eye. However, if the right eye is illuminated, both eyes show the pupillary response. If a lesion of the optic nerve leaves sufficient numbers of intact nerve fibers to carry information to the reflex center, the PLR will be present. However, the pupillary response could be slower and incomplete under such conditions. Similarly, a partial lesion of the oculomotor nerve may not be obvious when pupillary responses are tested. However, it is likely that such an animal will display a narrower palpebral fissure, pupillary dilation, and lateral strabismus in the eye of the affected side.

Self-evaluation

Answers can be found at the end of the chapter.

1 The tapetum lucidum is present in the:
   A Iris
   B Choroid
   C Retina
   D Ciliary body

2 Cell bodies of the photoreceptor cells are present in the:
   A Ganglion cell layer
   B Blind spot
   C Inner nuclear layer
   D Layer of rods and cones
   E Outer nuclear layer

3 The pupillary light reflex (PLR):
   A Refers to the pupillary dilation in response to low light
   B Does not require the oculomotor nerve
   C Cannot be induced in an eye with an optic nerve lesion
   D Elicits only a direct response in the eye that light is shown into

4 Most cone cells are in the area centralis:
   A True
   B False

5 Hyperpolarization of rod cells is caused by:
   A Closure of the cGMP-gated Na^+ channels
   B Opening of the cGMP-gated Na^+ channels
   C Increased activity of Na^+–K^+ pumps
   D Closure of nongated K^+ channels

6 In darkness, photoreceptors are depolarized because of increased levels of cGMP.
   A True
   B False

7 When the left eye is illuminated, which lesion is likely to result in the presence of the direct PLR, but the absence of the consensual response?
   A A lesion of the left optic nerve
   B A lesion of the optic chiasm
   C A lesion of the left optic tract
   D A lesion of the right oculomotor nerve

8 The pretectal nucleus mediates which of the following:
   A Visual information to the primary visual cortex
   B Pupillary dilation in response to dim light
   C Pupillary constriction in response to light
   D Body and ocular reflex

9 Complete loss of the visual field of the left eye would most likely result from:
   A A lesion of the right optic nerve
   B A lesion of the left optic nerve
   C A lesion of the left visual cortex
   D A lesion of the right oculomotor nerve

10 The dark current is generated by photoreceptors in response to:

    A Light

    B Darkness

11 A dog shows the following clinical signs: pupillary dilation of the right eye, lateral strabismus of the right eye, and drooped right eyelid. The lesion likely involves:

    A Pons

    B Midbrain

    C Medulla oblongata

    D Spinal cord

12 What cells give rise to axons of the optic nerve?

    A Photoreceptors

    B Bipolar cells

    C Ganglion cells

    D Lateral geniculate nucleus

    E Medial geniculate nucleus

Suggested reading

Evans, H.E. (ed.) (1993) *Miller's Anatomy of the Dog*, 3rd edn. W.B. Saunders, Philadelphia.

Gamlin, P.D. and Clarke, R.J. (1995) The pupillary light reflex pathway of the primate. *Journal of the American Optometric Association* 66:415–418.

Glickstein, M., King, R.A., Miller, J. and Berkley, M. (1967) Cortical projections from the dorsal lateral geniculate nucleus of the cat. *Journal of Comparative Neurology* 130:55–75.

Howard, D.R. and Breazile, J.E. (1973) Optic fiber projections to dorsal lateral geniculate nucleus in the dog. *American Journal of Veterinary Research* 34:419–424.

Hultborn, H., Mori, K. and Tsukahara, N. (1978) The neuronal pathway subserving the pupillary light reflex. *Brain Research* 159:255–267.

Koch, S.A. and Rubin, L.F. (1972) Distribution of cones in retina of the normal dog. *American Journal of Veterinary Research* 33:361–363.

Laties, A.M. and Sprague, J.M. (1966) The projection of optic fibers to the visual centers in the cat. *Journal of Comparative Neurology* 127:35–70.

Mowat, F.M. Peterson-Jones, S.M., Willamson, H., Luthert, P.J., Ali R.R. and Bainbridge, J.W. (2008) Topographical characterization of cone photoreceptors and the area centralis of the canine retina. *Molecular Vision* 14:2518–2527.

Answers

1	B	**7**	D
2	E	**8**	C
3	C	**9**	B
4	A	**10**	B
5	A	**11**	B
6	A	**12**	C

8 Motor System

Etsuro E. Uemura
Iowa State University, Ames, IA, USA

The motor system directs the voluntary control of muscles. It is the system that enables animals to walk, run, bark, eat, or bite if necessary. The motor system includes the cerebral motor cortex, basal nuclei, cerebellum, brainstem, spinal cord, and peripheral nerves. They work together to integrate signals initiated by the motor cortex into motor patterns. Locomotion relies on three key components of body movements: **voluntary**, **reflex**, and **rhythmic**. Voluntary movements are under central control and can even vary between performance of the same purposeful task. They also improve with experience and learning. Reflex movements represent the stereotyped local motor responses to sensory stimuli. Such local reflexes are part of the system that maintains proper muscle tone and posture that is essential for voluntary movements. Reflex movements are modulated by the central motor centers. Voluntary movements depend also on the neural control of locomotion, triggered by central pattern generators in the spinal cord. They produce coordinated patterns of rhythmic activity and descending motor signals are not required to control every aspect of muscle activity. This enables efficient use of upper motor regulation of locomotion.

Voluntary motor control

1 What are upper motor neurons and lower motor neurons? Where are they located?

2 Where is the primary motor area of the cerebral cortex? What motor tracts originate from there?

3 What roles are played by the basal nuclei in goal-directed movement?

4 Name the motor nuclei in the brainstem that play a key role in voluntary motor control and explain how they control lower motor neurons?

5 List the descending motor tracts that play a key role in voluntary movements and explain their origin, termination sites, location in the spinal cord, and functions.

6 Explain the modulatory role of the cerebellum in goal-directed movement, maintenance of posture, and equilibrium.

7 What is the basis of ataxia and hypermetria?

8 What is the role of a motor unit in voluntary movements?

Voluntary movement is directed by the primary motor cortex (Figure 8.1). However, the task of the motor cortex in synthesizing numerous signals into patterns of action requires coordination of the entire cerebral cortex, basal nuclei, and cerebellum (Figure 8.2). The motor cortex and brainstem motor centers give rise to the descending motor tracts that control motor neurons innervating skeletal muscles. These motor tracts also act on the local reflex circuitries to maintain posture and muscle tone, and on the central pattern generator in the spinal cord to initiate, modify, or terminate locomotor activity. Through this organization, the motor system directs the voluntary control of muscles, from the simplest movements to the most complex. Even the simplest movement is highly integrated and requires inputs from different areas of the central and peripheral nervous systems.

Cerebral cortex

The cerebral cortex initiates voluntary movements. In the dog, the **primary motor area** is represented by the postcruciate gyrus and the rostral suprasylvian gyrus. The area may extend into the precruciate gyrus. For the motor cortex to initiate goal-directed movements, it relies on information from other areas of the cerebral cortex, including the current position of the body,

Dukes' Physiology of Domestic Animals, Thirteenth Edition. Edited by William O. Reece, Howard H. Erickson, Jesse P. Goff and Etsuro E. Uemura.
© 2015 John Wiley & Sons, Inc. Published 2015 by John Wiley & Sons, Inc.
Companion website: www.wiley.com/go/reece/physiology

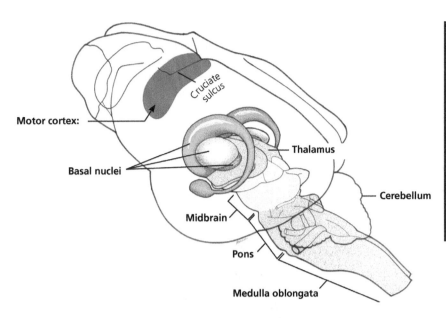

Figure 8.1 The relative position of the cerebral motor cortex, basal nuclei, thalamus, midbrain, pons, medulla oblongata, and cerebellum. The primary motor cortex, which initiates voluntary muscular action, is represented by the postcruciate gyrus and the rostral suprasylvian gyrus. The motor area may extend into the precruciate gyrus. The cerebral cortex gives rise to the corticospinal, corticonuclear, and corticopontine tracts. The midbrain gives rise to the rubrospinal tract, the pons to the pontine reticulospinal tract, and the medulla oblongata to the medullary reticulospinal tract.

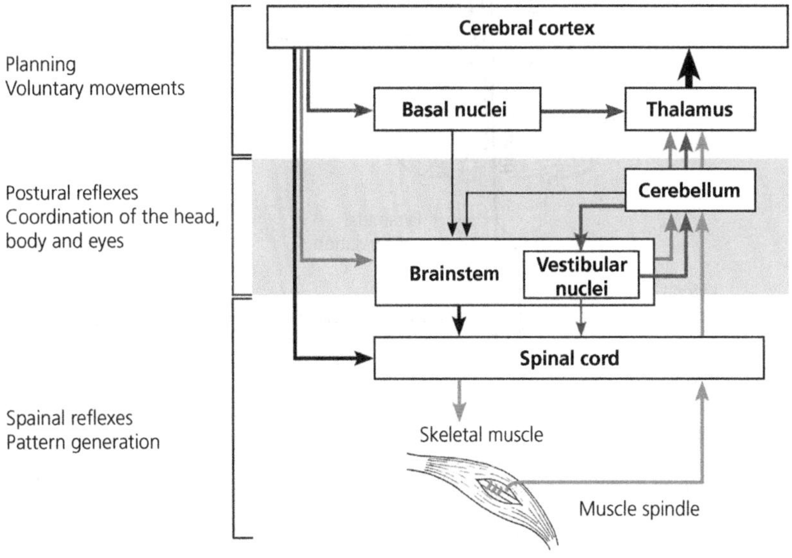

Figure 8.2 The motor centers that influence the spinal motor neurons. Almost every region of the cerebral cortex is able to regulate the primary motor cortex via the basal nuclei and cerebellum. The basal nuclei execute cortical motor outputs by sending efferents to the brainstem (e.g., reticular formation and red nucleus), which gives rise to the descending motor tracts that control lower motor neurons in the spinal cord. The cerebrum also influences the cerebellum via the brainstem. The vestibular nuclei work with the cerebellum to maintain stable eye and body position in response to changes in head position.

the expected goal and strategy to reach that goal, and memories associated with past experiences. The entire cerebral cortex feeds signals to the basal nuclei and the cerebellum (Figure 8.2). In turn, both areas provide feedback to the primary motor cortex. This enables the primary motor cortex to facilitate or inhibit lower motor neurons, via its descending motor tracts, in the spinal cord and brainstem.

The cerebral motor cortex gives rise to three descending motor tracts: the corticonuclear, corticopontine, and corticospinal (Figure 8.3). Their axons enter the gray matter, where they influence lower motor neurons primarily via **interneurons**. The **corticonuclear tract** descends to reach its target nuclei in the brainstem. This tract mediates such voluntary actions as eye movements, mastication, facial expression, swallowing, neck movement, and tongue movement. The **corticopontine tract**

terminates in the pons and synapses with neurons that send their axons, as the pontocerebellar fibers, to the contralateral cerebellum. This is one of several ways the cerebellum monitors cerebral motor activities. The **corticospinal tract** is a crossed pathway, as most of its fibers cross (75% or so in dogs) at the pyramidal decussation and descend as the **lateral corticospinal tract** in the contralateral side of the spinal cord. The remaining fibers stay in the ipsilateral side of the spinal cord and descend as the **ventral corticospinal tract**. However, the fibers of the ventral corticospinal tract do cross back when they reach the level of the lower motor neurons they innervate. As a result, each cerebral hemisphere controls the contralateral side of the body. The corticospinal tract is more developed in primates than in other animals. In dogs, the lateral corticospinal tract terminates approximately 50% of its axons in the cervical, 30% in the thoracic, and 20% in the lumbosacral cord segments. The ventral corticospinal tract descends to the mid-thoracic cord segments. In humans, the corticospinal tract is essential for precise and refined activities of individual muscles of the extremities. It provides the nonpostural, modifiable movements that are the basis of acquired motor skills.

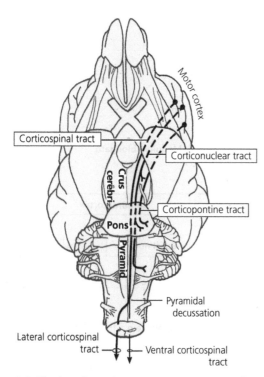

Figure 8.3 The three descending motor tracts: corticospinal, corticonuclear, and corticopontine. The corticonuclear tract terminates in all the cranial motor nuclei of the brainstem, whereas the corticospinal tract descends to the spinal cord. The corticopontine tract terminates in the pons. Some of the corticonuclear fibers and all the corticospinal fibers that arrive at the medulla form the pyramid at the ventral surface of the medulla oblongata, and are therefore referred to as the pyramidal tract.

Brainstem motor nuclei

Three key motor nuclei in the brainstem are the red nucleus of the midbrain, pontine and medullary reticular formation, and vestibular nuclei in the medulla oblongata (Table 8.1 and Figures 8.1 and 8.4). The **red nucleus** gives rise to the rubrospinal tract, which is functionally similar to the lateral corticospinal tract. In animals, the rubrospinal tract is a key motor tract for voluntary movement. The primary role of this tract is to control the flexor motor system and fine movements of the extremities.

The **reticular formation** gives rise to the pontine and medullary reticulospinal tracts. These descending motor tracts maintain the muscle tone necessary for supporting the body against gravity, as well as postural adjustment and synergic movements of the body. The **pontine reticulospinal tract** descends in the ventral funiculus of the spinal cord. It facilitates spinal motor neurons (alpha, gamma) that supply the extensor muscles, but it simultaneously inhibits motor neurons to the flexor muscles (Figure 8.5B). Thus, stimulation of the pontine reticular formation has pronounced effects on the ipsilateral extensor muscles. The **medullary reticulospinal tract** descends in the lateral funiculus of the spinal cord. It opposes the pontine reticulospinal tract by inhibiting spinal motor neurons (alpha, gamma) that supply the extensor muscles and simultaneously facilitates motor neurons for flexor muscles. Thus the reticular formation plays a vital role in coordination of the extensor and flexor muscles. This reticular action is the basis for the maintenance of posture, muscle tone, and spinal reflexes. The **vestibular nuclei** in the medulla oblongata give rise to two descending tracts, the medial and lateral vestibulospinal tracts. They descend in the ventral funiculus of the spinal cord (Figure 8.5) They maintain balance of the body by facilitating lower motor neurons for extensor muscles and inhibiting lower motor neurons for flexor muscles.

Descending motor tracts to the spinal cord can be divided into two groups based on their preference in controlling axial muscle, proximal muscles of the limbs, or distal muscles of the limbs. A group of tracts that descend in the lateral funiculus (e.g., lateral corticospinal, rubrospinal) primarily control lower motor neu-

Table 8.1 Descending motor tracts.

Tract	Origin	Location (funiculus)	Crossed or uncrossed	Destination	General effect
Lateral corticospinal	Cerebral cortex	Lateral	Crossed	Entire cord*	
Rubrospinal	Red nucleus	Lateral	Crossed	Entire cord	Facilitate flexion but inhibit extension
Medullary reticulospinal	Medullary RF	Lateral	Bilateral	Entire cord	
Pontine reticulospinal	Pontine RF	Ventral	Uncrossed	Entire cord	
Tectospinal	Rostral colliculus	Ventral	Crossed	Cervical	Facilitate extension but inhibit flexion
Lateral vestibulospinal	Vestibular nuclei	Ventral	Uncrossed	Entire cord	
Medial vestibulospinal	Vestibular nuclei	Ventral	Uncrossed	Cervical and upper thoracic	

*Terminates approximately 50% of its axons in the cervical, 30% in the thoracic and 20% in the lumbosacral cord segments.
RF, reticular formation.

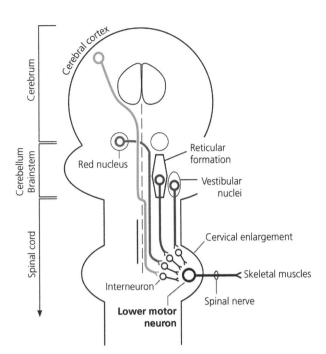

Figure 8.4 Upper motor neurons are located in the primary motor cortex, red nucleus of the midbrain, reticular formation, and vestibular nuclei. They give rise to the descending motor tracts (see Table 8.1), which influence lower motor neurons in the brainstem (not shown) and the spinal cord. The descending tracts influence lower motor neurons primarily via interneurons.

rons for distal muscles. One exception is the medullary reticulospinal tract from the medullary reticular formation. It controls lower motor neurons for axial and proximal limb muscles. The other group of motor tracts descends in the ventral funiculus. They, like the medullary reticulospinal tract, control lower motor neurons for axial muscles and proximal limb muscles. The descending motor tracts have traditionally been classified into pyramidal and extrapyramidal tracts. The corticospinal and corticonuclear tracts are collectively referred to as the **pyramidal tract**, because these tracts form the pyramid at the ventral surface of the medulla oblongata (Figure 8.3). All other descending motor tracts for voluntary movements are referred to as the **extrapyramidal tract**. The pyramidal tracts are less well developed in domestic animals than in the primate. In domestic animals, the extrapyramidal tracts play a more important role in locomotion. Pyramidal and extrapyramidal motor tracts descend in the lateral or ventral funiculus of the spinal cord (Table 8.1 and Figure 8.5).

Upper and lower motor neurons

Motor neurons are classified as upper motor neurons and lower motor neurons based on their location and target tissue. Cortical motor neurons are commonly referred to as **upper motor neurons**, but the red nucleus of the midbrain, vestibular nuclei, and motor neurons of the reticular formation are also considered

upper motor neurons (Figure 8.4). Upper motor neurons are responsible for voluntary muscle control, regulation of muscle tone, and maintenance of posture against gravity. They do not innervate skeletal muscle directly, but exercise their influence on the lower motor neurons by way of their descending motor tracts. **Lower motor neurons** are located in the cranial and spinal motor nuclei. Their axons, unlike upper motor neurons, leave the central nervous system (CNS) and innervate skeletal muscles (Figure 8.4). Lower motor neurons include the spinal alpha, gamma, and visceral motor neurons as well as motor neurons of the cranial motor nuclei. In a clinical context, however, only alpha motor neurons are often referred to as lower motor neurons.

Clinical correlations

In the dog, bilateral lesions of the red nucleus may induce hypokinesia (Greek *kinesis*, movement), a condition of reduced motor function or activity. However, voluntary motor control is most likely unimpaired. Lesions involving the medullary reticular formation or descending medullary reticulospinal tract may cause unopposed excitatory influence of the pontine reticular formation on the spinal lower motor neurons. Under this condition, voluntary movement of muscles may be weak (paresis), myotatic reflex may be pronounced (hyperreflexia), and muscle tone may be increased (hypertonia). A lesion of the vestibular nuclei, vestibular nerve, or vestibular receptor is likely to induce head tilt, circling, and falling to the side of the lesion. Abnormal nystagmus (i.e., nystagmus that occurs while the head is motionless) may also appear. These clinical signs are caused by the lack of vestibular control on the vestibulospinal tracts that exert excitatory influence on extensor muscles and inhibitory influence on flexor muscles.

Basal nuclei and goal-directed movements

The **basal nuclei** consist of the caudate nucleus, putamen, and globus pallidus. They are located deep inside the cerebrum. The basal nuclei coordinate complex movements of the body by influencing the cerebral motor cortex and other major motor centers (e.g., red nucleus, reticular formation) in the brainstem (Figure 8.2). The primary afferents of the basal nuclei come from wide areas of the cerebral cortex. The basal nuclei, in return, modulate cerebral motor outputs by acting on the primary motor cortex via the thalamus. This feedback to the cerebral cortex enables the basal nuclei to participate in not only the regulation of voluntary movements but also the learning of motor skills. Efferents of the basal nuclei also reach the brainstem motor centers. This connection, which operates in concert with the cerebellum, initiates well-coordinated voluntary movements.

Studies on monkeys have shown that the changes in neuronal activity of the basal nuclei occur prior to firing of the neurons of the motor cortex and prior to the movement of the body. The importance of the basal nuclei in motor planning and initiating voluntary movements can be seen in patients with Parkinson's disease. These patients with damaged basal nuclei show rigidity,

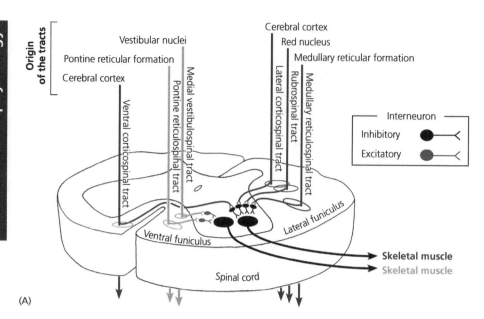

(A)

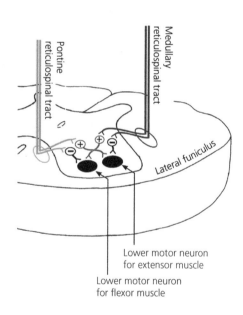

(B)

Figure 8.5 (A) The descending motor tracts are located in the white matter. Only the tracts on the right side of the spinal cord, with the exception of the ventral corticospinal tract, are shown in the diagram. Not all the tracts occupy an area independent from the others. For example, the areas occupied by the lateral corticospinal tract and rubrospinal tract may overlap in the lateral funiculus. (B) Two descending tracts (pontine and medullary reticulospinal) are illustrated with interneurons. The medullary reticulospinal tract in the lateral funiculus is excitatory to flexors and inhibitory to extensors. In contrast, the pontine reticulospinal tract in the ventral funiculus is excitatory to extensors and inhibitory to flexors. This contrasting functional diversity reflects spinal interneurons [excitatory (+), inhibitory (–)] that mediate motor signals to lower motor neurons.

rhythmical tremors at rest, and slowed initiation and execution of intended movement. Such observations suggest that the basal nuclei are an important part of the complex processes that execute planning, initiation and coordination of specific motor sequences. Experimental studies have also shown that the effect of the basal nuclei in general is inhibitory to many of their target nuclei. Subsequently, a motor system becomes active when this inhibitory effect of the basal nuclei is released. Thus, proper application and removal of inhibitory control is crucial in resting, standing, and walking. Any malfunctions of the basal nuclei lead to deficits in movement of the body, such as extraneous unwanted movements or difficulty with initiating intended movements.

Cerebellar modulation of voluntary movements

Since voluntary movements initiated in the cerebral cortex require the highest degree of synergy, the cerebellum is in intimate contact with the cerebrum, brainstem, and spinal cord (Figure 8.2). The cerebellum can be viewed as having a carbon copy of the pattern of cerebral motor activity. One way the cerebellum monitors efferents of the cerebral motor cortex is via the corticopontine tract and pontocerebellar fibers that project cerebral motor signals to the contralateral cerebellum. The cerebellum also monitors the position of the head, neck, eyes, trunk, and extremities by receiving signals from **proprioceptors** in the muscle and joints. Thus, the internal organization enables the cerebellum to (i) assess disparities between intended motor actions of the cerebral cortex and muscular response in progress and (ii) correct any disparity while a movement is in progress by influencing the motor cortex and motor centers in the brainstem. The motor centers include the red nucleus, reticular formation, and vestibular nuclei (Table 8.1). These motor centers give rise to the descending tracts that influence lower motor neurons. Thus, the cerebellum functions as an error-correcting device for goal-directed movements.

Clinical correlations

Damage to the cerebellum does not result in paralysis or diminished sensation, but rather a loss of spatial accuracy and smooth execution of movements. Cerebellar lesions also reduce muscle tone and affect balance. The cerebellum continues to develop through gestation and several days after birth. Thus, *in utero* infection with, for example, herpesvirus can lead to a loss of neurons and subsequent cerebellar hypoplasia. In cats, *in utero* infection with panleukopenia virus also induces similar cerebellar hypoplasia. These animals display **ataxia** (i.e., lack of voluntary coordination of muscle movements) and **intention tremors** (i.e., a disorder characterized by a broad, coarse, and low-frequency tremor) of the head and body. Such clinical signs become obvious as the animals start to ambulate, but are unlikely to progress over time. When the initiation of each successive movement is delayed, rapid alternating movements cannot be performed. On the other hand, when termination of each movement is delayed by a slow response of antagonist muscles, the result is an error in timing and overshooting (**hypermetria**). When a dog with hypermetria reaches a dish to drink water, the head overshoots and hits the edge of the dish instead of the water. The gait of animals with ataxia is characterized by unsteady walking and the animal spreads its feet apart in order to stabilize its posture (wide stance). A lesion of the cerebellar area that has reciprocal connections with the vestibular system affects the ability to maintain equilibrium and eye movements that occur in response to changes in head position.

Motor unit

Each skeletal muscle fiber receives only one motor end plate, forming the neuromuscular synapse, but the number of muscle fibers innervated by a single alpha motor neuron varies greatly from a half dozen to hundreds. This functional unit of a single alpha motor neuron and all the muscle fibers it innervates is referred to as a **motor unit**. Each motor unit has a unique contractile force, determined by the number of muscle fibers it innervates. The number of muscle fibers innervated by a single motor neuron decreases as the need for fine control of a muscle increases. Thus, a single motor neuron innervates only a dozen or fewer extraocular muscle fibers. In contrast, larger motor units generally innervate larger muscles that generate powerful force and each motor neuron innervates hundreds and thousands of muscle fibers. The motor system utilizes motor units effectively to generate appropriate contractile force for any given task. The order of recruitment of motor units is determined by the size of the neuronal cell bodies. When the force needed is minor, smaller motor neurons are activated first. This is because the threshold for depolarization reflects neuronal size, i.e., the first neurons to fire are smallest in size due to their low threshold for synaptic activation and the last to fire are the largest in size because of their high threshold.

Reflex motor control

1 Explain the stretch and flexor reflexes, and their roles in maintenance of posture.
2 Describe the differences between the monosynaptic and polysynaptic reflex and list the spinal reflexes that utilize such pathways.
3 What is the role of the gamma loop in reflex motor control?

A reflex is a relatively simple involuntary response to a specific sensory stimulus. It is an integral part of maintaining muscle tone and posture. The spinal cord and brainstem contain the necessary neural circuitries that not only mediate local reflexes but also maintain muscle tone. A reflex is either monosynaptic or polysynaptic in type. The **monosynaptic reflex** is the simplest reflex. It requires peripheral sensory neurons that bring sensory signals from sensory receptors to the spinal cord and central motor neurons that respond to sensory signals by triggering contraction of skeletal muscles. One example of a monosynaptic reflex is the stretch reflex, commonly demonstrated by the knee-jerk (Figure 8.6). The monosynaptic reflex shows the importance of the connection between Ia sensory fibers (see Table 1.2)

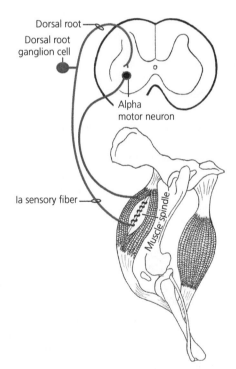

Figure 8.6 The quadriceps reflex requires a minimum of two neurons (one sensory and one motor). Sensory neurons have their cell bodies in the dorsal root ganglion, while cell bodies of motor neurons are in the ventral horn. Sensory fibers (Ia type) enter the spinal cord to synapse with lower motor neurons in the ventral horn. Axons of lower motor neurons leave the cord to innervate the skeletal muscle. A deficit in reflex reaction or an abnormal reflex suggests a lesion of sensory or motor components, such as peripheral nerves, spinal cord, upper motor neurons or their descending tracts, or skeletal muscle. Thus, the reflex test is of diagnostic value if assessed with other neurologic examinations.

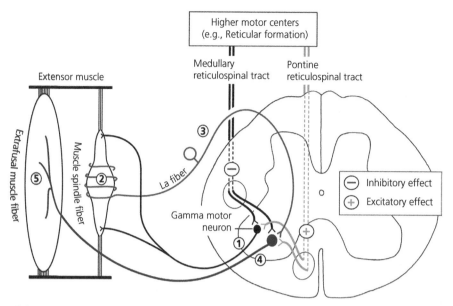

Figure 8.7 Activation of alpha motor neurons via the gamma loop. The intrafusal muscles of the muscle spindle are innervated by primary sensory and gamma motor neurons. This dual innervation allows the higher motor centers to modify sensitivity of the muscle spindle via the gamma motor neurons. (1) The gamma motor neuron is activated by higher motor centers (e.g., via pontine reticulospinal tract). (2) Activation of the gamma motor neuron induces contraction of the intrafusal muscle fibers. (3) Such contraction leads to increase in firing of sensory fiber Ia. (4) Sensory fiber Ia increases firing of the alpha motor neuron. (5) Extrafusal muscle fibers contract in response to discharge of the alpha motor neuron. Excitatory and inhibitory interneurons that interpose between the descending motor tract and motor neurons in the ventral horn are not illustrated.

innervating muscle spindles and the alpha motor neurons in the spinal cord. The CNS utilizes this pathway to modulate the sensitivity of the muscle spindle. Stimulation of gamma motor neurons by descending motor fibers stretches intrafusal muscle fibers and increases firing of Ia sensory fibers innervating the muscle spindle (Figure 8.7). In response to increased activation of Ia sensory fibers, alpha motor neurons in the spinal cord trigger muscle contraction. This neural circuit composed of gamma motor neurons, Ia primary sensory fibers, and alpha motor neurons is referred to as the **gamma loop**. Thus, the CNS modulates stretch reflexes and muscle tone by modulating the gamma loop.

The gamma loop is also critical for keeping the muscle spindle functional even when a skeletal muscle contracts and shortens its length. Muscle spindles are located in the perimysium. They are not only surrounded by extrafusal muscle fibers but also lie parallel to them. Thus, muscle spindles are in an ideal location to monitor changes in the tension and length of extrafusal muscle fibers as they undergo contraction and relaxation. However, if intrafusal muscle fibers remain at the same length during muscle contraction, a slack intrafusal muscle fiber would be useless for detecting the change in muscle length. However, this does not happen. The descending motor fibers innervate both alpha and gamma motor neurons. As the extrafusal muscle fibers contract, the gamma motor neurons also contract the intrafusal muscles, maintaining their proper length (Figure 8.8). Thus, muscle spindles continue to monitor changes in tension and muscle length even as the muscle undergoes contraction and shortening.

Clinical correlations

Local neural circuitries are under the influence of the cerebral cortex and motor centers in the brainstem (e.g., red nucleus, reticular formation). Consequently, a lesion of the spinal cord often induces changes in muscle tone and the myotatic reflex caudal to the lesion. Thus, examining limbs by passive movement encounters increased resistance (i.e., hypertonia) and the myotatic reflex can be exaggerated (i.e., hyperreflexia). These effects are most pronounced in the extensor muscles. The mechanism responsible for spasticity and its associated hypertonia and hyperreflexia is poorly understood. It has been speculated that such a condition reflects increased activation (or release from inhibitory input) of gamma motor neurons, and subsequent increase in activity of type Ia afferents of muscle spindles (Figure 8.7). This leads to excitation of associated alpha motor neurons and their skeletal muscle fibers.

Maintenance of posture and muscle tone

The motor system maintains posture by (i) providing a tonic excitatory bias to motor circuits that excite extensor muscles and (ii) modulating the stretch reflex. The stretch reflex induces contraction of extensor muscles whenever they are stretched by postural changes. Extensor muscles are primarily antigravity muscles, and they are excited by the descending motor tracts in the ventral funiculus of the spinal cord (Figure 8.5B). Any lesion that disrupts the descending motor tracts affects posture and the animal may fall toward the side of the lesion.

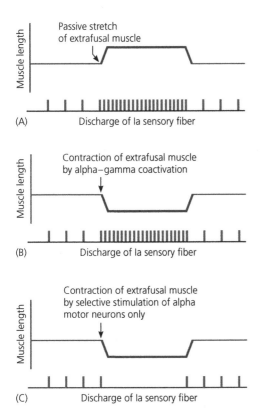

(A) Passive stretch of extrafusal muscle

Muscle length

Discharge of Ia sensory fiber

(A)

(B) Contraction of extrafusal muscle by alpha–gamma coactivation

Muscle length

Discharge of Ia sensory fiber

(B)

(C) Contraction of extrafusal muscle by selective stimulation of alpha motor neurons only

Muscle length

Discharge of Ia sensory fiber

(C)

Figure 8.8 Descending motor fibers innervate both alpha and gamma motor neurons, enabling intrafusal muscle fibers to maintain proper length in response to contraction of extrafusal muscle fibers. (A) Passive stretching of the muscle by tapping its tendon stretches intrafusal muscle fibers and increases firing of Ia sensory fibers. (B) Voluntary contraction of the extrafusal muscle fibers triggers alpha–gamma coactivation. Even though the extrafusal muscle fibers shorten as they contract, simultaneous contraction of the intrafusal muscle fibers adjust their length accordingly, enabling them to detect the change in the extrafusal muscle fibers. (C) Experimental stimulation of alpha motor neurons (i.e., no alpha–gamma coactivation) triggers muscle contraction, but the intrafusal muscle fibers fail to detect the change in the extrafusal muscle lengths.

Why is the **stretch reflex** involved in maintenance of posture and muscle tone? Animals face the pull of gravity, requiring the continuous contraction of skeletal muscles to keep the body upright. When gravitational pull on the body stretches the extensor muscles, their muscle spindles are also stretched, exciting their sensory fibers. Efferents of the muscle spindle stimulate alpha motor neurons in the spinal cord, contracting the extensor muscles. This feedback system keeps each muscle at precisely the right tone. The importance of the stretch reflex in postural maintenance was shown in a study on the stabilizing influence of the ankle joint. In this study, human subjects standing on a movable platform were subjected to induced forward or backward body sway by sliding the platform backward or tilting it upward (Figure 8.9). When posture is destabilized by forward sway in sliding the platform backward, the extensor muscle of the ankle (i.e., gastrocnemius) stretches, triggering a stretch reflex that extends the ankle. The ankle extension stabilizes posture in this

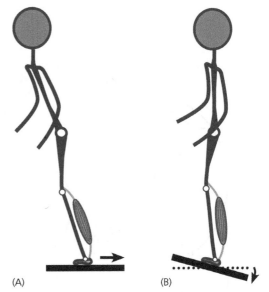

(A)   (B)

Figure 8.9 (A) Unexpected backward sliding of the platform tilts the body forward. Stretch reflex induced by stretching the gastrocnemius muscle maintains balance. This stretch reflex is enhanced and its latency shortened following repeated trials. (B) When ankle rotation is induced directly by tilting the platform, the stretch reflex is suppressed and the ankle does not extend. Adapted from Nashner (1976).

situation. However, when ankle rotation is induced directly by tilting the platform, the stretch reflex is suppressed, and the ankle does not extend. If the direct ankle rotation induces the stretch reflex, posture becomes unstable by extension of the ankle. Thus it appears that the stretch reflex can be enhanced or suppressed depending on whether the reflex serves to stabilize or destabilize posture. Such modulation of the stretch reflex is under the control of the descending tracts from the higher motor centers.

Most spinal reflex arcs involve sensory, motor and additional neurons known as interneuerons. **Interneurons** interpose the sensory and motor neurons. Some interneurons are excitatory and some are inhibitory to their target neurons. Spinal interneurons are located in the gray matter of the spinal cord. The interneurons may cross the midline of the spinal cord to terminate on the contralateral motor neurons. Interneurons give versatility to the reflex arc by connecting the proper afferent and efferent neurons. For example, the animal withdraws the limb subjected to pain, but extends the contralateral limb at the same time (i.e., **crossed extensor reflex**) (Figure 8.10). In this example, sensory input excites neurons in the cord that inhibit the antagonists (extensors) of the flexor muscles of that limb. This organization of neurons is called reciprocal innervation, and occurs in many kinds of reflexes. Maintaining posture (i.e., supporting the body against gravity) requires extension of all four limbs induced by a local spinal reflex and upper motor neurons that modify the activity of alpha and gamma motor neurons. When one limb is flexed, the opposite limb must extend to support the increased weight on that limb. This ipsilateral flexion and contralateral extension reflex helps maintain posture.

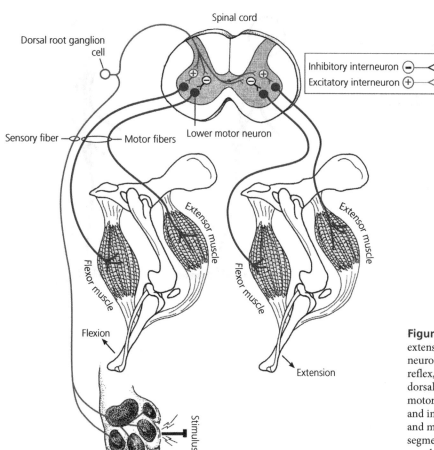

Inhibitory interneuron ⊖—<
Excitatory interneuron ⊕—<

Figure 8.10 The flexor reflex with crossed extensor thrust involves a minimum of three neurons linked in series. Just like the monosynaptic reflex, the cell bodies of sensory neurons are in the dorsal root ganglion and the cell bodies of lower motor neurons are in the ventral horn. Excitatory and inhibitory interneurons interpose the sensory and motor neurons. This illustration shows only the segmental circuit; however, spinal reflexes are mostly intersegmental (i.e., involve several segments of the spinal cord).

Rhythmic motor control

> **1** What are the two phases of the step cycles of locomotion?
>
> **2** What is the role of the central pattern modulator in locomotion?

Walking can be defined as a method of locomotion using the four legs, alternately, to provide both support and propulsion, with at least one foot being in contact with the ground at all times. The gait cycle is used to describe the complex activity of locomotion, from initial placement of the supporting heel on the ground to when the same heel contacts the ground for a second time. Each step cycle of locomotion consists of two phases: (i) the **swing phase**, where the foot is off the ground and swinging forward and (ii) the **stance phase**, where the foot is planted on the ground and the leg is moving backward. The swing phase is mediated by flexor muscles and the stance phase by extensor muscles. A cat walking on a treadmill shows reciprocal bursts of electrical activity from flexors during the swing phase and from extensors during the stance phase of walking.

This rhythmic pattern of walking is dependent on groups of spinal interneurons that act as a **central pattern generator** located in the thoracolumbar spinal cord. The central pattern generator induces rhythmic and repetitive contraction and relaxation of flexor and extensor muscles. Descending motor inputs (e.g., from the cerebral cortex) can act on these spinal circuits to initiate, modify, or terminate locomotor activity. The midbrain is also a site for initiating locomotor activity. For example, electrical stimulation of the locomotor area of the midbrain triggers the stepping action of animals on a treadmill. Speed of stepping is proportional to the intensity of electrical stimulation, and animals walk faster as the intensity of electrical stimuli increases. However, no descending motor tracts are known to originate in the locomotor area of the midbrain. In animals, stimulation of the midbrain locomotor area excites the medullary reticular formation and lesioning of the medullary reticulospinal tract effectively blocks the locomotive effect of the midbrain. Such an observation suggests that the medullary reticular formation mediates locomotor signals from the midbrain to the central pattern generators in the spinal cord.

Sensory feedback plays a key role in generating the rhythmic step cycle of swing and stance phases. When the extending limb (stance phase) reaches a certain point, the sensory receptor signals to the central pattern generator, which then changes from stance phase to swing phase. In the cat, it appears there is at least one central pattern generator for each limb and they are coupled to each other for coordinated rhythmic movement. As mentioned previously, the basic rhythmic pattern of the central pattern generator is independent of the higher motor centers. Thus, a cat with disrupted descending motor tracts has no problem walking on a treadmill with support. However, such a cat has no voluntary motor control of walking and the cat simply follows the speed of the treadmill. Thus, the motor system that directs goal-directed movements works in tandem with the central pattern generator. This unique design allows efficient use of upper motor regulation of locomotion. As the basic rhythmic movements of the four limbs are generated by spinal central pattern generators, there is no need for descending motor signals to control every aspect of muscle activity, but only to modulate the activity of the spinal pattern modulators. This simplifies the regulatory role of higher motor centers on local circuitries pre-programmed for generating a basic rhythmic pattern of locomotion.

Self-evaluation

Answers can be found at the end of the chapter.

1 A lesion involving lower motor neurons results in:
   A Hypermetria
   B Hyperreflexia
   C Muscle atrophy
   D Sensory deficit

2 Motor tracts descending in the ventral funiculus are:
   A Excitatory to lower motor neurons for extensor muscles
   B Excitatory to lower motor neurons for flexor muscles
   C Inhibitory to lower motor neurons for extensor muscles
   D Inhibitory to lower motor neurons for both extensor and flexor muscles

3 Which statement is correct for the muscle spindle.
   A It is made of extrafusal muscles surrounded by connective tissue capsule
   B It is made of extrafusal muscles with no connective tissue capsule
   C It is made of intrafusal muscles surrounded by connective tissue capsule
   D It is made of smooth muscles surrounded by connective tissue capsule

4 The stretch reflex pathway is made of:
   A Sensory neurons only
   B Motor neurons only
   C Sensory and motor neurons
   D Sensory neurons, motor neurons, and interneurons

5 Motor tracts in ventral funiculus controls axial and proximal muscles.
   A True
   B False

6 The flexor reflex is an example of the monosynaptic reflex.
   A True
   B False

7 The pyramid of the medulla oblongata carries descending fibers of the:
   A Corticospinal tract
   B Medullary reticulospinal tract
   C Corticopontine tract
   D All of the above

8 Gamma motor neurons are:
   A Present in the dorsal horn of the spinal cord
   B Much larger than alpha motor neurons
   C Large motor neurons innervating extrafusal muscle fibers
   D Small motor neurons innervating intrafusal muscle fibers

9 The gamma loop is made of:
   A Ia primary sensory fibers and alpha motor neurons
   B Ia primary sensory fibers and extrafusal muscle fibers
   C Gamma motor neurons, Ia primary sensory fibers, and alpha motor neurons
   D Gamma motor neurons and intrafusal muscle fibers

10 Rhythmic pattern of walking relies on the central pattern generator in the:
   A Cerebral motor cortex
   B Basal nuclei
   C Cerebellum
   D Thoracolumbar spinal cord

11 Stance phase of the step cycle represents where the foot is off the ground and swinging forward.
   A True
   B False

12 Axons of the alpha motor neurons of the spinal cord:
   A Are not myelinated
   B Pass through the dorsal root to innervate the smooth muscle
   C Terminate in skeletal muscle fibers as motor end plates
   D Terminate in intrafusal fibers of muscle spindles

13 Passive stretching of the muscle by tapping its tendon stretches intrafusal muscle fibers and decreases firing of Ia sensory fibers.
   A True
   B False

Suggested reading

Dietz, V. (2003) Spinal cord pattern generators for locomotion. *Clinical Neurophysiology* 114:1379–1389.

Drew, T. (1996) Role of the motor cortex in the control of visually triggered gait modification. *Canadian Journal of Physiology and Pharmacology* 74:426–442.

Ijspeert, A.J. (2008) Central pattern generators for locomotion control in animals and robots: a review. *Neural Networks* 2:642–653.

Jankowska, E. and Lundbeg, A. (1981) Interneurons in the spinal cord. *Trends in Neurosciences* 4:230–233.

Leblond, H., Menard, A. and Gossard, J.P. (2001) Corticospinal control of locomotor pathways generating extensor activities in the cat. *Experimental Brain Research* 138:173–184.

Nashner, L.M. (1976) Adapting reflexes controlling the human posture. *Experimental Brain Research* 26:59–72.

Schubert, M., Curt, A., Colombo, G. and Berger, W. (1996) Voluntary control of human gait: conditioning of magnetically evoked motor responses in a precision stepping task. *Experimental Brain Research* 126:583–588.

Answers

1	C	8	D
2	A	9	C
3	C	10	D
4	C	11	B
5	A	12	C
6	B	13	B
7	A		

9 Vestibular System

Etsuro E. Uemura

Iowa State University, Ames, IA, USA

The vestibular system maintains stable eye and body position in response to changes in head position. This system does so by sensing head motion and regulating lower motor neurons innervating the body and extraocular eye muscles. When the head turns to one side, body position is maintained by activating the descending vestibular influence on extensor muscles. The vestibular system also drives the eyes in the opposite direction, so that a stable retinal image can be maintained. However, the vestibular system is not the only system that plays such a role. Proprioceptive and visual information are also important for maintaining equilibrium. Proprioceptors in muscles and joints signal position and movement of body parts, and vision also signals position of the head and body relative to the environment. For example, a reflex known as the righting reflex enables a cat to land right side up when it falls. In this reflex, the first compensatory response of the body involves movement of the head toward its normal position, followed by other reflexive body movements. Excessive or prolonged stimulation of the vestibular system may result in nausea and even vomiting. The neural pathways that trigger such vestibular effects seem to be efferent fibers of the vestibular nuclei that project to visceral centers in the brainstem.

Vestibular organ

1 What is the vestibular organ? Where is it located?

2 Describe the morphology of the vestibular organ and its sensory receptors.

3 What is the difference between the crista ampullaris and maculae in their orientation of sensory hair cells? How do such morphological differences relate to their functions?

4 Explain what is meant by the morphological polarization of sensory cells.

5 What receptors of the vestibular organ are sensitive to head rotation? What is the reason for their sensitivity?

6 What receptors of the vestibular organ are sensitive to linear head motion? What is the reason for their sensitivity?

The vestibular organ is located in the osseous labyrinth of the temporal bone (see Figure 6.1). The vestibular organ is composed of two chambers, the **utricle** (Latin *utriculus*, a small sac) and **saccule** (Latin *saccule*, a small sac), and three ducts, the **semicircular ducts**, that join at the utricle (Figure 9.1). Each semicircular duct also bears an enlargement, the **ampulla**. These chambers and ducts are made of a thin connective tissue sheath covered on both sides with simple squamous epithelium. The vestibular organ contains **endolymph**, which has a high concentration of K^+ and a low concentration of Na^+. Filling the space between the vestibular organ and its bony cavity is fluid called **perilymph**. It is similar to cerebrospinal fluid and has a high Na^+ and low K^+ concentration. Semicircular ducts in each ear are arranged in three orthogonal planes in space.

The vestibular organ in the inner ear houses sensory receptors that detect the spatial orientation of the head. There are two types of vestibular sensory receptors, the macula and the crista ampullaris. The **crista ampullaris** (Latin *crista*, ridge; *ampulla*, a jug) is located in each ampulla of the semicircular ducts and detects angular acceleration and deceleration. The **macula** (Latin *macula*, a spot; this receptor appears as a small spot) is located in the utricle and saccule and responds primarily to linear acceleration or deceleration, and gravity.

Dukes' Physiology of Domestic Animals, Thirteenth Edition. Edited by William O. Reece, Howard H. Erickson, Jesse P. Goff and Etsuro E. Uemura.
© 2015 John Wiley & Sons, Inc. Published 2015 by John Wiley & Sons, Inc.
Companion website: www.wiley.com/go/reece/physiology

The crista ampullaris runs transversely across each ampulla (Figures 9.1 and 9.2A). The sensory receptor cells are separated from one another by supporting cells. The sensory receptor cells are also called **sensory hair cells** because they have hair-like structures, comprising a kinocilium and numerous stereocilia, at the apical surface (Figure 9.2B). Sensory hair cells are arranged in an orderly pattern. The kinocilium attaches to one margin of the apical cell surface and stereocilia occupy the remaining apical surface. Because of this unique arrangement of kinocilium and stereocilia, a sensory hair cell is often substituted by an arrow in illustrations, the head of the arrow pointing to the kinocilium and the tail representing the stereocilia (Figure 9.2C). The stereocilia are also oriented in rows of ascending height, with the tallest stereocilia lying next to the kinocilium. Each stereocilium is connected to its neighbor by a small filament, the tip link (Figure 9.3A). Within each ampulla, the sensory hair cells are supported by the connective tissue crista, which extends across the base of the ampulla. Arising from the crista and completely encapsulating the stereocilia is a gelatinous structure, the cupula. The **cupula** (Latin *cupula*, small inverted cup) attaches to the roof of the ampulla, forming a fluid-tight partition. Angular acceleration induced by rotational head movements causes the endolymph in the semicircular ducts to be displaced. Such displacement of the endolymph pushes the cupula to one side or the other, bending the stereocilia of the sensory hair cells in the same direction. Bending the stereocilia affects the firing rate of the vestibular nerve fibers synapsing with sensory hair cells.

The macula is a sensory receptor located in the utricle and saccule. Structural features of sensory cells of the macula are similar to those of the crista ampullaris (Figure 9.4). The kinocilium and stereocilia project into the statoconial (also known as the otolith) membrane. It is composed of a gelatinous substance similar to the cupula of the crista ampullaris. However, unlike the cupula, statoconial membrane is covered by heavy crystals of calcium carbonate called **statoconia** (or otoconia) (Greek *ous*, ear; *konis*, dust). These crystals are about three times as dense as the surrounding endolymph and they function as an inertial mass within the receptor. The statoconial membrane has a narrow central depression, the **striola**, that bisects the underlying macula.

Orientation of sensory cells

In the crista ampullaris of the lateral semicircular duct, the sensory hair cells are all arranged with their kinocilia on the side of the utricle (Figure 9.5). In contrast, the anterior and posterior semicircular ducts have their hair cells arranged with the kinocilia on the side away from the utricle. Sensory cells of the macula are arranged in an orderly pattern (Figure 9.6). However, their

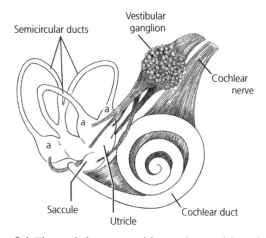

Figure 9.1 The vestibular portion of the membranous labyrinth consists of three semicircular ducts, the utricle and the saccule, each of which houses a vestibular receptor. The vestibular nerve originates from the crista ampullaris in the ampulla (a) and the macula of the saccule and utricle. Attached to the saccule is the cochlear duct that contains the sensory receptor, the organ of Corti, for hearing.

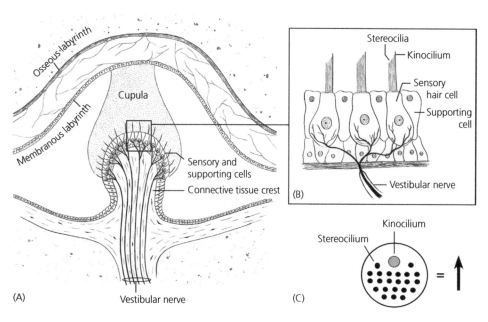

Figure 9.2 (A) Section of the ampulla showing the crista ampullaris. It consists of sensory hair cells, supporting cells, cupula, and connective tissue crest. Stereocilia and kinocilium are embedded in a gelatinous flap, the cupula. (B) Each sensory hair cell has a single long kinocilium and numerous stereocilia at the apical end. (C) Dorsal view of a sensory hair cell. A sensory cell is substituted by an arrow to illustrate the unique morphological arrangement of a kinocilium and stereocilia. The head of the arrow points to the position of the kinocilium, and the tail represents stereocilia.

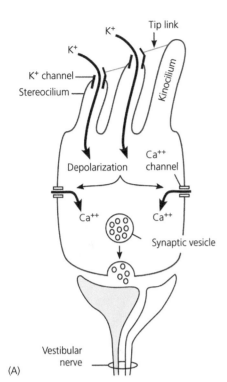

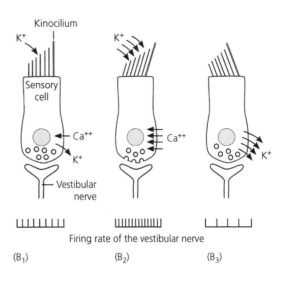

Firing rate of the vestibular nerve

(B_1) (B_2) (B_3)

Figure 9.3 (A) Sensory cells have mechanically gated K^+ channels in the apical portions of the stereocilia. Bending the stereocilia toward the kinocilium results in the opening of these K^+ channels, allowing influx of K^+ into the cell and depolarizing the cell membrane. This opens voltage-gated Ca^{2+} channels at the base of the sensory cells, triggering an influx of Ca^{2+}. Increase in intracellular Ca^{2+} leads synaptic vesicles to release their neurotransmitter into the synaptic clefts. (B_1) Sensory hair cells maintain resting potential when kinocilium and stereocilia are in an upright position. Bending the stereocilia modifies the response of vestibular sensory cells and their afferent fibers as shown in (B_2) and (B_3). (B_2) Bending the stereocilia toward the kinocilium opens K^+ channels of the stereocilia, resulting in influx of K^+ into the cell. Subsequent Ca^{2+} influx leads to release of transmitter from the sensory hair cell and increases the firing rate of the vestibular nerve. (B_3) Bending the stereocilia away from the kinocilium is thought to open K^+ channels in the basolateral portions of the sensory cells. This causes outflow of K^+, hyperpolarization of the cell, and decrease in release of neurotransmitter. As a result, the vestibular nerve decreases its firing rate.

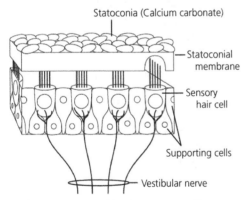

Figure 9.4 The macula resembles the crista ampullaris except that the otolith membrane of the macula contains heavy crystal of calcium carbonate.

stereocilia do not face in a single direction. Sensory cells of the utricle are polarized so that kinocilia are always on the side toward the striola, a curved dividing ridge that runs through the middle of the macula. In contrast, kinocilia of saccular sensory cells are oriented on the side away from the striola. The striola curves

through the macula. As a result sensory cells of the maculae are polarized in many different directions. This arrangement makes utricular and saccular sensory cells directionally sensitive to a wide variety of linear head movements and positions.

Transduction of vestibular stimulus

1 Explain how the morphological polarization of sensory cells relates to receptor potentials of the vestibular sensory cells.

The sensory hair cells maintain resting potential when kinocilia and stereocilia are in an upright position (Figure 9.3B_1). Movements of the stereocilia toward the kinocilium cause the sensory hair cell membrane to depolarize, resulting in an increased firing rate of the vestibular nerve fibers (Figure 9.3B_2). When the stereocilia are deflected away from the kinocilium, the sensory hair cell is hyperpolarized and the firing rate of the vestibular nerve fibers decreases (Figure 9.2B_3). The mechanisms underlying the depolarization and hyperpolarization of the sensory hair cells depend on the K^+-rich endolymph that

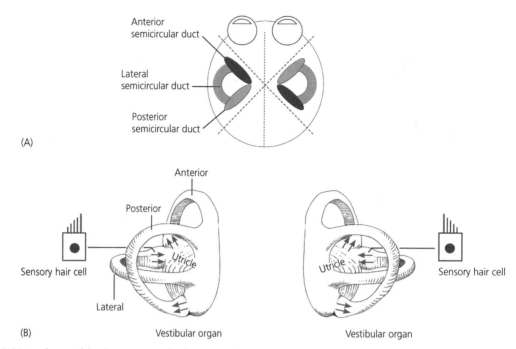

Figure 9.5 (A) Dorsal view of the three semicircular ducts in each inner ear. The lateral semicircular ducts are in a horizontal plane. The anterior and posterior ducts lie in a vertical plane and are approximately at right angles to one another. Furthermore, the anterior semicircular duct of one side is roughly parallel to the posterior semicircular duct on the other side. (B) In the ampulla of the lateral semicircular duct, the sensory hair cells are all arranged with their kinocilia on the side of the utricle. However, in the ampulla of the anterior and posterior semicircular ducts, the hair cells are arranged with the kinocilia on the side away from the utricle. Only two sensory hair cells are illustrated in each ampulla. The unique arrangement of sensory hair cells in each ampulla causes the vestibular nerve to either increase or decrease in firing rate depending on the direction of head rotation.

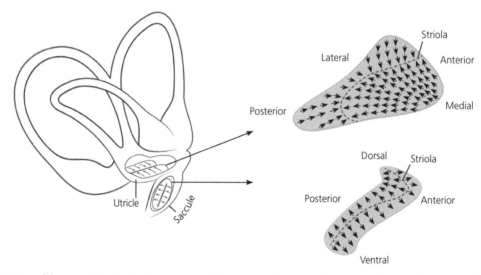

Figure 9.6 Orientation of the macula in the utricle and saccule. When the head is in upright position, the macula in the utricle is oriented horizontally and the macula in the saccule is oriented vertically. Sensory cells of the maculae are arranged in an orderly pattern. All sensory cells in the utricle have kinocilia on the side toward the striola, a curved dividing ridge that runs through the middle of the macula. However, sensory cells in the saccule have kinocilia on the side away from the striola.

bathes the apical portion of sensory hair cells. Deflection of the stereocilia toward the kinocilium causes the tip links to stretch, opening mechanically gated K^+ channels in the apical portions of the stereocilia. This allows K^+ to flow into the cell from the endolymph and depolarizes the cell membrane. This depolarization, in turn, opens voltage-gated calcium channels at the base of the hair cells, allowing Ca^{2+} to enter the cells. The rise in intracellular Ca^{2+} causes synaptic vesicles to release their transmitter into the synaptic clefts. Vestibular nerve fibers respond by undergoing depolarization and increasing their rate of firing.

A rise in intracellular Ca^{2+} also activates Ca^{2+}-activated K^+ channels at the basolateral area of sensory cells. K^+ leaves the sensory cell at the basolateral area due to the low K^+ content of the intercellular space. The outflow of K^+ hyperpolarizes the sensory cells, closing the Ca^{2+} channels. As the cell hyperpolarizes and intracellular Ca^{2+} transients dissipate, the Ca^{2+}-activated K^+ channels partially close, but due to the continued K^+ influx through K^+ channels of stereocilia the membrane depolarizes, initiating another cycle of Ca^{2+} influx through Ca^{2+}-activated channels. This continues as long as deflection of the stereocilia is maintained toward the kinocilium.

When the kinocilium and stereocilia return to their resting position (Figure 9.3B$_1$), Ca^{2+} channels close and Ca^{2+}-activated K^+ channels at the basolateral area of sensory cells close; however, since vestibular nerve fibers fire spontaneously at about 90 spikes per second, it is likely that some Ca^{2+} channels of the sensory hair cells are open at all times, causing a slow constant release of neurotransmitter. Deflection of the stereocilia away from the kinocilium results in hyperpolarization of the sensory cells (Figure 9.3B$_3$). This process may involve the opening of K^+ channels, allowing K^+ to flow out of the sensory cells into the interstitial space. Hyperpolarization decreases the rate at which the neurotransmitter is released by the sensory hair cells. This leads to a decrease in the firing rate of vestibular nerve fibers.

Detection of head movement

1 What is the structural and functional basis for detecting head movement (angular, linear) and head tilt?

Angular acceleration and deceleration

The three semicircular ducts of each vestibular organ detect angular acceleration and deceleration whenever an animal changes its rate of angular motion during turning or tilting of the head and/or body. When the head is still, the endolymph and the cupula remain still and nerve fibers of the crista ampullaris in each ear fire at the same rate (Figure 9.7). When the head rotates, the endolymph in the semicircular duct lags behind the turning motion because of inertia. The inertia of the endolymph places a shear force on the cupula, which bends the kinocilia. If the shear force bends the stereocilia toward the kinocilium, the firing of the vestibular nerve increases. In contrast, bending the stereocilia away from the kinocilium leads to decreased firing of the vestibular nerve. If the rotation is brief, the resting tonic rate is quickly resumed. If the rotation is sustained, the friction of the endolymph on the walls of the membranous labyrinth results in acceleration of endolymph movement until the velocity of the endolymph equals the rotational velocity of the head, resulting in removal of the shear exerted on the cupula. The tonic firing rate is then resumed as if the head were not rotating. When head rotation stops quickly, the endolymph that gained momentum during the initial head rotation does not stop immediately. As a result, the momentum of the endolymph places a shearing force

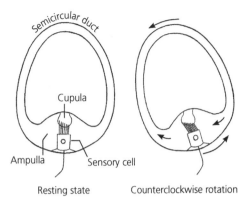

Figure 9.7 Shear force is exerted on the cupula by the endolymph when the head starts rotating. This causes kinocilia and stereocilia to bend in a specific direction depending on the direction of head rotation. For example, counterclockwise rotation of this semicircular duct causes endolymph in the semicircular duct to be displaced, pushing the cupula and stereocilia in the opposite direction.

on the cupula in the opposite direction, bending the stereocilia. Such an excessive vestibular stimulation will induce a sensation of dizziness. As soon as the friction of the walls slows the movement of the endolymph, the cupula returns to its nonrotational position, and the tonic rate of discharge will resume.

The lateral semicircular duct on each side of the head is in a horizontal plane. The anterior semicircular duct on one side lies approximately in the same vertical plane as the posterior duct on the opposite side (Figure 9.5A). Interestingly, the hair cells of the right and left semicircular ducts in a given plane are oppositely polarized. Thus, the sensory hair cells in the lateral semicircular ducts are arranged with their kinocilia on the side of the utricle (Figure 9.5B). In contrast, the sensory hair cells in the anterior and posterior semicircular ducts are arranged with the kinocilia on the side away from the utricle. Because of this unique orientation of the semicircular ducts and their sensory hair cells in each ear, turning the head in any one plane results in different firing responses from sensory hair cells in the complementary right and left semicircular ducts. For example, when the head turns counterclockwise, the endolymph in the lateral semicircular ducts lags behind the turning motion of the head because of inertia. As a result, endolymph in the left ampulla will bend stereocilia of the sensory hair cells in the direction of the kinocilia, exciting vestibular nerve fibers innervating them. In contrast, endolymph in the right ampulla pushes stereocilia away from the kinocilia, hyperpolarizing the vestibular nerve fibers innervating them and reducing their firing rate. Turning the head clockwise induces the opposite response from each lateral semicircular duct, causing the right vestibular nerve to increase its firing rate and the left to decrease its firing rate. Similarly, the anterior semicircular duct on one side and posterior semicircular duct on the other side generate contrasting firing of the vestibular nerve.

The lateral semicircular duct on each side works as a functional pair by responding oppositely to any head movement

(Figure 9.5). The anterior semicircular duct on one side and posterior semicircular duct on the other side do the same. Thus, directional head movement is coded by opposing vestibular signals. Since the vestibular nuclei on each side exchange fibers, they are able to detect head movement by comparing the relative discharge rates of right and left vestibular receptors. Such vestibular information is also processed by the cerebral cortex and cerebellum for further interpretation of head movement.

Head tilt

The maculae detect tilting of the head relative to gravity. They also respond to linear acceleration and deceleration. Side-to-side tilting is referred to as roll, and forward and backward tilting as pitch. At rest, the vestibular nerve fibers of the maculae have a moderate spontaneous firing rate (Figure 9.8). When the head tilts to one side or the other, the force of gravity slightly displaces the heavy statoconial membrane toward the tilted side. This places a shearing force on the kinocilia and stereocilia. If the head tilt is such that the movement of the statoconial membrane forces the stereocilia toward the kinocilia, the result is an increase in the tonic rate of discharge of the vestibular nerve. If the tilt is in the opposite direction, the result is a decrease in the tonic rate of discharge.

Linear acceleration and deceleration

The macula responds maximally to linear motion because of the inertia of the statoconial membrane during linear acceleration or deceleration of the head. If acceleration does not continue (i.e., velocity remains constant), the statoconial membrane returns to its usual position and the firing frequency of the vestibular nerve returns to the resting rate. During deceleration of the head, the heavy statoconia have momentum, exerting a shearing force on the hair cells until the momentum ceases. In linear movement, acceleration or deceleration is necessary to alter activity in the vestibular fibers. The crista ampullaris of the semicircular ducts may also serve partly to detect straight-line

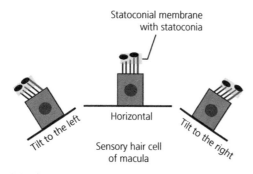

Figure 9.8 The maculae detect tilting of the head relative to gravity. They also respond to linear acceleration and deceleration. At rest, the vestibular nerve fibers of the maculae have a moderate spontaneous firing rate. When the head tilts to one side or the other, the force of gravity displaces the heavy statoconial membrane toward the tilted side. This places a shearing force on the kinocilia and stereocilia. Bending the stereocilia toward the kinocilium increases the firing rate of the vestibular nerve. Bending the stereocilia away from the kinocilium decreases the firing rate of the vestibular nerve.

movements, although to a lesser degree than they respond to angular acceleration. Conversely, the macula of the utricle and saccule are probably stimulated to some degree by rotation of the head.

The utricle and saccule in each inner ear operate as a functional unit. Sensory hair cells of the macula are arranged with kinocilia either facing the striola or on the side away from the striola (Figure 9.6). The striola curves through the macula, making the stereocilia and kinocilia polarized in many different directions. Thus, head tilt in any direction depolarizes some sensory cells and hyperpolarizes others, while causing no effect on some other groups. The orientation of the macula in each ear and the unique arrangement of their sensory hair cells enable the central nervous system (CNS) to detect motion of the head in any direction.

Vestibular nerve and central pathways

> **1** How does the vestibular system control eye movement and maintain equilibrium?
>
> **2** What is nystagmus and abnormal nystagmus?
>
> **3** Explain the vestibulo-ocular reflex.

The **vestibular nerve** innervates the crista ampullaris and the macula of the vestibular organ. Centrally, the vestibular nerve terminates in three areas of the CNS: the flocculonodular lobe, the vermis of the cerebellum, and the vestibular nuclei. The **vestibular nuclei** occupy the lateral ventricular wall of the rostral medulla oblongata (Figure 9.9B). The flocculonodular lobe and vestibular nuclei have a reciprocal connection by way of the caudal cerebellar peduncle (Figure 9.9A). The vestibular nerve on each side fires all the time in response to spontaneous firing of sensory cells. Firing frequency of the vestibular nerve is modulated by sensory hair cells, while firing of the vestibular nuclei is under the influence of the vestibular nerve, cerebellum, and proprioceptors. When the head is motionless, the firing pattern of the vestibular system on each side is balanced. When the head moves, the eyes move to maintain the field of view and the body adjusts to maintain posture. Such adjustments reflect changes in the firing pattern of the right and left vestibular receptors. When the head moves, signals to the vestibular nuclei on each side are no longer equal, as the vestibular nuclei receiving increased firing frequency dominate over the vestibular nuclei on the other side. This relative difference in firing of vestibular nuclei is the basis for triggering such reflexes as the vestibulospinal or vestibulo-ocular reflexes.

The vestibular nuclei have a reciprocal connection with the cerebellum (Figure 9.9A). Cerebellar Purkinje cells of the flocculonodular lobe are inhibitory to the vestibular nuclei. Inhibitory efferents reach the vestibular nuclei by way of the caudal cerebellar peduncle. Therefore, a unilateral lesion of the flocculonodular lobe or the caudal cerebellar peduncle frees the vestibular nuclei on the side of the lesion from cerebellar inhibition. As a result, the lesioned side fails to counter the vestibular

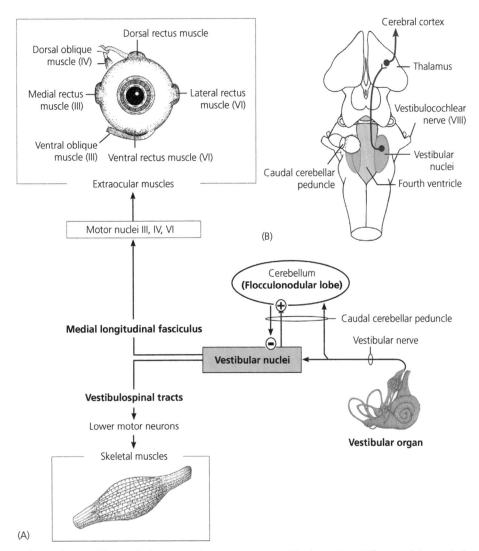

Figure 9.9 (A) The reflex pathways of the vestibular system that maintain eye and body position. Efferents of the vestibular organ reach the flocculonodular lobe, vermis (not shown), and vestibular nuclei. Vestibular efferents are excitatory (+) to the cerebellum. Flocculonodular efferents are inhibitory (–) to the vestibular nuclei. Efferents of the cerebellum and vestibular organ are integrated by the vestibular nuclei, which then regulates eye and body position. (B) Dorsal view of dissected brainstem showing the vestibulocochlear nerve (VIII) and vestibular nuclei of the medulla oblongata. The ascending pathway from the vestibular nuclei to the cerebral cortex via the thalamus comprises the vestibulo-thalamo-cortical pathway. This pathway is most likely for conscious perception of head and body orientation.

nuclei on the other side, triggering abnormal vestibular reflexes of the eyes and the body. The vestibular nuclei also work with the reticular formation. This enables the vestibular system to coordinate activities of muscles innervated by different segments of the spinal cord.

The vestibular nuclei give rise to (i) the descending vestibulospinal tracts that control lower motor neurons innervating the skeletal muscle of the trunk and extremities (Figure 9.9A), (ii) the ascending tract, the middle longitudinal fasciculus, that innervates the motor nuclei for the extraocular muscles (Figure 9.9A), and (iii) the vestibulo-thalamo-cortical tract (in cats) to the postcruciate and anterior suprasylvian gyri of the cerebral cortex (Figure 9.9B). The functional significance of vestibular projection to the cerebral cortex is unclear. It has been suggested that it plays a role in integration of vestibular and proprioceptive somatosensory signals important for motor performance. Electrophysiological studies in animals have demonstrated that many neurons in vestibular cortical areas respond to proprioceptive, visual and vestibular stimuli. These neurons are activated by moving visual stimuli as well as by rotation of the body (even with the eyes closed), suggesting that these cortical areas are involved in the perception of body orientation.

Vestibulospinal reflex

The vestibular control of skeletal muscles of the trunk and extremities is mediated by the descending **vestibulospinal tracts** (Figure 9.9A). These tracts descend in the ventral funiculus of the spinal cord and modulate the alpha and gamma motor neurons via spinal interneurons. They maintain balance of the body by facilitating lower motor neurons for extensor muscles and inhibiting lower motor neurons for flexor muscles. Although the vestibulospinal tracts do not mediate voluntary movements directed by the cerebral cortex, they are essential for highly skilled motor coordination.

Vestibulo-ocular pathway

The vestibular control of the extraocular muscles is mediated by the ascending medial longitudinal fasciculus. This tract originates in the vestibular nuclei and ascends in the brainstem to terminate in the motor nuclei of the oculomotor, trochlear, and abducent nerves. This vestibular regulation of the extraocular muscles enables an animal to keep its eyes on a target, by moving them in the opposite direction of head movement (Figures 9.9A and 9.10). This **vestibulo-ocular reflex** maintains a steady gaze while the head is moving. Such compensatory eye movement occurs for any direction of head movement, whether linear, rotational, or a combination of both. The vestibulo-ocular reflex can be inhibited voluntarily when an animal intends to focus on a moving object while turning the head in the same direction. Eye movements induced by the vestibular system are characterized by horizontal, vertical, and torsional movements. Horizontal eye movements are induced by the horizontal semicircular duct and utricle, while vertical eye movements are controlled by the vertical (i.e., anterior and posterior) semicircular ducts and the saccule. Torsional eye movements are induced by the vertical semicircular ducts and the utricle.

Clinical correlations

A lesion of the vestibular system is associated with head tilt, circling, and falling to the side of the lesion. This is caused by the lack of vestibular control on the vestibulospinal tracts that exert excitatory influence on ipsilateral extensor muscles. When injury to the brainstem involves the medial longitudinal fasciculus, there is no vestibulo-ocular reflex (i.e., no reflexive eye movement in response to head movement). A lesion involving the medial longitudinal fasciculus is suspected if there is an obvious deficiency in eye movement when the head is moved around. Blindness can be suspected when the eyes do not follow the examiner's finger, but the vestibulo-ocular reflex is present. Blindness due to lesions of the optic nerve can be tested by observing absence of the pupillary reflex to light. Lesions such as meningioma in the area of the orbital fissure may also induce loss of both voluntary eye movement (e.g., eyes fail to follow moving object) and vestibulo-ocular reflex (e.g., eyes fail to compensate when the head changes position). This is because the cranial nerves that innervate the extraocular muscles (oculomotor, trochlear and abducent) run through the orbital fissure.

Nystagmus

1 What is physiological nystagmus and how is it different from abnormal nystagmus?
2 Explain the anatomical basis of vestibular signs.

When the head moves slowly in any plane, the eyes maintain their gaze by turning slowly in a direction opposite to the head rotation. However, as the eyes reach the limit of rotation in the orbit, they move quickly in the direction of head rotation to return the eyes to a central position. The slow movement of the eyes maintains gaze as long as possible, while the quick movement serves to bring the eyes to a new visual field. If the head continues to rotate slowly, the slow phase reappears, followed by the quick phase. This combination of involuntary slow and quick movements of the eye is called **nystagmus**. The **direction of the nystagmus** is the direction of the **quick phase** (i.e., nystagmus to the right indicates that the quick eye movement is to the right).

Slow phase of nystagmus

The vestibulo-ocular reflex maintains a stable gaze. When the head is motionless, the eyes are motionless. This is because the right and left vestibular systems are in balance. The vestibular nerve on each side fires spontaneously at all times. This tonic discharge is modified by changes in head position, which triggers depolarization or hyperpolarization of sensory hair cells of the vestibular receptors. The reflexive eye movement reflects such change in firing patterns of the right and left vestibular organs.

When the head rotates in the horizontal plane, the endolymph displaces the cupula on one side, bending the stereocilia and kinocilia in one direction, while the cupula on the other side bends the stereocilia and kinocilia in the opposite direction (Figure 9.10A). The vestibular nuclei mediates vestibular signals to the ipsilateral motor nucleus of the oculomotor nerve and the contralateral motor nucleus of the abducent nerve, which also projects to the contralateral motor nucleus of the oculomotor nerve via the medial longitudinal fasciculus. Thus, the vestibular nuclei turn the eyes, via the oculomotor and abducent nuclei, slowly to the right or left depending on the direction of head rotation. For example, when the head turns counterclockwise (Figure 9.10A), the sensory receptor of the left lateral semicircular duct stimulates the left vestibular nuclei, whereas the sensory receptor of the right semicircular duct suppresses the right vestibular nuclei. The left vestibular nuclei trigger slow movement of the eye in the direction opposite to head rotation. This action is mediated by the right motor nucleus of the abducent nerve that innervates the lateral rectus muscle of the right eye and the left motor nucleus of the oculomotor nerve that innervates the medial rectus muscle of the left eye. During slow rightward eye movement, the leftward eye movement is prevented by inhibitory vestibular interneurons.

Quick phase of nystagmus

When the head starts to rotate counterclockwise (Figure 9.10A), the vestibular receptor stimulates the left vestibular nerve, increasing its firing rate. This leads to progressive excitation of the contralateral **excitatory burst neurons** in the parabducent nucleus of the reticular formation (Figure 9.10B). The excitatory

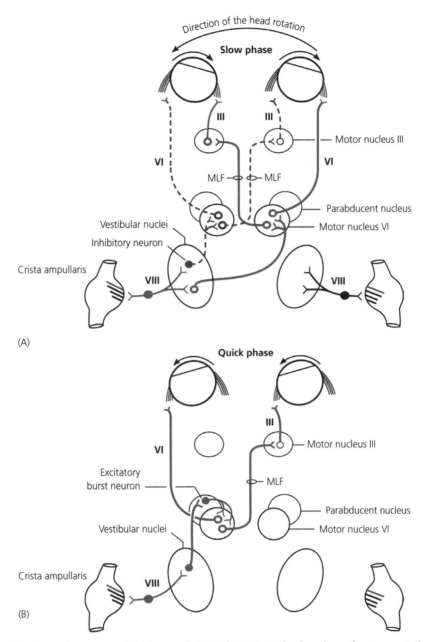

Figure 9.10 Slow and quick phases of nystagmus. (A) The neural circuit that initiates the slow phase of nystagmus. When the head turns counterclockwise, the left vestibular nerve is more excited than the right vestibular nerve. The left vestibular nuclei trigger the slow movement of the eye in the direction opposite to head rotation by stimulating the ipsilateral motor nucleus of the oculomotor nerve and contralateral motor nucleus of the abducent nerve. Leftward eye movement is inhibited by inhibitory vestibular interneurons to the left motor nucleus of the abducent nerve and the right motor nucleus of the oculomotor nerve. MLF, medial longitudinal fasciculus. (B) The neural circuit that initiates the quick phase of nystagmus. The quick phase of nystagmus triggered by the excitatory burst cells (shown in the left parabducent nucleus). The excitatory burst cells control the ipsilateral motor nucleus of the abducent nerve and the contralateral motor nucleus of the oculomotor nerve. The excitatory burst neurons require progressive vestibular stimulation before they reach firing threshold, thereby allowing time for completion of the slow phase.

burst neurons require progressive vestibular stimulation before they reach firing threshold potential. This delay before responding to vestibular efferents provides ample time for completion of the slow phase. On reaching the threshold potential, excitatory burst neurons discharge briefly and bring the left lateral and right medial recti into action by stimulating the ipsilateral motor nucleus of the abducent nerve and the contralateral motor nucleus of the oculomotor nerve. At the same time, inhibitory burst neurons in the parabducent reticular formation relax the opposite set of extraocular muscles by inhibiting contralateral excitatory burst neurons as well as the motor nucleus of the abducent nerve.

Clinical correlations

Abnormal nystagmus may appear when a lesion involves the vestibular organ, vestibular nerve, or vestibular nuclei. For example, a lesion of the right vestibular organ interferes with spontaneous firing of the right vestibular nuclei, resulting in loss of right vestibular control of the extraocular muscles. As a result, the normal left vestibular system dominates control of the extraocular muscles, triggering nystagmus even if the head is in a still position. Tonic signals from the right and left vestibular system are also the basis of the vestibulospinal reflex that maintains posture. Thus, a lesion of the vestibular receptor, vestibular nerve, or vestibular nuclei on one side removes excitation from the ipsilateral vestibulospinal tracts. The unopposed contralateral vestibulospinal tracts force the entire body to tip or fall toward the lesioned side. Such an animal may also display circular walking in the direction of the lesioned side.

Self-evaluation

Answers can be found at the end of the chapter.

1 Bending the stereocilia toward the kinocilium results in opening of:
   A Mechanically gated K⁺ channels in the stereocilia
   B Mechanically gated Na⁺ channels in the kinocilium
   C Ligand-gated K⁺ channels in the kinocilium
   D Ligand-gated Na⁺ channels in the stereocilia

2 The receptor that detects angular acceleration and deceleration of the head is the:
   A Organ of Corti
   B Macula in the saccule
   C Crista ampullaris
   D Macula in the utricle

3 The vestibular nuclei have a reciprocal connection with the flocculonodular lobe of the cerebellum.
   A True
   B False

4 Which statement is true?
   A The semicircular ducts are filled with endolymph
   B Each sensory hair cell has one kinocilium and numerous stereocilia at the basal cell surface
   C The cupula of the crista ampullaris is associated with statoconia (i.e., calcium carbonate)
   D The crista ampullaris is present in the utricle and saccule

5 The vestibulo-ocular reflex plays a role in keeping the gaze steady while the head is moving.
   A True
   B False

6 The cranial nerves innervated by the medial longitudinal fasciculus of the vestibular system are the:
   A II, III, and IV
   B III, IV, and V
   C IV, VI, and VII
   D III, IV, and VI
   E III, V, and VI

7 The vestibulospinal tracts facilitate lower motor neurons innervating:
   A Flexor muscles
   B Extensor muscles
   C Both extensor and flexor muscles

8 Nystagmus to the right means:
   A The quick phase of nystagmus is to the left
   B The quick phase of nystagmus is to the right
   C The slow phase of nystagmus is to the left
   D The slow phase of nystagmus is to the right

9 When the head continues to rotate clockwise, the direction of the nystagmus is to the:
   A Right
   B Left

10 An animal with a lesion of the right vestibular nerve is likely to fall or circulate to the:
   A Right
   B Left

11 The vestibulo-ocular reflex requires the medial longitudinal fasciculus.
   A True
   B False

Suggested reading

Carleton, S.C. and Carpenter, M.B. (1984) Distribution of primary vestibular fibers in the brainstem and cerebellum of the monkey. *Brain Research* 294:281–298.

De Lahunta, A. and Glass, E. (2009) *Veterinary Neuroanatomy and Clinical Neurology*, 3rd edn. Saunders Elsevier, St Louis, MO.

Dieterich, M. and Brandt, T. (1995) Vestibulo-ocular reflex. *Current Opinion in Neurology* 8:83–88.

Flock, A. and Goldstein, M.H. Jr (1978) Cupular movement and nerve impulse response in the isolated semicircular canal. *Brain Research* 157:11–19.

Ogawa, Y., Kushiro, K., Zakir, M., Sata, H. and Uchino, Y. (2000) Neuronal organization of the utricular macula concerned with innervation of single vestibular neurons in the cat. *Neuroscience Letters* 278:89–92.

Parker, D.E. (1980) The vestibular apparatus. *Scientific American* 243:118–135.

Schunk, K.L. (1988) Disorders of the vestibular system. *Veterinary Clinics of North America: Small Animal Practice* 18:641–665.

Wilson, V.J., Wylis, R.M. and Marco, L.A. (1967) Projection to the spinal cord from the medial and descending vestibular nuclei of the cat. *Nature* 215:429–430.

Answers

1 A		7 B	
2 C		8 B	
3 A		9 A	
4 A		10 A	
5 A		11 A	
6 D			

10 Autonomic Nervous System

Etsuro E. Uemura
Iowa State University, Ames, IA, USA

The autonomic nervous system (ANS) is designed to maintain homeostasis by controlling visceral organs and glandular secretions. The ANS regulates such functions as heart rate, digestion, respiratory rate, salivation, perspiration, pupillary dilation, micturition (urination), and sexual arousal. The ANS has two divisions, the sympathetic and parasympathetic. In general, these two systems work together, usually in antagonistic fashion, to maintain homeostasis of the body system. Most viscera receive a dual sympathetic and parasympathetic innervation, but some are innervated solely by the sympathetic division (e.g., sweat gland, vascular smooth muscle of skeletal muscle, skin, and arrector pili) or parasympathetic division (e.g., pupillary sphincter muscle, ciliary muscle). Unlike the somatic motor system that controls skeletal muscles, autonomic motor control must have slower and longer-lasting effects. Furthermore, certain viscera, such as the gastrointestinal tract and heart, are equipped with an intrinsic neural system that enables rhythmic movements. The role of the ANS in these organs is to modulate the intrinsic neural system. The ANS is under the control of the hypothalamus, which acts as an integrator for autonomic functions. Most autonomous functions are involuntary, but certain actions can work alongside some degree of conscious control. Hypothalamic control is mediated by the reticular formation, which comprises the central core of the brainstem, extending from the medulla oblongata to the midbrain. The reticular efferents reach the sympathetic and parasympathetic nuclei of the brainstem and spinal cord. The hypothalamus also controls the release of hormones from the hypophysis. Such neuronal and humoral influences are the basis for hypothalamic regulation of, for example, heart rate, respiration, blood pressure, body temperature, conjugate eye movement, locomotion, swallowing, vomiting, micturition and defecation, water balance, food intake, circadian rhythms, and emotion. The cerebral cortex has some influence on the ANS. For example, the sight of food triggers secretion of saliva and anticipation of a walk increases the heart rate of a dog.

Organization of the autonomic nervous system

1 What are the anatomical and functional differences between the central, peripheral, and autonomic nervous systems?

2 What are preganglionic and postganglionic neurons of the autonomic nervous system?

3 Where in the central nervous system (CNS) are the perikarya of sympathetic or parasympathetic preganglionic neurons located?

4 Explain the differences in location of the solely sympathetic and parasympathetic ganglia.

5 What tissues or organs are innervated sorely by the sympathetic division or parasympathetic division?

6 What are the differences between motor end plates of the neuromuscular synapse and axon varicosities of the autonomic fibers?

Neural influences are delivered to target tissues by the sympathetic and parasympathetic divisions (Figure 10.1). In dogs, the sympathetic fibers originate from the thoracic (T1–T13) and lumbar (L1–L3) spinal cord, whereas the parasympathetic fibers originate from the brainstem and sacral cord segments (S2–S3 in dogs) (Figure 10.2). The two systems generally complement each other. The sympathetic system functions in

Dukes' Physiology of Domestic Animals, Thirteenth Edition. Edited by William O. Reece, Howard H. Erickson, Jesse P. Goff and Etsuro E. Uemura.
© 2015 John Wiley & Sons, Inc. Published 2015 by John Wiley & Sons, Inc.
Companion website: www.wiley.com/go/reece/physiology

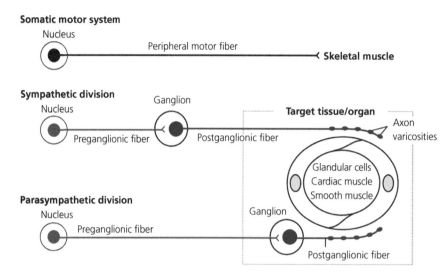

Figure 10.1 Organization of the autonomic nervous system. The sympathetic and parasympathetic divisions innervate visceral organ and glands. However, some tissues receive only sympathetic or parasympathetic innervation. Both divisions of the autonomic nervous system require a chain of two neurons between the nucleus of origin in the CNS and the peripheral targets.

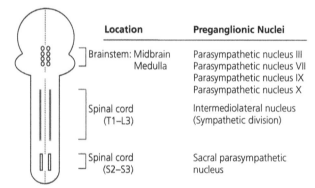

Figure 10.2 In both the sympathetic and parasympathetic systems, cell bodies of the preganglionic neurons are located in the CNS. Cell bodies of the sympathetic preganglionic neurons form the intermediolateral nucleus of spinal cord segments T1–L3. Cell bodies of the parasympathetic preganglionic neurons are located at two sites: the brainstem and sacral spinal cord segments S2 and S3 in dogs.

such a manner as to strengthen the body's defense against adverse conditions by expenditure of energy. The parasympathetic division, on the other hand, conserves and restores energy. A unique feature of the ANS is that both divisions require a two-neuron chain between the nucleus of origin in the CNS and the peripheral target organ. Synapse between the two neurons occurs outside the CNS, in ganglia. Using the ganglion as a point of reference, a presynaptic axon (i.e., axon from a neuronal cell body in the CNS) is called a **preganglionic fiber**. A postganglionic axon (i.e., axons from a neuronal cell body in the ganglion) is called a postganglionic fiber. The **postganglionic fibers** carry impulses to target tissues and organs. In both the sympathetic and parasympathetic divisions, preganglionic fibers are myelinated and postganglionic fibers are nonmyelinated.

Most visceral organs are innervated by both sympathetic and parasympathetic nerves. They have opposing actions, with the

sympathetic division preparing the body for emergency situations and the parasympathetic division conserving and restoring the energy sources of the body. Accordingly, the sympathetic system is often considered the "**fight or flight**" system, while the parasympathetic is the "**rest and digest**" system. However, their action is better viewed as complementary in nature rather than antagonistic. For example, the sympathetic and parasympathetic divisions continuously modulate the heart rate, in response to respiratory cycles.

Some tissues and organs are controlled primarily by one division (Table 10.1). Tissues innervated only by **parasympathetic fibers** include the sphincter muscle of the iris, ciliary muscle, and nasopharyngeal glands. Tissues innervated only by **sympathetic fibers** include the sweat glands (apocrine, merocrine), adrenal medulla, blood vessels, arrector pili, pancreatic islets, pineal gland, and pupillary dilator muscles. **Apocrine sweat glands** are supplied with adrenergic sympathetic postganglionic fibers. They secrete a viscous fluid that may contain pheromones. In contrast, the **merocrine** (or eccrine) sweat glands are innervated by sympathetic cholinergic postganglionic fibers. Merocrine glands are present in the skin of footpads. The **adrenal medulla** is innervated by sympathetic preganglionic fibers that synapse with chromaffin cells, the vestigial postganglionic neurons of the adrenal medulla. The majority of chromaffin cells release epinephrine and some norepinephrine. Most **blood vessels** are not innervated by the parasympathetic division, but are in a state of partial contraction maintained by sympathetic tone. Thus, blood vessels can be dilated or constricted by decreasing or increasing sympathetic stimulation, respectively. Without a compensatory increase in the sympathetic tone to arterioles, rising from a sitting position leads to a drop in blood pressure and fainting.

Tissues and organs respond differently to sympathetic and parasympathetic stimulation. For example, sympathetic stimulation during the fight or flight response induces vasoconstriction

Table 10.1 Innervation of tissues and organs by the autonomic nervous system.

Target organ and tissue	Sympathetic division	Receptor type	Parasympathetic division
Skin			
Apocrine sweat glands	Increase in secretion	β_2	—
Merocrine sweat glands	Increase in secretion	M_3	—
Arrector pili	Erection	α_1	—
Eye			
Iris: dilator muscle	Pupillary dilation	α_1	—
Sphincter muscle	—	—	Pupillary constriction
Ciliary muscle	—	—	Contraction (near vision)
Lung			
Bronchiolar muscle	Relaxation	β_2	Contraction
Heart			
SA node	Increase in heart rate	β_1	Decrease in heart rate
AV node and Purkinje fibers	Increase in conduction velocity	β_1	Decrease in conduction velocity
Atria, ventricle	Increase in contractility	β_1	Decrease in contractility
Arterioles			
Skin and mucosa	Constriction	α	—
Salivary glands	Constriction	α	—
Cerebral	Slight constriction	α	—
Skeletal muscle	Dilation	β_2	—
Coronary	Dilation	β_2	Slight dilation
Pulmonary	Dilation	β_2	—
Abdominal viscera	Constriction	α	—
Veins (systemic)	Constriction, Dilation	α, β_2	—
Gastrointestinal system			
Stomach, intestinal tract	Decrease in motility*	α_2, β_2	Increase in motility
Sphincters	Contraction	α_1	Relaxation
Gastric gland	Decrease in secretion	α_2	Increase in secretion
Gallbladder	Relaxation	β_2	Contraction
Liver	Glycogenolysis, gluconeogenesis	α_1, β_2	Glycogen synthesis
Pancreas			
Acini	Decrease in secretion	α	Increased secretion
Islets	Decrease in secretion	α_2	—
Adrenal medulla	Secretion of E and NE	N	—
Kidney	Renin secretion	β_2	—
Urinary bladder			
Detrusor muscle	Relaxation	β_3	Contraction
Trigone and sphincter	Contraction	α_1	Relaxation
Reproductive organs			
Penis	Ejaculation	α_1	Erection
Uterus (pregnant)	Contraction	α_1	Variable
Uterus (nonpregnant)	Relaxation	β_2	Variable
Glands			
Lacrimal	Slight secretion	α	Increase in secretion
Salivary	Slight viscous secretion	α	Increase in watery secretion
Nasopharyngeal	—	—	Secretion
Pineal	Melatonin synthesis	β	—

*Adrenergic fibers may synapse on (1) inhibitory α receptors on parasympathetic postganglionic cells of the myenteric plexus and (2) inhibitory β receptors on smooth muscle fibers.
E, epinephrine; NE, norepinephrine; N, nicotinic acetylcholine receptor.

that leads to increased blood pressure, increased heart rate, increased airflow through the lungs, and epinephrine release from the adrenal gland; however, vasodilation occurs in the heart, lungs, and skeletal muscles to supply needed oxygen. Parasympathetic effects are suppressed during the fight or flight response. As discussed in later sections of this chapter, these paradoxical sympathetic and parasympathetic effects reflect different types of adrenergic receptors (α-adrenergic, β-adrenergic) and cholinergic receptors (nicotinic, muscarinic) present in effector tissue and organs (Table 10.1).

Sympathetic division

1 What is the fight or flight response? What response would be expected in the various organs of the body?

2 Describe the sympathetic innervation of the head.

3 Describe the sympathetic innervation of smooth muscle and glands of the body.

4 Describe the sympathetic innervation of the thoracic, abdominal, and pelvic viscera.

5 What is the sympathetic effect on pupil diameter?

6 What is the sympathetic effect on vasculature of the skeletal muscle and skin?

7 What is Horner's syndrome? What causes this syndrome?

8 Where in the adrenal gland are postganglionic cells located?

Innervation of the head and neck

Sympathetic innervation of the head and neck is mediated by the **cranial cervical ganglia** (Figure 10.3). Preganglionic fibers from spinal cord segments T1–T5 (some fibers may even come from T6 and T7) join the vagosympathetic trunk to reach the cranial cervical ganglion. The postganlionic fibers leaving the cranial cervical ganglion continue as plexuses along the arteries of the head and neck regions. Postganglionic fibers from the cranial cervical ganglion innervate salivary glands, nasal glands, and smooth muscles (arrector pili, blood vessels, periorbit, eyelids, pupillary dilator) (Table 10.1). Postganglionic fibers from the cranial cervical ganglion also reach the carotid body, carotid sinus, and thyroid gland. Postganglionic fibers may also join the cranial laryngeal branches and pharyngeal branch of the vagus nerve.

Clinical correlations

A lesion affecting the sympathetic supply to the head is likely to induce the following clinical signs of **Horner's syndrome** on the affected side: miosis (i.e., small pupillary size), ptosis (i.e., drooping of the eyelid), enophthalmos (i.e., slight retraction of the eyeball), and partial prolapse of the third eyelid. **Miosis** results from loss of sympathetic control of the pupillary dilator muscle. **Ptosis** is caused by loss of tone in the smooth muscle of the eyelid. Ptosis leads to slight retraction of the eyeball (i.e., enophthalmos) and a partially protruded third eyelid. **Enophthalmos** reflects loss of tone in the periorbital smooth muscle that normally pulls the eyeball rostrally. The periorbital smooth muscle also attaches to the base of the third eyelid, maintaining its normal retracted position. Thus, partial **prolapse** results from loss of retraction of the third eyelid. In addition, slight retraction of the eye into the orbit (i.e., enophthalmos) displaces the third eyelid cartilage, also contributing to the partial protrusion of the third eyelid. This reflects the fact that the dog has no specific muscle that sweeps the third eyelid across the cornea, and the displacement of the third eyelid is passive. In addition to these clinical signs, a dog may display pink-colored and warmer skin (best seen in the ear) due to vasodilation. Horner's syndrome may be present when the animal suffers from (i) a middle ear infection, as sympathetic postganglionic fibers pass through the middle ear in proximity to the petrosal bone; (ii) severe avulsion of the brachial plexus (C7–T2) that damages the sympathetic preganglionic fibers to the cranial cervical ganglion; or (iii) spinal cord lesions that disrupt the reticulospinal tract from the medullary reticular formation that regulates the visceral motor neurons of the spinal cord.

Innervation of smooth muscles and glands of the body

The cranial cervical ganglion innervates blood vessels, arrector pili, and the lateral nasal gland in the head region (Figure 10.3). The sympathetic trunk ganglia caudal to T4 innervate the rest of the body wall and extremities (Figure 10.4). Postganglionic fibers join the spinal nerves by way of the rami communicantes to innervate blood vessels, sweat glands, and arrector pili. These structures do not receive parasympathetic innervation, so they are an exception to the dual innervation. Increased activity of the sympathetic system results in the contraction of arteriolar smooth muscles. This leads to an increase in peripheral vascular resistance and subsequent increase in blood pressure (Table 10.1). In contrast, decreased activity of the sympathetic system decreases vascular resistance due to relaxation of the arteriolar smooth muscle. Thus, decrease in sympathetic activity lowers blood pressure.

Innervation of the thoracic viscera

The thoracic viscera are primarily innervated by the cervicothoracic and middle cervical ganglia (Figure 10.3). The ansa subclavia may also contribute some fibers. Preganglionic fibers originate from spinal cord segments T1–T4. They reach postganglionic neurons in the **cervicothoracic ganglion** by way of the rami communicantes. Preganglionic fibers also ascend to the **ansa subclavia** and **middle cervical ganglion** where they synapse with postganglionic neurons. These fibers innervate the vasculature and smooth muscle of the respiratory airways and the lung. The sympathetic stellate cardiac nerve mediates relaxation of the smooth muscle of the respiratory airways and blood vessels, whereas the vagus nerve contracts the smooth muscle. Stimulation of the sympathetic fibers results in an increase in heart rate by increasing pacemaker activity of the sinoatrial (SA) node cells, impulse conduction at the atrioventricular (AV) node, and the contractile force of atrial and ventricular muscle fibers (Table 10.1).

Innervation of the abdominal and pelvic viscera

The abdominal and pelvic viscera are innervated by spinal cord segments T5–L3. To reach the celiac ganglion in the abdominal cavity, preganglionic fibers from the thoracic spinal segments caudal to T5 descend in the sympathetic trunk and emerge as the **greater thoracic splanchnic nerve** at the level of the T13 sympathetic trunk ganglion (Figure 10.5). From the celiac ganglion, postganglionic fibers accompany the arteries to the stomach, duodenum, pancreas, liver, gallbladder, spleen, and adrenal glands. Motility of the gastrointestinal tract is enhanced by parasympathetic fibers of the vagus nerve. However, how the sympathetic division controls the **gastrointestinal tract** is not clear. It has been speculated that adrenergic fibers synapse on inhibitory α-adrenergic receptors on parasympathetic

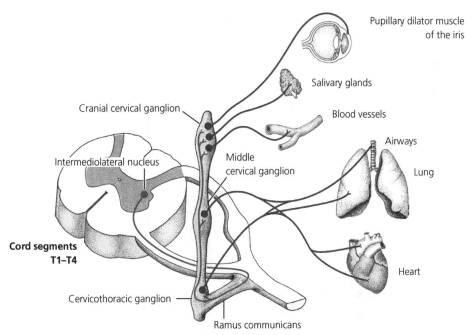

Figure 10.3 Sympathetic innervation of the head is mediated by the cranial cervical ganglion. Postganglionic fibers innervate the dilator muscle of the iris, salivary glands, and blood vessels. The thoracic viscera are innervated by postganglionic fibers from the cervicothoracic and middle cervical ganglia. The ansa subclavia (not shown) also contributes postganglionic fibers to the thoracic viscera.

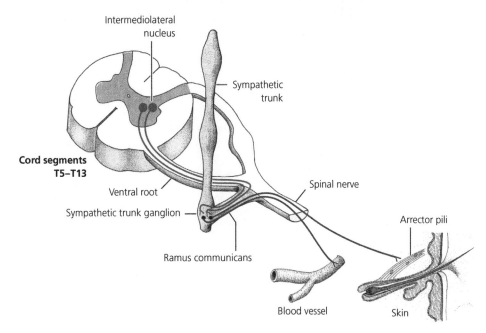

Figure 10.4 The sympathetic trunk ganglia at cord segments T5–T13 give rise to postganglionic fibers that innervate smooth muscles of the body except the head and neck.

postganglionic cells of the myenteric plexus and inhibitory β-adrenergic receptors on smooth muscle fibers. Thus, peristaltic action can be decreased by the sympathetic system.

The **adrenal medulla** receives sympathetic preganglionic fibers from cord segments T4 (or T5) to L1 (or L2). The adrenal medulla is composed of chromaffin cells, which are vestigial postganglionic neurons. Chromaffin cells secrete catecholamines (mostly epinephrine and some norepinephrine) into the

bloodstream in response to signals from sympathetic preganglionic neurons. Therefore, the sympathetic system regulates functions of endocrine cells in the adrenal gland. Preganglionic fibers from spinal segments L1–L3 reach the abdominal and pelvic ganglia via the sympathetic trunk (Figure 10.5). They either leave the sympathetic trunk ganglia at the level they enter or descend in the sympathetic trunk before exiting. Each sympathetic trunk ganglion of the lumbar segments gives rise to

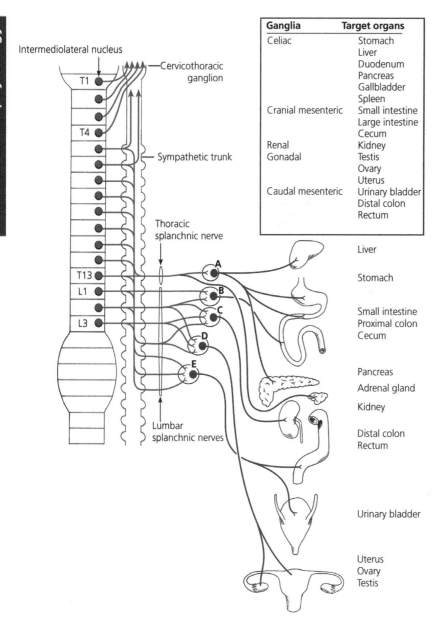

Ganglia	Target organs
Celiac	Stomach
	Liver
	Duodenum
	Pancreas
	Gallbladder
	Spleen
Cranial mesenteric	Small intestine
	Large intestine
	Cecum
Renal	Kidney
Gonadal	Testis
	Ovary
	Uterus
Caudal mesenteric	Urinary bladder
	Distal colon
	Rectum

Figure 10.5 The sympathetic fibers to the abdominal and pelvic visceral organs are supplied by the thoracic and lumbar splanchnic nerves. To reach the abdominal collateral ganglia, preganglionic fibers from the upper thoracic segments of the spinal cord descend in the sympathetic trunk to reach the T13 sympathetic trunk ganglion. They leave the sympathetic trunk, forming the thoracic splanchnic nerve. Preganglionic fibers from the L1–L3 cord segments either pass through the L1–L3 vertebral ganglia or descend in the sympathetic trunk to reach the sympathetic trunk ganglia caudal to L4. Each sympathetic trunk ganglion of the lumbar segment gives rise to a lumbar splanchnic nerve. A, celiac ganglion; B, cranial mesenteric ganglion; C, renal ganglion; D, gonadal ganglion; E, caudal mesenteric ganglion.

a **lumbar splanchnic nerve**. It is named after the level from which it arises. The first five lumbar splanchnic nerves supply one or more of the following collateral ganglia: celiac, cranial mesenteric, renal, and gonadal ganglia.

Parasympathetic division

> 1 How does the parasympathetic division respond to a fight or flight situation?
>
> 2 Describe the parasympathetic innervation of the head.
>
> 3 Describe the parasympathetic innervation of the thoracic, abdominal, and pelvic viscera.
>
> 4 What is the parasympathetic effect on pupil diameter and curvature of the lens?

The parasympathetic division of the ANS conserves and restores the energy sources of the body. For example, to conserve energy this division lowers blood pressure by slowing the heart rate and decreasing the force of contraction of the heart. To restore the energy sources, the parasympathetic division enhances digestive activity by increasing blood flow to the intestinal tract, increasing intestinal motility, and stimulating secretion of digestive enzymes. The parasympathetic division also mediates micturition by contracting the urinary bladder.

Origin of parasympathetic fibers

Cranial preganglionic fibers originate from the parasympathetic nuclei of the oculomotor (III), facial (VII), glossopharyngeal (IX), and vagus (X) nerves (Figure 10.6). Parasympathetic fibers of the **oculomotor nerve** innervate the iris and ciliary body of

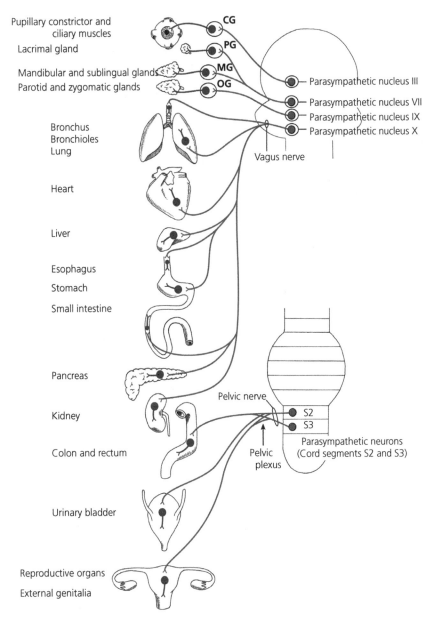

Figure 10.6 The parasympathetic innervation of the head and body. Cranial preganglionic fibers leave the brainstem as a part of cranial nerves III, VII, IX, and X. Postganglionic cell bodies are in the ciliary ganglion (CG), pterygopalatine ganglion (PG), mandibular ganglion (MG), and otic ganglion (OG). Spinal preganglionic fibers leave the sacral spinal cord (S2 and S3 in dogs) via the ventral roots and form the pelvic nerve. Parasympathetic ganglia for the pelvic viscera are located in either the plexus of the pelvic nerve on the wall of the rectum or the wall of the target organs. Only the intramural ganglia are shown in this illustration.

the eye. Activation of the parasympathetic fibers causes contraction of the pupillary sphincter muscle and the ciliary muscle. Thus, the pupil becomes smaller and the lens more convex, allowing greater refraction of light for near vision (see Figure 7.3). Parasympathetic fibers of the **facial nerve** innervate the salivary (mandibular, sublingual) and lacrimal glands. Parasympathetic fibers of the **glossopharyngeal nerve** innervate the parotid and zygomatic salivary glands. They induce watery secretion of saliva from the parotid and zygomatic

salivary glands. Parasympathetic fibers of the **vagus nerve** control the thoracic and abdominal viscera.

The **sacral outflow of the parasympathetic system** originates from cord segments S2 and S3 in dogs (Figure 10.6) and S1–S3 in cats. Preganglionic fibers are formed by the sacral parasympathetic nucleus located in the intermediate substance of the sacral cord. The preganglionic fibers course through the ventral root of the S2 and S3 spinal nerves, which together form the **pelvic nerve** located on the lateral wall of the distal rectum.

The pelvic nerve forms a plexus, which also receives the sympathetic fibers of the hypogastric nerve. Preganglionic fibers either terminate in the pelvic ganglia of the pelvic plexus or pass through the plexus to terminate in the terminal ganglia in the wall of the pelvic viscera. The pelvic nerve is essential for erection, ejaculation, urination, and defecation.

Clinical correlations

Clinical signs associated with a lesion of the facial nerve depend on the location of the lesion. A lesion of the facial nerve between the medulla oblongata and the middle ear may induce decreased tear production and potential development of keratitis (Greek keras, cornea; -itis, inflammation; i.e., corneal inflammation), loss of blinking and the palpebral reflex, and facial paresis (or paralysis) on the affected side of the face. If the lesion is more distally located (e.g., external to the stylomastoid foramen), tear production is not affected. A unilateral lesion of the vagus nerve is unlikely to cause any obvious clinical signs. However, bilateral cervical vagal disease is likely to induce paralysis of the larynx with inspiratory dyspnea (Greek dyspnoia, difficulty of breathing) that leads to cyanosis (Greek kyanos, blue; i.e., a bluish discoloration of skin and mucous membranes), altered vocalization, and dysphagia (Greek dys, difficult; phagein, to eat; i.e., difficulty in swallowing).

Neurotransmitters and their receptors

---

1 Classify the ANS divisions based on types of neurotransmitter released at the postsynaptic neurons.

2 What are the two classes of cholinergic receptors? Where are they located? What is their effect on postsynaptic neurons when they bind to acetylcholine?

3 What are the subtypes of muscarinic receptors? What are their functions?

4 What are the two classes of adrenergic receptors? Where are they found? What are their functions?

5 What receptor subtypes are responsible for sympathetic and parasympathetic effects on the heart and bronchioles of the lung?

6 What receptor subtypes are responsible for sympathetic and parasympathetic effects on the urinary bladder?

7 Describe the autonomic innervation of the adrenal gland and explain how this innervation is structurally and functionally unique.

Acetylcholine (ACh) is the sympathetic and parasympathetic preganglionic neurotransmitter. ACh is also a parasympathetic postganglionic neurotransmitter. Consequently, the parasympathetic division is often referred to as the **cholinergic division**. In contrast, sympathetic postganglionic fibers release norepinephrine, and the sympathetic division is referred to as the **adrenergic division**. The exception to this general rule is the merocrine (or eccrine) sweat glands, which are innervated by cholinergic sympathetic postganglionic fibers (Figure 10.7). Terminal portions of postsynaptic axons form a series of bead-like swellings (varicosities) (Figure 10.1). They are referred to as boutons en passage, and neurotransmitters are located in these varicosities. Axonal varicosities stay close to the surface of the effector cells, but structures similar to the neuromuscular synapse are, in general, not present.

Cholinergic receptors

Cholinergic receptors are classified into two types, nicotinic and muscarinic, based on their selective response to nicotine or muscarine (Figure 10.7). **Nicotinic acetylcholine receptors** (nAChR) are present at neuromuscular synapses and all autonomic ganglia. ACh binding to nAChR opens its ion channels, allowing influx of both Na^+ and K^+ according to the electrochemical gradient. Neurons are depolarized, as the driving force for Na^+ to enter the cell far exceeds that of K^+ to leave the cell. Activation of nicotinic receptors results in generation of excitatory postsynaptic potentials (EPSPs) of the postsynaptic neuron.

Muscarinic acetylcholine receptors (mAChR) are present in effector tissues innervated by parasympathetic postganglionic fibers. They are also present in the merocrine sweat glands innervated by cholinergic sympathetic fibers (Figure 10.7). There are several subtypes of muscarinic receptor (M_1, M_2, M_3, etc.) and all are coupled to G proteins linked to second messenger systems. ACh binding to mAChR leads to generation of either excitatory or inhibitory postsynaptic potentials (EPSPs or IPSPs). Postsynaptic response reflects the receptor subtype activated by ACh and subsequent opening of ligand-gated channels for specific ions. Thus, the action of ACh at a synapse depends on the muscarinic receptor subtypes present in the tissue. For example, M_2 receptors are present in the heart (Figure 10.8) and they respond to ACh released from parasympathetic postganglionic axons by decreasing heart rate and contraction force. In contrast, M_3 receptors in bronchioles and the urinary bladder respond to ACh by contracting bronchiolar and bladder smooth muscles (Figure 10.9). An anticholinergic drug, **atropine**, blocks parasympathetic effects. It is used to dilate the pupil or to suppress salivation and respiratory secretions.

Adrenergic receptors

Adrenergic receptors are of two types, **alpha** (α) and **beta** (β) (Table 10.1). α-**Adrenergic receptors** are mostly excitatory and induce vasoconstriction of most blood vessels, raising blood pressure, constricting sphincters of the gastrointestinal tract, contracting urethral smooth muscle, and dilating the pupils. β-**Adrenergic receptors** have several subtypes (e.g., β_1, β_2, β_3). β_1-Adrenergic receptors in the heart (cardiac muscle, pacemakers) increase heart rate and contraction force (Figure 10.8). Beta-blockers that act on the β_1 receptors of the heart reduce heart rate and prevent arrhythmias. The β_2-adrenergic receptor is present in smooth muscle

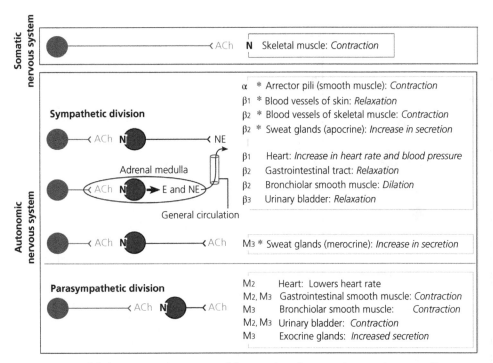

Figure 10.7 Neurotransmitters and their postsynaptic receptors of the somatic and autonomic nervous systems. Receptor type determines the effect of neurotransmitters on effector cells. ACh, acetylcholine; E, epinephrine; NE, norepinephrine; N, nicotinic cholinergic receptor; M, muscarinic cholinergic receptor; α, alpha-adrenergic receptor; β, beta-adrenergic receptor. Asterisks indicate tissues innervated solely by the sympathetic division.

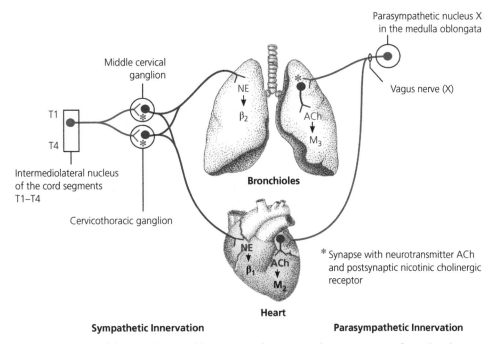

Figure 10.8 Autonomic innervation of the bronchioles and heart. Sympathetic preganglionic neurons are located in the intermediolateral nucleus of the spinal cord. Their axons terminate in the cervicothoracic and middle cervical ganglia. Parasympathetic preganglionic neurons are in the parasympathetic nucleus of the vagus nerve (X) and their axons terminate in the intramural ganglia of the lung and heart. Both sympathetic and parasympathetic preganglionic neurons release ACh, which binds to nicotinic ACh receptors of the postsynaptic neurons. Sympathetic postsynaptic fibers from the middle cervical and cervicothoracic ganglia release neurotransmitter norepinephrine (NE). NE binds to adrenergic β_2 receptors in the lung to relax bronchiolar smooth muscle and β_1 receptors in the heart to increase cardiac contraction and heart rate. The lung and heart also receive parasympathetic postsynaptic fibers that release ACh. In the lung, ACh binds to cholinergic M_3 receptors to constrict bronchiolar smooth muscle. In the heart, ACh binds to M_2 receptors to decrease cardiac contraction and heart rate.

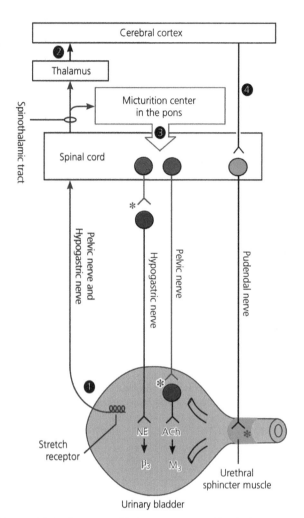

Figure 10.9 The urinary bladder is innervated by the hypogastric nerve (sympathetic) and pelvic nerve (parasympathetic), while the proximal urethra is under the control of the pudendal nerve (somatic). Sensory fibers of the hypogastric and pelvic nerves mediate signals from stretch receptors in the bladder wall that monitor the state of bladder distension. The bladder passively fills with urine without much increase in tension. The sequence of micturition is as follows. (1) When the bladder reaches near capacity, sensory fibers start to increase their activity. Sensory signals reach the thalamus and the pontine micturition center. (2) The thalamus projects to the somatosensory cerebral cortex for awareness of bladder distension, discomfort, and pain. (3) The micturition center initiates micturition by stimulating the pelvic nerve to initiate contraction of the bladder and inhibiting the pudendal nerve to relax the urethra. As the bladder becomes empty, sensory receptors in the bladder wall are no longer activated. Subsequently, the hypogastric, pelvic and pudendal nerves resume normal activity. This results in relaxation of the bladder wall and closure of the sphincter for refilling of urine. (4) The cerebral cortex is essential for awareness of bladder distension, discomfort, and pain. The cerebral cortex also initiates voluntary control of micturition. Thus, the external sphincter muscle is subject to both reflex and voluntary control. Asterisks indicate synapse with neurotransmitter ACh and postsynaptic nicotinic ACh receptors.

of the gastrointestinal tract. These β_2 receptors relax gastrointestinal smooth muscle. The β_2-adrenergic receptor is also present in the vascular smooth muscle of the heart and skeletal muscle, as well as bronchiolar smooth muscle. β_3-Adrenergic receptors are present in the urinary bladder and relax detrusor muscle in response to norepinephrine released from the sympathetic hypogastric nerve.

Micturition

> **1** What autonomic and somatic nerves innervate the urinary bladder and proximal urethra? What spinal cord segments give rise to these nerves?
>
> **2** Where is the micturition center located? What is its function?
>
> **3** What neurotransmitters are released and what receptors are present in the urinary bladder and the proximal urethra?
>
> **4** What clinical problems are expected in a dog with a lesion of the sacral spinal cord or pelvic nerve?

The urinary bladder in dogs is innervated by the sympathetic hypogastric nerve originating from cord segments L1–L3, the pelvic nerve from S2 and S3 (in dogs), and the pudendal nerve from S1 through S3. The urinary bladder fills with urine passively without much increase in pressure because of the adaptation of the detrusor muscle to stretch. While the bladder is filling, sacral sensory neurons innervating the bladder wall have low activity. As the bladder continues to fill and pressure increases, sensory signals of the hypogastric and pelvic nerves reflexively stimulate the motor neurons of the **hypogastric nerve** to relax the detrusor muscle and of the **pudendal nerve** to constrict the urethral sphincter muscle, preventing the passage of urine (Figure 10.9). Sensory signals also reach the pontine micturition center and the cerebral cortex.

When the bladder nears its urine-holding capacity, the pontine micturition center responds to sensory signals by triggering contraction of the detrusor muscle. This action is mediated by the **pontine reticulospinal tract** that excites both the **hypogastric nerve** and **pelvic nerve**, but inhibits the **pudendal nerve**. The hypogastric nerve, in response, releases norepinephrine that binds to adrenergic β_3 receptors, relaxing the detrusor muscle. The pelvic nerve releases ACh that binds to M_3 receptors, contracting the detrusor muscle. Pudendal nerve is inhibited by spinal inhibitory interneurons. Voluntary activation can override this micturition reflex by stimulating the pudendal motor neurons via the corticospinal tract. As the bladder is emptied, the pelvic nerve ceases firing and the pudendal nerve starts to discharge, contracting the urethral sphincter muscle.

The cerebral cortex is essential for awareness of bladder distension, discomfort, and pain. It also initiates voluntary control of micturition. This cortical control is mediated by the corticospinal tract that descends in the lateral funiculus of the spinal cord. The corticospinal tract innervates (i) lower motor neurons of the pudendal nerve innervating the urethral skeletal muscle of the external sphincter and (ii) abdominal muscles. The cortical involvement in micturition is the basis for house-training pets and territorial marking. Thus, the external sphincter muscle is subject to both reflex and voluntary control.

> **Clinical correlations**
>
> **A lesion of cord segments C1–L7** is frequently associated with compression of the spinal cord (e.g., disc herniation), fracture, or a vascular lesion. Micturition requires both the ascending spinothalamic tract and descending pontine reticulospinal tract. If these tracts are affected by a lesion, there will be neither bladder sensation nor voluntary micturition. The bladder fills until pressure within the bladder exceeds sphincter pressure. Although increase in abdominal pressure often leads to urine overflow, urinary retention is always high. The dog is unaware of either the bladder filling or urine overflow due to a lack of sensory signals reaching the cerebral cortex. A lesion of the corticospinal tract removes its effect on lower motor neurons of the pudendal nerve, resulting in hypertonicity of the external sphincter. As the bladder continues to extend, manually expressing urine becomes difficult and even dangerous. Excessive pressure within the bladder causes reflux of urine, increasing the risk of developing pyelonephritis (Greek *pyelos*, renal pelvis; *nephros*, kidney; *-itis*, inflammation; i.e., inflammation of the kidney). Furthermore, the bladder wall becomes extremely thin from over-stretching, and manual expression of urine may cause rupture of the bladder.
> **Lesions of the sacral cord segments** lead to overflow of urine because of an atonic distended bladder and low tone of the external sphincter of the urethra. Manual expression of urine can be performed with little resistance. The sacral cord segments or nerve roots could be lesioned by sacral fracture or ischemia. The animal shows absent or diminished perineal reflex. **Lesions of the pelvic nerve** lead to atonic bladder and the animal is incapable of voiding. This condition is a result of paralysis of the detrusor muscle accompanied by normal urethral resistance maintained by the pudendal nerve. As the bladder distends, urine overflows. The manual expression of urine can be performed with little resistance.

The colon and rectum, like the urinary bladder, are innervated by both the sympathetic and parasympathetic systems. The sympathetic innervation to the **internal anal sphincter** is excitatory, but it is inhibitory to the descending colon and rectum. Parasympathetic preganglionic fibers from the sacral plexus innervate the **striated external anal sphincter** via the sacral plexus and the pudendal nerve. Large lesions of the spinal cord cranial to the sacral cord segments are likely to affect voluntary control of defecation and may result in some fecal retention. However, gastrointestinal motility is also regulated by the intrinsic neurons of the myenteric plexus, and such cord lesions are unlikely to affect flow of bowel content and usually lead to involuntary evacuation.

Self-evaluation

Answers can be found at the end of the chapter.

1 Cell bodies of the sympathetic postganglionic neurons that play a role in pupillary dilation are located in the:
 A Intermediolateral nucleus
 B Cranial cervical ganglion
 C Ciliary ganglion
 D Cervicothoracic ganglion
 E Motor nucleus of the oculomotor nerve (III)

2 A tissue innervated solely by the sympathetic division is the:
 A Blood vessels of skeletal muscle
 B Gastrointestinal tract
 C Heart
 D Urinary bladder
 E Bronchiolar smooth muscle

3 Cell bodies of parasympathetic postganglionic neurons are located in the sympathetic trunk ganglia.
 A True
 B False

4 Which statement regarding the autonomic innervation of the adrenal medulla is true?
 A The adrenal medulla is innervated by both the sympathetic and parasympathetic divisions
 B The adrenal medulla is innervated only by the parasympathetic division
 C Sympathetic preganglionic neurons innervate chromaffin cells in the medulla
 D Chromaffin cells release ACh in response to their preganglionic stimuli

5 Pupillary contraction is mediated by:
 A Intermediolateral nucleus
 B Cranial cervical ganglion
 C Parasympathetic nucleus of the vagus nerve
 D Cervicothoracic ganglion
 E Parasympathetic nucleus of the oculomotor nerve

6 Horner's syndrome results from a lesion involving:
 A Vagus nerve
 B Cervicothoracic ganglion
 C Lumbar spinal cord
 D Pelvic nerve

7 The peripheral nerve that triggers contraction of the detrusor muscle of the bladder is the:
 A Hypogastric nerve
 B Pelvic nerve

C Pudendal nerve

D Vagus nerve

8 Absence of voluntary micturition associated with strong resistance to manual evacuation of bladder suggests that the lesion most likely involves:

A Spinal cord segments T3–T5

B Spinal cord segments S1–S3

C Hypogastric nerve

D Pudendal nerve

9 Sympathetic postganglionic neurons innervating the heart release the neurotransmitter _____ that binds to _____ receptors.

A Acetylcholine, muscarinic (M_2)

B Acetylcholine, nicotinic

C Norepinephrine, adrenergic (β_1)

D Norepinephrine, adrenergic (β_2)

E Norepinephrine, muscarinic (M_2)

10 A dog shows the following clinical signs: (i) pupillary dilation of the right eye, (ii) lateral strabismus of the right eye, and (iii) drooped right eyelid. The lesion likely involves:

A Pons

B Midbrain

C Medulla oblongata

D Spinal cord

11 Which of the following is not a feature of Horner's syndrome?

A Miosis

B Strabismus

C Ptosis

D Third eyelid protrusion

E Enophthalmos

Suggested reading

Andersson, P.O., Sjogren, C., Uvnas, B. and Uvnas-Moberg, K. (1990) Urinary bladder and urethral responses to pelvic and hypogastric nerve stimulation and their relation to vasoactive intestinal polypeptide in the anesthetized dog. *Acta Physiologica Scandinavica* 138:409–416.

Cummings, J.F. (1969) Thoracolumbar preganglionic neurons and adrenal innervation in the dog. *Acta Anatomica* 73:27–37.

De Lahunta, A. and Glass, E. (2009) *Veterinary Neuroanatomy and Clinical Neurology*, 3rd edn. Saunders Elsevier, St Louis, MO.

Federici, A., Rizzo, A. and Cevese, A. (1985) Role of the autonomic nervous system in the control of heart rate and blood pressure in the defence reaction in conscious dogs. *Journal of the Autonomic Nervous System* 12:333–345.

Marley, E. and Prout, G.I. (1968) Innervation of the cat's adrenal medulla. *Journal of Anatomy* 102:257–273.

Milner, P. and Burnstock, G. (1995) Neurotransmitters in the autonomic nervous system. In: *Handbook of Autonomic Nervous System Dysfunction* (ed. A.D. Korczyn), pp. 5–32. Marcel Dekker, New York.

Petras, J.M. and Faden, A.I. (1978) The origin of sympathetic preganglionic neurons in the dog. *Brain Research* 144:353–357.

Randall, W.C., Pace, J.P., Wechsler, J.S. and Kim, K.S. (1969) Cardiac responses to separate stimulation of sympathetic and parasympathetic components of the vagosympathetic trunk in the dog. *Cardiologia* 54:104–108.

Taira, N. (1972) The autonomic pharmacology of the bladder. *Annual Review of Pharmacology* 12:197–208.

Answers

1	B	7	B
2	A	8	A
3	B	9	C
4	C	10	B
5	E	11	B
6	B		

SECTION II

Body Fluids and Homeostasis

Section Editor: William O. Reece

11 Body Water: Properties and Functions

William O. Reece
Iowa State University, Ames, IA, USA

Water is the most abundant constituent of body fluids, comprising about 60% of total body weight. It is the solvent for the chemicals of the body, and the aqueous solutions formed from them become the media transported by diffusion to the cells of the body. The physical properties of water make it ideal for this transport function. It has a relatively high specific heat, whereby heat from the cells is absorbed with a minimum of temperature increase. Water also provides the lubrication necessary for minimizing friction associated with fluid flow, cell movement, and movement of body parts. In addition to these physical properties of water, an understanding of the physicochemical properties of aqueous solutions is fundamental when considering the many physiologic phenomena, which include maintenance of cell size, kidney function in the production of urine, respiratory gas movement, the generation of nerve impulses, capillary dynamics, and many more. In the practice of veterinary medicine, knowledge about solutions is utilized in planning treatment regimens for fluid replacement and electrolyte loss.

Physicochemical properties of solutions

1 How does facilitated diffusion differ from simple diffusion?
2 What parts of a cell membrane (protein or lipid) account for the diffusion of water-soluble substances? What parts are considered to be the pores?
3 How does active transport differ from facilitated diffusion?
4 Define osmosis.
5 Define a semipermeable membrane.
6 Define osmotic pressure and how it is determined.
7 How does a selectively permeable membrane differ from a semipermeable one?
8 As related to tone, how does effective osmotic pressure for a solution differ from a measured osmotic pressure?
9 What is the difference between hemoglobinemia and hemoglobinuria?

When H.F. Weisberg approached this topic, he seemed to have a feel for its basic importance when he quoted the following biblical verse (Proverbs 4:7): "Wisdom is the principal thing; therefore get wisdom: and with all thy getting get understanding." It is in this context that the physicochemical properties of solutions are presented, with emphasis on understanding.

Diffusion

Simple diffusion refers to the random movement of molecules, ions, and suspended colloid particles under the influence of **Brownian (thermal) motion.** Brownian motion is observed when light shines through air and dust particles are seen to move in a random motion. The movement of the dust particles is caused by their bombardment by air molecules. This same random motion occurs whether it is between air and dust or between two different

Dukes' Physiology of Domestic Animals, Thirteenth Edition. Edited by William O. Reece, Howard H. Erickson, Jesse P. Goff and Etsuro E. Uemura.
© 2015 John Wiley & Sons, Inc. Published 2015 by John Wiley & Sons, Inc.
Companion website: www.wiley.com/go/reece/physiology

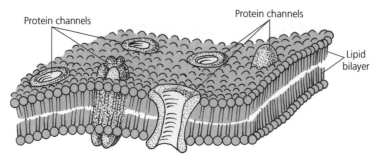

Figure 11.1 Structure of a cell membrane. The lipid bilayer is represented by a thin film of lipid that is two molecules thick. The protein channels (pores) may be composed of a single protein or a cluster of proteins. The channels may have specificity for certain substances, or they may be restrictive because of size. Virtually all water diffuses through the protein channels. Adapted from Reece, W.O. (2009) *Functional Anatomy and Physiology of Domestic Animals*, 4th edn. Wiley-Blackwell, Ames, IA.

metals placed side by side. Over time, the two metals will fuse with each. This is still simple diffusion. If a **concentration gradient** (differential) exists, molecules, ions, and colloidal particles tend to move from the area of their higher concentration to the area of their lower concentration. The movement is specific to each substance, i.e., Na^+ will diffuse from the area of its higher concentration to the area of its lower concentration regardless of the presence and concentrations of other substances. If the molecules and ions are dispersed equally, the random motion continues but does not accomplish net movement or flow; this represents a state of equilibrium. Energy is not required for simple diffusion.

Barriers to diffusion in the animal body are generally the membranes of cells. These consist of a lipid bilayer, which is a thin film of lipid only two molecules thick through which fat-soluble substances (especially carbon dioxide and oxygen) can readily diffuse (Figure 11.1). There might be **facilitated diffusion** for other substances, in which a carrier is required (Figure 11.2). However, facilitated diffusion for any substance still occurs from the area of its higher concentration to that of its lower concentration and, as in simple diffusion, energy is not required. Because cell membranes are predominantly lipid, they are relatively hydrophobic (water repelling), and the diffusion of water through the lipid bilayer proceeds with difficulty, but water can diffuse through protein channels. **Protein channels** (Figure 11.1) consist of large protein molecules interspersed in the lipid film; they provide structural pathways (**pores**) not only for water but also for water-soluble substances. Some substances may be excluded from diffusion through the pores because of their large size; conversely, diffusion may be facilitated because of other factors, such as a substance's relatively smaller size, its electrical charge (e.g., negative pore charge assists Na^+ diffusion), or the protein channel's specificity (e.g., specific ion channels). Other protein channels act as carrier proteins for the transport of substances in a direction opposite to their natural diffusion pathway. This is known as **active transport.** Whereas the transport of glucose into most cells of the body is accomplished by facilitated diffusion, exceptions exist in the lumens of the kidney tubules and intestines, where active transport is involved. In these locations, glucose is continually transported into the blood, where

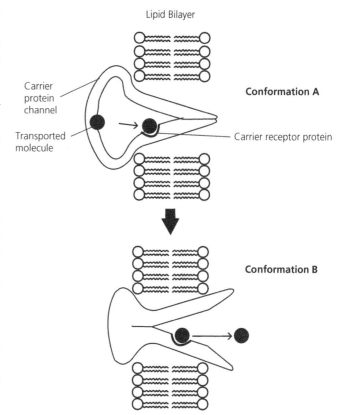

Figure 11.2 A postulated mechanism for facilitated diffusion. (A) The transported molecule enters the protein channel and binds with the receptor at the binding site. (B) Subsequent to binding, the protein channel undergoes a conformational change to open the channel on the opposite side, and the transported molecule is released, causing return of the protein channel to its original conformation. From Reece, W.O. (2009) *Functional Anatomy and Physiology of Domestic Animals*, 4th edn. Wiley-Blackwell, Ames, IA. Reproduced with permission from Wiley.

the concentration is high, from the lumen where its concentration may be minute. Loss of glucose from the body is prevented in these locations because of active transport. Active transport requires not only a carrier but also energy.

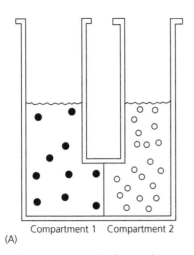 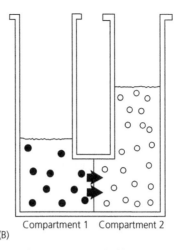

Compartment 1   Compartment 2   Compartment 1   Compartment 2
(A)   (B)

Figure 11.3 Osmosis. (A) Before osmosis. Equal volumes of aqueous solutions (solutes represented by black circles and open circles) are placed in compartments that are separated by a membrane permeable to water but not to the solutes (semipermeable membrane). The aqueous solution in compartment 1 has the highest concentration of water (lowest concentration of solute). (B) During osmosis. Osmosis (diffusion of water) occurs from compartment 1 to compartment 2 (highest water concentration to lowest water concentration) and the water level rises in compartment 2. From Reece, W.O. (2009) *Functional Anatomy and Physiology of Domestic Animals*, 4th edn. Wiley-Blackwell, Ames, IA. Reproduced with permission from Wiley.

Osmosis and osmotic pressure

The most abundant substance in the body that undergoes diffusion is water. Diffusion of water occurs throughout the body relatively easily. The amount diffusing into cells is usually balanced by an equal amount diffusing out. **Osmosis** is the process of diffusion of water through a semipermeable membrane from a solution of higher water concentration to a solution of lower water concentration. (It is important to note that it is the diffusion of water). A **semipermeable membrane** is one that is permeable (i.e., permits passage) to water but not to solutes. When comparing water concentrations of solutions, it is implied that the solution with the highest water concentration has the lowest solute concentration. A situation in which osmosis could occur is illustrated in Figure 11.3, where two different concentrations of water are separated by a semipermeable membrane. Net diffusion has occurred from the compartment with the highest water concentration, compartment 1, to the one with the lowest water concentration, compartment 2.

The quantitative measure of the tendency for water to diffuse is **osmotic pressure**. In the above example, this is the downward pressure that would have to be applied to the compartment with the lowest concentration of water (compartment 2) to prevent net diffusion of water from the compartment with the highest water concentration (compartment 1). In the animal body, osmotic pressure is a potential pressure because osmosis is not prevented when water imbalances exist. The number of **particles in a solution** (i.e., ions, molecules) determines its osmotic pressure; the greater the number of particles, the higher the osmotic pressure. For two aqueous solutions of NaCl separated by a membrane that permits diffusion of water but not NaCl, the highest osmotic pressure is measured for the solution with the highest concentration of NaCl (lowest concentration of water). Water will diffuse to the area of greatest osmotic pressure.

Table 11.1 Osmolality of several solutions as determined by vapor pressure lowering osmometry.*

Solution identification	Osmolality (mosmol/kg H$_2$O)
Bovine plasma	302
Bovine urine	1031
Bovine milk (skim)	272
Canine plasma	312
Canine urine	1904
Tap water	58

*Values obtained from student laboratory exercises.
Source: Reece, W.O. (2009) *Functional Anatomy and Physiology of Domestic Animals*, 4th edn. Wiley-Blackwell, Ames, IA. Reproduced with permission from Wiley.

Osmolar concentrations are used to express the osmotic strength of solutions (e.g., urine, plasma, NaCl). One mole of an undissociated (not ionized) substance is equal to 1 **osmole (osmol)**. If a substance dissociates into two ions (NaCl → Na$^+$ and Cl$^-$), 0.5 mol of the substance equals 1 osmol. The number of particles, not the mass of the solute, determines osmotic pressure. One liter of a solution that contains 300 mosmol of 0.3 mol/L glucose (which does not dissociate) exerts the same osmotic pressure as one that contains 300 mosmol of 0.15 mol/L NaCl. Similarly, the osmolality of a urine sample (many substances, both ionized and undissociated) measured as 300 mosmol exerts the same osmotic pressure as the previous solutions of glucose and NaCl.

A comparison of osmotic pressure for several solutions is shown in Table 11.1. Values were determined using an osmometer and are given in **osmolality (mosmol/kg H$_2$O)**. An osmometer is an instrument for measuring osmolality by freezing point depression or vapor pressure lowering (colligative properties). Values obtained are representative of diffusion through semipermeable membranes. Note that bovine urine has an osmotic pressure 3.3 times greater than that of bovine plasma (water concentration lower, solute concentration greater than bovine plasma). Canine urine has an osmotic pressure 6.1 times greater than that of canine plasma. Urine is formed from plasma, and canines have a greater potential for concentrating urine than bovines.

Tone of solutions

The membranes of the body vary in their permeability and allow certain solutes (as well as water) to diffuse through them. They are **selectively permeable membranes**. The measured osmotic pressure for a solution containing solutes that could diffuse through membranes would then not be an index for its tendency to cause osmosis. Instead, the **tone of a solution** is defined, which is the **effective osmotic pressure**. Only those particles (molecules, ions) for which the membrane is not permeable contribute to the tone. The principles of osmosis continue to prevail, except that now water diffuses to the greatest effective osmotic pressure. Figure 11.4 illustrates the tone of solutions. Two solutions of equal volumes and particle numbers are shown to be separated by a membrane that permits the passage of water and the particles in compartment 2. Each solution has the same measured osmotic pressure (same concentration of particles). Because compartment 1 has particles that cannot diffuse through the membrane, these particles are the ones that contribute to an effective osmotic pressure and, because the solution in compartment 2 has no effective osmotic pressure (because particles are diffusible), water diffuses to the greatest effective osmotic pressure, or from compartment 2 to compartment 1. In this example the net diffusion of water stops when the pressure resulting from the weight of the solution in compartment 2 opposes the diffusion resulting from the effective osmotic pressure in compartment 1.

From a practical standpoint, the tone of solutions that can be infused into the blood of animals is usually compared with the solution inside red blood cells (erythrocytes). The solution of erythrocytes is in osmotic equilibrium with plasma (the fluid part of blood). An infused solution is **hypotonic** if it has a lower effective osmotic pressure than the solution of erythrocytes, and it is **hypertonic** if it has a higher effective osmotic pressure than the solution of erythrocytes.

The effect of solutions with different tones on erythrocytes is illustrated in Figure 11.5. An erythrocyte placed in solution A enlarges. This solution must have a lower effective osmotic pressure than the erythrocyte solution (water diffuses to the higher effective osmotic pressure) and is classified as hypotonic to plasma. In solution B there is no change in the size of the erythrocytes. The solution in the beaker and in the erythrocyte must have the same effective osmotic pressure, and the beaker solution is classified as **isotonic** to plasma. The erythrocyte in solution C decreases in size, indicating a loss of erythrocyte water to the beaker solution. In this case the higher effective osmotic pressure is found in solution C (water diffuses to the higher effective osmotic pressure). The loss of water from erythrocytes caused by hypertonic solutions makes the cells wrinkled in appearance, and they are said to be **crenated**.

Table 11.2 presents the results of a laboratory exercise in which erythrocytes from a dog were placed in different concentrations of NaCl solutions. The 0.167 mol/L NaCl solution (0.977%) was considered isotonic for the erythrocytes of this dog (no change in volume). Both the 0.15 mol/L (0.877%) and 0.10 mol/L (0.585%) solutions were hypotonic (increased volume), while the 0.3 mol/L (1.76%) solution was decidedly hypertonic (decreased volume).

Erythrocytes vary in their ability to withstand **hemolysis** (rupture of erythrocytes with release of hemoglobin). Older

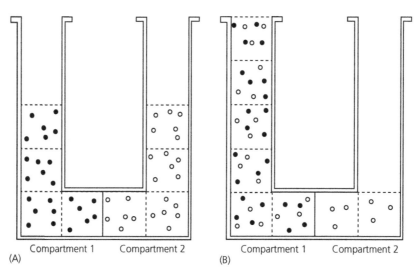

Figure 11.4 Hypothetical example of tone of solutions. (A) Before osmosis. Two aqueous solutions (solutes represented by black circles and open circles) of equal osmotic pressure are separated by a membrane permeable to water and open circle solutes (selectively permeable membrane). (B) During osmosis. Effective osmotic pressure is exerted only by black circle solute, and water diffuses from compartment 2 to compartment 1. At equilibrium, open circle solute has a new, lower concentration that is equal throughout compartments 1 and 2. Dashed lines represent divisions of equal volume. From Reece, W.O. (2009) *Functional Anatomy and Physiology of Domestic Animals*, 4th edn. Wiley-Blackwell, Ames, IA. Reproduced with permission from Wiley.

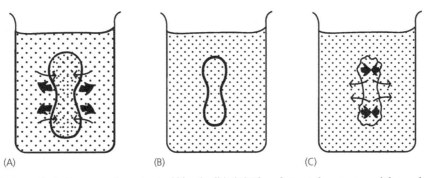

Figure 11.5 Effect of the tone of solution on erythrocytes (red blood cells). (A) The solution is hypotonic, and the erythrocyte expands. (B) The solution is isotonic, and no change occurs in erythrocyte size. (C) The solution is hypertonic, and the erythrocyte decreases in size. The thick arrows indicate the direction of cell volume change. The thin arrows indicate the direction of water diffusion. From Reece, W.O. (2009) *Functional Anatomy and Physiology of Domestic Animals*, 4th edn. Wiley-Blackwell, Ames, IA. Reproduced with permission from Wiley.

Section II: Body Fluids and Homeostasis

Table 11.2 Changes in volume of canine erythrocytes attributable to tone of suspending NaCl solution.*

Suspending solution		Volume change (percent)
Molarity	Percent	
0.3	1.76	−16.7
0.167	0.977	0.0
0.15	0.877	+2.0
0.10	0.585	+16.7

*Values obtained from student laboratory exercises.
Source: Reece, W.O. (2009) *Functional Anatomy and Physiology of Domestic Animals*, 4th edn. Wiley-Blackwell, Ames, IA. Reproduced with permission from Wiley.

Table 11.3 Osmotic fragility of erythrocytes from normal dogs (canine) and normal goats (caprine).*

Suspending solution (percent NaCl)	Normal dogs (percent hemolysis)	Normal goats (percent hemolysis)
0.85	0.0	0.0
0.75	0.6	2.1
0.65	0.7	88.0
0.60	1.7	93.6
0.55	14.0	97.7
0.50	67.4	97.7
0.45	94.4	97.7
0.40	95.7	100.0
0.35	100.0	100.0
0.30	100.0	100.0

*Values obtained from student laboratory exercises.
Source: Reece, W.O. (2009) *Functional Anatomy and Physiology of Domestic Animals*, 4th edn. Wiley-Blackwell, Ames, IA. Reproduced with permission from Wiley.

erythrocytes are more fragile and would be the first to hemolyze in solutions with reduced tone. Fragility of erythrocytes can also be increased by certain disease conditions or exposure to toxins and drugs. The degree of fragility can be determined by an **osmotic fragility test**. Blood from an animal is placed in NaCl solutions with decreasing concentration. The percent hemolysis is determined for each solution in comparison with a solution in which hemolysis would be expected to be 100%. The results of an osmotic fragility test for a normal dog (canine) are presented in Table 11.3, and are compared with those of a normal goat (caprine). It is apparent that goat erythrocytes are less resistant to hemolysis than dog erythrocytes when placed in solutions with increasing hypotonicity. Whereas dog erythrocytes are described as biconcave disks, goat erythrocytes are more spherical; therefore, expansion potential is minimal and hemolysis occurs earlier.

Solutions that cause erythrocytes to enlarge can be sufficiently hypotonic to cause hemolysis of the erythrocytes. Hemoglobin (red in color) in the erythrocyte imparts its color to the solution. Plasma from an animal in which hemolysis has occurred has some degree of redness, depending on the extent of the hemolysis (plasma is usually light yellow to colorless). When this occurs it is known as **hemoglobinemia**. Sometimes hemolysis occurs to such an extent that hemoglobin enters the kidney tubules and appears in the urine. In this condition, called **hemoglobinuria**, a red color is imparted to the urine.

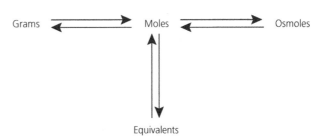

Figure 11.6 Pathways for the interconversion of grams, moles, osmoles, and equivalents. From Reece, W.O. (2009) *Functional Anatomy and Physiology of Domestic Animals*, 4th edn. Wiley-Blackwell, Ames, IA. Reproduced with permission from Wiley.

Interconversion of units of measurement

Solution composition and strength is variably expressed in moles, osmoles, and equivalents, and each has a reference to the weight in grams from which they can be derived. These units are related, and interconversions can be made and must proceed according to the pathways shown in Figure 11.6.

The problems listed below are frequently encountered when preparing solutions for infusion or when interpreting contents shown on labels for solutions commercially prepared. These will enhance your understanding and skill related to physico-chemical properties of solutions.

Question 1: How many grams would be needed to prepare 1 L of a 5% glucose solution?

Answer

Step 1: Percent solution = the concentration of solute in grams per 100 mL of aqueous solution. Accordingly, a 5% glucose solution would contain 5 g per 100 mL

Step 2: Because 1 L (1000 mL) is needed, the amount of glucose would be $(5 g \times 1000)/100 = 50 g$

Question 2: What is the molarity of a NaCl solution that contains 8.775 g/L?

Answer

Step 1: Molarity = g per L/molecular weight (MW)

Step 2: Molecular weight of NaCl = 58.5; therefore, molarity = $8.775/58.5 = 0.15 mol/L$

Question 3: What is the osmolarity of a 0.1 mol/L $CaCl_2$ solution?

Answer

Step 1: Osmolarity is a measure of osmotic pressure and is determined by numbers of particles

Step 2: One molecule of $CaCl_2$ when placed in solution would ionize and provide three particles (one Ca^{2+} and two Cl^-)

Step 3: The osmolarity (for molecules that ionize in solution) = number ions from molecule × molarity = $3 \times 0.1 = 0.3$ osmol = 300 mosmol (milliosmole)

Question 4: How many grams would be required to make 1 L of a 300 mosmol NaCl solution?

Answer

Step 1: 300 mosmol NaCl = 150 mmol/L NaCl = 0.15 mol/L NaCl

Step 2: g/L = molarity × MW = $0.15 \times 58.5 = 8.775 g$

Question 5: How many equivalents (mEq/L) of Na^+ and Cl^- are contained in a 0.15 mol/L solution of NaCl?

Answer

Step 1: NaCl is a monovalent molecule

Step 2: Eq for each ion = 1 (valence) × molarity = 0.15 Eq Na^+ and Cl^- = 150 mEq Na^+ + 150 mEq Cl^-

Question 6: How many equivalents (mEq/L) of Ca^{2+} and Cl^- are contained in a 0.1 mol/L solution of $CaCl_2$?

Answer

Step 1: $CaCl_2$ is a bivalent molecule

Step 2: Eq for each ion = 2 (valence) × molarity = $2 \times 0.1 = 0.2$ Eq Ca^{2+} and 0.2 Eq Cl^- = 200 mEq Ca^{2+} and 200 mEq Cl^-

Question 7: What is the osmolarity (mosmol/L) of a $CaCl_2$ solution labeled to contain 200 mEq Ca^{2+} and 200 mEq Cl^-?

Answer

Step 1: Convert milliequivalents to millimoles (mEq/valence = $200/2 = 100$ mmol/L $CaCl_2$

Step 2: Convert mmol/L to mosmol = 100 mmol/L × number of atoms per molecule (particles) = $100 \times 3 = 300$ mosmol

Distribution of body water

1 How do water and fluid differ from each other?

2 What percent of the body weight is water?

3 What are the two major body water compartments, and what percent of the body weight is represented by each?

4 Define interstitial fluid. What space does it occupy?

5 What substance gives interstitial water the characteristics of a gel?

6 Are intravascular fluid and plasma synonymous? Why would plasma volume have a greater value than plasma water?

The terms "water" and "fluid" are nearly the same but do differ inasmuch as a fluid, as found in the body, contains not only water but also solutes. The measurement of a compartment's volume usually includes the entire space occupied by the water and solutes. For example, blood plasma is a fluid, but its volume is slightly larger than the space occupied by the water it contains. For practical purposes, the compartments are referred to as **fluid compartments** because the fluid volume rather than the water volume is that which is usually measured.

Total body water and fluid compartments

Total body water (TBW) is the sum of the water contained in arbitrary divisions of its distribution among the intracellular and extracellular compartments. The extracellular compartment can be further divided into interstitial, intravascular, and transcellular compartments.

TBW is variable and depends mostly on the amount of fat in the body. Fat tissue is exceptional in its low water content (10% or less); thus, the total water content of a fat animal will be lower than that of a lean animal. In very lean cattle, about 70% of body weight is water, while in very fat animals TBW may account for only 40%. The average animal (neither fat nor lean) probably has water equivalent to 60% of its body weight.

Intracellular and extracellular fluid

About two-thirds of the body water is found within cells and this is the **intracellular fluid (ICF)**. The amounts given for percentage of body weight are average values and can vary. All water that is not in cells is considered to be **extracellular fluid (ECF)**, or outside the cells. This includes the **interstitial fluid (ISF)**, **intravascular fluid (IVF)**, and **transcellular fluid (TCF)**.

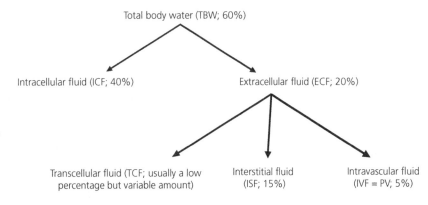

Figure 11.7 Total body water and its distribution among the fluid compartments. From Reece, W.O. (2009) *Functional Anatomy and Physiology of Domestic Animals*, 4th edn. Wiley-Blackwell, Ames, IA. Reproduced with permission from Wiley.

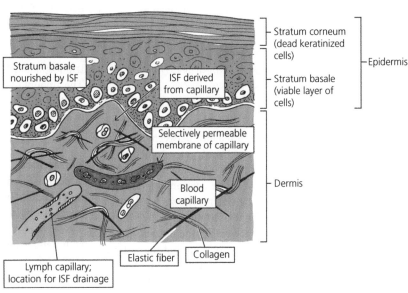

Figure 11.8 Schematic representation of the outer part of skin from a pig with special emphasis on the interstitial space, the space outside the capillaries and cells. The fluid of the interstitial space is interstitial fluid (ISF). Hyaluronic acid of the amorphous ground substance gives ISF the characteristics of a gel. An abnormal increase in ISF in this location is evident in a condition known as edema. Adapted from Reece, W.O. (2009) *Functional Anatomy and Physiology of Domestic Animals*, 4th edn. Wiley-Blackwell, Ames, IA. Reproduced with permission from Wiley.

Intravascular fluid is most often referred to as **plasma volume (PV)**. About 92% of the plasma volume is water and the remaining 8% is mostly protein. The division of TBW among the compartments is shown in Figure 11.7.

Interstitial fluid is fluid outside capillaries that immediately surrounds the cells. It is the environment of the cells. It occupies the **intercellular space** (also called **interstitial space** and **interstitium**) along with a number of **intercellular substances** (e.g., collagen, elastic fibers, fibroblasts, and plasma cells and mast cells). It is important to visualize the location of the interstitial space (Figure 11.8) relative to blood capillaries and body cells, particularly as it relates to edema (see Chapter 36). In addition to elastic and collagen fibers of the intercellular substance, an **amorphous** (without definite form or shape) **ground substance** is present; its principal component is **hyaluronic acid**. Hyaluronic acid is a highly hydrated gel that holds tissue fluid in its interstices. Because of the gel form, fluid is not observed to flow and accumulate in lower body parts, nor does fluid flow from a cut surface.

Transcellular fluid is the fluid found in body cavities. It includes intraocular fluid, cerebrospinal fluid, synovial fluid, bile, and fluids of the digestive tract. The most plentiful transcellular fluid is in the digestive tract, and its amount is greatest in ruminants because of the stomach compartments associated with fermentation.

Water movement between fluid compartments

Water molecules can rapidly penetrate most cell membranes. If an osmotic or hydrostatic pressure gradient exists between body fluid compartments, a shift of water will occur. If no appreciable hydrostatic pressure is involved, the result of water movement will be to equalize the osmoconcentration of the fluid compartments.

The response to an intravascular infusion of water would be to decrease the osmoconcentration of all compartments. This would happen with the intravascular infusion of any hypotonic solution having a lesser effective osmotic pressure than the ICF. Water would diffuse into the ICF compartment causing cellular overhydration. Infusion of a large volume could disrupt normal metabolic function and the condition of overhydration is known as **water intoxication**.

The infusion of an isotonic solution would become evenly distributed throughout the extracellular and intracellular compartments because no osmoconcentration differences would exist. The infusion of a hypertonic solution would present a greater effective osmotic pressure in the extracellular compartment than in the intracellular compartment and water would diffuse from the cells to the extracellular compartment. The infusion of a hypertonic solution has been useful in the treatment of head injuries to reduce the swelling (volume) often associated with head injuries.

Water balance

> 1 What is meant by water turnover?
>
> 2 What is the derivation of metabolic water? Why does 5 g of fat yield more metabolic water than 5 g of protein or carbohydrate?
>
> 3 What are examples of insensible water loss?
>
> 4 Why are excess water losses (e.g., diarrhea) more critical in young animals than in adults of the same species?

From day to day in any one animal the water content of the body remains relatively constant, with a balance between gains and losses. Water turnover is that amount of water gained by an animal to balance that which is lost. Typical values for lactating and nonlactating cows under moderate environmental conditions are shown in Table 11.4. The water turnover for the nonlactating cow is 29 L/day and for the lactating cow is 56 L/day. The water intake in both cases is equal to the output; there is water balance. The "pool size" stays constant, but the water in the pool changes (**water turnover**). The output of the lactating cow has increased, not only because of the obvious milk production, but also because of the greater fecal output associated with eating nearly twice as much and because of greater urine and vapor losses associated with increased metabolism.

Table 11.4 Daily water balance of Holstein cows eating legume hay (values in liters).

Balance	Nonlactating	Lactating
Intake		
Drinking water	26	51
Food water	1	2
Metabolic water	2	3
Total	29	56
Output		
Feces	12	19
Urine	7	11
Vaporized	10	14
Milk	0	12
Total	29	56

Source: Houpt, T.R. (2004) Water and electrolytes. In: *Dukes' Physiology of Domestic Animals*, 12th edn (ed. W.O. Reece). Cornell University Press, Ithaca, NY. Reproduced with permission from Cornell University Press.

Water gain

Water gains occur by ingestion of water in food and drink and from metabolic water. The food eaten by animals contains a variable amount of water; the usual drink is water or, in the very young, milk. **Metabolic water** is derived from the chemical reactions of cellular metabolism in the mitochondria. At the end of the electron transfer chain, hydrogen is combined with oxygen to form water; this is metabolic water as shown in Figure 11.9.

The metabolism of proteins, carbohydrates, and fats requires different amounts of cofactors, with the greatest amounts required for fats. Accordingly, the yield of metabolic water is greater for a certain amount of fat than for an equal amount of protein or carbohydrate. For example, the metabolic water yield from each of 100 g of protein, carbohydrate, and fat is 40, 60, and 110 mL, respectively. Energy in the form of adenosine triphosphate (ATP) is formed during the transfer of electrons. The amount of metabolic water formed varies but could be substantial under certain conditions. In domestic animals it is said to average about 5–10% of daily water gain, and it can approach 100% of the water gain for some small rodents.

Water loss

Water loss from the body is classified as either an insensible loss or a sensible loss. **Insensible losses** are associated with vapor losses and occur constantly by evaporation from the skin and by loss of water vapor in exhaled air. Inhaled air becomes saturated with water vapor in the respiratory passages and lungs, but there is no body mechanism to remove moisture from the respiratory gases before exhalation. **Sensible losses** are the visible losses; they are part of the urine, feces, and body secretions that leave the body and are not subject to evaporation. Sensible losses can become excessive in certain conditions, such as diarrhea, and threaten body stores of water.

Water requirements

No linear relationship exists between basal water needs and body weight. Accordingly, a 500-kg cow does not require 10 times more water than a 50-kg calf. However, the **basal daily needs** for water (that needed to maintain water balance) are related to caloric expenditure. Under **basal metabolism conditions** (e.g., resting animal, thermally neutral environment, fasting state), **caloric expenditure** is related linearly to body surface area. The cow might require only three to four times more water than the calf because her body surface area is three to four times greater. If the ECF (20% of body weight) is considered to be that from which emergency water is drawn, the 500-kg cow has 100 kg of fluid and the 50-kg calf has only 10 kg. Therefore, the cow has considerably more reserve on which to draw to supply basal needs for water than does the calf. In other words, the cow has ten times more reserve water to supply her needs, and her needs are only three to four times greater than the calf's. It is because of the more limited

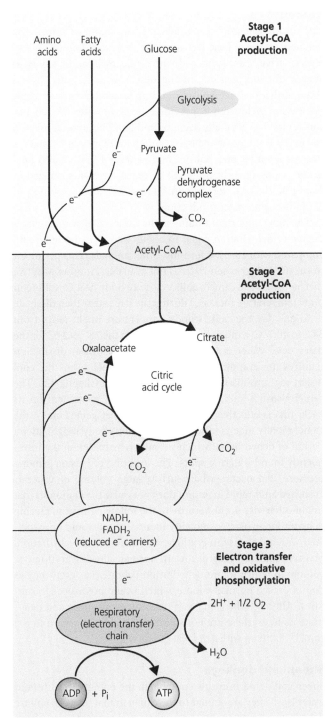

Figure 11.9 Catabolism of proteins, fats, and carbohydrates resulting in release of energy. Stage 3, via the electron transfer chain, provides for the oxidative phosphorylation of adenosine diphosphate (ADP) and the production of a high-energy substance, adenosine triphosphate (ATP). This is the location of oxygen consumption by the body and production of metabolic water. Adapted from Nelson, D.L. and Cox, M.M. (2000) *Lehninger Principles of Biochemistry*, 3rd edn. Worth Publishers, New York.

reserves associated with their relatively higher needs that calves become distressed more quickly in conditions of uncontrolled water loss (such as diarrhea). It should also be noted that because of the greater surface area relative to the body weight of calves, they will also lose body heat quicker than the cows.

Dehydration, thirst, and water intake

1 In dehydration, what is the immediate source (compartment) of water lost from the body?

2 For most animals, what is considered to be a severe loss of body water?

3 With continuing loss of water (dehydration), is there a proportionate loss of electrolytes?

4 Define thirst.

5 Where is the thirst center located?

6 How does dehydration stimulate thirst?

7 How does hypovolemia stimulate thirst?

8 How can thirst be temporarily relieved?

When water losses exceed water gains, a condition known as **dehydration** develops. The extent is variable and, when mild, physiologic mechanisms may be adequate to reestablish water balance via the thirst mechanism if water is available. Therapeutic measures (fluid replacement, treatment of underlying cause) may be necessary when water losses are moderate to severe and related to a disease condition.

Dehydration

In dehydration, the immediate source of water lost from the body is the ECF, followed by a shift from the intracellular to the extracellular fluid. A loss of water equal to 10% of body weight is considered to be severe for most animals. The concentrations of electrolytes (ions) in the body fluids do not continue to increase during dehydration, but are excreted by the kidney in proportion to the water loss. With continuing dehydration, water and electrolytes are depleted. Therefore, rehydration requires not only water but also appropriate electrolytes.

Stimulus for thirst

When water losses exceed water gain, there is an effort on the part of the kidneys to conserve water. Also, animals are provided with a **thirst mechanism** to recognize the need for water intake greater than that provided by food and metabolic water. **Thirst** is the conscious desire for water. Central to the thirst mechanism is a thirst center located in the hypothalamus of the brain and represented by thirst cells. The thirst cells are stimulated by an increase in their **osmoconcentration** (loss of water and increased salt concentration). Osmoconcentration of the thirst cells is a consequence of dehydration.

Another stimulus of thirst is the kidney hormone **angiotensin II**. This is formed in response to low blood pressure to bring about changes to increase blood pressure (e.g., salt retention, peripheral vasoconstriction, water ingestion). Loss of blood volume (**hypovolemia**), as in hemorrhage (an isotonic fluid loss), results in lowered blood pressure, and angiotensin II is formed. The thirst stimulation previously described causes an animal to drink water, which is subsequently absorbed, and blood volume and blood pressure are restored toward normal.

Relief of thirst

An experiment can be performed with a dog to show the effect of dehydration on thirst stimulation. A hypertonic NaCl solution is slowly injected intravenously, which increases the osmoconcentration of plasma and subsequently that of the thirst cells in the hypothalamus. After a few minutes, water that was previously offered to the dog and ignored is now consumed. The amount consumed is approximately equal to the amount that would have been needed to make the hypertonic plasma isotonic. Even though there was insufficient time for the water ingested to be absorbed, the dog's thirst was temporarily relieved because temporary relief can occur when the mouth and pharynx are wetted and when the stomach is distended following the ingestion of water. Both of these temporary relief methods help to prevent over-ingestion that would otherwise occur because a brief time is required after either method for water to be absorbed and to lower the osmoconcentration of thirst cells or to increase blood pressure, depending on what stimulus produced the thirst. Thirst is an important mechanism for maintaining water balance. Water must be adequately provided for animals or ill health, discomfort, and loss of production will be observed.

Adaptation to water lack

---

1 Why are Indian cattle breeds more tolerant of heat than European breeds?

2 How has the camel adapted to limited water availability?

3 Contrast the water-lack adaptive mechanisms of sheep and donkeys with each other and with the camel.

Throughout history, certain animals have had to adapt to conditions of water lack because of their habitat (little adaptation has been necessary, however, for cattle, swine, dogs, and cats). The problem is compounded by exposure to high temperatures. Indian cattle breeds (Zebu and Brahman) are more tolerant of heat than European breeds because of greater sweating (and hence cooling) and not because of any special water conservation mechanism. Adequate water must be provided. Camels, donkeys, and sheep, however, have adapted for coping with periods when water is not available.

Camels

The means whereby the dromedary (one-humped camel) has adapted to water lack has received the most interest. Many legends have been associated with this camel and its ability to survive for long periods in the desert without water. It was thought that the metabolism of hump fat, and the grater metabolic water yield from it, provided the extra water needed, but this notion has generally been discredited. The amount of fat in the hump is not great and even though more metabolic water is derived from fat metabolism, more energy (ATP) is also produced. Consequently, only half as much fat is metabolized as would be the case for protein and carbohydrate, resulting in about the same water production.

The most important finding is the camel's ability to endure a degree of dehydration equal to about 30% of its body weight, compared with 10–12% for most other animals. This permits it to survive longer when water is not available. Another adaptive mechanism is the camel's ability to store body heat (resulting in body temperature increase) during the day rather than dissipate it. In one day, the camel's body temperature might range from 34.2 to 40.7 °C, a much greater range than the 38–39.3 °C for the dairy cow. Water is thus conserved because heat dissipation requires the evaporation of water. The camel awaits the cool desert night to dissipate the stored heat (see Chapter 14). The camel also has summer fur, which is most prominent on its back; this is effective in reducing solar heat gain. Finally, the camel rapidly ingests water up to 25% of its body weight after a period of dehydration, which permits rehydration at the infrequently found watering spots. The lowering of plasma osmotic pressure that occurs when such a large volume of water is absorbed after rapid ingestion does not cause the hemolysis that might otherwise occur because of the following reason. During dehydration, plasma osmolality increases and would be associated with a decrease in erythrocyte volume. With rehydration, plasma osmolality returns toward normal, allowing erythrocyte volume to return to pre-dehydration volume (i.e., erythrocytes do not exceed normal volume, which would predispose to rupture). Although the camel can concentrate its urine and dehydrate its feces, these are not significant factors in regard to the camel's ability to withstand water deprivation.

Sheep and donkeys

Sheep and donkeys are also notable in their ability to withstand water lack. They are similar to the camel in that they can endure dehydration up to about 30% of their body weight. Also, sheep and donkeys are similar to the camel in being able to drink almost 25% of their body weight in water at one time without harmful effects. The sheep is protected from solar heat gain by its wool and excretes dry feces and relatively concentrated urine. The donkey dissipates heat by sweating more than the camel and sheep; its survival time is correspondingly less. Because sheep do not sweat as much as camels and donkeys, evaporative heat loss by way of the respiratory passages (panting) is a more important factor in sheep.

Self-evaluation

Answers can be found at the end of the chapter.

1 A different solution is placed on either side of a selectively permeable membrane. Water diffuses from side A to side B. Which side has the greater effective osmotic pressure for this to occur?
   A Side A
   B Side B

2 Solution 1 has a greater effective osmotic pressure than solution 2. Which one of these solutions has the greater tone?
   A Solution 1
   B Solution 2

3 Hyaluronic acid (a component of the intercellular substance):
   A Maintains an optimal pH of the ISF
   B Counteracts the effects of hyaluronidase
   C Is a highly hydrated gel that holds ISF in its interstices

4 Body fluid volumes were measured, and the values were reported as milliliters per kilogram of body weight but in a scrambled order with no body compartment identification. Total body water was reported as 610 mL/kg body weight and the compartment volumes were reported as 170, 230, 380, and 60. Select the series below that corresponds with the values shown.
   A ECF, ICF, ISF, PV
   B PV, ISF, ECF, ICF
   C ISF, ECF, ICF, PV
   D ECF, ICF, ISF, PV

5 The water requirement of a 1000-lb (454 kg) cow is about 30 L each day. If a calf weighs 100 lb (23 kg) and has about one-fifth the body surface area of the cow, what would be its approximate water requirement each day?
   A 30 L
   B 3 L
   C 6 L

6 The basal daily needs for water are directly related to:
   A Body weight
   B Caloric expenditure and body surface area
   C Animal color

7 More metabolic water is obtained from the metabolism of 100 g of fat than from 100 g of either protein or carbohydrate because:
   A Animals drink more when eating fat
   B More cofactors are reduced (and therefore need to be reoxidized) when fat is metabolized
   C 1 g of fat is heavier than 1 g of either protein or carbohydrate

8 Which one of the following solutions would cause a dog to begin drinking water (become thirsty) if it were infused into the dog's blood?
   A Hypertonic NaCl
   B Isotonic NaCl
   C Hypotonic NaCl

9 With continuing dehydration:
   A Only water is depleted
   B Only electrolytes are depleted
   C Both water and electrolytes are depleted

10 Which one of the following statements is correct as it relates to tolerance to dehydration?
   A Cattle have better tolerance than sheep
   B Sheep have better tolerance than cattle and pigs
   C Sheep, cattle, and pigs have the same tolerance
   D Pigs have better tolerance than sheep

Suggested reading

Houpt, T.R. (2004) Water and electrolytes. In: *Dukes' Physiology of Domestic Animals*, 12th edn (ed. W.O. Reece), pp. 12–25. Cornell University Press, Ithaca, NY.

Reece, W.O. (2004) Physiochemical properties of solutions. In: *Dukes' Physiology of Domestic Animals*, 12th edn (ed. W.O. Reece), pp. 3–11. Cornell University Press, Ithaca, NY.

Schmidt-Nielsen, K. (1997) *Animal Physiology: Adaptation and Environment*, 5th edn. Cambridge University Press, Cambridge, UK.

Vander, A.J., Sherman, J.H. and Luciano, D.S. (1994) *Human Physiology: The Mechanisms of Body Function*, 6th edn. McGraw-Hill, New York.

Answers

1 B	6 B
2 A	7 B
3 C	8 A
4 C	9 C
5 C	10 B

Section II: Body Fluids and Homeostasis

12 | The Composition and Functions of Blood

William O. Reece
Iowa State University, Ames, IA, USA

The blood vascular system evolved to provide for the transport of nutrients to the cells after they had become so numerous and so distant from the surface that diffusion was no longer adequate. The circulating medium came to be known as blood. The functions of blood are generally related to transport (e.g., nutrients, oxygen, carbon dioxide, waste products, hormones, heat, and immune bodies). There are additional functions of blood relating to its role in maintaining fluid balance and pH equilibrium in the body. Because blood must be maintained in a closed system for transport efficiency, it is provided with a mechanism for preventing blood loss if the normally closed system is opened.

General characteristics

1 What are the components of the hematocrit?
2 What accounts for the color of blood and for the color of plasma?

3 A dog weighs 10 kg and has a packed cell volume of 42% and a plasma volume of 500 mL. What is its blood volume expressed as percent of body weight?
4 Why is venous blood more acidic than arterial blood?
5 If the blood pH is measured to be 7.1 and the H^+ concentration has doubled, what is an approximate pH of that blood before the H^+ increase? Has the blood become more alkaline or more acidic?

Hematocrit

The relative proportion of cells to plasma is a clinically useful measure that can be determined by the hematocrit (Hct). When a column of blood is centrifuged, the components are separated according to their relative specific gravity. The cellular components (erythrocytes, leukocytes, and platelets, also known as thrombocytes) occupy the lower portion and, taken together, are known as the Hct. Plasma occupies the top portion and is the liquid component of blood, within which the cells and

Dukes' Physiology of Domestic Animals, Thirteenth Edition. Edited by William O. Reece, Howard H. Erickson, Jesse P. Goff and Etsuro E. Uemura.
© 2015 John Wiley & Sons, Inc. Published 2015 by John Wiley & Sons, Inc.
Companion website: www.wiley.com/go/reece/physiology

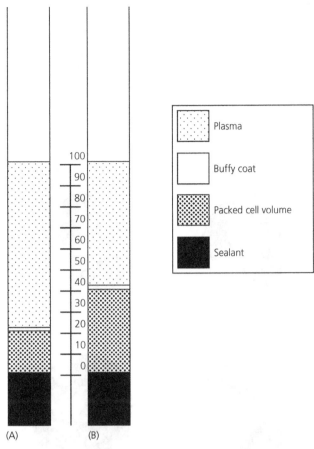

Figure 12.1 The microhematocrit as it might appear for an anemic (A) and a normal (B) animal. The buffy coat occupies an insignificant volume, and is not accounted for. Accordingly, in the normal hematocrit, the plasma volume would be noted as 60%. Adapted from Reece, W.O. (2009) *Functional Anatomy and Physiology of Domestic Animals*, 4th edn. Wiley-Blackwell, Ames, IA. Reproduced with permission from Wiley.

colloids are suspended and other transported substances are dissolved (Figure 12.1).

Blood color

The red color of blood is imparted by the hemoglobin contained within the erythrocytes. Gradations of color from bright red to bluish-purple are seen, depending on the degree of saturation of hemoglobin with oxygen. The greater the saturation, the brighter the red color. Plasma is yellow to colorless, depending on the quantity and species examined. Plasma that is ordinarily light yellow when observed in a test tube might be almost colorless in a capillary tube. The color of plasma results principally from the presence of **bilirubin**, a degradation product of hemoglobin. In cats, dogs, sheep, and goats, it is colorless or only slightly yellow. It is a darker yellow in the cow and even darker in the horse, which has a relatively high bilirubin concentration.

Blood volume

Blood volume (BV) is a function of lean body weight and is generally 8–10% of body weight. BV cannot be measured directly because exsanguination (removal of blood) results in the loss of only about 50% of the blood; the remainder is trapped in capillaries, venous sinuses, and other vessels. Erythrocyte volume and **plasma volume (PV)** can be measured by various techniques. If one or the other is measured, and the Hct is known, the BV can be calculated. For example, if the PV is 600 mL and the Hct is 40%, the PV represents 60% of the BV. BV is then determined by the following relationship:

$$BV = PV / (1 - Hct) = 600 / 0.60 = 1000 \text{ mL}$$

where the decimal equivalent of Hct is used. If these values were obtained from a 12.5-kg dog, the BV of 1000 mL translates to 80 mL/kg. Further calculation shows that this is the same as 8% of body weight if correction for specific gravity is not made and if 1 mL of blood is considered to weigh 1 g (80 mL = 80 g/1000 g = 0.08 = 8%).

Blood pH

Blood has a pH of about 7.4. Venous blood is slightly more acidic than arterial blood. Thus, if the arterial blood pH is 7.4, one would expect the venous blood pH to be about 7.36. The higher acidity of venous blood is related to the transport of carbon dioxide; higher concentrations of CO_2 exist in venous blood. The hydration of carbon dioxide in venous blood ($CO_2 + H_2O \leftrightarrow H_2CO_3 \leftrightarrow H^+ + HCO_3^-$) forms hydrogen ions, thus resulting in its higher acidity and lower pH.

The **pH symbol** is the chemical notation for the logarithm of the reciprocal of the **hydrogen ion concentration [H^+]** in gram-atoms per liter of solution. For monovalent substances, equivalent measurements are the same as gram-atom measurements; when the pH is 7.4, the [H^+] is 0.00000040 g-atoms of H^+ in 1 L of solution, or 40 nEq (nanoequivalents). When the [H^+] doubles (80 nEq) or halves (20 nEq), the pH changes by 0.3 units as follows:

pH	[H^+]
7.4	Normal
7.1	Double normal
7.7	Half normal
6.8	Four times normal

Even though the pH might seem to change very little, the [H^+] changes considerably. Therefore, the pH of the body fluids must be regulated precisely.

Leukocytes

1 How are leukocytes classified? Where are the various cells produced? What do segmented and band cells refer to?

2 Which one of the leukocytes seems to have the longest lifespan?

3 How do the numbers of red blood cells (RBCs) and white blood cells (WBCs) compare?

4 Which WBC predominates in the horse, dog, and cat? In the pig, cow, sheep, and goat?

5 Describe the movement of neutrophils from the circulation to sites of inflammation.

6 What is a principal function for each of the leukocytes?

7 Which WBC is classified as a mononuclear phagocytic system cell? Which mononuclear phagocytic system cell is in a fixed position in the liver?

8 Which one of the WBCs becomes more numerous in certain types of parasitisms?

9 Differentiate between the functions of lymphocyte T cells and B cells.

10 What are plasma cells and megakaryocytes?

11 Differentiate among leukopenia, leukocytosis, and leukemia.

12 What is meant by absolute numbers of leukocytes?

13 Define phagocytosis, pinocytosis, and endocytosis.

Classification and appearance

Leukocytes are classified as either **granulocytes**, containing granules in the cytoplasm, or as **agranulocytes**, containing few if any granules in the cytoplasm. There are three types of granulocytes, named according to which component of the hematoxylin and eosin (H&E) stain (hematoxylin, basic and colored blue; eosin, acidic and colored red) is taken up by their granules. **Neutrophils** are neither markedly acidophilic nor basophilic and incorporate both basic and acidic components into their granules. **Basophils** only accept the basic (hematoxylin) component, and **eosinophils** only accept the acidic (eosin) component. There are two types of agranulocytes: **monocytes** and **lymphocytes**. Granulocytes and monocytes are produced in the bone marrow from **myeloid stem cells** known as **myoblasts** and **monoblasts**, respectively. Lymphocytes originate from a lymphoid stem cell, known as a lymphoblast, in lymph tissue, such as lymph nodes, spleen, tonsils, and various lymphoid clusters in the intestine and elsewhere. The different types of leukocytes are shown in Figure 12.2 for humans; there are many similarities with those in animals.

The nuclei of the granulocytes assume various shapes as they proceed to maturity (Figure 12.3). The nuclei of the mature

Figure 12.2 Erythrocytes, leukocytes, and platelets (peripheral blood film, Wright's blood stain). (A) Polychromatophilic erythrocyte; (B) erythrocyte (mature); (C) platelets; (D) band neutrophil; (E) neutrophil (mature); (F) eosinophil; (G) basophil; (H) monocyte; (I) degenerating neutrophil; (J) large lymphocyte; (K) small lymphocyte. Adapted from Cormack, D.H. (2001) *Essential Histology*, 2nd edn. Lippincott Williams & Wilkins, Baltimore. Reproduced with permission from Lippincott Williams & Wilkins.

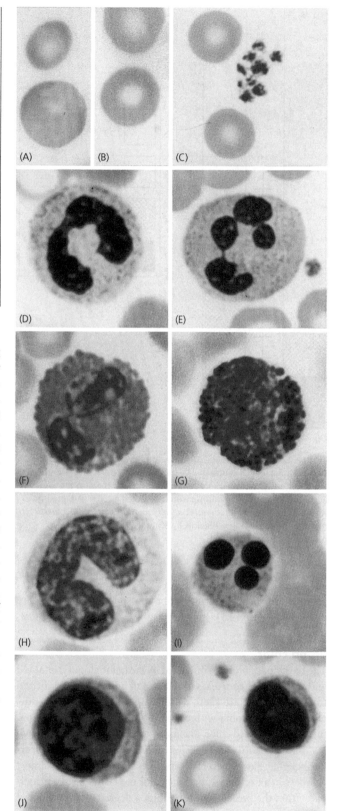

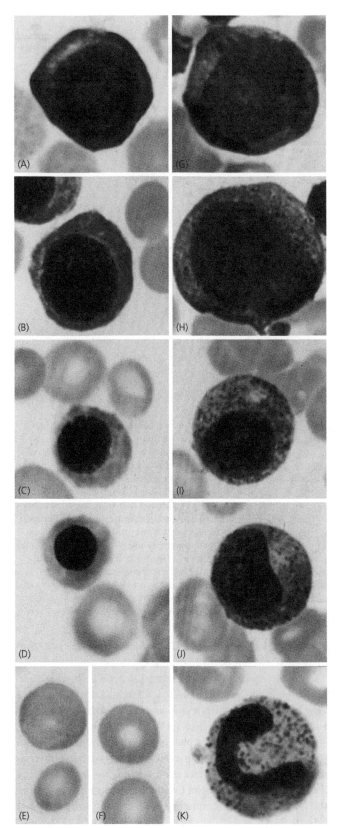

forms are generally divided into lobes or segments connected by filaments; these are sometimes called **segmented cells**. The younger forms have a nucleus that appears as a curved or coiled band without segmentation; these are known as **band cells**.

Lifespan and numbers

After their development, leukocytes are circulated in the blood until the time (relatively short) they leave the circulation to perform their extravascular function. Granulocytes can be present in the blood for 6–20 hours and are constantly leaving. Granulocyte time in the tissues varies considerably, but can be 2 or 3 days. Once granulocytes leave the blood, they do not normally return. They leave the body either from inflammatory sites or by way of the gastrointestinal, urinary, respiratory, or reproductive tracts. These organs are normally lined with neutrophils, which help prevent entry of organisms or foreign particles. Monocytes have a circulation time of 24 hours or less, but can remain in the tissues for several months. Many monocytes become fixed macrophages in the sinusoids of the liver, spleen, bone marrow, and lymph nodes; in this way they continue to function in the blood and lymph.

Lymphocytes recirculate repeatedly from the blood, to the tissues, to the lymph, and back to the blood. The **lymphocyte population** consists of **T cells** and **B cells**. Their lifespan varies, depending on classification. Generally T cells are long-lived (100–200 days), B cells are short-lived (2–4 days), and memory T and B cells are very long-lived (years).

The circulating leukocytes are considerably less numerous than erythrocytes. The numbers range from 7000 to 15,000 per microliter (µL) among the domestic animals (Table 12.1). To appreciate the volume from which the number is obtained, recall that a microliter (µL) is one-millionth of a liter, whereas a milliliter (mL) is one-thousandth of a liter. Accordingly, there are 1000 µL in 1 mL. The percentage distribution of the various types of leukocytes is not the same among the domestic species. There is a higher percentage of lymphoycytes than neutrophils among the cloven-hoofed animals (pig, cow, sheep, goat). The reverse (higher percentage of neutrophils than lymphocytes) is true for the horse, dog, and cat.

Figure 12.3 Microscopically recognizable stages of erythroid and granulocytic maturation (bone marrow film, Wright's blood stain). (A) Proerythroblast; (B) basophilic erythroblast; (C) polychromatophilic erythroblast; (D) normoblast; (E) polychromatophilic erythrocyte; (F) erythrocyte (mature); (G) myeloblast; (H) promyelocyte; (I) neutrophilic myelocyte; (J) neutrophilic metamyelocyte; (K) band neutrophil. Adapted from Cormack, D.H. (2001) *Essential Histology*, 2nd edn. Lippincott Williams & Wilkins, Baltimore. Reproduced with permission from Lippincott Williams & Wilkins.

Table 12.1 Total leukocytes per microliter of blood and percentage of each leukocyte.

Species	Total leukocyte count (per µL)	Neutrophil (%)	Lymphocyte (%)	Monocyte(%)	Eosinophil (%)	Basophil (%)
Pig						
1 day	10,000–12,000	70	20	5–6	2–5	<1
1 week	10,000–12,000	50	40	5–6	2–5	<1
2 weeks	10,000–12,000	40	50	5–6	2–5	<1
6 weeks and older	15,000–22,000	30–35	55–60	5–6	2–5	<1
Horse	8000–11,000	50–60	30–40	5–6	2–5	<1
Cow	7000–10,000	25–30	60–65	5	2–5	<1
Sheep	7000–10,000	25–30	60–65	5	2–5	<1
Goat	8000–12,000	35–40	50–55	5	2–5	<1
Dog	9000–13,000	65–70	20–25	5	2–5	<1
Cat	10,000–15,000	55–60	30–35	5	2–5	<1
Chicken	20,000–30,000	25–30	55–60	10	3–8	1–4

Source: Reece, W.O. and Swenson, M.J. (2004) The composition and functions of blood. In: *Dukes' Physiology of Domestic Animals*, 12th edn (ed. W.O. Reece). Cornell University Press, Ithaca, NY. Reproduced with permission from Cornell University Press.

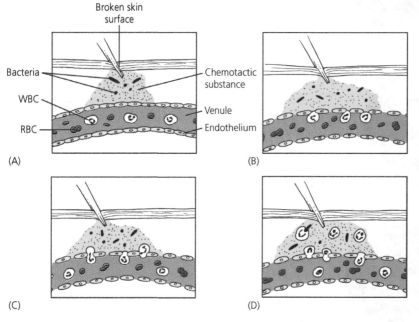

Figure 12.4 Mechanisms by which neutrophils are attracted to sites of injury. (A) Tissue injury and introduction of bacteria causes diffusion of a chemotactic substance to capillaries and venules. (B) Chemotactic substance increases endothelial porosity and adhesion of neutrophils to endothelium. (C) By a process known as diapedesis, the adhered neutrophils squeeze through endothelial pores. (D) Neutrophils proceed to injury site by ameboid movement and phagocytize bacteria and other debris. WBC, white blood cell; RBC, red blood cell. Adapted from Reece, W.O. (2009) *Functional Anatomy and Physiology of Domestic Animals*, 4th edn. Wiley-Blackwell, Ames, IA. Reproduced with permission from Wiley.

Function

As a group, the WBCs serve as a defense mechanism against bacterial, viral, and parasitic infections and proteins foreign to the body. Each of the WBCs has a specific role in this broad function.

Neutrophils

The cell membranes of certain cells can engulf particulate matter (e.g., bacteria, cells, degenerating tissue) and extracellular fluid and bring them into their cytoplasm. The ingestion of particulate matter is known as **phagocytosis**, the ingestion of extracellular fluid is **pinocytosis**, and both are forms of **endocytosis**.

Neutrophils have two types of granules in their cytoplasm. **Azurophilic granules** are the lysosomes of the neutrophil and supply enzymes to digest the ingested bacteria, viruses, and cellular debris. The other granules produce **hydrogen peroxide**, a

bactericidal substance, which is potentiated (made more active) by **peroxidase**, one of the lysosomal enzymes.

Substances within specific granules include **collagenase** and an iron-binding protein called **lactoferrin**. Lactoferrin has a very high affinity for ferric iron and can deprive phagocytized bacteria of the iron they need for further growth.

Neutrophils are highly phagocytic and this, coupled with their mobility, provides an effective body defense mechanism. Their numbers increase rapidly during acute bacterial infections. The mechanism by which neutrophils move from the blood to an inflammatory site is described as follows (Figure 12.4).

1 Degenerative products of inflamed tissue or bacterial cells can be **chemotactic** (chemically attracting) and diffuse through interstitial spaces to capillaries and venules.

2 Chemotactic substances increase porosity of these vessels and also provide for adhesion of neutrophils to endothelium (**margination**).

3 Neutrophils squeeze through endothelial openings (**diapedesis**).

4 Neutrophils proceed to inflammatory sites by **ameboid movement**.

This mechanism probably applies to the other leukocytes as well. When the neutrophils arrive at the inflamed site, they phagocytize bacteria and cell debris. The neutrophil lifespan is relatively short; dead neutrophils and their liquid is known as **pus**. The accumulation of pus within a connective tissue capsule is known as an **abscess**.

The leukocyte comparable to the neutrophil in birds is known as the **heterophil**.

Monocytes

Monocytes are usually the largest leukocyte seen on a stained blood film. They occur in normal blood to only a limited extent. Compared with other leukocytes, they have a copious cytoplasm. Circulating monocytes phagocytize bacteria, viruses, and antigen–antibody complexes from the bloodstream. However, their circulatory phagocytic function is not as pronounced as that which occurs in the tissues. The movement of neutrophils from capillaries and venules is accompanied by similar margination and diapedesis of monocytes. On entering the tissues, monocytes are transformed into **macrophages (large phagocytic cells)** and initially participate in the phagocytosis of bacterial cells. Macrophages kill phagocytized microbes by their acidic pH, bacteriostatic proteins, and degradative enzymes. They also produce hydrogen peroxide in greater quantity than neutrophils. Macrophages eventually predominate at the inflammatory site because of their longer lifespan. Also, they are attracted to some organisms that neutrophils ignore and they phagocytize the cellular debris that remains when inflammation subsides. The enzyme systems of monocytes are designed to degrade engulfed tissue debris from chronic inflammatory reactions, and monocyte numbers increase in chronic infections. They are especially valuable in the defense against long-term inflammation because of their larger size and longer lifespan. Lysosomes within the cytoplasm of neutrophils and monocytes help in the digestion of the phagocytized materials.

Monocytes are the cells that comprise the **mononuclear phagocytic system (MPS)**. The MPS was formerly known as the reticuloendothelial system. Its cells are either monocytes (intravascular) or are derived from monocytes (extravascular). The cells are mobile (macrophages) or become fixed in position (e.g., **Kupffer cells** in the liver sinusoids and others in the spleen and lymph nodes). The fixed cells are also phagocytic.

Eosinophils

On a stained blood film, eosinophils can be seen to have cytoplasmic granules that are red or reddish-orange (eosinophilic). These are about the same size as neutrophils. The granules con-tain several enzymes (e.g., **histaminase**) that dampen and terminate local inflammatory reactions of allergic origin. Eosinophils become more numerous in certain types of parasitisms. The parasitic forms are **opsonized** (attacked by antibodies) and the eosinophils discharge their granular contents onto the surface of the opsonized parasite, inflicting lethal damage.

In Cushing's disease there is oversecretion of adrenocorticosteroid hormones (see Chapter 51). When cortisol (an adrenocorticosteroid) is injected, this condition is simulated and the number of circulating eosinophils decreases. Cortisol reduces the eosinophil count by enhancing eosinophil diapedesis and by diminishing the release of eosinophils from the bone marrow. Cortisol production increases during stress, and lowered eosinophil blood counts have been associated with stress.

Basophils

Basophils of the blood are somewhat similar to the **mast cells** that are present in the interstitial spaces outside the capillaries. They seem to lack phagocytic power. Basophil granules contain histamine, bradykinin, serotonin, and lysosomal enzymes, substances that initiate an inflammatory response. Basophils and mast cells have receptors on their cell membranes for immunoglobulin E (IgE) antibodies (those associated with allergies). When the antibody on the cell membrane contacts its antigen, the basophil ruptures, releasing its granular contents, and the local vascular and tissue reactions of allergies are manifested. Basophils are rare in normal blood, and their distribution in blood is usually considered to be less than 1%.

Basophils enhance allergic reactions, whereas eosinophils tend to dampen them. There is a balance between their functions in that inflammatory reactions proceed quickly via basophils, and then are modified via eosinophils so that overreaction does not occur.

Lymphocytes

Lymphocytes can be classified morphologically as **small** or **large**. It is believed that large lymphocytes represent immature forms, whereas small lymphocytes represent more mature forms. Lymphocytes are involved in immune responses, and on this basis are classified as T cells or B cells. Both T and B cells are derived from **hematopoietic stem cells (lymphoblasts)** that differentiate to form lymphocytes. In mammals, shortly before or after birth, the site of early processing and differentiation of the stem cells for T lymphocytes is the thymus gland; for B lymphocytes, the sites are the fetal liver, spleen, and bone marrow. T cells are involved in **cell-mediated immunity**, which involves the formation of large numbers of lymphocytes to destroy foreign substances (antigens). The three different types of T cells are **cytotoxic T cells**, **helper T cells**, and **memory T cells**. Cytotoxic T cells are sometimes called killer cells. T-cell receptors bind to specific antigens, and cytotoxic substances are released into the foreign cell (e.g., bacteria, viruses, tissue cells) (Figure 12.5). Cytotoxic cells also attack cells of transplanted organs. Because cancer cells generate unique antigens when they become cancerous, cytotoxic T cells recognize the cancerous

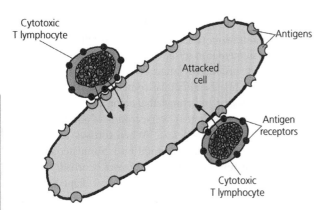

Figure 12.5 Mechanism by which sensitized cytotoxic T lymphocytes destroy a foreign cell. The attacked cell is killed by the release of cytotoxic and digestive enzymes from the T lymphocytes directly into the cytoplasm of the attacked cell. The T lymphocytes can proceed to other cells after their attack on a cell. Adapted from Reece, W.O. (2009) *Functional Anatomy and Physiology of Domestic Animals*, 4th edn. Wiley-Blackwell, Ames, IA. Reproduced with permission from Wiley.

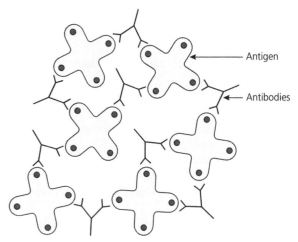

Figure 12.6 Antigen–antibody agglutination and precipitation. Antigens (molecules or cells) are grouped with other antigens by bivalent (two binding sites) antibodies. This causes them to agglutinate or precipitate. Adapted from Hall, J.E. (2011) *Guyton and Hall Textbook of Medical Physiology*, 12th edn. Saunders Elsevier, Philadelphia. With permission from Elsevier.

cells as foreign to the body and attack them. Helper T cells are the most numerous of the T cells. When helper T cells are activated, they assist in the activation of cytotoxic T cells and of B cells. Antigens ordinarily activate the cytotoxic T cells and B cells, but activation is more intense when assisted by helper T cells. Memory T cells are long-lived and respond to the same antigen when exposed at a later date.

B lymphoncytes were first discovered in birds, and early processing and differentiation was found to occur in the **bursa of Fabricius**, from which the name was derived (B for bursa). After exposure to an antigen, **activated B cells** proliferate and transform into **plasma cells** and a smaller number of **memory cells**. The **memory B cells** have a function similar to memory T cells and are readily converted to effector cells by a later encounter with the same antigen. B cells do not attack foreign substances directly, but instead the plasma cells produce large quantities of **antibodies (globulin molecules called immunoglobulins)** that inactivate the foreign substance. This type of immunity is known as **humoral immunity**. Antibodies can produce inactivation by causing **agglutination**, **precipitation**, **neutralization** (antibodies cover toxic sites), or **lysis** (rupture of the cell). Agglutination and precipitation reactions are shown in Figure 12.6.

A more common humoral method of immunity is represented by the **complement system**, which is composed of a number of enzyme precursors that are activated successively. From a small beginning, a large reaction occurs. Examples of **complement reactions** include (i) **opsonization**, in which foreign substances are covered by antibody and become vulnerable to phagocytosis by neutrophils and macrophages; and (ii) **chemotaxis**, in which the complement product attracts neutrophils and macrophages into the local region of the antigenic agent.

Lymphocytes comprise about two-thirds of the leukocytes in birds and in this regard are similar to the cloven-hoofed animals.

Diagnostic procedures

Diagnostic procedures related to WBCs include determination of their total number and distribution of the leukocyte types. The total number can be determined by dilution and subsequent counting, either manually in a hemacytometer or with an electronic counter. An increase in leukocyte numbers is called **leukocytosis**; this usually occurs in bacterial infections. A decrease in numbers is called **leukopenia**; this is usually associated with the early stages of viral infections. **Leukemia** is a cancer of WBCs and is characterized by leukocytosis. The determination of the percentage distribution of WBCs is known as a **differential white blood cell count**. In this procedure a smear is made of a blood drop which is subsequently stained. The cells are observed under a microscope, and the different types are counted and classified until a total of 100 has been tallied. The **relative number** for each type is then estimated as the percentage distribution in the blood (see Table 12.1).

The **absolute number** of leukocytes is calculated after the total number and differential count have been determined. The absolute number refers to the number per microliter for each leukocyte type. Determination of the absolute number can prevent misinterpretation of the differential count. For example, the total WBC count for a normal cow might be 9000/μL. The relative number could be 30% neutrophils and 60% lymphocytes, in which the absolute numbers would be 2700/μL (0.3×9000) and 5400/μL (0.60×9000), respectively. If traumatic reticuloperitonitis (hardware disease) is present, this same cow might have a total WBC count of 27,000/μL and a differential count of 70% neutrophils and 20% lymphocytes. A first interpretation might be that a lymphopenia exists (60% lymphocytes decreased to 20%). However, further calculation shows that the absolute number of lymphocytes remains the same (27,000/μL × 0.20 = 5400/μL), whereas the absolute number of neutrophils increases $(27,000/\mu L \times 0.70 = 18,900/\mu L)$. The neutrophil increase would indicate inflammation.

Erythrocytes

> 1 What chemical atom associated with hemoglobin binds loosely and reversibly with oxygen? How many molecules of O_2 can be transported by one molecule of hemoglobin?
>
> 2 What is the valence of iron before and after its binding with oxygen?
>
> 3 What are methemoglobin, myoglobin, and carbonmonoxyhemoglobin, and how do they differ from hemoglobin?
>
> 4 What is the average concentration of hemoglobin in the blood of domestic animals?
>
> 5 What is the physiologic name for the production of erythrocytes?
>
> 6 Where does RBC production occur during the postnatal, growth, and adult periods?
>
> 7 How does reticulocyte presence relate to lifespan of erythrocytes?
>
> 8 What substance controls the rate of erythropoiesis? Where is it produced?
>
> 9 How long does it take for new RBCs to enter the circulation after their formation begins?
>
> 10 If there are 7 million RBCs in each microliter of cow blood, how many would there be in 1 mL?
>
> 11 What are advantages of a discoid RBC shape? What is tolerance to RBC shape change known as?
>
> 12 Which domestic animal has the largest RBC? The smallest?
>
> 13 Which one of the erythrocyte indices is related to an erythrocyte's volume? What is the unit of expression? What is the unit of expression for the amount of hemoglobin in each RBC?

Hemoglobin and its forms

The principal component of erythrocytes is **hemoglobin (Hb)**, which makes up about one-third of the erythrocyte content, the remainder being water and stroma (structural components). The hemoglobin molecule (Figure 12.7) has a molecular weight of about 67,000 and is composed of four heme groups combined with one molecule of globin (the protein component). Globin is composed of four polypeptide chains, each containing one of the heme groups. Each heme group contains an iron atom that combines loosely and reversibly with one oxygen molecule. Therefore, one molecule of hemoglobin contains four molecules of oxygen. The iron atom of heme has a valence of +2 (Fe^{2+}, ferrous) regardless of whether molecular oxygen is combined with it. Because of the presence of hemoglobin, blood can transport about 60 times more oxygen than would be possible by its simple solution. Certain conditions cause the ferrous iron of heme to be oxidized to its ferric state. In one such condition, nitrate poisoning, the hemoglobin formed is known as **methemoglobin**, and it cannot transport oxygen. Another abnormal

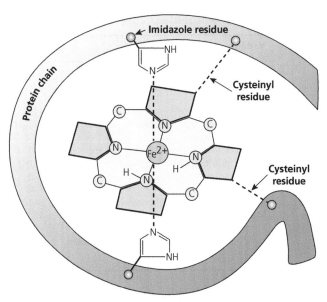

Figure 12.7 Schematic representation of one heme group and its associated polypeptide chain. Four of these combinations, at different orientations to each other, comprise hemoglobin. The heme is held to its specific polypeptide chain (one of four in the protein globin) by cysteine (an amino acid) bridges and by bonding of the iron to imidazole groups of histidine (an amino acid). Molecular oxygen binds with iron. Adapted from Conn, E.E. and Stumpf, P.K. (1963) *Outlines of Biochemistry*. John Wiley & Sons, New York.

form of hemoglobin is **carbonmonoxyhemoglobin** (sometimes called carboxyhemoglobin). As the name implies, carbon monoxide occupies the site normally occupied by oxygen. Hemoglobin has an affinity for carbon monoxide that is about 200 times greater than its affinity for oxygen. Thus, small concentrations of carbon monoxide compete more favorably for sites on Hb than normal concentrations of oxygen.

The hemoglobin of muscle is known as **myoglobin**. It differs from hemoglobin in that it has only one polypeptide chain and one associated heme group, so it can only combine with one molecule of oxygen instead of four. The concentration of hemoglobin in the blood of domestic animals averages about 12 g/dL (Table 12.2).

Erythropoiesis

The production of erythrocytes is known as **erythropoiesis**. Before birth, erythrocyte formation occurs in the liver, spleen, and bone marrow. During the postnatal, growth, and adult periods, erythropoiesis is restricted almost exclusively to the bone marrow. It seems that most bones are involved in erythropoiesis and the axial and appendicular skeletons account for about 35% and 65% of RBC production, respectively. This pattern has been observed in 1-year-old beagle dogs and can vary in other animals. The **axial skeleton** includes almost all bones except those of the limbs, which belong to the **appendicular skeleton**. The erythrocytes are continually formed and destroyed. Considering the large number of RBCs in the blood,

Table 12.2 Average values for several blood variables.

Variable	Horse*	Cow	Sheep	Pig	Dog	Chicken
Total RBC (×10⁶/μL)	9.0	7.0	12.0	6.5	6.8	3.0
Diameter of RBC (μm)	5.5	5.9	4.8	6.0	7.0	elliptic 7 × 12
Hct (%)	41.0	35.0	35.0	42.0	45.0	30.0
Sedimentation rate (mm/min)	2–12/10	0/60	0/60	1–14/60	6–10/60	1.5–4/60
Hemoglobin (g/dL)	14.4	11.0	11.5	13.0	15.0	9.0
Coagulation time (capillary tube method, min)	2–5	2–5	2–5	2–5	2–5	—†
Specific gravity (g/dL)	1.060	1.043	1.042	1.060	1.059	1.050
Plasma protein (g/dL)	6–8	7–8.5	6–8	6.5–8.5	6–7.8	4.5
Blood pH (arterial)	7.40	7.38	7.48	7.4	7.36	7.48
Blood volume (percent of body weight)	8–10	5–6	5–6	5–7	8–10	7–9
Mean corpuscular volume (MCV; fL)	45.5	52.0	34.0	63.0	70.0	115.0
Mean corpuscular hemoglobin (MCH; pg)	15.9	14.0	10.0	19.0	22.8	41.0
Mean corpuscular hemoglobin concentration (MCHC; %)	35.0	33.0	32.5	32.0	34.0	29.0

*Hot blooded.
†See section Species differences.
Source: data compiled from Swenson, M.J. (1993) Physiological properties and cellular and chemical constituents of blood. In: *Duke's Physiology of Domestic Animals*, 11th edn (eds M.J. Swenson and W.O. Reece). Cornell University Press, Ithaca, NY; and Jain, N.C. (1993) *Essentials of Veterinary Hematology*. Lea & Febiger, Philadelphia.

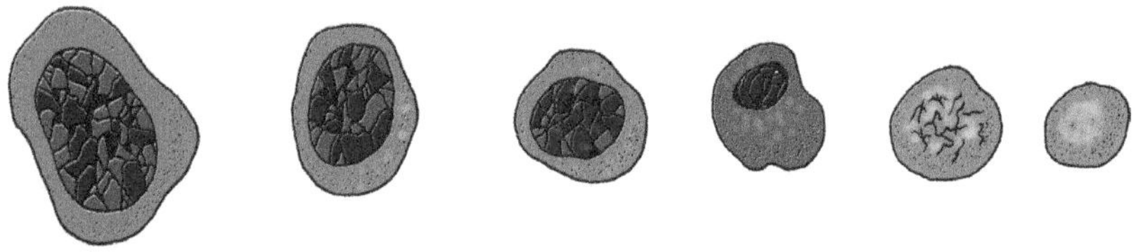

Rubriblast   Basophilic rubricyte   Polychromatophilic rubricyte   Metarubricyte   Reticulocyte   Erythrocyte

Figure 12.8 The stages of erythrocyte development. Adapted from Reece, W.O. (2009) *Functional Anatomy and Physiology of Domestic Animals*, 4th edn. Wiley-Blackwell, Ames, IA. Reproduced with permission from Wiley.

one should appreciate the dynamic aspect of this phenomenon. For example, approximately 35,000,000 erythrocytes are formed and destroyed in a 450-kg horse each second.

Erythrocytes are formed in the bone marrow from a foundation cell known as a **rubriblast**. Several intermediate forms are recognized in the genesis of the erythrocyte (Figure 12.8). The distribution of these forms can be studied by preparation and examination of bone marrow smears. Just before the developing erythrocyte's entrance into the circulation, the nucleus is expelled. The polyribosomes and ribosomes are retained and might still be apparent on stained smears for a day or so after their arrival in the circulation. If they are present, they are identified as **reticulocytes** because of the net-like appearance of the polyribosomes and ribosomes. **Polyribosomes (polysomes)** consist of several ribosomes joined together by the same messenger RNA molecule. During periods of rapid RBC production, reticulocyte numbers can increase. Reticulocytes are usually present in the blood of animals when the lifespan of erythrocytes is less than 100 days. The dog is an exception. Adult ruminants, and especially horses, with longer RBC lifespans do not have reticulocytes in the circulating blood in health. The nuclei of avian erythrocytes are not expelled before entry

into the circulation, and they persist throughout the life of the erythrocytes.

The rate of erythropoiesis seems to be controlled by the tissue need for oxygen. Reduced oxygen concentration at the tissue level results in the secretion of a hormone by the kidneys known as **erythropoietin**. Erythropoietin stimulates the bone marrow to begin formation of new erythrocytes. The lifespan of erythropoietin is less than 1 day; this short lifespan helps provide greater flexibility in the adjustment of erythrocyte numbers in order to regulate the tissue need for oxygen more precisely. New erythrocytes do not appear in the circulation until about 5 days after their formation begins. Thus, additional erythropoietin can be formed to allow continued production during the interim. When the new erythrocytes appear in the circulation, the tissue need for oxygen begins to be met and erythropoietin is no longer secreted.

Numbers

The number of erythrocytes can be determined by making known dilutions and counting the number of RBCs in a known volume using the counting chamber of a hemacytometer with the aid of a microscope. The Unopette© microcollection system

(Becton Dickinson and Company, Franklin Lakes, NJ) is widely used for this purpose. In addition to erythrocytes, leukocytes and platelets can also be enumerated with this system. Using various multiplication factors (which make allowance for dilution and for the limited volume that is counted), the number of RBCs per microliter of blood can be determined. More accurate determinations can be made using electronic counting equipment. A number of systems are available that are capable of counting erythrocytes, leukocytes, and platelets and of determining hemoglobin concentration. The cells are counted as they stream past a photoelectric cell in single file. A computer within provides print-outs of means, ranges, and call-outs for highs and lows. The erythrocyte indices are also calculated. Generally, there are about 7,000,000 RBCs per microliter of blood in the cow, pig, and dog (see Table 12.2). More RBCs are seen for hot-blooded horses (9,000,000/μL) and for sheep (11,000,000/μL). Values for the goat are not given in Table 12.2, but they average about 13,000,000/μL.

Shape

Erythrocytes are generally considered to be discocytes, with some degree of concavity. The dog's RBCs are typical biconcave disks, whereas the goat's RBCs are more spherical. The camel has elliptical RBCs, and the deer has RBCs that are somewhat sickle-shaped. The advantages of a discoid shape are (i) the provision of a larger surface area to volume ratio, (ii) minimal diffusion distance, and (iii) greater osmotic swelling (water intake) possible without threatening the integrity of the membrane.

The characteristic shape of erythrocytes is maintained by the molecular constitution of hemoglobin and by certain contractile proteins of the cell membrane. An altered shape, because of a difference in hemoglobin constitution, can result in disease such as sickle cell anemia in humans. A genetically induced substitution of the amino acid valine for the usual glutamic acid in the amino acid sequence of hemoglobin causes RBCs to assume a sickle shape, rather than the usual biconcave disk shape, when hemoglobin is deoxygenated. The altered shape makes the cells more vulnerable to destruction, and anemia results.

Erythrocytes are tolerant of shape changes as they circulate. Many variations are noted as they pass through the small lumen (duct) of capillaries or rebound from a collision with a vessel bifurcation (branch). This property of tolerance for shape change is known as **plasticity**.

Size

Among the domestic animals, dogs have erythrocytes with the largest diameter (7 μm), and sheep and goats have those with the smallest (4–4.5 μm). It seems that this was an adaptive feature, because RBCs of the smallest size are found in greater numbers. Because the sheep and goat were commonly found in regions of high altitude, with lower oxygen concentrations, the available hemoglobin was placed in a greater number of smaller packages so that a greater surface area would be available for diffusion.

Erythrocyte indices

The **erythrocyte indices** are determinations that are calculated after the erythrocytes (RBCs) have been enumerated and Hct and Hb concentration determined. There are three indices, and each relates to a value for a single RBC. Accordingly, the units are small and are shown for each as follows.

- **Mean corpuscular volume (MCV)** in femtoliters (fL); femto is one-quadrillionth (10^{-15}).
- **Mean corpuscular hemoglobin (MCH)** in picograms (pg); pico is one-trillionth (10^{-12}).
- **Mean corpuscular hemoglobin concentration (MCHC)** in g/dL (deciliter) or g percent.

Derivations of values are as follows (exponent manipulations completed but not included):

Mean corpuscular volume
$$MCV = (Hct/RBC) \times 10$$
Example: Hct = 42%; RBC = 7 million/μL
$$MCV = (42/7) \times 10 = 60 \, fL$$

Mean corpuscular hemoglobin
$$MCH = ([Hb]/RBC) \times 10$$
Example: [Hb] = 14 g/dL; RBC = 7 million/μL
$$MCH = (14/7) \times 10 = 20 \, pg$$

Mean corpuscular hemoglobin concentration
$$MCHC = ([Hb]/Hct) \times 100$$
Example: [Hb] = 14 g/dL; Hct = 42%
$$MCHC = (14/42) \times 100 = 33.3\%$$

The values for these indices are shown for each species in Table 12.2. The indices are valuable aids in the diagnosis of various anemias.

Lifespan

The lifespan of erythrocytes varies with species. Reported values for horses are 140–150 days. In adult ruminants (cattle, sheep, and goats) erythrocyte lifespan varies from 125 to 160 days, in pigs from 75 to 95 days, in dogs from 100 to 120 days, and from 70 to 80 days in cats. The lifespan of erythrocytes in chickens is 20–30 days.

Fate of erythrocytes

> 1 What cell accounts for removal of about 90% of aged RBCs? What are the organs where this occurs?
>
> 2 How can icterus (jaundice) occur during the degradation of hemoglobin?
>
> 3 How can hemoglobinemia and hemoglobinuria occur as a result of RBC destruction?

As erythrocytes age, several metabolic changes occur: the membrane becomes more rigid and fragile, and the discocyte converts to a poorly deformable spherocyte. Accordingly, some intravascular hemolysis of erythrocytes occurs (10%) and the

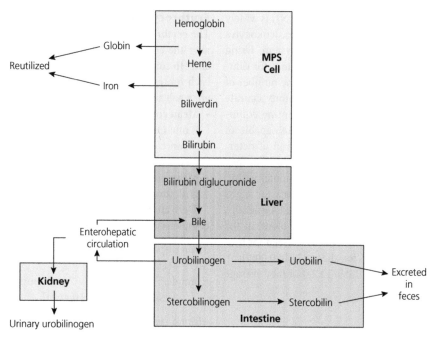

Figure 12.9 Degradation of hemoglobin starts in cells of the mononuclear phagocytic system (MPS). Iron released as shown is used preferentially for synthesis of new hemoglobin. Protein (globin) is degraded to amino acids and reutilized. Bilirubin released from MPS cells is insoluble and combines with a protein (known as free bilirubin) and is transported to the liver, where it is converted to bilirubin diglucuronide (soluble form of bilirubin). The soluble form enters the biliary system and is transported to the intestine. Bacterial reduction of bilirubin diglucuronide produces urobilinogen that may be recirculated via the enterohepatic circulation or further reduced to urobilin or stercobilinogen. Some of the recirculated urobilinogen bypasses the liver, enters the general circulation, and is excreted in the urine. Adapted from Reece, W.O. and Swenson, M.J. (2004) The composition and functions of blood. In: *Dukes' Physiology of Domestic Animals*, 12th edn (ed. W.O. Reece). Cornell University Press, Ithaca, NY. Reproduced with permission from Cornell University Press.

remainder of the aged RBCs (about 90%) is selectively removed from the circulating pool by cells of the MPS, mostly by the fixed cells in the spleen, liver, and bone marrow.

When erythrocytes are phagocytized by MPS cells, they undergo hemolysis within the phagocytic cell (**extravascular or intracellular hemolysis**), and the Hb, other proteins, and membrane lipids of the phagocytized RBCs are catabolized. A summary of Hb degradation that begins in this way is shown in Figure 12.9. The iron and globin are separated from heme, globin is degraded to its amino acids, and both iron and globin amino acids are reutilized. Iron is stored in the MPS cells in the form of **ferritin** and **hemosiderin** or is transferred to plasma, where it combines with a plasma protein, **apotransferrin**, to become **transferrin**. Transferrin circulates to the bone marrow, where the iron is used for the synthesis of new hemoglobin. During Hb synthesis, iron released from decomposing RBCs is used in preference to storage iron.

Heme is converted to **biliverdin** (a green pigment) and then reduced to bilirubin (a yellow pigment). **Free bilirubin** (water-insoluble) is released into the plasma, where it becomes bound to albumin (a plasma protein) and transported to the liver and "dumped." In the liver, the insoluble bilirubin conjugates with glucuronic acid to form **bilirubin glucuronide**, mainly diglucuronide, which is water-soluble. It is secreted into the bile in this form and enters the intestine. Bacteria within the large

intestine reduce bilirubin diglucuronide to **urobilinogen**. Most urobilinogen is excreted with the feces in the oxidized forms of **urobilin** or **stercobilin**, which are pigments that give feces its normal color. Part of the urobilinogen is reabsorbed into the enterohepatic circulation, from which most is re-excreted into the bile. Some of the absorbed urobilinogen bypasses the liver, enters the general circulation, and is excreted in the urine to become a part of the normal pigment of the urine as urobilin. Carbon monoixide (CO) is formed when the porphyrin ring of heme is opened. This is the only reaction in the body in which CO is formed and is excreted by the lungs.

Because of liver disease, free bilirubin combined with albumin might not be "dumped" and would continue to circulate and appear in high concentrations in the plasma and interstitial fluids. Also, if the bile duct becomes blocked, the bilirubin glucuronides (soluble bilirubin) could spill over into the plasma. Both of these conditions can produce a yellow color in the tissues known as **icterus**, or **jaundice**.

When erythrocytes are hemolyzed intravascularly, the Hb is first bound to **haptoglobin** (a plasma protein). This complex is rapidly removed by cells of the MPS, and the Hb is degraded as described above for extravascular hemolysis. Because the complex is a large molecule, it is not filtered through the kidney glomeruli. However, excessive intravascular hemolysis (hemolytic disease) can occur and sufficient

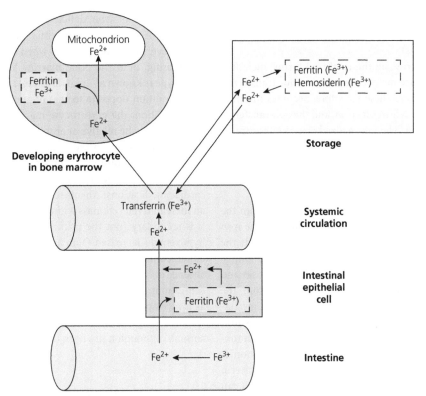

Figure 12.10 Summary of iron absorption, storage, and use. Iron must be in the ferrous (Fe^{2+}) oxidation state to be transported across membranes. Intracellular iron is bound to or incorporated into various proteins or other chelates in its ferric (Fe^{3+}) oxidation state to reduce its toxicity because free iron can catalyze free radicals from molecular oxygen and hydrogen ions and can have disastrous consequences for biological materials. Transported iron is bound to the protein apotransferrin and is known as transferrin. Iron is stored in tissues as either a diffuse, soluble, mobile fraction (ferritin) or as insoluble aggregated deposits (hemosiderin). Principal locations of iron storage are the liver and spleen, followed by the kidney, heart, skeletal muscle, and brain. In the bone marrow, all erythroid forms have surface membrane receptors for transferrin. When internalized, released iron is transported into the mitochondria of developing erythrocytes, where it is incorporated into the heme molecule or it combines with the protein apoferritin to be stored as ferritin. From Reece, W.O. and Swenson, M.J. (2004) The composition and functions of blood. In: *Dukes' Physiology of Domestic Animals*, 12th edn (ed. W.O. Reece). Cornell University Press, Ithaca, NY. Reproduced with permission from Cornell University Press.

haptoglobin might not be available. The plasma takes on a reddish appearance, and the condition is known as **hemoglobinemia**. The free Hb is then filtered at the glomeruli and enters the kidney tubules. Much of it is reabsorbed from the tubules, but can surpass the renal threshold for reabsorption and continue into the urine to give it a reddish color, a condition known as **hemoglobinuria**.

Iron metabolism

1 What is the oxidation state of the storage form of iron?

2 What is the oxidation state of iron for transfer across cell membranes?

3 What is the name of the transport form of iron?

4 Would iron in its transport form be toxic? If not, why not?

5 What are the normal limitations to iron absorption? Can iron toxicity occur as a result of excess ingestion and subsequent absorption?

Free iron (Fe^{3+}) catalyzes the separation of free radicals from molecular oxygen, and oxygen free radicals are toxic. To avoid toxicity, intracellular iron is either bound to or incorporated into various proteins. It is transported and stored in the protein-bound form in its **ferric (Fe^{3+}) oxidation state**. To be transported across membranes, iron must be in its **ferrous (Fe^{2+}) oxidation state**.

A large proportion of ingested iron is reduced to ferrous iron (Fe^{2+}) in the stomach. Within the duodenum and jejunum, most of the ferrous iron is absorbed into the intestinal epithelial cells. Iron absorption, transport, storage, and usage are summarized in Figure 12.10. From the intestinal cell, it enters the blood or can combine with a cellular protein (apoferritin) to become ferritin, a storage form of iron. Within 2 or 3 days, the ferritin is either converted back to its free form (Fe^{2+}) and absorbed into the blood or is cast into the intestinal lumen. The latter situation would be a result of the normal turnover of intestinal epithelial cells as they migrate from the crypts to the tips of the villi, from which they are exfoliated (shed into the lumen). The iron that enters the blood combines with apotransferrin (a plasma protein) to form transferrin. Combining with a protein prevents it from being excreted by the kidneys (the combination is poorly filtered at the glomerulus).

Within the bone marrow, all the erythroid forms, including reticulocytes, have surface membrane receptors for transferrin. Plasma transferrin binds to these receptors, becomes internalized by endocytosis, and releases its iron, and the apotransferrin is returned to the plasma. The internalized iron is either transported into the mitochondria of the developing erythrocyte, where it is incorporated into the heme molecule, or it combines with apoferritin to be stored as ferritin in its ferric (Fe^{3+}) oxidation state.

Two factors generally affect the absorption of iron from the intestinal epithelium into the blood: (i) the extent of the iron stores in the body, and (ii) the rate of erythropoiesis. If the requirement for iron increases and the iron stores are empty, absorption increases. If the requirement for iron decreases and the iron stores are adequate, absorption of iron from the intestine decreases. It seems that there is a self-limiting mechanism for iron absorption based on need. However, excess iron can be ingested and subsequently absorbed, inducing iron toxicity. The excretion of iron is minimal, so that regulation is unidirectional, i.e., controlled absorption. Iron with transferrin can be released to tissue cells anywhere so that excess iron can be deposited in all cells, especially those of the liver. Ferritin is a storage form of iron (see previous text). In addition, a more insoluble form, hemosiderin, accumulates in times of excess. The liver is the principal organ for iron storage. When liver stores are adequate the production of apotransferrin decreases, and when they are depleted the production of apotransferrin increases. Animals with iron-deficiency anemia have high concentrations of apotransferrin.

Anemia and polycythemia

---

1 Define anemia and polycythemia.
2 Without supplemental iron, why would anemia be common in baby pigs?
3 Differentiate between absolute and relative polycythemia.
4 What are some primary conditions that cause absolute polycythemia?

A reduction in the number of erythrocytes, the concentration of hemoglobin, or both is referred to as **anemia**, which can have several causes. It is called a **functional anemia** if erythropoietin production is not stimulated because of lack of exertion, whereby the tissues do not become hypoxic. Blood loss for any reason (e.g., trauma, parasitism) can also cause anemia. A common type of anemia in baby pigs is **iron-deficiency anemia**. This type is common in baby pigs because of their rapid growth and consequent need for greater blood volume, and also because of the lack of iron in their normal diet, which is sow's

milk. Because of iron deficiency, an insufficient quantity of hemoglobin is produced. Anemia can also occur from poor erythrocyte production, such as when certain nutritional factors are missing, or if the bone marrow has been poisoned. This latter type is known as **aplastic anemia**.

A condition opposite to that of anemia is **polycythemia**. In this condition, the erythrocyte mass is greatly increased. The condition may be relative or absolute. In **relative polycythemia**, there is an increase in red cell mass and a decrease in plasma volume. This is commonly encountered in conditions of shock and dehydration and in animals being treated with diuretic or cardiac medications. **Absolute polycythemia** is associated with an increased red cell mass without a decrease in plasma volume. It is secondary (not the primary condition) if associated with hypoxemia (decreased O_2 in arterial blood) or a tumor because either condition increases erythropoietin production. In the absence of hypoxemia or tumors, and when erythropoietin concentrations are normal or decreased, the condition is classified as a myeloproliferative disorder (increased bone marrow production) or **polycythemia vera**. Polycythemia vera is rare in animals, although it has been described in cats, dogs, and cattle.

Hemostasis: prevention of blood loss

---

1 What is the sequence of events from the time of vascular injury to a return to normal?
2 What is the principal chemical component of the clotting factors? Note the major sites of their synthesis.
3 What vitamin is required for the synthesis of several coagulation factors?
4 What chemical element is required for nearly all the hemostatic reactions?
5 What is the substance contained in the basement membrane of capillaries and throughout the interstitial space that provides for platelet adhesion?
6 What are the properties of vascular endothelium that prevent activation of platelets and procoagulants?
7 What is another name for platelets?
8 Study the fine structure of the platelet and relate its structure to the release of the granular contents.
9 What is the first response of platelets to disrupted endothelium and contact with subendothelial tissues?
10 In addition to collagen, what substance is required for the initial adhesion of platelets?
11 What is the principal messenger that is formed after platelet stimulation that will release Ca^{2+} from granule storage?
12 What is the role of aspirin in the blood coagulation scheme?
13 What is the platelet release reaction, and how is it initiated?
14 What is accomplished by platelet aggregation?
15 What are the four key reactions involved in the formation of a clot?
16 What is the relationship of the tenase and prothrombinase complexes to the formation of thrombin?

---

17 Know the difference between the extrinsic and intrinsic systems (tissue factor and contact activation pathways, respectively) and their relationship to each other.

18 In what way is the activation of factor X a focal point in the blood coagulation scheme?

19 What is the significance of factor XIII? What is its origin?

20 How is clot retraction accomplished? What is its function?

21 Once initiated, what prevents blood coagulation from spreading (clot growth)?

22 What is the role of plasmin? What is the principal plasminogen activator?

The effectiveness of blood function depends on its circulation within a closed system of vessels. The vessels might open because of disease or accident, and blood loss can be prevented or minimized by **hemostasis**. Hemostasis is a complicated process and the following summary is provided as an orientation to the details that follow.

When a blood vessel is damaged, endothelial cells are separated, the underlying collagen is exposed, and the surface loses its usual smoothness and nonwettability. Often the vessel is torn, cut, or separated and the hemostatic crisis is exacerbated. Regardless of the severity, platelets begin to contact the damaged surface. This initiates the adhesion process because the platelets develop projections and become sticky. The adhered platelets undergo a reaction in which aggregating agents are released and cause the accumulation of more platelets. When this occurs, blood coagulation soon becomes evident at the damaged site, and the platelet plug is strengthened by the formation of a fibrin meshwork. Clot retraction (reduction in size) occurs, and fibrinolysis (dissolution of fibrin) begins. Finally, the damaged vessel is repaired by connective tissue and endothelial cell growth, and there is a return to normal when the platelet–fibrin complex and other cell debris is removed (Figure 12.11).

Hemostatic components

A complex series of biochemical reactions make up the hemostatic process. The major contributors to the process are proteins, vascular endothelium, and platelets.

Proteins

The protein components of the blood coagulation pathway, their synonyms or common abbreviations, and site of synthesis are presented in Table 12.3. The designation of each factor with a roman numeral was described on first discovery and included factors I–XIII. As shown in Table 12.3, many still persist, but the identification of others was discontinued (e.g., VI was initially described but found later not to exist; IV identified Ca^{2+} and discontinued because it was not a protein). The major components now shown are proteins, and the list has grown because of continued discovery. These proteins are present in the blood or tissues and simply await an activation mechanism.

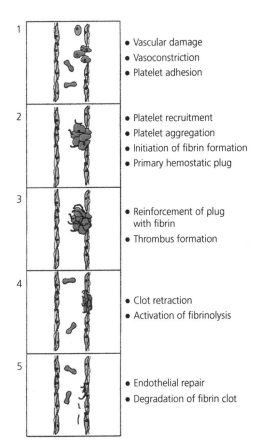

1
- Vascular damage
- Vasoconstriction
- Platelet adhesion

2
- Platelet recruitment
- Platelet aggregation
- Initiation of fibrin formation
- Primary hemostatic plug

3
- Reinforcement of plug with fibrin
- Thrombus formation

4
- Clot retraction
- Activation of fibrinolysis

5
- Endothelial repair
- Degradation of fibrin clot

Figure 12.11 The five major stages in the formation and dissolution of a blood clot, or thrombus, around the site of vascular injury, starting with the initiation of platelet activation after vascular damage and ending with endothelial repair. Adapted from Gentry, P.A. (2004) Blood coagulation and hemostasis. In: *Dukes' Physiology of Domestic Animals*, 12th edn (ed. W.O. Reece). Cornell University Press, Ithaca, NY. Reproduced with permission from Cornell University Press.

It is important to recognize that Ca^{2+} is required for nearly all the reactions and that vitamin K is required for production of prothrombin, protein C, protein S, and factors VII, IX, and X by the liver.

Vascular endothelium

The entire cardiovascular system is lined by a single layer of flattened cells known as the **endothelium**. It not only lines the heart, but also the vessels. At the capillary level, all that remains is the endothelial layer. Regardless of its location, it is underlain with a basement membrane that contains **collagen**. Collagen fibers are also present throughout the interstitial space. Collagen in the subendothelial tissue, as well as **fibronectin** released from endothelial cells, provide for the adhesion of platelets to the site of vascular injury.

As long as the endothelium is intact, the platelets and the proteins associated with blood coagulation (**procoagulants**) are not activated. The properties of the endothelium that prevent activation include (i) the negative charge on the endothelial cell surface that repels the negatively charged platelets; (ii) synthesis of inhibitors of platelet function (e.g., **prostacyclin**) and of fibrin formation

Table 12.3 The major components of the coagulation pathway (enzymes, protein cofactors, and substrates) involved in fibrin formation and fibrin degradation.

Component	Synonym	Site of synthesis
Fibrinogen	Factor I	Liver
Prothrombin	Factor II	Liver*
Thrombin		Plasma
Tissue factor	Thromboplastin	Vascular endothelium
Factor V		Vascular endothelium
Factor VII		Liver*
Factor VIII	Antihemophilic factor	Vascular endothelium
Factor IX	Christmas factor	Liver*
Factor X	Stuart factor	Liver*
Factor XI	Plasma thromboplastin antecedent	Liver
Factor XII	Hageman factor	Liver
Factor XIII	Fibrin stabilizing factor	Liver
von Willebrand factor	vWF	Vascular endothelium
Prekallikrein	PK, Fletcher factor	Liver
High-molecular-weight kininogen	HK, HMWK	Liver
Protein C		Liver*
Protein S		Liver*
Thrombomodulin	TM	Vascular endothelium
Plasminogen		Liver
Tissue-type plasminogen activator	t-PA	Liver
Urokinase-type plasminogen activator	uPA, prourokinase	Unknown

*Vitamin K dependent protein.
Source: Gentry, P.A. (2004) Blood coagulation and hemostasis. In: *Dukes' Physiology of Domestic Animals*, 12th edn (ed. W.O. Reece). Cornell University Press, Ithaca, NY. Reproduced with permission from Cornell University Press.

(e.g., **thrombomodulin**); and (iii) the generation of activators of fibrin degradation (e.g., **tissue plasminogen activator**).

Platelets

Platelets are also known as **thrombocytes**. An appreciation for the complexity of the platelet can be obtained from Figure 12.12. The band of microtubules that encircles the platelet contracts when platelets are activated and results in change of shape and extrusion of platelet granule contents into the open canalicular system and subsequent release from the platelet to its exterior. The granules (α granules and dense granules) contain many of the coagulation factors, other proteins, calcium, serotonin, adenosine disphosphate (ADP), and adenosine triphosphate (ATP), all of which assist or potentiate the coagulation process. Release of granule contents requires energy from the mitochondria and glycogen particles and ionized calcium from the dense tubular system, a component of the membrane system of the platelet.

Platelet reactions

Circulating platelets recruited at the site of vascular injury, where they undergo structural changes. These changes are associated with platelet reactions and, coupled with release of granule components, provide a highly reactive surface for the formation of thrombin and fibrin.

Platelet adhesion

The first response of platelets to disrupted endothelium and contact with subendothelial tissues is their adhesion or attachment to these surfaces. When this happens, a monolayer of platelets adheres to the site and they lose their discoid shape and form **pseudopods** as shown in Figure 12.13. The pseudopods permit greater contact with other platelets flowing by the site of damage and also with those already adhering to the disrupted

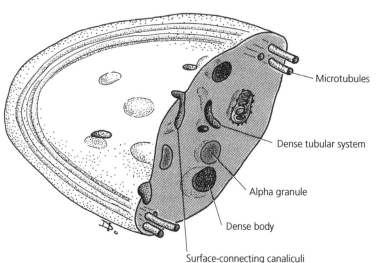

Microtubules

Dense tubular system

Alpha granule

Dense body

Surface-connecting canaliculi

Figure 12.12 Internal details of a platelet discernible at the electron microscope level. Dense bodies are also known as dense granules. Adapted from Cormack, D.H. (2001) *Essential Histology*, 2nd edn. Lippincott Williams & Wilkins, Baltimore. With permission from Lippincott Williams & Wilkins.

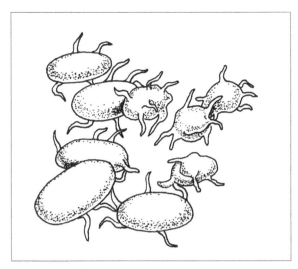

Figure 12.13 Platelet adhesion. This is the first response to blood vessel injury. The platelets lose their discoid shape and form sticky projections (pseudopods) for their continued adherence to the injured vessel and entrapment of other platelets. Adapted from Reece, W.O. (2009) *Functional Anatomy and Physiology of Domestic Animals*, 4th edn. Wiley-Blackwell, Ames, IA. Reproduced with permission from Wiley.

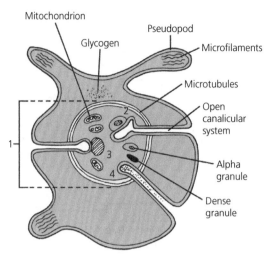

Figure 12.14 Platelet cross-section showing how microtubular contraction results in extrusion of platelet granule contents into the open canalicular system and release from the platelet. (1) Clustering of granules into center of the platelet after microtubular contraction; (2) contact of granule membrane with open canalicular system membrane; (3) fusion of granule membrane with open canalicular system membrane; (4) granule content extruded from open canalicular system. Adapted from MacIntyre, D.E. (1976) The platelet release reaction: association with adhesion and aggregation and comparison with secretory responses in other cells. In: *Platelets in Biology and Pathology*, Vol. 1 (ed. J.L. Gordon). Elsevier, Amsterdam. With permission from Elsevier.

endothelium and exposed subendothelium. The initial adhesion requires collagen that is present in the subendothelium and fibronectin from the endothelial cells. Continued adhesion results from **von Willebrand factor (vWF)** and fibronectin presence in platelet granules that are extruded from activated platelets.

Platelet activation

This is the means whereby platelets are stimulated to begin their further role in assisting hemostasis. The interaction of an **agonist** (e.g., collagen, thrombin, ADP) with its specific receptor on the platelet surface initiates the transmission of a signal through the cell membrane, which in turn activates **intracellular messengers**. Intracellular messenger activation results in the release of Ca^{2+} from storage pools into the platelet cytoplasm. The principal messenger, **thromboxane A$_2$ (TXA$_2$)** is produced from platelet membrane phospholipids after agonist interaction with membrane receptors. Aspirin blocks the formation of TXA$_2$, thus preventing the messenger from mobilizing Ca^{2+} from the granules to the cytoplasm.

Platelet release reaction

This event is initiated by the increase in intracellular calcium in response to the intracellular messenger, and granular contents are secreted. It involves clustering of granular content into the center of the platelet after microtubular contraction and, finally, granule content extrusion to the exterior from the **open canalicular system**. The mechanisms of release are illustrated in Figure 12.14.

Platelet aggregation

The exterior presence of the granule contents provides high concentrations of fibrinogen (needed to form fibrin), fibronectin and vWF (both needed for adhesion), factor V, and other proteins that assist conversion of prothrombin to thrombin at the platelet surface which, by piling platelets on each other, can lead to the formation of the primary platelet plug. After the release reaction, the platelets lose their individual integrity, lipoprotein membranes are fused, receptors are exposed for coagulation proteins (factors), and thus a highly reactive surface (platelet aggregates) is exposed for the formation of thrombin and fibrin.

Clot formation (blood coagulation)

Thrombin formation is the penultimate (next to last) stage in the formation of **fibrin**, which is insoluble and stabilizes the **platelet plug**. The stabilized platelet plug, formed by blood coagulation, is known as the **secondary hemostatic plug or clot**. Once the clot is formed, blood loss through the damaged endothelium is completely stopped. It was recognized previously that, after the platelet reactions, the stage was set for blood coagulation. Most of the proteins that participate in the hemostatic process circulate in plasma as inactive proenzymes, and each undergoes activation in sequence as coagulation proceeds. The sequence is referred to as a **cascade phenomenon** where each reaction represents an amplification point, and a small stimulus results in a larger response.

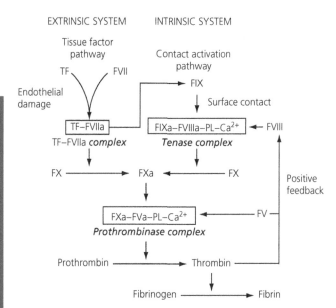

Figure 12.15 The two pathways by which factor (F)X activation can occur. In the extrinsic pathway (tissue factor pathway), activated FX (FXa) is generated by direct action of the tissue factor (TF)–FVIIa complex, whereas in the intrinsic pathway (contact activation pathway) FIXa must combine with FVIII, phospholipids (PL), and Ca^{2+} to form the tenase complex before FX can be activated at a physiologically relevant rate. The final common steps in fibrin formation involve formation of the prothrombinase complex, which activates prothrombin, allowing thrombin to convert fibrinogen to fibrin. From Gentry, P.A. (2004) Blood coagulation and hemostasis. In: *Dukes' Physiology of Domestic Animals*, 12th edn (ed. W.O. Reece). Cornell University Press, Ithaca, NY. Reproduced with permission from Cornell University Press.

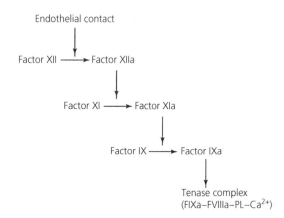

Figure 12.16 The contact phase for the activation of factor IX, initiated when factor XII is activated by contact with damaged endothelium. Factor XIIa activates factor XI (accelerated by prekallikrein and high-molecular-weight kininogen). Activated factor XI, in the presence of Ca^{2+}, activates factor IX (FIXa). FIXa, in association with other components of the tenase complex, allows the activation of factor X and FXa's association with the prothrombinase xomplex. PL, phospholipid. From Reece, W.O. (2009) *Functional Anatomy and Physiology of Domestic Animals*, 4th edn. Wiley-Blackwell, Ames, IA. Reproduced with permission from Wiley.

There are four key reactions involved in the formation of a clot: (i) activation of factor IX, (ii) activation of factor X, (iii) formation of thrombin, and (iv) fibrin formation (Figure 12.15). Activated factor IX (FIXa) is a component of the **tenase complex**, and activated factor X (FXa) is a component of the **prothrombinase complex**. These are key enzyme complexes assembled in close proximity on the surface of platelet aggregates. They accelerate the rate of biochemical cascade reactions resulting in the **generation of thrombin** (Figure 12.15).

Pathways to thrombin formation

The conversion of prothrombin to thrombin (the key enzyme in hemostasis) is catalyzed by the prothrombinase complex, comprising FXa, activated factor V (FVa), phospholipids, and Ca^{2+}. There are two separate activation mechanisms leading to the formation of the prothrombinase complex (see Figure 12.15), the **tissue factor pathway (extrinsic system)** and the **contact activation pathway (intrinsic system)**. The tissue factor pathway begins with a traumatized vascular wall or traumatized extravascular tissues that come in contact with the blood. The contact activation pathway begins with trauma to the blood itself or exposure of the blood to collagen from a traumatized blood vessel wall. The pathways are not independent of each

other and after blood vessel rupture, clotting occurs via both pathways simultaneously. **Tissue factor (TF)**, also known as **thromboplastin**, initiates the tissue factor pathway (see Figure 12.15), whereas contact of FXII and platelets with collagen in the vascular wall initiates the contact activation pathway (Figure 12.16).

Following vascular damage, TF and binding sites for FVII, FIX, and FX are exposed on the surface of endothelial cells. In the presence of Ca^{2+}, the TF–VIIa complex forms first and then activates FIX and FX (see Figure 12.15). Activated FIX (FIXa) can then become a part of the tenase complex without having FIX being activated via FXII in the contact activation pathway as shown in Figure 12.16. The rate of FXa formation by the proteolytic action of the tenase complex occurs at a much faster rate than that produced by the TF–VIIa complex acting alone and, accordingly, provides an amplification step in thrombin generation. In addition, the initial formation of thrombin accelerates FXa production by a positive feedback response that activates FVIII, a component of the tenase complex, and FV, a component of the prothrombinase complex (see Figure 12.15). The contact activation pathway is required to sustain thrombin formation at the site of severe trauma.

After activation of FX, there is a common pathway to the formation of thrombin, after which fibrin is formed from fibrinogen (see Figure 12.15).

Fibrin formation

The final step of blood coagulation is the conversion of **fibrinogen** (a plasma protein) to fibrin. This begins when thrombin has been formed. The first reaction produces fibrin monomers that spontaneously polymerize, and a loosely knit mesh is formed, held together by covalent peptide bonds. This polymer structure is permeable to blood flow and is referred to as soluble fibrin. The stabilization (formation of isopeptide bonds) of soluble fibrin to an insoluble fibrin clot is catalyzed by activated factor XIII (FXIIIa). Factor XIII is released from entrapped platelets, and its conversion to the active form is induced by thrombin in the presence of calcium. Stabilization renders fibrin more elastic and less subject to lysis.

Clot retraction

After stabilization, **clot retraction (shrinking of the clot)** occurs and is provided by the action of the platelet **contractile proteins, thrombosthenin, actin,** and **myosin.** These proteins are exposed when platelets are activated. The activation brings changes that activate thrombosthenin, actin, and myosin to react in a manner analogous to that which occurs during muscle contraction, and the clot retracts (serum is squeezed from the coagulum). Clot retraction permits greater blood flow in the damaged area while the tissue is being repaired. Failures of clot retraction can be associated with reduced platelet numbers.

Clot growth

Once blood coagulation has been initiated, the process extends into the surrounding blood; this is known as **clot growth.** Clot growth stops when blood flows fast enough to remove the thrombin that has been generated; this thrombin has not been otherwise absorbed by the fibrin that is formed and by the other activated factors. The thrombin and activated factors washed away by the blood are not effective because they have been diluted and because natural anticoagulant substances in plasma (e.g., antithrombin III) are present. These substances can prevent unwanted coagulation when procoagulants (substances favoring coagulation) are present in small quantities.

Fibrin degradation

After hemostasis has been established, the damaged vascular area is repaired by new tissue growth assisted by growth factors released from activated platelets. The fibrin that was formed to assist in the hemostatic process undergoes degradation (**fibrinolysis**) by a proteolytic enzyme called **plasmin** (Figure 12.17). **Plasminogen,** a protein present in plasma, becomes entrapped within the clot when it is formed. Plasminogen is activated to become plasmin by substances in blood and tissues known as plasminogen activators. The principal endogenous plasminogen activator is tissue-type plasminogen activator (t-PA), which is released from endothelial cells when they are stimulated by the presence of thrombin or by stasis of blood. Plasmin degrades the fibrin molecule into protein fragments known as **fibrin degradation products (FDPs).** When the outer surface of the fibrin clot is removed, fresh surfaces are exposed and degraded until clot removal is complete. The FDPs, platelets, and other cell debris are removed from the circulation by the MPS. Tissue-type plasminogen activator is produced commercially for human medical use to dissolve clots that are lodged in vessels and that block blood flow (e.g., coronary arteries).

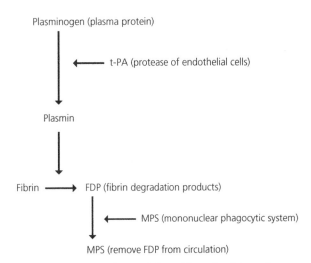

Figure 12.17 The degradation of fibrin (fibrinolysis). From Reece, W.O. (2009) *Functional Anatomy and Physiology of Domestic Animals,* 4th edn. Wiley-Blackwell, Ames, IA. Reproduced with permission from Wiley.

Prevention of blood coagulation

1 What are some preventatives against coagulation in the normal vascular system?

2 How does heparin prevent intravascular clotting?

3 What is the significance of mast cells? Why are there great numbers of them in the lung?

4 How do chelating agents prevent clotting in withdrawn blood?

In addition to procoagulants in the blood, there are also anticoagulants. Their presence balances and prevents coagulation that might otherwise occur because of small amounts of the procoagulants normally present. Also, when blood is withdrawn for analytical purposes or for storage, anticoagulants are added to the blood containers to prevent coagulation.

Prevention in normal circulation

The formation of thrombin occurs via a series of chemical reactions, so it is normal to have a small amount of thrombin in the circulation. The thrombin that is present could cause the conversion of fibrinogen (a normal plasma protein) to fibrin except that another protein, **antithrombin III,** blocks the action of thrombin on fibrinogen and also inactivates the thrombin that it binds.

In addition to antithrombin III action, coagulation in the normal vascular system is prevented by the **smoothness of the endothelium.** This prevents contact activation of factor XII, which is involved in the activation of factor IX in the intrinsic system (see Figure 12.16). Also, a **monomolecular layer of protein (net-negative charge)** is absorbed to the surface of the endothelium that repels clotting factors and platelets. When endothelial damage occurs, both the smoothness and the protein layer are lost at the damaged site.

Heparin, an anticoagulant, is produced by mast cells that reside in the pericapillary connective tissues. Mast cells are particularly abundant in the lungs because of the vulnerability of the lungs to emboli, which are clots that have broken loose from their original site and flow freely in the blood. The plasma concentration of heparin is normally low. The effectiveness of heparin in preventing normal intravascular clotting depends on its combining with antithrombin III to form a complex that removes not only thrombin but also factors IX, X, XI, and XII.

Because of the biological potency of thrombin, there are mechanisms that limit the rate and extent of thrombin generation around sites of vascular damage. One of these, the **anticoagulant protein C pathway**, involves the high-affinity binding of thrombin to **thrombomodulin (TM)**, a membrane protein of endothelial and peripheral blood cells. When bound to TM, thrombin loses its ability to activate platelets and to clot fibrinogen, and becomes an activator of protein C. Activated protein C destroys the activity of factors Va and VIIIa (thrombin modified FV and FVIII), which are cofactors in the prothrombinase and tenase complexes, respectively (see Figure 12.15).

Prevention in withdrawn blood

It is often desirable to prevent blood coagulation when blood is withdrawn from an animal for later examination and analysis. Anticoagulants are used for this purpose. **Chelating agents** are used most frequently; they bind the calcium ions so that they are not available for the coagulation process. Trisodium citrate, sodium oxalate, or ethylenediaminetetraacetic acid (sodium EDTA, disodium salt) is added in an appropriate quantity to the collection container and mixed with the withdrawn blood. Heparin is also available commercially and can be used to prevent coagulation of withdrawn blood. It is also used to prevent coagulation of blood in the body in certain disease conditions that predispose to clot formation.

Tests for blood coagulation

---

1 What is the range in minutes for normal coagulation times among domestic animals by the capillary tube method?

2 Why would low platelet counts be associated with delayed coagulation times?

3 How is dicoumarol associated with coagulation defects?

4 Why would liver disease be suspect as a cause of coagulation defects?

5 How is vWF associated with coagulation defects?

6 Why does blood withdrawn from birds, in which endothelial cell damage does not occur, coagulate with difficulty?

7 In the absence of the contact activation system, why do birds not show hemorrhagic problems?

Tests for blood coagulation are used to determine the adequacy of coagulation in an animal. Several techniques are available. Blood is withdrawn and subjected to standard methods, and the time interval is observed from withdrawal to coagulation. One of these is the capillary tube method, in which the blood is collected directly into a nonheparinized capillary tube. The tube is manually broken at 1-min intervals until the blood in the broken ends remains connected by a fibrin thread. The time in minutes for this to occur is the coagulation time (see Table 12.2 for normal values). A prolonged time interval indicates an inadequate mechanism in the body. Because platelets supply various factors to the coagulation mechanism, in addition to forming a platelet plug, estimation of their number is also helpful in assessing coagulation adequacy.

A common laboratory screening test is the one-stage prothrombin time. In this test, plasma is activated with a mixture of TF and phospholipids. Calcium is added, and the time to coagulation is determined. If clotting time is prolonged, there may be abnormalities in plasma FV, FVII, FX, prothrombin activity, or fibrinogen concentration.

Coagulation defects

Knowledge of the coagulation process is helpful in understanding coagulation defects when they occur. Vitamin K deficiency results in hemorrhage because of inadequate formation of prothrombin and factors VII, IX, and X. Also, dicoumarol interferes with the utilization of vitamin K and hence with prothrombin production.

Dicoumarol is a product of research on a hemorrhagic disease of livestock known as **sweet clover poisoning**. Both yellow and white sweet clover have a high coumarin content that is susceptible to metabolism by several common molds, with resultant dimerization of coumarin when mold growth occurs. Sweet clover hay is thick-stemmed and subject to incomplete drying when harvested and stored (bales, stacks, hay lofts). Mold growth is favored, and dicoumarol is produced. Because of its hemorrhagic properties, dicoumarol is commercially available in rodenticides, in which it is laced with rodent edibles. In human medicine a derivative of dicoumarol is used as a "blood thinner."

Other causes of coagulation defects are related to liver disease, platelet defects, and a complex problem known as disseminated intravascular coagulation, as well as those that are inherited. The most common inherited defects identified in domestic animals are those associated with factor IX activation and formation of the tenase complex. In this category, factor VIII (antihemophilic factor) deficiency is the most widespread. Other common inherited defects are deficiencies of factor IX and vWF. In the latter, platelet aggregates are poorly anchored to the damaged endothelium and are more susceptible to dislodgement by circulating blood. This deficiency is known as **von Willebrand disease (vWD)**.

Species differences

The interaction of activated platelets with damaged endothelium and coagulation proteins is a requirement among all animals for a normal hemostatic mechanism, even though platelet numbers and morphology may vary. The absence of factor XII (a component of the intrinsic mechanism) from the blood of marine mammals and reptiles prolongs the clotting time of their withdrawn blood.

In birds, the entire contact activation pathway appears to be absent, whereby activation of factor IX by that pathway does not occur. This is noticeable if blood is withdrawn atraumatically so that there is neither trauma to blood nor to endothelium. A coagulum will form but serum is extracted with difficulty. For this reason, when chemical analysis is desired, one should use an appropriate anticoagulant and harvest plasma (assuming plasma compatibility with the analysis). The blood will clot extremely rapidly if trauma to the vessel wall occurs during collection. In this case, the TF pathway is activated to form thrombin and associated enhancements to activate the tenase complex (see Figure 12.15). This is the reason that avian species have an intact coagulation mechanism, even though they do not have a functional contact activation system.

Plasma and its composition

> 1 What differentiates plasma from serum?
>
> 2 What is the concentration of protein in plasma?
>
> 3 What are the three major classes of plasma proteins?
>
> 4 Which one of the immunoglobulins is most abundant in normal animals?
>
> 5 What is meant by a state of equilibrium among plasma proteins, amino acids, and tissue proteins?
>
> 6 What plasma protein represents the major contribution to intravascular effective osmotic pressure? Why is this?
>
> 7 Which cation is most abundant in plasma? Which anion?
>
> 8 What is the concentration of glucose in the pig and dog? Is it lower in the ruminants and horse?

Plasma, the noncellular liquid part of blood, may be obtained from drawn blood in which coagulation has been prevented. When blood has been allowed to clot, the coagulation factors are effectively removed, and the liquid is known as serum. All the coagulation factors are present in plasma. Plasma is a complex fluid (containing numerous chemically active substances) that provides the medium of exchange between the blood vessels and the cells of the body. A number of these substances that are often referred to clinically are shown in Table 12.4 for several species. The major constituent of plasma is water (about 92–94%) and the percentage will vary depending mostly on the concentration of protein. Proteins are the most abundant of the substances dissolved or suspended in the water, and their concentration varies from 6 to 8 g/dL.

Plasma proteins

The three major classes of plasma proteins are **albumin, globulins** (α_1, α_2, β_1, β_2, γ), and **fibrinogen.** In humans, sheep, goats, and dogs, albumin predominates over the globulins; in horses,

pigs, cows and cats, the relative proportions of albumin and globulins are nearly equal.

The **gamma-globulins** include proteins called **immunoglobulins** (antibodies) and are produced by lymphocytes and plasma cells. There are five major isotypes of immunoglobulins, which are classified as IgG, IgE, IgA, IgM, and IgD. IgG is the most abundant immunoglobulin of normal animals. It crosses the dam's placental barrier to provide immunity to newborns in some species (primates and rodents) but not others. In the latter, transfer depends on the presence of IgG in colostrum and early ingestion by the newborn. IgE, IgA, IgM, and IgD provide the immune response to allergic conditions or parasitisms (release of histamine), the microorganisms present in the mouth and gastrointestinal tract (via colostrum), activation of the complement system, and clone formation of lymphocytes, respectively.

The **alpha and beta globulins** serve as the substrates for new substances and also perform transport functions (e.g., lactoferrin, a globulin that transports iron).

Origin

Plasma albumin, some of the globulins, and fibrinogen (and other coagulation factors) are formed in the liver. The balance of the globulins, including the gamma-globulins, is formed in the lymph nodes and mucosal tissues.

The plasma proteins, amino acids, and tissue proteins are in a state of equilibrium (Figure 12.18). When the amino acid concentration in tissue cells decreases below that of plasma, amino acids enter the cells and are used for synthesis of essential plasma and tissue proteins. The plasma proteins, formed mainly in the liver, may also be broken down into amino acids by MPS cells and made available for cellular protein synthesis. This occurs especially when the amino acid supply from digestive processes is inadequate. Plasma proteins do leak from capillaries into the interstitial fluid and are returned to the blood via the lymphatics. In this way, there is a 12- to 24-hour turnover (time within which all protein is leaked and returned).

Plasma proteins and colloidal osmotic pressure

The **plasma colloidal osmotic pressure** (also called **oncotic pressure**) is the **effective osmotic pressure of the plasma** (see Chapter 36). It is intimately associated with the balance of body fluids between the intravascular and interstitial fluid compartments. It arises because of the presence of the protein molecules and cations retained by the net negative charge of protein. The proteins are colloidal and nondiffusible. The effective osmotic pressure produced by these molecules opposes the hydrostatic pressure of blood in the capillaries and is responsible for reabsorption of fluid at the venous end of capillaries. The albumins account for about 80% of the plasma colloidal osmotic pressure because of their abundance and smaller molecular weight. The osmotic pressure that each protein fraction contributes is inversely related to the molecular

Table 12.4 Values (range) of some constituents of blood from mature domestic animals.

Constituent	Horse	Cow	Sheep	Pig	Dog	Chicken
Glucose (mg/dL)	60–110	40–80	40–80	80–120	70–120	130–270
		80–120 (calf)		80–120 (lamb)		
Nonprotein nitrogen (mg/dL)	20–40	20–40	20–38	20–45	17–38	20–35
Urea nitrogen (BUN) (mg/dL)	10–24	10–30	8–20	8–24	10–30	0.1–1.0
Uric acid (mg/dL)	0.5–1	0.1–2	0.1–2	0.1–2	0.1–1.5	1–2
						1–7 (laying hen)
Creatinine (mg/dL)	1–2	1–2	1–2	1–2.5	1–2	1–2
Amino acid nitrogen (mg/dL)	5–7	4–8	5–8	6–8	7–8	4–10
Lactic acid (mg/dL)	10–16	5–20	9–12		8–20	47–56
						20–98 (laying hen)
Cholesterol (mg/dL)	75–150	80–180	60–150	60–200	120–250	125–200
Bilirubin						
Direct (mg/dL)	0–0.4	0–0.3	0–0.3	0–0.3	0.06–0.1	
Indirect (mg/dL)	0.2–5	0.1–0.5	0–0.1	0–0.3	0.01–0.5	
Total (mg/dL)	0.2–6	0.2–1.5	0.1–0.4	0–0.6	0.10–0.6	
Electrolytes (mEq/L)						
Sodium	132–152	132–152	139–152	135–150	141–155	151–161
Potassium	2.5–5.0	3.9–5.8	3.9–5.4	4.4–6.7	3.7–5.8	4.6–4.7
Calcium	4.5–6.5	4.5–6.0	4.5–6.0	4.5–6.5	4.5–6.0	4.5–6.0
						8.5–19.5
						(laying hen)
Phosphorus	2–6	2–7	2–7	3–6	2–6	3–6
Magnesium	1.5–2.5	1.5–2.5	1.8–2.3	2–3	1.5–2.0	
Chlorine	99–109	97–111	95–105	94–106	100–115	119–130

Source: Reece, W.O. and Swenson, M.J. (2004) The composition and functions of blood. In: *Dukes' Physiology of Domestic Animals*, 12th edn (ed. W.O. Reece). Cornell University Press, Ithaca, NY. Reproduced with permission from Cornell University Press.

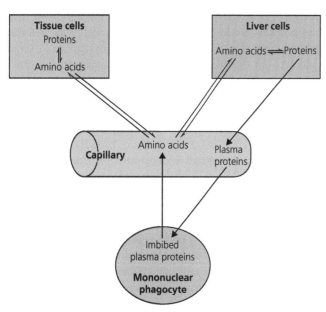

Figure 12.18 Reversible equilibrium among the tissue proteins, plasma proteins, and plasma amino acids. Adapted from Reece, W.O. and Swenson, M.J. (2004) The composition and functions of blood. In: *Dukes' Physiology of Domestic Animals*, 12th edn (ed. W.O. Reece). Cornell University Press, Ithaca, NY. Reproduced with permission from Cornell University Press.

weight and directly related to its concentration in terms of number of particles in the plasma (recall that osmotic pressure relates to particle numbers rather than mass). The molecular weights of fibrinogen, albumin, and globulins are approximately 300,000, 70,000, and 180,000, respectively. The molecular weight of fibrinogen is high and its plasma concentration is low, so its contribution to colloidal osmotic pressure is small. When the concentrations of globulins and albumin are nearly the same, albumin contributes two to three times as much osmotic pressure as globulins because there are two to three times more molecules (particles) in albumin than in an equal weight (concentration) of globulin.

Because of the many functions of plasma proteins, it is apparent that liver disease and resultant failure of adequate protein synthesis, or prolonged dietary protein deficiency, can lead to many body function problems.

Other plasma constituents

Oxygen, carbon dioxide, and nitrogen are the major gases of the atmosphere and are found in plasma. Their concentration in plasma depends on their concentration in the atmosphere and on their solubility in plasma. The major types of lipids in plasma are triglycerides, phospholipids, and cholesterol. The principal nonprotein nitrogen (NPN) compounds are amino acids, urea, uric acid, creatine, creatinine, and ammonium salts. Inorganic substances in the plasma are represented mainly by the electrolytes, including cations (Na^+, K^+, Ca^{2+}, Mg^{2+}) and anions (Cl^-, HCO_3^-, HPO_4^{2-}). Values for many of these constituents are shown in Table 12.4.

Self-evaluation

Answers can be found at the end of the chapter.

1 Intravascular hemolysis has occurred and hemoglobinemia is apparent, so:
   A Hemoglobinuria will never be present
   B Hemoglobinuria will always follow
   C Hemoglobinuria presence will depend on the amount of hemolysis
   Explain your choice for the correct answer.

2 Icterus is very visible in a dog. Which one of the following would indicate obstructive jaundice as being part of the problem?
   A Dark yellow urine
   B No urobilinogen in urine
   C Recent episode of hemolytic disesase
   Explain your choice for the correct answer.

3 Erythropoiesis associated with iron deficiency results in:
   A Microcytic hypochromic anemia
   B Microcytic hyperchromic anemia
   Explain your choice for the correct answer.

4 Which one of the following leukocytes is often increased in numbers in the presence of either local inflammatory reactions of allergic origin or certain types of parasitisms?
   A Neutrophils
   B Eosinophils
   C Monocytes
   D Lymphocytes
   Explain your choice for the correct answer.

5 Hematology data for two calves:

	Calf 1	Calf 2
RBC ($\times 10^6$/µL)	6.8	9.0
Hct (%)	23.0	33.0
Hb (g/dL)	7.0	11.5

Which calf has microcytic hypochromic anemia? (The other calf is normal.)
   A Calf 1
   B Calf 2
   Explain your choice for the correct answer.

6 Which one of the following cells might become more prevalent in circulating blood during a prolonged period of erythropoietin secretion?
   A Platelet
   B Monocyte
   C Reticulocyte
   D Eosinophil
   Explain your choice for the correct answer.

7 The ranges for the percentage of each leukocyte (relative) and absolute numbers of each leukocyte for cattle, based on a total leukocyte count of 7000–10,000/µL, are as follows.

	Relative	Absolute
Neutrophil	25–30	1750–3000
Lymphocyte	60–65	4200–6500
Monocyte	5	350–500
Eosinophil	2–5	140–500
Basophil	<1	<100

The total white blood cell count in week 1 for "Elsie" (the Borden cow) was 8000/µL and the distribution of neutrophils and lymphocytes was 30 and 60%, respectively. In week 2, Elsie's white blood cell count was 25,000/µL and the distribution was 70% for neutrophils and 20% for lymphocytes.
   A When was the distribution for neutrophils and lymphocytes normal (week 1, week 2)?
   B What is the absolute number of lymphocytes and neutrophils for each week?
   C When was there a leukocytosis (week 1, week 2)?
   D Was there a neutropenia shown in either week?
   E Was there a neutrophilic leukocytosis (neutrophilia) shown in either week?
   F Was there a lymphopenia shown in either week?
   G Was there a lymphocytosis shown in either week?

8 Which one of the following most closely approximates the number of erythrocytes in domestic animals?
   A 7,000,000/animal
   B 7,000,000/mL
   C 7000/µL
   D 7,000,000/µL

9 A Brown Swiss steer that weighs 1800 lb (817 kg) has a blood volume about 8% of its body weight? What is its blood volume in milliliters?

10 Arterial blood changes from bright red to a darker purplish color when it becomes venous blood. Which one of the following causes this?
   A Loss of oxygen
   B Gain of carbon dioxide

Suggested reading

Feldman, B.F., Zinkl, J.G. and Jain, N.C. (2000) *Schalm's Veterinary Hematology*, 5th edn. Lippincott Williams & Wilkins, Baltimore.

Gentry, P.A. (2004) Blood coagulation and hemostasis. In: *Dukes' Physiology of Domestic Animals*, 12th edn (ed. W.O. Reece). Cornell University Press, Ithaca, NY.

Section II: Body Fluids and Homeostasis

Jackson, M.L. (1987) Platelet physiology and platelet function: inhibition by aspirin. *Compendium on Continuing Education for the Practising Veterinarian* 9:627.

Jain, N.C. (1993) *Essentials of Veterinary Hematology.* Lea & Febiger, Philadelphia.

Reece, W.O. and Swenson, M.J. (2004) The composition and functions of blood. In: *Dukes' Physiology of Domestic Animals*, 12th edn (ed. W.O. Reece). Cornell University Press, Ithaca, NY.

Answers

1 C. With intravascular hemolysis, hemoglobin becomes free in the plasma. If not excessive, the free hemoglobin is bound to haptoglobin and the combination presents a molecular complex too large to be filtered at the glomerulus. With excessive hemolysis, there is insufficient haptoglobin and uncombined hemoglobin begins to be filtered. There is a limited capacity for endocytosis of hemoglobin by the tubular epithelium and hemoglobin can continue through the tubules and appear in the urine (hemoglobinuria). As water is reabsorbed from the tubules, hemoglobin concentration may increase to the point where the hemoglobin precipitates, causing acute renal failure.

2 B. Bilirubin is conjugated (made soluble) in the liver and transported to the small intestine via the bile duct. In the small intestine, bacterial action converts bilirubin to urobilinogen and finally to stercobilin. Some of the urobilinogen is reabsorbed into the portal circulation, and that part not recirculated to the intestine can be filtered at the glomerulus and appear in the urine. Bile duct obstruction would prevent the entry of conjugated bilirubin into the intestine and account for the absence of urobilinogen in the urine. Hemolytic disease would increase the concentration of free bilirubin, and unobstructed bile flow would permit its conjugated form to enter the small intestine with conversion to urobilinogen. Although bilirubin or its degradation products may give urine a darker color than normal, it is also recognized that other factors (e.g., concentrated urine) contribute to a darker color.

3 A. Iron deficiency causes a lag in hemoglobin synthesis. When 20% of hemoglobin is formed, DNA synthesis ceases and cell replication is discontinued. Because of the lag in hemoglobin synthesis, DNA synthesis and mitotic divisions continue, resulting in smaller cells (microcytic) that have less hemoglobin (hypochromic).

4 B. Eosinophils help dampen the inflammatory response associated with immediate-type hypersensitivity reactions by releasing histaminase to inactivate the histamine released by mast cells. They also attach to opsonized parasites and release their proteases onto the parasite surface, inflicting lethal damage.

5 A. Calf 1 has the microcytic hypochromic anemia according to the erythrocyte indices below:

	Calf 1	Calf 2
MCV (fL)	33.8	36.0
MCH (pg)	10.3	12.8
MCHC (%)	31.4	34.8

6 C. Reticulocyte numbers are often increased when there is an acute need for replenishment of erythrocytes (e.g., traumatic injuries causing rupture of the spleen). The continued erythropoietin secretion brings forth continued early release of reticulocytes into the circulating blood.

7 A. The respective absolute number for neutrophils and lymphocytes is 2400 and 4800/μL for week 1 and 17 500 and 5000/μL for week 2. Both values for week 1 are within the accepted range.

   B. Lymphocytes: week 1, 4800/μL; week 2, 5000/μL. Neutrophils: week 1, 2400/μL; week 2, 17 500/μL.

   C. Week 2 when the white blood cell count was 25 000/μL.

   D. No; the low value of 2400/μL is still within range.

   E. Yes; week 2 because 17 500/μL is beyond the range.

   F. No; the low value of 4800/μL is still within range.

   G. No; the high value of 5000/μL is still within range.

8 D

9 8% of 1800 pounds = 144 pounds of blood = 144 pints; 8 pints = 1 gallon, therefore 144/8 = 18 gallons.

10 A

13 Fundamentals of Acid–Base Balance

William O. Reece

Iowa State University, Ames, IA, USA

Acid–base balance in the body fluids is an impressive illustration of homeostasis and is one of the most vigorously regulated variables of the body. The relatively constant hydrogen ion concentration [H⁺] is the result of a balance between acids and bases. Under normal conditions, acids or bases are added continuously to the body fluids, either because of their ingestion or as a result of their production in cellular metabolism. In disease, an unusual loss or gain of acid or base may occur as a result of metabolic disease, insufficient respiratory ventilation, vomiting, diarrhea, or renal insufficiency. In many of these instances, fluid therapy is required for treatment. Therefore, a knowledge of acid–base physiology is essential in order to facilitate fluid and electrolyte therapy.

Introduction to acid–base balance

> 1 What are the respective changes in hydrogen ion concentration when the pH is increased and when the pH is decreased?
>
> 2 Is it an acid or a base that accepts and binds hydrogen ions from a solution?
>
> 3 How do the definitions of the terms "acidemia" and "alkalemia" differ from their respective counterparts of acidosis and alkalosis?
>
> 4 What is the chemical equation that is referred to as the hydration reaction?

The regulation of acid–base balance actually means regulation of [H⁺] in the body fluids. The [H⁺] is usually expressed in terms of pH, which is the negative log of the hydrogen ion concentration.

Relationship of pH to H⁺ concentration

The pH of the **extracellular fluid (ECF)** seldom varies from the normal value of 7.4. Relatively small pH changes are associated with correspondingly large changes in H⁺ concentration. For example, a pH of 7.4 represents a [H⁺] of 40 nEq/L. A decrease of pH from 7.4 to 7.1 (0.3 units) doubles the [H⁺] from 40 to 80 nEq/L. When the pH is increased from 7.4 to 7.7 (0.3 units), the [H⁺] is halved from 40 to 20 nEq/L. Enzymatic reactions in the cells of the body operate optimally within a very narrow range of pH. Therefore, mechanisms are present in the body to make corrections for the deviations that normally occur.

Terminology

Acids are defined as substances that donate hydrogen ions to a solution and **bases** are defined as substances that accept and bind hydrogen ions from a solution. An application of these definitions will assist in a better understanding and is presented in the section Hemoglobin and other proteins.

The normal range of blood pH may be assumed to be 7.35 to 7.45. Depression of pH below the normal range is known as **acidemia**; elevation above the normal range is called **alkalemia**. An acidemia is mildly abnormal when the pH varies between

Dukes' Physiology of Domestic Animals, Thirteenth Edition. Edited by William O. Reece, Howard H. Erickson, Jesse P. Goff and Etsuro E. Uemura.

Companion website: www.wiley.com/go/reece/physiology

7.20 and 7.35, and seriously abnormal when less than 7.20. An alkalemia is mildly abnormal when the pH varies between 7.45 and 7.60, and seriously abnormal when greater than 7.60.

A disturbance caused by the addition of excess acid or removal of base from the ECF is known as **acidosis**. If it is caused by the addition of excess base or the loss of acid, it is known as **alkalosis**.

The metabolism of most organic compounds containing carbon, hydrogen, oxygen, and nitrogen results in the formation of water, carbon dioxide, and urea. Carbon dioxide reacts with water to form carbonic acid, which dissociates to hydrogen and bicarbonate ions as follows:

$$CO_2 + H_2O \leftrightarrow H_2CO_3 \leftrightarrow H^+ + HCO_3^- \qquad (13.1)$$

This is a reversible reaction known as the **hydration reaction**. The hydration reaction will be referred to many times in renal and respiratory physiology. The reversal occurs when carbon dioxide is expired.

Maintenance of acid–base balance

1 What is the definition of a chemical buffer system?

2 What is the weak acid component and its conjugate base for each of the bicarbonate and phosphate chemical buffer systems?

3 Why is the bicarbonate buffer system regarded as the most important buffer system in the body?

4 Why is the phosphate buffer system of greater value in the intracellular fluid and the tubular fluid in the kidneys?

5 How is buffering by the imidazole group of hemoglobin associated with oxygenation and deoxygenation in the lungs?

6 After conversion to arterial blood in the lungs and in its return to the tissues, is hemoglobin in its basic form or its acidic form?

7 After loading of hydrogen ions from the tissue, and as it returns to the lungs, is hemoglobin in its basic form or in its acidic form?

8 What is the mechanism for the renal secretion of hydrogen ion that is associated with the bicarbonate buffer system?

9 What is the mechanism for the renal secretion of hydrogen ions associated with the phosphate buffer system?

10 What is the mechanism for the excretion of ammonium ions to accommodate for excess hydrogen ions and facilitate for limitations of the phosphate system?

Mechanisms for maintenance of the relatively constant [H⁺] in body fluids are provided by chemical buffer systems, the respiratory system, and the kidneys.

Chemical buffer systems

A **chemical buffer system** consists of a mixture of a weak acid and its conjugate base. An example is a solution of carbonic acid and bicarbonate ion. When a buffer system is present, the addition of an acid or base will result in a much smaller shift of pH than would occur if no buffers were present.

The **Henderson–Hasselbalch equation** describes the relationship between pH and the mixture of a weak acid and its conjugate base as follows:

$$pH = pK_a + \log \frac{\left[Base \right]}{\left[Acid \right]} \qquad (13.2)$$

As used in the Henderson–Hasselbalch equation, K_a is the **dissociation constant** for dissociation of the weak acid component. Thus, $pH = pK_a$ when base and acid are equal (i.e., the pH at which the ratio of base to acid is 1). This is illustrated by the titration curve for the bicarbonate buffer system in Figure 13.1.

An optimal buffer system for keeping the pH of the body fluids close to 7.40 would have pK_a close to 7.40 and be present in a high concentration. The following buffer systems may differ somewhat from these criteria, but possess their own uniqueness.

Bicarbonate buffer system

The weak acid component of the **bicarbonate buffer system** is H_2CO_3 and the conjugate base is HCO_3^-. They react with strong acid and strong base as follows:

$$HCl + NaHCO_3 \leftrightarrow H_2CO_3 + NaCl \qquad (13.3)$$

$$NaOH + H_2CO_3 \leftrightarrow NaHCO_3 + H_2O \qquad (13.4)$$

In equation 13.3, the basic component of the system reacts with an acid to form a weaker acid and a salt. In equation 13.4, the weak acid component reacts with a base to form a weaker base and water.

Total CO_2 of plasma exists in three forms: dissolved CO_2, carbonic acid, and bicarbonate ions. Dissolved CO_2 is in equilibrium with carbonic acid as expressed by the equation

$$CO_2 + H_2O \leftrightarrow H_2CO_3 \qquad (13.5)$$

The equilibrium of this equation is far to the left, and in plasma the concentration of dissolved CO_2 is about 1000 times higher than the concentration of carbonic acid. However, the concentration of dissolved CO_2 and carbonic acid is directly proportional to the partial pressure of CO_2 (Pco_2), and their sum, of which the concentration of dissolved CO_2 is the greater part, is related to Pco_2 by a constant, a, where a is equal to 0.03. Accordingly, because the concentration of H_2CO_3 is difficult to measure, as compared to the relative ease of measuring the partial pressure of CO_2, the Henderson–Hasselbalch equation is expressed as:

$$pH = pK_a + \frac{\left[HCO_3^- \right]}{a\,PCO_2} \qquad (13.6)$$

The pK_a of the bicarbonate buffer system is 6.1, so it does not appear to represent an optimal buffer system for blood with a

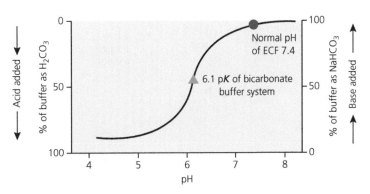

Figure 13.1 Titration curve for the bicarbonate buffer system. The pH (6.1) is equal to the pK when the base ($NaHCO_3$) and acid (H_2CO_3) are equal, which represents the greatest buffering power. Relative effectiveness of the system ranges between pH 5 and pH 7. Buffering power for the extracellular fluid is much less because normal pH is 7.4.

pH of 7.4. Nevertheless, the bicarbonate buffer system can be regarded as the most important buffer system in the body because the concentrations of its components can be independently regulated, i.e., the CO_2 concentration by the lungs and the bicarbonate concentration by the kidneys.

Phosphate buffer system

The phosphate buffer system is represented by NaH_2PO_4, the weak acid, and Na_2HPO_4, the conjugate base. They react with acid and base in a manner similar to the bicarbonate buffer system as follows:

$$HCl + Na_2HPO_4 \leftrightarrow NaH_2PO_4 + NaCl \qquad (13.7)$$

$$NaOH + NaH_2PO_4 \leftrightarrow Na_2HPO_4 + H_2O \qquad (13.8)$$

In the bicarbonate and phosphate reaction with a strong acid, a weaker acid and a salt of the strong acid are formed, and in reactions with a strong base, a weaker base and water are formed. The concentration of the phosphate buffers in the ECF is relatively low and is about one-sixth of that of the bicarbonate buffers. Accordingly, this buffer system plays a minor role in the blood. It is more important in the intracellular fluid (ICF) because of its greater concentration and the pK_a of the phosphate buffer system is 6.8. The intracellular pH generally is somewhat lower than the extracellular pH and therefore closer to the pK_a of the phosphate buffer. Also, the phosphate buffer system of the kidneys is effective in buffering the tubular fluid because (i) it becomes greatly concentrated in the tubular fluid due to the reabsorption of water in excess of phosphate and (ii) the pH of the tubular fluid generally becomes more acidic (carnivores) than the pH of the ECF, and therefore closer to the pK_a of the phosphate buffer system.

Hemoglobin and other proteins

Proteins are buffers because their molecules contain a large number of acidic and basic groups. The basic groups (RNH_2) act as buffers by accepting hydrogen ions forming cations (RNH_3^+). The plasma proteins are not a significant buffer for the blood, but the proteins of the body cells, coupled with the cellular phosphate buffers, and taken as an aggregate, are important to total body acid–base balance.

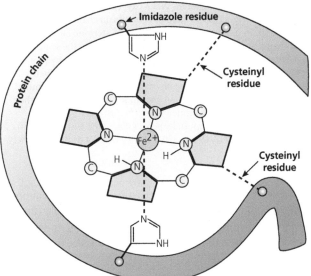

Figure 13.2 Schematic representation of one heme group and its associated polypeptide chain. Four of these combinations, at different orientations to each other, make up hemoglobin. The heme is held to its specific polypeptide chain (one of four in the protein globin) by cysteine (an amino acid) bridges and by bonding of the iron to imidazole groups of histidine (an amino acid). Molecular oxygen binds with iron. Adapted from Conn, E.E. and Stumpf, P.K. (1963) *Outlines of Biochemistry*. John Wiley & Sons, New York.

Hemoglobin is a complex iron-containing conjugated protein known as globin, a histone (Figure 13.2). Hemoglobin is a buffer because its molecule contains a large number of acidic and basic groups as described above and other types of buffering groups such as the **imidazole** groups of **histidine**. Histidine is an amino acid and has imidazole residues that bond with iron of the heme groups. Much of the buffering by oxyhemoglobin in the physiological range is done by the imidazole groups.

Hydrogen ions are accommodated by hemoglobin as follows:
1 Combination with the basic carboxyl groups, suppressing their ionization and forming dissociated groups:

$$R-COO^- + H^+ \leftrightarrow RCOOH \qquad (13.9)$$

2 Combination with imidazole groups of hemoglobin. The chemical buffering action of the imidazole groups of

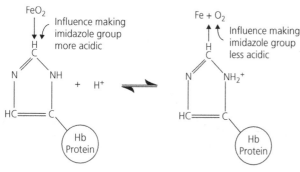

Figure 13.3 Schematic representation of the effect of oxygenation and deoxygenation of the chemical buffering action of the imidazole group ($C_3H_4N_2$) of hemoglobin. When oxygenated hemoglobin is deoxygenated (right) the β chains of hemoglobin change their shape (not shown). In their new conformation, the C-terminal histidines in the β chains react with the aspartates at position 94 in the same chain. This interaction raises the apparent pK of the imidazole group of the histidines, and hydrogen ions are taken up from solution. When deoxygenated hemoglobin is again oxygenated (left), the C-terminal histidines become free in solution once more; their pK falls and they give off hydrogen ions. Reprinted from *The ABC of Acid–Base Chemistry* by H.W. Davenport, by permission of the University of Chicago Press. © 1947, 1949, 1950, 1958, 1969, 1974 by the University of Chicago.

hemoglobin is affected by oxygenation and deoxygenation of hemoglobin. Imidazole groups become more acidic (donate H^+) when hemoglobin is oxygenated in the lungs, and become more basic (accept H^+) when hemoglobin is deoxygenated in the tissues (Figure 13.3).

Isohydric principle

The buffers of the blood and body fluids do not act independent of each other, but rather react in unison. When hydrogen ions are added to the ECF, each base of each buffer pair will bind hydrogen ions and share the acid load; the buffers buffer the buffers. This is known as the **isohydric principle**.

Role of the respiratory system

In addition to the chemical buffers that are involved with regulating pH of the body fluids, the respiratory system and kidneys are major contributors. The transport of carbon dioxide is facilitated by several reactions that effectively provide other CO_2 forms in addition to that which is in solution. Even though CO_2 is more soluble in water than O_2, the amount produced exceeds the amount that can be carried in solution. About 80% of CO_2 transport occurs in the form of bicarbonate (HCO_3^-). Its formation results from the hydration reaction (see equation 13.1) The equilibrium of the hydration reaction is far to the left in plasma and the plasma reaction accounts for little transport of CO_2. The hydration reaction is favored within erythrocytes because of the presence of the enzyme carbonic anhydrase and it proceeds with ease, forming H^+ and HCO_3^-. It would be a rate-limited reaction, however, if the reaction products (H^+ and HCO_3^-) were not removed. Removal is accomplished by chemical

buffering of the H^+ by imidazole groups and by diffusion of HCO_3^- out of the erythrocytes into the plasma. These reactions are shown in Figure 13.4. Not all the hydrogen ions are buffered, so venous blood has a lower pH than arterial blood. Also, because of the diffusion of HCO_3^- from erythrocytes to plasma, venous blood has a higher HCO_3^- concentration than arterial blood.

When the venous blood reaches the alveoli and the pressure difference favors diffusion of CO_2 in solution from the plasma to the alveoli, there is a prompt reversal of the hydration reaction with loss of CO_2. The venous blood becomes arterial blood and hemoglobin again becomes basic.

Hemoglobin is the most plentiful compound available for buffering H^+ formed during the hydration reaction. When hemoglobin is deficient, as in anemia, buffering of H^+ from all sources is jeopardized and acidemia results during periods of increased H^+ production, such as exertion.

Increased P_{CO_2} and increased H^+ concentration each stimulate increases in pulmonary ventilation (see Chapter 24). The response results in greater removal of CO_2 and associated reduction in hydrogen ions.

Role of the kidneys

The epithelial cells of the proximal tubules, distal tubules, and collecting ducts all secrete hydrogen ions. About 85% of hydrogen ions are secreted by the cells of the proximal tubule. Increases in ECF carbon dioxide cause increased H^+ secretion, and decreases in ECF carbon dioxide decrease H^+ secretion. Also, high intracellular pH (which includes tubular epithelial cells) associated with alkalemia and hypocapnia (low P_{CO_2}) depress H^+ secretion, and low intracellular pH caused by acidemia and hypercapnia (high P_{CO_2}) increase H^+ secretion (see section Hypokalemia and hyperkalemia).

The mechanism for the secretion of H^+ associated with the bicarbonate buffer system is shown in Figure 13.5. Carbon dioxide diffuses from the interstitial fluid into the tubular epithelial cell and hydration with water is facilitated by carbonic anhydrase to form carbonic acid. The equilibrium is to the right and carbonic acid dissociates forming HCO_3^- and H^+. The H^+ is secreted into the tubular lumen by a countertransport mechanism with Na^+ in the tubular lumen. The Na^+ is transported via active transport into the interstitial fluid (ISF). Electrical neutrality is maintained by the simultaneous movement of tubular Na^+ into the ISF with HCO_3^-. It should be noted that the HCO_3^- reabsorbed to the ISF is not the same HCO_3^- as in tubular fluid. Also, it should be noticed in Figure 13.5, that the H^+ transported to the tubular lumen combines with HCO_3^- to form H_2CO_3. Carbonic anhydrase on the luminal brush border surface of the proximal tubular epithelial cell promotes dissipation of H_2CO_3 to CO_2 and H_2O. Under normal balance conditions, the amount of H^+ secretion is about the same as the amount of HCO_3^- filtered at the glomerulus and the pH of the urine formed falls little. When the rate of HCO_3^- filtration exceeds the rate of H^+ secretion, all the secreted H^+

Section II: Body Fluids and Homeostasis

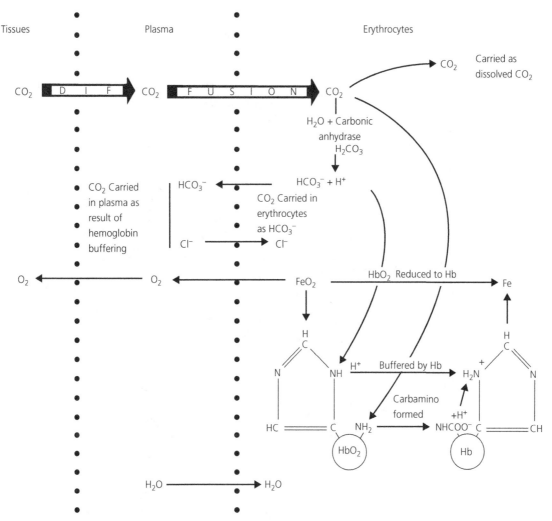

Figure 13.4 Schematic representation of the processes occurring when carbon dioxide diffuses from tissues into erythrocytes. The reactions shown as occurring in erythrocytes provide for the principal methods of transporting carbon dioxide from the cells to the lungs. Reprinted from *The ABC of Acid–Base Chemistry* by H.W. Davenport, by permission of the University of Chicago Press. © 1947, 1949, 1950, 1958, 1969, 1974 by the University of Chicago.

react with filtered HCO_3^-, and the bicarbonate that escapes reaction with H^+ appears in the alkaline urine.

Animals with advanced renal disease frequently become acidotic due to a reduced capacity for H^+ secretion and its associated reduced HCO_3^- reabsorption. Also, pharmacologic agents that inhibit carbonic anhydrase cause a reduction in H^+ secretion and HCO_3^- reabsorption, thereby contributing to acidemia.

When larger amounts of H^+ ions are secreted into the tubules and exceed tubular HCO_3^- buffering, they proceed to the distal nephrons. At these locations, the capacity to secrete H^+ ions is limited when the tubular pH is lowered to pH 4.5. Prior to this, the phosphate buffer system is important. Recall that the optimal buffer system is one where the pK_a of the system is close to the fluid being buffered and where the buffer is present in high concentration. In the proximal tubule, the concentration of the phosphate buffer components (HPO_4^{2-} and $H_2PO_4^-$) is very low

and therefore not a significant buffering factor. In the distal nephrons, the phosphate concentration in the tubular fluid is significantly increased due to reabsorption of water in excess of phosphate. Also, its pK_a of 6.8 is more adapted for acidic urine. The mechanism for the renal secretion of H^+ associated with the phosphate buffer system is shown in Figure 13.6.

The amount of available phosphate remains relatively constant, even in acidotic conditions, when the kidneys must excrete additional H^+ ions. To accommodate the additional H^+ ions, a large fraction of excess H^+ ions is excreted in the form of ammonium ions (NH_4^+). This process accommodates for the limitations of the phosphate system. The process begins in the liver with the NH_4^+ that is an end product of protein metabolism. If NH_4^+ is used in the synthesis of urea, H^+ ions are released and contribute to the urea load. However, some of this NH_4^+ is diverted from urea synthesis to the formation of glutamine. The

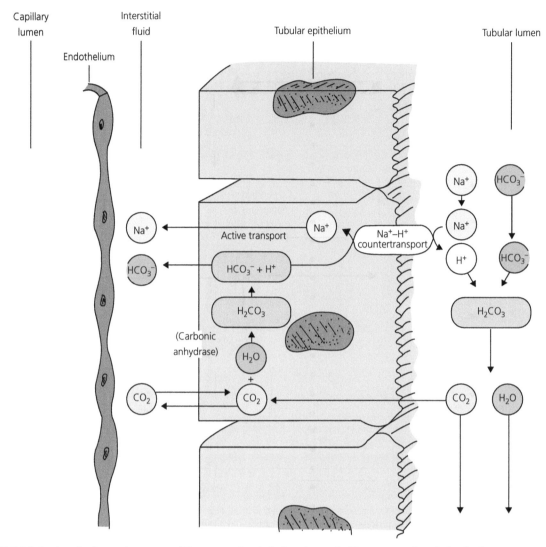

Figure 13.5 Mechanism for the renal secretion of H⁺ associated with the bicarbonate buffer system in the tubular fluid.

glutamine is carried by the circulation to the tubular epithelium of the kidney and is metabolized to α-ketoglutarate and ammonium. The NH_4^+ is then secreted into the urine, effectively removing H⁺ ions from the body. The further metabolism of α-ketoglutarate yields HCO_3^-, which is added to the blood. When there is a need to excrete more H⁺ ions, the production of glutamine in the liver rises, greatly increasing the amount of NH_4^+ excreted in the urine. Overall, excess H⁺ ions have been excreted and an equivalent amount of HCO_3^- returned to the blood. The process of excreting excess H⁺ ions in the form of ammonium ions is illustrated in Figure 13.7.

If instead of excess acid, there is an excess of base being released in body metabolism, this will result in a decrease in H⁺ ion secretion by renal tubules and collecting ducts, an increase in HCO_3^- excretion, and an alkaline urine. In this case, much less glutamine is formed and virtually no ammonium ions appear in the urine.

Intracellular potassium and hydrogen ion concentration relationships

1 How does hyperkalemia result from the response to maintain acid–base balance when blood becomes acidic?

2 How does hypokalemia result from the response to maintain acid–base balance when blood becomes alkaline?

3 What are the effects of hyperkalemia on nerve membrane potentials?

4 What are the effects of hypokalemia on nerve and muscle fiber membranes?

In this discussion, intracellular aspects will refer to all body cells and will include the renal tubular epithelial cells. **Normokalemia**, **hyperkalemia**, and **hypokalemia** refer to normal, increased, and decreased concentrations of plasma potassium ions, respectively.

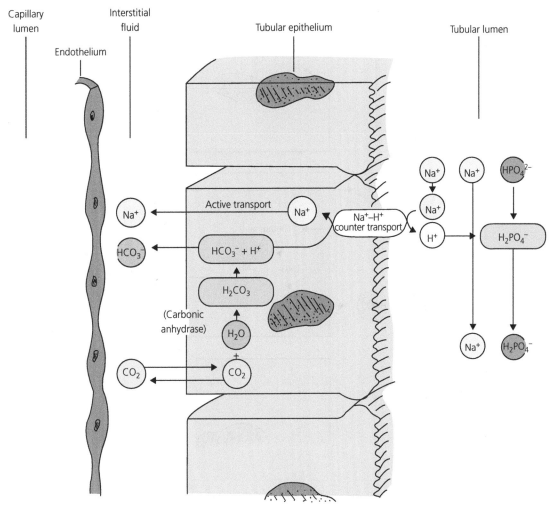

Figure 13.6 Mechanism for the renal secretion of H⁺ associated with the phosphate buffer system in the tubular fluid.

Normokalemia

Intracellular potassium concentration is normally high, approximating 140 mEq/L, whereas its extracellular concentration is normally about 5 mEq/L. Cells contain many large anions, such as proteins and organic phosphates, and therefore must contain a sufficient number of cations to maintain electrical neutrality. The major intracellular cation is K⁺ and, accordingly, it is primarily responsible for maintenance of electrical neutrality. Other intracellular cations in smaller amounts involved in maintaining electrical neutrality are Na⁺ and H⁺.

Hypokalemia and hyperkalemia

Hypokalemia is a decreased concentration of K⁺ ions in the ECF. This has an effect on nerve and muscle fiber membranes that prevents transmission of normal action potentials. Severe muscle weakness often develops. Hyperkalemia is an increased concentration of K⁺ ions in the ECF. High concentrations of potassium interfere with membrane potentials that may lead to cardiac toxicity, including weakness of contraction and arrhythmia.

Potassium is important in acid–base balance. In alkalemia, hydrogen ions leave the cells, entering the ECF in exchange for potassium ions that become intracellular. The hydrogen ion exchange for potassium ions leads to hypokalemia. The intracellular loss of hydrogen ions also occurs in the renal tubular epithelial cells whereby hydrogen ion secretion is decreased, permitting correction of alkalemia.

In acidemia, hydrogen ions enter the intracellular compartment in exchange for potassium ions that leave the cells to maintain electrical neutrality. The hydrogen ion exchange with potassium ions increases potassium ion concentration in the ECF that leads to hyperkalemia. The intracellular increase in hydrogen ions also occurs in the tubular epithelial cells. As a result, hydrogen ion secretion from the renal tubular epithelial cells increases and is associated with increasing bicarbonate return to the ECF, assisting correction of the acidemia (see Figure 13.5).

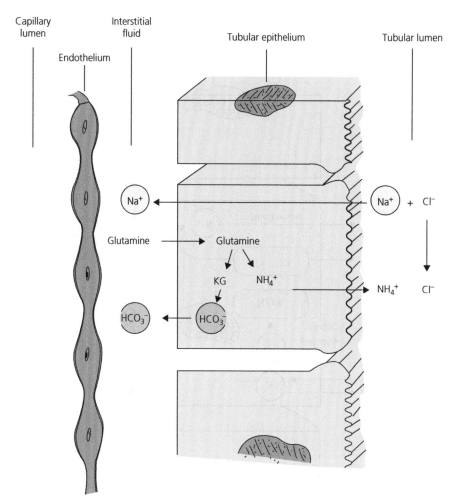

Figure 13.7 Mechanism for the secretion of H⁺ associated with the secretion of ammonium by the tubular epithelial cells and α-ketoglutarate (KG).

Acid–base balance disturbances

1 What are the acid–base disturbances known as that are associated with the buffer bases?

2 What are the acid–base balance disturbances that involve an abnormal increase or decrease of $P\text{CO}_2$?

3 What are some causes of metabolic acidosis and how do they contribute to the acidosis?

4 What are some causes of metabolic alkalosis and how do they contribute to the alkalosis?

5 What are some causes of respiratory acidosis and how do they contribute to the acidosis?

6 How can hyperventilation cause respiratory alkalosis?

The pH of the ECF is determined by the ratio of conjugate bases to their weak acids, as expressed for each buffer pair in the Henderson–Hasselbalch equation (see equation 13.2). The total amount of base in whole blood, including bicarbonate, hemoglobin, and the other bases of lesser importance, is called **buffer base**. These bases constitute the metabolic component that determines blood pH, and acid–base disturbances that involve primarily an abnormal decrease or increase of these bases are known as **metabolic acidosis** or **metabolic alkalosis**, respectively.

The weak acids in the blood, taken together, are usually measured in terms of dissolved carbon dioxide (i.e., $sP\text{CO}_2$). According to the isohydric principle, all other weak acids of the buffer pairs (mostly the acid form of hemoglobin) follow carbon dioxide changes. Acid–base disturbances that involve primarily an abnormal increase or decrease in $P\text{CO}_2$, which will usually be due to some problem of the respiratory system, are called **respiratory acidosis** or **respiratory alkalosis**, respectively.

With the development of any one of the above four processes, the first response is amelioration of the effect on pH by reaction with buffers in the blood and ISF. The second response is compensation in which the component not primarily affected by the initial disturbance is adjusted in order to bring blood pH back toward normal, For example, if the primary defect is respiratory acidosis, there will be renal compensation to excrete H^+ and return HCO_3^- to the ECF (see Figure 13.5). The compensation is complete if pH is returned to the normal range. Even though pH may be restored to the normal range, there may not be correction, in that the quantities of the respiratory or metabolic components may not have been restored to normal. Complete correction will have occurred when blood pH and the concentration of all acid–base components have been restored to normal.

Metabolic acidosis

The addition of strong acid to, or loss of base (bicarbonate) from, the ECF results in metabolic acidosis. Typical disease conditions that cause metabolic acidosis include:

1 ketosis and diabetes mellitus, in which β-hydroxybutyric acid and acetoacetic acid are produced;
2 renal acidosis, in which there is failure of bicarbonate reabsorption, and bicarbonate is lost in urine;
3 diarrhea, in which pancreatic juices and intestinal secretion containing bicarbonate are not reabsorbed and bicarbonate is lost.

In all these cases, there is loss of HCO_3^- and the pH is decreased. In accordance with the isohydric principle, the reduction in $[HCO_3^-]$ causes a decrease in all buffer bases of the ECF and red blood cells. Low blood concentration of buffer bases is called **hypobasemia**.

It is expected that plasma P_{CO_2} would rise as a result of production of CO_2 when added acid reacts with bicarbonate (see equation 13.3). The H_2CO_3 produced by this reaction is hydrated to CO_2 and H_2O (see equation 13.5). The respiratory control centers are very sensitive to change in P_{CO_2} and rapidly correct any deviation from the normal of 40 mmHg. If the fall in pH persists, the increased H^+ will act as a stimulus to the respiratory control center, whereby alveolar ventilation is increased resulting in a P_{CO_2} decrease (a reverse of the hydration reaction with loss of H^+). Respiratory adjustment of plasma P_{CO_2} will begin within a few minutes but may not be maximally developed for up to 24 hours.

Compensation by decreasing P_{CO_2} will bring the ratio of conjugate base to weak acid back to the normal value, but the hypobasemia will persist until the lost bicarbonate is replaced. Renal corrective action is required whereby hydrogen ions are excreted and plasma bicarbonate ions are restored (see Figure 13.5) by the secretion of H^+ by the renal tubule cells into the tubular fluid. This first ensures that all bicarbonate in the glomerular filtrate will be absorbed. The excess H^+ ions beyond those required to effect reabsorption of all bicarbonate ions will begin to acidify the urine. Most of the excess H^+ will be excreted from the body combined with urinary buffer bases. For each H^+ ion excreted, one HCO_3^- ion will be restored to the plasma (see Figure 13.6). This process will continue as long as the acidemia persists. In many severe diseases, however, renal action will not be sufficient to keep up with the release of acid products

within the body, and a serious acidemia will develop. Complete correction will be attained either when the disease has been terminated or as the result of vigorous acid-base therapeutic action.

Metabolic alkalosis

The gain of base (hydroxyl or bicarbonate ions) by the ECF or loss of strong acid from the ECF results in metabolic alkalosis and typically an alkalemia. Some common conditions associated with metabolic alkalosis include:

1 persistent vomiting, in which gastric acid is lost from the body;
2 potassium deficiency (hypokalemia), in which renal tubule cells secrete inappropriate amounts of hydrogen ions into the urine (see section Hypokalemia and hyperkalemia);
3 oxidation of ingested or injected salts of organic acids such as lactate or citrate;
4 injection of bicarbonate solution.

There is an increase in bicarbonate in the ECF with all these conditions, which secondarily results in an upward adjustment of all buffer bases, which is known as **hyperbasemia**. Most responses to metabolic alkalosis are corresponding but opposite to those found in metabolic acidosis. The hyperbasemia is accompanied by alkalemia. The rise in pH will depress pulmonary ventilation, and P_{CO_2} will rise (increasing the hydration of CO_2 and the production of hydrogen ions). Respiratory compensation will return pH toward normal, but the hyperbasemia will persist. Renal correction consists of decreased secretion of hydrogen ions and hence increased excretion of bicarbonate. The process will continue until the alkalemia is abolished.

Respiratory acidosis

If the rate of CO_2 production exceeds the loss of CO_2 by the lungs, respiratory acidosis develops. The primary change will be an increase in blood P_{CO_2} (**hypercapnia**) associated with the inability of the lungs to expire CO_2 at a normal rate. Common causes of respiratory acidosis include:

1 depression of the respiratory centers in the central nervous system;
2 abnormality of the chest wall or respiratory muscles that impedes bellows action of the thorax;
3 obstructions to gas movement or diffusion within the lung where either ventilation of the lung alveoli is diminished or diffusion between the alveoli and capillary blood is impeded.

The rise in P_{CO_2} represents a rise in carbonic acid, and buffer reactions occur with the nonbicarbonate bases, of which hemoglobin (Hb) is the most important as follows:

$$H_2CO_3 + Hb \leftrightarrow HCO_3^- + HHb \qquad (13.10)$$

The buffer action ameliorates the fall in pH caused by the rise in carbonic acid. Renal compensation becomes evident within a few hours and the low pH stimulates tubular cells to increase secretion of hydrogen ions into the urine with a concomitant increase in plasma bicarbonate. Renal compensation may require several days to bring the pH back into the normal range. Complete recovery of respiratory acidosis will not be possible until recovery from the pulmonary disease occurs.

Respiratory alkalosis

The loss of CO_2 may exceed the rate of production when there is hyperventilation, and respiratory alkalosis may occur. This is characterized by low plasma PCO_2 (**hypocapnia**) and alkalemia. Hyperventilation may be caused by some abnormal stimulus to the respiratory centers, either directly as in ammonia toxicity or indirectly via reflex from peripheral receptors due to **hypoxemia** (low PO_2). Plasma $[HCO_3^-]$ is unchanged initially by the fall in PCO_2, but buffer reactions with nonbicarbonate buffers occur immediately. Buffering by hemoglobin would occur as follows:

$$HHb + HCO_3^- \rightarrow Hb^- + H_2CO_3 \rightarrow CO_2 (removed) \qquad (13.11)$$

The $[HCO_3^-]$ falls and Hb proteinate ions rise by an equivalent amount. Renal compensation begins in a few hours and maximal capacity is reached after several days. Alkalemia depresses the rate of H^+ secretion by kidney tubule cells and excretion of filtered bicarbonate rises. With the fall of plasma bicarbonate, blood pH is returned toward normal. Final correction of the primary change in PCO_2 requires recovery from the cause of hyperventilation.

Evaluation of acid–base status

> 1 What are the blood variables involved in the assessment of acid–base disturbances?
>
> 2 When applied to the pH–bicarbonate diagram, what do the normal buffer line and the PCO_2 isobar represent?
>
> 3 What compensatory mechanism exists for respiratory alkalosis and respiratory acidosis? Study each in relation to the pH–bicarbonate diagram.
>
> 4 What compensatory mechanism exists for metabolic alkalosis and metabolic acidosis? Study each in relation to the pH–bicarbonate diagram?
>
> 5 What situations give credence for the use of anion-gap method for evaluating acid–base disorders?
>
> 6 What is the equation used to estimate plasma anion gap?

The blood variables involved in the assessment of the acid–base disturbances are pH, PCO_2, plasma $[HCO_3^-]$, and hemoglobin concentration. Two systems of clinical evaluation are frequently employed. One system uses the pH–bicarbonate diagram, which can be used to visualize and determine the types of acidosis or alkalosis and to approximate its severity. Analysis involves whole blood and includes the influence of hemoglobin as a blood buffer. Only pH and $[HCO_3^-]$ values are plotted. The other system uses whole blood values that can be plotted on the

Siggaard–Andersen alignment nomogram, and base excess is determined from the nomogram. In this system, base excess can be determined, if not otherwise provided, but visualization of the type of acidosis or alkalosis is not apparent. Most pH–blood gas analyzers can be adjusted for hemoglobin concentration and pH, PCO_2, and $[HCO_3^-]$, and base excess values are returned and can then be plotted on the pH–bicarbonate diagram. The Siggaard–Andersen nomogram would not provide further information. The pH–bicarbonate diagram is more instructional and provides better visualization of the type of acidosis or alkalosis and is therefore the one that will be explained more fully. If a base excess value is not otherwise provided, it can still be estimated from the pH–bicarbonate diagram by measurement of a vertical line drawn from the normal buffer line to the plot of the pH and bicarbonate values. The estimate would be determined by extrapolating the length of the vertical line to the bicarbonate scale on the diagram.

The pH–bicarbonate diagram

A **pH–bicarbonate diagram** that illustrates compensations that may occur is shown in Figure 13.8. Its components consist of a PCO_2 isobar and a normal buffer line. Any point along the PCO_2 isobar (shown for $PCO_2 = 40\,mmHg$) will represent possible combinations of bicarbonate concentration and pH that can exist when $PaCO_2$ remains at $40\,mmHg$. Points to the right or the left of the PCO_2 isobar represent respective deviations toward respiratory alkalosis ($PaCO_2$ decrease) and respiratory acidosis ($PaCO_2$ increase). The normal buffer line indicates a balance between metabolic acids and metabolic bases where points along the line represent possible combinations of bicarbonate concentration and pH that can occur as long as the metabolic acids and bases in the body fluids do not change. Points above or below the line represent respective deviations toward metabolic alkalosis and metabolic acidosis.

Compensatory mechanisms exist for all the previously discussed deviations. Renal compensation occurs for respiratory alkalosis and respiratory acidosis, and respiratory compensation occurs for metabolic alkalosis and metabolic acidosis. For each of the acid–base abnormalities that follows, on Figure 13.8 location 1 refers to development without compensation, and location 2 represents development with compensation.

Renal compensation for respiratory alkalosis (low $PaCO_2$) and respiratory acidosis (high $PaCO_2$)

1 *Respiratory alkalosis.* Any factor that increases pulmonary ventilation, decreases $PaCO_2$. Accordingly, hydrogen ion concentration is decreased, whereby renal tubular acid secretion and bicarbonate "reabsorption" are decreased and pH is returned toward normal (path A, Figure 13.8).

2 *Respiratory acidosis.* Any factor that decreases pulmonary ventilation, increases $PaCO_2$. Accordingly, hydrogen ion concentration is increased, whereby renal tubular acid secretion and bicarbonate "reabsorption" are increased and pH is returned toward normal (path B, Figure 13.8).

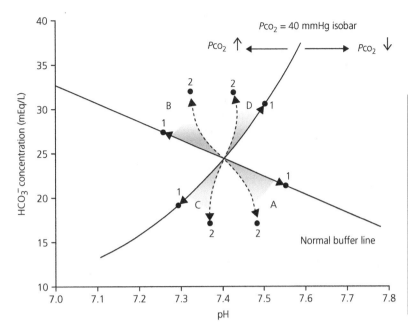

Figure 13.8 The pH–bicarbonate diagram. Arrows to locations 1 emanate from a central normal position and extrapolate to a pH and bicarbonate concentration without compensation. Dashed arrows to locations 2 extrapolate to a pH and bicarbonate concentration that results from compensation of the primary condition. (A) Renal compensation for respiratory alkalosis; (B) renal compensation for respiratory acidosis; (C) respiratory compensation for metabolic acidosis; (D) respiratory compensation for metabolic alkalosis.

Respiratory compensation for metabolic acidosis and metabolic alkalosis

1 *Metabolic acidosis.* Increase in hydrogen ion concentration resulting from increased metabolic acids stimulates pulmonary ventilation, whereby $Paco_2$ is decreased followed by a decrease in hydrogen ion concentration and pH returns toward normal (path C, Figure 13.8).

2 *Metabolic alkalosis.* Decrease in hydrogen ion concentration resulting from decreased metabolic acids decreases pulmonary ventilation, whereby $Paco_2$ is increased, followed by an increase in hydrogen ion concentration and pH returns toward normal (path D, Figure 13.8).

The shifts of pH and $[HCO_3^-]$ in acid–base disturbances that are not immediately compensated are the result of reaction of the added acid or base with chemical buffers. However, respiratory and renal compensation soon become effective.

In respiratory acidosis and alkalosis, renal compensation ameliorates the condition. If the primary problem were respiratory disease, correction will await recovery from the disease. If the primary problem were kidney disease, the renal adjustments of bicarbonate might be impaired, causing a more serious condition.

In many severe or prolonged diseases, the disturbance in acid–base balance would likely be only partially compensated. There are complex combinations of acidosis and alkalosis resulting from separate disease processes occurring simultaneously in the same animal.

The anion gap and acid–base status

Use of the pH–bicarbonate diagram for evaluation of acid–base status relies on the anaerobic collection of arterial blood and storage on ice until the time of analysis in a pH–blood gas analyzer. The anion-gap method offers a less precise but still useful way to clinically evaluate certain acid–base disorders when the pH–blood gas analyzer method is not available. This method is based on using plasma concentrations of sodium, potassium, chloride, and bicarbonate that are usually included in routine chemical panels. The concentrations of anions and cations in plasma must be equal to maintain electrical neutrality and in reality there is no "anion gap." The predominant cations in plasma are sodium and potassium and these are largely balanced by chloride and bicarbonate anions. There are unmeasured cations and anions normally present in plasma but these are not routinely included in measurements. The cations not included are calcium and magnesium and the anions are sulfates, phosphates, proteinate ions, and anions of organic acids. Therefore, there is an inequality in measured ions, with the cations exceeding the anions. Because the concentration of potassium varies very little, it may not be included in the calculation of the anion gap. The plasma anion gap is estimated as follows:

$$\text{Plasma anion gap} = [Na^+] - ([HCO_3^-] + [Cl^-]) \qquad (13.12)$$

Given respective values of 144, 24 and 108 mEq/L, the anion gap would be equal to 12 mEq/L. The values may range between 8 and 16 mEq/L.

The method is useful in the evaluation of metabolic acidosis. In ketosis, the excess ketone acids will react with bicarbonate (lowering its value), and their anions, acetoacetate and β-hydroxybutyrate, will accumulate (but are not measured). The anion gap will then increase far beyond its normal level because the measured bicarbonate has been decreased and replaced with anions not measured. However, if the cause of the metabolic acidosis involves the loss of both sodium and bicarbonate ions, there may be no change in the anion gap. This can occur in diarrhea. Also, if the loss of bicarbonate ions is balanced by a gain of chloride ions, no anion gap will be evident. This can occur in renal disease.

A modest decrease in anion gap occurs when unmeasured cations increase (e.g., hypercalcemia or hypermagnesemia), thereby reducing $[Na^+]$, or when unmeasured anions decrease (e.g., hypoproteinemia). In hypoproteinemic alkalosis, both $[HCO_3^-]$ and $[Cl^-]$ will increase in order to fill the protein gap.

In summary, a decrease in anion gap is best associated with hypoproteinemic alkalosis, whereas an increase is usually associated with some form of metabolic acidosis due to retention of acid (e.g., ketone acids, acetoacetic and β-hydroxybutyric acids).

Self-evaluation

Answers can be found at the end of the chapter.

1 According to the Henderson–Hasselbalch equation, the pH of body fluids decreases if the conjugate base/weak acid ratio decreases (more acid than base).
 A True
 B False

2 An increase in P_{CO_2} or hydrogen ion concentration in renal tubule epithelial cells increases the secretion of hydrogen ions into the tubular fluid.
 A True
 B False

3 Potassium-deficient states (hypokalemia) result in low intracellular potassium ion concentration and high intracellular hydrogen ion concentration. Accordingly:
 A The urine becomes more acidic (secretion of hydrogen ions) and the ECF becomes more alkaline (reabsorption of bicarbonate ions)
 B The urine and the ECF become more acidic
 C The urine and the ECF become more alkaline
 D The urine becomes more alkaline and the ECF becomes more acidic

4 When you are considering respiratory compensation for metabolic acidosis, think:
 A Increased hydrogen ion concentration, which stimulates ventilation, which reduces P_{CO_2}
 B Decreased hydrogen ion concentration, which "brakes" ventilation and P_{CO_2} accumulates

5 In respiratory compensation of metabolic acidosis, the pH of body fluids returns toward normal, but the CO_2 content of body fluids is _____ as a consequence of _____ respiration. Which one of the answers below has the respective words for the two blank spaces?
 A Increased, increased
 B Decreased, decreased

 C Increased, decreased
 D Decreased, increased

6–9 For questions 6–9, respectively, identify the primary acid–base disturbance and the compensating condition for Cases 1–4 as (A) metabolic acidosis, (B) metabolic alkalosis, (C) respiratory acidosis, or (D) respiratory alkalosis. To assist evaluation, refer to Figure 13.8.

	Case 1	Case 2	Case 3	Case 4
pH	7.24	7.20	7.60	7.50
P_{CO_2} (mmHg)	71	32	21	45
HCO_3^- (mEq/L)	33	12	17	35
Base excess (mEq/L)	+5	−15	−3	+13

Each of the conditions listed in questions 10–13 can lead to a primary acid–base disturbance. Identify the primary disturbance that can be produced for each as (A) metabolic acidosis, (B) metabolic alkalosis, (C) respiratory acidosis, or (D) respiratory alkalosis.

10 Diarrhea (pancreatic juice containing HCO_3^- not reabsorbed and so lost)

11 Abomasal torsion (hydrochloric acid in stomach not able to continue into duodenum, HCO_3^- accumulates in plasma)

12 Obstruction to gas movement in and out of lung

13 Hyperventilation caused by persistent hypoxemia

Suggested reading

Hall, J.E. (2011) Acid–base regulation. In: *Guyton and Hall Textbook of Medical Physiology*, 12th edn, pp. 379–396. Saunders Elsevier, Philadelphia.

Houpt, T.R. (2004) Acid–base balance. In: *Dukes' Physiology of Domestic Animals*, 12th edn (ed. W.O. Reece), pp. 162–177. Cornell University Press, Ithaca, NY.

Reece, W.O. (2004) Respiration in mammals. In: *Dukes' Physiology of Domestic Animals*, 12th edn (ed. W.O. Reece), pp. 138–139. Cornell University Press, Ithaca, NY.

Reece, W.O. (2009) The urinary system. In: *Functional Anatomy and Physiology of Domestic Animals*, 4th edn, pp. 344–347. Wiley-Blackwell, Ames, IA.

Answers

1 A		8 D, B
2 A		9 B, C
3 A		10 A
4 A		11 B
5 D		12 C
6 C, B		13 D
7 A, D		

14 Body Temperature and Its Regulation

William O. Reece
Iowa State University, Ames, IA, USA

Section II: Body Fluids and Homeostasis

The chemical reactions of the body, and therefore the functions of the body, depend on body temperature. An elevation of temperature accelerates the reactions, and a lowering of temperature depresses the reactions. To avoid fluctuations in function caused by temperature, mammals and birds have developed a means whereby body temperature is maintained at a relatively constant level regardless of the temperature of the surroundings. Mammals and birds are classified as **homeotherms, or warm-blooded animals. Poikilotherm (cold-blooded) animals** have a body temperature that varies with the temperature of the environment.

Body temperature

1 What factors can influence body temperature?

2 What is meant by core temperature?

3 Does a rectal temperature reading represent the temperature throughout the body?

4 What is meant by diurnal temperature?

5 Give an example of heat storage in an animal. What advantage is served by heat storage?

6 What is an approximate value for rectal temperature in common domestic animals?

An average body temperature is associated with each domestic animal species. These temperatures are shown in Table 14.1, along with their commonly observed ranges. The temperatures were obtained by rectal insertion of a thermometer in resting animals. A number of conditions can influence body temperature, including exercise, time of day, environmental temperature, digestion, and drinking of water.

Gradients of temperature

Different parts of the body can differ in temperature because of differences in metabolic rate, blood flow, or distance from the surface. For example, the liver and the brain can have a temperature that is higher than that of blood, and they are therefore cooled by blood circulation. The deep body temperature, or core temperature, is higher than the temperature of the limbs or even higher than the temperature observed rectally. However, **rectal temperature** represents a true steady state of temperature because it reaches equilibrium more slowly.

Diurnal temperature

Variations in temperature related to the time of day are designated as **diurnal temperatures.** Animals that are active during the day and sleep at night have body temperatures that are lower in the morning than in the afternoon. The opposite is true for **nocturnal (night-active) animals.** Also, as a water conservation measure, the body temperature of the camel is permitted to increase during the day so that the excess heat can be dissipated at night when the desert air is cool; this is known as heat storage. The temperature of a normal camel, watered every day and fully hydrated, varies by less than 2°C, between about 36 and 38°C (more water available for evaporation and less need for heat storage). When the camel is deprived of drinking water, however,

Dukes' Physiology of Domestic Animals, Thirteenth Edition. Edited by William O. Reece, Howard H. Erickson, Jesse P. Goff and Etsuro E. Uemura.
© 2015 John Wiley & Sons, Inc. Published 2015 by John Wiley & Sons, Inc.
Companion website: www.wiley.com/go/reece/physiology

Table 14.1 Average rectal temperatures of various species.

Animal	Average		Range	
	°C	°F	°C	°F
Stallion	37.6	99.7	37.2–38.1	99.0–100.6
Mare	37.8	100	37.3–38.2	99.1–100.8
Donkey	37.4	99.3	36.4–38.4	97.5–101.1
Camel	37.5	99.5	34.2–40.7	93.6–105.3
Beef cow	38.3	101	36.7–39.1	98.0–102.4
Dairy cow	38.6	101.5	38.0–39.3	100.4–102.8
Sheep	39.1	102.3	38.3–39.9	100.9–103.8
Goat	39.1	102.3	38.5–39.7	101.3–103.5
Pig	39.2	102.5	38.7–39.8	101.6–103.6
Dog	38.9	102	37.9–39.9	100.2–103.8
Cat	38.6	101.5	38.1–39.2	100.5–102.5
Rabbit	39.5	103.1	38.6–40.1	101.5–104.2
Chicken (daylight)	41.7	107.1	40.6–43.0	105.0–109.4

Source: Andersson, B.E. and Jonasson, H. (1993) Temperature regulation and environmental physiology. In: *Dukes' Physiology of Domestic Animals*, 11th edn (eds M.J. Swenson and W.O. Reece). Cornell University Press, Ithaca, NY.

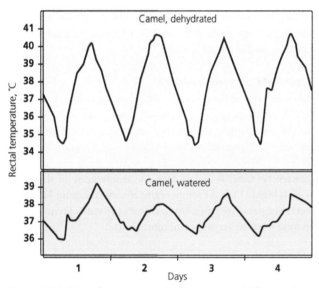

Figure 14.1 Diurnal temperatures in the watered and dehydrated camel. The rectal temperature elevations (heat storage) occur during the day, and the reductions occur at night. From Schmidt-Nielsen, K. (1963) Osmotic regulation in higher vertebrates. In: *The Harvey Lectures, 1962–1963*, Series 58. Academic Press, London.

its morning temperature can be as low as 34 °C and its highest temperature, in the late afternoon, can be nearly 41 °C (Figure 14.1).

Physiologic responses to heat

1 How can the diversion of blood to the skin result in loss of body heat? How can heat loss by this means be regulated?

2 What is the stimulus for allowing heat to be lost via the skin?

3 Where are thermosensitive cells located in the brain?

4 Are there any reflexes associated with heat gain or heat loss?

5 What percent of the heat produced in the body is normally lost by insensible means?

6 What type of sweat glands predominate in animals?

7 What is the principal function of the apocrine sweat glands?

8 Is sweating an important mechanism for heat loss among domestic animals? Which one of the domestic animals represents the greatest use of this means? The least?

9 What function is accomplished by panting? What is panting? How is hyperventilation prevented while panting? Is panting only observed in the dog?

10 Which domestic animals are most able to withstand extremes of heat?

11 What are factors associated with the pig's intolerance to heat?

12 How does the cat increase evaporative heat loss?

13 What is an approximate body temperature of birds? Why is pulmonary ventilation more likely to cool the body of birds than that of mammals?

Heat is produced constantly in the body as a result of metabolism. If there were not provisions for losing heat, the temperature of the body would increase to intolerable levels. Two principal means for losing heat are (i) radiation, conduction, and convection, and (ii) evaporation of water from the skin and respiratory passages. A third way considers the excretion of feces and urine that leave the animal at body temperature. Heat lost by excretion of feces and urine is small and is considered negligible. Under ordinary conditions, about 75% of the heat lost from the body is dissipated by radiation, conduction, and convection and is controlled mostly by vasomotor activity.

Circulatory adjustments

Inasmuch as circulating blood is a distributor of body heat, heat can be lost from the blood if blood is brought to the skin surface and exposed to a gradient for loss to the environment. A schematic section of the skin of the dog (Figure 14.2) illustrates the extensive network of blood vessels to the skin. The volume of blood circulating to the skin is controlled by sympathetic vasoconstrictor fibers to the blood vessels. An increase in tone results in constriction of blood vessels and diversion of blood from the surface, thereby conserving heat. A decrease in tone allows more blood to the surface. A stimulus for a decrease in tone, so that more heat can be lost from the body, is the temperature of the blood circulated to the brain. Thermosensitive cells in the rostral hypothalamus respond to warming by activating physiologic and behavioral heat loss mechanisms. Similarly, cooling of the same region stimulates other thermosensitive cells to evoke thermoregulatory responses for heat gain. Reflexes to inhibit vasoconstrictor tone also arise from thermoreceptors in the skin and other parts of the body.

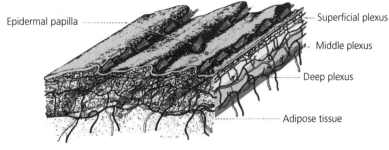

Figure 14.2 Schematic section of dog skin showing the extensive network of blood vessels and the location of insulating adipose tissue. Adapted from Evans, H.E. (1993) *Miller's Anatomy of the Dog*, 3rd edn. W.B. Saunders, Philadelphia.

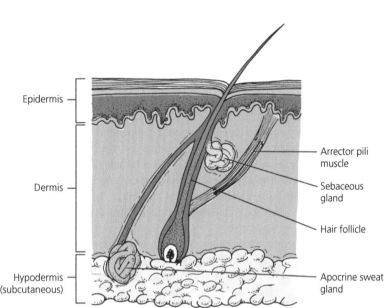

Figure 14.3 Schematic representation of apocrine and sebaceous glands and their association with a hair follicle. The secretory parts of the apocrine glands are located in the dermal and subcutaneous layers of the skin. The excretory ducts pass upward through the dermis and empty into the hair follicles above the ducts of the sebaceous glands. Adapted from Reece, W.O. (2009) *Functional Anatomy and Physiology of Domestic Animals*, 4th edn. Cornell University Press, Ithaca, NY.

Evaporative heat loss

Evaporation of water results in cooling. Loss of water by evaporation is referred to as **insensible water loss**; this includes water lost from the skin surfaces and water lost in the heated exhaled air. Normally about 25% of the heat produced in an animal at rest is lost when water is removed by insensible means.

Evaporative heat losses are increased by sweating and panting. The relative importance of sweating as a heat loss mechanism varies among species. Generally, the function of sweat glands as dissipaters of body heat is less effective in domestic animals than in humans.

There are two types of sweat glands: **apocrine** and **eccrine**. Eccrine sweat glands are those typically found in humans, but are sparse among domestic animals. In the dog and cat they occupy only the foot pad location. This area does not subserve thermoregulation, but provides a moist surface and subsequent improved traction. Horses, cattle, sheep, dogs, and cats have apocrine sweat glands disseminated over the body surface (Figure 14.3). The composition, volume, stimulus for secretion, and function of apocrine sweat varies among species. In the dog, and perhaps in other species, apocrine sweat is a proteinaceous, white, odorless, milky fluid that is formed slowly and continuously. On the skin surface, it mixes with sebum from the sebaceous glands to form a protective emulsion that acts as a physical and chemical barrier. Characteristic animal odors arise from the action of bacterial flora on apocrine secretions. Heat loss from sweating (thermoregulatory function) is probably greatest in the horse, followed (in order) by cattle, sheep, dogs, cats, and swine.

The panting mechanism is effective in dissipating the heat load because greater amounts of air are forced over moist surfaces (see Chapter 25). Panting is most effective in the dog, but is also observed in the other domestic animals. Essentially, panting is an increase in dead space ventilation without change in respiratory alveolar ventilation. A decreased tidal volume is associated with the increased respiratory frequency of panting; in this way, hyperventilation of the alveoli is prevented.

In cattle, panting is accompanied by increased salivation, and the salivary secretion promotes cooling by evaporation. Salivary secretion loss by evaporation and drooling (physical loss to the exterior of the body) can result in metabolic acidosis because of loss of bicarbonate and phosphate buffers contained in ruminant saliva.

Increases in sweating and panting are brought about by increased blood temperature, subsequent adjustments by the hypothalamus, and reflexes produced by local heating of the skin.

Section II: Body Fluids and Homeostasis

Responses to extremes of heat

Different animal species differ in their ability to withstand heat. The humidity of the air becomes a factor: as humidity increases, evaporation from insensible losses is reduced and less cooling occurs. Of all domestic animals, cattle and sheep seem to be the most able to withstand extremes of heat. Open-mouth panting and sweating occur as the temperature increases, and these animals can withstand temperatures as high as 43 °C (109 °F) with humidity above 65%.

The pig cannot tolerate a temperature above 35 °C (95 °F) with humidity above 65%. The intolerance of pigs to heat is recognized by transporters of livestock. During periods of heat, the transport of pigs is usually delayed until night, and they often are hosed with water. Pigs do not sweat copiously, and their small mouth makes them ineffective at panting. In addition, they often have substantial subcutaneous fat.

When the relative humidity is above 65%, the cat cannot withstand prolonged exposure to an environmental temperature of 40 °C (104 °F) or higher. In addition to panting, the cat can increase evaporative losses by spreading saliva over its hair coat. Because the dog is effective at panting, it can withstand extreme environmental temperatures better than the cat, but it is in danger of collapse when its rectal temperature reaches 41 °C (106 °F).

In birds, the air sacs are extensions of the lungs that extend into the body cavities. The body temperature of birds is about 41 °C (106 °F). Pulmonary ventilation air is more likely to cool the body of birds than that of mammals because of the larger gradient and because of the closeness of the air to the body organs (via air sacs, see Chapter 26). It seems that prolonged exposure of a hen to an air temperature of 38 °C (100 °F) is unsafe if the relative humidity is above 75%. A rectal temperature of 45 °C (113 °F) is the upper limit of safety in the chicken.

Physiologic responses to cold

1   How are responses to cold activated?
2   What is accomplished by the countercurrent flow of blood in the limbs of animals?
3   What are some behavioral responses for reducing heat loss?
4   What is piloerection?
5   Which farm animals have the lowest critical temperature?
6   What is accomplished by shivering?
7   What is the role of thyroid hormone in adaptation to cold?

Cold activates body heating mechanisms, just as excess heat activates body cooling mechanisms. With excess cooling, heat is either conserved by reducing heat loss or is generated to compensate for that which is lost. The physiologic responses to cold are activated by blood temperature and local reflexes, as are the responses to heat.

Reduction of heat loss

In an attempt to reduce heat loss, animals instinctively curl up when they lie down. This behavioral response reduces the surface area exposed to the cold. To increase the insulation value of their hair or fur, **piloerection** occurs. In this process the hair is made to become more erect by the arrector pili muscle of the hair follicle (see Figure 14.3). With sustained exposure to cold, the hair coat thickens and the amount of subcutaneous fat increases.

In contrast to vasodilation, which occurs to accommodate heat loss, the peripheral vessels are constricted by an increase in vasoconstrictor tone. Heat is also conserved by the arrangement of the deep blood vessels that supply the legs of animals. Blood returning in the veins from the colder legs is close to the warmer blood in the arteries directed to the legs. Because of the temperature differences, heat is transferred from the arteries to the veins; this decreases the gradient for heat loss from the arterial blood to the environment. This arrangement of blood vessels is known as a **countercurrent system**.

Increase in heat production

When the ability to reduce heat loss is not adequate to maintain a normal body temperature, heat must be produced. The temperature to which body temperature decreases before heat generation begins is known as the **critical temperature**. Among farm animals, cattle and sheep have the lowest critical temperature, which means that they are better suited to withstand cold.

Shivering is one means by which heat is generated. Shivering is a generalized rhythmic contraction of muscles. Because 30–50% of the energy of muscle contraction is converted to heat, the seemingly spasmodic contraction of muscle serves a useful purpose.

Other methods are used to generate heat in addition to shivering. **Epinephrine** and **norepinephrine** are both released in increased amounts in the cold. **Brown fat** is an important source of thermogenesis (see section Brown fat versus white fat). Epinephrine and norepinephrine are the stimuli for increased metabolism of brown fat. In addition to hibernating animals, brown fat is also found in newborn mammals. Epinephrine and norepinephrine have calorigenic effects on other cells as well, and the calorigenic effects are potentiated by thyroid hormone. **Thyroid hormone** is secreted in increased amounts during periods of cold.

Hibernation

1   What is the favored definition of hibernation? Is a greatly reduced core temperature a necessary component of hibernation?
2   Is the bear considered to be a true hibernator?
3   Is hibernation characteristic of homeotherms or of poikilotherms?
4   What prevents hibernators from freezing? Is there periodic awakening from hibernation?
5   What is brown fat?

Hibernation is the act of resting in a dormant state in a protected burrow. This definition has recently returned to favor. Formerly, it was proposed that

> Hibernation is the assumption of a state of greatly reduced core temperature by a mammal or a bird which has its active body temperature near 37 °C, meanwhile retaining the capability of spontaneously rewarming back to the normal homeothermic level without absorbing heat from its environment (Menaker, 1962).

According to the former definition, bears were not considered to be true hibernators because their core body temperature was not greatly reduced. The core body temperature of bears is reduced by only 6.8 °C during their dormancy, as opposed to a reduction of 20–30 °C by animals that were considered to be true hibernators. The lesser reduction in body temperature of the bear is now believed to be a biologic protection for hibernating bears; accordingly, they are considered true hibernators. Because of their large body mass, it is thought that too much time would be involved in their revival to activity if their body temperature were lowered by 20–30 °C. The longer revival time would make them easy victim to another cannibalistic bear that had revived.

The characteristics of hibernation are as follows.

1 Hibernation is a process involving warm-blooded animals.
2 The process is autonomous: the animal induces and reverses it by some self-contained mechanism.
3 The process is radical: changes involve not only overt physiologic functioning, but also cellular and subcellular changes.
4 All physiologic functions continue, but at a reduced rate.
5 During the process, body temperature is lowered significantly to a level compatible with survival for the species.

Awakening from hibernation

Hibernating animals awake from their dormant state periodically. For example, the kidneys continue to form urine and the animal has a need to urinate. A protective mechanism against profound cooling also exists in winter hibernators. If the body temperature declines to levels near freezing, the animal awakes and rapidly rewarms.

Brown fat versus white fat

Brown fat is a connective tissue with a color that results from cytochrome pigments and a high density of mitochondria. It is typically found in hibernating animals and in smaller species. It is also present in the newborn of many species and disappears within the first few months of life. Its usual location is in the subcutaneous region between the scapulae (shoulder blades) and in the region of the kidneys as well as within the myocardium. The ability of hibernators to elevate their body temperature from reduced levels to the temperature necessary for arousal (nonshivering thermogenesis) is facilitated by their depots of brown fat. Brown fat differs from white fat not only in color, but also in metabolic characteristics. When brown fat cells are stimulated, they consume oxygen and produce heat at a high rate.

Hypothermia and hyperthermia

1 What is hypothermia?
2 How can hypothermia occur in anesthetized animals?
3 What is fever? What are its beneficial effects?
4 Where is the need for fever sensed?
5 What are the characteristics of heat stroke? How can its associated hyperthermia be relieved?

Reduction of the deep body temperature below normal in nonhibernating homeotherms is known as **hypothermia**; **hyperthermia** is the reverse.

Hypothermia

Hypothermia can readily occur during central nervous system anesthesia because the hypothalamic response to cold blood is depressed. It normally occurs as a result of prolonged exposure to cold, coupled with an inability of the heat-conserving and heat-generating mechanisms to keep pace. Tolerance to lowered body temperatures varies among species. In dogs, death can occur when the rectal temperature approximates 25 °C (77 °F). Hypothermia in any animal can become life-threatening unless environmental conditions improve or external heat is provided.

It is important to monitor body temperature during and after procedures requiring anesthesia because of the depressed hypothalamic response. External heat sources are often fitted to surgical tables for the maintenance of body temperature. When these are used, there must be assurance that local injury to skin does not occur. When animals do not recover quickly after anesthesia (e.g., pentobarbital anesthesia), monitoring body temperature and provision of external heat is extremely important.

Fever

Fever is an elevation of deep body temperature that is brought on by microorganism-caused disease. Fever is usually beneficial because immunologic mechanisms are accelerated and the high temperature induced is detrimental to the microorganisms, but it can be damaging if allowed to become excessive. In fever, the set point of the hypothalamus is elevated and the body senses that the blood is too cold, so heat-conserving and heat-generating mechanisms are recruited. Shivering and a feeling of coolness are characteristics of the beginning of fever. Fever is generally self-limiting; maximum temperatures of 41 °C (106 °F) can be approached.

Heat stroke and impaired evaporation

Hyperthermia exclusive of fever can be associated with **heat stroke**. In this condition, heat production exceeds the evaporative capacity of the environment and occurs when the humidity is high. Hyperthermia can also develop when the evaporative mechanisms become impaired as a result of loss of body fluid

Section II: Body Fluids and Homeostasis

or reduced blood volume. Antipyretic drugs (effective against fever) are ineffective in reducing body temperature in heat stroke and impaired evaporation conditions, and relief is obtained only by whole-body cooling.

Self-evaluation

Answers can be found at the end of the chapter.

1 The average rectal temperature in a healthy cow should be about:
   A 98.6°F
   B 101.5°F
   C 104.0°F
   D 106.5°F

2 Variations in temperature related to the time of day are known as:
   A Diurnal temperatures
   B Core temperatures
   C Poikilotherms
   D Ambient temperatures

3 What part of the brain has a temperature regulating center?
   A Medulla
   B Thalamus
   C Hypothalamus
   D Cerebral cortex

4 Which sweat gland type predominates among the domestic animals?
   A Eccrine
   B Apocrine

5 Which one of the following animals has the greatest heat loss from sweating?
   A Sheep
   B Cats
   C Dogs
   D Horses
   E Pigs

6 Which of the following domestic animals are best able to withstand extremes of heat?
   A Horse
   B Dog
   C Pig
   D Cattle and sheep

7 Which of the following domestic animals are best able to withstand cold?
   A Horse
   B Dog

   C Pig
   D Cattle and sheep

8 Piloerection is a response to:
   A Heat
   B Cold
   C Watching television

9 A true hibernator:
   A Is not represented by the bear
   B Abandons homeothermy in cold weather but will awaken if body temperature approaches freezing or some other higher set point
   C Abandons homeothermy in the cold and may freeze if body temperature becomes lower than freezing
   D Maintains a constant body temperature even while it sleeps through cold weather

10 Fever has no beneficial effects.
   A True
   B False

Suggested reading

Andersson, B.E. and Jonasson, H. (1993) Temperature regulation and environmental physiology. In: *Dukes' Physiology of Domestic Animals*, 11th edn (eds M.J. Swenson and W.O. Reece). Cornell University Press, Ithaca, NY.

Folk, G.E. Jr, Larson, A. and Folk, M.A. (1976) Physiology of hibernating bears. In: *Bears: Their Biology and Management* (eds M.R. Pelton, J.W. Lentfer and G.E. Folk), pp. 373–380. Proceedings of the Third International Conference on Bear Research and Management, June 1974. International Union for Conservation of Nature and Natural Resources, Morges, Switzerland.

Menaker, M. (1962) Hibernation–hypothermia: an annual cycle of response to low temperature in the bat *Myotis lucifugus*. *Journal of Cellular and Comparative Physiology* 59:163–173.

Nakayama, T., Hammel, H.T., Hardy, J.D. and Eisenman, J.S. (1963) Thermal stimulation of electrical activity of single units of the preoptic region. *American Journal of Physiology* 204:1122–1126.

Robertshaw, D. (2004) Temperature regulation and the thermal environment. In: *Dukes' Physiology of Domestic Animals*, 12th edn (ed. W.O. Reece). Cornell University Press, Ithaca, NY.

Answers

1	B	6	D
2	A	7	D
3	C	8	B
4	B	9	B
5	D	10	B

SECTION III

The Kidneys and Urinary System

Section Editor: William O. Reece

15 The Renal System: Structures and Function

William O. Reece

Iowa State University, Ames, IA, USA

Two major functions of the kidneys are excretion of metabolic waste products and regulation of the volume and composition of the body's internal environment, the extracellular fluid (ECF). In this regard it has been said that the composition of the body fluids is determined not by what the mouth takes in but by what the kidneys keep. Other essential functions are secretion of hormones and hydrolysis of small peptides. The hormones participate in the regulation of systemic and renal dynamics, red blood cell production, and calcium, phosphorus and bone metabolism. Small peptide hydrolysis conserves amino acids, detoxifies toxic peptides, and regulates effective plasma levels of some peptide hormones. Because of these multiple functions, there are many clinical signs associated with renal disease.

Gross anatomy of the kidneys and urinary system

1 Why are the kidneys considered retroperitoneal structures?

2 Differentiate between the renal hilus and the renal pelvis.

3 Differentiate between ureter and urethra.

4 What is the functional boundary between the bladder and urethra?

5 What are the medullary portions of the collecting tubules known as?

6 What differentiates the external sphincter from the internal sphincter?

The kidneys are paired organs suspended from the dorsal abdominal wall by a peritoneal fold and the blood vessels that serve them. They are located slightly cranial to the mid-lumbar region (Figure 15.1). Because they are separated from the abdominal cavity by their envelope of peritoneum, they are called **retroperitoneal** structures. Blood is carried to each kidney by a renal artery, and venous blood is conveyed away from each kidney by a renal vein. The renal artery arises directly from the aorta, and the renal vein empties directly into the caudal vena cava (Figure 15.2).

The kidney is described as a bean-shaped structure for most domestic animals. In the horse, however, it is described as heart-shaped, and in cattle it is lobulated (Figure 15.3). If a mid-sagittal cut is made through the kidney (Figure 15.4), an outer cortex and an inner medulla are visible. The striations of the medulla are formed by the anatomic arrangement of the major parts that occupy the medulla, the **loop of Henle** of long-looped nephrons and the medullary portion of the **collecting tubules** (see section The nephron). The medullary portions of the collecting tubules are known as **collecting ducts**. The **renal hilus** is the indented area on the concave edge of the kidney through which the ureter, blood vessels, nerves, and lymphatics enter or leave. The **renal pelvis** (see Figure 15.4) is the expanded origin of the ureter within the kidney. The final discharge of urine from the many collecting ducts is received by the renal pelvis. The **ureter** is a muscular (smooth muscle) tube that conveys urine from the renal pelvis to the urinary bladder. The urinary bladder is a hollow muscular (smooth muscle) organ that varies in size depending on the amount of urine it contains at any one time. The smooth muscle of the urinary bladder is known as the **detrusor muscle**.

The **neck of the bladder** is the caudal continuation of the bladder leading to the urethra. The smooth muscle in the neck is mixed with a considerable amount of elastic tissue and functions as an **internal sphincter**. The **urethra** is the caudal continuation of the neck of the bladder. It conveys the urine from the bladder to the exterior (Figure 15.5). The **external sphincter** lies beyond the neck; it is composed of skeletal

Dukes' Physiology of Domestic Animals, Thirteenth Edition. Edited by William O. Reece, Howard H. Erickson, Jesse P. Goff and Etsuro E. Uemura.

© 2015 John Wiley & Sons, Inc. Published 2015 by John Wiley & Sons, Inc.

Companion website: www.wiley.com/go/reece/physiology

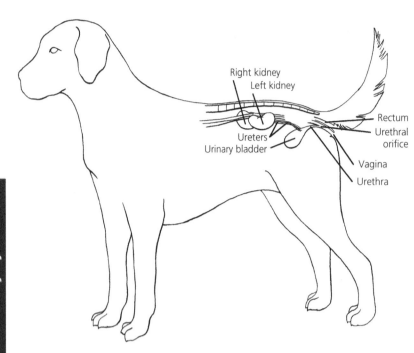

Figure 15.1 Side view of female dog showing general location of kidneys, ureters, urinary bladder, urethra, urethral orifice, and vagina. From Reece W.O. (2009) *Functional Anatomy and Physiology of Domestic Animals*, 4th edn. Wiley-Blackwell, Ames, IA. Reproduced with permission from Wiley.

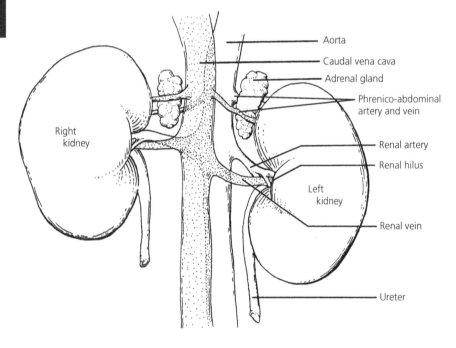

Figure 15.2 Ventral view of canine kidneys showing renal arteries, veins, and ureters and their positions relative to the aorta, vena cava, and adrenal glands. From Reece W.O. (2009) *Functional Anatomy and Physiology of Domestic Animals*, 4th edn. Wiley-Blackwell, Ames, IA. Reproduced with permission from Wiley.

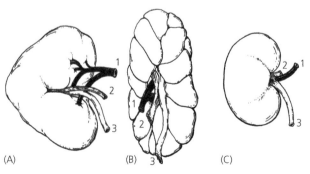

Figure 15.3 Right kidney, ventral view. (A) Horse, (B) cow, (C) sheep. These represent heart-shaped, lobulated, and bean-shaped kidneys, respectively. (1) Renal artery; (2) renal vein; (3) ureter. From Reece W.O. (2009) *Functional Anatomy and Physiology of Domestic Animals*, 4th edn. Wiley-Blackwell, Ames, IA. Reproduced with permission from Wiley.

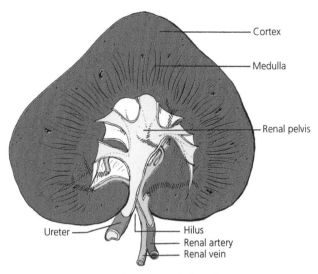

Figure 15.4 Mid-sagittal plane of horse kidney showing cortex, medulla, renal pelvis, hilus, ureter, renal artery, and renal vein. Adapted from Reece W.O. (2009) *Functional Anatomy and Physiology of Domestic Animals*, 4th edn. Wiley-Blackwell, Ames, IA. Reproduced with permission from Wiley.

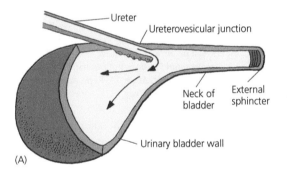

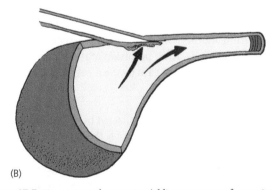

Figure 15.5 Ureterovesicular junction (oblique entrance of ureter into the urinary bladder). (A) Urine is conveyed to the urinary bladder from the renal pelvis by peristalsis and enters at the ureterovesicular junction. (B) During micturition (emptying of the urinary bladder), urine is directed through the neck of the bladder to the urethra. Urine does not reenter the ureter because the ureterovesicular junction is closed by the hydrostatic pressure of urine associated with contraction of the detrusor muscle of the bladder wall. Adapted from Reece W.O. (2009) *Functional Anatomy and Physiology of Domestic Animals*, 4th edn. Wiley-Blackwell, Ames, IA. Reproduced with permission from Wiley.

muscle that encircles the urethra at this point. The functional boundary between the bladder and the urethra is represented by this sphincter.

The nephron

> 1 Do large-breed dogs have significantly greater numbers of nephrons than small-breed dogs?
>
> 2 Besides their location, what differentiates juxtamedullary nephrons from cortical nephrons?
>
> 3 Will the tubular fluid from both cortical and juxtaglomerular nephrons be subjected to medullary influence associated with concentrating the urine?
>
> 4 What is the progressive order of vessels as blood enters the afferent arterioles and exits via renal veins?
>
> 5 What are the components of the nephron (in order) from the glomerulus to the inner medullary collecting duct?
>
> 6 Be aware where the distal tubule begins and the location of its output. Is the influence of the distal tubule in the cortex or in the medulla?

The functional unit of the kidney is the **nephron**. An understanding of nephron function is essential for understanding kidney function. Nephron numbers vary considerably among species, and approximate numbers for several species are given in Table 15.1. Within a species, nephron numbers are relatively constant. Considering the differences in size among various breeds of dogs, it might be thought that the kidneys of large-breed dogs would contain more nephrons than the kidneys of small-breed dogs. This is not the case, however, and the larger kidney size in large dogs is compensated for by their having larger nephrons rather than more nephrons.

The mammalian kidney has two principal types of nephrons, identified by (i) the location of their glomeruli and (ii) the depth of penetration of the loops of Henle into the medulla. Those nephrons with glomeruli in the outer and middle cortices are called superficial or **corticomedullary nephrons**. They are associated with a short loop of Henle that extends to the junction of the cortex and medulla or into the outer zone of the medulla.

Table 15.1 Approximate number of nephrons in each kidney for several domestic animals and humans.

Species	Nephrons
Cattle	4,000,000
Pig	1,250,000
Dog	415,000
Cat	190,000
Human	1,000,000

Source: Reece, W.O. (2009) *Functional Anatomy and Physiology of Domestic Animals*, 4th edn. Wiley-Blackwell, Ames, IA.

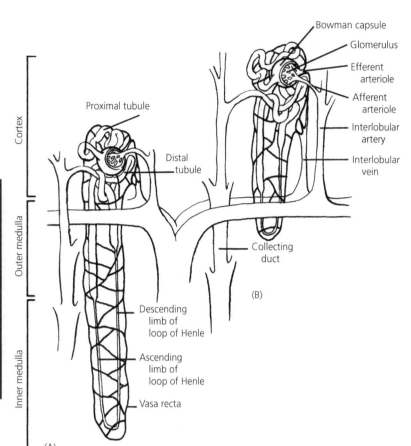

Figure 15.6 Types of mammalian nephrons: (A) juxtamedullary (long-looped) nephron; (B) cortical nephron. From Reece W.O. (2009) *Functional Anatomy and Physiology of Domestic Animals*, 4th edn. Wiley-Blackwell, Ames, IA. Reproduced with permission from Wiley.

Those nephrons with glomeruli in the cortex close to the medulla are known as **juxtamedullary nephrons**. Juxtamedullary nephrons are associated with long loops of Henle that extend more deeply into the medulla; some extend as deep as the renal pelvis. The relationship of each nephron type to the cortex and medulla is shown in Figure 15.6. The juxtamedullary nephrons are those that develop and maintain the osmotic gradient of the interstitial fluid of the medulla, from low to high in outer to inner medulla, respectively. The percentage of nephrons having long loops of Henle (juxtamedullary nephrons) varies among animal species and ranges from 3% in the pig to 100% in the cat. In humans the percentage of long-looped nephrons is about 14%. It is important to note, however, that the tubular fluid of all nephrons (cortical and juxtamedullary) is emptied into shared collecting ducts that proceed through the medulla to the renal pelvis. Thus, regardless of the influence of different nephron types on the tubular fluid, the final output of each nephron is subjected to the same factors affecting urine concentration (medullary influence).

Nephron components

A typical nephron and its component parts are shown in Figure 15.7. The **glomerulus** is the tuft of capillaries through which filtration is accomplished. The glomerular capillaries are covered by epithelial cells and the total glomerulus is encased by Bowman's capsule, which collects the glomerular filtrate for transport through the nephron tubules and ducts. The **afferent arteriole** conducts blood to the glomerulus, and the **efferent arteriole** conducts blood away from the glomerulus. Blood leaving through the efferent arterioles is redistributed into another bed of capillaries known as the **peritubular capillaries**; these perfuse the nephron tubules. The vasa recta are capillary branches from the peritubular capillaries associated with the long-looped nephrons. After perfusion of the kidneys, blood is returned to the caudal vena cava by the renal veins.

Nephron tubules and ducts

Filtrate from the glomerulus is collected by **Bowman's capsule** and is subsequently directed through the convoluted (coiled) proximal tubules, which lie in the cortex of the kidney. The proximal tubule is continued by the **loop of Henle**, which dips into the medulla. The loop of Henle consists of a **descending limb** and an **ascending limb**. The ascending limb returns to its glomerulus of origin in the cortex where its end has a thickened segment known as the **macula densa**. Beyond the macula densa, the tubule is known as the **distal tubule**, which resides entirely in the renal cortex, and it ends with its respective connecting tubule that empties into a **cortical collecting tubule**. A cortical collecting tubule is not unique to a single nephron because it receives tubular fluid from the convoluted portion of several

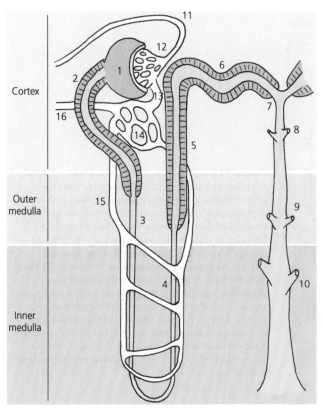

Figure 15.7 The functional nephron with blood supply. A juxtamedullary nephron is shown so as to display the vasa recta. (1) Bowman's capsule; (2) proximal tubule; (3) descending limb of loop of Henle; (4) thin ascending limb of loop of Henle; (5) thick ascending limb of loop of Henle; (6) distal tubule; (7) connecting tubule; (8) cortical collecting tubule; (9) outer medullary collecting duct; (10) inner medullary collecting duct; (11) afferent arteriole; (12) glomerulus; (13) efferent arteriole; (14) peritubular capillaries; (15) vasa recta; (16) to renal vein. Thick ascending limb of loop of Henle becomes distal tubule when it passes between the afferent and efferent arterioles at the glomerulus (location of macula densa). Adapted from Reece W.O. (2009) *Functional Anatomy and Physiology of Domestic Animals*, 4th edn. Wiley-Blackwell, Ames, IA. Reproduced with permission from Wiley.

distal tubules. When the collecting tubule turns away from the cortex and passes down into the medulla, it is known as a collecting duct. Successive generations of collecting ducts coalesce to form progressively larger collecting ducts. The tubular fluid is finally discharged from the larger collecting ducts into the pelvis of the kidney, and is conveyed from there by the ureters to the urinary bladder for storage until discharge through the urethra. A summary of nephron component parts encountered by glomerular filtrate as it becomes tubular fluid and finally urine with final discharge through the urethra is shown in Figure 15.8.

Loop of Henle

The loop of Henle is composed of three segments: the **thin descending limb**, the **thin ascending limb**, and the **thick ascending limb**. Their relative thicknesses are a result of differences in the epithelial cells and do not refer to changes in lumen

diameter. The descending thin segment of each loop is continuous with the ascending thin segment at the hairpin curve. The descending limbs of cortical nephrons only go as deep as the outer aspect of the outer medulla. The juxtamedullary nephrons are the long-looped nephrons and have descending limbs that can extend to the renal pelvis. The thin segment of the descending limb is a straight tubule continuous from the proximal tubule and is followed after its hairpin turn by the thin ascending limb. The thick segment of the ascending limb is a straight tubule continuous from the thin ascending limb. The thick segment of the ascending limb of the loop of Henle returns in its ascent to its glomerulus of origin, passes between the afferent and efferent arteriole, and proceeds from there as the distal tubule to its cortical collecting tubule.

The juxtaglomerular apparatus

1 What is the collective name of the thickened tubular epithelial cells making contact with its glomerulus of origin?
2 What is the name of the specialized smooth muscle cells that make contact with the thickened tubular epithelium of the thick ascending limb that is making contact with its glomerulus of origin?
3 What is the name of the cells outside the glomerulus and between the cells noted in items 1 and 2 above?
4 What are the three components of the juxtaglomerular apparatus?
5 What is the function of the juxtaglomerular apparatus?

When the thick segment of the ascending limb of the loop of Henle returns to its glomerulus of origin in the cortex, it was noted that it passes in the angle between the afferent and efferent arterioles and continues as the distal tubule (Figure 15.9). The side of the tubule that faces the glomerulus comes in contact with the arterioles; the contact epithelial cells of the tubules are more dense than the other epithelial cells and are collectively called the **macula densa**. The macula densa marks the beginning of the distal tubule. The smooth muscle cells of the afferent arteriole that makes contact with the macula densa are specialized smooth muscle cells and are called **juxtaglomerular (JG) granular cells**. The JG granular cells have secretory granules that contain **renin**, a proteolytic enzyme.

The space between the macula densa and the afferent and efferent arterioles as well as the space between the glomerular capillaries is known as the **mesangial region** and consists of **mesangial cells** and **mesangial matrix** (Figure 15.9). Mesangial cells secrete the matrix, secrete the glomerular basement membrane, provide structural support, have phagocytic activity, and secrete prostaglandins. Mesangial cells also exhibit contractile activity and can influence blood flow through glomerular capillaries. Those cells located between the macula densa and the arterioles are known more specifically as **extraglomerular mesangial cells**, or **lacis cells**.

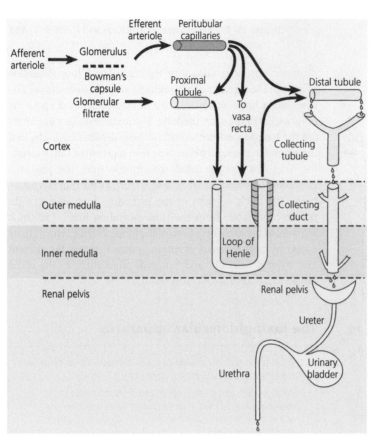

Figure 15.8 Summary of kidney blood flow and tubular fluid flow as it applies to the nephron. The fraction of plasma filtered at the glomerulus enters Bowman's capsule as glomerular filtrate. It continues through the nephron tubules and ducts as tubular fluid. The tubular fluid is subjected to reabsorption and secretion and enters the renal pelvis as urine. After removal of the filtration fraction of plasma at the glomerulus, the remaining blood that enters the efferent arteriole is distributed via peritubular capillaries to the proximal tubules, vasa recta, and distal tubules for exchanges with the tubular fluid. Urine is finally evacuated from the urinary bladder by micturition. Adapted from Reece W.O. (2009) *Functional Anatomy and Physiology of Domestic Animals*, 4th edn. Wiley-Blackwell, Ames, IA. Reproduced with permission from Wiley.

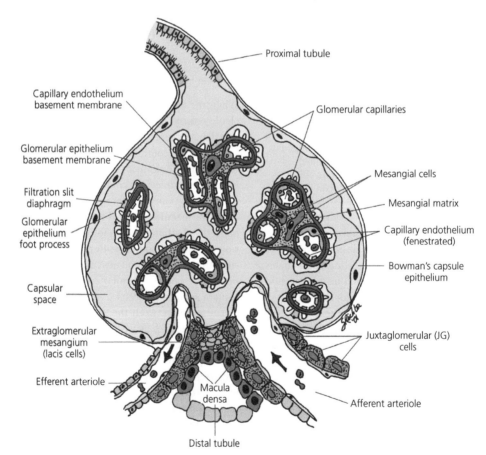

Figure 15.9 The juxtaglomerular (JG) apparatus. The JG apparatus is located at the junction of the distal tubule and its glomerulus of origin. It is associated with regulation of blood flow and filtration fraction for the nephron and with the secretion of renin, an enzyme involved in the formation of angiotensin II. Structures within the capsular space (Bowman's capsule) appear as independent structures because of the transverse section view. Structurally, they are continuous with each other and with the afferent and efferent arterioles. Adapted from Reece W.O. (2009) *Functional Anatomy and Physiology of Domestic Animals*, 4th edn. Wiley-Blackwell, Ames, IA. Reproduced with permission from Wiley.

Because of their intimacy and functional relationship, the three components of the JG apparatus are (i) the macula densa, (ii) the JG granular cells, and (iii) the extraglomerular mesangial cells. The JG apparatus is involved in feedback mechanisms that assist regulation of renal blood flow and glomerular filtration rate.

Innervation

> 1 What division of the autonomic nervous system provides innervation to the kidneys?
>
> 2 What structures are innervated?
>
> 3 What changes are invoked by efferent renal sympathetic nerve activity (ERSNA)?
>
> 4 What is the significance of renal sympathetic nerves having functionally specific groups of fibers versus a homogeneous group of fibers?
>
> 5 Are sensory (afferent) fibers intermixed with motor (efferent) fibers in the renal nerves?
>
> 6 What is a renorenal reflex?
>
> 7 What is the response to obstruction to ureteral flow in the right ureter?

Innervation to the kidney is provided by the **sympathetic (adrenergic) division** of the **autonomic nervous system**. The postganglionic renal nerves enter the hilus of the kidney in association with the renal artery and vein and provide adrenergic innervation to the renal vasculature, all segments of the nephron, and the JG granular cells. **Efferent renal sympathetic nerve activity (ERSNA)** produces marked changes in renal hemodynamics, tubular ion and water transport, and renin secretion. Although the renal sympathetic nerves were previously considered to be a homogeneous group of fibers, it is now known that the above effects of stimulation are mediated by functionally specific groups of fibers separately innervating the renal vessels, tubules, and JG granular cells.

Although the autonomic nervous system is described as a motor (efferent) system, there are sensory (afferent) fibers intermixed with the motor fibers. Accordingly, the renal nerves are the communication link between the central nervous system and the kidneys. Renorenal reflexes via afferent input from sensory receptors in the kidneys allow total renal function to be self-regulated and balanced between the two kidneys.

Renorenal reflex control of renal function

Renorenal reflexes are defined as responses occurring in one kidney as a result of intervention on the same (ipsilateral) or the opposite (contralateral) kidney that are mediated by neurohumoral mechanisms. Two classes of renal sensory receptors have been identified: (i) **renal mechanoreceptors** responding to increases in intrarenal pressure, and (ii) **renal chemoreceptors** responding to renal ischemia and/or changes in the chemical environment of the **renal interstitium**.

Afferent renal nerves exert a tonic inhibition of contralateral ERSNA, promoting water and sodium excretion from the opposite kidney. Therefore, renal sensory receptors form the basis for renorenal reflexes which, with afferent and efferent neural pathways, serve as a self-regulating or feedback system to balance renal excretory function between the two kidneys.

Renal pelvis pressure increases when there is obstruction to ureteral flow of urine. The mechanosensitive neurons are activated at pressures below the pain sensation threshold and their afferent renal nerves lead to a reflex decrease in contralateral ERSNA followed by a contralateral diuresis and natriuresis. The ipsilateral impairment of urine flow and solute excretion is compensated by an increase in contralateral urine flow and solute excretion, resulting in unchanged total urine flow and solute excretion.

Overview of urine formation

> 1 What are the three processes associated with urine formation?
>
> 2 What is the difference between plasma, glomerular filtrate, and urine?
>
> 3 Follow the pathway of fluid from plasma in the afferent arteriole through the several components of the nephron to its final discharge from the urethra.
>
> 4 Define RBF, RPF, GFR, and FF. Which variable (RBF, RPF, GFR, or FF) represents the largest volume? What is an approximate value for the percentage of glomerular filtrate that is excreted as urine?

From plasma to urine

The three processes involving the nephrons, collecting ducts, and their blood supply in urine formation are glomerular filtration, tubular reabsorption, and tubular secretion. As a result of glomerular filtration, an ultrafiltrate of plasma known as **glomerular filtrate** appears in the Bowman's capsule. Glomerular filtrate becomes **tubular fluid** when it enters the nephron tubules because of the compositional changes that begin to occur immediately as a result of reabsorption from the tubular lumen and secretion into the tubular lumen (Figure 15.10). Tubular reabsorption and tubular secretion continue throughout the length of the nephrons and collecting ducts, so that tubular fluid does not become urine until it enters the renal pelvis. With the possible exception of mucus addition in the horse, there are no compositional changes in urine beyond the collecting ducts.

Distribution of blood at the glomerulus

Renal blood flow (RBF) refers to the rate at which blood flows to the kidneys. Inasmuch as plasma is the fluid part of the blood, from which the glomerular filtrate is formed, **renal plasma flow (RPF)** refers to that part of the RBF that is plasma. As long as there continues to be an RBF, a glomerular filtrate will be formed from the plasma at the glomerulus. The rate at which it is formed is known as the **glomerular filtration rate (GFR)** and is measured in milliliters per minute. RBF and RPF are also measured in milliliters per minute, and the ratio of GFR to RPF is referred to as the **filtration fraction (FF)**. The FF is the fraction (or percentage) of plasma flowing through the glomerulus that becomes glomerular filtrate. The blood that continues into the

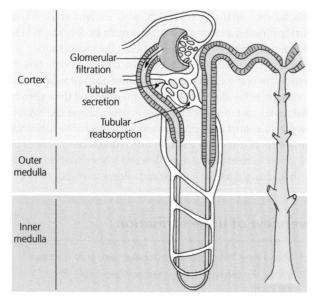

Figure 15.10 Functional nephron and processes involved in urine formation. The arrows indicate the origins and destinations of the three processes associated with the formation of urine. After glomerular filtration, glomerular filtrate enters the proximal tubule and becomes tubular fluid. Tubular secretion is directed from the peritubular capillaries into the tubules, and tubular reabsorption is directed from the tubules into the peritubular capillaries. Tubular reabsorption and tubular secretion occur throughout the length of the nephron. Adapted from Reece W.O. (2009) *Functional Anatomy and Physiology of Domestic Animals*, 4th edn. Wiley-Blackwell, Ames, IA. Reproduced with permission from Wiley.

Table 15.2 Approximate values for several kidney function variables in an 11.35-kg (25-lb) dog in a normal state of hydration.

Variable	Value
Cardiac output (mL/min)	1500
Blood flow to kidneys (% of cardiac output)	20
Renal blood flow (mL/min)	300
Renal plasma flow* (mL/min)	180
Glomerular filtration rate (mL/min)	45
Filtration fraction (decimal equivalent)	0.25
Urine volume in 24 hours[†] (mL)	681
Glomerular filtrate volume in 24 hours (mL)	64,800
Volume of urine as percent of filtrate	1.05
Filtrate reabsorbed (%)	98.95

*Based on plasma portion of hematocrit being approximately 60%.
[†]Calculated from average rate for dogs being 60 mL/kg per 24 hours.
Source: Reece, W.O. (2009) *Functional Anatomy and Physiology of Domestic Animals*, 4th edn. Wiley-Blackwell, Ames, IA.

efferent arterioles has an increased value for packed cell volume and protein concentration because a fraction of the plasma has been filtered and has entered the tubules. The protein concentration is higher because it is virtually prevented from being filtered with the other plasma components.

An example for the relationships of RBF, RPF, GFR, FF and the percentage of urine formed relative to the amount of filtrate formed in 24 hours is shown in Table 15.2.

Self-evaluation

Answers can be found at the end of the chapter.

1 As it affects urine concentration, the outcome is influenced by:
  A Cortical nephrons
  B Juxtamedullary nephrons
  C Both cortical and juxtamedullary nephrons
  Explain your answer.

2 The thin descending limb, the thin ascending limb, and the thick ascending limb of the loop of Henle:
  A Have the same lumen diameter
  B Have the same epithelial cell thickness
  C Have a lumen diameter corresponding to the limb being thin or thick
  Explain your answer.

3 Innervation to the kidney is provided by:
  A A homogeneous group of motor (efferent) fibers
  B Functionally specific groups of fibers with both motor (efferent) and sensory (afferent) activity
  C Functionally specific groups of fibers with only motor (efferent) activity
  Explain your answer.

4 The following values were obtained in a renal physiology laboratory where RBF, RPF, GFR, and FF were being measured but their identity has been lost: 16 mL/min per kg; 3.36 mL/min per kg; 8.64 mL/min per kg; 0.35. Their reassigned identity should be:
  A GFR, RBF, FF, RPF
  B RBF, GFR, RPF, FF
  C RBF, GFR, FF, RPF
  D RPF, RBF, FF, GFR
  Explain your answer.

5 What would be the response of a renoreneal reflex following a left ureteral obstruction?
  A A mechanoreceptor response would occur only after pain was apparent
  B The impairment of urine flow from the left ureter does not involve afferent (sensory) fiber intervention
  C Mechanoreceptors in the left kidney activate a reflex to increase activity of the right kidney
  Explain your answer.

Suggested reading

Dibona, G.F. (2000) Differentiation of vasoactive renal sympathetic nerve fibers. *Acta Physiologica Scandinavica* 168:195–200.

Dibona, G.F. and Kopp, U.C. (1997) Neural control of renal function. *Physiological Reviews* 77:75–197.

Reece, W. (2004) Kidney function in mammals. In: *Dukes' Physiology of Domestic Animals*, 12th edn (ed. W.O. Reece), pp. 73–106. Cornell University Press, Ithaca, NY.

Reece, W. (2009) *Functional Anatomy and Physiology of Domestic Animals*, 4th edn. Wiley-Blackwell, Ames, IA.

Answers

1 C. The tubular fluid of all nephrons, both cortical and juxtamedullary, is emptied into shared collecting ducts that proceed through the medulla to the renal pelvis. Thus, regardless of the influence of different nephron types on the tubular fluid, the final output of each nephron is subjected to the same factors affecting urine concentration (medullary influence).

2 A. The relative thickness is a result of differences in the epithelial cells and does not refer to changes in lumen diameter.

3 B. It is now known that the effects of stimulation are mediated by functionally specific groups of fibers separately innervating the renal vessels, tubules, and JG granular cells. Also, although the autonomic nervous system is described as a motor (efferent) system, there are sensory (afferent) fibers intermixed with the motor fibers that serve as a communication link between the central nervous system and the kidneys.

4 B. Renal blood flow is the greatest value, followed by renal plasma flow. Glomerular filtration rate is that part of renal plasma flow that becomes glomerular filtrate. Filtration fraction is the fraction of renal plasma flow that becomes glomerular filtrate.

5 C. Mechanosensitive neurons are activated from the left ureter and their afferent renal nerves lead to a reflex increase in the efferent renal sympathetic nerve activity of the right kidney and the impairment of urine flow and solute excretion in the left kidney is compensated by an increase of urine flow and solute excretion in the right kidney, resulting in unchanged total urine flow and solute excretion.

Section III: The Kidneys and Urinary System

16 Glomerular Filtration and Tubular Transport

William O. Reece

Iowa State University, Ames, IA, USA

Two important functions of the kidneys are to filter the plasma and either return filtered substances to the plasma or excrete them with the urine. The former function is described as glomerular filtration and the latter as tubular transport.

Glomerular filtration

1 How do the capillary beds of the glomeruli and peritubular capillaries differ? Which one resembles the arterial end of a muscle capillary and which one represents the venous end?

2 What factors associated with the intravascular lysis of erythrocytes would give rise to hemoglobinuria and/or acute renal shutdown?

3 How does efferent arteriolar constriction increase the FF?

4 How does poor kidney perfusion relate to greater access to filtration of large molecules?

5 Describe the tubuloglomerular feedback mechanism for the regulation of RBF and GFR.

6 What is the role of renin in the autoregulation of RBF and GFR?

Formation of the filtrate

The kidneys have the functional counterpart of two capillary beds, represented by the glomeruli and the peritubular capillaries. The glomeruli are considered to be a high-pressure system (high hydrostatic pressure favoring filtration), and the peritubular capillaries, which are perfused with blood coming from the glomerular capillary bed, are considered to be a low-pressure system (low hydrostatic pressure favoring reabsorption). As such, the glomeruli are similar to the arterial end of a typical muscle capillary, and the peritubular capillaries are similar to the venous end.

The formation of urine begins when an **ultrafiltrate of plasma** passes through the fenestrated capillary endothelium, the glomerular basement membrane, and the glomerular epithelium of Bowman's capsule into the capsular space of Bowman's capsule (Figure 16.1). Energy for this filtration process is provided by the heart in the form of **hydrostatic pressure (HP)** within the glomerular capillaries and is opposed by the **colloidal osmotic pressure (COP)** of plasma proteins plus the HP of the filtrate.

The dynamics of filtration are illustrated in Figure 16.1. According to the values shown, there is net filtration because the capillary HP of 60 mmHg exceeds the combined values for capillary COP of 32 mmHg and Bowman's capsule space HP of 18 mmHg (60 – [32 + 18] =10 mmHg). Although some filtration of protein (a potential source of COP in Bowman's capsule) occurs (as in muscle capillaries), the filtrate does not accumulate as it does in muscle because the HP in Bowman's capsule causes filtrate to flow away from the capsule and through the nephron tubules. Therefore COP in Bowman's capsule space is negligible.

Nature of the filtrate

The glomerular filtrate is called an ultrafiltrate of plasma because the larger components (colloids and blood cells) are not filtered. Practically speaking, it is similar to plasma and interstitial fluid, except that it has a lower protein concentration than either of them.

Because of its fenestrations (see Figure 16.1), the capillary endothelium of the glomerulus is more porous than muscle capillary endothelium, and larger molecules are more readily filtered. Protein molecules are relatively restricted from filtration (similar to their restriction in muscle capillaries) because of their large molecular size, but they may not be excluded altogether. Proteins with a molecular weight of 70,000 and above

Dukes' Physiology of Domestic Animals, Thirteenth Edition. Edited by William O. Reece, Howard H. Erickson, Jesse P. Goff and Etsuro E. Uemura.

© 2015 John Wiley & Sons, Inc. Published 2015 by John Wiley & Sons, Inc.

Companion website: www.wiley.com/go/reece/physiology

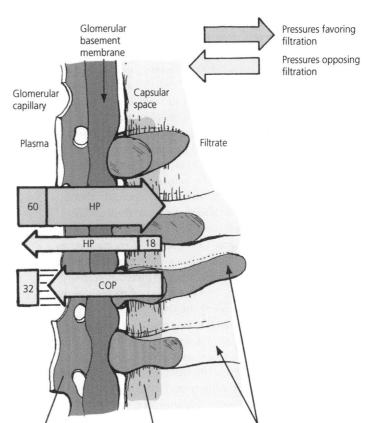

Figure 16.1 Dynamics of glomerular filtration in mammals. Bowman's capsule is separated from the glomerulus by a glomerular membrane, through which filtration occurs. The extent of filtration is determined by the difference between the pressures favoring filtration and those opposing filtration. In this illustration, filtration occurs because 60 − (32 + 18) =10 mmHg. Values greater or less than 10 mmHg would correlate with more or less filtration, respectively. Pressure values (60, 32, 18) are in mmHg. HP, hydrostatic pressure; COP, colloidal osmotic pressure. Adapted from Reece, W.O. (2009) *Functional Anatomy and Physiology of Domestic Animals*, 4th edn. Wiley-Blackwell, Ames, IA.

are virtually excluded from the filtrate. Albumin, the smallest of the plasma proteins, has an average molecular weight of about 69,000 and 0.2–0.3% of its plasma concentration can appear in the filtrate. Hemoglobin has a molecular weight of about 68,000 and, when unbound, it appears in filtrate at a concentration equal to about 5% of its unbound concentration in plasma. The hemoglobin in plasma that arises from normal intravascular lysis of erythrocytes is bound by **plasma haptoglobin** (a plasma protein) so that the combined size prevents leakage at the glomerulus. If excessive intravascular lysis occurs, plasma haptoglobin becomes saturated and unbound hemoglobin begins to appear in the urine, a condition known as **hemoglobinuria**. If tubular hemoglobin concentration rises too high, coupled with continued water reabsorption from the tubules, hemoglobin can precipitate and block tubules. Blocked tubules can cause **acute renal shutdown**.

Factors that influence filtration

The GFR can be varied by changes in the diameter of the afferent or efferent arterioles. Dilation of the afferent arteriole increases the blood flow to the glomerulus, which in turn increases the HP and the potential for filtration. Constriction of the efferent arteriole increases the glomerular HP, just as blockage of a vein increases the HP in capillaries behind it. At the same time, it reduces **renal blood flow (RBF)**. Neural and humoral factors are also capable of affecting these diameter changes. These will be discussed at appropriate points in the chapter.

For any given molecular size, positively charged molecules are more readily filtered than negatively charged molecules. This is because of electrostatic repulsion by anionic sites in the glomerular basement membrane that are composed mostly of **proteoglycans**. These negatively charged proteoglycans repel similarly charged molecules. In the physiologic pH range, plasma albumin molecules are polyanionic; in addition to their large molecular size, this is an important aspect in restricting their filtration. Poor perfusion of the kidneys cans result in a change in the electrostatic charge of the glomerular membrane, and molecules previously restricted from filtration can be filtered and gain entrance to the capsular space.

Autoregulation

In normal day-to-day situations, with varying levels of activity, RBF and **glomerular filtration rate (GFR)** remain relatively constant within a wide range of mean systemic arterial pressure. Between 80 and 130 mmHg, changes in RBF and GFR are minimal. This phenomenon, intrinsic to the kidney and independent of renal nerve activity, is termed **autoregulation**.

One explanation relates to a myogenic stretch receptor response in the afferent arteriole, whereby increased blood pressure would increase the stretch and the arteriole would respond by contracting. In this way, RBF would be decreased and glomerular HP reduced. The reduced glomerular HP would reduce GFR. A reduction in blood pressure would cause less tension, and the blood vessel would dilate, thereby increasing RBF and glomerular HP resulting in increased GFR.

A closely related mechanism for autoregulation is known as **tubuloglomerular feedback**. It has two components that act together to control GFR: (i) an afferent arteriolar feedback mechanism and (ii) an efferent arteriolar feedback mechanism. **Macula densa cells** (see Figure 15.9, Chapter 15) sense changes in volume delivery to the distal tubules. Decreased GFR slows the flow rate in the loop of Henle that allows increased reabsorption of sodium and chloride ions in the ascending limb of the loop of Henle, thereby decreasing the concentration of sodium chloride at the macula densa cells. This results in a signal from the macula densa decreasing resistance to blood flow in the afferent arterioles which raises glomerular HP, helping to return GFR to normal. The signal from the macula densa also increases release of renin from the juxtaglomerular (JG) cells of the afferent and efferent arterioles (major storage sites for renin). **Renin**, an enzyme, increases the formation of angiotensin I, which is converted to angiotensin II by **angiotensin-converting enzyme (ACE)**. **Angiotensin II** constricts the efferent arterioles, thereby increasing glomerular HP and glomerular filtration, assisting the return of GFR toward normal. The production of angiotensin II continues because of the conversion of plasma **angiotensinogen** (produced in the liver) to angiotensin I by renin and its subsequent conversion to angiotensin II by ACE (Figure 16.2). Although ACE is derived mainly from the capillary endothelium of the lung, because of its vascularity, it is also derived in the kidney endothelium and other organ beds.

Next to vasopressin, angiotensin II is the second most potent vasoconstrictor produced in the body. It is rapidly destroyed in the peripheral capillary beds by a number of enzymes called angiotensinases. Although not related to autoregulation, angiotensin II stimulates the secretion of aldosterone, which causes reabsorption of Na+. This becomes a factor in ECF volume regulation.

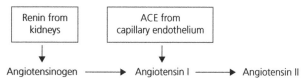

Figure 16.2 The conversion of angiotensinogen to angiotensin II. Plasma angiotensinogen is produced in the liver. It is converted to angiotensin I by renin released from the juxtaglomerular cells of the afferent and efferent arterioles. Angiotensin I is converted to angiotensin II by angiotensin-converting enzyme (ACE) derived from capillary endothelium.

Tubular transport

> 1 Why is reabsorption of fluid from tubules into the peritubular capillaries analogous to reabsorption that occurs at the venous end of a muscle capillary?
>
> 2 How do reductions in peritubular capillary HP and elevations in peritubular capillary COP relate to greater tubular reabsorption?
>
> 3 What are the three mechanisms whereby 65% of Na+ reabsorption occurs in the proximal tubules?
>
> 4 What are the mechanisms and location that account for 25% of Na+ reabsorption?
>
> 5 What is important about the flexibility accorded Na+ reabsorption in the distal nephron?
>
> 6 What accounts for 65% of water reabsorption in the proximal tubules? Note the limitations for urea and other nonactively reabsorbed solutes.
>
> 7 What are the mechanisms for the reabsorption of proteins and peptides?
>
> 8 What are the two methods associated with H+ secretion? How is K+ secretion related to dietary intake of K+?
>
> 9 What is the relationship of transport maximum to diabetes mellitus?
>
> 10 What is the significance of the property of the proximal tubule known as glomerulotubular balance?

Tubular transport refers to all phenomena associated with tubular fluid throughout the nephron and collecting ducts. Transport from Bowman's capsule to the renal pelvis is accomplished by a difference in HP (high in Bowman's capsule, low in renal pelvis). Tubular reabsorption involves transport of water and solute from tubular fluid to peritubular capillaries. Tubular secretion is associated with transport of solute from **peritubular capillaries** to the tubular fluid. The directions and structures traversed for both reabsorption and secretion are shown in Figure 16.3.

Capillary dynamics in peritubular capillaries

Reabsorption of fluid from tubules into the peritubular capillaries is analogous to the reabsorption that occurs at the venous end of a muscle capillary. In other words, in contrast to the filtration that occurs at the glomerulus, peritubular capillary dynamics favor reabsorption. This occurs because the protein not filtered at the glomerulus now contributes to a greater COP in the peritubular capillary than the COP in the tubular fluid. Also, a reduction in peritubular capillary HP lessens this force that would be counteractive to the gain in COP. It is important to associate reductions in peritubular capillary HP and elevations in peritubular capillary COP with greater tubular reabsorption.

Tubular reabsorption

Substances important to body function, such as Na+, glucose, and amino acids, enter tubular fluid by filtration at the glomerulus. Because of their relatively small molecular size, they pass easily through the glomerular membrane, and their concentrations in the glomerular filtrate are about equal to their concentrations in

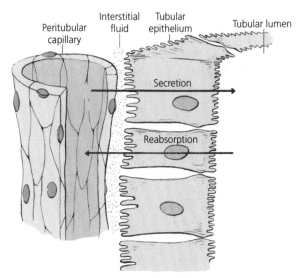

Figure 16.3 Structures that separate tubular fluid in the tubular lumen from plasma in peritubular capillaries. The energy requirement for reabsorption and secretion processes is provided by the Na⁺/K⁺-ATPase ("sodium pump") located in the basolateral membrane of proximal tubule epithelial cells. Adapted from Reece, W.O. (2009) *Functional Anatomy and Physiology of Domestic Animals*, 4th edn. Wiley-Blackwell, Ames, IA.

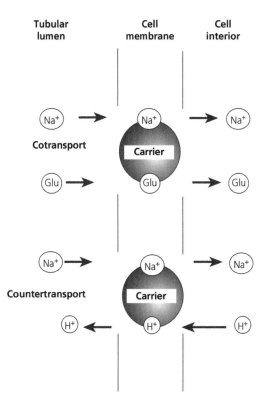

Figure 16.4 Membrane transport mechanisms. Cotransport is the transport of two compounds through a membrane in the same direction, with the flow of one (Na⁺) down its preexisting gradient carrying the other (glucose) against a gradient. Countertransport also couples the transport of one compound (Na⁺, as above) to transport of the other (H⁺) in an opposite direction. From Reece, W.O. (2009) *Functional Anatomy and Physiology of Domestic Animals*, 4th edn. Wiley-Blackwell, Ames, IA.

plasma. Unless these substances are returned to the blood, they are excreted in the urine and lost from the body. In order that Na⁺, glucose, and amino acids from the tubular fluid may be returned to the blood, energy is supplied by the **Na⁺/K⁺-ATPase pump (sodium pump)** on the basal and lateral surfaces of the tubular epithelial cells. Simultaneous transport of two or more compounds on the same carrier in the same direction (e.g., Na⁺ plus glucose, or Na⁺ plus amino acid) is known as **cotransport**. **Countertransport** refers to the movement of a compound in one direction, driven by the movement of a second compound in the opposite direction (e.g., Na⁺–H⁺ countertransport). These two mechanisms are illustrated in Figure 16.4.

Sodium absorption

About 65% of Na⁺ reabsorption occurs in the proximal tubule by three major mechanisms. The energy requirement for each is derived from the Na⁺/K⁺-ATPase located in the basal and lateral borders of the proximal tubule epithelial cells. The direction of transport is thus from the nephron proximal tubule to the peritubular capillaries. Recall that reabsorption is favored at this location because of the capillary dynamics (i.e., increased COP, decreased HP) distal to the glomerulus. The reabsorption of Na⁺ is accompanied by anions to maintain electrical neutrality. About 75% of the anions are Cl⁻ and 25% are HCO₃⁻.

When Na⁺ is actively transported from the tubular epithelial cells (directed to the peritubular capillaries), a chemical and electrical gradient (**electrochemical gradient**) is created between the epithelial cells and the proximal tubule lumen. The luminal membrane contains carrier proteins specific for Na⁺ coupled with either glucose or an amino acid (cotransport).

Because of the electrochemical gradient and the cotransport mechanism, Na⁺ readily diffuses (facilitated diffusion) from the tubular lumen into the epithelial cell along with its coupled solute (glucose or amino acid). The peritubular space has become electropositive because of Na⁺ transport to that space. In order to maintain electrical neutrality, Cl⁻ ions readily diffuse from the tubular lumen to the peritubular space through the tight junctions between tubular epithelial cells.

A second mechanism for the reabsorption of Na⁺ is countertransport with H⁺. The epithelial cells of the proximal and distal tubules, and collecting ducts all secrete H⁺ ions that result from the hydration of CO₂ within the epithelial cells, which produces H⁺ and HCO₃⁻. However, about 85% of H⁺ ions are secreted by the cells of the proximal tubule. The HCO₃⁻ ions in the cells that produced the H⁺ diffuses through the basolateral membranes into the peritubular space to maintain electrical neutrality with the Na⁺ that was countertransported with the H⁺.

A third mechanism for Na⁺ reabsorption is known as chloride-driven Na⁺ transport and occurs in more distal portions of the proximal tubules. At this location, there is more HCO₃⁻ being reabsorbed into the peritubular space as anion rather than Cl⁻, and the Cl⁻ concentration increase in the tubule creates a gradient for its diffusion into the peritubular space through the "leaky" tight junctions. This is accompanied by diffusion of Na$^+$ through the tight junctions in the same direction to maintain electrical neutrality.

The three mechanisms described account for about 65% of Na$^+$ reabsorption with the remaining 35% continuing beyond the proximal tubules. About 25% of the tubular load of Na$^+$ is reabsorbed in the ascending thick segment of the loop of Henle (medullary and cortical). Sodium entry occurs via a Na$^+$–K$^+$–2Cl$^-$ carrier in the luminal membrane (cotransport). All four sites on the carrier must be occupied for net transport into the cell. Once in the cell, Na$^+$ is actively extruded across the basolateral surfaces by the Na$^+$/K$^+$-ATPase, and Cl$^-$ diffuses passively to maintain electrical neutrality. Na$^+$–K$^+$–2Cl$^-$ cotransport in the loop of Henle is inhibited by the so-called loop diuretics such as furosemide (diuretics increase output of urine).

The remaining 10% of filtered Na$^+$ is presented to the distal nephron. The mechanism for active Na$^+$ reabsorption in the distal convoluted and connecting tubules of the distal nephrons is coupled with the cotransport of Cl$^-$. Beyond the connecting tubules, Na$^+$ reabsorption in the collecting ducts is not coupled with Cl$^-$ reabsorption, but rather occurs via **conductive Na$^+$ channels**. The tight junctions in this location are tighter and not only limit the ability of Cl$^-$ to accompany Na$^+$, but also prevent the Na$^+$ pumped into the basolateral spaces from leaking back into the tubular lumen. A characteristic of the conductive Na$^+$ channel is that an increased amount of Na$^+$ will be reabsorbed by the collecting duct if an increased load is delivered. Na$^+$ reabsorption via the conductive Na$^+$ channel in the collecting duct is stimulated by the hormone **aldosterone**, whereby Na$^+$ reabsorption is increased. This is an accommodation for **hypovolemia** and its associated declining blood pressure. The Na$^+$ increase is followed by reabsorption of water by osmosis, thereby returning blood volume and in turn blood pressure toward normal.

Glucose and amino acid reabsorption

Glucose and amino acids are reabsorbed by cotransport (Figure 16.5). They are coupled with specific carriers that require Na$^+$ binding and diffuse to the cell interior because of the electrochemical gradient for Na$^+$. Inside the cell, the Na$^+$ and glucose or amino acids separate from the carrier. The Na$^+$ is then actively transported by Na$^+$/K$^+$-ATPase to the peritubular space, and presumably specific carriers are present for facilitated diffusion of glucose and amino acids into the peritubular space. It is likely that several specific Na$^+$–amino acid carriers are present in the luminal membrane for amino acid transport.

Transport of water and nonactively reabsorbed solutes

After the movement of solute (Na$^+$, Cl$^-$, HCO$_3^-$, glucose, amino acids) into the peritubular space, an osmotic gradient is established whereby a greater effective osmotic pressure is present in the peritubular space. In response to the greater effective osmotic pressure in the peritubular space, water diffuses from the tubular lumen through the tight junctions

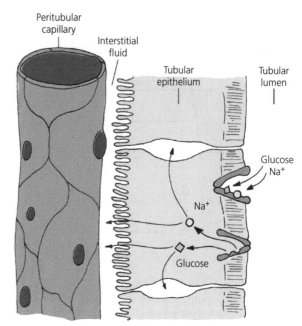

Figure 16.5 Transport of Na$^+$ from tubular lumen into the tubular epithelial cell and its cotransport with glucose. The protein carrier conformation permits binding of Na$^+$ and glucose from the lumen. Carrier conformational change permits Na$^+$ and glucose release into the epithelial cytoplasm. Once released, the carrier returns to its original conformation for binding of more Na$^+$ and glucose. The Na$^+$ released into the tubular epithelial cytoplasm is actively transported through the basal and lateral borders of the cells into the interstitial fluid and diffuses from there into the capillaries. Glucose follows the same pathways except that it is not actively transported. Amino acids are also cotransported with Na$^+$ similar to that of glucose. Adapted from Reece, W.O. (2009) *Functional Anatomy and Physiology of Domestic Animals*, 4th edn. Wiley-Blackwell, Ames, IA.

(paracellular) and tubular cells (transcellular) into the peritubular space.

The reabsorption of about 65% of the Na$^+$ and its accompanying anions from the proximal tubules accounts for most of the effective osmotic pressure in the peritubular space. Accordingly, 65% of the water is reabsorbed from the proximal tubule (an additional amount for the other osmotically active substances, i.e., glucose, amino acids). As the water is reabsorbed, urea and other nonactively reabsorbed solutes are concentrated in the tubular lumen. A chemical concentration gradient is established for urea and other nonactively reabsorbed solutes, and they are reabsorbed down their concentration gradient. The extent of their reabsorption is dependent on the permeability of the proximal tubular epithelium for the solute. The permeability of the proximal tubular epithelium for urea is much less than that for water, and thus more than half of the amount of urea in the glomerular filtrate continues beyond the proximal tubule.

Reabsorption of proteins and peptides

It has been noted that proteins with a molecular weight of less than about 69,000 have the potential to become part of the glomerular filtrate. Because they are important nutrients, most of these proteins are reabsorbed in the proximal tubule and are not lost in the urine. However, a small quantity of protein is present in normal urine. The protein concentration in random samples of urine from 157 dogs with no evidence of urinary tract disease averaged 23 mg/dL. The protein in urine from normal dogs has been reported to contain 40–60% albumin. Other components include all fractions of globulins. For example, if a 9.5-kg beagle formed 500 mL of urine in 24 hours, the amount of protein lost in that 24 hours would be about 115 mg.

Proteins (and polypeptides) are reabsorbed by endocytosis and subsequently degraded by cellular lysosomes to their constituent amino acids. The amino acids presumably move from inside the cell to the peritubular space by facilitated diffusion.

Small peptides are hydrolyzed at the luminal brush border of the proximal tubule and the resultant amino acids taken into the cell by the cotransport mechanism of the luminal membrane. Small-peptide hydrolysis is a high-capacity mechanism capable of returning to the body large amounts of amino acids that might otherwise be lost in the urine as peptides or fail to be reabsorbed into the cell by endocytosis.

Other substances

Krebs cycle intermediates (i.e., lactate and citrate) are reabsorbed as well as the plasma cations and anions Ca^{2+}, Mg^{2+}, K^+, and phosphate. Water-soluble vitamins present in plasma would otherwise be lost in the urine if mechanisms for reabsorption were not present.

Tubular secretion

Several substances are transported from the peritubular capillaries into the interstitial fluid and then to the tubular lumen via the tubular epithelial cells. The countertransport of H^+ that accompanies Na^+ reabsorption in the proximal and distal tubules is one example (see Figure 16.4). H^+ secretion continues in the distal nephron but does not appear to be coupled with Na^+ reabsorption. Distal nephron H^+ secretion is primarily an active process and occurs in the intercalated cells of the collecting duct.

Renal K^+ transport is unique in that it is reabsorbed in some parts of the tubule and secreted in others. When dietary potassium intake is extremely low there is greater reabsorption of K^+ in the distal nephron, and when dietary potassium intake is high there is greater K^+ secretion. A number of organic acids and bases are secreted by nonspecific mechanisms. Penicillin is lost from the body fluids because of tubular secretion. A longer-acting penicillin that has been developed persists in the body for longer periods because its rate of secretion has been slowed.

Transport maximum

For substances such as glucose that are associated with a carrier for their transport from tubular lumen to peritubular fluid, there is a maximum rate at which they can be reabsorbed: this is known as the tubular **transport maximum** (T_m). When the T_m for the substance in a nephron is exceeded, the substance will appear in the urine. In the disease known as **diabetes mellitus**, the movement of glucose from plasma into body cells is impaired because of the lack of insulin. Glucose concentration in plasma therefore increases, causing the plasma and tubular loads of glucose to increase. When the increased tubular load exceeds the availability of carrier molecules for glucose reabsorption, the excess glucose continues its flow through the tubules into the urine. Because glucose is retained within the tubules, it contributes to the effective osmotic pressure of the tubular fluid, and water remains in the tubular fluid. Thus, in diabetes mellitus, glucose can be detected in the urine and a greater volume of urine is formed. Because greater amounts of water are lost from the body in the urine, the afflicted animal drinks more water to compensate for the urine loss. Increased urine formation is known as **diuresis**; when it is caused by retention of water in the tubules, because of the increased effective osmotic pressure in the tubular lumen, it is known as **osmotic diuresis**.

Glomerulotubular balance

The amount of filtrate reabsorbed by the proximal tubule is consistently a certain percentage of the filtrate (about 65% for water and NaCl) rather than a constant amount for each unit of time. This property of the proximal tubule to reabsorb a consistent fractional amount of glomerular filtrate is known as **glomerulotubular balance**. If the GFR is low, only a fractional amount of filtrate is reabsorbed in the proximal tubule (rather than most of it), and the remaining fraction (about one-third) continues to the distal nephron where the regulatory processes are given a chance to operate. If the GFR is high, the additional amount of filtrate does not continue to the distal nephron but, rather, only about one-third of it, and the limited capacity for regulation is not overloaded.

Self-evaluation

Answers can be found at the end of the chapter.

1 Which one of the following would have the highest values for hematocrit and plasma protein concentration?
   A Blood in the afferent arterioles
   B Tubular filtrate
   C Blood in the efferent arteriole
   Explain your choice for the correct answer.

2 Generally speaking, protein molecules are normally restricted from filtration through the glomerular membrane because of:
   A Their size and polyanionic nature
   B Their molecular shape
   C Their combination with cations
   Explain your choice for the correct answer.

3 A plasma glucose concentration of 300 mg/dL and a urinalysis that is positive for glucose has been found in a dog. Which one of the following would be a likely clinical sign?

A Stranguria

B Polyuria and polydipsia

C Hematuria

Explain your choice for the correct answer.

4 Because of a decrease in GFR, the tubular fluid in the loop of Henle has been slowed allowing greater reabsorption of sodium and chloride ions in the ascending loop of Henle. The macula densa senses the decrease in sodium concentration. Which one of the following responses occurs?

A Afferent arteriole dilation, release of renin, and efferent arteriole dilation

B Afferent and efferent arteriole constriction

C Afferent arteriole dilation, release of renin, and efferent arteriole constriction

Explain your choice for the correct answer.

5 Hemoglobin that arises from intravascular lysis of erythrocytes:

A Remains as free hemoglobin in the plasma and is subject to filtration

B Will be bound to haptoglobin (a plasma protein) regardless of the extent of hemolysis and because of the larger molecular weight it is excluded from filtration

C Will be bound to haptoglobin as long as the lysis is not severe, but if lysis is excessive, haptoglobin becomes saturated and unbound hemoglobin may be filtered and appear in urine, a condition known as hemoglobinuria

Suggested reading

Hall, J.E. (2011) Urine formation by the kidneys: I. Glomerular filtration, renal blood flow, and their control. In: *Guyton and Hall Textbook for Medical Physiology*, 12th edn, pp. 303–322. Saunders Elsevier, Philadelphia.

Reece, W. (2004) Kidney function in mammals. In: *Dukes' Physiology of Domestic Animals*, 12th edn (ed. W.O. Reece), pp. 73–106. Cornell University Press, Ithaca, NY.

Reece, W. (2009) The urinary system. In: *Functional Anatomy and Physiology of Domestic Animals*, 4th edn, pp. 312–358. Wiley-Blackwell, Ames, IA.

Answers

1 C. Loss of plasma volume from the blood that perfuses the glomeruli via the afferent arterioles and retention of protein would cause the efferent arteriole blood to have a higher hematocrit and protein concentration.

2 A. Plasma albumin is the smallest of the plasma proteins and its molecular weight is just above the threshold that virtually excludes filtration through the fenestrations and slit pores. The filtration barrier is further characterized by negatively charged groups. In the physiologic pH range, plasma albumin molecule are polyanionic and their filtration is effectively impeded.

3 B. The high plasma glucose concentration coupled with glucose in the urine implies that the renal threshold for glucose has been surpassed and filtered glucose remains in the tubules. The tubular glucose contributes to a greater effective osmotic pressure in the tubule and water is retained in the tubule and becomes an obligated water loss with the glucose excretion. The greater water loss causes increased thirst and more frequent urination.

4 C. To accomplish the required increase in GFR, the first response is afferent arteriole dilation which increases glomerular HP. This is followed by release of renin from the juxtaglomerular cells of the afferent and efferent arterioles. Renin is converted to angiotensin II, a potent vasoconstrictor, causing efferent arteriole constriction, thereby increasing glomerular HP and assisting the return of GFR to normal.

5 C

17 Maintenance of Extracellular Fluid Hydration

William O. Reece

Iowa State University, Ames, IA, USA

Countercurrent mechanism

> **1** What is the function of the countercurrent mechanism?
>
> **2** What characteristics of the descending limb of the loop of Henle would cause the osmolality of the tubular fluid at the hairpin turn to be high?
>
> **3** What factors in the thin and thick segments of the ascending limb of the loop of Henle cause the tubular fluid to become diluted before it enters the distal tubule?
>
> **4** How does the recirculation of urea assist the countercurrent multiplier system?
>
> **5** What would happen to the vertical medullary gradient in the medulla if the countercurrent exchanger system did not exist?
>
> **6** During periods of diuresis, how does urea contribute to medullary washout?

The many functions of water and its importance have been presented (see Chapter 11). A principal function of the kidneys is to regulate the volume and composition of the body's internal environment, the extracellular fluid (ECF). The beginning of that process was discussed in Chapter 16. This chapter will discuss the means whereby the tubular fluid is subjected to processing that will allow either the conservation or the elimination of water in order to maintain constant hydration of the ECF.

The function of the countercurrent system is to prepare the interstitial fluid (ISF) of the renal medulla so that the tubular fluid of the proximal tubules entering the medullary loop of Henle can be modified before its return to the distal tubule. Modification of the tubular fluid (after it leaves the proximal tubule) for the conservation or elimination of water depends on the existence of a very high osmolality in the ISF of the renal medulla. The osmolality increases with distance from the cortex, reaching a maximum in the innermost parts of the medulla. The maximum value varies by species. In the dog, it is about 2400 mosmol/kg H_2O, compared with plasma osmolality of about 300 mosmol/kg H_2O. The high osmolality exists because of the **countercurrent mechanism**. It is established by the activities of the loops of Henle and is maintained by the special characteristics of the blood supply to the medulla (the **vasa recta**).

A countercurrent system of tubules or vessels exists where the inflow of fluid runs parallel to, counter (opposite) to, and in close proximity to the outflow for some distance. These characteristics are common to the anatomic arrangements of the loops of Henle and the vasa recta. Accordingly, the countercurrent mechanism in the kidney comprises two countercurrent systems: the **countercurrent multiplier** (loops of Henle) and the **countercurrent exchanger** (vasa recta).

Countercurrent multiplier system

The countercurrent multiplier is represented in Figure 17.1 by the (i) descending limb, (ii) thin segment of the ascending limb, and (iii) thick segment of the ascending limb of the loop of Henle. The osmolality of the tubular fluid changes as it progresses through the loop of Henle because of the permeability characteristics of the loop of Henle limbs and segments coupled with active cotransport of NaCl in the thick segment of the ascending limb. In the descending limb (impermeable to solutes, permeable to water), water diffuses by osmosis to the higher osmotic pressure of the ISF, and solute concentration (mostly NaCl) increases while approaching the hairpin turn of the loop of Henle. The thin segment of the ascending limb is permeable to NaCl and impermeable to water. Therefore, water remains in the tubule and NaCl diffuses (because of concentration gradient) to the ISF. In the thick segment of the ascending limb, NaCl is actively transported (cotransport) to the ISF and water continues to be retained. While the osmolality of the tubular fluid entering the descending limb is 300 mosmol/kg H_2O, the tubular fluid leaving the ascending limb and entering the distal tubule has been diluted (osmolality

Dukes' Physiology of Domestic Animals, Thirteenth Edition. Edited by William O. Reece, Howard H. Erickson, Jesse P. Goff and Etsuro E. Uemura.
© 2015 John Wiley & Sons, Inc. Published 2015 by John Wiley & Sons, Inc.
Companion website: www.wiley.com/go/reece/physiology

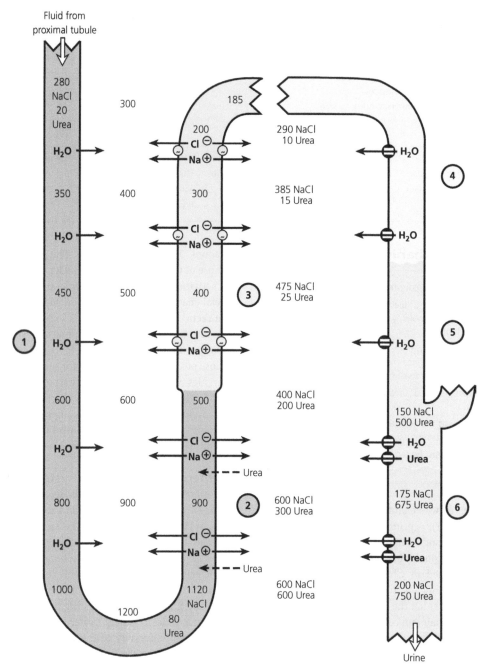

Figure 17.1 Countercurrent multiplication in the loop of Henle and recirculation of urea. Values shown (in mosmol/kg H$_2$O) are hypothetical but approximate those of humans under conditions of low water intake. Single numbers represent total osmolality. Identified numbers (NaCl, urea) represent specific contribution to total osmolality. Transport of NaCl and urea at the level of the thin segment of the ascending limb of the loop of Henle is by simple diffusion. Active transport of Na$^+$ in the ascending thick limb is coupled with the transport of Cl$^-$ (cotransport). Water channels (also urea) on the right are open (influence of antidiuretic hormone). In this example, urine is being concentrated. Circled numbers identify locations as follows: (1) descending limb of the loop of Henle; (2) thin segment of ascending limb of loop of Henle; (3) thick segment of ascending limb of loop of Henle; (4) cortical collecting duct; (5) outer medullary collecting duct; (6) inner medullary collecting duct. See text for details. From Reece, W.O. (2009) *Functional Anatomy and Physiology of Domestic Animals*, 4th edn. Wiley-Blackwell, Ames, IA. Reproduced with permission from Wiley.

185 mosmol/kg H$_2$O). Variations in tubular fluid osmolality (described in upcoming sections) that determine whether the urine is dilute or concentrated occur in the distal tubule and collecting ducts.

The vertical osmotic gradient in the ISF (lower in outer medulla, higher in inner medulla and at hairpin turn) is established and maintained by (i) continued active transport of NaCl by the thick segment of the ascending limb, (ii) concen-

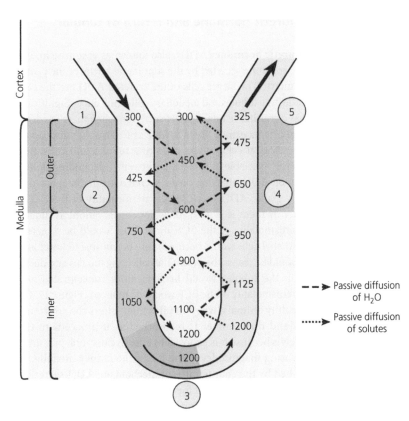

Figure 17.2 Countercurrent exchange in vasa recta. Values (in mosmol/kg H_2O) approximate those of humans. Blood enters from the cortex near (1) with an osmolality of about 300 and descends through an increasingly hypertonic peritubular fluid in the medulla (2). Water diffuses out and solute diffuses in until the hairpin turn is reached (3). The blood then ascends through decreasing hypertonicity, and water diffuses in and solute diffuses out (4). When blood returns to the cortex (5), the osmolality is only slightly higher than when it entered the vasa recta. From Reece, W.O. (2009) *Functional Anatomy and Physiology of Domestic Animals*, 4th edn. Wiley-Blackwell, Ames, IA. Reproduced with permission from Wiley.

Section III: The Kidneys and Urinary System

tration of tubular fluid in the descending limb, and (iii) passive diffusion of NaCl from the lumen of the thin segment of the ascending limb into the inner medullary ISF.

Role of urea

In addition to NaCl, urea also contributes to the high solute concentration in the ISF of the kidney medulla. The presence of urea is accomplished by a recirculation mechanism for urea between the collecting ducts and the loop of Henle (see Figure 17.1). **Recirculation** means that urea diffuses from the inner medullary collecting ducts into the ISF, and from there diffuses into the lumens of the thin segments of the ascending limbs of the loops of Henle. Diffusion occurs because of the permeability of these nephron parts for urea and because of concentration differences (high to low concentration). After the entrance of urea into the loops of Henle, it is retained there because of membrane impermeability until it again arrives at the inner medullary collecting ducts, which have a variable permeability depending on the amount of antidiuretic hormone (ADH) (see section Concentration of urine). The recirculation mechanism and high concentration of urea in the medulla not only assist the countercurrent multiplier system and osmotic gradient, but also ensure excretion of urea when urine output is low. For example, if urine is formed at the rate of 2 mL/min and it has a urea concentration of 2 mg/mL, then 4 mg of urea would be excreted each minute. If, however, urine formation is reduced to 1 mL/min (greater reabsorption of water), the concentration of urea is increased to 4 mg/mL and

excretion is maintained at 4 mg/min. The concentration of urea remains high in the collecting ducts because the concentration is also high in the ISF (diffusion from the collecting ducts limited by concentration difference).

Countercurrent exchanger system

A countercurrent exchanger is a countercurrent system in which transport between outflow and inflow is entirely passive. The vasa recta act as countercurrent exchangers (Figure 17.2). They are permeable to water and solutes throughout their length. In the descending limbs, water is drawn by osmosis from the plasma of the vasa recta to the hyperosmotic ISF (created by countercurrent multiplier), and the solutes diffuse from the ISF into the vasa recta. In the ascending limbs, solutes diffuse back into the ISF, and water is drawn by osmosis back into the vasa recta. The net result is that the solutes responsible for the vertical medullary gradient are mostly retained in the ISF of the medulla. The vasa recta carry away slightly more solutes than are brought into them.

An increased rate of medullary blood flow would reduce the time for diffusion of solute from the ascending limb back to the ISF, and the blood leaving the ascending limb would have a higher concentration of solute. The result would be a gradual loss, or washout, of the medullary gradient, referred to as **medullary washout**. Medullary loss of solute is normally prevented because the blood flow to the vasa recta is reduced (vasa recta comprise 10–20% of kidney blood flow) and it is often characterized as sluggish. All the excess salt removed from the medullary ISF by the vasa recta must be replaced by the loops of Henle for the osmotic gradient to be maintained. If countercurrent blood flow in the vasa recta did not exist, and blood from the descending limbs of the vasa recta returned directly to the renal vein instead of counterflowing into the ascending limb, the solute of the renal medulla would be quickly removed instead of being retained.

Medullary washout

Loss of medullary gradient (loss of solute concentration) reduces the ability to concentrate tubular fluid on its descent through the medullary collecting ducts. In addition to the reduced and sluggish blood flow in the vasa recta, medullary washout can also be caused by diuretics that block active NaCl cotransport in the thick segments of the ascending limbs of the loops of Henle. Examples of these diuretics are furosemide and ethacrynic acid, known as loop diuretics. They produce diuresis because increased delivery of NaCl (because of blocked reabsorption) to the distal nephrons increases the effective osmotic pressure within the tubules and prevents reabsorption of a proportional amount of water. Also, failure to reabsorb NaCl from the loops of Henle into the medullary interstitium decreases the osmoconcentration of the medullary interstitial fluid (washout), reducing its potential for reabsorbing water from the tubular fluid of the medullary collecting ducts.

A contribution to medullary washout is also provided by urea during periods of diuresis. Increased urine flow increases the clearance of urea whereby a greater amount of urea filtered is excreted. A lesser amount is thus recirculated and the contribution of urea to medullary osmolality is decreased, which further diminishes the ability to concentrate tubular fluid in the collecting ducts.

Concentration of urine

> **1** What are the factors that contribute to the low osmolality of the tubular fluid at the end of the distal tubule?
>
> **2** What are the target cells of ADH?
>
> **3** How responsive is the rate of ADH secretion to deviations in plasma osmolality?
>
> **4** What would the urine-to-plasma osmolal ratio be if the osmolality of the innermost region of the medulla was 1200 mosmol and there was an extreme need for water conservation?

At the end of the distal tubule, and before the fluid enters the cortical collecting tubules and ducts, the osmolality is about 150 mosmol. Tubular fluid entering the distal tubules has an osmolality lower than that of plasma because of the removal of Na^+ and Cl^- that occurred in the ascending limb of the loops of Henle along with the simultaneous retention of water in the tubules. Also, there is continued active transport of NaCl and low permeability for water and urea in the distal tubule.

Antidiuretic hormone and return of tubular water

Antidiuretic hormone (ADH), also known as **vasopressin**, is a peptide hormone secreted by the supraoptic nuclei of the posterior pituitary. The target cells of the secreted ADH are the cortical collecting tubules and medullary collecting ducts. Significant changes occur in the rate of ADH secretion when there are deviations in plasma osmolality of as little as 1% in either direction.

The epithelial cells of the collecting tubules and collecting ducts have a variable permeability for water, depending on the amount of ADH that has been secreted from the posterior pituitary gland. ADH increases the permeability of these cells for water. If there is a need for water conservation, as judged by hyperosmolality of the ECF, more ADH would be secreted. The epithelial cells would become more permeable to water and water would be reabsorbed from the collecting tubules and ducts. Water in the tubules would become more concentrated and the hyperosmolality of the ECF would be reduced (Figure 17.3).

In healthy animals, when tubular fluid enters the collecting tubules and ducts, water is reabsorbed as it proceeds to the renal pelvis because it is exposed to effective osmotic pressures of increasing magnitudes in the ISF of the kidney medulla, as established by the countercurrent mechanism. ADH secretion is consistent with the need for water conservation. In extreme cases of water conservation, it would be possible for the osmolality of the tubular fluid, and hence that of the urine, to approach the osmolality of the ISF in the innermost region of the medulla. In the dog, this would approach 2400 mosmol and the urine-to-plasma osmolal ratio (2400/300) would be approximately 8:1. The urine would have a concentration eight times that of plasma. Some desert rodents (e.g., kangaroo rat) attain a urine-to-plasma osmolal ratio of about 16:1. This ratio represents an extreme adaptation for body water conservation. Environmental water is not available for desert animals (water gain mostly metabolic water), and water losses are minimized for survival. Table 17.1 compares the percentage of long-looped nephrons (loops of Henle extending deeply into the medulla) and **relative medullary thickness** of different animals. The relative medullary thickness is derived from measurements of the depth of the medulla from the corticomedullary junction to its innermost depth, which protrudes into the renal pelvis. Relative medullary thickness is believed to be a better predictor of urine concentrating ability than percentage of long-looped nephrons. As judged by freezing point depression (solute particles lower the freezing point of solutions), the kangaroo rat has the greatest concentrating capacity for urine. Compared with humans, it seems that its innermost medullary osmolality would be about four times that of humans, or about 4800 mosmol.

Other factors affecting ADH release

ADH release from the posterior pituitary is influenced by other factors in addition to hydration of the ECF. Cold environments inhibit ADH release, so urine production and water intake

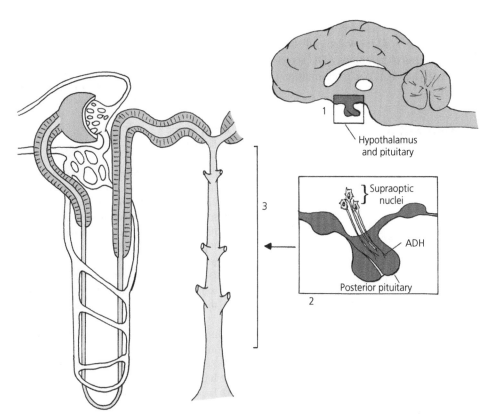

Figure 17.3 Relationships among the hypothalamus, posterior pituitary, and kidneys in the regulation of extracellular hydration. (1) Extracellular dehydration detected by osmoreceptors in the hypothalamus. Boxed area shows location in the brain of the area in (2). (2) ADH (neurosecretion of supraoptic nuclei in hypothalamus) secreted into blood in response to dehydration. (3) Cortical collecting tubules and medullary collecting ducts are targets of ADH, causing increased reabsorption of water. Adapted from Reece, W.O. (2009) *Functional Anatomy and Physiology of Domestic Animals*, 4th edn. Wiley-Blackwell, Ames, IA. Reproduced with permission from Wiley.

Table 17.1 Relationship of structure to concentrating capacity in mammalian kidneys.

Animal	Kidney size* (mm)	Long-looped nephrons (%)	Relative medullary thickness[†]	Maximum freezing point depression in urine (°C)
Beaver	36	0	1.3	0.96
Pig	66	3	1.6	2
Human	64	14	3	2.6
Dog[‡]	40	100	4.3	4.85
Cat	24	100	4.8	5.8
Rat	14	28	5.8	4.85
Kangaroo rat	5.9	27	8.5	10.4
Jerboa	4.5	33	9.3	12
Psammomys	13	100	10.7	9.2

*Kidney size = cube root of the product of the dimensions of the kidney.
[†]Relative medullary thickness = medullary thickness in millimeters = 10/kidney size.
[‡]Beeuwkes and Bonventre (1975) have shown that the dog kidney does contain short-looped or corticomedullary nephrons; therefore, long-looped nephrons comprise fewer than 100% of the nephrons.
Source: Schmidt-Nielsen, B. and O'Dell, R. (1961) Structure and concentrating mechanism in the mammalian kidney. *American Journal of Physiology* 200:1119–1124. Reproduced with permission from The Americal Physiological Society.

increase. The need for water intake results from thirst induced by water loss from diuresis. The need for water availability in cold weather is apparent. Ethyl alcohol inhibits ADH secretion, and dehydration is a consequence of alcohol consumption (not a factor for domestic animals).

Urine concentration failure

1 How would urinalysis differentiate between diabetes insipidus and diabetes mellitus?

2 Why is polydipsia a clinical sign of both diabetes insipidus and diabetes mellitus?

3 What are some causes of impaired urine concentrating ability associated with chronic renal failure?

Hypotonic tubular fluid entering the collecting tubules and ducts could be excreted as urine if water were not reabsorbed. This happens in **diabetes insipidus**, in which there is either an absence of ADH or severely decreased amounts of ADH. Animals with this condition have clinical signs of **polyuria** (formation and excretion of a large volume of urine) and **polydipsia** (excessive thirst manifested by excessive water intake). The urine formed is dilute and has a lower-than-normal specific gravity. Animals with **diabetes mellitus** may also show polyuria and polydipsia. Polyuria in this disease is caused by an osmotic diuresis because of the presence of glucose in the urine (failed to be reabsorbed) and is not caused by a lack of ADH. The urine specific gravity would likely be higher than normal and would test positive for glucose. As in diabetes insipidus, polydipsia is a compensation for the polyuria to overcome the water deficit.

In addition to diabetes insipidus, other kidney disease processes are characterized by decreased concentrating ability. Impaired concentrating ability is notable in **chronic renal failure**. Reasons cited are as follows.

1 Because of a loss of nephron numbers, more solute (Na^+, Cl^-) fails to be reabsorbed, thereby contributing to osmotic diuresis.

2 Hypertonicity in the medullary ISF is not maintained (medullary washout) because of loss of medullary tissues, decreased blood flow in the vasa recta, and decreased Na^+ and Cl^- cotransport from the thick segment of the ascending limb of the loop of Henle.

3 Damage to cells in the collecting tubules and collecting ducts makes them less responsive to ADH.

Self-evaluation

Answers can be found at the end of the chapter.

1 Which one of the following nephron parts is associated with the establishment of a high salt concentration in the medulla of the kidney?
   A Bowman's capsule
   B Proximal tubule
   C Loop of Henle
   D Distal tubule

2 Loss of solute (Na^+, Cl^-) and retention of water that occurs in the ascending limb of the loop of Henle causes the tubular fluid to be _____ as compared with plasma.
   A Hypotonic
   B Hypertonic
   C Isotonic

3 With regard to the tubular transport of urea:
   A It is actively transported from the proximal tubule so that about one-third to one-half of its presence continues to the loop of Henle
   B It is essentially trapped within the nephron tubules throughout their length so that it can be excreted
   C It plays no part in osmoconcentration of the ISF of the renal medulla
   D During the process of its being excreted, there is recirculation of some from the inner medullary collecting ducts to the ascending thin limb of the loop of Henle

4 Which one of the following is not associated with diabetes mellitus?
   A Increased urine formation
   B Renal threshold for glucose is exceeded
   C Increased thirst
   D Lack of antidiuretic hormone (ADH)

5 When antidiuretic hormone from the posterior pituitary is released in greater amounts, what will happen to the fluid in the collecting ducts of the kidney?
   A It will become more dilute
   B It will remain the same
   C It will become more concentrated

6 Detection of increased osmoconcentration of the ECF by osmoreceptors in the hypothalamus would result in:
   A More concentrated urine
   B More dilute urine
   C No change in urine concentration

7 Which part of the loop of Henle has the lowest osmolality (greatest dilution)?
   A Ascending thin limb
   B Descending thin limb
   C Ascending thick limb
   D Hairpin loop

8 Where in the loop of Henle does urea permeability begin and end?
   A Begins and ends in the thin ascending limb
   B Begins in the thin ascending limb and ends at the end of the thick ascending limb
   C Begins and ends in the thick ascending limb
   D There is permeability for urea throughout the loop of Henle

9 Movement of solute and water between the vasa recta and the ISF occurs by:
   A Passive diffusion for water and urea and active transport for NaCl
   B Passive diffusion for water and NaCl and active transport for urea
   C Passive diffusion for water, urea, and NaCl

10 A diuretic that interferes with the cotransport of NaCl in the thick segment of the ascending limb of the loop of Henle would:

A Decrease the osmolality of the tubular fluid

B Predispose (tendency for) to medullary washout

C Further concentrate the medullary ISF

D Reduce the excretion of urea

Suggested reading

Hall, J.E. (2011) Urine concentration and dilution: regulation of extracellular fluid osmolarity and sodium concentration. In: *Guyton and Hall Textbook of Medical Physiology*, 12th edn, pp. 345–360. Saunders Elsevier, Philadelphia.

Reece, W. (2004) Kidney function in mammals. In: *Dukes' Physiology of Domestic Animals*, 12th edn (ed. W.O. Reece), pp. 73–106. Cornell University Press, Ithaca, NY.

Reece, W. (2009) The urinary system. In: *Functional Anatomy and Physiology of Domestic Animals*, 4th edn, pp. 312–358. Wiley-Blackwell, Ames, IA.

Answers

1 C	6 A
2 A	7 C
3 D	8 A
4 D	9 C
5 C	10 B

Section III: The Kidneys and Urinary System

18 Kidney Regulation of Extracellular Volume and Electrolytes

William O. Reece
Iowa State University, Ames, IA, USA

One of the two major functions of the kidneys is to regulate the volume and composition of the body's internal environment, the extracellular fluid (ECF). This chapter focuses on details of how this is accomplished. It will rely not only on knowledge presented in previous chapters of Section III, but also on Chapter 11 in Section II. Review of these chapters will be helpful in understanding the presentation in this chapter.

Regulation of extracellular fluid osmolality and volume

1 What is the response to hyperosmolality with regard to thirst and antidiuretic hormone (ADH) release? What would be the response to hypoosmolality?

2 How is the regulation of [Na$^+$] related to ECF volume expansion and ECF volume depletion?

3 Where are the principal receptors located that respond to acute changes in blood volume?

4 What are the three levels of ERSNA activity in response to hypovolemia (study Figure 18.3)?

5 What are the effects of the left atrial stretch reflex initiated by hypervolemia?

6 What is the stimulus for the release of ANP in hypervolemia and what is its role in reducing intravascular volume?

7 What action of diuretics promotes diuresis?

The ability to retain water in the ECF is due to its effective osmotic pressure. Since about 90% of the effective osmotic pressure of the ECF is due to Na$^+$ and its associated anions, the central role played by Na$^+$ must be recognized when one is considering the regulation of **ECF osmolality (osmoregulation)** and **ECF volume (volume regulation)**. In osmoregulation the ratio of Na$^+$ to water (**osmoconcentration**) is being regulated, and in volume regulation the absolute amounts of Na$^+$ and water that are present are being regulated.

Osmoregulation

From day to day in any one animal, the water content of the body is relatively constant. There is water balance because water intake is equal to water excretion. Water excretion without water intake would cause ECF hyperosmolality, and water intake without water excretion would cause hypoosmolality. To prevent either, the plasma osmolality is maintained within narrow limits by appropriate adjustments of water excretion and intake. These adjustments are governed by centers in the hypothalamus that influence both the secretion of ADH (water excretion) and **thirst** (water intake).

In the event of water load (intake exceeds excretion) the ECF is diluted, causing hypoosmolality. The response of **osmoreceptors** in the hypothalamus would be to inhibit the secretion of ADH and subsequently increase water excretion, returning the osmolality to normal.

When water loss exceeds water intake, the ECF is concentrated, resulting in **hyperosmolality**. A water deficit requires prevention of water loss and also requires water intake for correction. Hyperosmolality of the ECF stimulates greater secretion of ADH so that water excretion is suppressed. The major defense against hyperosmolality is the stimulation of thirst, so that the animal seeks water for ingestion (Figure 18.1). The osmoreceptors respond to effective osmotic pressure in the ECF, hence the osmolality increase can only be due to substances restricted from diffusion into the osmoreceptor cells. Because Na$^+$ predominates in this regard, the osmoreceptor cells have been referred to as sodium receptors. Osmolality increase due to urea (freely diffusible) would not contribute to effective

Dukes' Physiology of Domestic Animals, Thirteenth Edition. Edited by William O. Reece, Howard H. Erickson, Jesse P. Goff and Etsuro E. Uemura.
© 2015 John Wiley & Sons, Inc. Published 2015 by John Wiley & Sons, Inc.
Companion website: www.wiley.com/go/reece/physiology

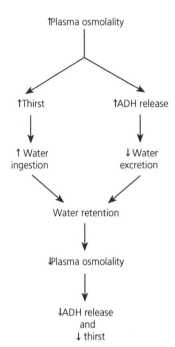

Figure 18.1 Cycle of events for the relief of hyperosmolality. Increased thirst is the predominant factor for the correction of hyperosmolality. ADH, antidiuretic hormone. From Reece, W.O. (2004) Kidney function in mammals. In: *Dukes' Physiology of Domestic Animals*, 12th edn (ed. W.O. Reece). Cornell University Press, Ithaca, NY. Reproduced with permission from Cornell University Press.

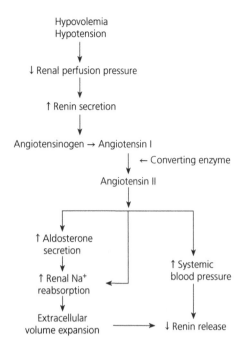

Figure 18.2 Renin–angiotensin–aldosterone system response to hypovolemia and hypotension. From Reece, W.O. (2004) Kidney function in mammals. In: *Dukes' Physiology of Domestic Animals*, 12th edn (ed. W.O. Reece). Cornell University Press, Ithaca, NY. Reproduced with permission from Cornell University Press.

osmotic pressure and subsequent stimulation of the osmoreceptors. When defects occur in the ability to concentrate urine, as in diabetes insipidus (lack of ADH), water losses increase and are followed by a simultaneous increase in plasma osmolality. This activates the thirst mechanism, promoting water intake, and prevents hyperosmolality that might otherwise occur from the excessive excretion of water (Figure 18.1).

Volume regulation

The maintenance of normal plasma volume, which varies directly with ECF volume, is essential for adequate tissue perfusion and is closely related to the regulation of sodium balance. Na^+ loading (excess) tends to produce ECF volume expansion (because of the increase in effective osmotic pressure and associated water retention), and Na^+ excretion by the kidneys rises in an attempt to lower the volume toward normal. Conversely, the kidneys retain Na^+ in the presence of ECF volume depletion. Change in volume is the signal that allows urinary Na^+ excretion to vary as needed with fluctuations in Na^+ intake.

Renin–angiotensin–aldosterone system

Because of its role in blood volume homeostasis, a review of the **renin–angiotensin–aldosterone system** and its effects is presented. The **juxtaglomerular (JG) granular cells** of the afferent arteriole of each glomerulus secrete the proteolytic enzyme renin. Renin converts plasma **angiotensinogen** (produced in the liver) to **angiotensin I**. Angiotensin I is converted to

angiotensin II by **angiotensin converting enzyme**, which is located in vascular endothelial cells. The lung is a major contributor to conversion because of its vascularity.

The major effects of angiotensin II reverse the ECF volume reduction and hypotension that are usually responsible for its production. Within the kidney, angiotensin II promotes Na^+ reabsorption and subsequent water retention. Na^+ reabsorption is stimulated directly by angiotensin II in the early proximal tubule and indirectly by enhanced secretion of aldosterone from the adrenal cortex. Aldosterone stimulates Na^+ reabsorption in the cortical and medullary collecting ducts. Systemically, angiotensin II causes arteriolar vasoconstriction, which increases vascular resistance and elevates systemic blood pressure. A summary of the renin–angiotensin–aldosterone system response to hypovolemia and hypotension is shown in Figure 18.2.

Receptors of volume change

Peripheral receptors in the cardiovascular system that respond to volume change are pressure receptors and include arterial baroreceptors (aortic arch and carotid sinus) and **cardiac baroreceptors** (walls of the atria and ventricles). While there may be interaction among these receptors, the principal receptors responding to acute changes in blood volume are those in the left atrium of the heart. Vagal afferents from these receptors provide a neural link between the heart as a sensor of blood volume and the kidney as an effector organ that varies excretion of water and sodium to maintain body fluid (blood) volume homeostasis.

Efferent renal sympathetic nerve activity

The effects of **efferent renal sympathetic nerve activity (ERSNA)** are mediated by functionally specific groups of fibers separately innervating the JG granular cells, the nephron tubules, and the renal vasculature (see section Innervation in Chapter 15). The responses of these groups to ERSNA are graded: with increasing intensity, renin secretion from the JG granular cells increases first, followed by increased renal tubular reabsorption of sodium, and lastly by renal vasoconstriction which decreases **renal blood flow (RBF)** and increases vascular resistance. It has been mentioned that these effects can override autoregulatory responses.

Hypovolemia

In **hypovolemia (volume depletion)**, decreasing vagal afferent stimulation from receptors in the left atrium increases ERSNA and the above responses are associated with resumption of normovolemia by increasing NaCl and water reabsorption (Figure 18.3). The following discussion relates to maximum responses but one must recognize that gradations exist.

Renin secretion is the first response to be recruited by increased ERSNA and is followed by the generation of angiotensin II. Angiotensin II promotes renal NaCl and water retention and therefore expansion of the plasma volume according to the earlier discussion. Correction of declining

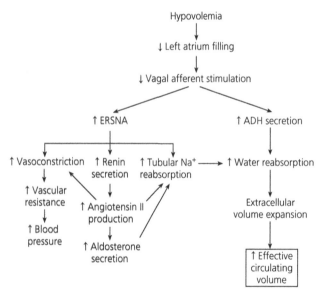

Figure 18.3 Renal and cardiovascular responses induced by the sympathetic division of the autonomic nervous system in response to reduced circulating volume (hypovolemia). Efferent renal sympathetic nerve activity (ERSNA) responses are graded depending on the severity of hypovolemia. Accordingly, renin secretion is the first response, followed by tubular Na⁺ reabsorption, and finally vasoconstriction to alleviate declining blood pressure associated with hypovolemia. ADH, antidiuretic hormone. From Reece, W.O. (2004) Kidney function in mammals. In: *Dukes' Physiology of Domestic Animals*, 12th edn (ed. W.O. Reece). Cornell University Press, Ithaca, NY. Reproduced with permission from Cornell University Press.

systemic blood pressure, associated with hypovolemia, is also provided by angiotensin II via arteriolar vasoconstriction, which elevates systemic vascular resistance.

ERSNA directly increases renal tubular sodium reabsorption as the second response of recruitment. This is followed by increased water reabsorption and ECF volume expansion.

ERSNA sufficient to influence the renal vasculature is the last element to be recruited for correction of hypovolemia and associated hypotension. Responses are renal vasoconstriction with decreases in RBF and increased vascular resistance. Also, there is contraction of the glomerular mesangial cells. Afferent arterioles are constricted more than efferent arterioles by ERSNA, thereby reducing RBF and glomerular hydrostatic pressure, while at the same time diverting blood from the kidneys to restore systemic blood pressure. However, kidney function can continue due to the simultaneous recruitment of tubular reabsorption and renin secretion.

Hypervolemia

In **hypervolemia (volume expansion)**, myocardial cells in the left atrium are stretched and a reflex is initiated whose afferent limb is in the vagus nerves. The efferent limb for the diuretic response results in suppression of ADH release and that for the natriuretic response results in suppression of ERSNA. In addition to suppression of ADH release as a factor in the diuretic response, suppression of ERSNA also contributes substantially to the diuresis produced by left atrial distension (decreased Na⁺ reabsorption). Taken together, diuresis and natriuresis reduce the volume expansion that was the stimulus for initiation of the reflex to reestablish normovolemia.

Myocardial cells of the atria release **atrial natriuretic peptide (ANP)** when they are stretched during volume expansion. In addition to natriuresis and diuresis, the other biologic actions of ANP that tend to reduce intravascular volume, and accordingly the stimulus that resulted in its release, are as follows:

1 relaxation of vascular smooth muscle;
2 reduction of cardiac output by shift of fluids from the intravascular compartment to the extravascular compartment;
3 inhibition of the renin–angiotensin–aldosterone system;
4 inhibition of the sympathetic nervous system;
5 action on the central nervous system to modulate vasomotor tone, thirst, and ADH release.

Many of the actions of ANP counterbalance those of the renin–angiotensin–aldosterone system and it is believed that the two systems may act in a concerted manner to regulate body fluid and cardiovascular activity.

Normovolemia

Normal volume regulation (normovolemia) is probably maintained according to autoregulatory mechanisms (see section Autoregulation in Chapter 16). The response to a reduction in ECF volume that accompanies reduced Na⁺ intake depends on the severity of the reduction. Accordingly, renin secretion (and associated effects of angiotensin II production), proximal tubule

Na$^+$ reabsorption, and systemic vasoconstriction are recruited, in that order, by enhanced ERSNA (see Figure 18.3). These events provide for antinatriuresis and antidiuresis and restoration of the declining ECF volume and blood pressure. With volume expansion associated with increased Na$^+$ intake, left atrial stretch results in a reflex whereby ADH secretion is reduced and ERSNA is decreased. These events provide for natriuresis and diuresis with reduction of ECF volume and a return to normovolemia. Beyond the limits of autoregulation of Na$^+$ deficiency or excess, the mechanisms described for hypovolemia and hypervolemia can override the autoregulatory mechanisms.

Diuretics and volume adjustment

A **diuretic** is an agent that increases the rate of urine volume output and are useful drugs for the treatment of conditions where ECF loss is needed, for example edema and hypertension. **Increased urine output (diuresis)** is secondary to **increased sodium output (natriuresis)** caused by the action of the diuretic in inhibiting the reabsorption of NaCl in various nephron tubule locations. Retention of NaCl in the tubules increases the effective osmotic pressure in the tubules, which in turn causes retention of a volume of water that might otherwise have been reabsorbed and now becomes urine. Potassium, calcium, and magnesium, in addition to chloride, are other solutes associated secondarily with sodium reabsorption, and the renal output of these may be increased by some of the diuretics.

Several classes of diuretics exist that differ in their site and mechanism of action. A listing of these is shown in Table 18.1. The loop diuretics are most effective with regard to amount of NaCl and water excretion. One of these, **furosemide**, has already been mentioned (see section Tubular transport in Chapter 16) as it related to inhibition of the Na$^+$-K$^+$-2Cl$^-$ cotransport mechanism in the thick ascending limb of the loop of Henle. Two others in this class are ethacrynic acid and bumetanide. Refer to Table 18.1 for the other classes of diuretics (with names of some commonly used drugs), sites of action, mechanism of action, and percent filtered Na$^+$ that is excreted. **Osmotic diuretics** are substances that inhibit water and solute reabsorption by increasing effective osmotic pressure of tubular fluid. They are represented by mannitol, a nonreabsorbable polysaccharide. Their site of action is mainly in the proximal tubule. They produce a relative diuresis, whereby water is lost in excess of Na$^+$ and K$^+$. All the diuretics involve some degree of Na$^+$ excretion, associated with water loss.

Regulation of extracellular fluid electrolytes

1 How is the ECF [Na$^+$] regulated?

2 Why is the regulation of ECF [K$^+$] critically controlled?

3 What provides for the regulation of ECF [K$^+$] and what is the stimulus for its production?

4 What is the role of parathyroid hormone following its secretion in response to low ECF [Ca^{2+}]?

5 What is the effect of parathyroid hormone on phosphate excretion?

Sodium concentration

About 65% of Na$^+$ reabsorption occurs in the proximal tubules, about 25% in the ascending thick segment of the loop of Henle (medullary and cortical), and the remaining 10% is presented to

Section III: The Kidneys and Urinary System

Table 18.1 Classes of diuretics, tubular sites of action, mechanisms of action, and percentage of filtered Na$^+$ excreted.

Class of diuretic	Site of action	Mechanism of action	Percentage of filtered Na$^+$ excreted
Loop diuretics Furosemide Ethacrynic acid Bumetanide	Thick ascending limb of loop of Henle	Inhibit Na$^+$-K$^+$-2 Cl$^-$ cotransport in luminal membrane	Up to 25
Thiazide diuretics Chlorothiazide	Distal tubule and connecting tubule	Inhibit Na$^+$-Cl$^-$ cotransport in luminal membrane	Up to 3–5
Competitive inhibitors of aldosterone* Spironolactone	Cortical collecting tubule	Inhibit action of aldosterone on tubular receptor, decrease Na$^+$ reabsorption and decrease K$^+$ secretion	Up to 1–2
Osmotic diuretics Mannitol	Mainly proximal tubule	Inhibit water and solute reabsorption by increasing effective osmotic pressure of tubular fluid	Minimal
Carbonic anhydrase inhibitors† Acetazolamide	Proximal tubule	Inhibit H$^+$ secretion and HCO$_3^-$ reabsorption, which reduces Na$^+$ reabsorption	Minimal

*Referred to as potassium-sparing diuretics.
†Produces NaCl and H$_2$CO$_3$ loss. Diuresis is modest but useful where concurrent metabolic alkalosis is present because excess HCO$_3^-$ in urine tends to restore acid–base balance.
Source: Reece, W.O. (2004) Kidney function in mammals. In: *Dukes' Physiology of Domestic Animals*, 12th edn (ed. W.O. Reece). Cornell University Press, Ithaca, NY.

the distal nephron. The mechanism for active Na$^+$ reabsorption in the distal convoluted and connecting tubules of the distal nephrons is coupled with the cotransport of Cl$^-$. Beyond the connecting tubules, Na$^+$ reabsorption in the collecting tubules and collecting ducts is not coupled with Cl$^-$ reabsorption, but rather occurs via conductive Na$^+$ channels. The tight junctions are tighter and not only limit the ability of Cl$^-$ to accompany Na$^+$ but also prevent Na$^+$ pumped into the basolateral spaces from leaking back into the tubular lumen. The unidirectional Na$^+$ reabsorption via the conductive Na$^+$ channel in the collecting tubules and collecting ducts is influenced by **aldosterone** concentrations. In the complete absence of aldosterone, seemingly 10% of the tubular load of Na$^+$ (and associated anions) could be lost in the urine. Conversely, with excess aldosterone, the last vestige of the tubular load of Na$^+$ can be reabsorbed.

Even though aldosterone is associated with Na$^+$ reabsorption, it is not a regulator of ECF Na$^+$ concentration. This lack of regulation by aldosterone in dogs is illustrated in Figure 18.4. In this instance, the aldosterone system has been blocked, and it is noted that plasma Na$^+$ concentration remains stabilized near normal, even though sodium intake increases. In another experiment with dogs, the aldosterone system is left intact and the **ADH–thirst system** is blocked (Figure 18.5). This latter experiment shows that plasma Na$^+$ concentration increases in proportion to increases in sodium intake and, coupled with the former experiment, demonstrates that ECF Na$^+$ concentration is regulated by the ADH–thirst system (as in osmoregulation) and not by aldosterone.

Potassium concentration

Average values for intracellular fluid (ICF) and ECF concentrations of K$^+$ are 140 mEq/L and 5 mEq/L, respectively. The large concentration difference of K$^+$ across membranes of 135 (140 − 5) mEq/L is maintained by the **Na$^+$/K$^+$-ATPase system** and is critical for the excitability of nerve and muscle cells, and also for the contractility of cells. Accordingly, regulation of the K$^+$ concentration in the ECF is very sensitive; a rise in [K$^+$] of a few tenths of a milliequivalent per liter causes urinary excretion to increase sevenfold.

Because there is no regulation of dietary K$^+$ intake, K$^+$ balance involves changing K$^+$ output to match K$^+$ input, and this is regulated primarily by changing the amount of K$^+$ excreted in urine. About 10% of the tubular load of K$^+$ is delivered to the distal nephron regardless of K$^+$ input and output, so K$^+$ balance occurs almost exclusively in the collecting ducts of the distal nephrons. With high K$^+$ intake, secretion exceeds reabsorption and K$^+$ is excreted in urine in order to maintain K$^+$ balance in the ECF.

The regulation of K$^+$ concentration in the ECF is accomplished by aldosterone and an increase in plasma K$^+$ concentration is the major stimulus for aldosterone secretion. After its secretion, aldosterone facilitates K$^+$ excretion into the tubular lumen of the collecting ducts as follows:

1 increases the activity of the Na$^+$/K$^+$-ATPase and its associated transport of K$^+$ into the tubular cells from the peritubular fluid,

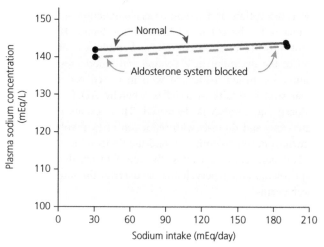

Figure 18.4 Response of canine plasma sodium concentration to increasing sodium intake in cases where the aldosterone system is blocked and where the ADH–thirst system is intact. Adapted from Reece, W.O. (2004) Kidney function in mammals. In: *Dukes' Physiology of Domestic Animals*, 12th edn (ed. W.O. Reece). Cornell University Press, Ithaca, NY. Reproduced with permission from Cornell University Press.

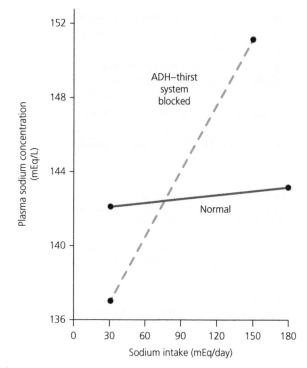

Figure 18.5 Response of canine plasma sodium concentration to increasing sodium intake in cases where the ADH–thirst system is blocked and the aldosterone system is intact. Courtesy of Dr David B. Young, University of Mississippi School of Medicine, Jackson. Reproduced with permission of D. Young.

whereby the concentration gradient for diffusion from the tubular cell into the lumen of the collecting ducts is increased;

2 stimulates Na$^+$ reabsorption from the lumen of the collecting ducts into the cell, which increases the transepithelial

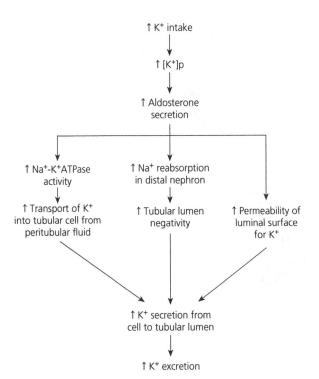

Figure 18.6 Pathways whereby plasma potassium concentration ($[K^+]_p$) is restored after an increase in potassium intake. From Reece, W.O. (2004) Kidney function in mammals. In: *Dukes' Physiology of Domestic Animals*, 12th edn (ed. W.O. Reece). Cornell University Press, Ithaca, NY. Reproduced with permission from Cornell University Press.

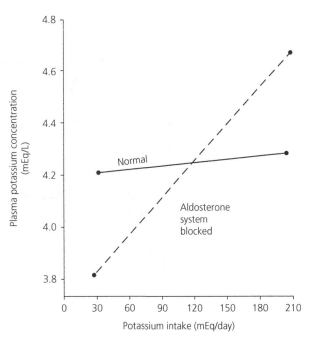

Figure 18.7 Response of canine plasma K^+ concentration to increasing potassium intake when the aldosterone system is blocked: plasma K^+ concentration increases simultaneously with increases in potassium intake. Courtesy of Dr David B. Young, University of Mississippi School of Medicine, Jackson. Reproduced with permission of D. Young.

potential difference (lumen negative), whereby the electrical gradient for diffusion of K^+ from the tubular cell into the tubular lumen is increased;

3 increases the permeability of the tubular lumen membrane for K^+, thereby facilitating diffusion from the tubular cell into the lumen.

Potassium excretion following increased potassium intake is illustrated in Figure 18.6.

The role of aldosterone in the regulation of ECF K^+ concentration is shown in Figure 18.7. In the experiment depicted in this figure, dogs with intact adrenal glands were given increasing amounts of potassium after the aldosterone feedback system was blocked. Plasma K^+ concentration increased simultaneously with increases in K^+ intake.

Calcium concentration

About half of plasma Ca^{2+} is bound to albumin and is not filtered at the glomerulus. The other half exists as ionic Ca^{2+}, and some is bound to citrate, bicarbonate, or phosphate. Most of the filtered Ca^{2+} (80–85%) is reabsorbed from the proximal tubule and medullary portions of the loop of Henle. The reabsorption in these parts is passive, following gradients established by NaCl and water.

Regulation of Ca^{2+} occurs primarily in the distal tubule and the connecting tubule. **Parathyroid hormone (PTH)**, secreted by the parathyroid glands, acts on the kidney tubules to increase the reabsorption of Ca^{2+}, while at the same time promoting the excretion of phosphorus. PTH is secreted in response to low concentrations of Ca^{2+} in the ECF. Another role of the kidney in response to a decreasing Ca^{2+} concentration in the ECF involves the formation of the active form of **vitamin D (1,25-dihydroxycholecalciferol)**, also known as **calcitriol** (Figure 18.8) PTH controls the formation of active vitamin D by the kidney. Active vitamin D promotes Ca^{2+} absorption from the intestine.

Magnesium concentration

A lesser percentage of Mg^{2+} (about 25%) is protein bound so that about 75% is filtered. The proximal tubule accounts for 25–30% of its reabsorption, and most of the remainder is reabsorbed from the loop of Henle. Alterations that occur in Mg^{2+} excretion are due to changes in the loop of Henle reabsorption. Specific factors that regulate plasma Mg^{2+} concentration have not been identified. It is believed that there may be a direct effect of plasma Mg^{2+} concentration on tubular function and its subsequent reabsorption.

Phosphate concentration

About 80–95% of filtered phosphate is reabsorbed, and most reabsorption occurs in the proximal tubule. There is a specific **Na$^+$–phosphate cotransporter** in the luminal membrane for transport from the lumen into the cell. After cell entry, phosphate diffuses across the basolateral membrane into the peritubular fluid.

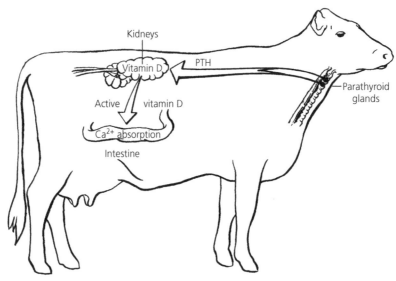

Figure 18.8 Relationship between parathyroid hormone (PTH), the kidneys, and calcium ion homeostasis in the cow. PTH from the parathyroid gland activates vitamin D in the kidney; activated vitamin D promotes absorption of Ca^{2+} from the intestine. From Reece, W.O. (2009) *Functional Anatomy and Physiology of Domestic Animals*, 4th edn. Wiley-Blackwell, Ames, IA. Reproduced with permission from Wiley.

Two factors appear to regulate phosphate transport: the plasma phosphate concentration and PTH. Virtually no phosphate is excreted with a low phosphate load, and this is believed to be due to increased Na^+–phosphate cotransport activity. With a high phosphate load, urinary excretion increases because of a direct effect of phosphate concentration and also because of increased PTH secretion that promotes excretion of excess phosphate.

Self-evaluation

Answers can be found at the end of the chapter.

1 The renin–angiotensin–aldosterone system is effective in the adjustments needed for the correction of:
   A Hypovolemia
   B Hypervolemia
   Explain your choice for the correct answer.

2 Volume receptors in the left atrium are stretched during hypervolemia that results from increased Na^+ intake. Which one of the following is influential in the return to normal?
   A Aldosterone
   B Inhibition of ERSNA and release of ANP
   C ADH
   Explain your choice for the correct answer.

3 Extracellular fluid Na^+ concentration is regulated by:
   A Osmoreceptor–ADH system and thirst mechanism
   B Aldosterone mechanism
   Explain your choice for the correct answer.

4 Detection of increased osmoconcentration of the ECF by osmoreceptors in the hypothalamus would by followed by:

   A Secretion of ADH, more dilute urine, suppression of thirst, and loss of water
   B Secretion of ADH, more concentrated urine, stimulation of thirst, and water retention
   Explain your choice for the correct answer.

5 Which one of the following hormones promotes the tubular reabsorption of Na^+ and the tubular secretion of K^+?
   A Antidiuretic hormone
   B Secretin
   C Aldosterone
   D Oxytocin
   Explain your choice for the correct answer.

Suggested reading

Dibona, G.F. (2000) Neural control of renal function. *Physiological Reviews* 77:75–197.

Hall, J.E. (2011) Renal regulation of potassium, calcium, phosphate, and magnesium: integration of renal mechanisms for control of blood volume and extracellular fluid volume. In: *Guyton and Hall Textbook of Medical Physiology*, 12th edn, pp. 361–378. Saunders Elsevier, Philadelphia.

Reece, W. (2009) Kidney function in mammals. In: *Dukes' Physiology of Domestic Animals*, 12th edn (ed. W.O. Reece), pp. 73–106. Cornell University Press, Ithaca, NY.

Answers

1 A. Renal hypoperfusion as a consequence of hypovolemia contributes to the secretion of renin, which results in the production of angiotensin II. Angiotensin II directly stimulates Na^+ reabsorption

(and hence water reabsorption) in the proximal tubules, and because it also stimulates aldosterone secretion Na^+ is reabsorbed from collecting ducts (stimulated by aldosterone) which also results in water reabsorption. The reabsorption of water helps restore blood volume.

2 B. Whereas aldosterone and antidiuretic hormone would further increase the hypervolemia, inhibition of efferent renal sympathetic nerve activity (ERSNA) and release of atrial natriuretic peptide (ANP) would provide for natriuresis and diuresis with return to normovolemia.

3 A. Na^+ and its associated anions comprise about 90% of the ECF effective osmotic pressure. Any increase in Na^+ concentration stimulates the osmoreceptors to cause increased secretion of ADH and also stimulation of thirst. The combination of water conservation by ADH and water intake by thirst reduces the plasma Na^+ concentration back to normal. Low Na^+ concentration reduces ADH secretion, and water is lost, thereby increasing plasma Na^+ concentration.

4 B. Because of the osmoconcentration, there is a need for water conservation and water intake. Antidiuretic hormone will provide the water conservation by decreasing urine output, and the urine would be more concentrated. At the same time, thirst would be stimulated and water intake increased.

5 C. In its role of regulating the K^+ concentration of the ECF, aldosterone exerts its activity in the cortical collecting tubules and medullary collecting ducts. In this regard, aldosterone is secreted in response to elevated K^+ concentrations in the ECF. Although Na^+ reabsorption is coupled with K^+ secretion, aldosterone is not involved with the regulation of Na^+ concentration.

Section III: The Kidneys and Urinary System

19 Micturition, Characteristics of Urine, and Renal Clearance

William O. Reece

Iowa State University, Ames, IA, USA

Claudius Galen (AD *c*.130–*c*.200), a Greek physician and writer on medicine, was the first to demonstrate that urine was formed in the kidneys and transmitted from them to the bladder by the ureters. Before this time there was much speculation about how fluid taken by mouth passed from the intestine to the bladder.

Sir **William Bowman (1816–1892)** published his theory of urinary secretion and his discovery of the capsule surrounding the **malpighian body (glomerulus)**, which he showed to be continuous with the urinary tubule, in 1842. He believed that water alone was secreted at the malpighian body and that the dissolved constituents were secreted by the epithelium of the urinary tubules. According to his view, the quantity of water secreted at the capsule approximated urine volume. In 1874, **Rudolph Heidenhain (1834–1897)** revived Bowman's theory and indicated that urine is formed by the combined secretory activities of the glomerular capillary tufts and of the renal tubules. Thereafter, the secretory theory was referred to as the **Bowman–Heidenhain theory**.

The so-called modern theory of urine formation was proposed by **Arthur Cushny (1866–1926)** in 1917. He concluded that ultrafiltration (not secretion) occurred at the glomerulus and that tubular reabsorption accounted not only for water but also for other plasma constituents. The fluid reabsorbed was considered to be of constant composition, resembling protein-free plasma. Cushny rejected tubular secretion.

There were many other views of urine formation during this period and all of them contributed to our present-day understanding of urine formation that recognizes glomerular filtration, tubular reabsorption of a fluid of varying composition, and tubular secretion. The preceding chapters were developed in this context and the present chapter summarizes aspects of urine elimination and characteristics, and describes a method for the evaluation of kidney performance associated with renal clearance.

Micturition

> 1 What prevents backflow of urine from the bladder to the ureters?
> 2 How are the sacral spinal cord and brainstem reflexes coordinated to allow for storage of the urine while it is formed?
> 3 What are the events associated with the initiation and maintenance of micturition?
> 4 Do the sympathetics have a role in micturition?
> 5 How do spinal injuries relate to urinary incontinence?
> 6 What term describes the clinical sign associated with FUS?

During the formation of urine, the tubular fluid flows through the tubules because of a hydrostatic pressure (HP) difference that exists between **Bowman's capsule** and the renal pelvis. The HP in Bowman's capsule is about 15–20 mmHg, and there is almost no HP in the renal pelvis.

Transport of urine to the urinary bladder

Urine is transported from the renal pelvis to the urinary bladder by peristalsis in the ureters. The ureters enter the urinary bladder at an oblique angle to form a functional valve, the **ureterovesicular valve** (see Chapter 15). Once urine has entered the bladder, its backflow into the ureters is prevented as the bladder fills.

The urinary bladder is a hollow muscular (smooth muscle) organ that varies in size depending on the amount of urine it contains at any one time. Emptying of the bladder is accomplished by contraction of the bladder musculature, which is

Dukes' Physiology of Domestic Animals, Thirteenth Edition. Edited by William O. Reece, Howard H. Erickson, Jesse P. Goff and Etsuro E. Uemura.
© 2015 John Wiley & Sons, Inc. Published 2015 by John Wiley & Sons, Inc.
Companion website: www.wiley.com/go/reece/physiology

Section III: The Kidneys and Urinary System

arranged in three sheets. The muscle sheets converge on the neck of the bladder in such a way that their contraction also shortens and widens the neck, decreasing urethral resistance. Passive tension of elastic elements in the mucosa ordinarily keep the lumen of the neck closed.

The epithelial cell lining of the bladder, known as **transitional epithelium**, accommodates for the change in bladder size. When the bladder is empty the cells appear to be piled on one another, giving it a stratified appearance. A transition occurs on filling so that the piled-up appearance gives way to a thinner epithelial stratification.

The urethra is the caudal continuation of the neck of the bladder. It conveys the urine from the bladder to the exterior. The **external sphincter** lies beyond the bladder; it is composed of skeletal muscle that encircles the urethra at this point. The functional boundary between the bladder and the urethra is represented by this sphincter.

Escape of urine while the bladder is filling is prevented by contraction of the external sphincter and by tension passively exerted by elastic elements within the mucosa. When the external sphincter relaxes and the bladder muscle contracts, urine is expelled from the bladder.

Micturition reflexes

Micturition is the physiologic term for emptying of the bladder. The bladder is allowed to fill before emptying because of reflexes having control centers in the sacral spinal cord and brainstem. Receptors in the bladder wall are stretched during filling and have the reflex ability (activation of sacral spinal cord reflex center) of allowing urine to be evacuated through the neck of the bladder and external sphincter. However, the brainstem reflex center prevents the contraction of the bladder and relaxation of the external sphincter that would otherwise occur. Normal filling occurs, and the cerebral cortex is aroused when the bladder is sufficiently full. Voluntary control intervenes, and micturition is permitted when appropriate. Once micturition proceeds, complete emptying is ensured because of another reflex (brainstem) activated by **flow receptors** in the urethra. As long as urine is flowing, bladder contraction continues until there is no further flow (bladder is empty).

The parasympathetic nerves are the sole motor supply to the detrusor muscle of the bladder. The sympathetic nerves have no effect on micturition, but seem to constrict the neck of the bladder during ejaculation, thus directing the ejaculate through the penile urethra without backflow into the bladder.

Behavioral and practical aspects

The following keen observations that describe micturition are quoted from a book written over 90 years ago. The word "horse," as used herein, may refer to the male or collectively to both sexes.

> At the moment the bladder wall begins to contract, it is assisted by the abdominal muscles and a fixed diaphragm. The flow is never so powerful in the female as in the male, the final expulsion of the last drops from the urethra of the latter being effected by the rhythmical contraction of the perineal muscles and by the accelerator urinae. During the act both the horse and mare stand with the hind-legs extended and apart, resting on the toes of both hind feet, thereby sinking the posterior part of the body. The male animal also often advances the fore-legs in order to avoid their being splashed; in this position the penis is protruded, and the tail raised and quivering. The streams which flow from the two sexes are very different in size, depending on the relative diameters of the urethral canal. The mare after urinating spasmodically erects the clitoris, the cause of which is difficult to see; it may be due to the passage of a hot alkaline fluid over a remarkably sensitive surface. The horse can, under ordinary circumstances, pass urine only when standing still, though both sexes can defecate while trotting; but in a condition of oestrum the mare can empty her bladder while cantering. In the ox the urine simply dribbles away, owing to the curved character of the urethral canal, and is directed towards the ground by the tuft of hair found on the extremity of the sheath. The ox can pass his urine while walking. The cow arches her back to urinate, but instead of extending her hind-limbs, as does the mare, she brings them under her body, at the same time raising the tail.
>
> The upright position is essential to micturition; no horse of either sex can evacuate the bladder while lying down – a point of extreme importance in practice. Further, it will be remembered that the fundus of an over-distended bladder hangs into the abdominal cavity, and is thus on a lower level than the urethra; this contributes to the difficulty of emptying an over-distended organ. As a horse cannot micturate at work, it is obvious that opportunity for this should be regularly afforded, or much suffering must result.
>
> Smith, F. (1921) *Manual of Veterinary Physiology*, 5th edn. Alex. Eger, Chicago.

Descriptive terms

Urinary continence is the normal condition of storing urine in the bladder while it fills. Continence is maintained by continuous tone of the external sphincter muscle and by closure of the neck of the bladder, which is augmented by elastic tissue. An incontinent animal dribbles urine at frequent intervals instead of permitting the bladder to fill. Spinal injuries cranial to the sacrum are frequently the cause; in such injuries, the brainstem reflexes do not effectively prevent emptying, and thus emptying is initiated by the sacral reflexes as the bladder fills.

Polyuria refers to increased urine output, **oliguria** means decreased output, and **anuria** describes the condition of no output. **Dysuria** is a term used to describe difficult or painful micturition. **Stranguria** is slow, dropwise, painful discharge of urine caused by spasm of the urethra and bladder. Stranguria is a clinical sign of **feline urologic syndrome (FUS)**, caused by obstruction of the urethra by a plug consisting of struvite (magnesium ammonium phosphate) crystals and mucoid material.

Characteristics of mammalian urine

> 1 Why is urine normally yellow in color?
>
> 2 What appears to be the purpose for the secretion and presence of mucus in horse urine?
>
> 3 What is the principal nitrogenous constituent of mammalian urine and where is it formed?

Section III: The Kidneys and Urinary System

Urinalysis is a very important diagnostic procedure consisting of an evaluation of several physical and chemical properties of urine, estimation of its solute concentration, and microscopic examination of urine sediment. It requires a mastery of laboratory techniques and thoughtful interpretation. It is beyond the scope of this book to provide detailed information for urinalysis, and only some general characteristics of urine are considered.

Laboratory evaluation

Composition

Urine is formed to keep the composition of the **extracellular fluid (ECF)** constant and, generally, most substances that are present in ECF are also present in urine. Also, the composition of urine varies depending on whether substances are being conserved or excreted.

Color

Urine is usually yellow in color. The yellow color is derived from **bilirubin** excreted into the intestine and reabsorbed into the portal circulation as **urobilinogen**. Much of the urobilinogen is re-excreted by the liver into the intestine, but urobilinogen that bypasses the liver can be excreted by the kidneys into the urine. The various bilinogens are colorless but are spontaneously oxidized on exposure to oxygen. Thus urobilinogen, when partially oxidized, is known as **urobilin**, and it is largely responsible for the yellow color of urine.

Odor

The odor of urine is characteristic for a species and is probably influenced by diet. A dietary example is the characteristic odor imparted to human urine after the ingestion of asparagus as caused by the formation of **asparagine** (the amide form of the amino acid aspartic acid). Among animals, species differences are readily recognized when one enters an enclosure housing a particular species.

Consistency

Urine has a watery consistency in most species. Horse urine is somewhat thick and syrupy, however, because of the secretion of **mucus** from glands in the pelvis of the kidneys and the upper part of the ureters. The urine of the horse has high concentrations of carbonates and phosphates, which seem to precipitate on standing. The secretion of mucus provides a carrier for the precipitated carbonates and phosphates and prevents their collection in the renal pelvis. The combination of the precipitated carbonates and phosphates gives the appearance of pus and could be erroneously described as such.

Nitrogen component

The principal nitrogenous constituent of mammalian urine is **urea**. Urea is formed by the liver from ammonia, which is produced during amino acid metabolism. The body expends considerable energy in producing urea so that the toxicity of

Table 19.1 Volumes and specific gravities of urine.

Animal	Volume (mL/kg body weight per day)	Specific gravity (mean and range)
Cat	10–20	1.030 (1.02–1.040)
Cattle	17–45	1.032 (1.030–1.045)
Dog	20–100	1.025 (1.016–1.060)
Goat	10–40	1.030 (1.015–1.045)
Horse	3–18	1.040 (1.025–1.060)
Sheep	10–40	1.030 (1.015–1.045)
Swine	5–30	1.012 (1.010–1.050)
Human	8.6–28.6	1.020 (1.002–1.040)

Source: Reece, W.O. (2009) *Functional Anatomy and Physiology of Domestic Animals*, 4th edn. Wiley-Blackwell, Ames, IA. Reproduced with permission from Wiley.

ammonia can be avoided. Compared with ammonia, urea is relatively nontoxic at normal concentrations.

Amount and specific gravity

The amount of urine excreted daily varies with diet, work, external temperature, water consumption, season, and other factors. Marked pathologic variations may occur. The specific gravity of urine varies with the relative proportion of dissolved matter and water. In general, the greater the volume, the lower the specific gravity. Volume and specific gravities for several domestic animals and humans are shown in Table 19.1.

Renal clearance

1 What are the features of creatinine that make it useful in the renal clearance formula for measuring kidney function?

2 Why do diseased kidneys have a lower renal clearance than normal kidneys?

3 Would a plasma concentration for creatinine of 6 mg/dL be of concern?

4 Why are osmolal clearance values useful for evaluating diuretics?

Renal clearance is a measurement of the kidney's ability to remove substances from the plasma. Clearance measurements have been used to determine elements of kidney function discussed previously (see Chapter 15): renal blood flow (RBF), renal plasma flow (RPF), glomerular filtration rate (GFR), and filtration fraction (FF). As a measure of the kidney's ability to remove substances from the plasma, renal clearance measurements can also be used for the evaluation of kidney disease.

Renal clearance can be determined by the following general formula:

$$C_x = \frac{U_x \dot{V}}{P_x}$$

where C_x indicates clearance of substance x (mL/min), U_x concentration of x in urine (mg/mL), $\dot{V}$ rate of urine formation (mL/min), and P_x concentration of x in plasma (mg/mL). Thus, if $U_x = 130$ mg/mL, $\dot{V} = 1$ mL/min, and $P_x = 2$ mg/mL, then $C_x = (130 \times 1)/2 = 65$ mL/min. Note that $U_x \dot{V}$ (130 mg/mL × 1 mL/min) is the rate at which substance x is excreted.

Accordingly, dividing the excretion rate by the concentration of the substance in plasma (130 mg/min divided by 2 mg/mL = 65 mL/min) gives the amount of plasma that would be needed (completely cleared) each minute to provide the quantity that is excreted. This value does not imply that 65 mL of the RPF is completely cleared of x and that the remainder continues through the kidney with none extracted. Rather, it means that every milliliter of the RPF contributes some x to that which is excreted, but the amount excreted in the urine each minute would require all of x in 65 mL of the RPF.

Creatinine clearance application

Creatinine clearance is a useful clinical assessment for the evaluation of kidney disease. In many animals (e.g., dog, cat, sheep, cattle), creatinine is filtered freely, is not reabsorbed, and is not secreted. Its measurement provides an estimate of kidney function. The **endogenous creatinine clearance method** is most often used for the evaluation of kidney disease. It is endogenous in that it uses the amount that is normally present in blood.

Creatinine is a nitrogenous byproduct of muscle metabolism. The major reaction that produces creatinine is the spontaneous loss of phosphoric acid from **creatine phosphate** in muscle. Creatinine production is independent of protein metabolism. The amount produced depends on the mass of muscle in the body and is very consistent from day to day. Because it is constantly produced, it is constantly excreted, and normal plasma creatine concentrations are 0.5–2.0 mg/dL. High plasma concentrations of creatinine are a first indication of kidney disease.

Creatinine clearance is essentially a measure of GFR and can be used clinically for the assessment of kidney function because creatinine clearance is directly related to functional renal mass. Accordingly, loss of nephron numbers by kidney disease can be confirmed by a corresponding decrease in creatinine clearance. Diseased kidneys have a lower renal clearance value for creatinine than a normal kidney because the excretion rate is diminished as a result of reduced filtration (fewer functional nephrons) and, because it is not cleared, the plasma concentration would be correspondingly higher. A decrease in excretion rate coupled with increased plasma concentration of creatinine results in lower values for creatinine clearance. Normal values for endogenous creatinine clearance in the dog are between 2 and 4 mL/min per kg body weight.

To understand creatinine clearance as a measure of kidney function, consider the following.

1 The concentration of creatinine in the glomerular filtrate is the same as the concentration of creatinine in the plasma (because it is filtered freely).
2 Water is reabsorbed from the tubules but creatinine stays (also, no creatinine is added by tubular secretion) and becomes more concentrated.

Table 19.2 Determination of GFR by the endogenous creatinine clearance method in a healthy 14-kg dog.*

Collected data
$\dot{V}$ = urine flow rate = 280 mL ÷ 1440 min = 0.194 mL/min
$[U_{cr}]$ = urine creatinine concentration = 150 mg/dL = 1.5 mg/mL
$[P_{cr}]$ = plasma creatinine concentration = 0.6 mg/dL = 0.006 mg/mL

Calculations
$[U_{cr}]\dot{V}$ = creatinine excretion rate = 1.5 mg/mL × 0.194 mL/min = 0.291 mg/min
$C_{cr} = [U_{cr}]\dot{V}/[P_{cr}]$ = 0.291 mg/min ÷ 0.006 mg/mL = 48.5 mL/min
GFR = C_{cr}/kg body weight = 48.5 mL/min ÷ 14 kg = 3.46 mL/min per kg

*Normal values for endogenous creatinine clearance in dogs: 2.98±0.96 mL/min per kg body weight.
Source: Reece, W.O. (2009) *Functional Anatomy and Physiology of Domestic Animals*, 4th edn. Wiley-Blackwell, Ames, IA. Reproduced with permission from Wiley.

3 The excreted creatinine represents all that was present when filtered.
4 The plasma concentration of creatinine represents its concentration in the filtrate as the filtrate was formed.
5 The filtrate volume can be determined by dividing the urine concentration of creatinine by its plasma concentration.
6 The volume per unit of time (mL/min) is obtained by appropriate application of the urine flow rate.

Creatinine clearance (C_{cr}) as determined by the endogenous method would consider the following:

1 collection of urine for 24-hour period (shortened periods could be used);
2 volume collected divided by 1440 (number of minutes in 24 hours) to determine urine flow rate ($\dot{V}$) in mL/min;
3 determination of creatinine concentration for urine $[U_{cr}]$ and for plasma $[P_{cr}]$;
4 the product of urine concentration $[U_{cr}]$ and $\dot{V}$ provides the excretion rate ($[U_{cr}]\dot{V}$);
5 the quotient obtained from $[U_{cr}]\dot{V} \div [P_{cr}]$ is further divided by the animal's weight in kilograms to provide an estimation of the GFR in mg/min per kg.

An example of the determination of kidney function by the endogenous creatinine clearance method in a healthy 14-kg dog is provided in Table 19.2.

Other applications of renal clearance

The renal clearance concept can be applied to substances other than creatinine for studies of kidney function in addition to assessment of kidney health status. Renal clearance measurements are made for determining RPF and GFR. Values for GFR and RPF are used to calculate the FF (GFR/RPF = FF), and the value determined for RPF, when coupled with the hematocrit (Hct), can be used to calculate RBF (RPF/PCV = RBF). These assessments were first presented in Chapter 15. In addition, it is useful in physiologic and pharmacologic studies for determining the fraction of substances reabsorbed, determining whether substances are reabsorbed or secreted, for quantitative estimates of the ability to concentrate urine in different animals (**solute-free water clearance**), and **osmolal clearance** which provides a quantitative estimate of solute excretion. Osmolal clearance estimates are of value in evaluating the action of diuretics. Increased values indicate that the water loss is associated with solute loss, which is the purpose for using diuretics.

Self-evaluation

Answers can be found at the end of the chapter.

1 Tubular fluid is transported from Bowman's capsule to the renal pelvis by:
   A Action of cilia
   B Peristalsis
   C Hydrostatic pressure gradient
   D Bucket brigade

2 The principal nitrogenous constituent of mammalian urine is:
   A Amino acids
   B Uric acid
   C Urea
   D Ammonia

3 The most probable reason for the abundant secretion of mucus in the kidney pelvis and upper part of the ureter in the horse is that it:
   A Provides a carrier for the carbonates and phosphates and prevents their collection in the renal pelvis
   B Prevents irritation from highly alkaline urine
   C Reduces friction for passage of urine

4 A renal clearance for urea of 50 mL/min means that:
   A 50 mL of the RPF are completely cleared of their urea, and the remainder continue through the kidney with none extracted
   B 50 mL of filtrate are formed each minute, and all of the urea is excreted
   C Each milliliter of the RPF contributes urea to that which is excreted, but the amount excreted in the urine each minute would require all of the urea in 50 mL of the RPF

5 Creatinine clearance evaluations provide an estimate of:
   A Functional renal mass
   B Amount of protein metabolism
   C Muscle mass
   D Ability to concentrate urine

6 Which division of the autonomic nervous system is associated with micturition?
   A Sympathetic
   B Parasympathetic
   C Both sympathetic and parasympathetic

7 Which one of the following statements about creatinine is *not* true?
   A The amount produced depends on the mass of muscle in the body and is very constant from day to day
   B Creatinine is a nitrogenous byproduct of muscle metabolism
   C Creatinine production depends on the amount of protein metabolism and therefore is variable
   D High plasma concentrations of creatinine are a first indication of kidney disease

8 Sacral center reflex emptying of the urinary bladder (without brainstem and cerebral cortex control):
   A Cannot occur without integration with the brainstem center
   B Will be near normal except will lack voluntary inhibition and facilitation by the cerebral cortex
   C Will be frequent and incomplete

9 Which one of the following terms most accurately describes a clinical sign of feline urologic syndrome (FUS)?
   A Stranguria
   B Oliguria
   C Polyuria
   D Anuria

10 The usual yellow color of urine is derived from:
   A Carotene
   B Uric acid
   C Bilirubin
   D Urea

Suggested reading

Reece, W. (2004) Kidney function in mammals. In: *Dukes' Physiology of Domestic Animals*, 12th edn (ed. W.O. Reece), pp. 73–106. Cornell University Press, Ithaca, NY.

Answers

1	C	6	B
2	C	7	C
3	A	8	C
4	C	9	A
5	A	10	C

20 Kidney Function in Birds

William O. Reece
Iowa State University, Ames, IA, USA

With regard to urine formation and elimination, birds have many similarities to mammals, but major differences are notable. Similarities include glomerular filtration followed by tubular reabsorption and tubular secretion whereby the filtrate is modified. Also, bird urine can have an osmolality that is above or below that of plasma. Differences from mammals include the presence of two major nephron types, the presence of a renal portal system, formation of uric acid instead of urea as the major end product of nitrogen metabolism, and post-renal modification of ureteral urine.

To understand renal physiology of birds, it is important to review the anatomy of the avian urinary organs and relate form with function.

Gross anatomy

1 Visualize the division of the kidneys into lobes and lobules and the structural detail of a lobule.

2 What are the two nephron types associated with avian kidneys?

3 Where is the location of each nephron type within a lobule?

4 What is lacking in the reptilian nephron that makes it incapable of concentrating urine?

5 Where are the loops of Henle of the mammalian nephrons located within a lobule?

6 What structures are located in the medullary cone?

7 Would the tubular fluid from reptilian nephrons be exposed to the osmotic gradient in the medullary cone on its exit from the kidney?

8 What is the origin and distribution of renal portal blood?

9 What structure controls the amount of renal portal blood that perfuses the kidney?

Avian kidneys are paired retroperitoneal structures that are closely fitted to the bony depressions of the fused pelvis. Each kidney is divided into cranial, middle, and caudal lobes. Ureters transport urine from the kidneys to the **cloaca**, which is the common collection site for the digestive, reproductive, and urinary organs (Figure 20.1). Each lobe is composed of lobules, as shown in Figure 20.2. A lobule somewhat resembles a mushroom, with its cortex corresponding to the cap of the mushroom and its smaller medulla corresponding to the stem.

Nephron types

Avian kidneys are characterized by having two major nephron types, reptilian and mammalian (Figure 20.3). The **reptilian-type nephrons** are located in the cortex and lack loops of Henle. An intermediate segment that connects the proximal and distal tubules and which is believed to represent a primitive nephron loop has been described. Reptilian-type nephrons are not capable of concentrating urine.

The **mammalian-type nephrons** have well-defined loops of Henle that are grouped into a **medullary cone** (see Figure 20.2), the part of the lobule that corresponds to the stem of a mushroom. Other structures in the medullary cone are **collecting ducts** and **vasa recta**, all of which enter at the wider cortical end of the cone. The extent of the vasa recta is shown in Figure 20.4.

Renal portal system

A unique feature of the avian kidney is the **renal portal system**, which supplies a portion of the blood that perfuses the tubules. Venous blood arriving by this means derives from the hindlimbs via the external iliac and sciatic veins (Figure 20.5). The renal portal blood enters the kidney from its periphery, supplying

Dukes' Physiology of Domestic Animals, Thirteenth Edition. Edited by William O. Reece, Howard H. Erickson, Jesse P. Goff and Etsuro E. Uemura.
© 2015 John Wiley & Sons, Inc. Published 2015 by John Wiley & Sons, Inc.
Companion website: www.wiley.com/go/reece/physiology

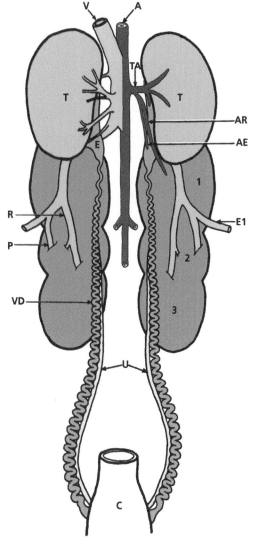

Figure 20.1 Ventral view of organs and associated structures of the dorsal abdominal cavity of a cockerel. A, abdominal aorta; AE, epididymal artery; AR, cranial renal artery; C, cloaca; E, epididymis; EI, external iliac vein; P, caudal renal portal vein; R, renal vein; T, testis; TA, testicular artery; U, ureters; V, posterior vena cava; VD, ductus deferens; 1, 2 and 3, cranial, middle, and caudal lobes of the left kidney, respectively. Adapted from Hodges, R.D. (1974) *The Histology of the Fowl*. Academic Press, New York. Reproduced with permission from Elsevier.

afferent blood to the peritubular capillaries. Within the peritubular capillaries, it is mixed with efferent arteriolar blood coming from the glomeruli (Figure 20.6). The mixture perfuses the tubules and proceeds to the central vein of the lobule. It is estimated that the renal portal system supplies half to two-thirds of the blood to the kidney.

A **renal portal valve** (smooth muscle sphincter) is located at the juncture of the right and left renal veins and their associated iliac veins (see Figure 20.5). The valves receive both adrenergic and cholinergic nerve fibers. Sympathetic innervation is stimulatory and results in valve closure, whereas parasympathetic stimulation is inhibitory and facilitates valve opening. Closure

of the valves would have the potential of diverting more blood to the renal portal system. The renal portal system appears to be a greater capacity system and allows greater blood flow to the kidneys when birds are frightened or are fleeing. Engorgement of the renal portal veins is sometimes mistaken for perirenal hemorrhage on necropsy examination because of the surface location of these veins.

Formation of urine

1 Under control conditions, which nephron type provides the greatest volume of filtrate?
2 Would the tubular fluid from reptilian nephrons be exposed to the osmotic gradient in the medullary cone on its exit from the kidney?
3 What would be an approximate osmolality of ureteral urine when birds are dehydrated?

Renal plasma flow (RPF) and **glomerular filtration rate (GFR)** appear to be autoregulated within a broad range of blood pressures (110 to 60 mmHg in the domestic fowl). It is believed that renal arteriolar smooth muscle response to stretch (pressure) is the likely mechanism of autoregulation. Regardless of usual autoregulatory mechanisms, GFR is variable and changes as needed for varying urinary output of water and sodium.

There is some evidence that the avian kidney can alternate between the use of reptilian-type and mammalian-type nephrons, depending on the need for water conservation. For example, when birds are given a salt load (and thus the need to conserve water for diluting the added salt), a majority (about 80%) of the reptilian-type nephrons shut down to zero filtration.

Concentration of avian urine

The avian proximal tubule absorbs about 70% of the filtered volume of water, which depends on active sodium reabsorption. Regulation of water reabsorption occurs in the collecting ducts where urine more concentrated than plasma can be produced and it is associated with a countercurrent mechanism similar to that in mammals.

A corticomedullary osmotic gradient exists in the peritubular fluid of the medullary cone that is established by the loops of Henle of the mammalian-type nephrons and maintained by the vasa recta. The osmotic gradient permits the excretion of urine that has an osmolality greater than that of plasma. All tubular fluid, whether from nephrons of the reptilian or the mammalian type, is exposed to the osmotic gradient because of the exit of the collecting ducts through the medullary cone to join the common ureteral branch.

The renal response to the **antidiuretic hormone of birds, arginine vasotocin,** like that in mammals, consists of an increased permeability of the collecting ducts to water. The tubular fluid reaches osmotic equilibrium with the peritubular interstitial fluid surrounding the tubules, thus becoming hyperosmotic to plasma as collecting ducts pass through the medullary cone. Urea (1–10%

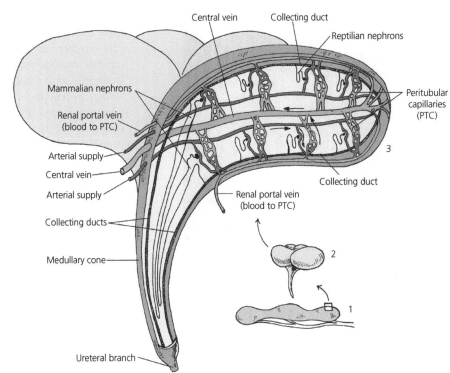

Figure 20.2 Arrangement of reptilian and mammalian nephrons within a lobule. (1) An avian kidney with its three lobes; (2) a lobule from a lobe; (3) the inner structure of a lobule. Reptilian nephrons do not have loops of Henle. Mammalian nephrons are located near the medullary cone and extend their loops of Henle into the cone. The tubular fluid from both nephron types are received by common collecting ducts that also extend into the medullary cone where it is exposed to interstitial fluid concentration gradients similar to those of mammalian kidneys. All urine from a lobule leaves by a common ureteral branch. Adapted from Reece, W.O. (1997) *Physiology of Domestic Animals*. Williams & Wilkins, Baltimore. Lippincott Williams & Wilkins © 1997.

Section III: The Kidneys and Urinary System

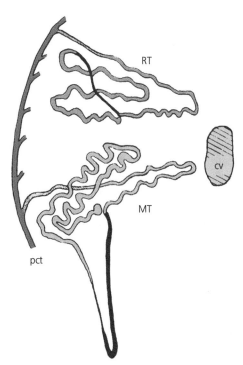

Figure 20.3 The location of avian reptilian-type (RT) and mammalian-type (MT) nephrons relative to an intralobular central vein (cv) and a perilobular collecting tubule (pct). The intermediate segment of the RT nephron and nephron loop of the MT nephron are shown in black. The finely stippled areas are beginnings of collecting tubules, also known as ducts. Adapted from Johnson, O.W. (1979) Urinary organs. In: *Form and Function in Birds*, Vol. 1 (eds A.S. King and J. McClelland). Academic Press, San Diego, CA. Reproduced with permission from Elsevier.

of total urinary nitrogen) plays virtually no role in the establishment of hypertonicity of the medullary cone interstitial fluid in birds. The hypertonicity is most likely created by NaCl transport from the thick ascending limbs of the loops of Henle. The maximum concentration that urine can attain is close to the concentration of the interstitial fluids at the tip of the medullary cone. In birds with free access to water, urine osmolality is nearly isosmotic with plasma (320 mosmol/kg H_2O). During dehydration, osmotic concentration can increase to about 600 mosmol/kg H_2O with a urine to plasma osmolal ratio of 1.60 : 1.

Composition of urine

1 What is the principal nitrogenous constituent of avian urine?

2 What is the value of having two sources of blood perfusing the tubules?

3 What is the value of having uric acid precipitated in the tubules?

4 What organs in birds are sites for the conversion of ammonia to uric acid?

5 How do the effects of angiotensin II in birds vary from the effects in mammals?

6 What is the role of aldosterone on the kidney?

7 What are the effects of atrial natriuretic peptide?

8 What hormone is involved in the regulation of calcium and phosphorus?

9 Where is the major location for the post-renal modification of ureteral urine?

10 What is the apparent function of mucus that is present in avian feces?

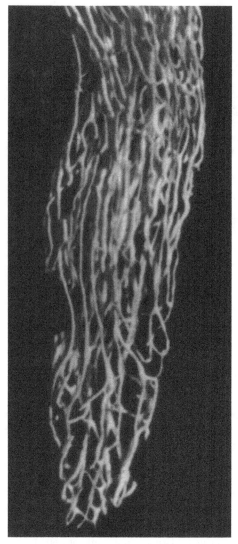

Figure 20.4 The vasa recta and associated capillary plexus from an avian kidney medullary cone. "Microfil" injection via ischiadic artery. From Johnson, O.W. (1979) Urinary organs. In: *Form and Function in Birds*, Vol. 1 (eds A.S. King and J. McClelland). Academic Press, San Diego, CA. Reproduced with permission from Elsevier.

Uric acid formation and excretion

The metabolism of proteins and amino acids results in the production of nitrogenous end products. Among the many different kinds of animals, ammonia, urea, or uric acid accounts for two-thirds or more of the total nitrogen excreted. Accordingly, animals are divided into three groups, depending on whether their main nitrogenous excretory product is ammonia, urea, or uric acid.

Because ammonia is a very toxic substance, it must be either excreted rapidly or converted to a substance that is less toxic, such as urea or uric acid. **Ammonia excretion** is encountered only in animals that are entirely aquatic, whereby the ammonia can be quickly discharged into their aquatic environment. The **urea excreting group** is found among mammals and among amphibians.

In reptiles and birds, **uric acid** is formed instead of urea because these animals develop in egg shells that are impervious to water. The excretion of urea obligates water excretion (because of its effective osmotic pressure), and because there is only limited water in eggs it must be conserved. Once uric acid reaches a certain concentration, it precipitates. As a precipitate (no effective osmotic pressure), there is no water obligated in its excretion. If urea were excreted it would be necessary to eliminate that liquid urine formed, and this is not possible within eggs.

Just as urea is formed in the liver of mammals from ammonia, so uric acid is formed in the liver of birds from ammonia. The kidneys of birds are also a site for the formation of uric acid. Uric acid precipitates in the tubules because the extra blood from the renal portal system that perfuses the tubules leads to greater tubular secretion and consequently greater tubular concentration. The greater amounts in the tubules exceed uric acid solubility and it precipitates. Uric acid continues in the tubules in its precipitated form as urate and appears in the urine as a white coagulum. Because uric acid is no longer in solution, it does not contribute to the effective osmotic pressure of the tubular fluid, and obligatory water loss is avoided.

Excretion of electrolytes

Birds have considerable control over tubular reabsorption of Na$^+$ and Cl$^-$, and the fraction of that filtered to that which is excreted may vary from less than 0.5 to 30%. Hormones involved in producing the varied amounts of sodium chloride excreted are **angiotensin II**, **aldosterone**, and **atrial natriuretic peptide**.

The presence of a complete **renin–angiotensin–aldosterone system** in birds is well established. It appears that the physiologic effects of angiotensin vary with osmoregulatory status. When there is salt and volume depletion, angiotensin II stimulates a reduction in GFR, antidiuresis, and antinatriuresis. When there is salt and volume loading, the response to angiotensin II becomes natriuretic and diuretic. In mammals, angiotensin II stimulates only antinatriuresis and antidiuresis.

Aldosterone is presumed to have an action on the kidney similar to that in mammals, whereby it is associated with sodium reabsorption coupled with potassium secretion. Aldosterone is likely the principal regulator of plasma potassium concentration. In chickens, urinary potassium concentrations are elevated (40 mEq/L) when plasma concentrations are elevated by dehydration, and decreased (6 mEq/L) when plasma concentrations are lowered by water loading.

Birds secrete **atrial natriuretic peptide (ANP)** from the atria of the heart. ANP has natriuretic and diuretic activity in birds similar to its function in mammals.

Under normal conditions, the avian kidney reabsorbs more than 98% of filtered calcium. Reabsorption depends on the presence of **parathyroid hormone (PTH)** and is coupled with the excretion of phosphate. PTH inhibits phosphate reabsorption and stimulates its secretion. The dual action of PTH on calcium reabsorption and phosphate excretion assists in the maintenance of an appropriate calcium/phosphorus ratio.

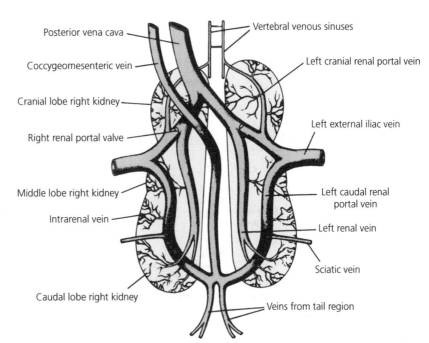

Figure 20.5 The veins associated with the renal portal system of birds. Blood arrives from the hindlimbs via the external iliac and sciatic veins. Also shown is a renal portal valve. Its closure has potential for diverting more blood to the renal portal system. Adapted from Sturkie, P.D. (1986) Kidneys, extrarenal salt excretion, and urine. In: *Avian Physiology*, 4th edn (ed. P.D. Sturkie). Springer-Verlag, New York. Reproduced with permission from Elsevier.

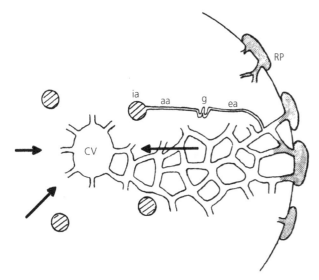

Figure 20.6 Intralobular blood flow. Intralobular artery (ia) supplies afferent arterioles (aa) supplying blood to glomeruli (g). Blood leaving the glomeruli via efferent arterioles (ea) enters the peritubular capillaries and mixes with blood from branches of the renal portal (RP) veins. Peritubular blood enters the central vein (CV) of each lobule. Arrows indicate direction of blood flow. From Johnson, O.W. (1979) Urinary organs. In: *Form and Function in Birds*, Vol. 1 (eds A.S. King and J. McClelland). Academic Press, San Diego, CA. Reproduced with permission from Elsevier.

Modification of ureteral urine

Post-renal modification of ureteral urine is possible because of its exposure to membranes of the **cloaca**. It is also exposed to membranes of the colon and ceca because of retrograde flow caused by reverse peristalsis. The cloaca functions mainly as a storage organ, and the major post-renal modification of ureteral

urine takes place in the colon. Water reabsorption from the colon follows the active reabsorption of Na⁺. NaCl and water reabsorption does occur from the ceca and could involve urine water if retrograde flow progressed to that location.

Urine characteristics

Bird urine unmixed with feces is cream colored and contains thick mucus. Precipitated uric acid is mixed with the mucus. Mucus secretion probably facilitates transport of the precipitated solutes similar to the mucus in equine urine.

The avian salt gland

> 1 What birds have modified nasal glands known as salt glands?
> 2 Where are the glands located?
> 3 What is the function of salt glands?
> 4 Do the salt glands function continuously like the kidneys?

All birds have glands in the head known as **nasal glands,** which in many species produces a nonserous, nonmucoidal secretion having uncertain function. In those species with a marine lifestyle, these glands are well developed and are capable of producing copious secretions containing high concentrations of NaCl. Because of their osmoregulatory function in these species, they have been called **salt glands.** Functional salt glands have been reported in many representatives of 13 orders of birds including ostriches, penguins, pelicans, ducks, geese, hawks, eagles, and gulls.

Avian salt glands are derived embryologically from invaginations in the nasal epithelium that persist as the main ducts of the gland. They are paired and are composed of tubular lobes (Figure 20.7A,B) that are parallel and run the length of the

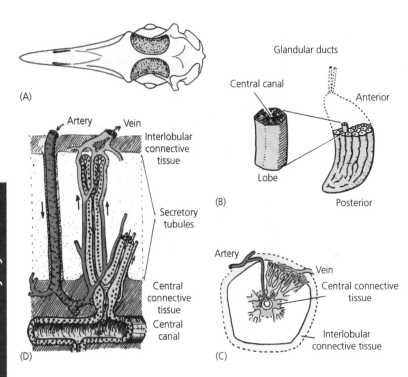

Figure 20.7 The avian salt gland. (A) Skull of the herring gull (*Larus argentatus*) from above showing the position of the salt glands. (B) Gross structure of the salt gland. (C) Transverse section through a lobe of the salt gland. (D) Circulation in the salt gland showing opposing directions of flow in the secretory tubules and in the capillaries. The tubules branch repeatedly, but only two ramifications are shown. Reproduced with permission from Fänge, R., Schmidt-Nielsen, K. and Osaki, H. (1958) The salt gland of the herring gull. *Biological Bulletin* 115:162–171.

gland. Each lobe has a central canal that is continuous with a duct of the gland. The secretion is formed in secretory tubules, arranged radially around the central canal of each lobe and are continuous with it (Figure 20.7C,D). The epithelial cells comprising the tubules are responsible for the secretion process. The blood flow to the gland forms a network of capillaries that course along the tubules to the periphery of the lobes where veins collect the blood near the surface (Figure 20.7C,D).

The salt glands have a structure entirely different from that of the kidney and can excrete a salt solution of up to twice the concentration of sea water. These glands secrete the excess salt when food with high salt content is ingested or when sea water is drunk. The salt secretion flows through the salt gland ducts into the nasal cavity, runs out through the nares, and drips from the tip of the beak. The salt glands secrete only NaCl and none of the other substances excreted by the kidneys. They function only when there is a salt load; otherwise they are at rest.

Self-evaluation

Answers can be found at the end of the chapter.

1 Which one of the following nephron components is lacking in reptilian nephrons?
  A Proximal tubule
  B Loop of Henle
  C Distal tubule
  D Collecting duct

2 Renal portal system blood is:
  A Venous blood
  B Arterial blood

3 Reptilian nephron tubular fluid bypasses the medullary cones where it could otherwise become concentrated.
  A True
  B False

4 The avian nephron associated with the countercurrent mechanism is the:
  A Reptilian type
  B Mammalian type

5 Renal portal blood enters the vascular supply perfusing the renal tubules at the level of the:
  A Glomerulus
  B Peritubular capillaries
  C Vasa recta

6 The principal nitrogenous component of avian urine is:
  A Ammonia
  B Urea
  C Uric acid

7 Uric acid precipitates in the renal tubules in order to:
  A Avoid ammonia toxicity
  B Avoid obligation of water excretion
  C Lubricate the renal tubules
  D Have a better mix with feces

8 Ammonia is converted to uric acid in birds:
  A In the liver
  B In the kidneys
  C In the liver and kidneys

9 The location for the greatest post-renal modification of ureteral urine is the:
  A Colon
  B Cloaca
  C Ceca

10 The salt glands (nasal glands):
  A Secrete only NaCl and serve an extrarenal osmoregulatory function
  B Are active continuously
  C Function similar to kidneys

Suggested reading

Goldstein, D.L. and Skadhauge, E. (2000) Renal and extrarenal regulation of body fluid composition. In: *Sturkie's Avian Physiology*, 5th edn (ed. G.C. Whittow). Academic Press, San Diego, CA.

Hodges, R.D. (1974) *The Histology of the Fowl*. Academic Press, New York.

Johnson, O.W. (1979) Urinary organs. In: *Form and Function in Birds*, Vol. 1 (eds A.S. King and J. McClelland). Academic Press, San Diego, CA.

Shoemaker, V.H. (1972) Osmoregulation and excretion in birds. In: *Avian Biology*, Vol. 2 (eds D.S. Farner and J.R. King). Academic Press, New York.

Sturkie, P.D. (1986) Kidneys, extrarenal salt excretion, and urine. In: *Avian Physiology*, 4th edn (ed. P.D. Sturkie). Springer-Verlag, New York.

Answers

1	B	6	C
2	A	7	B
3	B	8	C
4	B	9	A
5	B	10	A

Section III: The Kidneys and Urinary System

SECTION IV

Respiration

Section Editor: William O. Reece

21 Overview of the Respiratory System

William O. Reece
Iowa State University, Ames, IA, USA

Respiration is the means by which animals obtain and use oxygen and eliminate carbon dioxide. Several separate issues are involved in this process, including the chemical factors associated with oxygen uptake and carbon dioxide production, mechanical and physical aspects concerned with ventilation of the lungs, transport of gases between the lungs and blood and between the blood and tissues, and the regulation of ventilation. The goal of this chapter is to provide an orientation to the respiratory system for the discussions that follow in subsequent chapters.

Respiratory apparatus

1 How are the nostrils of the horse adapted to the need for greater air intake?

2 What functions are served by the conchae?

3 Where is the olfactory epithelium located?

4 List the openings to the pharynx.

5 What is the function of the pharynx and syrinx?

6 What is the function of tracheal rings? Why are they incomplete dorsally?

7 What are the subdivisions of the trachea (in order from largest to smallest)?

8 Where does most of the diffusion of gas between air and blood occur?

9 Describe the pleura and mediastinal space.

10 What structures lie within the mediastinal space?

11 What happens to mediastinal pressure when intrapleural pressure decreases?

The **respiratory apparatus** consists of the lungs and pleura and the air passages leading to the lungs, including the nostrils, nasal cavities, pharynx, larynx, trachea, bronchi, and bronchioles.

The lungs and pleura

The lungs are the principal structures of the respiratory system. They are paired structures and occupy all space in the thorax that is not otherwise filled. When the thorax expands in volume, the lungs also expand; this provides for airflow into the lungs. Air is an excellent radiographic contrast media because it is radiolucent (relatively penetrable by X-rays). Therefore, air-filled lungs provide good contrast for thoracic structures (normal and pathologic) that are radiopaque (relatively impenetrable by X-rays). Dorsal–ventral and lateral view radiographs of a normal canine thorax are shown in Figure 21.1. The radiopaque objects (heart and blood vessels) appear superimposed on the radiolucent background of air. The heart and blood vessels are visible because the blood contained within is relatively radiopaque. The blood vessels appear as branching white tubes.

The lungs have an almost friction-free movement within the thorax because of the **pleura**, a smooth serous membrane. The pleura consists of a single layer of cells fused to the surface of a connective tissue layer. It envelops both lungs (**visceral pleura**). The pleura for the right and left lung meet near the midline, and here it reflects upward (dorsally), turns back on the inner thoracic wall, and provides for its lining (**costal pleura**). The space between the respective visceral pleura layers as they ascend to the dorsal wall is known as the **mediastinal space**. Within the mediastinal space are the venae cavae, thoracic lymph duct, esophagus, aorta, and trachea (Figure 21.2). The mediastinal space is intimately associated with the **intrapleural space** (space between visceral and costal pleura); thus, pressure changes in the intrapleural space are accompanied by similar changes in the mediastinal space. Also, pressure changes within the mediastinal space are accompanied by changes within the mediastinal structures, provided that their walls are responsive to relatively low-pressure distensibility.

Section IV: Respiration

Dukes' Physiology of Domestic Animals, Thirteenth Edition. Edited by William O. Reece, Howard H. Erickson, Jesse P. Goff and Etsuro E. Uemura.
© 2015 John Wiley & Sons, Inc. Published 2015 by John Wiley & Sons, Inc.
Companion website: www.wiley.com/go/reece/physiology

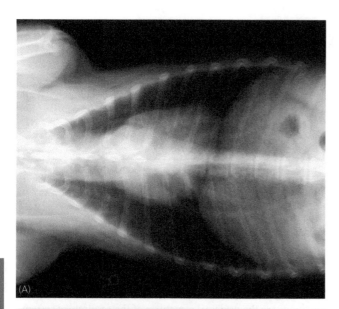

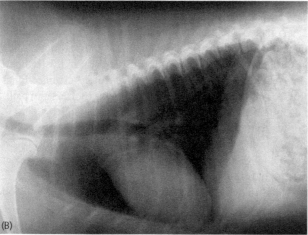

Figure 21.1 Radiographs of healthy canine thorax. (A) Dorsal–ventral view; (B) lateral view. The heart and major blood vessels are visible because blood is relatively radiopaque. Blood in lesser blood vessels gives a slightly cloudy appearance to the lung field as compared with the clear appearance of air in the trachea. Radiographs courtesy of Dr Elizabeth Riedesel, Iowa State University, College of Veterinary Medicine, Veterinary Clinical Sciences Department, Radiology Section. Adapted from Reece, W.O. (2009) *Functional Anatomy and Physiology of Domestic Animals*, 4th edn. Wiley-Blackwell, Ames, IA. Reproduced with permission from Wiley.

Airways to the lungs

The **nostrils (nares)** are the paired external openings to the air passages (Figure 21.3). The nostrils are the most pliable and dilatable in the horse and the most rigid in the pig. Nostril dilatation is advantageous when more air is required, as in running, and in situations in which breathing is not done through the mouth. The horse is a runner and open-mouth breathing is not characteristic, therefore dilatable nostrils are advantageous.

The nostrils provide the external openings for the paired **nasal cavities**. The nasal cavities are separated from each other

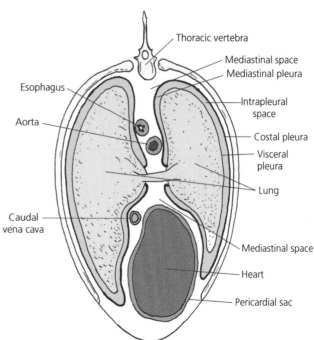

Figure 21.2 Schematic transverse section of equine thorax showing the relationships of the visceral, costal, and mediastinal pleura. The aorta, esophagus, venae cavae, and thoracic lymph duct (not shown) are within the mediastinal space. The esophagus, venae cavae, and lymph duct (soft structures) respond by increasing and decreasing pressures within their lumens, associated with similar changes in intrapleural and mediastinal spaces. From Reece, W.O. (2009) *Functional Anatomy and Physiology of Domestic Animals*, 4th edn. Wiley-Blackwell, Ames, IA. Reproduced with permission from Wiley.

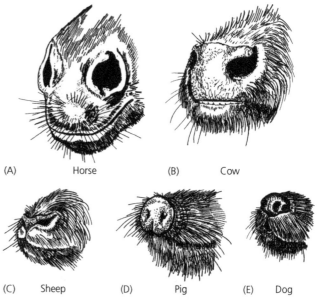

Figure 21.3 The nostrils of several domestic animals: (A) horse; (B) cow; (C) sheep; (D) pig; (E) dog. From Frandson, R.D., Wilke, W.L. and Fails, A.D. (2003) *Anatomy and Physiology of Farm Animals*, 6th edn. Lippincott Williams & Wilkins, Baltimore. Reproduced with permission from Lippincott Williams & Wilkins.

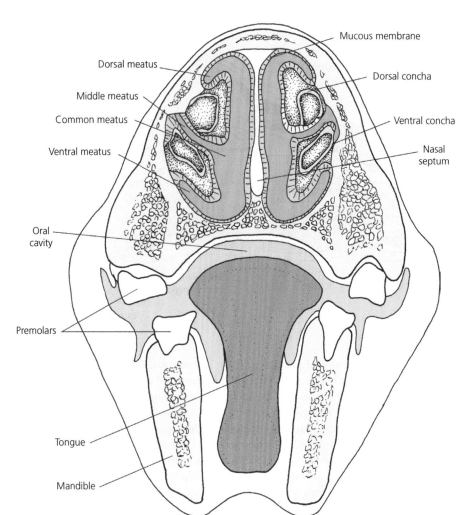

Figure 21.4 Transverse section of the head of a horse showing the division of the nasal cavities. The airways are noted as the dorsal, middle, ventral, and common meatus. The conchae consist of turbinate bones covered by a highly vascularized mucous membrane. It can be seen that incoming air is exposed to a large surface area for adjustment of its temperature and humidity. Adapted from Reece, W.O. (2009) *Functional Anatomy and Physiology of Domestic Animals*, 4th edn. Wiley-Blackwell, Ames, IA. Reproduced with permission from Wiley.

Section IV: Respiration

by the **nasal septum** and from the mouth by the **hard and soft palates**. In addition, each nasal cavity contains mucosa-covered turbinate bones (**conchae**) that project to the interior from the dorsal and lateral walls, separating the cavity into passages known as the common, dorsal, middle, and ventral meatus (Figure 21.4). The mucosa of the turbinates is well vascularized and serves to warm and humidify inhaled air. Another function, mainly of the conchae, that is often overlooked involves cooling the arterial blood that supplies the brain. Arteries that supply blood to the brain divide into many smaller arteries at its base and then rejoin before entering. These smaller arteries are bathed in a pool of venous blood that comes from the walls of the nasal passages, where it has been cooled. As a result, brain temperature might be 2 or 3°C lower than body core temperature. The brain is the most heat-sensitive body organ, so this cooling method is particularly important during times of extreme activity. The mouth breathing that occurs when the environmental air is extremely cold seems to be reflexive, which might prevent the overcooling of the brain that could otherwise occur if all the inhaled air traversed the meatus and

had contact with the conchae. The **olfactory epithelium** is located in the caudal portion of each nasal cavity, and greater perception of odors (a nonrespiratory function) is achieved by **sniffing** (i.e., fast, alternating, and shallow inspirations and expirations).

The **pharynx** is caudal to the nasal cavities and is a common passageway for air and food (Figure 21.5). The openings to the pharynx include two posterior nares, two eustachian tubes, a mouth (oral cavity), a glottis, and an esophagus. The opening from the pharynx leading to the continuation of the respiratory passageway is the **larynx**, the organ of phonation (sound production) in mammals. Sound is produced by the controlled passage of air, which causes vibration of vocal cords in the larynx. The organ of phonation in birds is called the **syrinx**; this is located where the trachea divides to form the bronchi.

The **glottis** is the slit-like opening between the vocal cords and is the site of insertion of an endotracheal (within the trachea) tube for providing assisted ventilation and for administration of inhalant anesthetics. Extending craniad from the larynx is the

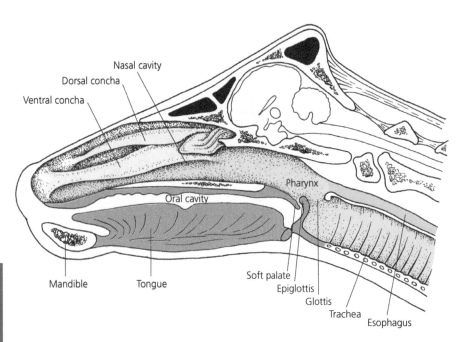

Figure 21.5 Mid-sagittal section of the head of a cow with nasal septum removed. The stippled area represents the pathway for air through the nasal cavity, pharynx, larynx, and trachea. The glottis is the opening to the larynx that is continued caudally by the trachea. Adapted from Reece, W.O. (2009) *Functional Anatomy and Physiology of Domestic Animals*, 4th edn. Wiley-Blackwell, Ames, IA. Reproduced with permission from Wiley.

epiglottis. It is a leaf-shaped plate of cartilage covered with mucous membrane that is located at the root of the tongue and is passively bent over the larynx during the act of swallowing, thereby preventing the entrance into the trachea of a bolus of food. A cranial view of the glottis and epiglottis as they would appear with the mouth open and the tongue extended is shown in Figure 21.6. In this view, the soft palate (caudal extension of the hard palate) has been hyperextended with the maxilla (upper jaw). When placing an endotracheal tube, the soft palate is often seen ventral to the epiglottis with usual mouth opening and must be lifted by manipulation of the endotracheal tube to expose the glottis. Figure 21.7 shows an endotracheal tube in place relative to the structures encountered.

The **trachea** is the primary passageway for air to the lungs. It is continued from the larynx cranially and divides caudally to form the right and left bronchi. The tracheal wall contains cartilaginous rings to prevent collapse of the tracheal airway (Figure 21.8). Each tracheal ring is incomplete (not joined dorsally), which permits variations in diameter that are regulated by the tracheal smooth muscle. This diameter can increase during times of greater ventilatory requirements.

The right and left bronchi and their subdivisions continue all the way to the **alveoli**, the final and smallest subdivision of the air passages (Figure 21.9). The subdivisions of the trachea to the alveoli, from the largest to the smallest, comprise bronchi, bronchioles, terminal bronchioles, respiratory bronchioles, alveolar duct, alveolar sac, and alveoli.

Pulmonary alveoli

The **pulmonary alveoli** are the principal sites of gas diffusion between the air and blood. The separation of air and blood, and thus the diffusion distance, is minimal at the alveolar level. The alveolar epithelium and the capillary endothelium are

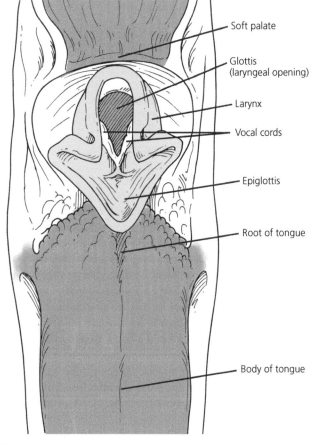

Figure 21.6 Cranial view of canine glottis (opening to the larynx, between vocal cords) and epiglottis (cranial extension from the larynx). The soft palate is not shown in the location that would be seen with usual mouth-opening techniques. Adapted from Reece, W.O. (2009) *Functional Anatomy and Physiology of Domestic Animals*, 4th edn. Wiley-Blackwell, Ames, IA. Reproduced with permission from Wiley.

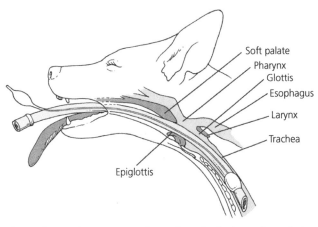

Figure 21.7 Schematic view of an endotracheal tube in place relative to the structures encountered. Adapted from Reece, W.O. (2009) *Functional Anatomy and Physiology of Domestic Animals*, 4th edn. Wiley-Blackwell, Ames, IA. Reproduced with permission from Wiley.

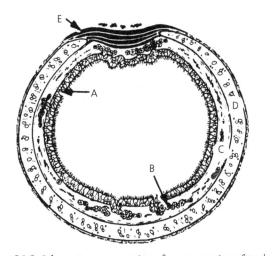

Figure 21.8 Schematic representation of a cross-section of trachea. (A) Pseudostratified epithelium lines the lumen; (B) glands in the lamina propria; (C) glands in the submucosa; (D) cartilage; (E) band of smooth muscle. The tracheal muscle and the cartilage form most of the tracheal wall. From Dellmann, H.D. (1993) *Textbook of Veterinary Histology*, 4th edn. Lea & Febiger, Philadelphia. With permission from Wiley.

intimately associated (Figure 21.10). Here, venous blood from the **pulmonary arteries** becomes arterial blood and is returned to the left atrium by the **pulmonary veins**. The darker purple color of venous blood becomes bright red arterial blood during the resaturation of hemoglobin with new oxygen that has diffused from the alveoli. During the seventeenth century, Richard Lower showed that the change in blood color occurred in the lungs because of the influence of fresh air. The idea that the diffusion of oxygen and carbon dioxide between blood and air was separate from a secretion process was proven by August and Marie Krogh. (August Krogh won the Nobel prize in 1920 for his studies of the capillaries.)

Factors associated with breathing

1 What are the mechanical activities associated with inspiration? What are some conditions for active expiration?

2 Differentiate between abdominal and costal breathing. When is either accentuated?

3 What are some commonly referred to states of breathing?

4 Know the subdivision of lung volume. What is the difference between a lung volume subdivision and a lung capacity subdivision?

5 When expansion of the lungs is restricted, how is adequate ventilation maintained?

6 What are some factors that affect respiratory frequency?

Many factors of breathing terminology must be understood for one to observe, describe, and measure individual animal behavior related to respiration.

Respiratory cycles

A **respiratory cycle** consists of an inspiratory phase followed by an expiratory phase. **Inspiration** involves an enlargement of the thorax and lungs, with an accompanying inflow of air. The thorax enlarges by contraction of the **diaphragm** (the musculotendinous separation between the thorax and abdomen) and by contraction of external **intercostal muscles** (muscles located between the ribs) (Figure 21.11). Diaphragmatic contraction enlarges the thorax in a caudal direction, and external intercostal muscle contraction enlarges the thorax in a craniad and outward direction. Under normal breathing conditions, inspiration requires greater effort than expiration, and sometimes expiration might seem to be passive. **Expiration** can become quite an active process, particularly during times of accelerated breathing and also when there are impediments to the outflow of air. The internal intercostal muscles contract to assist in expiration. Other skeletal muscles can aid in either inspiration or expiration, such as the abdominal muscles. When contracted, these muscles force the abdominal viscera forward to press on the diaphragm, which in turn decreases thoracic volume.

The **respiratory pattern** or **waveform**, when recorded, varies little among mammalian species. The inspiratory and expiratory phases of the cycles are generally smooth and symmetrical. An exception to this general statement is the horse, in which there are two phases during inspiration and two phases during expiration (Figure 21.12). This species difference may be due to a time delay in the firing of the late inspiratory neurons. These neurons are described in Chapter 24.

Complementary breathing cycles are characterized by a deep rapid inspiration followed by expiration of longer duration. They occur normally in many species but apparently not in the horse. This type of cycle has frequently been called a **sigh**. As it naturally occurs, it is probably a compensatory mechanism for poor ventilation. In laboratory exercises where ventilation is impaired by the addition of dead-space volume, not only do respiratory frequency and tidal volume increase but also the number of

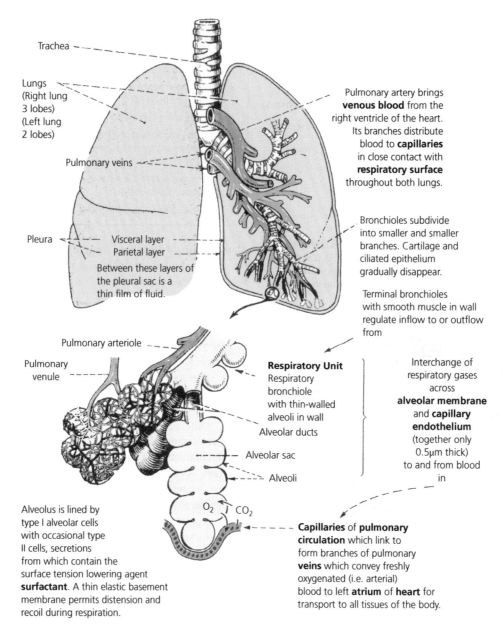

Trachea

Lungs
(Right lung
3 lobes)
(Left lung
2 lobes)

Pulmonary veins

Pleura
Visceral layer
Parietal layer
Between these layers of
the pleural sac is a
thin film of fluid.

Pulmonary artery brings
venous blood from the
right ventricle of the heart.
Its branches distribute
blood to **capillaries**
in close contact with
respiratory surface
throughout both lungs.

Bronchioles subdivide
into smaller and smaller
branches. Cartilage and
ciliated epithelium
gradually disappear.

Terminal bronchioles
with smooth muscle in wall
regulate inflow to or outflow
from

Pulmonary arteriole

Pulmonary
venule

Respiratory Unit
Respiratory
bronchiole
with thin-walled
alveoli in wall

Alveolar ducts

Alveolar sac

Alveoli

Interchange of
respiratory gases
across
alveolar membrane
and **capillary
endothelium**
(together only
0.5μm thick)
to and from blood
in

Alveolus is lined by
type I alveolar cells
with occasional type
II cells, secretions
from which contain the
surface tension lowering agent
surfactant. A thin elastic basement
membrane permits distension and
recoil during respiration.

O_2 CO_2

Capillaries of **pulmonary
circulation** which link to
form branches of pulmonary
veins which convey freshly
oxygenated (i.e. arterial)
blood to left **atrium** of **heart** for
transport to all tissues of the body.

Figure 21.9 Schematic representation of lung subdivisions. Adapted from Mackenna, B.R. and Callander, R. (1997) *Illustrated Physiology*, 6th edn. Churchill Livingstone, Edinburgh. With permission from Elsevier.

complementary breathing cycles increase. Anesthetists often create complementary cycles at regular intervals by manually compressing the rebreathing bag.

Types of breathing

There are two **types of breathing**: abdominal and costal. **Abdominal breathing** is characterized by visible movements of the abdomen, in which the abdomen protrudes during inspiration and recoils during expiration. Normally the abdominal type of breathing predominates. The other type is called **costal breathing**; it is characterized by pronounced rib movements. During painful conditions of the abdomen such as peritonitis, in which movement of the viscera would aggravate the pain, costal

breathing can predominate. Similarly, during painful conditions of the thorax such as pleuritis, abdominal breathing might be more apparent. Binding of the thorax to minimize the outward and craniad expansion of the thorax requires greater diaphragmatic effort, and subsequent movement of abdominal viscera accentuates the abdominal type of breathing.

States of breathing

In addition to the different types of breathing, there are variations in breathing relating to the frequency of breathing cycles, depth of inspiration, or both. **Eupnea** is the term used to describe normal quiet breathing, with no deviation in frequency or depth. **Dyspnea** is difficult breathing, in which visible effort is required to breathe.

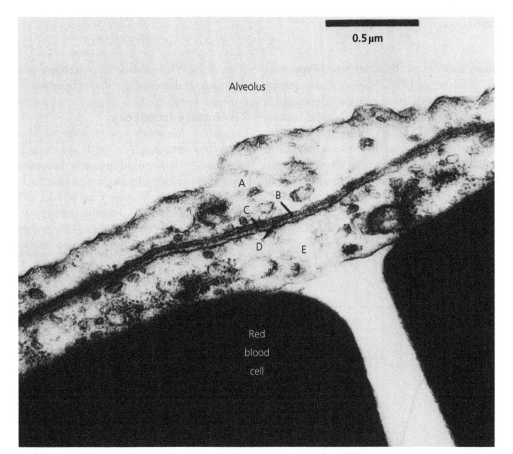

Figure 21.10 Electron micrograph of a mouse lung showing an attenuated portion of alveolar epithelium and its proximity to capillary endothelium. The respiratory membrane (without alveolar fluid layer) is composed of (A) alveolar epithelium, (B) alveolar epithelial basement membrane, (C) interstitial space, (D) capillary endothelial basement membrane, and (E) capillary endothelium. From Reece, W.O. (2004) Respiration in mammals. In: *Dukes' Physiology of Domestic Animals*, 12th edn (ed. W.O. Reece). Cornell University Press, Ithaca, NY. Reproduced with permission from Cornell University Press.

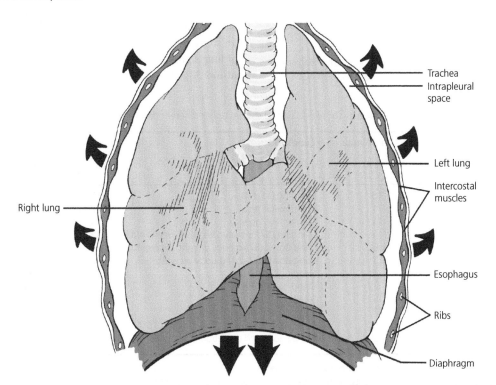

Figure 21.11 Schematic of the thorax during inspiration (ventral view). Shown are the directions of enlargement (arrows) when the diaphragm and inspiratory intercostal muscles contract during inspiration. Adapted from Reece, W.O. (2009) *Functional Anatomy and Physiology of Domestic Animals*, 4th edn. Wiley-Blackwell, Ames, IA. Reproduced with permission from Wiley.

The animal is usually aware of this breathing state. **Hyperpnea** refers to breathing characterized by increased depth, frequency, or both, and is noticeable after physical exertion. The animal is not acutely conscious of this state. **Polypnea** is rapid shallow breathing, somewhat similar to panting. Polypnea is similar to hyperpnea in regard to frequency, but is unlike hyperpnea in regard to depth. **Apnea** refers to a cessation of breathing. However, as used clinically, it generally refers to a transient state of cessation of breathing. **Tachypnea** is excessive rapidity of breathing, and **bradypnea** is abnormal slowness of breathing.

Respiratory frequency

Respiratory frequency refers to the number of respiratory cycles each minute. It is an excellent indicator of health status, but must be interpreted properly because it is subject to numerous variations. In addition to variations observed among species, respiratory frequency can be affected by other factors, such as body size, age, exercise, excitement, environmental temperature, pregnancy, degree of filling of the digestive tract, and state of health. Pregnancy and digestive tract filling increase frequency because they limit the excursion of the diaphragm during inspiration. When expansion of the lungs is restricted, adequate ventilation is maintained by increased frequency. For example, when cattle lie down, the large rumen pushes against the diaphragm and restricts its movement, and respiratory frequency is seen to increase.

Respiratory frequency usually increases during disease. Thus, frequency is a useful determinant of health status, but the frequency for a species under various conditions must be known so that this parameter can be interpreted properly (Table 21.1). Values are meaningful only when obtained unobtrusively from animals at rest.

Lung sounds

It is obvious from Figure 21.9 that considerable branching of the pulmonary airways occurs. Although the branches may have smaller diameters than the parent branch, the combined cross-sectional area of the branches shows an increase over that of the parent. Consequently, the velocity of airflow diminishes progressively from the trachea toward the bronchioles. Listening for lung sounds with the aid of a stethoscope is termed **auscultation**. A good-quality stethoscope should be used in quiet

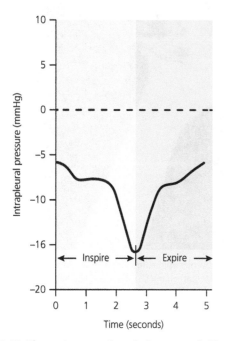

Figure 21.12 The respiratory cycle in the horse recorded by measuring intrapleural pressure. Note the two phases during inspiration and the two phases during expiration. Adapted from McCutcheon, F.H. (1951) The mammalian breathing mechanism. *Journal of Cellular and Comparative Physiology* 37:447–476.

Table 21.1 Respiratory frequency for several animal species under different conditions.*

Animal	No. of animals	Condition	Cycles/min	
			Range	Mean
Horse	15	Standing (at rest)	10–14	12
Dairy cow	11	Standing (at rest)	26–35	29
	11	Sternal recumbency	24–50	35
Dairy calf	6	Standing (52 kg body weight, 3 weeks old)	18–22	20
	6	Lying down (52 kg body weight, 3 weeks old)	21–25	22
Pig	3	Lying down (23–27 kg body weight)	32–58	40
Dog	7	Sleeping (24°C)	18–25	21
	3	Standing (at rest)	20–34	24
Cat	5	Sleeping	16–25	22
	6	Lying down, awake	20–40	31
Sheep	5	Standing, ruminating, 1.3 cm wool, 18°C	20–34	25
	5	Same sheep and conditions except 10°C	16–22	19

*Data from veterinary student laboratory assignments.
Source: Reece, W.O. (2004) Respiration in mammals. In: *Dukes' Physiology of Domestic Animals*, 12th edn (ed. W.O. Reece). Cornell University Press, Ithaca, NY.

surroundings. The high-velocity turbulent airflow in the trachea and bronchi produces the lung sounds heard through a stethoscope in a normal animal. Laminar low-velocity flow in the bronchioles produces no sound. To amplify the sounds, deep respiratory efforts can be produced by placing a plastic bag loosely over the muzzle of the animal.

The term **breath sound** applies to any sound that accompanies air movement through the tracheobronchial tree. Breath sounds vary randomly in intensity over a broad range depending on whether the sounds are produced over the larger airways or over the remaining lung parenchyma.

Adventitious sounds are extrinsic to the normal sound production mechanism of the respiratory tract and are abnormal sounds superimposed on the breath sounds. Adventitious sounds are further classified as crackles and wheezes. Diseases resulting in edema or exudates within the airways can result in crackles. Wheezes suggest airway narrowing (e.g., bronchoconstriction, bronchial wall thickening, external airway compression).

With the exception of laminar low-velocity flow in the bronchioles (noted above), the absence of respiratory sounds implies that nonfunctional lung tissue is beneath the stethoscope.

Pulmonary volumes and capacities

> 1 What is the difference between pulmonary volumes and pulmonary capacities?
> 2 What is the definition of vital capacity?
> 3 What is the functional residual capacity?

Conventional descriptions for lung volumes are either associated with the amount of air within them at any one time or with the amount associated with a breath. **Tidal volume** is the amount of air breathed in or out during a respiratory cycle. It can increase or decrease from normal, depending on ventilation requirements. Tidal volume is probably used more frequently than other terms. **Inspiratory reserve volume** is the amount of air that can still be inspired after inhaling the tidal volume, and **expiratory reserve volume** is the amount of air that can still be expired after exhaling the tidal volume. **Residual volume** is the amount of air remaining in the lungs after the most forceful expiration. Also, some part of the residual volume remains in the lungs after they have been removed from the thorax during slaughter or for postmortem examination. Because of the remaining residual volume, excised lung sections float in water. Consolidation of lung tissue, as occurs in pneumonia, causes them to sink.

Sometimes it is useful to combine two or more of these volumes. Such combinations are called capacities. Total lung capacity is the sum of all volumes. Vital capacity is the sum of all volumes over and above the residual volume; it is the maximum amount of air that can be breathed in after the most forceful expiration. **Inspiratory capacity** is the sum of the tidal and inspiratory reserve volumes. **Functional residual capacity** is

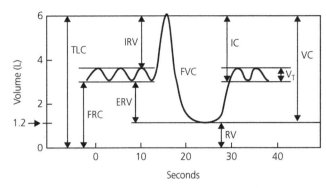

Figure 21.13 Subdivisions of lung volumes and capacities. TLC, Total lung capacity; FRC, functional residual capacity; ERV, expiratory reserve volume; IRV, inspiratory reserve volume; RV, residual volume; IC, inspiratory capacity; V_T, tidal volume; VC, vital capacity; FVC, forced vital capacity. From Cloutier, M.M. and Thrall, R.S. (2004) The respiratory system. In: *Physiology*, 5th edn (eds R.M. Berne, M.N. Levy, B.M. Koeppen and B.A. Stanton). Mosby, St Louis, MO. With permission from Elsevier.

the sum of the expiratory reserve volume and the residual volume. This is the lung volume that is ventilated by the tidal volume. It serves as the reservoir for air and helps to provide constancy to the blood concentrations of the respired gases. The relationships of pulmonary volumes and capacities are illustrated in Figure 21.13.

Self-evaluation

Answers can be found at the end of the chapter.

1 Which one of the following is associated with cooling of blood that provides a cooling mechanism for the brain?
   A Pharyngeal mucosa
   B Conchae mucosa
   C Tracheal mucosa
   Explain your choice for the correct answer.

2 The darker purple color of venous blood is due to:
   A Decreased concentration of carbon dioxide
   B Increased concentration of carbon dioxide
   C Decreased concentration of oxygen
   D Increased concentration of oxygen
   Explain your choice for the correct answer.

3 Which type of breathing predominates during normal quiet breathing?
   A Abdominal
   B Costal
   Explain your choice for the correct answer.

4 Which one of the respiratory volumes is associated with the amount of air breathed in or out during a respiratory cycle?
   A Inspiratory reserve volume
   B Tidal volume
   C Residual volume
   Explain your choice for the correct answer.

5 Which one of the following breathing states is characterized by increased depth, frequency, or both, and is noticeable after physical exertion?

A Dyspnea

B Hyperpnea

C Polypnea

Explain your choice for the correct answer.

Suggested reading

Dellman, H. (1993) *Textbook of Veterinary Histology*, 4th edn. Lea & Febiger, Philadelphia.

Frandson, R., Wilke, W. and Fails, A. (2009) *Anatomy and Physiology of Farm Animals*, 7th edn. Wiley-Blackwell, Ames, IA.

Mackenna, B. and Callander, R. (1997) *Illustrated Physiology*, 6th edn. Churchill Livingstone, Edinburgh.

Answers

1 B. The arterial blood supplying the highly vascularized conchae is cooled by the inhaled air in the spaces of the conchae. The arterial blood that was cooled is now venous blood that returns to the base of the brain where it enters a pool. Arteries that supply blood to the brain divide into a large number of smaller arteries that are then bathed in the cooled venous pool and rejoin before entering the brain, thereby providing a cooling mechanism.

2 C. The color of blood has nothing to do with carbon dioxide, but rather with the presence of hemoglobin. When hemoglobin is saturated with oxygen, it is bright red. With increasing loss of oxygen saturation it becomes darker and more purple in color.

3 A. Costal breathing is characterized by pronounced rib movements and would be prominent during painful conditions of the abdomen such as peritonitis. Abdominal breathing is characterized by visible movements of the abdomen and normally predominates. It only gives way to costal breathing when abdominal breathing is painful.

4 B. Inspiratory volume is the amount of air that can still be inspired after inhaling the tidal volume. Residual volume is the amount of air remaining in the lungs after the most forceful expiration. Tidal volume is the amount of air that is either breathed in or out during a respiratory cycle.

5 B. Dyspnea is difficult breathing, in which visible effort is required to breathe. Polypnea is rapid shallow breathing. It is similar to hyperpnea in regard to frequency, but is unlike hyperpnea in regard to depth.

22 Physical and Mechanical Aspects of Respiration

William O. Reece

Iowa State University, Ames, IA, USA

The gases of concern in respiratory physiology are oxygen, carbon dioxide, nitrogen, and water vapor. All these gas molecules are present in the atmosphere and in body fluid solutions. Basic principles of physicochemical properties of solutions still apply but are now applied to gas molecules.

Physical principles of gas exchange

1 When oxygen and carbon dioxide are subjected to the same pressure in the body fluids, which one will transport the greater quantity of their respective gas?

2 How would you define partial pressures? See Table 22.1 for how they are used.

3 Can individual gases in the body fluids diffuse independent of other gases, regardless of their partial pressure?

4 Does blood subjected to 400 mmHg have four times more oxygen than the same blood subjected to 100 mmHg? Explain.

5 Why is the partial pressure of oxygen in alveolar gas ($P_{A}O_2$) less than the partial pressure of oxygen that is being inhaled?

6 Why is the total of partial pressures in closed spaces (e.g., peritoneal cavity) less than the total of partial pressures in arterial blood and in alveolar air?

7 Why is there a decrease in both Pa_{O_2} and Pa_{CO_2} in hyperpnea associated with thickening of the pulmonary membrane (e.g., pulmonary interstitial edema)?

Physics of gases

Several physical laws are helpful in the study of gases. **Boyle's law** relates pressure to volume. If the mass and temperature of a gas in a chamber remain constant but the pressure is increased or decreased, the volume of the gas varies inversely with the pressure, e.g., if the pressure is increased, the volume is decreased.

Charles' law notes the effect of temperature on gas volume. If the pressure of a given quantity of gas remains constant but the temperature is varied, the volume of the gas increases directly in proportion to the increase in the temperature, e.g., if the temperature is increased, the volume of the gas is increased.

Finally, a very important law to understand is **Henry's law**, which relates to the volumes of gases that dissolve in water. Specifically, the quantity of gas dissolved in water at equilibrium is affected by the pressure of the gas to which the water is exposed and also by the solubility coefficient of the gas and is directly proportional to each:

$$Volume = Pressure \times Solubility\ coefficient$$

The gases of concern for the body water of animals are carbon dioxide, oxygen, and nitrogen. Carbon dioxide is the most soluble of these gases, being about 22 times more soluble than oxygen. Nitrogen is the least soluble, being about half as soluble as oxygen. The effect of Henry's law is shown for oxygen and carbon dioxide in Figure 22.1.

Partial pressures

The **partial pressure** of gas is a common concept associated with respiratory physiology. It may be defined as the pressure exerted by a given gas in a mixture of gases. The sum of the partial pressures of each of the gases in a mixture is always equal to the total pressure. Specific partial pressures are identified by symbols appended to P, which is the physiological designation for partial pressure. For example, the designation of the partial pressure of oxygen would be Po_2. Further particularization is achieved with the use of additional symbols. Arterial, venous, and alveolar descriptions are commonly used and referred to by the symbols a, v, and A, respectively. The partial pressure of CO_2

Dukes' Physiology of Domestic Animals, Thirteenth Edition. Edited by William O. Reece, Howard H. Erickson, Jesse P. Goff and Etsuro E. Uemura.
© 2015 John Wiley & Sons, Inc. Published 2015 by John Wiley & Sons, Inc.
Companion website: www.wiley.com/go/reece/physiology

Table 22.1 Symbols common to respiratory physiology.

Symbol	Definition
P	Partial pressure
P_{O_2}	Partial pressure of oxygen
P_{aO_2}, P_{vO_2}, P_{AO_2}	Arterial, venous, and alveolar P_{O_2}, respectively
P_{CO_2}	Partial pressure of carbon dioxide
P_{aCO_2}, P_{vCO_2}, P_{ACO_2}	Arterial, venous, and alveolar P_{CO_2}, respectively
P_{N_2}	Partial pressure of nitrogen
P_{H_2O}	Partial pressure of water vapor (gas phase of H_2O)
V	Volume of gas
$\dot{V}$	Volume of gas per unit time
V_T, V_D, V_A	Tidal, dead space, and alveolar V, respectively
V_E, V_I	Expired and inspired V, respectively
MRV	Minute respiratory volume (total volume of gas moved in or out of airways and alveoli in 1 min
Q	Volume of blood
$\dot{Q}$	Volume of blood per unit time
$\dot{V}/\dot{Q}$	Ventilation–perfusion ratio

Source: Reece, W.O. (2004) Respiration in mammals. In: *Dukes' Physiology of Domestic Animals*, 12th edn (ed. W.O. Reece). Cornell University Press, Ithaca, NY. Reproduced with permission from Cornell University Press.

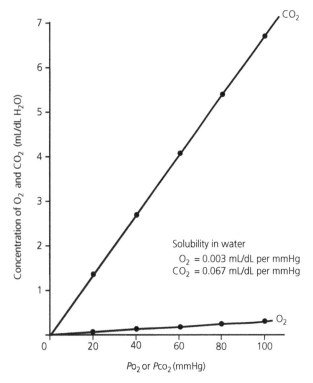

Figure 22.1 Relative solubilities of carbon dioxide and oxygen in water. From Reece, W.O. (2004) Respiration in mammals. In: *Dukes' Physiology of Domestic Animals*, 12th edn (ed. W.O. Reece). Cornell University Press, Ithaca, NY. Reproduced with permission from Cornell University Press.

in arterial blood is designated as either P_{aCO_2} or arterial P_{CO_2}. The symbols and their definitions are provided in Table 22.1.

The partial pressure of a gas is found by multiplying its concentration by the total pressure. For example, dry air contains 20.94% O_2. The total pressure for air at sea level (barometric pressure) is 760 mmHg. The P_{O_2} is the product of its percentage composition and total pressure of the mixture ($P_{O_2} = 0.2093 \times 760$ mmHg = 159 mmHg).

Gases exhibit net movement by simple diffusion in response to pressure differences. Net diffusion occurs from areas of high pressure to areas of lower pressure, and this applies to gases in a gas mixture, gases in a solution, and gases moving from the gas phase into the dissolved state (application of Henry's law). Regardless of the total pressure for the gas mixture, each individual gas diffuses independently, i.e., diffusion from its high partial pressure to its low partial pressure.

There is a tendency for students to believe that high partial pressures of oxygen in blood are related to large volumes of oxygen. That this is not correct may be explained by Henry's law, whereby the quantity of gas dissolved in water at equilibrium is affected not only by the pressure of the gas to which the water is exposed, but also by its solubility. Henry's law applies to the water of the blood and not to the hemoglobin within. Because the solubility of oxygen (0.003 mL/dL per mmHg) is quite low, it is apparent that oxygen in solution represents a small portion of the oxygen present in blood. Accordingly, a P_{aO_2} of 400 mmHg does not imply that four times more oxygen is present in blood than when the P_{aO_2} is 100 mmHg. It would have four times more if solubility were the only factor. However, hemoglobin absorbs oxygen (removes it from solution) and is virtually saturated with oxygen when the P_{aO_2} is 100 mmHg. About 20 mL of oxygen is present in each 100 mL of blood when the hemoglobin concentration is approximately 15 g/dL (amount varies with species) and the P_{aO_2} is 100 mmHg. Therefore, the additional pressure increase to 400 mmHg would only increase the oxygen content of the blood by its solubility in water (0.3 mL/100 mmHg), or 0.9 mL oxygen in addition to the 20 mL oxygen in the blood that is represented by the first 100 mmHg, because hemoglobin is saturated at 100 mmHg.

It is difficult to visualize a partial pressure for water. One must remember that water has a gas phase known as vapor. The vapor pressure of water is caused by the molecules of water at the surface tending to escape into the gas above the liquid. When the temperature of the water is increased, the tendency of the water molecules to escape is also increased. The symbol for water vapor pressure is P_{H_2O}, and at a barometric pressure of 760 mmHg, P_{H_2O} is equal to 47 mmHg at 37 °C and 52 mmHg at 39 °C. The average deep body temperature in many of the domestic animals is 39 °C.

Partial pressures of gases in the lungs, blood, and tissues

The approximate composition (and corresponding partial pressures) of dry atmospheric air at sea level (760 mmHg) is as follows: 20.93% O_2 (P_{O_2}, 159 mmHg); 0.03% CO_2 (P_{CO_2},

Table 22.2 Total and partial pressures (in mmHg) of respiratory gases in humans at rest (sea level).

Gases	Venous blood	Alveolar air	Arterial blood	Tissues
Oxygen	40	109	100	30 or less
Carbon dioxide	45	40	40	50 or more
Nitrogen	569	564	569	569
Water vapor	47	47	47	47
Total	701	760	756	696

Source: Reece, W.O. (2009) *Functional Anatomy and Physiology of Domestic Animals*, 4th edn. Wiley-Blackwell, Ames, IA. Reproduced with permission from Wiley.

0.23 mmHg); 79.0% N_2 (P_{N_2}, 600 mmHg). Values for the partial pressure of these gases in the tissues, blood, and pulmonary alveoli are presented for humans in Table 22.2. Note that alveolar air P_{O_2} (109 mmHg) is much reduced from the above value of 159 mmHg for dry air that is inhaled. This reduction is the result of three factors: (i) oxygen is being consumed by the tissues (lowering blood oxygen) and thus oxygen constantly leaves the alveoli and enters venous blood as it becomes arterial; (ii) the air is humidified, creating a P_{H_2O} of 47 mmHg at 37 °C, which in turn dilutes the oxygen present in the alveoli; and (iii) CO_2 constantly enters the alveoli from venous blood and this also dilutes the oxygen present.

Increased ventilation could increase the alveolar P_{O_2} because the replacement with atmospheric air, which contains more oxygen than alveolar air, would be more rapid. Under these conditions, one observes that arterial P_{O_2} increases because of the greater partial pressure difference. Also worthy of note are the following, which are demonstrated in Table 22.2.

1 There may be a difference between arterial P_{O_2} and alveolar P_{O_2} ($P_{aO_2} < P_{AO_2}$) because some of the blood leaving the lung has been shunted (does not receive oxygen). A **shunt** is defined as any mechanism by which blood that has not been through ventilated areas of lung is added to the systemic arteries. The effect may be small in healthy animals.

2 Alveolar P_{CO_2} and arterial P_{CO_2} are the same because of the greater diffusion coefficient for CO_2 and also because the small arteriovenous difference in P_{CO_2} results in an imperceptible change from shunted blood.

3 Nitrogen is in virtual equilibrium throughout the system because it is neither consumed nor produced.

4 Water vapor pressure is the same throughout the system because the gases remain at 100% humidification.

5 Whereas the sum of the partial pressure in the alveolar air and arterial columns total approximately that of the atmosphere (760 mmHg), the venous and tissue columns do not. They are less by approximately the amount of oxygen that is consumed. Absorption of gas from closed spaces

(peritoneal and pleural cavities) into venous blood occurs because of partial pressure differences in oxygen between venous blood and the closed spaces. This phenomenon is observed when the peritoneal cavity is surgically entered and a slight inrush of air occurs.

6 Each gas diffuses in response to its own partial pressure difference and is independent of the other gases. Simple diffusion occurs because of the random motion of molecules from an area of their higher concentration to an area of their lower concentration.

The direction of diffusion in response to differences in partial pressures is shown for oxygen and carbon dioxide in Figure 22.2.

Factors affecting gas diffusion

Diffusion between alveolar gas and blood is separated by the respiratory membrane (see Figure 21.10, Chapter 21, Overview of the Respiratory System). In general, the respiratory membrane is composed of alveolar epithelium, alveolar epithelium basement membrane, interstitial space, capillary endothelium basement membrane, and capillary endothelium. The distance for diffusion between alveolar gas and blood, as shown in Figure 21.10, probably represents a minimum. Pulmonary separation can become greater, depending on the interposition of cells and the amount of interstitial space. Diffusion through tissues is described as follows:

$$\dot{V}_{gas} = \frac{A \cdot D(P_1 - P_2)}{T}$$

where the rate of diffusion ($\dot{V}_{gas}$) is proportional to the surface area (A), the difference in gas partial pressure between the two sides ($P_1 - P_2$) and a diffusion coefficient (D) and is inversely proportional to the tissue thickness (T). The diffusion coefficient for carbon dioxide through the respiratory membrane is about 22 times more than that for oxygen. Also, as the distance of diffusion increases, as in pulmonary interstitial edema, the diffusion rate decreases. Under this condition, one may notice greater ventilatory efforts in an attempt to compensate for the hypoxemia (decreased oxygen concentration in arterial blood) that has developed because of the reduced rate of diffusion for oxygen. Blood-gas analysis of arterial blood would show reduced partial pressure for both oxygen and carbon dioxide. Because of the decrease in diffusion rate due to distance, one might have expected an increase in carbon dioxide; however, because its diffusion coefficient is much greater than that for oxygen, the increased ventilation overcompensates for diffusion decrease due to distance and a decrease in P_{aCO_2} is observed. Another feature worth noting is the direct relationship of surface area to diffusion rate. Small mammals have very high oxygen requirements in comparison with large mammals because the basal oxygen requirement is more nearly proportional to body surface

Section IV: Respiration

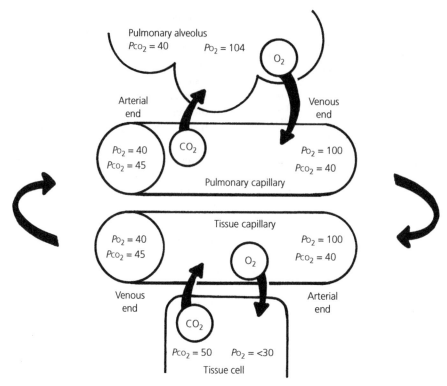

Figure 22.2 Direction of diffusion for oxygen (O_2) and carbon dioxide (CO_2) as shown by arrows. In the pulmonary alveolus the P_{CO_2} is 40 mmHg and the P_{O_2} is 104 mmHg; at the arterial end of the pulmonary capillary the P_{O_2} is 40 mmHg and the P_{CO_2} is 45 mmHg, whereas at the venous end the P_{O_2} is 100 mmHg and the P_{CO_2} is 40 mmHg; at the venous end of the tissue capillary the P_{O_2} is 40 mmHg and the P_{CO_2} is 45 mmHg, whereas at the arterial end the P_{O_2} is 100 mmHg and the P_{CO_2} is 40 mmHg; and in the tissue cell the P_{CO_2} is 50 mmHg and the P_{O_2} is <30 mmHg. From Reece, W.O. (2009) *Functional Anatomy and Physiology of Domestic Animals*, 4th edn. Wiley-Blackwell, Ames, IA. Reproduced with permission from Wiley.

area than to body weight. Small mammals, however, have about the same proportion of lung volume to body weight as large mammals. They have greater lung efficiency for the given volume because of a greater number of smaller alveoli, which increases surface area for diffusion. The efficiency of the lungs is decreased when alveolar walls are destroyed (e.g., emphysema), thus reducing surface area and diffusion rate.

Up to this point, only diffusion between alveolar air and blood has been mentioned. It must be understood that the same principles apply for diffusion between the blood and the body tissues. The differences between arterial and venous blood are a reflection of gas diffusion that occurs in the lung and other body tissues. Diffusion of gases in the body results from the generation of pressure differences according to the above diffusion-rate equation. With the exception of pressure difference, the other factors of the equation are somewhat fixed under normal conditions. Diffusion occurs because oxygen is consumed by the tissues, which lowers the P_{aO_2}, and CO_2 is produced by the tissues, which increases the P_{vCO_2}. As fresh air is brought into the lungs, a gradient is generated to replenish oxygen in the blood and to remove the carbon dioxide that has accumulated.

Mechanics of respiration

1 Why is intrapleural pressure always less than intrapulmonic pressure?

2 Why are animals with the condition of pneumothorax unable to inflate their lungs?

3 How does the mediastinal pressure assist return of blood to the heart and also regurgitation in ruminants?

4 How do the properties of surfactant assist inspiration and expiration?

5 How do changes in the amount or composition of surfactant affect lung compliance?

6 What is the relationship between lung compliance values and livestock feeding efficiency?

7 Why is the selection of an endotracheal tube important as related to airway resistance?

Respiratory pressures

Air flows in and out of the lungs in response to pressure differences created by increase or decrease of thoracic volume, respectively (Figure 22.3).

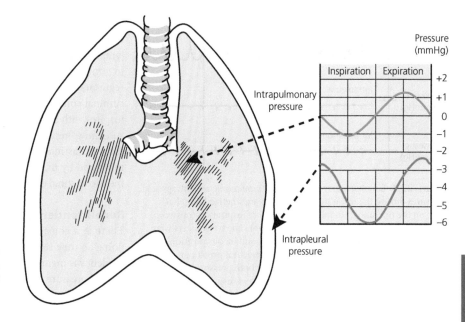

Figure 22.3 Intrapleural and intrapulmonic (intrapulmonary) pressures associated with inspiration and expiration. Adapted from Ganong, W.F. (2001) *Review of Medical Physiology*, 20th edn. McGraw-Hill, New York.

Section IV: Respiration

Intrapulmonic pressure

Intrapulmonic pressure refers to the air pressure in the lungs and the passages leading to them. The intrapulmonic pressure quickly equals the pressure of the atmosphere after the thoracic volume stabilizes because of free communication between the interior of the lungs and the outside. During inspiration the intrapulmonic pressure becomes slightly subatmospheric because the enlargement of the thorax and lungs is a little more rapid than the inrush of air. During expiration the intrapulmonic pressure becomes slightly greater than atmospheric pressure because the thorax decreases in size and allows the lungs to decrease in size (recoil tendency) and compress the air within them. The air moves out in response to this compression. It can thus be seen that pressure differences create the actual movement of air. Intrapulmonic pressure has also been referred to as **alveolar** or **intra-alveolar pressure**.

Intrapleural pressure

Intrapleural pressure refers to the pressure in the thorax outside the lungs (including the mediastinum). It has sometimes been called **intrathoracic pressure**. An intrapleural space is quite minimal and the lungs occupy most of the thoracic cavity not otherwise occupied. The intrapleural pressure is always less than the intrapulmonic pressure. This holds true not only during normal breathing but also under conditions of forceful expiration and under conditions of positive-pressure ventilation (forced-air inflation). Intrapleural pressure is less than intrapulmonic pressure because the lung is adhered to the thoracic wall by the liquid layer between the visceral and parietal pleura. Expansion of the thorax is followed by expansion of the lungs. However, the lungs always have a recoil tendency because (i) the surface tension of the fluid lining the inside of the alveoli

is always pulling the alveolar surface into the smallest possible size and (ii) the elastic forces (elastin and collagen fibers) tend to recoil the lungs at all times. The inward recoil of the lung tissue pulls on the liquid layer between the visceral and parietal pleura causing a hydrostatic pressure that is subatmospheric.

Under conditions of normal breathing, intrapulmonic pressure becomes only slightly negative (−1 mmHg) during inspiration and only slightly positive (+1 mmHg) during expiration. A simultaneous recording of intrapleural pressure would probably show a value of about −2 mmHg at the end of expiration and a value of about −6 mmHg at the end of inspiration (Figure 22.4). All of these are relative to atmospheric pressure.

Pneumothorax

In the condition called pneumothorax (Figure 22.5), air enters the space between the visceral and parietal pleura, breaks the adhesion, and eliminates the potential for inflating the lungs. Animals with a complete mediastinum (e.g., dog, where right and left lung are separated) will have lung collapse only on the side where air enters. The lungs collapse because of the elastic and surface tension forces. Attempts by the animal to inhale will be unsuccessful, and death from **asphyxia** will result.

Pressure in the mediastinal space

It is important to understand the relationship of the mediastinal structures to the intrapleural pressure. These structures are enveloped by a mediastinal pleura. A subatmospheric intrapleural pressure is transmitted to the mediastinal structures, i.e., the vena cava and the esophagus (Figure 22.6). This has important consequences of a helpful nature. During inspiration, when the intrapleural pressure becomes more negative to atmospheric pressure, the transmission of reduced pressure to the vena cava

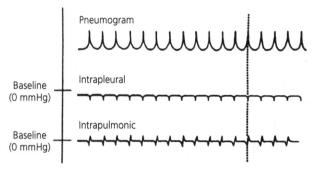

Figure 22.4 Simultaneous recording of intrapulmonic and intrapleural pressures during the respiratory cycle of an anesthetized dog. Each peak on the pneumogram indicates the end of inspiration (upsweep) and the beginning of expiration (downsweep). The transducers were not equally calibrated. Dashed line shows simultaneous position of pens at end of inspiration. Note that (i) intrapleural pressure remains subatmospheric at the end of expiration, (ii) both pressure measurements have their greatest negativity at the end of inspiration, and (iii) intrapulmonic pressure sharply becomes positive at the moment expiration begins. Drawn from actual recording. From Reece, W.O. (2004) Respiration in mammals. In: *Dukes' Physiology of Domestic Animals*, 12th edn (ed. W.O. Reece). Cornell University Press, Ithaca, NY. Reproduced with permission from Cornell University Press.

and the thoracic lymph duct assists the flow of blood and lymph to the heart. Because of valves in these vessels, the blood and lymph do not flow back when the pressure becomes less negative to atmospheric pressure during expiration. During the study of regurgitation in ruminants, it has been shown that entry of ruminal content into the esophagus is assisted when the animal inspires with a closed glottis. This creates a greater than normal subatmospheric intrapleural pressure, which is transmitted to the mediastinal structures. The intrapleural pressure can be measured by means of an appropriate transducer placed within the mediastinal esophagus.

Recoil tendency of lungs

There is a constant tendency for the lungs to collapse, and in doing so they recoil inward from the thoracic wall. This recoil tendency is mentioned in the previous explanation of why intrapleural pressure is always less than intrapulmonic pressure. The recoil tendency is due to (i) stretching of elastin and collagen fibers by lung inflation and (ii) surface tension of fluid lining the alveoli. The stretching of elastic fibers is easy to visualize as a force that contributes to recoil.

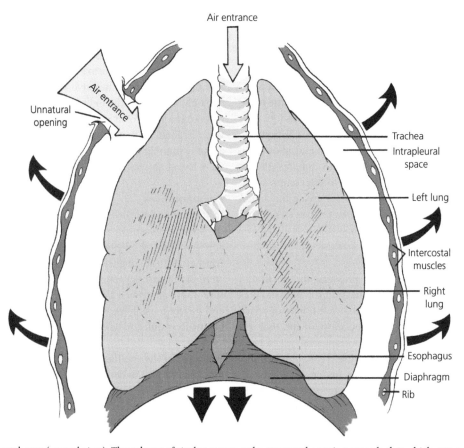

Figure 22.5 Pneumothorax (ventral view). The volume of air that enters at the unnatural opening exceeds that which enters the trachea when the intrapleural volume is increased during inspiration. The intrapleural pressure reduction is then not sufficient to permit lung inflation. The dark arrows show the directions of thoracic enlargement when the diaphragm and inspiratory intercostal muscles contract during inspiration. Adapted from Reece, W.O. (2009) *Functional Anatomy and Physiology of Domestic Animals*, 4th edn. Wiley-Blackwell, Ames, IA. Reproduced with permission from Wiley.

Surface tension

Surface tension, which is less easily visualized, is a manifestation of attracting forces between atoms or molecules. Identical atoms or molecules exert equal attractions for each other, whereas unlike atoms or molecules may have more or less attraction for each other (Figure 22.7).

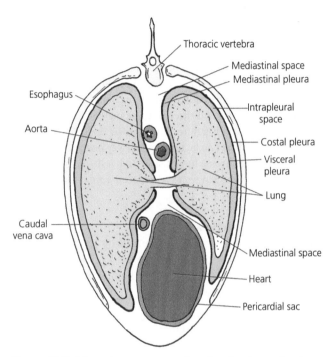

Figure 22.6 Schematic transverse section of equine thorax showing the relationships of the visceral, costal, and mediastinal pleura. The aorta, esophagus, venae cavae, and thoracic lymph duct (not shown) are within the mediastinal space. The esophagus, venae cavae, and lymph duct (soft structures) respond by increasing and decreasing pressures within their lumens, associated with similar changes in intrapleural and mediastinal spaces. Adapted from Reece, W.O. (2009) *Functional Anatomy and Physiology of Domestic Animals*, 4th edn. Wiley-Blackwell, Ames, IA. Reproduced with permission from Wiley.

The effect of surface tension on pulmonary alveoli can be explained by **Laplace's law**, represented as $P = 2T/r$, where pressure (P) inside the alveolus is directly related to the tension (T) exerted on its inner surface and inversely related to its internal radius (r). Tension in the wall of the alveolus tends to contract it, and the pressure inside the alveolus tends to expand it. When there is no movement of the alveolus, there is equilibrium between the forces of expansion and contraction. If the surface tension in the alveolus remains the same, regardless of the radius, then the pressure required to inflate increases as the radius decreases and decreases as the radius increases. Accordingly, one would observe that a greater pressure would be required to begin inspiration (because the radius is smallest) and that small alveoli (with their greater pressure) would empty into larger alveoli. These untenable situation would occur if the surface tension remained the same, regardless of radius. This is not the case, however, because of pulmonary surfactant.

Surfactants

Surfactants are surface-active substances for which water molecules have a lesser attraction. Because of this property the surfactant molecules accumulate at the surface (see Figure 22.7C) and a reduction in surface tension occurs. This results from the reduction in the number of water molecules at the surface (displaced by surfactant molecules) and also because the surfactant molecules have a lesser attraction for each other and for water molecules. Accordingly, the surface-tightening effect and the downward pull are reduced.

Pulmonary surfactant is a lipoprotein complex containing about 30% protein and 70% lipid. Most of the lipid fraction is composed of the phospholipid dipalmitoyl lecithin. Surfactant is synthesized by the type II alveolar epithelial cells (secretory cells). This fact places alveolar epithelium in the category of an active metabolic unit and not simply a passive membrane for the exchange of oxygen and carbon dioxide. It is estimated that the lung may account for as much as 8–10% of the basal oxygen

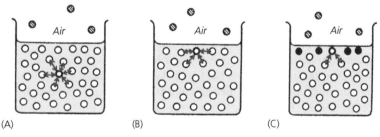

Figure 22.7 Surface tension. (A) Water molecules (open circles) below the surface of water standing in a beaker have equal attraction for each other in all directions. (B) Water molecules at the water–air interface do not have equal attracting forces. Note that the air molecules (shaded circles) are fewer in number and are less able to exert an upward force. Therefore the water molecules on the surface have more molecules pulling them down than up and they dive downward, creating a pull on the surface. Further, the attraction from molecules to the side causes a tightening of that surface. When translated to the inner aspect of a sphere (such as an alveolus), one can visualize that the sphere would be reduced in size by the tightening effect. (C) Accumulation of surfactant (solid circles) at the surface has the effect of reducing surface tension. Adapted from Comroe, J.H. Jr. *Physiology of Respiration*, 2nd edn. Copyright © 1974 by Year Book Medical Publishers, Inc., Chicago. Reproduced with permission from Elsevier.

Section IV: Respiration

consumption of the body. Surfactant is formed relatively late in human fetal life and in some animal species. However, the time of its formation is not known for most of the domestic species. In the premature human infant, surfactant deficiency at birth leads to a respiratory distress syndrome characterized by dyspnea, cyanosis, and expiratory grunts. There are clinical, pathological, and biochemical resemblances to human respiratory distress syndrome among some animal species. The syndrome in animals has been described most completely for horses and swine, in which it has been called barker syndrome. The name is derived from the noise associated with the expiratory grunts. The syndrome does not correlate with premature birth of foals and piglets. Although the primary cause may differ, development of the syndrome among human infants, foals, and piglets appears to involve a failure in the production of surfactant.

At the end of expiration, when the alveoli have assumed their smallest radius, it appears that increased pressure would be required to begin the next inspiration and thus inflate the alveoli. According to Laplace's law, this would be true if the surface tension factor remained the same at all stages of inflation. However, as the alveolar radius is reduced, the pulmonary surfactant becomes more compressed on the surface, is more active as a surface-active agent, and therefore reduces the surface tension. Inspiration is assisted because the reduction in surface tension tends to counteract the effect of reducing alveolar radius with regard to pressure needed to inflate the alveoli. It also stabilizes the alveoli so that small alveoli do not empty into larger alveoli. At the end of inspiration the alveoli will have expanded. For any initial amount of surfactant, the surfactant is diluted at the surface and is thus less surface active. The surface tension at this point will have been increased. Physiologically, this provides an upper limiting factor to inspiration and assists the elastin and collagen fibers in providing recoil necessary for expiration.

Lung compliance

Lung compliance is a measure of the distensibility of the lungs and is determined by measurement of the lung volume change for each unit of pressure change. The standard units for pulmonary compliance are milliliters (or liters) per centimeter of water. If a compliance value in a particular animal has decreased over a period of time (greater pressure for same volume expansion), the tissues of the lung must be more rigid and less distensible or certain abnormalities may have further reduced the expansibility of the thorax. Factors that affect compliance are those conditions that destroy lung tissue or cause it to be fibrotic or edematous or that in any way impede lung expansion.

Changes in surfactant (amount or composition) affect compliance values, and lack of surfactant is associated with decreased compliance. When the alveoli enlarge during inspiration, the distance between surfactant molecules is increased (separation).

With reduction in alveolar size during expiration, the surfactant molecules return to their more compressed state (recombination). For surfactant, molecular separation is accomplished with greater difficulty than molecular recombination so that a pressure measurement for a given lung volume during inspiration is greater (decreased compliance) than for the same lung volume during expiration.

Metabolic cost of breathing

An expenditure of energy is associated with breathing and is related to the muscle contractions necessary for expanding the lungs. During the expansion of the lungs there is muscle work associated with overcoming (i) the elastic and surface tension forces, (ii) the nonelastic forces (rearrangement of tissues), and (iii) airway resistance. All three of these may be increased during disease. Surfactant failures and fibrosis or stiffening of the tissues affect the first two factors, and airway obstruction affects the third. During chronic lung disease in livestock, more energy is required for breathing and a reduced feed efficiency can be measured.

Resistance to airflow

The resistance to airflow is determined by the same factors that govern the flow of liquids in tubes. A modification of **Poiseuille's law** for laminar flow of liquids in rigid smooth cylindrical tubes is as follows:

$$\text{Resistance} = \frac{8\eta l}{\pi r^4}$$

where η is the coefficient of viscosity, l is the length of the tube, and r is the radius of the tube. This equation renders some approximation of resistance, even though respiratory tubes are not smooth, cylindrical, and rigid. If the length is increased four times, then the pressure must be increased four times to maintain constant airflow. If the radius of the tube is halved, however, then the pressure must be increased 16 times to maintain constant flow. For situations that require endotracheal intubation, this points out the necessity of selecting an endotracheal tube that is of maximum size compatible with the existing airway and an adapter that is similar in diameter to the endotracheal tube.

It has been pointed out that resistance to airflow is one of the factors associated with the work of breathing. Resistance is greater during expiration than it is during inspiration because the expansion of the lungs during inspiration pulls upon the airways in a manner that assists their greater opening, whereas some degree of compression of the airways occurs during expiration. During many instances of pulmonary distress, the expiratory phase is more exaggerated than the inspiratory phase due to greater compression associated with increased expiratory muscle contraction needed to overcome added resistance.

Self-evaluation

Answers can be found at the end of the chapter.

1 Does blood with a hemoglobin concentration of 15 g/dL and subjected to 400 mmHg have four times more oxygen than the same blood subjected to 100 mmHg?
   A Yes
   B No
   Explain your choice for the correct answer.

2 Diffusion distance of the respiratory membrane has increased because of pulmonary interstitial edema and diffusion of oxygen and carbon dioxide is impeded. A greater respiratory effort is then needed in an attempt to compensate for the decreased diffusion rate. Which one of the following would reflect the arterial blood gas analysis for oxygen and carbon dioxide?
   A Pao_2 increases and $Paco_2$ increases
   B Pao_2 decreases and $Paco_2$ decreases
   C Pao_2 decreases and $Paco_2$ increases
   Explain your choice for the correct answer.

3 Differentiate between intrapulmonic and intrapleural pressures. Describe their changes relative to each other during a respiratory cycle (inspiration followed by expiration). How does inspiration assist blood flow return to the heart? Explain.

4 What are surfactants? How do they assist respiration during inspiration and during expiration (relate to Laplace's law, $P = 2T/r$)? Explain.

5 A lung compliance value has decreased from the time that it was first measured. This means that:
   A A greater effort is required to expand the lungs
   B Less effort is required to expand the lungs
   Explain your choice for the correct answer.

Suggested reading

Comroe, J. Jr (1974) *Physiology of Respiration*, 2nd edn. Year Book Medical Publishers, Inc., Chicago.

Reece, W. (2004) Respiration in mammals. In: *Dukes' Physiology of Domestic Animals*, 12th edn (ed. W.O. Reece), pp. 114–148. Cornell University Press, Ithaca, NY.

Reece, W. (2009) *Anatomy and Physiology of Domestic Animals*, 4th edn. Wiley-Blackwell, Ames, IA.

Answers

1 B. The blood exposed to 100 mmHg has oxygen in solution and oxygen combined with hemoglobin. Hemoglobin is virtually saturated with oxygen when the PaO2 is 100 mmHg and any increase in pressure beyond 100 mmHg will only increase the oxygen content by that which is in solution. Therefore, the additional pressure increase to 400 mmHg would only increase the oxygen content by its solubility in water (0.3 mL/100 mmHg or 0.9 mL oxygen) in addition to the 20 mL oxygen in the blood that is represented by the first 100 mmHg because hemoglobin is saturated with oxygen at 100 mmHg.

2 B. Blood-gas analysis of arterial blood would show reduced partial pressures for both O_2 and CO_2. Because of the decrease in diffusion rate due to distance, one might have expected an increase in CO_2; however, because its diffusion coefficient is much greater than that for O_2 (22 times greater), the increased ventilation overcompensates for diffusion decrease due to distance and a decrease in $PaCO_2$ is observed.

3 Intrapulmonic pressure refers to the air pressure in the lungs and the passages leading to them. Intrapleural pressure refers to the pressure in the thorax outside the lungs (including the mediastinum). During inspiration, thoracic volume increases and intrapleural pressure decreases. The lungs respond to the decreased pressure by expansion of their volume and intrapulmonic pressure decreases. Air flows inward. During expiration, thoracic volume decreases, intrapleural pressure becomes less negative, the lungs recoil (elasticity and surface tension forces), and intrapulmonic pressure increases. Air flows outward. Intrapleural pressure is always less than intrapulmonic. During inspiration, the mediastinal pressure also becomes more negative. The soft structures within the mediastinal space (caudal and cranial venae cavae) also expand, reducing luminal pressure and providing an assist to blood flow to the heart.

4 Surfactants are surface-active substances that have little or no attraction from water molecules and they accumulate at the surface. According to Laplace's law, the pressure to expand the alveoli is directly related to the tension in the alveolar walls and inversely related to their radius. Without surfactant, initiating inspiration would be difficult because of the small radius coupled with no change in tension. With surfactant, surface tension is reduced at end-expiration (beginning of inspiration) because surfactant is more concentrated at the surface due to the reduced surface area. Accordingly, less pressure is required to expand the alveoli. At end-inspiration (beginning of expiration), surfactant molecule concentration is reduced (surface tension increased) and an assist is given to recoil of the lungs during expiration.

5 A. Lung compliance is a measure of the distensibility of the lungs and is determined by measurement of the lung volume change for each unit of pressure change. If a compliance value in a particular animal has decreased over a period of time (greater pressure for same volume expansion), the tissues of the lung must be more rigid and less distensible.

23 Pulmonary Ventilation and Transport of Gases

William O. Reece
Iowa State University, Ames, IA, USA

Ventilation is generally regarded as the process by which gas in closed places is renewed or exchanged. As it applies to the lungs, it is a process of exchanging the gas in the airways and alveoli with gas from the environment. The main function of ventilation is to replenish oxygen and to remove carbon dioxide.

Pulmonary ventilation

1 What is the hydration reaction?

2 Apart from its role in ventilating the alveoli, what are further functions of physiologic dead space ventilation?

3 How is physiologic dead space compensated when it may be increased under certain conditions?

4 What is meant by a mismatch of ventilation and blood flow that might be occasioned during anesthesia and represented by low $\dot{V}/\dot{Q}$ lung units?

5 Is the generalized vasoconstriction that occurs at high altitudes in cattle and chickens activated by the P_{O_2} of the alveolar gas or the P_{O_2} of pulmonary arterial blood?

Ventilation terminology

Total ventilation is the volume of gas moved in or out of the airways and alveoli over a certain period of time. **Minute ventilation** is the total volume of gas moved in or out of the airways and alveoli in 1 min. It is determined by the relationship:

$$\dot{V}_E = fV_T$$

where $\dot{V}_E$ is the minute ventilation (expired), f is respiratory frequency in cycles per minute, and V_T is the average tidal volume. Minute ventilation is also referred to as the **minute respiratory volume (MRV)**.

Normoventilation refers to normal ventilation in which a $P_{A_{CO_2}}$ of about 40 mmHg is maintained. **Hyperventilation** refers to alveolar ventilation increased beyond the metabolic needs and a $P_{A_{CO_2}}$ below 40 mmHg. Hyperventilation causes **respiratory alkalosis**. **Hypoventilation** is alveolar ventilation decreased below metabolic needs and a $P_{A_{CO_2}}$ above 40 mmHg. Acute hypoventilation causes **respiratory acidosis**. Respiratory alkalosis and respiratory acidosis are disturbances of acid–base equilibrium where the pH of blood [H⁺] is increased or decreased, respectively, from normal. Hydrogen ion concentration is influenced by CO_2 according to the **hydration reaction** whereby the combination of CO_2 with water yields H_2CO_3, which dissociates to H⁺ and HCO_3^- as follows:

$$CO_2 + H_2O \leftrightarrow H_2CO_3 \leftrightarrow H^+ + HCO_3^-$$

The reactions are reversible and CO_2 increase and decrease are associated with an increase and decrease, respectively, of hydrogen ions.

The tidal volume is used to ventilate not only the alveoli, but also the airways leading to the alveoli. Because there is little or no diffusion of oxygen and carbon dioxide through the membranes of most of the airways, they compose part of what is called **dead space ventilation**. The other part of dead space ventilation is made up of alveoli with diminished capillary perfusion. Ventilating these alveoli is ineffective in producing changes in blood gases. Ventilation of nonperfused alveoli and the airways, because neither accomplish exchange of the respiratory gases, is referred to as physiologic dead space.

Dukes' Physiology of Domestic Animals, Thirteenth Edition. Edited by William O. Reece, Howard H. Erickson, Jesse P. Goff and Etsuro E. Uemura.
© 2015 John Wiley & Sons, Inc. Published 2015 by John Wiley & Sons, Inc.
Companion website: www.wiley.com/go/reece/physiology

Physiologic dead space is defined as the volume of gas that is inspired but which takes no part in gas exchange in the airways and alveoli. Therefore, the tidal volume (V_T) has a dead space component (V_D) and an alveolar component (V_A) or $V_T = V_D + V_A$.

Physiologic dead space ventilation is a necessary part of the process of ventilating the alveoli and is not totally wasted. It assists in tempering and humidifying inhaled air and in the cooling of the body under certain conditions, such as when panting is necessary. During panting, the respiratory frequency increases and the tidal volume decreases, so that alveolar ventilation remains approximately constant.

Physiologic dead space may be increased under certain conditions, and it will be observed that tidal volume, respiratory frequency, or both increase in order to keep alveolar ventilation constant. It may also be observed that the frequency of complementary breaths increases as a compensation for added dead space. The limits of compensation must be recognized when dead space is added in the form of tubes and breathing devices. **Panting**, which represents increased dead-space ventilation, is an important temperature-regulating mechanism in many species. During panting the respiratory frequency is increased and the tidal volume is decreased so that alveolar ventilation remains relatively constant in order to maintain constancy of Pa_{CO_2}. However, hyperventilation can occur in animals exposed to severe heat stress and result in respiratory alkalosis.

Ventilation and perfusion relationships

The partial pressures of oxygen and carbon dioxide in the blood are related not only to alveolar ventilation but also to the amount of blood that perfuses the alveoli. The relationship of these two factors to each other is referred to as the **ventilation/perfusion ratio** and is abbreviated $\dot{V}_A/\dot{Q}$. A normal ventilation/perfusion ratio implies that there is a balance between ventilation and perfusion of the alveoli, so that exchange of oxygen and carbon dioxide between the alveoli and blood is optimal (Figure 23.1A). Deviations from normal are known as **mismatching of ventilation and blood flow** within the lung.

Now consider the meaning of ratio deviations from normal that lie between the extremes. A value less than normal (low $\dot{V}_A/\dot{Q}$) means that ventilation has declined but that perfusion remains adequate (Figure 23.1B). A ventilation/perfusion ratio with a value greater than normal (high $\dot{V}_A/\dot{Q}$) means that ventilation is exceeding perfusion (Figure 23.1C). Figure 23.1B and Figure 23.1C represent extremes. Within the lung at any one time there may exist an uneven distribution of blood flow and ventilation so that areas of low $\dot{V}_A/\dot{Q}$, normal $\dot{V}_A/\dot{Q}$, and high $\dot{V}_A/\dot{Q}$ represent different lung units. For animals at rest and in the standing position, the dorsal aspects have a higher ventilation/perfusion ratio, resulting in high $\dot{V}_A/\dot{Q}$ lung units; the ventral aspects have a lower ventilation/perfusion ratio, resulting in low $\dot{V}_A/\dot{Q}$ lung units. It is likely that with greater activity a

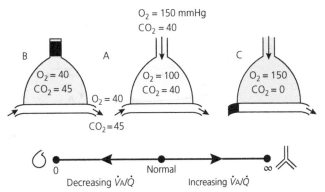

Figure 23.1 Extremes of ventilation–perfusion ratio. Normal gas exchange is seen in (A) where the balance of ventilation and blood flow is such that the alveolar P_{O_2} is 100 mmHg and the P_{CO_2} is 40 mmHg. In (B), ventilation has been completely obstructed, the ventilation–perfusion ratio is nil, and the alveolar gas tensions are those of mixed venous blood. In (C), blood flow has been stopped, the ventilation–perfusion ratio is infinitely high, and alveolar gas tensions are those of inspired gas. The line at the bottom shows the way the ventilation–perfusion ratio changes between these two extremes (the symbol on the left shows the right ventricle and the symbol on the right shows the trachea). From West, J.B. (1990) *Ventilation/Blood Flow and Gas Exchange*, 5th edn. Blackwell Scientific Publications, Oxford. Reproduced with permission from Wiley.

resumption of more equal matching of ventilation and perfusion occurs.

Blood leaving the lungs is a mixture from all lung units (low, normal, and high $\dot{V}_A/\dot{Q}$) as shown in Figure 23.2. The high $\dot{V}_A/\dot{Q}$ units may have a slightly greater oxygen content than blood from normal and low $\dot{V}_A/\dot{Q}$ units but, because of their restricted blood flow, a greater amount of blood (**shunted blood**) is forced to perfuse low $\dot{V}_A/\dot{Q}$ units where ventilation is reduced. Accordingly, the contribution of the high $\dot{V}_A/\dot{Q}$ units to oxygenation is not sufficient to compensate for the lesser contribution to oxygenation by low $\dot{V}_A/\dot{Q}$ units and Pa_{O_2} and oxygen content of systemic blood is less than blood from perfectly matched ventilation and perfusion.

Mismatches of ventilation and blood flow are probably the most common cause of **hypoxemia**. Chronic obstructive lung diseases, such as **chronic bronchitis** and **alveolar pulmonary emphysema** (alveoli unduly distended or with ruptured walls), are productive of mismatching of ventilation and blood flow throughout the lung. The initial restriction to airflow by chronic bronchitis produces low $\dot{V}_A/\dot{Q}$ lung units, and the emphysema that follows produces high $\dot{V}_A/\dot{Q}$ lung units. A diversity of lung units will be present, and hypoxemia is a predominant feature.

Mismatches can be accentuated under conditions of prolonged inactivity associated with anesthesia. Deeper than normal inflation is regularly induced to reestablish patency in alveoli where their excursions have been limited. Also, if

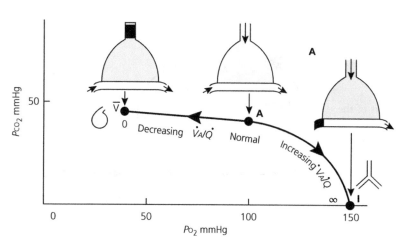

Figure 23.2 A ventilation/perfusion ratio ($\dot{V}A/\dot{Q}$) line where $\bar{v}$ represents the P_{O_2} and P_{CO_2} of mixed venous blood when ventilation is blocked ($\dot{V}A/\dot{Q} = 0$) and where I represents the P_{O_2} and P_{CO_2} of alveolar gas when perfusion is blocked ($\dot{V}A/\dot{Q} = $ infinity). Mismatches of ventilation and perfusion within lung units at any point on the line influence oxygenation of the blood accordingly. From West, J.B. (1990) *Ventilation/Blood Flow and Gas Exchange*, 5th edn. Blackwell Scientific Publications, Oxford. Reproduced with permission from Wiley.

prolonged recovery periods are characteristic of the anesthetic, animals are regularly turned from one side to the other. The lower portions of the lung have a tendency to inadequate ventilation which, when coupled with adequate blood flow, results in low $\dot{V}A/\dot{Q}$ lung units. Rotation provides for resumption of alveolar filling.

Hypoxic vasoconstriction

When the P_{O_2} of alveolar gas is reduced, the smooth muscle cells in the walls of the small arterioles contract in the hypoxic region. This **vasoconstriction** has the effect of directing blood flow away from hypoxic regions of lung to regions that have adequate oxygenation. The response is activated by the P_{O_2} of the alveolar gas, not the P_{O_2} of pulmonary arterial blood. The mediator of the vasoconstriction is not known, but it is believed that cells in the perivascular tissue release a vasoconstrictor substance in response to hypoxia.

Generalized pulmonary vasoconstriction occurs at altitudes above 2100 m where ambient P_{O_2} is less than 100 mmHg. The generalized pulmonary vasoconstriction leads to a rise in pulmonary arterial pressure and a substantial increase in work for the right heart. Right ventricular failure may follow, with a subsequent increase in central venous pressure and a predisposition to edema. Pulmonary vascular smooth muscle responses vary with species, cattle and chickens being the most responsive domestic species and therefore potentially susceptible to generalized severe hypoxic pulmonary hypertension leading to right heart failure. Cattle raised at high altitudes commonly have a condition referred to as **brisket disease** because of the accumulation of edematous fluid in the region of the brisket, the location in cattle where overt edema is most likely to develop with right heart failure. Chickens are also susceptible to right ventricular failure at high altitude, and meat-type chickens, particularly growing males, which have a high oxygen requirement, are affected most severely. Overt edema in chickens is located in the peritoneal cavity, and the accumulation of fluid within that cavity is known as **ascites**. When caused by pulmonary hypertension, the condition is called **hypoxic ascites**.

Oxygen transport

1 How many molecules of oxygen can one molecule of hemoglobin transport?

2 Does the intake of oxygen by hemoglobin in the lungs and the yield of oxygen to tissues involve a valence change of iron?

3 If it were not for hemoglobin, how much more blood would be needed to accommodate the tissue needs?

4 With a hemoglobin concentration of 15 g/dL what amount (volumes percent) of oxygen is yielded when going from 100 mmHg (P_{aO_2}) to 40 mmHg (P_{vO_2})? How does this compare with an anemic animal (7.5 g/dL)?

5 What is the means whereby anemic animals compensate for preventing severe reductions of P_{vO_2} (the oxygen buffer function of hemoglobin)?

6 What is the significance of the lower part of the dissociation curve being steep?

7 What is the significance of shifts of the oxygen–hemoglobin curve to either the right or the left?

General comments about hemoglobin

Hemoglobin is the red pigment of blood. When it is saturated with oxygen, it is bright red; as it loses oxygen, it becomes purplish. The **hemoglobin molecule**, a chromoprotein, consists of a pigment component called **heme** and a **protein**. The protein component is composed of four **polypeptide chains** (globin subunits), each containing one heme. Each heme group contains an iron atom in the ferrous state, which combines loosely and reversibly with one oxygen molecule. Therefore, one molecule of hemoglobin contains **four iron atoms** and can transport **four molecules of oxygen**. The exchange of oxygen does not involve a change in valence of iron (ferrous to ferric). Electron shifts occur in groups close to iron during oxygen delivery and uptake. The electron shifts influence oxygen binding and hydrogen ion balance. Greater detail about hemoglobin and its different forms are presented in Chapter 12.

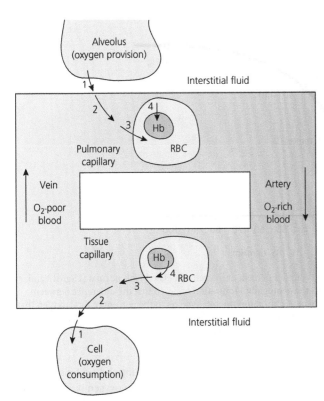

Figure 23.3 General scheme of oxygen transport showing diffusion process. Diffusion occurs because of the presence of pressure gradients. In this diagram, blood is oxygenated at the top and deoxygenated at the bottom; blood flow is clockwise. See text for further explanation. Hb, hemoglobin; RBC, red blood cell. From Reece, W.O. (2004) Respiration in mammals. In: *Dukes' Physiology of Domestic Animals*, 12th edn (ed. W.O. Reece). Cornell University Press, Ithaca, NY. Reproduced with permission from Cornell University Press.

General scheme of oxygen transport

The transport of oxygen from alveoli to hemoglobin and from hemoglobin to tissues occurs via diffusion gradients. When oxygen-poor blood arrives at the lungs, the process of diffusion is from alveoli to erythrocytes. Reversal of the process occurs when oxygen-rich blood arrives at the tissues.

The **transport of oxygen** is illustrated in Figure 23.3. The process of oxygen uptake by hemoglobin proceeds as follows: oxygen passes from air in the alveolus to successive solution in interstitial fluid (1), plasma (2), and erythrocyte fluid (3), and finally to combination with hemoglobin (4). The process of oxygen yield to the cells proceeds in the reverse direction. Diffusion of oxygen away from interstitial fluid lowers the P_{O_2} of the erythrocyte fluid and, just as an increased P_{O_2} increases the saturation of hemoglobin with oxygen, decreased P_{O_2} causes desaturation of hemoglobin.

Quantitative aspects

Most of the oxygen in blood is that which is combined with hemoglobin; relatively little is dissolved in water. The solubility coefficient of oxygen in water allows only 0.003 mL to be dissolved in each 100 mL of blood for each millimeter of mercury partial pressure. For an arterial P_{O_2} of 100 mmHg, this amounts to 0.3 mL of oxygen dissolved in each 100 mL of blood.

The volume of oxygen combined with hemoglobin in each deciliter of blood is the product of hemoglobin concentration (in grams per deciliter), volume of oxygen with each gram of hemoglobin (milliliters per gram), and oxygen saturation (decimal fraction) at the partial pressure of its measurement. For example, if the hemoglobin concentration in blood is 15 g/dL and hemoglobin is 97.5% saturated at 100 mmHg, and 1.34 mL oxygen combines with each gram of hemoglobin when it is fully saturated, then 15 g/dL × 1.34 mL/g × 0.975 = 19.6 mL/dL of oxygen is combined with hemoglobin in each 100 mL of blood (19.6 volumes percent or vol%).

Of the total amount of oxygen transported by 100 mL of blood (0.3 mL in solution +19.6 mL with hemoglobin =19.9 mL), it can be seen that only 1.5% is carried in solution, whereas 98.5% is combined with hemoglobin. If hemoglobin were not present, it would take 66.3 times more blood to transport the same amount of oxygen.

The oxygen–hemoglobin dissociation curve

The loading and unloading of oxygen from hemoglobin are best described by the oxygen–hemoglobin dissociation curve (Figure 23.4). The following points should be remembered.

1 The amount of oxygen associated with hemoglobin is related, but is not directly proportional (as was the amount in solution), to the pressure of dissolved oxygen in the water of the red blood cell and plasma.

2 Before the combination of oxygen with hemoglobin, there must be oxygen in solution; similarly, after its removal from hemoglobin, oxygen is again in solution so that it may diffuse to the consuming cells (the oxygen unloads because P_{O_2} in solution is lowered) (see Figure 23.3).

In addition to a scale for percent saturation of hemoglobin, Figure 23.4 also has scales for volumes percent of oxygen (volumes [in milliliters] of oxygen per 100 mL of blood) associated with hemoglobin when the hemoglobin concentration of blood is normal (15 g/dL) or reduced (7.5 g/dL), as in anemia. In this way, the amount of oxygen transported by anemic blood may be compared with normal blood. A study of Figure 23.4 will show the following.

1 At a P_{O_2} of 100 mmHg (the approximate P_{O_2} of arterial blood), hemoglobin is about 97.5% saturated with oxygen. Hemoglobin will transport about 19.6 vol% when the hemoglobin concentration is 15 g/dL and about 9.8 vol% when the hemoglobin concentration is 7.5 g/dL.

2 When the P_{O_2} is 40 mmHg (approximately the P_{O_2} of venous blood), hemoglobin is still about 72% saturated with oxygen. It will transport about 14.5 vol% when the hemoglobin concentration is 15 g/dL, and about 7.25 vol% when the hemoglobin concentration is lowered to 7.5 g/dL.

3 In going from a P_{O_2} of 100 mmHg to one of 40 mmHg, about 5 vol% of oxygen is yielded by 100 mL of blood when the

Section IV: Respiration

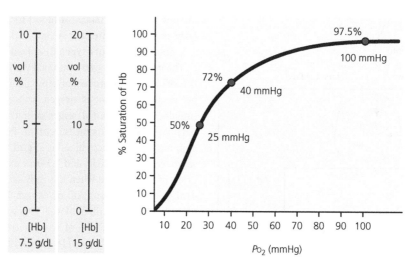

Figure 23.4 The oxygen–hemoglobin dissociation curve for human blood. Volumes percent of oxygen associated with normal (15 g/dL) and half normal (7.5 g/dL) hemoglobin concentrations [Hb] are shown relative to the hemoglobin saturation scale, so that the difference between hemoglobin saturation and volume of oxygen transported can be seen. The hemoglobin saturation scale refers to the percent of total oxygen that hemoglobin is capable of binding. From Reece, W.O. (2004) Respiration in mammals. In: *Dukes' Physiology of Domestic Animals*, 12th edn (ed. W.O. Reece). Cornell University Press, Ithaca, NY. Reproduced with permission from Cornell University Press.

hemoglobin concentration is 15 g/dL, and about 2.5 vol% is yielded when the hemoglobin concentration is 7.5 g/dL. The former value (5 vol%) reflects oxygen consumption under normal resting conditions.

4 For blood to yield 5 vol% of oxygen when an animal is anemic (7.5 g/dL of hemoglobin), it appears that the Po_2 of blood would have to be reduced to about 25 mmHg. Reductions of this magnitude are unusual in the living animal, however, because cardiac output increases in order to transport more oxygen than would otherwise be available.

5 The P_{50} for this curve is about equal to 25 mmHg. P_{50} is a notation for the associated Po_2 when hemoglobin is 50% saturated with oxygen. It is the same regardless of the concentration of hemoglobin. P_{50} changes when the dissociation constant for hemoglobin changes (oxygen–hemoglobin dissociation curve shifts right or left). P_{50} values normally given for human blood are 26 or 27 mmHg.

The fraction of oxygen given up by blood as it passes through the tissue capillaries is known as **fractional extraction** or **percent extraction**. In the above example, where blood with a hemoglobin concentration of 15 g/dL carries about 20 vol% of oxygen and yields about 5 vol% of oxygen, the fractional extraction is ¼ . In the example of the anemic animal (hemoglobin concentration of 7.5 g/dL) this would become about ½ .

It can be seen that under normal conditions hemoglobin will set an upper limit on the Po_2 in the tissues at approximately 40 mmHg, which is referred to as the **oxygen buffer function of hemoglobin**. The dissociation of oxygen from hemoglobin is such that the Po_2 of blood must fall to about 40 mmHg in order to supply the minimal need of 5 vol% of oxygen at the tissue level; values below 40 mmHg do not provide the desirable oxygen tension for optimum cell function. It is known that the prolonged provision of oxygen at high

oxygen tension is detrimental to lung cells (cells that are intimately exposed to oxygen without the oxygen buffer function of hemoglobin). Also, the maintenance of end-capillary Po_2 close to 40 mmHg assists the diffusion of oxygen into the tissue cells by providing a gradient for diffusion. Because the lower part of the dissociation curve is steep, large amounts of oxygen can be withdrawn from hemoglobin with little reduction in Po_2 from 40 mmHg, and the diffusion gradient for oxygen will be maintained.

The association of oxygen with hemoglobin and its dissociation from hemoglobin are not stable under all conditions. Different conditions change the equilibrium of the reaction between hemoglobin and oxygen that form oxyhemoglobin. This equilibrium is represented by the oxygen–hemoglobin dissociation curve: when the equilibrium changes, shifts in the curve can be observed (Figure 23.5). When the curve shifts to the right, it denotes a decreased affinity of hemoglobin for oxygen. Under these conditions more oxygen is yielded for each reduction in Po_2. Similarly, a shift to the left denotes an increased affinity of hemoglobin for oxygen, and less oxygen is yielded for each reduction in Po_2. Increases in hydrogen ion and carbon dioxide cause the curve to shift to the right (decreased affinity for oxygen); therefore a shift to the right would be expected at the level of the tissue capillaries where arterial blood becomes venous blood because hydrogen ions and carbon dioxide are being produced. This shift to the right is appropriate because it provides a greater yield of oxygen at the tissues where it should be unloaded because oxygen is being consumed. When the blood reaches the lungs, where both CO_2 and hydrogen ion concentrations are lowered, a shift of the curve to the left is appropriate so that hemoglobin has a greater affinity for oxygen and oxygen uptake is facilitated. The effect of CO_2 and hydrogen ions on

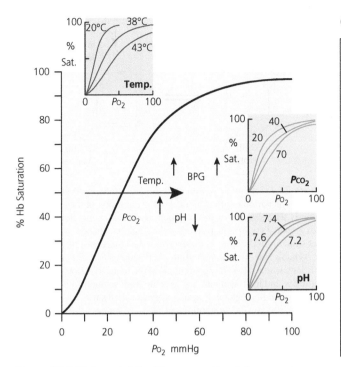

Figure 23.5 Rightward shift of the oxygen dissociation curve by increases in H^+, P_{CO_2}, temperature, and 2,3-bisphosphoglycerate (BPG). From West, J.B. *Respiratory Physiology: The Essentials*, 7th edn. © 2004, Lippincott Williams & Wilkins, Baltimore. Reproduced with permission from Lippincott Williams & Wilkins.

the ability of hemoglobin to yield or receive oxygen is referred to as the **Bohr effect**. Other factors noted to cause shifts in the curves are the temperature of the blood and the concentration of 2,3-bisphosphoglycerate (2,3-BPG) within the red blood cell. There is a greater need for oxygen during hyperthermia, and because increases in blood temperature cause the curve to shift to the right, greater yields of oxygen are provided to the tissues at these times. The normal fractional extraction for avian blood is about ½ in contrast to ¼ for mammalian blood. The higher body temperature of these animals (41 °C vs. 39 °C) assists in the provision of easier oxygen yield. 2,3-BPG is normally present in the blood, but its concentration varies under different conditions; 2,3-BPG concentration is known to increase during conditions of chronic hypoxia. During prolonged exposure to a hypoxic environment, the oxygen–hemoglobin dissociation curve is shifted to the right (induced by 2,3-BPG), and the dissociation of oxygen from hemoglobin is promoted. The initial response in many/most species is a leftward shift due to hypoxemia-induced hyperventilation. Increased 2,3-BPG then helps to shift the curve to the right, back toward the original position. The magnitude of the shift caused by hypoxia is not as large at the P_{O_2} of oxygen loading (upper part of curve) as it is at the P_{O_2} of oxygen unloading (steep part of curve), so that a near-normal affinity for loading occurs coupled with greater ease of unloading, and an overall advantage is obtained.

Carbon dioxide transport

1 Why does the reaction of carbon dioxide with plasma proteins not provide a significant amount of carbon dioxide transport?

2 Why does the hydration reaction of carbon dioxide not provide a significant amount of carbon dioxide transport?

3 How does carbonic anhydrase in erythrocytes favor the transport of carbon dioxide?

4 What happens to the H^+ and HCO_3^- that forms from the hydration reaction? How does their removal from the formation site facilitate their continued formation and thus greater carbon dioxide loading by venous blood?

5 What are the two means by which hydrogen ions are accommodated by hemoglobin?

6 How does the chloride shift assist in the maintenance of electrical neutrality?

7 How does the oxygenation of hemoglobin assist the unloading of carbon dioxide from the blood to the alveoli?

8 Does the unloading of oxygen from hemoglobin in the tissue capillaries make hemoglobin more basic?

9 How is carbon dioxide production related to oxygen consumption in the respiratory quotient equation?

General scheme of carbon dioxide transport

A schematic illustration of carbon dioxide transport is shown in Figure 23.6. This scheme considers the following points.

1 Carbon dioxide is highly soluble in body fluids and, because of pressure gradients, readily diffuses from its production site, the body cells, through interstitial fluid, to the plasma of venous blood of the tissue capillaries.

2 At this point, carbon dioxide is transported not only by that which is in solution, but also by reactions that occur in plasma, and by reactions that occur in red blood cells.

3 The venous blood circulates to the pulmonary capillaries and, because of pressure gradients that favor unloading of carbon dioxide, the carbon dioxide in solution diffuses from the pulmonary capillaries to the alveoli. This is followed by a reversal of the reactions that accommodated the prior loading of carbon dioxide in plasma and red blood cells.

4 The venous blood now becomes arterial blood that exhibits a reduction in the partial pressure of carbon dioxide whereby diffusion gradients will again favor loading of carbon dioxide from its site of production.

Carbon dioxide in plasma

Carbon dioxide that diffuses to plasma from the cells not only will exist as dissolved carbon dioxide but also will combine with terminal amino groups of plasma proteins to form carbamino compounds and will be hydrated to form ionization products of carbonic acid. The reactions with the amino groups is as follows:

$$R-NH_2+CO_2 \leftrightarrow R-N\begin{matrix}H\\|\\COOH\end{matrix} \leftrightarrow R-N\begin{matrix}H\\|\\COO^-\end{matrix}+H^+$$

Section IV: Respiration

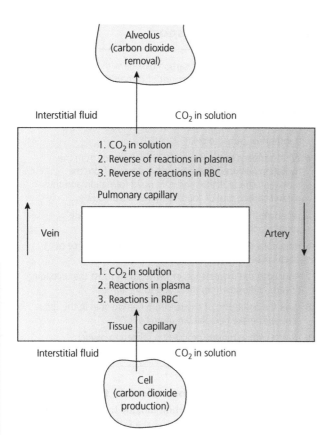

Figure 23.6 General scheme of carbon dioxide transport showing diffusion process. Diffusion occurs because of pressure gradients. Blood flow is clockwise; carbon dioxide is taken up by blood from cells at bottom and removed from blood by the lungs at top. The numbered processes are listed in order of their occurrence. The reactions in plasma and the RBC are those associated with hydration of carbon dioxide, formation of carbamino compounds, and the buffering of hydrogen ions. These reactions are relatively minimal in plasma. The last carbon dioxide molecule to move into plasma solution from tissue cells is the first to leave at the alveolus. RBC, red blood cell. From Reece, W.O. (2009) *Functional Anatomy and Physiology of Domestic Animals*, 4th edn. Wiley-Blackwell, Ames, IA. Reproduced with permission from Wiley.

This reaction does not account for a significant amount of transport because there are relatively few free or terminal amino groups on plasma proteins capable of combining with carbon dioxide.

The hydration of carbon dioxide, forming ionization products of carbonic acid, proceeds as follows:

$$CO_2 + H_2O \leftrightarrow H_2CO_3 \leftrightarrow H^+ + HCO_3^-$$

The equilibrium of the hydration reaction in plasma is far to the left. In fact, the concentration of carbon dioxide in plasma is about 1000 times greater than the concentration of carbonic acid. In summary, the reactions that occur in plasma with carbon dioxide comprise only about 10% of carbon dioxide transport.

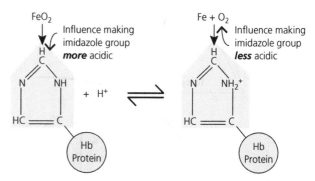

Figure 23.7 Schematic representation of the effect of oxygenation and deoxygenation on the chemical buffering action of the imidazole group ($C_3H_4N_2$) of hemoglobin. When oxygenated hemoglobin is deoxygenated (right), the β chains of hemoglobin change their shape (not shown). In their new conformation, the C-terminal histidines in the β chains react with the aspartates at positions 94 in the same chain. This interaction raises the apparent pK of the imidazole group of the histidines, and hydrogen ions are taken up from solution. When deoxygenated hemoglobin is again oxygenated (left), the C-terminal histidines become free in solution once more; their pK falls and they give off hydrogen ions. Reprinted from *The ABC of Acid–Base Chemistry* by H.W. Davenport, by permission of the University of Chicago Press. © 1947, 1949, 1959, 1958, 1969, 1974 by the University of Chicago.

Carbon dioxide in erythrocytes

Carbon dioxide readily diffuses into erythrocytes, and reactions with water and amino groups are more significant than in plasma. There are greater numbers of terminal amino groups on hemoglobin than there are on plasma proteins, so that this form of carriage is more prominent. Also, the hydration reaction is facilitated by the presence of **carbonic anhydrase**, an enzyme found within erythrocytes. The carbonic acid that is formed ionizes to produce hydrogen ions and bicarbonate ions. Even though the equilibrium of the hydration reaction favors the formation of hydrogen ions and bicarbonate ions, it is rate-limited if the ionization products are not removed. However, the ionization products are removed by the buffering of hydrogen ions by hemoglobin and by the diffusion of bicarbonate ions from the erythrocytes to the plasma.

Hydrogen ions are accommodated by hemoglobin as follows.
1 Combination with basic carboxyl groups, suppressing their ionization and forming undissociated groups:

$$R — COO^- + H^+ \leftrightarrow R — COOH$$

The electrical neutrality of the carboxyl groups was previously maintained by sodium and potassium ions.
2 Combination with imidazole groups of hemoglobin (Figure 23.7).

As noted earlier, electrical neutrality before buffering is maintained by sodium and potassium ions in balance with the carboxyl groups. After ionization of the carboxyl groups is suppressed by hydrogen ions, electrical neutrality of sodium and potassium ions is maintained by bicarbonate ions formed from the hydration reaction facilitated by carbonic anhydrase

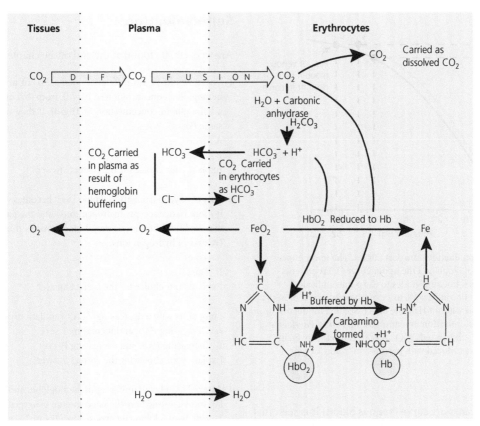

Figure 23.8 Schematic representation of the processes occurring when carbon dioxide diffuses from tissues into erythrocytes. The reactions shown as occurring in erythrocytes provide the principal methods of transporting carbon dioxide from the cells to the lungs. Reprinted from *The ABC of Acid–Base Chemistry* by H.W. Davenport, by permission of the University of Chicago Press. © 1947, 1949, 1959, 1958, 1969, 1974 by the University of Chicago.

and chloride ions resulting from suppression of hydrogen ions. As bicarbonate ions accumulate with continued hydration of carbon dioxide, they diffuse from the erythrocytes to the plasma because of a concentration gradient. Sodium and potassium ions do not readily diffuse, and electrical neutrality is then maintained by chloride ions that diffuse from the plasma (where they are in relatively higher concentration) to the erythrocytes. This transfer of chloride ions is known as the **chloride shift**. The reactions of carbon dioxide within erythrocytes are schematically represented by Figure 23.8.

The chemical reactions within erythrocytes associated with carbon dioxide transport, and the imbalance of osmotic particles (Na^+ and K^+ retained in erythrocytes), cause an increase in the effective osmotic pressure of erythrocyte fluid, causing inward diffusion of water. An observation of slightly increased erythrocyte size in venous blood as compared with their size in arterial blood is explained by this phenomenon.

When venous blood reaches the capillaries of the lung, the carbon dioxide in solution in plasma begins to diffuse toward the alveoli. All the reactions that had previously accommodated carbon dioxide transport are now reversed, so that carbon dioxide may be lost at the lung. The reverse reactions are facilitated because hemoglobin is becoming oxygenated. Oxygenated hemoglobin is more acidic (acids donate H^+ to solutions) and, accordingly, releases hydrogen ions. These hydrogen ions combine with bicarbonate ions to form carbonic acid, which in turn is dehydrated to carbon dioxide and water. The effect of oxygen on hydrogen ion and carbon dioxide loading and unloading from hemoglobin is known as the **Haldane effect**. The loss of oxygen from hemoglobin in the tissue capillaries makes hemoglobin more basic (bases accept H^+ from solutions) and hydrogen ions are received, facilitating the hydration reaction and loading of carbon dioxide.

Carbon dioxide transport curves

The amount of carbon dioxide transported in all its forms (carbon dioxide in solution, reactions with protein, and with hemoglobin) varies with changes in partial pressure of carbon dioxide and is illustrated by carbon dioxide transport curves (Figure 23.9).

Oxygen–hemoglobin dissociation curves are shifted to the right or left by several factors (see Figure 23.5). In the upper

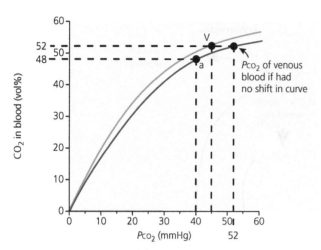

Figure 23.9 Carbon dioxide transport curves. The lower curve (a) represents arterial blood and the upper curve (V) represents venous blood. Dashed lines are guides to the points indicated. Extension of dashed line at 52 vol% to P_{CO_2} (mmHg) axis represents hypothetical location without Haldane effect. See text for details. From Reece, W.O. (2004) Respiration in mammals. In: *Dukes' Physiology of Domestic Animals*, 12th edn (ed. W.O. Reece). Cornell University Press, Ithaca, NY. Reproduced with permission from Cornell University Press.

carbon dioxide transport curve (venous blood) it is seen that, for every increment of P_{CO_2}, a greater volume of CO_2 is transported in venous blood than in arterial blood. This happens because of the Haldane effect, whereby loss of oxygen from arterial blood provides for greater accommodation of carbon dioxide. When arterial blood becomes venous blood, the P_{CO_2} is about 5 mmHg higher and contains about 4 vol% more carbon dioxide than arterial blood. If it were not for the Haldane effect, allowing for a greater accommodation of carbon dioxide, the P_{CO_2} in venous blood would be about 12 mmHg higher than that in arterial blood (rather than 5 mmHg higher) in order to transport the added 4 vol% of carbon dioxide.

It is instructive to relate volumes percent of oxygen consumed and volumes percent of carbon dioxide removed to the **respiratory quotient** (RQ), which is defined as follows:

$$RQ = \frac{CO_2 \text{ production}}{O_2 \text{ consumption}}$$

Substituting the value for oxygen consumption from the oxygen–hemoglobin association curve for arterial blood of 5 vol% of oxygen and the value for carbon dioxide production from the carbon dioxide transport for arterial blood of 4 vol% of carbon dioxide, it is found that RQ = 4 vol%/5 vol% = 0.8. This represents a respiratory quotient that is common for intermediary metabolism, wherein the diet is balanced for carbohydrates, fats, and proteins.

Self-evaluation

Answers can be found at the end of the chapter.

1 There would be no difference in the P_{O_2} of arterial blood with a hemoglobin concentration of 10 g/dL from that of arterial blood with a hemoglobin concentration of 15 g/dL if they were exposed to the same P_{O_2}.
 A True
 B False
 Explain your choice for the correct answer

2 Loss of oxygen from arterial blood as it becomes venous blood makes it more basic (accepts hydrogen ions) and the gain of oxygen as the venous blood becomes arterial blood makes the blood more acidic (release of hydrogen ions).
 A True
 B False
 Explain your choice for the correct answer.

3 Lung units with a decreasing $\dot{V}_A/\dot{Q}$ ventilation/perfusion ratio have:
 A Decreasing P_{AO_2} and increasing P_{ACO_2}
 B Increasing P_{AO_2} and decreasing P_{ACO_2}
 Explain your choice for the correct answer.

4 Arterial blood containing 5 g/dL hemoglobin and exposed to a P_{O_2} of 500 mmHg would have the same amount of oxygen as blood containing 10 g/dL hemoglobin and exposed to a P_{O_2} of 250 mmHg (hemoglobin saturation equals 100% at a P_{O_2} of 250 mmHg).
 A True
 B False
 Explain your choice for the correct answer.

Suggested reading

Hall, J.E. (2011) Transport of oxygen and carbon dioxide in blood and tissue fluids. In: *Guyton and Hall Textbook of Medical Physiology*, 12th edn, pp. 495–504. Saunders Elsevier, Philadelphia.

Hlastala, M.P. and Berger, A.J. (1996) *Physiology of Respiration*. Oxford University Press, New York.

West, J.B. (1990) *Ventilation/Blood Flow and Gas Exchange*, 5th edn. Blackwell Scientific Publications, Oxford.

West, J.B. (2008) *Pulmonary Pathophysiology*, 7th edn. Wolters Kluwer/ Lippincott Williams & Wilkins, Baltimore.

Answers

1 A. Regardless of the amount of hemoglobin present, there will be no difference in P_{O_2} when both bloods are exposed to the same P_{O_2}. However, there would be a difference in the amount of oxygen transported whereby the blood with 15 g/dL would transport more than the blood with 10 g/dL.

2 A. When venous blood reaches the capillaries of the lung, the carbon dioxide in solution in plasma begins to diffuse toward the alveoli. All

the reactions that had previously accommodated carbon dioxide transport are now reversed, so that carbon dioxide may be lost at the lung. The reverse reactions are facilitated because hemoglobin is becoming oxygenated. Oxygenated hemoglobin is more acidic (acids donate H^+ to solutions) and, accordingly, release hydrogen ions. The hydrogen ions combine with bicarbonate ions to form carbonic acid, which in turn is dehydrated to carbon dioxide and water. When arterial blood arrives at the tissue capillaries, oxygen is lost from hemoglobin and it becomes more basic (bases accept H^+ from solutions) and hydrogen ions are received, facilitating the hydration reaction and loading of carbon dioxide.

3 A. For $\dot{V}A/\dot{Q}$ to decrease from normal implies that alveolar ventilation is reduced to a greater degree than perfusion. Accordingly, $P_{A O_2}$ is decreased and $P_{A C O_2}$ is increased, so that blood perfusing this unit will reflect these changes.

4 B. Even though the hemoglobin in both bloods is completely saturated with oxygen, the amount of oxygen in the blood with 5 g/dL hemoglobin would be less than the amount in the blood with 10 g/dL because the amount is related to the amount of hemoglobin. The P_{O_2} of 500 mmHg versus 250 mmHg does not imply doubling the amount of oxygen. Since both bloods are saturated with oxygen, very little more would be contained in the blood with P_{O_2} of 500 mmHg.

24 Regulation of Respiration

William O. Reece

Iowa State University, Ames, IA, USA

Pulmonary ventilation is regulated closely to maintain the concentrations of hydrogen ions, carbon dioxide, and oxygen at relatively constant levels while meeting the needs of the body under varying conditions. If either the hydrogen ion or the carbon dioxide concentration increases or if the oxygen concentration decreases, their levels will be returned to normal by increasing ventilation. Conversely, if either the hydrogen ion or carbon dioxide concentration decreases or if oxygen concentration increases, pulmonary ventilation will be decreased. This regulatory mechanism is controlled by changes in tidal volume, frequency of respiratory cycles, or both.

Regulation of respiration

> 1 Which region within the respiratory center is associated with inspiratory activity?
>
> 2 What are the roles of the ventral respiratory group and the pneumotaxic center?
>
> 3 How might complementary breaths be associated with the apneustic center?

The respiratory center

The rhythmic pattern of breathing and the adjustments that occur therein are integrated within portions of the brainstem known as the **respiratory center** (Figure 24.1). Unlike many centers, it is not a collection of circumscribed nuclei but rather consists of regions within the medulla and pons associated with specific respiration-related functions. Four specific regions have been identified: (i) the **dorsal respiratory group (DRG)** in the dorsal medulla, (ii) the **ventral respiratory group (VRG)** in the ventral medulla, (iii) the **pneumotaxic center (PC)** in the rostral portion of the pons, and (iv) the **apneustic center** in the caudal pons.

Neurons of the DRG are primarily associated with inspiratory activity and generate the basic rhythm of breathing. Output from the DRG is relayed via the phrenic nerve to the diaphragm to provide for its contraction and the inspiratory phase of the breathing cycle that follows. Input to the DRG is relayed via the vagal and glossopharyngeal nerves. Mechanoreceptors in the lung are stimulated during lung inflation and relay impulses via the vagus nerves to the DRG and these play an important role in lung inflation-induced termination of inspiration (see section Hering–Breuer reflexes). The vagal and glossopharyngeal nerves also relay information to the DRG from peripheral chemoreceptors (e.g., skin, muscle, joints).

The VRG has neurons that are associated with both inspiratory and expiratory activity but it is primarily responsible for expiration. If expiration is considered to be passive during normal quiet breathing, the expiratory neurons are not active; however, during exercise, when expiration becomes an active process, the expiratory neurons are active. The inspiratory neurons of the VRG serve to give an assist to inspiratory activity begun by the DRG and at the same time inhibit the VRG expiratory group neurons during the inspiratory phase of the breathing cycle. It is likely that the inspiratory neurons of the VRG are also more active during exercise. The PC inhibits inspiration and therefore regulates inspiratory volume and respiratory rate.

The primary function of the PC is to limit inspiration, thereby controlling the duration of the filling phase of the respiratory cycle. The pneumotaxic signal that controls the filling phase may be strong or weak. The effect of a strong signal is to increase

Dukes' Physiology of Domestic Animals, Thirteenth Edition. Edited by William O. Reece, Howard H. Erickson, Jesse P. Goff and Etsuro E. Uemura.
© 2015 John Wiley & Sons, Inc. Published 2015 by John Wiley & Sons, Inc.
Companion website: www.wiley.com/go/reece/physiology

Section IV: Respiration

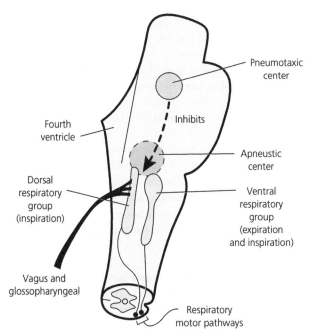

Figure 24.1 Components of the respiratory center. The pneumotaxic and apneustic centers are located in the pons, and the dorsal and ventral respiratory groups are located in the medulla. Modified from Figure 41-1 in Hall, J. (2011) *Guyton and Hall Textbook of Medical Physiology*, 12th edn. Saunders Elsevier, Philadelphia. With permission from Elsevier.

the respiratory rate whereby both inspiration and expiration are shortened and which are coupled with a lesser tidal volume. The converse is true for a weak PC signal.

The apneustic center is the least understood of all the regions of the respiratory center; consequently, there is no consensus as to its role. Whereas the PC is concerned with the termination of inspiration, the apneustic center is believed to be associated with deep inspirations (**apneusis**). Perhaps **complementary breaths (sighs)** are manifestations of apneustic center activity.

Neural control of ventilation

> 1 What are the two components of the Hering–Breuer reflexes? Which one of the components can be used to initiate an inspiration in unresponsive animals?
>
> 2 Why is endotracheal intubation difficult in lightly anesthetized animals?
>
> 3 How does a greater negativity of intrapleural pressure created by thoracic enlargement assist the flow of blood to the heart?

Hering–Breuer reflexes

The basic rhythm of respiration may be modified so that the breathing rate, depth, or both are changed. The reason for the modification is to change the rate of ventilation in response to body needs. Afferent impulses to the respiratory center from several receptor sources have been identified. The most noteworthy of these among many of the animals are the **Hering–Breuer**

reflexes. The receptors for these reflexes are located in the lung and particularly in the bronchi and bronchioles.

There are two components to the Hering–Breuer reflexes: (i) the inspiratory-inhibitory or inflation reflex and (ii) the inspiratory or deflation reflex. The nerve impulses generated by the receptors of the Hering–Breuer reflexes are transmitted by fibers in the vagus nerves to the respiratory center. The effect of inflation-receptor stimulation is to inhibit further inspiration (stimulation of neurons in the DRG) and to stimulate expiratory nerves in the VRG. The inspiratory or deflation reflex component is activated at some particular point of deflation. The deflation receptors might not be activated to bring about the next inspiration during eupnea, but they might be active when deflation is more complete. Deflation reflex receptor stimulation can be elicited in anesthetized dogs by manual compression of the thorax, which is followed immediately by inspiration. Practical use of this reflex is appropriate for respiratory depressed or unresponsive animals to promote more adequate ventilation in the former or to initiate ventilation in the latter. During exercise when tidal volume and frequency are increased, it would appear that the deflation reflex is more active in order to hasten the beginning of the next inspiration.

In addition to the receptors located in the lung, there are other peripherally located receptors that assist in modifying the basic rhythm. Stimulation of receptors in the skin is excitatory to the respiratory center, and deeper than usual inspiration may be noted. Perhaps their excitation to the inspiratory area is through the apneustic center, inasmuch as inspiratory gasps are occasionally seen. Advantage is taken of these receptors when stimulation of breathing is desired in newborn animals. Rubbing the skin with a rough cloth often starts the breathing cycles. An assist to ventilation needed during muscle activity is obtained from receptors located in tendons and joints. They will be stimulated when muscle contraction causes movement. It is also believed that when impulses are directed to skeletal muscles from the cerebral cortex, collateral impulses go to the brainstem and stimulate the respiratory center to increase alveolar ventilation. This mechanism might account for increases in ventilation that are not explainable by mere observation of changes in carbon dioxide, oxygen, and hydrogen ion concentration in the blood.

Upper air passage reflexes

A number of respiratory reflexes are initiated in the upper air passages. Stimulation of the mucous membrane in these regions causes reflex inhibition of respiration. A striking example of this reflex is the inhibition of respiration that occurs during swallowing. Another example is seen in diving birds and mammals when they submerge. Stimulation of the mucous membrane of the larynx in the unanesthetized animal causes not only inhibition of respiration but, usually, also powerful expiratory efforts (coughing). Similarly, stimulation of the nasal mucous membrane frequently leads to sneezing. Obviously the function of all these reflexes is to protect the delicate respiratory passages and the depths of the lungs from harmful substances (irritating gases, dust, food particles) that otherwise might be inspired. To make the protection more certain, the glottis is closed and the bronchi may be constricted. Endotracheal intubation is often difficult in lightly anesthetized animals because of reflex closure of the glottis.

Baroreceptor modification of respiration

The principal function of afferent impulses from baroreceptors in the carotid and aortic sinuses is to regulate the circulation. However, the same receptors are also able to modify respiration. The receptors are constantly generating impulses that increase in frequency when blood pressure increases and which decrease in frequency when blood pressure decreases. These impulses to the respiratory center are inhibitory in nature, and respiratory frequency decreases when impulse frequency increases. It is believed that the function of this response is to modify the return of blood to the heart. For example, when blood pressure is reduced, respiration increases and flow of blood to the heart is facilitated. The effect of increased respiratory excursions, as evidenced by thoracic enlargement, is to provide a greater negativity of intra-pleural pressure. Reduction in intrapleural pressure is transmitted to the mediastinal space, which aids in the expansion of the vena cava and lowers the blood pressure within. The larger blood pressure difference that is created between the vena cava and the peripheral veins assists in the flow of blood to the heart.

Voluntary control of respiration

Ordinary respirations proceed quite involuntarily. However, it is a matter of everyday experience that they may be altered voluntarily within wide limits; they may be hastened, slowed, or stopped altogether for a while. If respirations are entirely inhibited voluntarily, there soon comes a time when one must breathe again; the cells of the respiratory center escape from the inhibition. Phonation and related acts and the use of the abdominal press in the expulsive acts of defecation, urination, and parturition are examples of more or less complete voluntary control of the respiratory movements.

Humoral control of respiration

1 Do increases in $Paco_2$ and hydrogen ion concentration increase pulmonary ventilation?
2 Does an increased Pao_2 increase pulmonary ventilation?
3 What are the respective renal compensations for respiratory alkalosis and respiratory acidosis?
4 What are the respective respiratory compensations for metabolic acidosis and metabolic alkalosis?
5 Why is the respiratory center response to respiratory acidosis greater than the response to metabolic acidosis?
6 Do the carotid and aortic bodies respond to the partial pressures of oxygen and carbon dioxide or to the amount of oxygen and carbon dioxide?
7 Why are the carotid and aortic body responses to Pao_2 not as effective as a stimulus for oxygen lack in anemic animals?
8 Under what conditions would oxygen partial pressure via the carotid and aortic bodies be important as a drive to increase ventilation?

In addition to the rather direct neural impingement on the respiratory center that has just been described, there are also blood chemicals that modify the basic rhythm. Inasmuch as these factors are present in the blood, this control mechanism may be referred to as **humoral control**. Specifically, the chemicals referred to are carbon dioxide, oxygen, and hydrogen ions. Their concentrations in arterial blood change alveolar ventilation as follows.

1 An increase in Pco_2 causes alveolar ventilation to increase; a decrease in Pco_2 causes alveolar ventilation to decrease.
2 An increase in hydrogen ion concentration causes alveolar ventilation to increase; a decrease in hydrogen ion concentration causes alveolar ventilation to decrease.
3 A decrease in Po_2 causes alveolar ventilation to increase; an increase in Po_2 causes alveolar ventilation to decrease.

Respiratory role in acid–base balance

The interactions of carbon dioxide, oxygen, and hydrogen ion concentrations on respiration are quite apparent under certain conditions, and because of the role of the respiratory system in acid–base balance, a brief description is instructive here. A detailed discussion is presented in Chapter 13. A pH–bicarbonate diagram that illustrates the compensations that may occur is shown in Figure 24.2. Its components consist of a Pco_2 isobar and a normal buffer line. Any point along the Pco_2 isobar (shown fo $Pco_2 = 40$ mmHg) would represent possible combinations of bicarbonate concentration and pH that can exist whe $Paco_2$ is normal (40 mmHg). Points to the right or left of the $Pco_2 = 40$ mmHg isobar represent respective deviations toward respiratory alkalosis ($Paco_2$ decrease) and respiratory acidosis ($Paco_2$ increase). The normal buffer line indicates a balance between metabolic acids and metabolic bases where points along the line represent possible combinations of bicarbonate concentration and pH that can occur as long as the metabolic acids and bases in the body fluids are normal. Points above or below the line represent respective deviations toward metabolic alkalosis and metabolic acidosis.

Compensatory mechanisms exist for all the above-mentioned deviations. Renal compensation for respiratory alkalosis (low $Paco_2$) and respiratory acidosis (high $Paco_2$) occurs as follows.

1 *Respiratory alkalosis.* Because of decreasing $Paco_2$, renal tubular acid secretion and bicarbonate "reabsorption" are decreased and pH is returned toward normal (path A, Figure 24.2).
2 *Respiratory acidosis.* Because of increasing $Paco_2$, renal tubular acid secretion and bicarbonate "reabsorption" are increased and pH is returned toward normal (path B, Figure 24.-2).

Respiratory compensation for metabolic acidosis and metabolic alkalosis occurs as follows.

3 *Metabolic acidosis.* The hydrogen ions from increased metabolic acids stimulate respiration whereby $Paco_2$ is decreased (causing hydrogen ion concentration to decrease) and pH returns toward normal (path C, Figure 24.2).

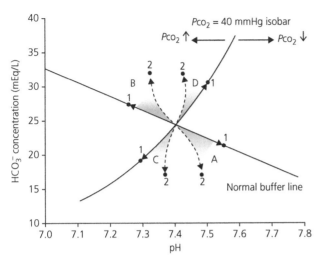

Figure 24.2 Compensations for the development of acid–base balance abnormalities. Location 1 refers to development without compensation, and location 2 refers to development with compensation. Respiratory alkalosis (A) with decreased P_{CO_2}: renal compensation with decreased H^+ secretion and HCO_3^- reabsorption (lesser pH increase than would have occurred without renal compensation). Respiratory acidosis (B) with increased P_{CO_2}: renal compensation with increased H^+ secretion and HCO_3^- reabsorption (lesser pH decrease than would have occurred without renal compensation). Metabolic acidosis (C) with increased extracellular fluid $[H^+]$: increased $[H^+]$ stimulates ventilation; P_{CO_2} decreases and pH increases (lesser pH decrease than would have occurred without respiratory compensation). Metabolic alkalosis (D) with decreased extracellular fluid $[H^+]$: decreased $[H^+]$ "brakes" ventilation; P_{CO_2} increases and pH decreases (lesser pH increase than would have occurred without respiratory compensation).

4 *Metabolic alkalosis*. Because metabolic acids (hydrogen ions) are decreased, a braking effect (described later) on respiration occurs whereby Pa_{CO_2} increases (causing hydrogen ion concentration to increase) and pH returns toward normal (path D, Figure 24.2).

The association of carbon dioxide with the hydrogen ion concentration and pH just described is by way of the hydration reaction:

$$CO_2 + H_2O \leftrightarrow H_2CO_3 \leftrightarrow H^+ + HCO_3^- \qquad (24.1)$$

Central chemoreception

Chemosensitive areas near the ventral surface of the medulla are highly sensitive to changes in hydrogen ion concentration of the interstitial fluid of the brain (Figure 24.3). The chemoreceptors in these areas are excitatory to the respiratory center, causing increases in tidal volume and in frequency. Whereas hydrogen ions diffuse poorly through the blood–cerebrospinal fluid barrier and the blood–brain barrier, carbon dioxide is freely diffusible and indirectly exerts its influence on ventilation through the intermediary of hydrogen ions after hydration (see equation 24.1). Therefore, whenever the Pa_{CO_2} increases, the P_{CO_2} of both the interstitial fluid of the medulla and the cerebrospinal fluid

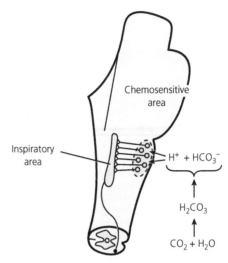

Figure 24.3 The chemosensitive area of the brainstem respiratory center. The chemosensitive area is stimulated by hydrogen ions, which are formed by the conversion of carbon dioxide through the hydration reaction. Modified from Figure 41-2 in Hall, J. (2011) *Guyton and Hall Textbook of Medical Physiology*, 12th edn. Saunders Elsevier, Philadelphia. With permission from Elsevier.

increases, forming hydrogen ions through hydration. Because of the barriers to hydrogen ion diffusion, the respiratory center response to respiratory acidosis (increased Pa_{CO_2}) is greater than the response to metabolic acidosis (increased hydrogen ion concentration).

Peripheral chemoreception

Up to this point, the chemical control of alveolar ventilation has been discussed only in terms of its direct effect on the medulla (the chemosensitive area) via carbon dioxide and hydrogen ions. It should be noted that oxygen does not exert its hyperpneic influence in that area. The anatomical entities known as the **carotid and aortic bodies**, found in the region of the bifurcation of the carotid arteries and the arch of the aorta, respectively, are chemoreceptors. They detect changes in the partial pressures of carbon dioxide and oxygen and hydrogen ion concentration and affect the respiratory center by transmission of impulses in afferent nerve fibers of the glossopharyngeal nerves (from the carotid bodies) and vagus nerves (from the aortic arch). Although the medulla is the principal location for detection of changes in carbon dioxide and hydrogen ion concentrations, it has been shown that the carotid and aortic body chemoreceptors supply about 50% of the ventilator drive in response to changes in Pa_{CO_2}. Denervation of the carotid bodies in most of the domestic animals (dogs, cats, sheep, goats, ponies, cattle) causes chronic hypoventilation (Pa_{CO_2} increased by 5–10 mmHg), indicating that the carotid bodies supply an important part of the tonic drive to resting ventilation in normoxic conditions. Carotid and aortic body chemoreceptors, however, are the only places where the partial pressure of oxygen is detected. These small organs are highly perfused with blood, and the oxygen needed for baseline activity is obtained from the oxygen in solution. The arteriovenous difference in oxygen content across the

Section IV: Respiration

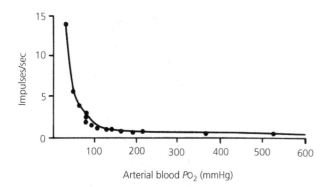

Figure 24.4 Effect of arterial oxygen partial pressure on the number of impulses per second from the carotid body to the respiratory center. The impulses are excitatory. From Reece, W.O. (2004) Respiration in mammals. In: *Dukes' Physiology of Domestic Animals*, 12th edn (ed. W.O. Reece). Cornell University Press, Ithaca, NY. Reproduced with permission from Cornell University Press.

carotid body is too small for measurement. It should be emphasized that stimulation of the receptors is accomplished by the partial pressure of oxygen and carbon dioxide rather than by the amount of oxygen and carbon dioxide. Arterial blood with half as much hemoglobin may have a Po_2 of 100 mmHg, even though it has only half as much oxygen as normal blood (see Figure 23.4, Chapter 23). Any increased respiratory frequency in anemic animals would not be brought about by the oxygen-lack mechanism because the carotid and aortic bodies are responding to the partial pressure of oxygen and not to the amount. Similarly, persons suffering from carbon monoxide poisoning (severe oxygen lack) do not experience a corresponding increase in respiratory frequency because the Po_2 remains normal.

Nerve impulse transmission by the carotid and aortic bodies to the respiratory center varies with the Po_2 perfusing them, as mentioned above. This is illustrated for the carotid bodies by Figure 24.4. Note that the impulse discharge rate is increased most significantly in the Po_2 range 20–60 mmHg and declines rapidly after 60 mmHg. The oxygen–hemoglobin dissociation curve (see Figure 23.4, Chapter 23) shows that hemoglobin is still about 90% saturated with oxygen at a partial pressure of 60 mmHg. Therefore, no serious oxygen lack is present and little change in ventilation occurs.

It is apparent that oxygen regulation is not normally needed. Hemoglobin is nearly saturated at an Po_2 of 100 mmHg, and there would be no advantage to a higher partial pressure. Also, alveolar ventilation can be reduced to about half normal and hemoglobin will retain considerable saturation. Accordingly, it is generally recognized that the leading chemical factor in normal regulation of ventilation resides with carbon dioxide. A ready response is obtained from relatively small changes in its partial pressure. However, regulation by Po_2 becomes more important in pneumonia, pulmonary edema, and the pneumonconioses, where ventilation–perfusion mismatches develop and where gases are not as readily diffusible through the respiratory membrane. Decreased diffusion is more readily noticed for

oxygen than for carbon dioxide because of the smaller diffusion coefficient for oxygen. Furthermore, hyperventilation caused by oxygen lack may reduce Pco_2 and hydrogen ion concentration, whereby they become ineffective in stimulating increased ventilation. The oxygen-lack mechanism continues to function and provides the drive to increase ventilation.

Related regulation factors

> 1 What is the braking effect and what is its significance?
> 2 How is the braking effect minimized during adaptation to high altitude?
> 3 How would you recognize grouped breathing and Cheyne–Stokes breathing?
> 4 How does increased cardiac output and splenic contraction assist the respiratory response to exercise?

Braking effect

It is important to recognize that the accumulation of those substances (carbon dioxide and hydrogen ions) produced by the cells increases ventilation in order to eliminate them and that a reduction in the amount of the substance consumed (oxygen) increases ventilation so that the supply will be replenished. It is just as important to also recognize that reduction of carbon dioxide and hydrogen ions decreases ventilation. This decreased ventilation, in turn, prevents their extreme loss, which otherwise would cause drastic changes in body fluid pH. In other words, hyperventilation might lower the carbon dioxide concentration, and consequently the hydrogen ion concentration, to a point where the body fluids are too alkaline (respiratory alkalosis). This effect, whereby reduced concentrations of carbon dioxide and hydrogen ions decrease alveolar ventilation, is known as the **braking effect**. It can be observed to some extent with increased concentrations of oxygen, but the effect is time dependent and far more subtle. This situation whereby respiratory alkalosis is prevented by the braking effect develops during ascent to high altitudes with reduced oxygen. The braking effects of carbon dioxide and hydrogen ions are most apparent for the first several days, but adaptation reduces their influence so that ventilation can further increase to compensate for the reduced oxygen in the atmosphere. Adaptation is accomplished by renal compensation (see Figure 24.2), whereby hydrogen ions are retained and pH returns toward normal and the braking effect is minimized. The further increase in ventilation provided for by adaptation allows an increase in Pao_2 because of the decrease in $Paco_2$.

Periodic breathing

Breathing is considered abnormal when normal respiratory cycles and frequency patterns do not occur. The cycles sometimes occur in rapid succession (in pairs, triplets, or quadruplets) and are followed by varying intervals of apnea. This has

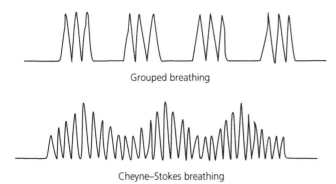

Grouped breathing

Cheyne–Stokes breathing

Figure 24.5 Drawings that illustrate pneumograms of periodic breathing. In grouped breathing, cycles appear in clusters of two or three. In Cheyne–Stokes breathing, cycles alternately wax and wane. From Reece, W.O. (2004) Respiration in mammals. In: *Dukes' Physiology of Domestic Animals*, 12th edn (ed. W.O. Reece). Cornell University Press, Ithaca, NY. Reproduced with permission from Cornell University Press.

been referred to as **grouped breathing** (Figure 24.5). This may be common with head injuries and is frequently observed in animals anesthetized with pentobarbital.

Another form of periodic breathing is known as **Cheyne–Stokes breathing**. This is not frequently reported in veterinary medicine. Perhaps it is unrecognized. It is characterized by successive occurrence of the respiratory cycles in a waxing and waning pattern (Figure 24.5). This breathing pattern is believed to be caused by a delay in the time from perfusion of the lungs with blood to the subsequent arrival of that blood at the brain. In other words, the chemoreceptors may sense an increased P_{aCO_2} and ventilation would be increased. Blood then equilibrates with the hyperventilated lungs, and the P_{aCO_2} is lowered. When this blood reaches the brain, it exerts a braking effect on ventilation and the P_{aCO_2} increases. The pattern of breathing is successively repeated because hyperventilation occurs again with the rise in P_{aCO_2}. In normal breathing, circulation time between the lungs and the brain is relatively short; P_{aCO_2} remains relatively constant, and respiratory cycles are of equal duration.

Another explanation for Cheyne–Stokes breathing postulates that some part of the respiratory control mechanism (possibly a chemoreceptor) has an increased gain so that the response to a stimulus causes an overly large ventilatory response, which in turn produces a larger than normal fall in P_{aCO_2}. The braking effect is initiated and is followed by an oscillatory change in ventilation and blood gases.

Responses to exercise

Exercise and other forms of exertion place a stress on the respiratory system. The response in animals varies considerably, most notably due to prior conditioning and/or health status. This topic is presented in greater detail in Chapter 41. Because of the impingement of exercise on respiration, a brief summary is presented here.

During exercise, oxygen consumption and carbon dioxide production increase. The ventilation rate increases to match these changes. Therefore, during moderate exercise with good preconditioning, little change can be noted in P_{aO_2}, P_{aCO_2}, and arterial pH. However, there is an increase in P_{CO_2} due to greater carbon dioxide production. The increased ventilation is likely due to the activation of joint and muscle receptors because P_{aCO_2} not P_{vCO_2} is the factor that influences ventilation. Cardiac output increases during exercise, resulting in increased pulmonary blood flow. Accordingly, more pulmonary capillaries are perfused (and distended) resulting in more gas exchange. The distribution of blood flow in the lung becomes more uniform, which decreases ventilation–perfusion inequalities where they may have existed. An assist to gas transport during exercise in many animals, most notably the dog and horse, is provided by splenic contraction, whereby a concentrated mass of erythrocytes is forced into the circulation. The response to exercise is different for animals that lack preconditioning and/or are otherwise compromised by health problems (e.g., anemia). This may also apply to a lesser degree in animals with good preconditioning when exertion increases beyond a moderate level. We now notice increased P_{aO_2} and P_{vO_2}, and decreased P_{aCO_2}. These changes are consistent with further increases in ventilation and cardiac output. Also noticed is a decrease in arterial pH (increased hydrogen ion concentration) associated with lactic acid production from anaerobic glycolysis. The increased ventilation is stimulated by the increased hydrogen ion concentration because increased P_{aO_2} and decreased P_{aCO_2} are braking effects to ventilation. The increased cardiac output provides for the transport of greater quantities of oxygen than would otherwise be available, which contributes to the increases in P_{aO_2} and P_{vO_2}.

Self-evaluation

Answers can be found at the end of the chapter.

1 Which one of the Hering–Breuer reflexes would be helpful in initiating an inspiration in an over-anesthetized or otherwise unresponsive dog?
   A Inspiratory-inhibitory reflex (inflation reflex)
   B Inspiratory reflex (deflation reflex)
   Explain your choice for the correct answer.

2 Which sequence of events is the means whereby afferent impulses from baroreceptors in the carotid and aortic sinuses are able to modify respiration and thereby assist return of blood flow to the heart?
   A Blood pressure decrease, increased respiration, increased intrapleural pressure negativity, expansion of the vena cava
   B Blood pressure increase, increased respiration, intrapleural pressure becomes more positive, no change in vena cava
   Explain your choice for the correct answer.

3 Breathing was delayed for 2 min following cessation of hyperventilation with a respirator (braking effect). Before breathing resumes,

cyanosis was very apparent. An arterial blood sample taken just before breathing resumed showed the P_{CO_2} to be 35 mmHg, the pH to be 7.45, and the P_{O_2} to be 40 mmHg. The stimulus for the resumption of breathing was:

A Carbon dioxide

B Hydrogen ion

C Oxygen

Explain your choice for the correct answer.

4 During the development of carbon monoxide poisoning or as observed in anemic (nonexerted) animals:

A Ventilation of the lungs is increased because of hypoxemia

B Ventilation of the lungs is not increased because the P_{O_2} of arterial blood remains normal

C Carbon monoxide does not interfere with oxygen transport and there is no deficiency of hemoglobin

Explain your choice for the correct answer.

5 A calf breathing room air has a pulmonary ventilation rate of 26 L/min. It is placed on a gas mixture, and the rate becomes 22 L/min. The gas mixture most likely is:

A Oxygen enriched

B Carbon dioxide enriched

Explain your choice for the correct answer.

Suggested reading

Hall, J. (2011) *Guyton and Hall Textbook of Medical Physiology*, 12th edn. Saunders Elsevier, Philadelphia.

Reece, W. (2004) Respiration in mammals. In: *Dukes' Physiology of Domestic Animals*, 12th edn (ed. W.O. Reece). Cornell University Press, Ithaca, NY.

Reece, W. (2009) *Functional Anatomy and Physiology of Domestic Animals*, 4th edn. Wiley-Blackwell, Ames, IA.

Answers

1 B. The inspiratory-inhibitory reflex prevents overinflation of the lungs and is activated at the height of inspiration. The inspiratory reflex initiates inspiration at the end of expiration. Compression of the thorax in a nonbreathing dog stimulates the receptors that respond to limiting expiration and that begins the next inspiration.

2 A. When blood pressure is reduced, respiration increases and the thorax is enlarged, providing a greater negativity of intrapleural pressure. The reduction in intrapleural pressure is transmitted to the mediastinal space, which aids in the expansion of the vena cava, lowering the blood pressure within. The lower vena cava pressure assists blood flow to the heart from the more positive pressure in the peripheral veins.

3 C. The P_{CO_2} of 35 mmHg continues to be hypocapnic as a result of the hyperventilation and as such would exert some degree of "braking." Hydrogen ion increase stimulates increased ventilation and the pH of 7.45 (slightly alkaline) reflects some degree of H^+ decrease, so is not a stimulus. The P_{aO_2} of 40 mmHg is a definite stimulus for ventilation and, coupled with the clinical sign of cyanosis (indicates hypoxemia), would account for the resumption of breathing.

4 B. Carotid and aortic bodies are the only places where the P_{O_2} is detected. Stimulation of the receptors is accomplished by the P_{O_2} rather than by the amount of oxygen. Anemic animals may have a decreased amount of hemoglobin but the P_{O_2} in arterial blood may still be 100 mmHg. Accordingly, an increased frequency in anemic animals would not be brought about by the oxygen-lack mechanism because the carotid and aortic bodies are responding to the P_{O_2} and not the amount of oxygen.

5 A. The effect of added oxygen would be a reduction in pulmonary ventilation as opposed to stimulation by oxygen lack. Carbon dioxide enrichment would increase ventilation inasmuch as it is regarded as the leading chemical factor in normal regulation of ventilation.

25 Other Functions of the Respiratory System

William O. Reece

Iowa State University, Ames, IA, USA

Respiratory clearance, panting, and purring are important topics related to serving the respiratory system. Respiratory clearance is the means whereby inhaled materials are processed by the body to minimize harmful outcomes. It has been noted that inspired air, by its intimate contact with blood that circulates to the brain, serves to cool the brain. Also, overall body cooling is served by panting, which is highly developed in the dog. Although the function of purring may not be as apparent, it is common to the feline family and has been studied. Greater detail will be presented for each of these topics and will conclude with terminology common to respiratory pathophysiology.

Respiratory clearance

1 What is meant by respiratory clearance?

2 What are the physical forces that provide for deposition of particles on a mucous membrane?

3 What is the difference between upper respiratory clearance and alveolar clearance?

4 What is the size of particles that are deposited by Brownian motion?

5 What provides for the proximal movement of the mucous blanket?

6 What is the process of development of alveolar phagocytes?

7 How are inhaled particles transported from alveoli to lymph nodes that are in series with lymph vessels that drain from the lungs?

8 What is an example of a pneumoconiosis observed in cats and dogs living in industrialized cities?

The surface area of the inner aspects of the lungs is about 125 times larger than the surface area of the body, and therefore the lungs represent an important route of exposure for many environmental substances. The inhalation of certain agricultural chemicals is a significant health hazard for which precautionary measures to prevent inhalation have been developed. Furthermore, the importance of inhaled particles is apparent when considering the exposure of livestock to the aerosols emanating from feedlot dust or other confinement sources. The aerosols can be combined with bacteria and viruses, so their prompt removal can help to prevent diseases caused by them. Similarly, the removal of irritant substances prevents lung disease and protects lung efficiency.

The removal of particles that have been inhaled into the lungs is called **respiratory clearance**. There are two types, upper respiratory clearance and alveolar clearance, and each depends on the depth to which particles have been inhaled.

Physical forces

Three physical forces operate within the respiratory system to cause settlement of particles from the inhaled air, just as they do to cause settlement of dust from the environmental air outside the body. The settlement of particles on a mucous membrane is referred to as **deposition**. These physical forces are as follows.

1 **Gravitational settling (sedimentation)** causes deposition of particles simply because of the force of gravity and the mass of particles. This provides for deposition in the nasal cavity and the tracheobronchial tree.

2 **Inertial forces** cause deposition in the nasal cavity, the pharynx, and the tracheobronchial tree. Since this deposition involves the factor of velocity, it probably promotes earlier deposition than gravitational settling. It becomes more of a factor at points of branching of the airways where the direction of flow changes. Inertial forces and gravitational settling are probably the most important deposition factors.

Dukes' Physiology of Domestic Animals, Thirteenth Edition. Edited by William O. Reece, Howard H. Erickson, Jesse P. Goff and Etsuro E. Uemura.
© 2015 John Wiley & Sons, Inc. Published 2015 by John Wiley & Sons, Inc.
Companion website: www.wiley.com/go/reece/physiology

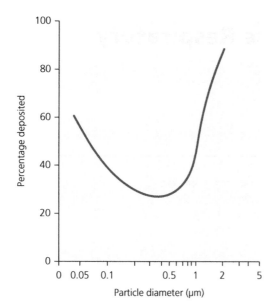

Figure 25.1 Percentage of inhaled particles of unit density deposited in the lung according to their size. Particles in the range of 0.1–1.0 μm are those least affected by combined Brownian motion, sedimentation, and inertial impaction. Adapted from Reece, W.O. (2004) Respiration in mammals. In: *Dukes' Physiology of Domestic Animals*, 12th edn (ed. W.O. Reece). Cornell University Press, Ithaca, NY. Reproduced with permission from Cornell University Press.

Particle deposition increases with increased particle size and increased density for both gravity and inertia.

3 **Brownian motion** accounts for deposition of submicron particles. These very small particles show random motion that is imparted by air molecule bombardment. This factor becomes significant where there is a relatively large area of intimate surface such as in the very small airways and alveoli.

Particle size

The fraction of inhaled particles that is retained in the respiratory system and the depth to which the particles penetrate before deposition are closely related to particle size. Large particles settle on the mucosa of the upper respiratory tract, and smaller particles penetrate more deeply into the lungs. For unit-density particles, those larger than 10 μm are essentially all removed in the nasal cavity. The deposition of particles proximal to the respiratory bronchioles decreases as particle size becomes smaller and is almost zero at diameters of 1 μm or less. Particles that penetrate to the alveolar air spaces (see Figure 21.9, Chapter 21) are generally smaller than 1–2 μm in diameter. Particle deposition is least when the diameters are between 0.3 and 0.5 μm, but begins to increase again when diameters are less than 0.3 μm (Figure 25.1) because particles less than 0.3 μm diameter are more susceptible to Brownian movement.

Upper respiratory tract clearance

Once deposited, particles are cleared (removed) according to the location of their deposition. **Upper respiratory tract clearance** refers to the removal of particles that have been

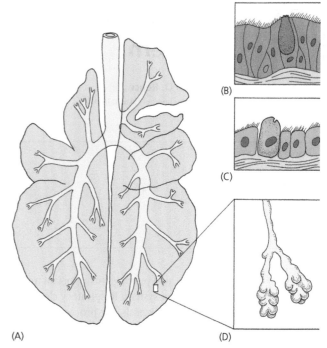

Figure 25.2 Contributors to the moving mucous blanket of the bronchial tree. The moving mucous blanket is directed toward the pharynx by the action of the ciliated cells, and the secretion is provided by the goblet cells of the bronchi, the Clara cells of the bronchioles, and alveolar fluid. (A) Outline of the bovine lung superimposed over the bronchial tree. (B) Pseudostratified epithelium of the bronchi, composed of secretory (goblet) cells, ciliated cells, and basal cells. (C) Cuboidal epithelium of the terminal bronchioles, composed of ciliated cells and secretory (Clara) cells. (D) The terminal bronchiole is the most distal air passage free of alveoli. Adapted from Reece, W.O. (2009) *Functional Anatomy and Physiology of Domestic Animals*, 4th edn. Wiley-Blackwell, Ames, IA. Reproduced with permission from Wiley.

deposited at points proximal to the alveolar ducts. **Alveolar clearance** refers to the removal of particles that have been deposited within the alveoli. Upper respiratory tract clearance is dependent on the proximal movement of a blanket of mucinous fluid. The movement is provided by the ciliary activity of the columnar epithelium lining the tracheobronchial mucous membrane. The components of the mucous blanket are derived from three sources: (i) the film of fluid covering the alveolar membrane, (ii) the apocrine mucus-secreting cells that line the respiratory bronchioles, and (iii) the goblet cells of the tracheobronchial mucosa proximal to the respiratory bronchioles (Figure 25.2). The rate of transport of the mucinous fluid is about 15 mm/min. When the mucous blanket and its contents reach the pharynx, it is ultimately swallowed. This is the means whereby inhaled materials appear in the feces.

Alveolar clearance

Several concepts of alveolar clearance have been developed, as outlined here.

1 There may be specialized absorptive sites near the alveolar ducts. It has been observed that visible deposits of particulate

matter accumulate there. There are distal branches of the lymphatics at that location, and the accumulated particulates and fluid may be awaiting their entry into those lymphatics.

2 There may be a continuous flow of alveolar fluid to the bronchial epithelium, where it is then conveyed onward by the **moving mucous blanket**. It is believed that the fluid flow is facilitated by the mechanical action of breathing and its associated changes in alveolar surface area (increase with inspiration, decrease with expiration). The result is that the cells and the particulate matter on the surface are moved out of the alveoli during expiration while the lower fluid layer follows the changes in surface area with each respiratory cycle. This is similar to the accumulation of driftwood on the beach as water moves toward and recedes from the shore.

3 There is a general consensus that **phagocyte activity** is the most important process for clearance of inhaled insoluble particles and microorganisms. The current view is that alveolar phagocytes develop from monocytes that arrive at the alveolar wall from a capillary and migrate through the epithelial lining to enter the lumen of an alveolus. Once in the alveolus, they transform to **macrophages** and phagocytize large amount of particulate material. These macrophages have frequently been referred to as **dust cells** because of particles noted within their cytoplasm. The process by which macrophages move from the alveoli to the moving mucous blanket is not clearly understood. It may be by random travel or by mechanical and directional assistance derived from alveolar fluid flow.

4 Although alveolar epithelial cells are not considered to be phagocytic, endocytosis does occur and particles may appear within the cytoplasm of these cells. Through normal cell turnover, **desquamation** occurs and they become **free cells** in the alveoli. Their subsequent movement to the moving mucous blanket would provide a clearance mechanism similar to that of macrophages, except that the quantity cleared is less. This mechanism of endocytosis, followed by desquamation and movement to the moving mucous blanket, is the important one in birds.

5 An inhaled particle may be **solubilized** by the alveolar fluid and cleared from the alveolus by absorption. However, a lack of permeability of the alveolar epithelium for the substance would virtually exclude its absorption.

6 It is well known that inhaled particles may be found in **lymph nodes** that are in series with **lymph vessels** that drain from the lungs. For material to enter these vessels, it must first be absorbed or transported from the alveolar epithelium to the interstitial space. It is known that terminal lymphatics are present in the interstitial space distal to the level of alveolar ducts. Inasmuch as lymphatic capillaries are highly permeable, it is no problem for particles to enter their interior. Once the particles have entered the lymph capillaries, they are directed to the lymph nodes where they are either blocked by size or phagocytized by the mononuclear phagocyte system of the lymph nodes.

It has been noted already that phagocytosis facilitates the removal of particles by the alveolar clearance mechanism. It should also be recognized that phagocytosis by macrophages renders particles incapable of irritating or otherwise injuring the alveolar surface epithelium and also prevents penetration of dust particles into the lung interstitial space.

The fate of particles that settle on the alveolar surface may be summarized according to four possibilities.

1 Particles may be transported to the mucous blanket of the tracheobronchial mucosa and thence to the pharynx, where they may be swallowed. This possibility includes free particles on the surface and those that have been phagocytized by macrophages or internalized by endocytosis into alveolar epithelial cells that subsequently desquamate.

2 Particles may be transported to the **satellite lymph nodes** that are in series with lymph vessels that serve the lungs (from which some may escape into the blood).

3 Particles may be dissolved and transferred in solution into either the lymph or the blood.

4 Some particles may fail to be phagocytized or may not be soluble. Instead, they may stimulate a local connective tissue reaction and be **sequestered (isolated)** within the lung. In this event a **pneumoconiosis** may develop from continued exposure. This is a fibrous induration of the lung resulting from inhalation of certain dusts. Examples are **asbestosis** and **silicosis**. Also, dogs and cats that live in highly industrialized cities may show signs of **anthracosis** caused by the inhalation of coal dust.

Panting

> 1 Tidal volume consists of dead space volume and alveolar volume. Which one of these components is regulated to satisfy metabolic needs and which one is regulated to satisfy body temperature needs?
>
> 2 What are the three patterns of panting?
>
> 3 What pattern of panting would provide for the least cooling?
>
> 4 How do patterns 2 and 3 differ in providing the greatest cooling?
>
> 5 What is the greatest source of water for evaporation from the nasal mucosa of the dog?

Panting is prevalent among many animal species, and panting in the dog is described in this section. Perhaps it is similar in the other animals when it occurs. The respiratory center of the dog responds not only to the usual stimuli but also to body core temperature. The integration of these inputs permits the respiratory center to respond to metabolic needs by regulating alveolar ventilation and to dissipation of heat by regulating dead-space ventilation. Dead-space ventilation is increased by panting, which provides for cooling of the body by evaporation of water from the mucous membranes of the tissues involved. Studies have shown that there are three patterns of panting:

1 inhalation and exhalation through the nose;
2 inhalation through the nose, exhalation through the nose and mouth;
3 inhalation through the nose and mouth and exhalation through the nose and mouth.

Passage of air through the nasal cavity allows for more intimate association of air and mucosa than movement of air in the open mouth. Accordingly, it is reasoned that if, during panting, air moved in and out through the mouth only, the tongue and oral surfaces would not humidify the air sufficiently. Correspondingly larger volumes of air would need to be moved to provide cooling equivalent to that of fully saturated air. This would increase the expenditure of energy, and the heat load would increase. If air moved in and out only through the nose, the heat and water vapor added to the air during inhalation would be partially recovered by the body during exhalation. This is because of a countercurrent exchange system that would operate between the airstream and the nasal surfaces. Body cooling in this instance would be lessened.

It can be seen that the least cooling is accomplished by nasal inhalation and exhalation (pattern 1). This pattern has been observed in resting dogs when the ambient temperature was below 26 °C and also when they ran at slow speeds in the cold. Patterns 2 and 3 are observed when dogs rest quietly at ambient temperatures above 30 °C and during exercise, except when exercise occurs at very low temperatures. Air directed through the nose and out the mouth accomplishes the greatest cooling, but where greater tidal volume is needed inhalation through the mouth and nose is necessary. There appears to be continual oscillation between patterns 2 and 3. The proportion of time that pattern 3 is used instead of pattern 2 increases as temperature and activity are increased; pattern 3 is associated with greater alveolar ventilation requirements.

By changing the relative amounts of air exhaled through the nose or through the mouth, the dog can modulate the amount of heat dissipated without changing frequency or tidal volume. The advantage of a constant frequency is that added energy is not then needed to change from the intrinsic panting frequency (about 300 pants per minute) of the respiratory system. A change in tidal volume, especially an increase, could be undesirable because of its effect on hyperventilation and subsequent respiratory alkalosis. Apparently, this extreme may be prevented by ensuring that cooling is achieved by change in air direction (from pattern 1 to pattern 2). Tidal volume increase may be achieved when needed by a change from pattern 1 or 2 to pattern 3.

The airflow characteristics described for panting imply that the nasal mucosa, rather than the oral surfaces and the tongue, is the principal site of evaporation. Accordingly, an adequate supply of water must be provided to the nasal mucosa, and this may be derived from glandular secretions (nasal and orbital), vascular transudate, or both. The secretion from the lateral nasal glands has been studied to determine whether these glands serve to supply additional water during panting. There are two of these glands, one in each maxillary recess. Each gland empties through a single duct that opens about 2 cm inside the nostril. This rostral location is advantageous for caudal distribution of secretion when the airflow is directed into the nose and out through the mouth. The rate of secretion increases with increasing ambient temperature. An increase from 25 to 40 °C increases the amount secreted 40 times. It has been suggested that this role of the lateral nasal glands is analogous to that of sweat glands in humans.

Purring

> 1 How many times per second does alternating activation of the diaphragm and intrinsic laryngeal muscles occur during both inspiration and expiration?
>
> 2 How are each of the 25 successive sounds produced with 1 s of purring during both inspiration and expiration?
>
> 3 What would seem to be the function of purring?

Purring is noted in some members of the feline family and is both audible and palpable in most domestic cats. The following explanation of purring is derived from a reported study in the domestic cat. The study used electromyographic and tracheal pressure recording techniques and showed that the purr results from a highly regular, alternating activation of the diaphragm and intrinsic laryngeal muscles at a frequency of 25 times per second during both inspiration and expiration. The study showed that purring probably results from some oscillating mechanism within the central nervous system. Each repeated cycle has three phases: (i) glottal closing, (ii) initiation of glottal opening and sound production, and (iii) complete glottal opening (low glottal resistance and high airflow).

Glottal closing occurs when the adductor muscles of the larynx contract (i.e., the vocal cords become approximated). Each of the 25 successive sounds associated with 1 s of purring is produced when a pressure difference created on either side of the closed glottis is dissipated at the time when glottal opening begins (i.e., there is a sudden separation of the vocal cords). Glottal opening may be passive, but there is speculation that contraction of the laryngeal abductor muscles during inspiration occurs simultaneously with contraction of the diaphragm.

During the inspiratory phase of the respiratory cycle, there is also intermittent contraction of the diaphragm. In other words, diaphragmatic contraction alternates with laryngeal adductor contraction (glottal closure). The alternating contractions of the laryngeal adductors and of the diaphragm prevent extreme negativity in tracheal pressure at the time of glottal closure and also promote inspiratory flow during the time the glottis is open. Airflow during inspiration is provided by the intermittent contraction of the diaphragm and the lung expansion that follows. Repeated cycling and sound production continue until inspiration is complete.

During the expiratory phase of the respiratory cycle, the recoil tendency of the lungs creates tracheal pressure that is greater than pharyngeal pressure when the glottis is closed. When the laryngeal adductors relax, the glottis opens, the higher tracheal pressure forces air through the vocal cords, a sound is produced, the glottis closes (the vocal cords become approximated), tracheal pressure increases, and the cycle repeats until expiration is completed.

The reason for purring in cats is not known. It is known to occur at times when they are contented, when they are sick, and when they are sleeping. It seems possible that the intermittent nature of the inspiratory and expiratory phases of the respiratory cycle when a cat is purring may provide improved ventilation and prevent atelectasis during times of shallow breathing. In other words, purring may provide a function similar to complementary breaths.

Pathophysiology terminology

> 1 Is cyanosis a sign of hypercapnia or improper oxygenation of blood?
>
> 2 What is asphyxia?
>
> 3 What is the usual cause of atelectasis?

Hypoxia

Hypoxia is a decrease below normal Po_2 in air, blood, or tissue, short of anoxia. **Anoxia** literally means "without oxygen" and should not be used when the condition may be one of decreased Po_2, for which the term "hypoxia" is more appropriate. **Hypoxemia** is a decrease in the oxygen concentration of the arterial blood. Four types of hypoxia are recognized.

1 **Ambient hypoxia:** the arterial blood is insufficiently saturated with oxygen because of a low Po_2 in the atmosphere being breathed. This occurs naturally at high altitudes.

2 **Anemic hypoxia:** there is a decrease in the oxygen capacity of the blood because of a shortage of functioning hemoglobin. The Po_2 in arterial blood and the percentage saturation of hemoglobin are normal. Oxygen delivery to the tissues may be inadequate. Anemic hypoxia occurs after hemorrhage, in various anemias, and when some of the hemoglobin is changed to methemoglobin or is combined with carbon monoxide.

3 **Stagnant hypoxia,** also known as **ischemic hypoxia:** blood flow through the whole body or a tissue is diminished. The oxygen content of arterial blood is normal, but the tissues fail to receive enough oxygen because of diminished blood flow.

4 **Histotoxic hypoxia:** the cells are unable to use the oxygen that is supplied. The amount of oxygen in arterial blood is normal, but because the cells are unable to use it, the amount is above normal in venous blood.

Other terms

Hypercapnia and **hypocapnia** are increased and decreased $Paco_2$, respectively, in arterial blood and are indicative of hypoventilation and hyperventilation. **Cyanosis** is a bluish or purplish coloration of the skin and mucous membranes. The color reflects the degree of deoxygenation of hemoglobin. When observed throughout the body, it relates to improper oxygenation of blood. When seen locally, it is probably caused by blood flow obstruction.

Asphyxia is a condition of hypoxia combined with hypercapnia. Breathing into a closed space provides a good example, and this results in what is commonly called suffocation.

Hyperbaric oxygenation is the provision of oxygen to the body at relatively high partial pressure. The Po_2 may be extreme to the point that oxygen toxicity occurs. When this happens, there is a marked elevation of the Po_2 in the cells (**hyperoxia**) and the activity of many enzymes involved in tissue metabolism is affected.

Atelectasis is failure of the alveoli to open or remain open and usually involves one or more relatively small areas of lung. The usual cause of atelectasis is occlusion of the bronchus or bronchiole that supplies the area. This results most often from plugs of mucus or purulent exudate. When the bronchus closes, the air contained in the alveoli at the time is absorbed and the airless alveoli collapse because of the surrounding pressures. Also, breathing high oxygen mixtures lowers/removes nitrogen which normally acts as an alveolar stent. Thus, during high oxygen breathing, all the gas may be absorbed from alveoli, and they become atelectatic.

Pneumonia is an acute inflammation of the lung that occurs in all species from a variety of causes. In the first stage the capillaries are distended with blood and the alveoli become filled with serous fluid. The serous fluid becomes mixed with erythrocytes, various leukocytes, and fibrin. Final resolution involves liquefaction of the alveolar debris, its removal, and regeneration of the alveolar epithelium.

Self-evaluation

Answers can be found at the end of the chapter.

1 Which one of the following forms of particle deposition becomes more of a factor at points of airway branching?
   A Gravitational settling
   B Inertial forces
   C Brownian motion
   Explain your choice for the correct answer.

2 Which one of the following alveolar clearance concepts would favor the development of a pneumoconiosis?
   A Internalized by alveolar epithelial cells that subsequently desquamate
   B Transport to satellite lymph nodes
   C Are neither soluble nor fail to be phagocytized
   Explain your choice for the correct answer.

3 Which pattern of panting provides for the greatest cooling?
   A Inhalation and exhalation through the nose
   B Inhalation through the nose, and exhalation through the nose and mouth

C Inhalation through the nose and mouth and exhalation through the nose and mouth

Explain your choice for the correct answer.

4 Which type of hypoxia defines the condition where the cells are unable to use the oxygen that is supplied?

A Anemic hypoxia

B Ischemic hypoxia

C Histotoxic hypoxia

Explain your choice for the correct answer.

5 Which one of the following terms best describes asphyxia?

A Hypoxia combined with hypercapnia

B Atelectasis

C Pneumonia

Explain your choice for the correct answer.

Suggested reading

Blatt, C., Taylor, C. and Habel, B. (1972) Thermal panting in dogs: the nasal gland, a source of water for evaporative cooling. *Science* 177:804–805.

Morrow, P. (1973) Alveolar clearance of aerosols. *Archives of Internal Medicine* 133:101–108.

Reece, W. (2004) Respiration in mammals. In: *Dukes' Physiology of Domestic Animals*, 12th edn (ed. W.O. Reece), pp. 114–148. Cornell University Press, Ithaca, NY.

Answers

1 B. Inertial forces account for deposition of particles not previously deposited by gravitational settling. It involves the factor of velocity and directional change associated with airway branching.

2 C. Pneumoconiosis develops because the particles are not removed from the lung and they stimulate a local tissue reaction and become sequestered within the lung, and with continued exposure a pneumoconiosis may develop.

3 C. Cooling involves evaporation of water and the nasal mucosa is the principal site rather than the oral surfaces and the tongue. Adequate supply of water is derived from nasal and orbital glandular secretions. These are in a rostral location and their secretion is advantageous when airflow is directed into the nose and out through the mouth. The greatest surface area exposure occurs when both inhalation and expiration occur through the nose and mouth.

4 C. Histotoxic hypoxia occurs when the cells are unable to use the oxygen that is supplied. Ischemic hypoxia also has normal arterial oxygen content but the tissues fail to receive it because of diminished blood flow. Anemic hypoxia applies to a decrease in the oxygen capacity of the blood because of a shortage of functioning hemoglobin.

5 A. Asphyxia is a decrease below the normal amount of oxygen in the blood coupled with an increased carbon dioxide. It is also known as suffocation. Atelectasis is a failure of the alveoli to open or remain open that usually involves one or more relatively small areas of the lung. Pneumonia is an acute inflammation of the lung.

26 Respiration in Birds

John W. Ludders

College of Veterinary Medicine, Cornell University, Ithaca, NY, USA

The class Aves consists of 27 orders, 168 families and approximately 10,000 species worldwide. Birds, representing the only clade of dinosaurs to have survived the Cretaceous–Paleogene extinction event 65.5 million years ago, inhabit every continent on this planet and live in a wide range of environmental niches, some inhospitable to humans.

In 1981 Dr John B. West led the American Medical Research Expedition to the summit of Mount Everest to obtain data on human respiratory physiology at extreme altitudes. As expedition members climbed toward the mountain's summit (8848 m), some with oxygen cylinders strapped to their backs, they looked up at the cobalt blue sky and saw a flock of bar-headed geese (*Anser indicus*) flying over the Himalayan peaks at more than 9375 m (30,750 feet) during their annual migration between the Indian Subcontinent and the South–Central Asian Lakes. How can birds extract sufficient oxygen at such high altitudes and be able to maintain bodily functions while meeting the demands of exercising muscle? In large part the answer is the avian pulmonary system, so unlike the mammalian pulmonary system, and very efficient at gas exchange.

Humans have been fascinated with birds for millennia probably because of their ability to fly and their inherent beauty. Humans have also had a more practical interest in birds as a source of food. In the process of domesticating and selecting for certain desirable production characteristics, such as rapid weight gain or high egg-laying capability, a number of structural and functional changes have occurred in domesticated species that are not seen in their wild counterparts. For example, a line of turkeys selected for rapid weight gain have lower lung volume and gas exchange surface area compared to turkeys not so selected. Layer chickens also have a smaller lung volume relative to body weight, a lower oxygen diffusing capacity, and a greater blood–air capillary volume ratio than their wild ancestor, the red jungle fowl. Thus when studying avian physiology it is important to keep in mind that important physiological differences exist between wild and domesticated birds.

Avian respiratory anatomy

1 How does the avian trachea differ from the mammalian trachea? What are the functional implications of these anatomic differences?

2 What are the possible consequences for an anesthetized intubated bird if the cuff of an endotracheal tube is overinflated?

3 How many orders of branching of the bronchi occur prior to reaching the gas-exchange surfaces of the avian lung?

4 What is another name for a tertiary bronchus?

5 What role do the air sacs play in ventilation?

6 During ventilation, do birds have a volume of gas that is equivalent to tidal volume?

7 How might the air sacs be used to help ventilate a bird that has an upper airway obstruction?

8 What are the two types of tertiary bronchial (parabronchial) tissue that may be found in avian lungs?

9 Where does gas exchange occur in the avian lung?

10 What two factors contribute to gas exchange efficiency in birds?

Dukes' Physiology of Domestic Animals, Thirteenth Edition. Edited by William O. Reece, Howard H. Erickson, Jesse P. Goff and Etsuro E. Uemura.
© 2015 John Wiley & Sons, Inc. Published 2015 by John Wiley & Sons, Inc.
Companion website: www.wiley.com/go/reece/physiology

The avian pulmonary system consists of two functionally separate and distinct components: one for ventilation (trachea, bronchi, air sacs, thoracic skeleton, and muscles of respiration), and one for gas exchange (parabronchial lung).

Trachea

As in mammals, the avian trachea conducts air from the nares and mouth to the bronchi while warming, moisturizing, and screening particulate matter from inspired gas. Anatomically, however, significant differences exist between the avian trachea and the mammalian trachea. Avian tracheal cartilages are complete rings unlike the incomplete C-shaped rings of mammals. From one class of birds to another, unlike in mammals, there are tremendous variations in tracheal anatomy that have significant implications for ventilation. For example, emu and ruddy ducks have an inflatable sac-like diverticulum that opens from the trachea and the males of many waterfowl species have a tracheal bulbous expansion. Some penguins and petrels have a double trachea, while other classes of birds have complex tracheal loops or coils that may be located in the caudal neck, within the keel, or within the thorax and keel (Figure 26.1). With their relatively long necks, not to mention tracheal loops and coils, the typical bird trachea is 2.7 times longer than that of a comparably sized mammal, but it is also 1.29 times wider so resistance to airflow through the trachea in birds is comparable to that in mammals (see Poiseuille's law for laminar flow,

Chapter 22). Tracheal volume, on the other hand, is about 4.5 times greater than that of comparably sized mammals. The impact of the larger tracheal dead-space volume is reduced in at least three ways: (i) birds have a relatively low respiratory frequency (approximately one-third that of mammals) so that minute tracheal ventilation rate is only about 1.5–1.9 times greater than that of comparably sized mammals (see ventilation formulas, Chapter 23); (ii) tidal volume in birds is about 1.7 times larger than that of a comparably sized mammal; and (iii) the large expansible volume and greater compliance of the respiratory system means that birds expend less energy when breathing compared with mammals, so they are able to overcome any limitations imposed by the larger tracheal dead space.

Bronchi

Mammals have many orders of bronchial branching leading to the gas-exchange area of the lung (the alveoli), but the bronchial system of birds consists of only three orders of branching before the gas-exchange surfaces are reached: a primary bronchus (extrapulmonary and intrapulmonary), secondary bronchi, and tertiary bronchi, more commonly referred to as parabronchi (Figure 26.2).

Primary bronchi

Each primary bronchus enters a lung ventrally and obliquely at the junction of the cranial and middle thirds of the lung, then passes dorsolaterally to the lung surface where it turns caudally

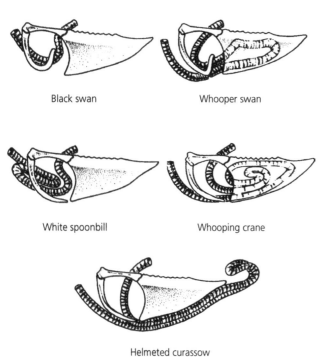

Black swan   Whooper swan

White spoonbill   Whooping crane

Helmeted curassow

Figure 26.1 Tracheal loops found in birds: black swan (*Cygnus atratus*); whooper swan (*Cygnus cygnus*); white spoonbill (*Platalea leucorodia*); whooping crane (*Grus americana*); helmeted curassow (*Crax pauxi*). Adapted from McLelland, J. (1989) Larynx and trachea. In: *Form and Function in Birds* (eds A.S. King and J. McLelland), Vol. 4, pp. 69–103. Academic Press, New York. Reproduced with permission from Elsevier.

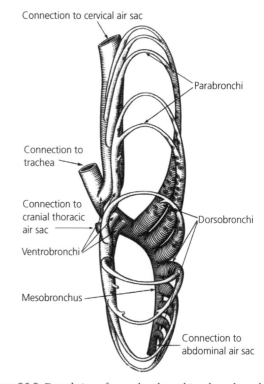

Figure 26.2 Dorsal view of secondary bronchi and parabronchi in the right lung of a goose. From Brackenbury, J.H. (1987) Ventilation of the lung–air sac system. In: *Bird Respiration*, Vol. I (ed. T.J. Seller). CRC Press, Boca Raton, FL. Image provided by Professor J.H. Brackenbury. Reproduced with permission from Taylor & Francis.

in a dorsally curved course until it opens at the caudal lung margin into the abdominal air sac. The primary bronchi have a well-developed layer of smooth muscle consisting of an internal circular smooth muscle layer and a longitudinally oriented layer of smooth muscle. In response to stimuli such as acetylcholine, pilocarpine, and histamine, these smooth muscles can change the internal diameter of the primary bronchus.

Secondary bronchi

Any bronchus arising from a primary bronchus is a secondary bronchus. In most birds the secondary bronchi are arranged into four groups: medioventral, mediodorsal, lateroventral, and laterodorsal secondary bronchi. The medioventral secondary bronchi arise from the primary intrapulmonary bronchus close to where it enters the lung, while the mediodorsal, lateroventral, and laterodorsal secondary bronchi arise from the caudal

curved portion of the primary intrapulmonary bronchus. Depending on the species, between the medioventral group of secondary bronchi and the three remaining groups is a section of primary bronchus, the **intrapulmonary bronchus or mesobronchus**, that is devoid of secondary bronchi. Many of the medioventral and lateroventral secondary bronchi open into the cervical, clavicular, and cranial thoracic, or abdominal air sacs.

Tertiary bronchi (parabronchi)

The tertiary bronchus (parabronchus) and its mantle of surrounding tissue is the basic unit for gas exchange (Figure 26.3). Parabronchi are long narrow tubes that display a high degree of anastomosis. There is a network of smooth muscle surrounding the entrances to the parabronchi that appears to be controlled by the **vagus nerve**, because when it is electrically stimulated the smooth muscle contracts and narrows the openings to the

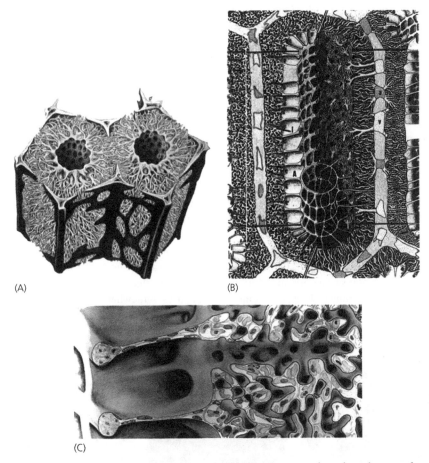

(A)

(B)

(C)

Figure 26.3 Three-dimensional drawings of parabronchi, atria and infundibula. (A) Two parabronchi and surrounding tissue consisting of air capillaries and blood capillaries where gas exchange occurs. (B) Single parabronchus cut longitudinally; on the left side are atria (A) with infundibula (I) departing from them and the three-dimensional air capillary meshwork arising from the infundibula. On the right side, within the inter-parabronchial septa are the arterioles (dense stippling) from which the capillaries originate and run radially toward the lumen. The infundibula lie between the capillaries, which are surrounded by a well-developed three-dimensional air capillary network. (C) Cross-section of atria and infundibula. Two circular smooth muscle bundles bound the opening leading from the parabronchus into the atrium; atria are separated by septa running horizontally and vertically. Originating from each atrium are a few infundibula that pass perpendicularly into the parabronchial mantle. At the far right an infundibulum is shown in longitudinal section with air capillaries arising from it at all levels. The air capillaries cross-link and interlace with blood capillaries. The very thin epithelium of the air capillaries and its surfactant film are shown as a single dark line. From Duncker, H.-R. (1974) Structure of the avian respiratory tract. *Respiration Physiology* 22:1–19, with permission from Elsevier Science and Professor Duncker; digital images kindly provided by Professor Duncker.

parabronchi. The inner surfaces of the tubular parabronchi are pierced by numerous pentagonal or hexagonal openings into chambers called atria that are separated from each other by inter-atrial septa (Figure 26.3C). The inter-atrial septa are covered by a thin epithelial layer with a core of densely packed bundles of smooth muscle that frame the atrial openings. Since the avian lung is richly innervated with vagal and sympathetic nerves, it is possible that afferent and efferent neural pathways exist for controlling pulmonary smooth muscle and thus varying airflow through the parabronchial lung.

Air capillaries and peri-parabronchial mantle

In each atria and arising from the atrial surface opposite the parabronchial opening are funnel-shaped ducts (infundibula) that lead to air capillaries (Figure 26.3C). The air capillaries, which are 3–20 μm in diameter depending on the species, form an anastomosing three-dimensional network that is intimately interlaced with a similarly structured network of blood capillaries (Figure 26.4); gas exchange occurs within this mantle of interlaced air and blood capillaries. The surface area for gas exchange varies from species to species, from a low of about 10 cm²/g body weight in the domestic chicken to a high of 87 cm²/g in the hummingbird. In bats, the only flying mammal, the surface area is 63 cm²/g, while in shrews and humans the value is 33 and 18 cm²/g, respectively. Thickness of the blood–gas barrier is also important as it affects gas diffusion across the barrier (see factors affecting gas diffusion, Chapter 22); as the barrier thickness increases, gas diffusion decreases. The most meaningful estimator of diffusing capacity (or conductance) of the blood–gas barrier is its **harmonic mean thickness** (τ_{ht}), defined as the mean of the reciprocal of the barrier thickness at each point in the barrier. The harmonic mean thickness in domestic chickens and hummingbirds is 0.318 and 0.099 μm, respectively, while in bats, shrews and humans it is 0.219, 0.338, and 0.620 μm, respectively. The greater surface area and thinner mean harmonic thickness of the avian lung make it an extremely efficient gas exchanger, more so than the mammalian lung.

Types of parabronchial tissue

The avian lung consists of two types of parabronchial tissue (Figure 26.5): (i) **paleopulmonic parabronchial tissue** is found in all birds and consists of parallel stacks of profusely anastomosing parabronchi (Figure 26.5A); and (ii) **neopulmonic parabronchial tissue** consisting of a meshwork of anastomosing parabronchi located in the caudolateral portion of the lung, its degree of development being species dependent (Figure 26.5B,C). Penguins and emu have only paleopulmonic parabronchi. Pigeons, ducks, and cranes have both paleopulmonic and neopulmonic parabronchi, with the neopulmonic parabronchi accounting for 10–12% of total lung volume. In fowl-like birds and songbirds the neopulmonic parabronchi are more developed and may account for 20–25% of total lung volume. Paleopulmonic and neopulmonic parabronchi are histologically indistinguishable from each other, but the direction of gas flow differs within the two types.

Through anatomic and physiologic studies using latex rubber casts and gas washout techniques, the specific volume (respiratory gas volume per unit of body mass) of the avian respiratory system is estimated to be between 100 and 200 mL/kg, but the volume of gas in parabronchi and air capillaries accounts for only 10% of the total specific volume. By comparison, a dog's specific volume is 45 mL/kg, and pulmonary gas volume in the mammalian lung is 96% of the total specific volume. Because the ratio of residual gas volume (i.e., gas in the lungs) to tidal volume is so much smaller in birds than in mammals, it has been suggested that cyclic changes in direction of paleopulmonic parabronchial gas flow, such as reversal of gas flow, would adversely affect gas exchange. The unidirectional flow of gas within the paleopulmonic lung solves this problem (see section Mechanics of ventilation). In addition, it appears that the volume of parabronchial gas available for gas exchange may be larger than anatomic studies indicate, possibly because of factors such as the effect of cardiac-generated pulses in the pulmonary capillaries, somewhat analogous to the effects of high-frequency ventilation.

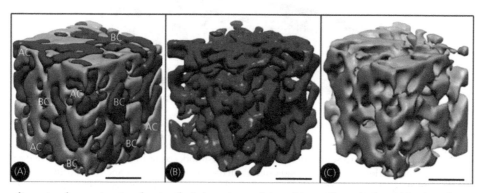

Figure 26.4 Three-dimensional reconstruction showing the intimate intertwining of air capillaries (AC) and blood capillaries (BC) in the paleopulmonic lung of the ostrich (*Struthio camelus*). (A) Combined three-dimensional reconstruction of blood capillaries (red) and air capillaries (cyan). (B) Three-dimensional reconstruction showing the blood capillaries. (C) Three-dimensional reconstruction of air capillaries. Scale bars, 20 μm. From Maina, J.N. (2009) Three-dimensional serial section computer reconstruction of the arrangement of the structural components of the parabronchus of the ostrich, *Struthio camelus*, lung. *Anatomical Record* 292:1685–1698. Reproduced with permisiosn from Wiley.

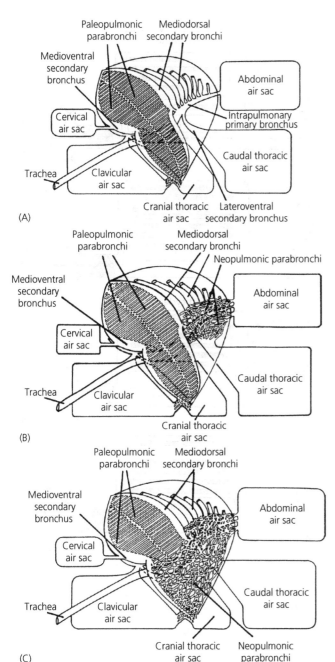

Figure 26.5 Drawings of paleopulmonic and neopulmonic parabronchial lungs (right lungs). (A) The paleopulmonic lung found in penguins and emus. (B) The paleopulmonic and neopulmonic lung found in storks, ducks and geese. (C) The paleopulmonic and more highly developed neopulmonic lung found in chickens, sparrows and other songbirds. From Fedde, M.R. (1980) Structure and gas-flow pattern in the avian respiratory system. *Poultry Science* 59:2642–2653. Reproduced with permission from *Poultry Science*.

Air sacs

Birds have nine air sacs: two cervical, an unpaired clavicular, two cranial thoracic, two caudal thoracic, and two abdominal air sacs. Histologically, the air sacs are thin-walled structures composed of simple squamous epithelium covering a thin layer

of connective tissue; they are poorly vascularized and for this reason do not significantly contribute to gas exchange. To varying extent, depending on the species, diverticula from the air sacs aerate the cervical vertebrae, some of the thoracic vertebrae, vertebral ribs, sternum, humerus, pelvis, and head and body of the femur, and possibly the pectoral muscles.

Functionally, the air sacs serve as bellows to the lungs by providing tidal airflow to the relatively rigid avian lung. Based on their bronchial connections, air sacs are grouped into a cranial group consisting of cervical, clavicular, and cranial thoracic air sacs, and a caudal group consisting of caudal thoracic and abdominal air sacs. The volume of the air sacs is distributed approximately equally between the cranial and caudal groups. During ventilation all air sacs are effectively ventilated, with the possible exception of the cervical air sacs, and the ratio of ventilation to volume is similar for each air sac.

In domestic species, such as chickens, ventilation is much reduced when birds are placed in dorsal recumbency. A number of factors may contribute to this phenomenon, not the least of which may be heavy breast muscles or the weight of abdominal viscera either increasing the work of ventilation or compressing the abdominal air sacs. The latter would reduce their volume and thus their effective tidal volume and flow of gas across the gas-exchange surfaces of the lung. However, recent studies involving red-tailed hawks have shown that ventilation is unaffected when these birds are positioned in dorsal recumbency. This supports the contention that domestication and selection for certain desirable production characteristics in domestic fowl have resulted in a number of structural and functional changes that may affect ventilation, but which are not observed in wild species.

Mechanics of ventilation

1 What are the consequences for a bird if thoracic movement, especially that of the keel (sternum), is impeded during restraint for physical examination? What might be the consequences of obesity on ventilation? What might be the consequences of body position on ventilation such as when a bird is turned on to its back?

2 In birds, does inspiration require active contraction of the muscles of ventilation? Does expiration require active contraction of the muscles of ventilation?

3 In birds, what would be the pulmonary consequence of relaxing the muscles of ventilation as can occur during anesthesia?

4 What mechanisms control the direction of gas flow within the avian pulmonary system? Would positive pressure ventilation adversely affect gas flow and gas exchange?

5 Describe the two types of parabronchi and the direction of gas flow in each.

Muscles of respiration and the thoracic skeleton

Birds do not possess a muscular diaphragm, but depend on cervical, thoracic and abdominal muscles for inspiration and expiration, both of which are active processes requiring muscular

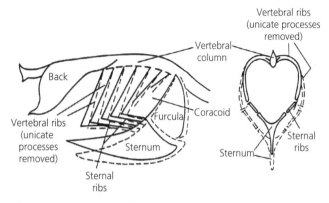

Figure 26.6 Changes in the position of the thoracic skeleton during breathing in a bird. The solid lines represent thoracic position at the end of expiration while the dotted lines show the thoracic position at the end of inspiration. From Fedde, M.R. (1986) Respiration. In: *Avian Physiology* (ed. P.D. Sturkie), 4th edn, pp. 191–220. Springer-Verlag, New York. Reproduced with permision from Springer.

activity. During inspiration, the inspiratory muscles contract and the internal volume of the thoracoabdominal cavity increases (Figure 26.6). Since air sacs are the only significant volume-compliant structures within the body cavity, their volume also increases. As pressure within the air sacs becomes negative relative to ambient atmospheric pressure, air flows from the atmosphere into the pulmonary system (Figure 26.7). As a result of inspiratory valving (see next paragraph), during inspiration there is little or no flow in the ventrobronchi that connect the parabronchi and the intrapulmonary bronchus (mesobronchus) and, as a result, inspired gas flows caudally through the meso-bronchus. A portion of the gas crosses the neopulmonic lung and continues into the caudal thoracic and abdominal air sacs, while a portion goes to the dorsobronchi and thence across the paleo-pulmonic lung. During contraction of the expiratory muscles the internal volume of the thoracoabdominal cavity decreases, pressure within the air sacs increases, and gas flows out of the caudal thoracic and abdominal air sacs, crosses the neopulmonic lungs to the paleopulmonic lungs, and thence out the ventro-bronchi and trachea to the environment. Gas flow from the cranial air sacs does not pass back through the parabronchi but goes directly to the ventrobronchi, the trachea and thence the environment. During expiration there is little or no flow in the intrapulmonary bronchus (mesobronchus) as a result of expiratory valving (see next paragraph).

During inspiration and expiration the direction of gas flow in the paleopulmonic parabronchi is unidirectional, but in the neopulmonic parabronchi it is bidirectional. Although poorly understood, the mechanisms responsible for the unidirectional flow of gas through the intrapulmonary bronchus, the secondary bronchi, and the paleopulmonic parabronchi are probably governed by processes that create **aerodynamic valves**, which are not mechanical valves such as valve leaflets or tissue dams. Aerodynamic valving occurs during both inspiration and expiration, but the controlling factors for each

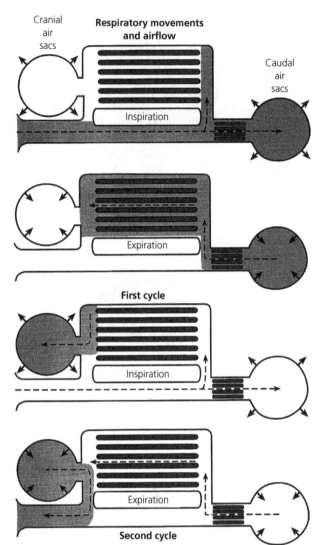

Figure 26.7 Pathway of airflow associated with inspiration and expiration in birds. The same bolus of air (darkened area) is followed through two respiratory cycles. It can be seen that ventilation of the parabronchial mantle is accomplished during inspiration and during expiration. Air going to the caudal air sacs ventilates the neopulmonic mantle, and as it leaves it ventilates both neopulmonic and paleo-pulmonic mantles. When the cranial air sacs expand during inspiration, they are filled by air that has passed through the parabronchial mantles. Cranial air sac air is then directed to the exterior during expiration without ventilating parabronchial mantles. Modified from Scheid, P., Slama, H. and Piiper, J. (1972) Mechanisms of unidirectional flow in parabronchi of avian lungs: measurements in duck lung preparations. *Respiratory Physiology* 14:83–95. Reproduced with permission from Elsevier.

appear to vary. **Inspiratory valving** occurs primarily as a consequence of gas convective inertial forces (gas flow and density), and the accelerating effects of a constriction in the primary bronchus just cranial to where the ventrobronchi arise. Additional factors involved in inspiratory valving include the orientation of secondary bronchial and air sac orifices in relation to the direction of gas flow, and pressure differences between the cranial and caudal groups of air sacs. The net effect is that the inspired gas stream continues straight along the axis of the primary bronchus and intrapulmonary bronchus (mesobronchus) rather than turning into the ventro-bronchi and the cranial air sacs. **Expiratory valving**, or that mechanism directing gas from the caudal thoracic and abdominal air sacs to and through the dorsobronchi and then the parabronchi, is not influenced by gas density but by dynamic compression of the intrapulmonary bronchus, a phenomenon affected by viscous resistance and gas flow. Dynamic compression occurs when pressure in the air sacs is greater than the pressure in the lumen of the intrapulmonary bronchus. As a result of this pressure gradient the diameter of the bronchus tends to narrow or collapse. In addition, the greater the gas flow, the greater the pressure exerted on the bronchus. In general, the efficiency of both inspiratory and expiratory valving decreases at low flows.

Gas exchange

1 What physiologic model best describes gas exchange in the avian lung?
2 Do air sacs significantly contribute to gas exchange?
3 Do birds have a volume of gas that is equivalent to mammalian alveolar gas?

The gas-exchange efficiency of the avian lung is greater than that of the mammalian lung. The **cross-current model** has been used historically to describe the relationship between gas and blood flows within the avian lung; this model has also been the basis for mathematically modeling gas exchange (Figure 26.8). Three-dimensional computer reconstruction of the avian lung provides evidence that a **counter-current mechanism** also exists within the avian lung, but its contribution to gas exchange remains to be elucidated (Figure 26.9). In birds there is no equivalent of alveolar gas because parabronchial gas continuously changes in composition as it flows along the length of the parabronchus. The degree to which oxygen is extracted from respired gas and added to capillary blood, and carbon dioxide removed from the blood and added to respired gas, depends on where along the length of the parabronchus and for how long blood contacts the blood–gas interface. The efficiency of the avian lung can be put into perspective by considering what happens to the partial pressures of carbon dioxide and oxygen both in respired gas as it flows through the lung and in blood as it perfuses the lung. As gas flows along the parabronchus it receives carbon dioxide and gives off oxygen so that gas at the inflow end of the parabronchus has the lowest partial pressure of carbon dioxide and gas at the outflow end of the parabronchus has the highest partial pressure of carbon dioxide; the reverse is true for oxygen. The overall result is that in end-parabronchial gas the partial pressure of carbon dioxide (PE_{CO_2}) can exceed the partial pressure of carbon dioxide in

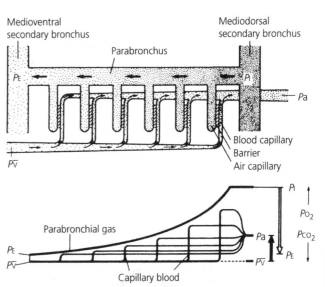

Figure 26.8 Cross-current model for avian parabronchial gas exchange. (*Top*) Schematic of a parabronchus with radially departing air capillaries. Blood capillaries are also shown running from the periphery toward the lumen of the parabronchus and contacting the air capillaries for only a small fraction of the parabronchial length. (*Bottom*) Partial pressure profiles of the gas phase from the initial parabronchial values (PI) to end-parabronchial values (PE), and partial pressure profiles in blood of the blood capillaries showing that arterial blood (Pa) is derived as a mixture from all capillaries. The arrows at right show the overlap in the ranges of gas (open arrow) and blood (closed arrow) partial pressures (i.e., PCO_2 is lower and PO_2 higher in blood than respective values in parabronchial gas), a phenomenon that cannot occur for arterial blood exposed to alveolar gas in the mammalian lung. From Scheid, P. and Piiper, J. (1987) Gas exchange and transport. In: *Bird Respiration*, Vol. 1 (ed. T.J. Seller), pp. 97–129. CRC Press, Boca Raton, FL. Reproduced with permission from Taylor & Francis.

arterial blood (Pa_{CO_2}), and the partial pressure of oxygen (PE_{O_2}) can be lower than the partial pressure of oxygen in arterial blood (Pa_{O_2}). This potential overlap of blood and gas partial pressure ranges for carbon dioxide and oxygen (something that cannot occur in the mammalian alveolar lung) demonstrates the high gas exchange efficiency of the avian lung. For a number of reasons, however, this gas-exchange efficiency usually is not apparent under resting conditions (Table 26.1), but becomes readily apparent under conditions of stress or exercise such as hyperthermia, hypoxia, or during flight at altitude.

A number of factors can limit gas-exchange efficiency in the avian lung, including mismatching of ventilation and perfusion, diffusion barriers, and inhomogeneities within the lung. The movement of gas within the parabronchi is by convective flow, while diffusion is the primary gas transport mechanism in the air capillaries. However, in a study of ducks that inhaled iron oxide particles (particles with a diffusion coefficient three orders of magnitude less than that of nitrogen or oxygen), the particles were found in atria and infundibula suggesting that some degree of convective transport occurs at this level. Nonetheless, anything that increases barriers to diffusion will adversely affect gas exchange.

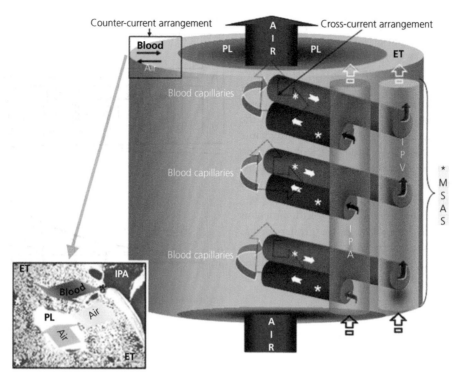

Figure 26.9 A schematic diagram showing the cross-current and counter-current relationships between air and blood in the lung of the ostrich. The cross-current arrangement occurs as a result of the perpendicular orientation between the flow of air along the parabronchial lumen (PL) (deep blue vertical arrow) and that of venous blood into the exchange tissue (ET) from the periphery (dashed arrows). The counter-current relationship occurs as a result of the flow of air from the parabronchial lumen (PL) into the air capillaries and that of venous blood flowing from the periphery of the parabronchus. The exchange tissue is supplied with venous blood by inter-parabronchial arteries (IPA) that give rise to arterioles (stars) that terminate in blood capillaries. Oxygenated blood flows into the intra-parabronchial venules (asterisks) that drain into inter-parabronchial veins (IPV) and thence into the pulmonary vein which returns blood to the heart. The arrangement of the inter-parabronchial arteries and veins along the parabronchus forms a multicapillary serial arterialization system (MSAS) where respiratory gases are exchanged at infinitely many points where the air and blood capillaries contact. (*Inset*) The cross-current orientation between bulk airflow along the parabronchial lumen (PL) (large green arrow) and that of venous blood inwards (large red arrow), and the counter-current arrangement between flow of air outwards (large white arrow) and venous blood flow inwards (large red arrow) are shown on a toluidine blue stained, transversely cut section. From Maina, J.N. (2009) Three-dimensional serial section computer reconstruction of the arrangement of the structural components of the parabronchus of the ostrich, *Struthio camelus*, lung. *Anatomical Record* 292: 1685–1698, with permission of the author. Reproduced with permission from Wiley.

Table 26.1 Gas exchange variables in awake resting birds.

Variable	Common starling (*Sturnus vulgaris*)	Pigeon (*Columba* sp.)	Black duck (*Anas rubripes*)	Domestic fowl (*Gallus* sp.)	Muscovy duck (*Cairina moschata*)	Pekin duck (*Anas* sp.)
Weight (kg)	0.08	0.38	1.03	1.6	2.16	2.38
M_{O_2} (mmol/min)	0.13	0.35	0.84	1.09	—	1.67
F_{resp} (min^{-1})	92	27	27	23	10	8–15
V_T (mL)	0.67	7.5	30	33	69	16–98
V_E (L/min)	0.061	0.204	0.79	0.760	0.700	0.807–0.910
Q (L/min)	—	0.127	—	0.430	0.844	0.423–0.973
Pa_{O_2} (mmHg)	—	95	—	87	96	93–100
Pa_{CO_2} (mmHg)	—	34	—	29	36	34–36

M_{O_2}, oxygen consumption; F_{resp}, respiratory frequency; V_T, tidal volume; V_E, minute ventilation; Q, cardiac output.
Source: adapted from Powell, F.L. and Scheid, P. (1989) Physiology of gas exchange in the avian respiratory system. In: *Form and Function in Birds*, Vol. **4** (eds A.S. King and J. McLelland), pp. 393–437. Academic Press, New York. Reproduced with permission from Elsevier.

Gas exchange, flight and altitude

Flight is the ability to produce lift, to accelerate, and to maneuver at various speeds. In terms of energy expenditure, it is the most demanding form of locomotion in animals and exerts the most demands on the respiratory system; its energetic demands are beyond those attainable by non-flying animals. For example, a pigeon running on a treadmill has an oxygen consumption of 27.4 mL/min; while flying at 19 m/s, oxygen consumption is 77.8 mL/min. However, at high speeds the energy cost per unit of distance covered is less than that of other forms of locomotion, thus it is the most efficient form of locomotion.

Smaller, agile passerine birds can attain speeds of 15–40 kph, while swifts, pigeons and loons can attain speeds of 90–150 kph (56–93 mph) and falcons (albeit during dives on prey) have been clocked at more than 180 kph (≥112 mph). Although these flight speeds may seem slow by comparison to commercial jet flight, we gain a different perspective when speed is scaled to body size. A Boeing 747-400 jet has a length of 71 m and cruises at 963 kph or 268 m/s, thus traveling 3.8 times its own length in 1 s. By comparison, a swift flying at 40 kph covers 100 of its body lengths in 1 s. An athletic human covers five body lengths in 1 s; the cheetah, the fastest land mammal, covers 18 body lengths per second.

As previously mentioned, birds can fly at very high altitudes as documented by high-altitude encounters between aircraft and birds. A Rüppell's griffon (*Gyps rueppelli*), a type of vulture, was sucked into a jet engine at 11,485 m (37,680 feet) over the West African country of Côte d'Ivoire. Whooper swans (*Cygnus cygnus*) have been detected flying at 8500 m (27,887 feet). Bar-headed geese (*Anser indicus*) migrate over the Himalayas at altitudes of more than 9375 m (30,750 feet), an altitude at which barometric pressure is approximately 31.1 kPa (233 mmHg), approximately one-third of that at sea level, and the Po_2 in the cold dry air is 6.5 kPa (48.8 mmHg). If during migration the geese maintain constant body core temperatures of about 41 °C, and the inhaled air is warmed to body temperature and is fully saturated with water vapor, the Po_2 in the air reaching the air capillaries where gas exchange occurs would barely exceed 4.9 kPa (36.6 mmHg). What makes it possible for birds to fly – to exercise! – in this inhospitable environment? A number of contributing factors include the high gas-exchange efficiency of the avian lung (the ability to extract more oxygen from a given volume of air compared with a mammal), the ability to preserve cerebral blood flow in the face of very low arterial partial pressures of carbon dioxide, and enhanced delivery of oxygen by hemoglobin to tissues.

$Paco_2$ and cerebral blood flow

Cerebral blood vessel diameter and its effect on cerebral blood flow is influenced by $Paco_2$. High partial pressures of CO_2 in arterial blood cause cerebral vasodilatation and an increase in cerebral blood flow, while low partial pressures cause vasoconstriction and a decrease in cerebral blood flow. Mammals can tolerate CO_2 partial pressures down to 20 mmHg, but below this the resistance to cerebral blood flow is so high that blood perfusion of the brain is compromised and can result in cerebral ischemia. Birds, however, are able to maintain cerebral blood flow at $Paco_2$ values of 8–10 mmHg. This is an obvious survival advantage for birds that fly at altitude because it allows them to hyperventilate so as to meet their oxygen demands while preserving cerebral perfusion.

Avian hemoglobin

Hemoglobin, strictly speaking, is not part of the respiratory system, but is crucial for blood to transport oxygen from the lungs to all tissues of the body. In most vertebrates hemoglobin is composed of four subunits, each of which has its own binding site for oxygen. There are some significant differences between avian hemoglobin and hemoglobin found in other vertebrates (Table 26.2). In adult birds there are two different types of hemoglobin, hemoglobin A and D, each varying from the other in their affinity for oxygen. Hemoglobin A is often the more prevalent form and has a lower affinity for oxygen than hemoglobin D. Lower affinity means that oxygen dissociates more

Table 26.2 Characteristics of avian blood that influence oxygen transport, especially as they relate to flight at altitude.

Bird	Altitude (m)	Percent HbD	Oxygen affinities of Hb	P_{50} (mmHg)
Rüffell's griffon	11,278	16	HbD/D' > HbA' > HbA	16.4
Bar-headed goose	>8848	10	HbD > HbA	27.2
Andean goose	6000	4–40	Both HbD and HbA are high affinity	33.9
Golden eagle	7500	35	HbD > HbA	
Northern goshawk	4000	15	HbD > HbA	
Pigeon		0		29.5
Parakeet		0		
Macaw		0		
Duck			HbA > HbD	35.2–42.6
Turkey			HbA > HbD	33.4

HbA, hemoglobin A; HbD, hemoglobin D.
Source: adapted from Lewis, S. (1996) *Avian Biochemistry and Molecular Biology*, pp. 82–99. Cambridge University Press, Cambridge. Reproduced with permission from Cambridge University Press.

readily from hemoglobin as arterial blood becomes venous blood. In general, avian hemoglobin shows more cooperativity with oxygen than does hemoglobin in other vertebrates. Cooperativity is the phenomenon whereby the binding of one molecule of oxygen with hemoglobin facilitates the binding of the next molecule of oxygen and so on up to binding four oxygen molecules by a hemoglobin molecule. Cooperativity accounts for the sigmoidal shape of the oxygen–hemoglobin binding curve and the degree of cooperativity that a hemoglobin molecule possesses is expressed by the Hill coefficient. A low Hill coefficient indicates that the hemoglobin has weak cooperativity, whereas a number approaching the number of binding sites in a hemoglobin molecule (four per molecule) indicates strong cooperativity. A generally accepted Hill coefficient for mammalian hemoglobin is 2.8, while that for avian hemoglobin has been observed to be above the theoretical limit of 4. The advantage of this high cooperativity is that it increases the delivery of oxygen to tissues.

Another feature of avian hemoglobin is its interaction with inositol pentaphosphate and inositol tetraphosphate (in mammals the principal organic phosphate is bisphosphoglycerate or BPG, formerly referred to as DPG), which shifts the oxygen–hemoglobin dissociation curve to the right thus decreasing the affinity of hemoglobin for oxygen, which enhances oxygen delivery to tissues. The presence of two types of hemoglobin, both with different oxygen affinities, means that erythrocytes have a greater range of oxygen partial pressures over which oxygen can be bound and released. This hemoglobin arrangement is advantageous for those species of birds that must cope with large variations in the partial pressure of oxygen. For example, high-altitude flying birds and penguin species encounter hypoxic conditions, but the conditions differ in that high-altitude flyers, such as bar-headed geese, contend with prolonged hypoxia during sustained flight whereas penguins experience transient but frequent hypoxia during dives. The P_{50} of hemoglobin, the partial pressure of oxygen at which hemoglobin is 50% saturated with oxygen, is lower in birds that live at extreme altitudes where the partial pressures of oxygen are very low, and in diving birds such as penguins. A low P_{50} means that the hemoglobin has a high affinity for oxygen thus favoring the uptake of oxygen, an obvious advantage under hypoxic conditions. The hemoglobin–oxygen affinity ($P_{50} = 28$ mmHg, pH 7.5) in emperor penguins (*Aptenodytes forsteri*) is similar to that in bar-headed geese ($P_{50} = 27.2$ mmHg). In emperor penguins this P_{50} allows increased oxygen at low blood Po_2 during dives and more complete depletion of the respiratory store of oxygen.

Carbon dioxide also affects the binding of oxygen to hemoglobin through processes known as the Bohr effect. The first process involves pH in that the hydration of carbon dioxide results in the formation of carbonic acid which, when it dissociates, yields hydrogen ions that more readily bind with oxyhemoglobin than deoxyhemoglobin. In the lungs, where carbon dioxide is low (and pH is high), the binding of oxygen by hemoglobin is favored. At the level of tissues, where carbon dioxide and

hydrogen ions are prevalent (pH is low), the unloading of oxygen is favored where it is needed – at the tissues. The other process in the Bohr effect that occurs in mammals, but to a lesser degree in birds, involves the binding of carbon dioxide with hemoglobin, more so with deoxyhemoglobin than oxyhemoglobin, to form carbamino compounds that produce small increases in P_{50}. In birds the strong binding of the organic phosphates to hemoglobin prevents this CO_2 Bohr effect.

Gas exchange and diving

Some species of diving birds are truly remarkable divers. Probably the consummate avian diver is the emperor penguin (*Aptenodytes forsteri*) which has attained depths in excess of 540 m (1772 feet, where ambient pressure is more than 54.6 atm or 41,496 mmHg or 5.5 MPa) and dive durations of up to 28 min. True, marine mammals reach greater depths, for example southern elephant seals (*Mirounga leonina*) achieve depths of 1653 m (5422 feet) with dives lasting up to 120 min. Sperm whales (*Physeter macrocephalus*) have been recorded to dive to 2035 m (6675 feet) with dives lasting up to 83 min. In December 2010, a human competitive free diver (without fins or diving assists) set a record of 101 m (331 feet) in a dive that lasted 4.17 min. Focusing on the emperor penguin, what makes it possible for this nonflying bird to exercise and hunt for food at such extreme depths?

For a diving animal the depth and duration of a dive depend on stores of oxygen accumulated just prior to the start of the dive. These oxygen stores are located in the respiratory system, blood and muscle and depend on the respiratory air volume, blood volume, hemoglobin concentration, muscle mass and myoglobin concentration. The distribution of total oxygen stores varies between deep and shallow divers; in animals that dive deeper and longer, the contribution of the oxygen stored in the respiratory system is less than the oxygen stored in the blood and muscle compartments. Less reliance on the respiratory oxygen store in deep divers decreases the need for gas exchange at depth. Other physiologic mechanisms also facilitate deep dives of long duration, such as bradycardia, efficiency of swimming, and hypoxemic tolerance.

Bradycardia, a heart rate significantly less than that of an animal at rest, does occur in birds, but the cause differs depending on the species and conditions under which heart rate is measured. During free voluntary dives by the emperor penguin, bradycardia occurs as a result of the classic Scholander–Irving dive response, especially when dives exceed these birds' aerobic dive limit (ADL). Resting heart rate in these penguins is about 73 beats/min; during free voluntary dives exceeding the ADL, heart rates of 41 beats/min have been recorded; during a dive that lasted 18 min the heart rate was 6 beats/min. These observations in emperor penguins contrast with the absence of true bradycardia in diving ducks, cormorants, and other penguin species in which the bradycardia occurred as a result of forced submergence, thus being induced by stress. Diving bradycardia preserves the respiratory and blood oxygen stores by decreasing tissue perfusion and oxygen uptake, and by isolating muscle from the circulation.

Enhanced anaerobic capacity and **hypoxemic tolerance** are also essential for longer dives. This was exemplified in the emperor penguin that set a dive duration record of 28 min. After the dive the bird required 6 min before it stood up from a prone position, another 20 min before it began to walk, and 8 hours before it dived again.

The depletion rate of the large myoglobin-bound oxygen store in muscle is conserved due to the efficiency of swimming. In emperor penguins, hypothermia does not appear to play a role in oxygen utilization as core body temperature is maintained during dives. The emperor penguin has a diving respiratory volume of 117 mL/kg, blood volume of 100 mL/kg, hemoglobin concentration of 18 g/dL, muscle mass of 25% of body mass, and myoglobin concentration of 6.4 g/100 g muscle; the total body oxygen store is 65–68 mL/kg, of which 31–33% is in the respiratory system, 30% in blood, and 36–39% in muscle.

Control of ventilation

> 1 What respiratory control mechanisms are similar among birds and mammals?
>
> 2 What respiratory control mechanisms are unique to birds?
>
> 3 What are intrapulmonary chemoreceptors and what role do they have in regulating respiration?

Ventilation and breathing pattern are regulated to meet the demands imposed by changes in metabolic activity (e.g., rest and flight) as well as other demands on the system imposed by a wide range of sensory inputs (e.g., heat and cold), forebrain-controlled behavior, and emotional inputs. It must be kept in mind that birds do not have a diaphragm and as such do not have a phrenic nerve. It is assumed that there is a central respiratory control center in the avian brain, but this has not been unequivocally demonstrated. As in mammals, the central pattern generator appears to be located in the pons and medulla oblongata, with facilitation and inhibition coming from higher regions of the brain. Bilateral vagotomy in birds results in a slow deep-breathing pattern just as in mammals, indicating that output from the central pattern generator may be controlled in a similar manner in both birds and mammals. It also appears that the chemical drive on respiratory frequency and inspiratory and expiratory duration depend on vagal afferent feedback from receptors in the lung as well as on extrapulmonary chemoreceptors, mechanoreceptors, and thermoreceptors.

Chemoreceptors

Central chemoreceptors affect ventilation in response to changes in arterial P_{CO_2}, and hydrogen ion concentration. Peripheral extrapulmonary chemoreceptors, specifically the carotid bodies, are influenced by P_{aO_2} and increase their discharge rate as P_{aO_2} decreases, thus increasing ventilation; they transiently decrease their rate of discharge as P_{aO_2} increases or when P_{aCO_2} decreases. These responses are the same as those observed in mammals.

Unlike mammals, birds have a unique group of peripheral receptors located in the lung called intrapulmonary chemoreceptors (IPC) that are acutely sensitive to carbon dioxide and insensitive to hypoxia. The IPC affect rate and volume of breathing on a breath-to-breath basis by acting as the afferent limb of an inspiratory-inhibitory reflex that uses as the afferent signal the timing, rate, and extent of CO_2 washout from the lung during inspiration. As P_{CO_2} in the lung decreases, the receptors become stimulated and increase their rate of discharge. As the rate of discharge increases, ventilation decreases, so these receptors may serve to fine tune the pattern of ventilation in birds. Their exact location within the lung is in question (some believe that they are uniformly distributed throughout the lung while others believe that they are located primarily in the caudal portion of the paleopulmonic lung), but some of their characteristics have been elucidated. Some receptors have peak activity at the beginning of inspiration, others during expiration, and others are biphasic. They are sensitive to both static and dynamic changes in P_{CO_2} in their microenvironment and can follow rapid changes in P_{CO_2} up to rates of 160 cycles per second. The signals from the receptors appear to be conducted by small myelinated afferent fibers with a conduction velocity of approximately 7 m/s. These receptors have been shown to be inhibited by inhalant anesthetics such as halothane.

Mechanoreceptors

Peripheral mechanoreceptors, probably located in the walls of the air sacs or in the tissues surrounding the air sacs, are sensitive to inflation of the respiratory system and insensitive to hypoxia or hypercarbia. However, P_{CO_2} does influence the volume dependence of inspiratory duration and expiratory duration in birds, which suggests that the duration of inspiration and expiration are a function of both mechanical and chemical feedback through convergence of these inputs on a rhythm-generating mechanisms in the brainstem.

Arterial and carotid baroreceptors are located at the base of the aorta and in the wall of the common carotid artery and they can influence ventilation. An increase in blood pressure causes hypoventilation while a decrease in blood pressure results in hyperventilation.

Proprioceptors, receptors located in joints and muscles and that influence ventilation in mammals, have not been identified in birds.

Thermoreceptors

Thermoreceptors are located centrally and peripherally, with the hypothalamus integrating temperature information from these sources. In birds, spinal thermoreceptors are of primary importance, but ambient temperature, through its effect on peripheral receptors, can cause either panting or shivering. For birds, the major route of heat loss is through evaporation from respiratory tract surfaces, so the respiratory system must balance gas exchange with evaporative heat loss. During heat stress in birds, respiratory frequency markedly increases while tidal volume decreases, the net effect being a sixfold to sevenfold increase in minute ventilation. In some birds (ostrich, Bedouin fowl, rock partridge, Pekin duck, pigeon), this large increase in minute ventilation does not result in a change in arterial blood gases and pH. The respiratory control system functions to maximize ventilation of the upper airway dead space thus enhancing evaporative water loss and cooling the body, but without overventilating the parabronchi.

There may be species differences in CO_2 responsiveness depending on the ecological niche occupied by a given species. The CO_2 responsiveness of IPC in chickens, ducks, emu and pigeons appears to be greater than IPC of burrowing owls, a species that lives underground where the concentration of CO_2 is higher than that for above-ground birds.

Pulmonary defense mechanisms

> 1 What is the mucociliary escalator?
>
> 2 What is the relationship between the radius of a sphere and surface tension? How does this concept apply to biological structures such as air capillaries (see Chapter 7)?
>
> 3 What is the function of surfactant in mammals and birds? Does it have a similar function in birds and mammals?
>
> 4 What would be the consequences for gas exchange if there were no surfactant?
>
> 5 What processes govern transudation and what are the consequences for gas exchange if transudation occurs in air capillaries?

The avian lung must deal with a number of challenges that constantly threaten to disrupt the anatomic features that make it such an efficient gas exchanger. The lung must be able to eliminate a variety of inhaled particles, and preserve function in the face of forces inherent in the anatomic design of the lung. Birds have a number of mechanical and biological mechanisms for protecting the respiratory system.

Mucociliary transport

Histologically, the trachea consists of four layers including a mucous membrane consisting of simple and pseudostratified, ciliated, columnar epithelium with large numbers of simple alveolar mucous glands composed of typical mucus-secreting cells. The primary bronchi are lined with low columnar, pseudostratified epithelium containing goblet cells, intraepithelial mucous alveoli, and projecting ridges with cilia. Thus in both the trachea and bronchi there is a layer of protective mucus that traps inhaled particulate matter. This mucous layer and the cilia

move trapped material toward the oropharynx (**mucociliary escalator**) where it can be swallowed and excreted from the body. For a short distance the secondary bronchi have the same histologic structure as the primary bronchus, but subsequently consist of simple squamous epithelium with single small circular bands of smooth muscle covered by ciliated epithelium.

Phagocytosis

Within a parabronchus at the level of the atria there is loose connective tissue at the base of the inter-atrial septa and the floor of the atria that may contain clusters of macrophages. The epithelium continuously lining the atria, infundibula, and air capillaries consists of three cell types: granular cells (granular pneumocytes), squamous atrial cells, and squamous respiratory cells. It has been demonstrated that both epithelial cells and macrophages phagocytize inhaled particles in the avian lung and that the particulate matter is eventually transported to the gut and excreted in the feces. However, wandering macrophages are rarely found in the healthy avian respiratory tract and for this reason it is assumed that they are not a primary defense against inhaled particles. Rather the inhaled particles appear to be trapped in the trilaminar substance found on the parabronchial atria and infundibula, then phagocytized by the epithelial cells which may release the particles into the interstitium where macrophages phagocytize the particles, but the fate of the particles from this site is unknown.

The **granular cells** appear to be analogous to type II pneumocytes of the mammalian pulmonary alveolus as they contain characteristic osmiophilic lamellar bodies, the precursor to **surfactant**. They are confined to the luminal surface of the head and stalk of the inter-atrial septa and they possess short blunt microvilli that extend from their apical surface. The squamous atrial cells line the major portion of the atria and, depending on the species and the level of air pollution, possess branched microvilli that extend from their apical cytoplasm and surfactant is sandwiched between the tentacle-like microvilli. These cells produce a surfactant which spreads as a trilaminar substance (see next section) and unevenly coats the surfaces of the atria, but they also transport small airborne particles to underlying macrophages. At the floor of the atria the epithelium transforms into the very flat squamous respiratory cells that continue into, and completely line, the infundibula and air capillaries. These cells have a smooth surface with single microvilli and they too produce and are completely covered with surfactant.

Trilaminar substance

The law of Laplace ($P = \gamma/r$, where P represents opening pressure, γ surface tension, and r radius of tubule), when applied to the small-diameter air capillaries, indicates that high surface tensions occur and generate significant negative pressure across the blood–gas barrier. Two phenomena could occur that would adversely affect gas exchange: (i) influx of fluid (transudation) into the air capillaries, or (ii) the air capillaries would collapse. The high surface tension associated with the small radius of curvature of the air capillaries causes a lower hydrostatic pressure in the air capillaries relative to the hydrostatic pressure in the blood capillaries. This hydrostatic pressure gradient favors the movement (transudation) of fluid from blood capillaries to air capillaries. This pressure is counteracted by the osmotic pressure of plasma proteins in blood and by the surfactant that spreads over the surface of the air capillaries and reduces their surface tension so that transudation does not normally occur. Any fluid in the blood–gas interspace or in the air capillaries would, of course, interfere with gas exchange by increasing the diffusion distance between the lumen of the air capillary and the blood capillary.

In birds, surfactant is a lipoproteinaceous material that forms a **trilaminar substance** unique to birds. It covers the surfaces of the atria, infundibula and air capillaries (sometimes weakly so depending on the species), but it is also found in outgrowths of squamous respiratory cells that form at the abluminal surface of the cells and extend through clefts between blood capillaries to reach other air capillaries. In addition to this network, squamous respiratory cells appear to project parallel processes, retinacula, that bridge to the opposite side of air capillaries. The overall result is an intricate intercapillary anastomosing network that firmly anchors the air capillary system to the blood capillaries and forms the structural basis for the rigid avian lung that changes by only about 1.4% during the respiratory cycle; this network also structurally maintains the integrity and stability of the blood–gas interface. This structural arrangement suggests that the trilaminar substance lining the air capillary surfaces may be of less importance in preventing collapse of the air capillaries by reducing surface tension, but of more importance in preventing transudation of fluid from blood into the air capillaries.

Collapse of the air capillaries is prevented by structural features of the avian lung. Air and blood capillaries possess structural elements that preserve their anatomic and gas exchange integrity. These elements form an interdependent, tightly coupled network of tension and compression in the avian lung that gives the lungs rigidity while strengthening the air and blood capillaries, thus preserving their anatomic integrity and function.

Applied physiology and practical concerns

> 1 During general anesthesia, what anesthesia-related factors would cause a bird to hypoventilate?
>
> 2 Does mechanical ventilation of an anesthetized bird adversely affect gas exchange? Why or why not?
>
> 3 Could a fracture of the avian humerus adversely affect pulmonary function? How?
>
> 4 A general inhalant anesthetic is usually delivered via the trachea, but if a bird's trachea is obstructed, what route could be used to deliver the inhalant anesthetic?

- The fully conscious, healthy, unmedicated bird obviously compensates for the larger tracheal dead space. However, under the depressant effects of anesthetic drugs, ventilation is depressed and a greater percentage of minute ventilation becomes dead-space ventilation. Furthermore, aerodynamic valving becomes considerably less effective at the low airway flows encountered in anesthetized spontaneously breathing birds. The consequence is that ventilation is less efficient in anesthetized birds.

- Because both inspiration and expiration require muscle activity, anything that depresses muscle function also adversely affects ventilation. For example, anesthetic drugs generally cause muscle relaxation and the degree of relaxation depends on the anesthetic used, depth of anesthesia, and physical condition of the bird. In like manner, anything that impairs thoracic movement, especially movement of the sternum (such as improper physical restraint), will impair ventilation. This may be more true in domesticated species than in wild related species.

- Control of breathing and the consequent regulation of arterial P_{CO_2} and HCO_3^- concentration influence eggshell calcification. In laying hens, anything that causes hyperventilation, such as heat stress or being moved to high altitude, results in parabronchial hyperventilation that causes hypocapnia. The low CO_2 results in less bicarbonate being available to interact with calcium, the final result being thinner eggshells. Management techniques that elevate plasma bicarbonate concentration may benefit eggshell formation.

- During anesthesia and surgery it may be necessary to provide positive-pressure ventilation manually or by a mechanical ventilator, but this artificial ventilation does not adversely affect gas exchange. Indeed, during positive-pressure ventilation the direction of gas flow within the avian lung may be reversed, but such a reversal does not affect gas exchange because the efficiency of the cross-current model does not depend on the direction of gas flow.

- Because of the flow-through nature of the avian respiratory system, it is possible to ventilate birds by continuously flowing gas through the trachea and lungs and out through a ruptured or cannulated air sac. This same technique can be used to induce and maintain inhalational anesthesia in birds by flowing anesthetic gas through a cannula inserted into an air sac, across the lung and out the trachea. Air sac cannulation and unidirectional ventilation can also be used to ventilate an apneic bird or a bird with an obstructed airway.

- The air sacs of birds, especially the caudal thoracic and abdominal air sacs, are susceptible to a variety of diseases because of the pathway that inspired gas follows through the respiratory system. Inspired particulate matter (environmental pollutants, infectious agents) tends to settle out in the caudal portions of the respiratory system such as the caudal thoracic and abdominal air sacs, near the origin of the medio-dorsal secondary bronchi and their associated paleopulmonic parabronchi, and the neopulmonic parabronchi.

- Placing a bird on its back during physical examination or anesthesia may adversely affect ventilation, especially if the bird has heavy pectoral muscles or is overconditioned as is often the case with domestic poultry. A number of factors may contribute to this phenomenon, not the least of which is the weight of the abdominal viscera compressing the abdominal air sacs thus reducing their effective volume. If a bird must be placed in this position, such as for anesthesia and surgery, then ventilation should be assisted by either instituting mechanical ventilation or unidirectional ventilation.

- During the processing of poultry, birds are shackled, electrostunned and exsanguinated, and the carcasses are immersed in a scalding tank to assist with defeathering. At this time there may be a variable amount of respiratory activity due to improper stunning, incomplete exsanguination, or agonal gasping that results in aspiration of water with its contaminants and which is distributed to the air sacs. Although the air sacs are removed during evisceration, the diverticula that extend to the wing, thigh, and pectoral areas remain and become part of edible tissue.

- During inhalational anesthesia hypoventilation is common and respiratory arrest is not uncommon. When apnea occurs the bird can be artificially ventilated either by mechanical means (mechanical ventilator or by intermittently squeezing the reservoir bag on the breathing circuit) or by gently pumping the sternum, thereby expanding and compressing the thoracoabdominal cavity.

- Injections of drugs or other substances into the intraperitoneal cavity can be inadvertently injected into the air sacs with disastrous consequences for the bird. Whenever injecting substances by this route the operator must always first draw back on the syringe plunger so to ascertain if the needle is in an air sac (in which case air will be easily aspirated) or in the peritoneal cavity.

Self-evaluation

Answers can be found at the end of the chapter.

1 A slightly overweight pet goose is induced to anesthesia with isoflurane, an inhalant anesthetic (delivered in 95% oxygen). It is then intubated and anesthesia is maintained with isoflurane. During anesthesia, the goose is positioned on its back for radiographs. While so positioned, an arterial blood sample is collected for pH and blood gas analysis. The results (pH 7.27, Pa_{CO_2} 69 mmHg, and Pa_{O_2} 366 mmHg) indicate that the bird is hypoventilating. Give at least four reasons why the bird is hypoventilating.

2 During inspiration in a bird, the pressure within the air sacs:
  A Decreases relative to ambient atmospheric pressure
  B Increases relative to ambient atmospheric pressure
  C Does not change relative to ambient atmospheric pressure

3 During expiration in a bird, the pressure within the air sacs:
  A Decreases relative to ambient atmospheric pressure
  B Increases relative to ambient atmospheric pressure
  C Does not change relative to ambient atmospheric pressure

4 Which of the following statements most accurately describes avian air sacs?
  A The air sacs are highly vascular membranes that significantly contribute to gas exchange
  B The air sacs receive inspired air before it crosses the paleopulmonic and neopulmonic lung tissues
  C The volume of the air sacs is unaffected by body position
  D The air sacs do not have a significant gas-exchange function and only serve to provide a tidal flow of gas across the lung tissue

5 The flow of gas across the paleopulmonic lung occurs during:
  A Inspiration
  B Expiration
  C Both inspiration and expiration

6 The flow of gas across the neopulmonic lung occurs during:
  A Inspiration
  B Expiration
  C Both inspiration and expiration

Suggested reading

Bernhard, W., Gebert, A., Vieten, G. et al. (2001) Pulmonary surfactant in birds: coping with surface tension in a tubular lung. *American Journal of Physiology* 281:R327–R337.

Brown, R.E., Brain, J.D. and Wang, N. (1997) The avian respiratory system: a unique model for studies of respiratory toxicosis and for monitoring air quality. *Environmental Health Perspectives* 105:188–200.

Gleeson, M. and Molony, V. (1989) Control of breathing. In: *Form and Function in Birds* (eds A.S. King and J. McLelland), Vol. 4, pp. 439–484. Academic Press, London.

Maina, J.N. (2006) Development, structure, and function of a novel respiratory organ, the lung–air sac system of birds: to go where no other vertebrate has gone. *Biological Reviews of the Cambridge Philosophical Society* 81:545–579.

Maina, J.N. (2007) Spectacularly robust! Tensegrity principle explains the mechanical strength of the avian lung. *Respiratory Physiology and Neurobiology* 155:1–10.

Maina, J.N., Jimoh, S.A. and Hosie, M. (2010) Implicit mechanistic role of the collagen, smooth muscle, and elastic tissue components in strengthening the air and blood capillaries of the avian lung. *Journal of Anatomy* 217:597–608.

Meir, J.U. and Ponganis, P.J. (2009) High-affinity hemoglobin and blood oxygen saturation in diving emperor penguins. *Journal of Experimental Biology* 212:3330–3338.

Ponganis, P.J., Meir, J.U. and Williams, C.L. (2011) In pursuit of Irving and Scholander: a review of oxygen store management in seals and penguins. *Journal of Experimental Biology* 214:3325–3339.

Sachs, G., Traugott, J., Nesterova, A.P. et al. (2012) Flying at no mechanical energy cost: disclosing the secret of wandering albatrosses. *PLOS ONE* 7(9):e41449.

Scheuermann, D.W., Klika, E., De Groodt-Lasseel, M.H. et al. (1997) An electron microscopic study of the parabronchial epithelium in the mature lung of four bird species. *Anatomical Record* 249:213–225.

Wideman, R.F., Forman, M.F., Hughes, J.D. et al. (1998) Flow-dependent pulmonary vasodilation during acute unilateral pulmonary artery occlusion in jungle fowl. *Poultry Science* 77:615–626.

Answers

1 The inhalant anesthetic depresses the central nervous system (CNS), including the respiratory control centers, so that the CNS is less responsive to CO_2. In general, inhalant anesthetics produce muscular relaxation, so the inspiratory and expiratory muscles of respiration are also relaxed. The result is a decreased tidal volume, decreased minute ventilation, and increased dead-space ventilation. As minute ventilation decreases so too does the effectiveness of aerodynamic valving, thus further reducing the effectiveness of ventilation. With the bird on its back, the abdominal viscera compress both the abdominal and caudal thoracic air sacs thus reducing tidal volume and minute ventilation.

2 A. During inspiration the volume of the thoracic and abdominal cavities increases, thus generating negative pressures. Since the air sacs are the only compliant structures within the body cavity, they too expand and the pressure within them decreases relative to atmospheric pressure and gas flows into the pulmonary system.

3 B. During expiration, the pressure within the air sacs increases relative to atmospheric pressure and gas flows out of the pulmonary system. During expiration the volume of the thoracic and abdominal cavity decreases, thus generating positive pressures. Since the air sacs are the only compliant structures within the body cavity, they too decrease in volume and the pressure within them increases relative to atmospheric pressure and gas flows out of the pulmonary system.

4 D. The air sacs are thin, membranous, relatively avascular structures that do not participate in gas exchange to any significant extent. Their purpose is to provide a tidal flow of gas across the gas-exchange surfaces. When a bird is placed on its back, the abdominal contents can compress the abdominal air sacs and thus decrease tidal volume.

5 C. Gas flows across the paleopulmonic lung during both inspiration and expiration.

6 C. As in the paleopulmonic lung, gas flow across the neopulmonic lung occurs during both inspiration and expiration.

Section IV: Respiration

SECTION V

Muscle Physiology

Section Editor: William O. Reece

27 Physiology of Skeletal Muscle

William O. Reece

Iowa State University, Ames, IA, USA

The most visible aspect of muscle function is that which is related to locomotion. Animals are able to stand and lie down, graze in pastures, run when threatened, or compete at racetracks. Other functions not so visible, but necessary for overall body function, include muscles for respiration, digestion, parturition, blood and lymph circulation, swallowing, and generation of body heat.

Overview of muscle physiology

> **1** What is the difference between the origin and the insertion of a skeletal muscle?
>
> **2** What is the difference between a flexor and an extensor skeletal muscle?
>
> **3** What is the difference between an adductor and an abductor skeletal muscle?

Muscle is a contractile tissue and accomplishes diverse functions by shortening and pulling on other structures. In addition to shortening, muscle has other properties that include **excitability**, the capacity to receive and respond to a stimulus, **extensibility**, the ability to be stretched, and **elasticity**, the ability to return to original shape after being stretched. There are three types of muscle fibers in the animal body: skeletal, smooth, and cardiac. Each is characterized not only by microscopic structural differences but also by their location, function, and innervation.

Arrangement and location

A primary consideration in determining what muscles accomplish is their fiber arrangement. Accordingly, the muscle fibers might be arranged in sheets, sheets rolled into tubes, bundles, rings (sphincters), or cones, or they might remain as discrete fibers or clusters for more precise or less forceful action. The emptying of visceral structures (e.g., urinary bladder, stomach, heart) or conveyance of intestinal contents or organ secretions, as provided by smooth and cardiac muscle, is accomplished because of their intimate association with the affected part. Apart from the skeletal muscle sphincters, the effects of skeletal muscle may be noted at a point some distance from their location. This means that their contraction must be transmitted somehow to the affected part, whereby one end of the muscle must be relatively fixed or anchored and the other end must be attached directly or by a tendon to the moveable part. Accordingly, the anatomic description of a skeletal muscle sometimes refers to its **origin** and **muscle insertion**, the origin being the least moveable end and the insertion the most moveable end. Contraction of skeletal muscle brings the origin and the insertion closer together and, when attachments involve two bones, one or both of the bones will move.

Types of movement

Skeletal muscles are often described according to the type of movement performed and are strategically located to best serve the structure they affect. They are **flexors** if they are located

Section V: Muscle Physiology

on the side of the limb toward which the joint bends when decreasing the joint angle. They are **extensors** if they are located on the side of the limb toward which the joint bends when increasing the joint angle. **Adductors** are muscles that pull a limb toward the median plane, and **abductors** pull a limb away from the median plane. **Sphincters** are arranged circularly to constrict body openings. Lack of adduction occasionally occurs in the hindlimb of cows after parturition or calving. The adductor muscles are supplied by the obturator nerves (one to each leg), each of which passes through an opening (obturator foramen) in the birth canal. Injury of the nerves during the calving process can be followed by the inability to adduct one or both of the hindlegs and is identified as obturator paralysis.

Skeletal muscle

> **1** What is the explanation for the greater number of capillaries and mitochondria associated with red fibers?
>
> **2** Which fiber type is associated with sustained flight?
>
> **3** Which fiber type is associated with the pectoralis muscle of chickens and pheasants (rapid reaction, short duration)?

Fiber types

Individual skeletal muscles can be observed by gross anatomic inspection and by dissection and comprise the major portion of the muscle mass of the animal body. Skeletal muscle fibers can be classified into three types: (i) red or dark (type I; slow twitch); (ii) white or pale (type II; fast twitch); and (iii) intermediate with characteristics between those of red and white fibers (Figure 27.1). Most skeletal muscles are probably a mixture of these three types but in some animals the red, and in others the white, predominates. Multiple peripherally arranged nuclei are present in each fiber (Figure 27.2).

Red fibers

The crimson red pectoralis muscle (breast muscle) of pigeons contrasts sharply with the white color of the chicken pectoralis muscle. In birds, the amount of red pigmentation in the pectoralis muscle

can be correlated directly with the ability to sustain flight. Geese, ducks, and pigeons are known for their sustained flight and have a predominance of red pectoralis muscle fibers. Red fibers are also known as **slow twitch fibers**. The reddish appearance is due to the large amounts of myoglobin, the transporter of oxygen. A large number of mitochondria and capillaries are present in red fibers (see Figure 27.1) and, coupled with the substantial amounts of

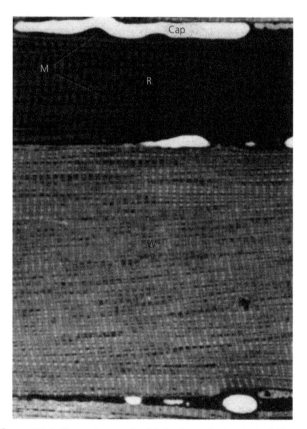

Figure 27.1 Photomicrograph of skeletal muscle showing red fibers (R) and white fibers (W). Red fibers have more mitochondria (M) packed between their myofibrils, especially in association with capillaries (cap). From Cormack, D.C. (1987) *Ham's Histology*, 9th edn. J.B. Lippincott, Philadelphia. With permission from Lippincott Williams & Wilkins.

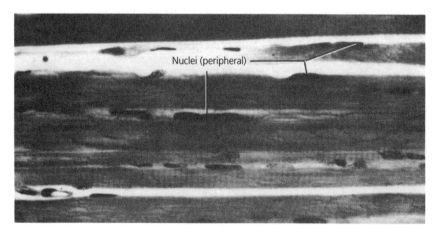

Figure 27.2 Photomicrograph of a longitudinal section of skeletal muscle fibers. Note the striations and the multiple peripherally located nuclei. From Cormack, D.C. (1987) *Ham's Histology*, 9th edn. J.B. Lippincott, Philadelphia. With permission from Lippincott Williams & Wilkins.

myoglobin, support the greater oxidative metabolism needed for sustained flight or other activities of this nature (e.g., horses in competition or sustained running to a destination).

White fibers

White fibers are also known as **fast twitch fibers** and are characteristic of the white pectoralis muscle of the chicken and pheasant. These are muscles that react rapidly and with short duration and consist of large fibers with great strength of contraction. They have an extensive sarcoplasmic reticulum for rapid release of energy via the glycolytic process. There is a less extensive blood supply and fewer mitochondria because oxidative metabolism is of secondary importance.

Skeletal muscle harnessing

> 1 What is the organization of the connective tissue components from within outward?
> 2 What is a muscle bundle?

Muscle tissue, in addition to muscle cells (muscle fibers), contains a connective tissue component that provides for harnessing. The whole muscle is wrapped in an outer connective tissue sheath known as the **epimysium**, and any given muscle is composed of muscle bundles, each containing a collection of muscle fibers (Figure 27.3). Connective tissue extensions from the epimysium, known as the **perimysium**, surround the muscle bundles. Extensions from the perimysium, known as the **endomysium**, surround each of the muscle fibers and are attached to the **sarcolemma** (muscle fiber membrane). The muscle fiber is the contractile unit that shortens, and the pull that it exerts is transmitted by endomysium, perimysium, and epimysium to the tendon or aponeurosis that is attached to a bone, thereby causing its movement.

Some muscles seem to arise directly from a bone, and their attachment could be considered a fleshy **attachment**. These

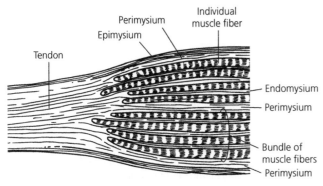

Figure 27.3 Longitudinal section of a muscle. The connective tissue elements of muscle are continuous with a tendon. Adapted from Ham, A.W. (1974) *Histology*, 7th edn. J.B. Lippincott, Philadelphia. Reproduced with permission from Lippincott Williams & Wilkins.

muscle fibers, however, do have a short tendinous attachment to the periosteum of the bone.

Microstructure of skeletal muscle

> 1 What is a muscle fiber?
> 2 Are the sarcomeres of a myofibril in alignment with the sarcomeres of all the myofibrils of the muscle fiber?
> 3 Which one of the myofilaments projects from the Z line into the sarcomere that it separates?
> 4 Which one of the myofilaments occupies the central location when viewing the spatial arrangement?
> 5 What is the ratio of actin to myosin?
> 6 Are the tubules of the sarcotubular system located within the myofibrils or outside the myofibrils?
> 7 How is the sarcoplasmic reticulum oriented relative to the T tubules?
> 8 Which one of the sarcotubular system tubules contains extracellular fluid?
> 9 Which one of the sarcotubular system components is a storage site for calcium ions?

Skeletal muscle cells are more commonly known as muscle fibers because of their elongated shape. Individual fibers generally range from 5 to 100 μm in diameter and 10 to 30 cm in length and may not extend the full length of a whole muscle. However, they may be attached end to end to form longer structures. Each has its own wrapping of endomysium that also contains an associated rich capillary network.

The division of muscles into smaller and smaller parts, ending in **myofibrils**, is shown in Figure 27.4. Depending on the diameter of the muscle fiber, there might be several hundred to several thousand myofibrils within one muscle fiber. Each myofibril has striations or banding. The further division of myofibrils into repetitive units (**sarcomeres**) and their components is shown in Figure 27.5. Sarcomeres contain protein **myofilaments** called **actin** and **myosin**, which by their arrangement give rise to striations (Figure 27.5B). Inasmuch as the striations are characteristic of the muscle fiber, it is apparent that the sarcomeres of a myofibril are in alignment with the sarcomeres of all the other myofibrils of the muscle fiber. The **Z line** is located at each end of a sarcomere and is common to both sarcomeres that it separates. Actin filaments project from the Z line into the sarcomeres that it separates (Figure 27.5B). Thus, each sarcomere has actin filaments projected toward its center from each end. The actin of two sarcomeres common to the same Z line compose an **I band**. The myosin filaments are centrally located within a sarcomere and, coupled with the overlay of actin filaments, provide the dark banding (**A band**) of the characteristic striations (Figure 27.6). The actin and myosin filaments have a regular spatial arrangement to each other, as shown in the cross-section of a myofibril (Figure 27.5C), which has a 2 : 1 ratio of actin to myosin. A longitudinal section of the spatially arranged

Section V: Muscle Physiology

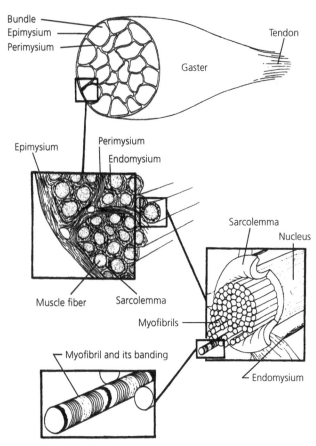

Figure 27.4 The division of muscles into smaller parts, ending in myofibrils. From Feduccia, A. and McCrady, E. (1991) *Torrey's Morphogenesis of the Vertebrates*, 5th edn. John Wiley & Sons, New York. Reproduced with permission from Wiley.

myofilaments shows cross-linkages extending from the myosin filaments toward the actin filaments (Figure 27.5D). During muscle-fiber shortening, the actin filaments appear to slide deeper into the myosin filaments.

Sarcotubular system

Skeletal muscle fibers contain a network of tubules known as the sarcotubular system. These tubules are located within the muscle fiber, but are outside the myofibrils. The sarcotubular system is composed of two separate tubule sets, with each set having a different arrangement among the myofibrils (Figure 27.7). The tubules arranged parallel to the myofibrils and which encircle them are known as the **sarcoplasmic reticulum**. The tubules arranged transversely (right angles) to the myofibrils are known as **T tubules**. T tubules extend transversely from one side of the fiber to the other. They open to the outside of the fiber (surface of the sarcolemma), and therefore their lumens contain extracellular fluid. The T-tubule openings are regularly spaced throughout the length of the muscle fiber because of their orientation to each sarcomere. Similarly, their openings are regularly spaced around the circumference of the fiber so that all myofibrils are intimately served by the sarcotubular system.

In reference to a sarcomere, the T tubules are located near the junction of the actin filaments with the myosin filaments. Therefore, each sarcomere is close to two T tubules (see Figure 27.7). The individual tubules (**sarcotubules**) of the sarcoplasmic reticulum are located regularly throughout the length of the muscle fiber between the T tubules, and they in turn contain intracellular fluid. The T tubules do not open into the sarcoplasmic reticulum; instead the bulbous ends of the

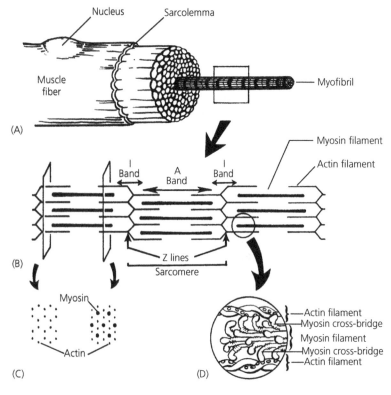

Figure 27.5 The division of myofibrils into sarcomeres. (A) Cross-section of a muscle fiber. (B) Longitudinal arrangement of myofilaments within sarcomeres. (C) Spatial arrangement of the myofilaments within a sarcomere. (D) Further details of the relationship between actin and myosin molecules. From Reece, W.O. (2009) *Functional Anatomy and Physiology of Domestic Animals*, 4th edn. Wiley-Blackwell, Ames, IA. Reproduced with permission from Wiley.

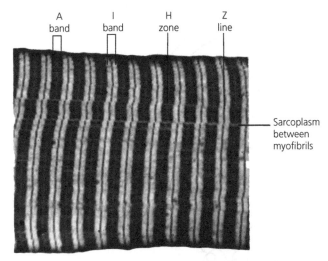

A band   I band   H zone   Z line

Sarcoplasm between myofibrils

Figure 27.6 Photomicrograph of a longitudinal section of a skeletal muscle fiber showing the characteristic banding. From Cormack, D.C. (2001) *Essential Histology*, 2nd edn. Lippincott Williams & Wilkins, Baltimore. With permission from Lippincott Williams & Wilkins.

sarcoplasmic reticulum are closely associated with the T tubules (Figure 27.8). The point of closeness of a T tubule with the bulbous ends of two adjoining sarcoplasmic reticula is known as a **triad**. The principal function of the sarcotubular system is to provide a means for conduction of an impulse from the surface of the muscle fiber to its innermost aspects. The sarcoplasmic reticulum is an important storage site for calcium ions and has a prominent role in the initiation and termination of muscle contraction. It has an anastomosing channel-like structure that surrounds each myofibril (see Figure 27.7).

The neuromuscular junction

1 Where does the terminal branch of a motor neuron make contact with a skeletal muscle fiber?

2 What is the action of calcium ions when they enter the terminal bulb of an axon?

3 What is the neurotransmitter that is stored in the membrane-bound vesicles within the terminal branch of the axon?

4 What is the synaptic cleft?

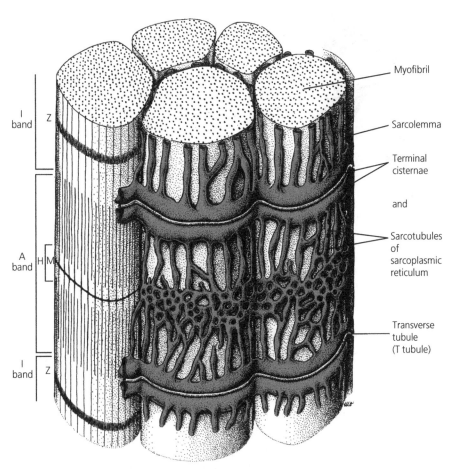

I band   Z

A band   H M

I band   Z

Myofibril

Sarcolemma

Terminal cisternae

and

Sarcotubules of sarcoplasmic reticulum

Transverse tubule (T tubule)

Figure 27.7 Diagram of part of a mammalian skeletal muscle fiber showing the sarcoplasmic reticulum that surrounds myofibrils. Two transverse (T) tubules supply a sarcomere and are in close association with the sarcoplasmic reticulum. The T tubules open to the surface of the sarcolemma. From Cormack, D.C. (2001) *Essential Histology*, 2nd edn. Lippincott Williams & Wilkins, Baltimore. With permission from Lippincott Williams & Wilkins.

Section V: Muscle Physiology

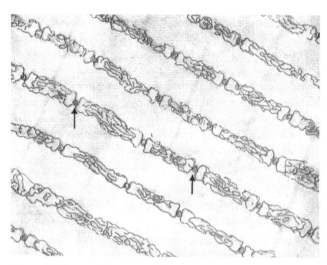

Figure 27.8 Sarcoplasmic reticulum in the extracellular spaces between the myofibrils, showing a longitudinal system paralleling the myofibrils. Also shown in cross-section are T tubules (arrows) that lead to the exterior of the fiber membrane and which are important for conducting the electrical signal into the center of the muscle fiber. From Fawcett, D.W. (1981) *The Cell*. W.B. Saunders, Philadelphia. With permission from Elsevier.

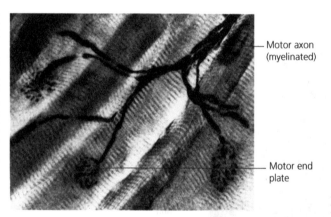

Figure 27.9 Photomicrograph showing the distribution of terminal branches from a nerve fiber to individual muscle fibers to compose a motor unit. A motor end plate is a small flattened mound on the muscle fiber surface formed by the axon terminal branch and its myelin covering. From Cormack, D.C. (2001) *Essential Histology*, 2nd edn. Lippincott Williams & Wilkins, Baltimore. With permission from Lippincott Williams & Wilkins.

A motor neuron can have a number of terminal branches, with each one ending on a separate muscle fiber (Figure 27.9). A **motor unit** consists of a motor neuron and the muscle fibers that it innervates. The largest motor units, in which one axon supplies many muscle fibers, are found in the limbs and postural muscles. The smallest motor units, in which one axon may supply only a few muscle fibers, are found in association with eye movements.

The end bulb of each terminal branch makes contact with an individual muscle fiber at a specialized area known as the **neuromuscular junction** (Figure 27.10) and occurs at the approximate midpoint of the muscle fiber. The terminal branch of the axon does not actually make contact with the muscle fiber

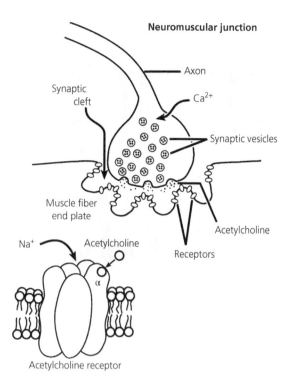

Figure 27.10 Schematic of the neuromuscular junction and the associated acetylcholine receptor channel. From Bailey, J.G. (2004) Muscle physiology. In: *Dukes' Physiology of Domestic Animals*, 12th edn (ed. W.O. Reece). Cornell University Press, Ithaca, NY. Reproduced with permission from Cornell University Press.

but is separated from it by a gap approximately 50 nm wide known as the **synaptic cleft**, a term derived from the word "synapse." A neurotransmitter, **acetylcholine (Ach)**, is stored in the membrane-bound vesicles within the terminal branch of the axon (see Figure 27.10). The neuromuscular junction functions as an amplifier for the spinal or cranial motor neuron action potential. Voltage-gated Ca^{2+} and Na^+ channels are opened when the action potential reaches the neuromuscular junction. An influx of calcium ions enters the terminal bulb of the axon, increasing the calcium ion concentration 10–100 times. Calcium ions trigger the binding of synaptic vesicles to the plasma membrane of the terminal bulb and the release of ACh into the synaptic cleft. ACh diffuses into invaginations of the muscle fiber sarcolemma located immediately below the synaptic cleft and is bound to ACh receptors at that site.

Depolarization of muscle fibers

1 What chemical begins depolarization of a muscle fiber and what is the direction of propagation from the neuromuscular junction?

2 Beginning with depolarization of the sarcolemma, what is the route of depolarization whereby it arrives at every sarcomere in the myofibril?

3 What enzyme hydrolyzes the neurotransmitter that initiated depolarization?

4 How does succinylcholine cause relaxation (prevents muscle contraction) of muscle?

Acetylcholine begins depolarization of muscle fibers by increasing the permeability of the sarcolemma for Na^+ ions, whereby the action potential is propagated by the opening and closing of Ca^{2+} and Na^+ channels and it proceeds in all directions from the neuromuscular junction, located centrally on the muscle fiber. The action potential is conducted into all parts of the muscle fiber beginning with the T tubules. The T tubules serve as communication links between the sarcolemma and the myofibrils within each muscle fiber. When a stimulus is received and depolarization of the sarcolemma begins, it continues in the T tubules and because of their close association with the sarcoplasmic reticulum, they also are depolarized and calcium ions (stored in the sarcoplasmic reticulum) are released into the cytosol of the muscle fiber, allowing contraction to begin. The signal which has caused depolarization has proceeded from the sarcolemma, into the T tubules, sarcoplasmic reticulum, myofibrils, and every sarcomere in the myofibril within milliseconds. Thus, all the myofibrils within a muscle fiber will contract at the same time and a more synchronized contraction results.

Almost immediately after its release, ACh is hydrolyzed by the enzyme **acetylcholinesterase (AChE)** into acetic acid and choline. The next action potential propagated to the muscle fiber must await a new action potential at the neuromuscular junction. AChE is present in large amounts in the synaptic cleft's small size and this, coupled with the limited diffusion distance of ACh in the synaptic cleft, accounts for the rapid hydrolysis of ACh.

Neuromuscular block

A low concentration of calcium in the extracellular fluid (hypocalcemia) is recognized clinically in dairy cows after calving (parturient paresis or milk fever) as a state of semi-paralysis caused by partial neuromuscular block. This happens because fewer calcium ions are available to trigger the binding of synaptic vesicles to the axon end-bulb plasma membrane and release of ACh. Because ACh release begins depolarization of the sarcolemma, the lowered amount depresses the continuation of depolarization.

Hypocalcemia in the bitch may be recognized clinically after whelping as **eclampsia** or **puerperal tetany**. There appears to be a difference in function of the neuromuscular junction between the cow and the bitch, whereby it is blocked by hypocalcemia in cows leading to paresis, but not blocked in the bitch. In the bitch, there is a deficit of calcium ions, the voltage-gated Ca^{2+} and Na^+ channels become more permeable to sodium ions, and inward flow of sodium changes the membrane potential, thereby requiring a stimulus of lesser magnitude to depolarize. The nerve fiber becomes more excitable, discharging repetitively, rather than remaining in the resting state, causing tetanic muscle contractions.

Muscle relaxants

Induced relaxation of muscle is clinically useful for procedures requiring cessation of muscle contraction (e.g., surgical procedures, immobilization). **Muscle relaxants** commonly used for this purpose are **curare** and **succinylcholine**.

The active substance in curare, D-tubocurarine, blocks the effects of ACh by binding to ACh receptors. The conformational change of the ACh receptors that would have allowed opening of the Ca^{2+} and Na^+ channels and generation of post-synaptic action potentials are blocked, and skeletal muscle paralysis results. Curare has been used as a muscle relaxant for some surgical procedures. Another muscle relaxant that has been more useful clinically is succinylcholine. Because its structure is similar to ACh, it binds with ACh receptors but does not allow opening of the Ca^{2+} and Na^+ channels, and postsynaptic action potentials are blocked thereby preventing muscle contraction. Succinylcholine is not hydrolyzed by AChE but by nonspecific cholinesterases in plasma. The rate of hydrolysis is rather rapid although slow compared with hydrolysis by AChE. The amount of nonspecific cholinesterase varies among animal species, so that the length of induced relaxation will vary.

Skeletal muscle contraction

1 How is the natural attraction between actin and myosin inhibited during relaxation?

2 What are the three major components of the actin filament?

3 What causes the active sites on the actin and tropomyosin strands to be uncovered? How are calcium ions involved?

4 What "cocks" the myosin cross-bridge heads prior to their attachment to the active sites on actin?

5 What causes detachment of myosin cross-bridge heads from the actin myofilaments?

6 What provides for the rephosphorylation of ADP? Why is this referred to as oxidative phosphorylation?

7 What is the primary fuel for muscle contractions during prolonged endurance exercise?

8 What is the cause of physiologic contracture? Is this known as muscle cramping?

9 What is tetany?

10 What is the function of treppe?

Muscle activity involves repeated cycles of contraction and relaxation. Contraction, or shortening, occurs when calcium ions are released from the sarcoplasmic reticulum into the myofibrils. This is followed by relaxation after the calcium ions are rapidly returned by active transport to the sarcoplasmic reticulum. Another cycle begins when calcium ions are again released following the next depolarization of the sarcolemma. These cycles are referred to as **excitation–contraction coupling**.

Mechanical changes of actin and myosin

The contraction process involves an interaction between the actin and the myosin myofilaments. There is a natural attraction between actin and myosin for each other that involves active sites on the actin molecule. Attraction is inhibited during relaxation because the active sites are covered, but when calcium ions enter the myofibril the active sites are uncovered. The relative location of the actin and myosin myofilaments to each other

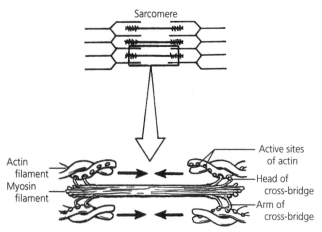

Figure 27.11 The components of the actin and myosin myofilaments associated with contraction of the sarcomere. Arrows indicate the direction of actin movement during contraction (shortening of myofibrils). From Reece, W.O. (2009) *Functional Anatomy and Physiology of Domestic Animals*, 4th edn. Wiley-Blackwell, Ames, IA. Reproduced with permission from Wiley.

within a sarcomere is shown in Figure 27.11. The projecting portions of the myosin molecules (**cross-bridges**) attach to the active sites during contraction and bend toward the center, causing the actin to slide toward the myosin molecule center.

The actin filament has three major components (all protein): **actin**, **tropomyosin**, and **troponin** (Figure 27.12A). Actin and tropomyosin are arranged in helical strands interwoven with each other. Troponin is located at regular intervals along the strands and contains three proteins, two of which bind actin and tropomyosin together and a third which has an affinity for calcium ions. Active sites (places where myosin cross-bridges attach) are located on the actin strands and are normally covered by the tropomyosin strands (Figure 27.12B). When calcium ions bind to the troponin complex, a conformational change occurs between the actin and tropomyosin strands that causes the active sites to be uncovered. The uncovered sites favor activation of the natural attraction that exists between actin and myosin and allows attachment of myosin cross-bridge heads (Figure 27.12C). The mechanics of contraction and relaxation are shown in Figure 27.13.

Energy changes

The energy changes that permit attachment and detachment of the myosin cross-bridge heads are synchronized with the mechanical changes of the actin molecule during contraction and relaxation. These are summarized as follows and illustrated in Figure 27.14.

1 **Adenosine triphosphatase (ATPase)** of the myosin cross-bridge heads hydrolyzes ATP to adenosine diphosphate (ADP) and inorganic phosphate (P_i), leaving the ADP and P_i bound to the heads. Energy from the hydrolysis of ATP "cocks" the heads so that they increase their angle of attachment to the cross-bridge arm and become perpendicular to the active sites of the actin myofilaments (Figure 27.14A).

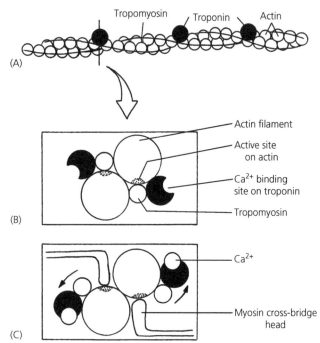

Figure 27.12 Conformational changes of the actin filament after calcium binding. (A) The actin filament with its three proteins, actin, troponin, and tropomyosin. The vertical line indicates the cross-section location for (B) and (C). (B) The active sites on actin are covered by tropomyosin. (C) Ca^{2+} binds to troponin, resulting in a conformational change that exposes the active sites on actin. Myosin cross-bridge heads attach to actin active sites, and myofibril contraction begins. From Reece, W.O. (2009) *Functional Anatomy and Physiology of Domestic Animals*, 4th edn. Wiley-Blackwell, Ames, IA. Reproduced with permission from Wiley.

2 After depolarization of the sarcotubular system, calcium ions diffuse from the sarcoplasmic reticulum into myofibrils and bind to the troponin complexes, whereby actin myofilaments are uncovered; calcium ions are returned rapidly to the sarcoplasmic reticulum once the shortening process begins (ATP is required for return). The natural attraction of myosin to actin is now permitted, and the "cocked" heads bind with active sites (Figure 27.14B).

3 Binding with actin causes conformational changes in the cross-bridge heads ("uncocking") and they bend (tilt) toward the cross-bridge arms (toward the center of the sarcomere), pulling actin with it. The energy is derived from previous ATP hydrolysis (Figure 27.14C).

4 Tilting of the cross-bridge heads causes release of ATP and P_i and sites on the heads are exposed for binding of new ATP. The binding of new ATP causes detachment of myosin cross-bridge heads from actin myofilaments (Figure 27.14D).

The ATPase of myosin cross-bridge heads then hydrolyzes ATP as before, cocking the heads; the process is repeated when the next neuromuscular transmission causes depolarization of the sarcotubular system. Repetition of the process causes the actin myofilaments to be pulled further into the center, thus shortening the sarcomere.

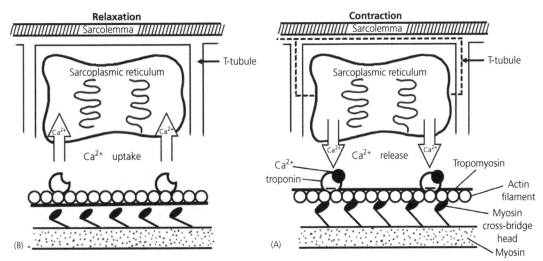

Figure 27.13 A cycle of contraction followed by relaxation. (A) The dashed line indicates transfer of depolarization from the sarcolemma and T tubules to the sarcoplasmic reticulum. Depolarization is followed by Ca^{2+} release from the sarcoplasmic reticulum with diffusion to the myofibrils. Ca^{2+} binds to troponin, removing blocking action of tropomyosin. Myosin cross-bridge heads attach to active sites on actin and bend toward center of myosin molecule. (B) ATP binds to myosin cross-bridge heads, causing their detachment from actin. Ca^{2+} is returned to the sarcoplasmic reticulum using energy supplied by ATP. Removal of Ca^{2+} from troponin restores blocking action of tropomyosin. From Reece, W.O. (2009) *Functional Anatomy and Physiology of Domestic Animals*, 4th edn. Wiley-Blackwell, Ames, IA. Reproduced with permission from Wiley.

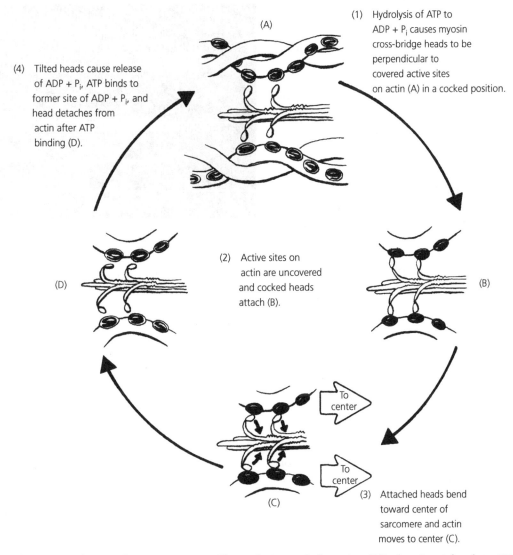

Figure 27.14 The sequence of actin and myosin interaction. This results in muscle shortening. ATP, adenosine triphosphate; ADP, adenosine diphosphate; P_i, inorganic phosphate. From Reece, W.O. (2009) *Functional Anatomy and Physiology of Domestic Animals*, 4th edn. Wiley-Blackwell, Ames, IA. Reproduced with permission from Wiley.

Source of energy

The immediate energy for muscle contraction is thus derived from ATP, forming ADP and P_i. The amount of ATP in muscle fibers is limited, and rephosphorylation of ADP must occur so that contraction can continue. This is accomplished by the transfer from **creatine phosphate (CP)**, which is about five times more plentiful than ATP, according to the following reaction:

$$CP + ADP \xrightarrow{\text{kinase}} C + ATP$$

Because the amount of CP is also limited, the necessary rephosphorylation of creatine (C) to CP and ADP is ultimately derived from intermediary metabolism within the muscle fiber and from the associated reoxidation of reduced cofactors that occurs in the electron transfer chain of the mitochondria. This process is an aerobic system known as **oxidative phosphorylation**.

Aerobic metabolism is important as an energy source for muscle contractions of animal athletes and for endurance exercise required of migrating animals, where repetitive skeletal muscle contractions continue for hours or days. The primary fuel for muscle contractions during prolonged endurance exercise is fatty acids rather than glucose. The fatty acids are broken down to acetyl-CoA and enter the citric acid cycle resulting in the formation of ATP.

Muscle contraction is 50–70% efficient in regard to accomplishment of work. The nonwork portion is dissipated as heat. This heat source is important to the body for the maintenance of body temperature. When at rest, body cooling may result in shivering, which is an attempt to generate heat by muscle contraction.

Contraction versus contracture

Muscle shortening can occur in the absence of action potentials. This type of shortening is referred to as **rigor** or **physiologic contracture**, as opposed to contraction. The actin and myosin filaments remain in a continuous contracted state because sufficient ATP is not available to bring about relaxation (see previous section). Contracture that occurs after death is referred to as **rigor mortis**. However, in this case lack of ATP for relaxation endures, and relaxation only occurs as a result of postmortem autolysis caused by lysosomes 12–24 hours after death. Those muscles that were most active just before death are those that develop rigor mortis first (i.e., greater exhaustion of ATP and CP associated with greater muscle activity). The generation of new ATP via intermediary metabolism is no longer available.

Contraction strength

Contraction strength varies and is achieved by motor unit summation or by wave summation. The stimulation of one motor unit causes a weak contraction, whereas the stimulation of a large number of motor units develops a strong contraction. This is known as **motor unit summation**. All gradations of contraction strength are possible, depending on the number of motor units stimulated. Increasing the strength of contraction by **wave summation** occurs when the frequency of contraction

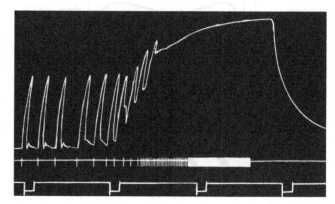

Figure 27.15 Increasing muscle strength by increasing the frequency of contraction. This is known as wave summation. Tetany occurs when individual contractions are fused and cannot be distinguished from each other. From Carlson, A.J. and Johnson, V. (1953) *The Machinery of the Body*, 4th edn. University of Chicago Press, Chicago. Reproduced with permission from University of Chicago Press.

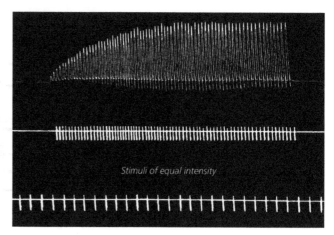

Stimuli of equal intensity

Figure 27.16 The staircase phenomenon of skeletal muscle. This is also known as treppe. Successive stimuli of the same intensity produce contractions of increasing strength. From Carlson, A.J. and Johnson, V. (1953) *The Machinery of the Body*, 4th edn. University of Chicago Press, Chicago. Reproduced with permission from University of Chicago Press.

is increased. When a muscle is stimulated to contract before the muscle has relaxed, the strength of the subsequent contraction, as measured by the height of a lifted load, is increased. When the frequency is sufficient such that the individual muscle twitches become fused into a single prolonged contraction, the strength is at a maximum; this condition is known as **tetany** (Figure 27.15).

Muscles seem to "warm up" to a maximum contraction state. This can be shown by applying stimuli of equal intensity a few seconds apart to a muscle. Each successive muscle twitch has slightly more strength than the preceding one, until optimal contraction strength is reached (Figure 27.16). This phenomenon is referred to as **treppe**, or the **staircase phenomenon**. Successive stimulations are believed to provide an increasing concentration of calcium ions in the sarcoplasm during the initial contractions of rested muscles.

Self-evaluation

Answers can be found at the end of the chapter.

1 Cardiac muscle cells have separations between adjacent cells known as intercalated disks. Their function is to:
   A Regenerate new cells
   B Provide a location for neuromuscular junctions
   C Provide low electrical resistance and thus facilitate depolarization from one cell to the next
   D Release Ca^{2+} for initiation of muscle contraction

2 Pelvic delivery of an unusually large calf has caused a cow to be down and unable to bring her hindlegs together. Obturator nerve paralysis is suspected, and the affected muscles are classified as:
   A Abductors
   B Adductors
   C Extensors
   D Flexors

3 Which one of the following is the smallest component of a skeletal muscle?
   A Sarcomere
   B Myosin
   C Myofibril
   D Muscle fiber

4 The sarcotubular system:
   A Is located within muscle fibers but outside of myofibrils
   B Is a system within each of the myofibrils
   C Has no direct communication (openings) with extracellular fluid
   D Consists of a nerve fiber and the muscle fibers that it innervates

5 Conduction of depolarization from the surface of a muscle fiber to its inner aspects is accomplished by the:
   A Neuromuscular junction
   B Actin filaments
   C Endomysium
   D Sarcotubular system

6 Which tubule set of the sarcotubular system releases Ca^{2+} when depolarized for its diffusion to the myofibrils?
   A Transverse tubules
   B Sarcoplasmic reticulum

7 What chemical begins the depolarization of skeletal muscle fibers after a nerve impulse initiates its release?
   A Ca^{2+}
   B Acetylcholine
   C Succinylcholine
   D Acetylcholinesterase

8 The Ca^{2+} released from the sarcoplasmic reticulum begins the contraction process by:
   A "Cocking" the myosin filament cross-bridge heads
   B Rephosphorylating ADP
   C Exposing actin filament cross-bridge binding sites
   D Facilitating ACh release from the neuromuscular junction

9 Myosin cross-bridge heads detach from actin active sites when the cross-bridge heads bind:
   A Ca^{2+}
   B ATP
   C Creatine phosphate
   D $ADP + P_i$

10 Rigor mortis is an example of _____, which results from a depletion of _____ and a failure of cross-bridge heads to _____ to/from actin. (Select appropriate combination below.)
   A Contraction; Ca^{2+}; attach
   B Relaxation; Ca^{2+}; attach
   C Contracture; ATP; detach
   D Contraction; ATP; detach

Suggested reading

Bailey, J.G. (2004) Muscle physiology. In: *Dukes' Physiology of Domestic Animals*, 12th edn (ed. W.O. Reece), pp. 871–885. Cornell University Press, Ithaca, NY.

Hall, J.E. (2011) Excitation of skeletal muscle: neuromuscular transmission and excitation–contraction coupling. In: *Guyton and Hall Textbook of Medical Physiology*, 12th edn, pp. 83–88. Saunders Elsevier, Philadelphia.

Reece, W. (2009) Muscle. In: *Functional Anatomy and Physiology of Domestic Animals*, 4th edn, pp. 206–229. Wiley-Blackwell, Ames, IA.

Section V: Muscle Physiology

Answers

1 C	6 B
2 B	7 B
3 B	8 C
4 A	9 B
5 D	10 C

28 Physiology of Smooth Muscle

William O. Reece
Iowa State University, Ames, IA, USA

Smooth muscle is so named because it has no visible striations. **Myofilaments** are present and are composed of the contractile proteins **actin** and **myosin**, as in skeletal muscle. However, the filaments are more loosely organized than those in skeletal muscle, which accounts for the lack of visible striations. Smooth muscle is an important functional part of many organs, including the contractile aspect of the intestines, urinary bladder, ureter, blood vessels, uterus, the iris and ciliary muscles of the eye, and the arrector pili muscles that cause hair on the skin to erect. These structures receive innervation from the autonomic nervous system but some may also respond, directly or indirectly, to stretch or extracellular fluid change (e.g., acidosis or alkalosis).

Smooth muscle functions in some sites by performing active contractions (e.g., **peristalsis**) and in other sites with states of sustained contraction called **tone**. In the intestine, tone is maintained constantly and peristalsis inconstantly. The size of arterioles depends on tone of the encircling smooth muscle, which assists in regulating blood pressure.

Smooth muscle types

> **1** What is the difference between multiunit smooth muscle and single-unit smooth muscle?
>
> **2** Which smooth muscle type would be associated with peristaltic waves?
>
> **3** What is the purpose of gap junctions between cell membranes of single-unit smooth muscle?

There are two general types of smooth muscle that vary according to their location, function, organization into sheets or bundles, and characteristics of innervation. These general types are (i) **multiunit smooth muscle** and (ii) **single-unit smooth muscle** (also known as unitary and visceral) (Figure 28.1).

Multiunit smooth muscle

This type of muscle is found in the ciliary body and iris of the eye, the arrector pili muscle of skin hair, and the walls of large arteries. It is composed of discrete smooth muscle fibers. Each muscle fiber is innervated separately and contracts only when it receives synaptic stimuli. Therefore, each fiber can contract independent of the others. Conduction of impulses from one cell to the next does not exist. The individual cells may exist in bundles, but not in sheets.

Single-unit (visceral) smooth muscle

The term "single-unit" does not mean single muscle fibers but rather a large mass of muscle fibers. In this type of smooth muscle, large areas of muscle tissue contract simultaneously and are responsible for **peristaltic waves** of contraction that move intestinal contents from one end of the digestive tract to the other. These waves also occur in the uterus and ureters. Harnessing of single-unit smooth muscle occurs in the following manner.

1 Cell membranes of the fibers within a sheet of fibers are adherent to each other at multiple points, whereby the force generated by one muscle fiber can be transmitted to the next.

2 There are also **gap junctions** between cell membranes that allow ions to flow freely from one muscle fiber to the next. This allows actions potentials to travel from one fiber to the next causing the muscle fibers to contract together.

Dukes' Physiology of Domestic Animals, Thirteenth Edition. Edited by William O. Reece, Howard H. Erickson, Jesse P. Goff and Etsuro E. Uemura.
© 2015 John Wiley & Sons, Inc. Published 2015 by John Wiley & Sons, Inc.
Companion website: www.wiley.com/go/reece/physiology

Microstructure of smooth muscle

> 1 What are dense bodies that are associated with smooth muscle fibers?
>
> 2 What is the ratio of actin to myosin in smooth muscle?
>
> 3 What is the counterpart of skeletal muscle T tubules in smooth muscle?

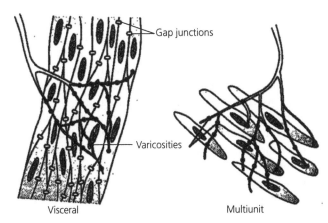

Figure 28.1 Multiunit and visceral smooth muscle types. Autonomic motor neurons synapse with individual multiunit smooth muscle fibers and with several single-unit smooth muscle fibers. Varicosities distributed along the terminal axons of both fiber types contain transmitter substance within their vesicles. Gap junctions between visceral smooth muscle fibers allow free ion flow from one muscle fiber to the next. From Hall, J.E. (2011) *Guyton and Hall Textbook of Medical Physiology*, 12th edn. Saunders Elsevier, Philadelphia. With permission from Elsevier.

The individual cells are spindle-shaped and have a centrally located nucleus (Figure 28.2), in contrast to skeletal muscle fibers that have multiple, peripherally located nuclei. Smooth muscle fibers are referred to as **fusiform** or **spindle-shaped** because they tend to be wide along the middle portion of the fiber and tapered at the ends. The tapered portion of each fiber lies adjacent to the wide portion of the neighboring fibers (see Figure 28.2). This arrangement permits adjacent fibers to be packed closely together, which is most favorable for contractile function.

The arrangement of the myofilaments within a single muscle fiber is shown in Figure 28.3. Note the presence of **dense bodies** that are points of attachment for actin thin filaments. Some dense bodies are scattered throughout the cytoplasm attached to an intermediate filament that links several dense bodies together, while others are attached to the sarcolemma. The dense bodies are rigid stable structures that retain their original shape and attachment during contraction. In this manner, the dense bodies correspond to the **Z lines** of skeletal muscle. Because actin attaches to the fiber sarcolemma-associated dense bodies, smooth muscle fibers develop a wrinkled appearance along their borders when contracted (see Figure 28.3).

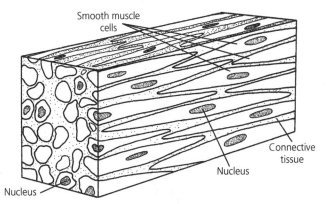

Figure 28.2 Smooth muscle cells exposed in longitudinal and cross-sectional planes. The cells are characteristically spindle-shaped and have a centrally located nucleus. From Reece, W.O. (2009) *Functional Anatomy and Physiology of Domestic Animals*, 4th edn. Wiley-Blackwell, Ames, IA. Reproduced with permission from Wiley.

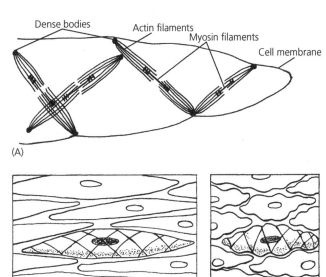

Figure 28.3 Contraction of smooth muscle. (A) Physical structure of smooth muscle. Dense bodies attach either to the cell membrane or to an intracellular structural protein that links several dense bodies together. The dense bodies are functionally similar to Z lines. (B) A translucent view of a relaxed smooth muscle cell. (C) A translucent view of a contracted smooth muscle cell. Dense bodies not shown in (B) and (C). From Reece, W.O. (2009) *Functional Anatomy and Physiology of Domestic Animals*, 4th edn. Wiley-Blackwell, Ames, IA. Reproduced with permission from Wiley.

Interspersed among the actin filaments in the muscle fiber are myosin thick filaments. The myosin filaments have a diameter more than twice that of the actin filaments and the ratio of actin to myosin is 15 : 1 instead of 2 : 1 as in skeletal muscle. The actin filaments from two separate dense bodies extend toward each other and surround a myosin filament (see Figure 28.3), thereby providing a contractile unit that is similar to a contractile unit of skeletal muscle (i.e., the sarcomere).

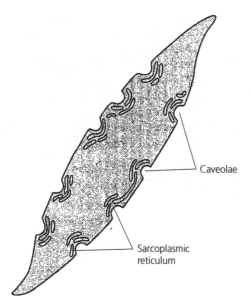

Figure 28.4 Sarcoplasmic tubules in a large smooth muscle fiber showing their relation to invaginations in the cell membrane called calveolae. From Hall, J.E. (2011) *Guyton and Hall Textbook of Medical Physiology*, 12th edn. Saunders Elsevier, Philadelphia. With permission from Elsevier.

T tubules are absent in smooth muscle fibers, but there are numerous invaginations in the fiber membrane called **calveoli** (Figure 28.4). It is believed that they may have a function similar to T tubules in that they are in close proximity to portions of rudimentary sarcoplasmic reticuli found in smooth muscle fibers.

Smooth muscle contraction

> **1** What is calmodulin?
>
> **2** What is the action of myosin kinase?
>
> **3** What "cocks" the myosin cross-bridge heads?
>
> **4** What is accomplished by the regulatory chain of myosin cross-bridge heads after they are "cocked" and repetitive binding with uncovered active sites of actin?
>
> **5** What is the action of myosin phosphatase that causes repetitive binding to stop?

A big difference between skeletal muscle and smooth muscle is that skeletal muscle contracts and relaxes rapidly and smooth muscle contraction is prolonged and often of a tonic nature.

Excitation–contraction coupling in smooth muscle

Smooth muscle does not have the tropomyosin–troponin complex, the protein that covers active sites on the actin filament in skeletal muscle. Further, the active sites are uncovered when troponin combines with calcium ions. Instead of the tropomyosin–troponin complex, smooth muscle contains another protein known as **calmodulin**, a regulatory protein similar to the

tropomyosin–troponin complex, but which differs in the manner in which contraction is initiated. The sequence in smooth muscle whereby activation of the myosin cross-bridge heads supports contraction is as follows.

1 After the influx of calcium ions following depolarization of the fiber membrane, the calcium ions bind with calmodulin.

2 The **calcium–calmodulin** combination binds with and activates **myosin kinase** (phosphocreatine kinase in skeletal muscle), a phosphorylating enzyme.

3 Each of the **myosin cross-bridge heads** has what is called a **regulatory chain** that becomes phosphorylated in response to myosin kinase.

4 When the regulatory chain is phosphorylated ($ADP + P_i \rightarrow ATP$), the head is "cocked" and has the ability to bind repetitively with the uncovered active sites on the actin filament.

5 Repetitive binding with the actin active sites continues through the entire cycling process, with each binding adding to the muscle fiber contraction and development of tension.

6 Relaxation of contracted smooth muscle fibers requires the presence of the enzyme **myosin phosphatase** located in the intracellular fluid of the smooth muscle fiber. Myosin phosphatase splits the phosphate from the regulatory chain on the cross-bridge heads, the heads detach, whereby repetitive binding stops and contraction ceases.

7 Variations in the amount of time for contraction and maintenance of tension are probably determined by the amount of myosin phosphatase in the fibers.

Contrasts between smooth and skeletal muscle contraction

> **1** What are the reasons for the slower cycling of myosin cross-bridge head attachment and detachment?
>
> **2** How is ATPase activity related to attachment of myosin cross-bridge heads to actin?
>
> **3** Why is less energy required to sustain contraction tension in smooth muscle?
>
> **4** What are some reasons why the maximum force of contraction attained by smooth muscle can be greater than that of a skeletal muscle?

Aside from the structural differences, there are functional differences relating to the characteristics of contraction between smooth muscle and skeletal muscle.

1 The cycling of cross-bridge head attachment and detachment to actin sites is much slower in smooth muscle. The sarcoplasmic reticulum is rudimentary in smooth muscle fibers and calcium ions must enter the fiber from the extracellular fluid. Also, the Ca^{2+} pumps are in the fiber membrane and are much slower than those in the sarcoplasmic reticulum of skeletal muscles.

2 Cross-bridge heads have less ATPase activity (provides energy for attachment of cross-bridge heads to actin) in smooth muscle, thereby reducing movements of the cross-bridge heads and slowing the rate of cycling.

3 Much less energy is required to sustain contraction tension in smooth muscle because slow attachment and detachment cycling requires only one molecule of ATP for each cycle, regardless of its duration. Maintenance of tonic contractions (e.g., intestines, urinary bladder) without cycling provides energy economy for the body.

4 The maximum force of contraction attained by smooth muscle can be greater than that of skeletal muscle because of the prolonged attachment of myosin cross-bridge heads to the actin filaments. Also, smooth muscle tissue has much more **extracellular material** (i.e., collagen, elastin) than skeletal muscle. Each smooth muscle fiber is surrounded by a **basal lamina** and **reticular fibers** that when coupled with the extracellular material helps to organize the force produced by individual smooth muscle fibers into a combined effort, as in peristalsis of the gut and contractions of the uterus. In this regard, smooth muscle has the ability to produce a contractile force comparable to that of skeletal muscle.

Smooth muscle contraction stimuli

1 How does the innervation by autonomic nerve fibers to single-unit smooth muscle differ from that of skeletal muscle?

2 Are acetylcholine (parasympathetic) and norepinephrine (sympathetic) secreted by the same fiber?

3 What contributes to the simultaneous contraction of large areas of single-unit smooth muscle fibers?

4 Are multiunit smooth muscle fibers stimulated by stretch?

Autonomic nervous system

Neuromuscular junctions found in skeletal muscle fibers do not occur in smooth muscle. The autonomic nerve fibers innervating single-unit smooth muscle branch diffusely on top of a sheet of muscle fibers. Instead of making direct contact, there are multiple **varicosities** (similar to a terminal bulb of presynaptic neurons) distributed along the nerve fiber with vesicles containing the transmitter substance, either **acetylcholine** or **norepinephrine**. They are never secreted by the same fiber. Smooth muscle fibers are usually innervated by both sympathetic and parasympathetic nerve fibers, each having opposite effects on the muscle fibers. Some smooth muscle fibers may be innervated by only one division of the autonomic nervous system (e.g., blood vessels).

Smooth muscle cells normally have a certain level of **tone**, and the amount of released neurotransmitter determines whether the muscle fibers will contract further or relax. The neurotransmitter released by the varicosities diffuses over a large area and affects numerous single-unit smooth muscle fibers. In this way, large areas of smooth muscle contract simultaneously, with electrical stimuli being transmitted repeatedly among neighboring fibers by way of **gap junctions**. These allow action potentials to travel from one fiber to the next, causing muscle fibers that are not otherwise directly affected by the diffused neurotransmitter to contract together. This kind of activity is common in the large peristaltic waves of contraction that move intestinal contents from one end of the digestive tract to the other and similar peristaltic waves that occur in the uterus and the ureters.

Stimuli other than autonomic

The membrane of single-unit smooth muscle fibers is sensitive to mechanical stimuli. Stretching the membrane of these fibers leads to depolarization and consequently contraction, whereby contractile tension can be propagated or maintained over a large area of muscle tissue. With autoregulation of blood flow in arterioles, a rise in blood pressure causes stretch of the encircling smooth muscle that stimulates contraction. This maintains a fairly constant blood flow in the tissue they supply.

Multiunit smooth muscle is found in the ciliary body and the iris of the eye, in the ductus deferens, and the walls of large arteries. In these units of smooth muscle, each muscle fiber is innervated separately and contracts only when it receives synaptic stimuli.

In addition to the above stimuli, smooth muscle may be affected directly or indirectly by changes in oxygen concentration, pH, or ion concentrations in the extracellular fluid.

Self-evaluation

Answers can be found at the end of the chapter.

1 Smooth muscle is innervated by somatic nerves (spinal and cranial nerves) instead of autonomic nerves.
A True
B False

2 Single-unit (visceral) smooth muscle refers to a large mass of muscle fibers whereas multiunit smooth muscle refers to single muscle fibers.
A True
B False

3 Dense bodies in smooth muscle fibers are points of attachment for myosin (thick) filaments.
A True
B False

4 T tubules are absent in smooth muscle fibers but a similar function is associated with structures known as calveoli.
A True
B False

Section V: Muscle Physiology

5 Smooth muscle is characterized by rapid contraction and relaxation rather than prolonged contraction that is often of a tonic nature.

A True

B False

6 Smooth muscle does not have the tropomyosin–troponin complex found in skeletal muscle but contains another protein known as calmodulin that initiates contraction in the same manner as the tropomyosin–troponin complex.

A True

B False

7 Each myosin cross-bridge head composes a regulatory chain that is phosphorylated in response to myosin kinase and "cocks" the myosin cross-bridge heads.

A True

B False

8 The cycling of cross-bridge attachment and detachment to actin sites is much slower in smooth muscle than in skeletal muscle.

A True

B False

9 Neuromuscular junctions found in skeletal muscle fibers are also associated with smooth muscle fibers.

A True

B False

10 The autoregulation of blood flow in arterioles is an example of the sensitivity of single-unit smooth muscle fibers to mechanical stimuli, whereby a rise in blood pressure causes stretch of encircling smooth muscle that stimulates contraction.

A True

B False

Suggested reading

Bailey, J.G. (2004) Muscle physiology. In: *Dukes' Physiology of Domestic Animals*, 12th edn (ed. W.O. Reece), pp. 887–889. Cornell University Press, Ithaca, NY.

Hall, J.E. (2011) Excitation and contraction of smooth muscle. In: *Guyton and Hall Textbook of Medical Physiology*, 12th edn, pp. 91–98. Saunders Elsevier, Philadelphia.

Reece, W. (2009) Muscle. In: *Functional Anatomy and Physiology of Domestic Animals*, 4th edn, pp. 222–223. Wiley-Blackwell, Ames, IA.

Answers

1	B		6	B
2	A		7	A
3	B		8	A
4	A		9	B
5	B		10	A

29 Physiology of Cardiac Muscle, Muscle Adaptations, and Muscle Disorders

William O. Reece
Iowa State University, Ames, IA, USA

Cardiac muscle

> **1** Why are cardiac muscle fibers considered a functional syncytium rather than a morphological syncytium?
>
> **2** What is the predominant source of energy when engaged in aerobic metabolism?
>
> **3** What is the function of gap junctions?

Cardiac muscle is found only in the heart and over the lifetime of a domestic animal contracts millions of times, demonstrating its properties of endurance. Cardiac muscle, like skeletal muscle, is striated, and has a similar organization of sarcomeres with actin and myosin filaments. There are differences, however, in how the fibers are organized and innervated that allow their coordinated function. Greater detail of heart function is described in Section VI. However, in order to compare the three types of muscle, a description of the fundamental properties of cardiac muscle is included herein.

Morphological differences

In contrast to skeletal muscle, cardiac muscle fibers do not fuse into a single multinucleated fiber during embryonic development. Cardiac muscle fibers are typically uninucleated, with the nucleus centrally placed within each fiber rather than peripherally as in skeletal muscle (Figure 29.1). Cardiac myocytes branch or bifurcate during embryonic development and bind to myocytes in adjacent chains. However, the fibers do not fuse and remain separated as distinct fibers with their respective sarcolemma throughout development.

Because the fibers do not fuse with each other they do not form a morphological syncytium, but because of their branching and bifurcations they form a **functional syncytium** that will allow coordinated contraction. The dark, dense cross-bands found on the ends of cardiac muscle fibers are called **intercalated disks** (see Figure 29.1), which are continuous with the sarcolemma and are intercellular junctions.

The diameter and length of mature cardiac muscle fibers are approximately 15 μm and 85–100 μm, respectively. Mature skeletal muscles have a larger diameter (0.1–0.5 mm) and a longer length (10–30 cm).

Energy sources

Mitochondria make up about 40% of the cytoplasmic volume compared with only about 2% in skeletal muscle. This reflects the reliance of cardiac muscle on aerobic metabolism. Cardiac muscle cells stop contracting after about 30 s of oxygen deprivation. There are numerous lipid droplets in cardiac muscle fibers that contain triglycerides, the storage form of fatty acids, which are the predominant energy source when engaged in aerobic metabolism.

Gap junctions and action potentials

Gap junctions present within the intercalated disks allow communication between the cytoplasm of adjacent end-to-end fibers, and permit the free diffusion of ions and action potentials. As a result of their end-to-end location, action potentials are conducted rapidly in a direction parallel to the longitudinal axis. Thus because of the gap junctions and intercalated disks all cardiac muscle fibers are electrically connected, whereas skeletal

Section V: Muscle Physiology

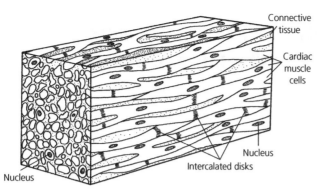

Figure 29.1 Cardiac muscle fibers exposed in longitudinal and cross-sectional planes. Note elongated branching fibers with irregular contours at their junctions with other fibers. From Reece, W.O. (2009) *Functional Anatomy and Physiology of Domestic Animals*, 4th edn. Wiley-Blackwell, Ames, IA. Reproduced with permission from Wiley.

muscle fibers must be separately stimulated by a motor neuron to form an action potential.

Action potentials in cardiac muscle tissue spread from fiber to fiber, which allows depolarization to spread through the entire heart, leading to coordinated virtually simultaneous contraction of all the cardiac muscle fibers in a heart chamber and permitting the movement of large volumes of blood through the cardiovascular system. This is why cardiac muscle tissue is considered to be a functional syncytium.

Excitation–contraction coupling

> 1 How does the source of calcium ions for muscle contraction in cardiac muscle differ from that in skeletal muscle?
>
> 2 Can a very high concentration of calcium ions in the extracellular fluid be detrimental?
>
> 3 How do the catecholamines affect cardiac muscle?

Recall that **excitation–contraction coupling** is the mechanism by which the action potential causes the myofibrils of muscle to contract. In cardiac muscle, as in skeletal muscle, the action potential spreads to the interior of the cardiac muscle fiber via the T tubules to the membranes of the sarcoplasmic reticulum (SR), followed by release of Ca^{2+} into the sarcoplasm of the sarcoplasmic reticulum. This is followed by muscle contraction. Differences exist in cardiac muscles that are related to Ca^{2+} release. In skeletal muscle, the SR provided all the Ca^{2+} to provide full contraction strength. However, the T tubules of cardiac muscle have a diameter much greater than that of the T tubules in skeletal muscle; therefore, in addition to the Ca^{2+} released into the sarcoplasm by the SR, a large quantity of extra Ca^{2+} also diffuses into the sarcoplasm from the T tubules at the time of the action potential. In addition, the inner aspect of the T tubules contains a large quantity of mucopolysaccharides that are electronegatively charged and which bind an abundant store of Ca^{2+} derived from extracelluar fluid (ECF). This is

facilitated because the openings of the T tubules directly communicate with ECF surrounding the fibers. Therefore, the strength of contraction of cardiac muscle is dependent on the concentration of Ca^{2+} in the ECF, which is not the case for skeletal muscle because all the Ca^{2+} is released from the SR inside the fiber and the strength of contraction is affected very little by the ECF Ca^{2+} concentration.

An increase in the ECF concentration of Ca^{2+} increases contractile force, but a very high concentration leads to cardiac arrest during systole (contraction) due to **rigor** (contraction without action potentials) of cardiac muscle fibers.

Catecholamines (i.e., epinephrine and norepinephrine) increase the movement of calcium ions into cardiac muscle fibers as well as increase the sensitivity of the contractile mechanism to the presence of calcium ions.

Muscle adaptations

> 1 Is regeneration of cardiac muscle fibers possible? What happens if they die?
>
> 2 How does hypertrophy differ from hyperplasia?
>
> 3 Does increase in cardiac muscle size involve hypertrophy or hyperplasia?
>
> 4 What is denervation atrophy?

Muscle is the most adaptive tissue in the animal body. Individual muscle fibers of skeletal, cardiac, and smooth muscle increase in size as a normal response to chronic mechanical stress, as with regular exercise. Similar stress in skeletal and smooth muscle causes division of muscle fibers through mitosis to produce new fibers. A decrease in size can occur in all three muscle types in response to disuse or disease.

Hypertrophy and hyperplasia

An increase in individual muscle-fiber size is referred to as **hypertrophy**. It is common in skeletal, cardiac, and smooth muscle fibers. Postnatal growth of skeletal muscle fibers is not accomplished by an increase in the number of muscle fibers but rather by the addition of myofibrils to the periphery and addition of sarcomeres to the tendinous ends.

An increase in the number of muscle fibers is called **hyperplasia**. Regeneration of skeletal-muscle fibers is possible from so-called **satellite fibers**, but this requires an intact endomysium for successful repair. Cardiac muscle fibers can increase in size in the same way as in skeletal muscle, in that it involves hypertrophy and not hyperplasia.

Regeneration of cardiac-muscle fibers does not occur, because there is no counterpart to the satellite cells of skeletal muscle. If myocardial fibers die, they are replaced by fibrous noncontractile scar tissue. Smooth-muscle organs can increase their size not only by hypertrophy but also by hyperplasia, which accounts for considerable regenerative ability.

Atrophy

A decrease in the size of a muscle is referred to as **atrophy**. When a body part has been immobilized for a period of time, the muscles become smaller (referred to as **disuse atrophy**). Loss of the nerve supply to a muscle results in **denervation atrophy**. This was formerly a common condition in harnessed draft horses. The presence of the collar presses on the suprascapular nerve that supplies the two major muscle masses of the shoulder blade. The resulting denervation causes the muscle of the shoulder to atrophy, resulting in a condition known as **sweeney** (also called **shoulder slip**).

Muscle disorders

> 1 What is the general mechanism whereby tetanus neurotoxin produces muscular spasm?
>
> 2 Is the expression of tetanus similar in all animal species?
>
> 3 What is the predisposing condition causing exertional rhabdomyolysis?
>
> 4 Does the acute form of exertional rhabdomyolysis occur in working dogs and racing greyhounds?
>
> 5 What are the dominant clinical signs of bovine parturient paresis? What is its cause?
>
> 6 Milk fever in the cow and eclampsia in the bitch are caused by hypocalcemia. Why are the clinical signs different?
>
> 7 What stress factors contribute to dark cutting beef?

The overview of muscle physiology at the beginning of Chapter 27 alluded to the multitude of body functions associated with muscles. Accordingly, it is not surprising that there are a large number of infectious, nutritional, and metabolic diseases that are manifested by muscle disorders. Only a few will be briefly considered in which muscle disorders are a distinguishing feature.

Tetanus

Tetanus is a bacterial disease caused by a potent neurotoxin elaborated by the organism *Clostridium tetani*. The neurotoxin reaches the central nervous system and prevents release of an inhibitory transmitter (glycine). The resulting sensitivity to the excitatory impulses, unchecked by inhibitory impulses, produces generalized muscular spasm (**tetany**). Tetanus in humans has been called lockjaw because the masseter muscles that close the mouth are stronger than the muscles that open the mouth and the jaws remain in a closed position. Expression of tetanus in animals varies somewhat among species. In the horse, tonic spasms of skeletal muscles are extensive. Beginning first at the head or in muscles of the hindlimbs, they extend either slowly or rapidly until the condition becomes generalized. Spasms may be limited to a definite group of muscles, such as muscles of the jaw, causing difficulty in prehension and mastication and drooling of saliva because of difficulty in swallowing. The clinical signs described for the horse are somewhat similar in other species but more distinctive in cattle, with extension of the head and neck, tucked-up abdomen, and extended tail.

Exertional rhabdomyolysis

Exertional rhabdomyolysis (ER) is a specific disease of horses characterized by a suddenly developing muscle pain or cramping of the hindlimbs. At one time, ER was considered a single entity, described as azoturia, tying up, or Monday morning disease. Several different myopathies are now recognized that have similarities in clinical presentation.

The disease occurs only in well-nourished animals and appears during exercise after a period of idleness, typically when individuals at regular work are kept idle with no exercise and no reduction in diet for 2–5 days, whereby an attack may develop in 15 min to 1 hour after exercise is resumed. This predisposing condition is the most essential causative influence. The intensity of exercise or work is of little significance when it occurs.

Clinical signs generally occur within 30 min after leaving the stable: sweating begins, the gait becomes stiff, and the animal is reluctant to move. Signs of distress include recumbency, pawing, and stretching. Firm, painful, lumbar and gluteal musculature are common signs. Urine is red/brown and often described as coffee-colored. The exercise induces muscle necrosis that results in the release of creatine kinase (CK) and myoglobin into the circulation. Excessive myoglobinuria may cause renal tubular damage and acute renal failure.

Acute ER may be sporadic and occur on a single occasion, or chronic where recurrent episodes occur repeatedly in susceptible horses. The acute episodes are identical regardless of their being sporadic or recurrent. Recurrent ER is seen frequently in thoroughbreds, standardbreds, and Arabian horses. It is likely due to abnormal regulation of intracellular calcium in skeletal muscle.

Acute ER occurs in racing greyhounds and working dogs where severe cases are characterized by muscle ischemia after exercise or excitement. The avascularity and lactic acidosis bring forth clinical signs and outcomes similar to equine ER.

Some nonexercise-associated rhabdomyopathies are nutritional myopathies, associated with vitamin E and selenium deficiency, and a genetic myopathy known as polysaccharide storage myopathy (PSSM).

Bovine parturient paresis (milk fever)

Parturient paresis is a paralysis and loss of consciousness leading to coma in dairy cows that have recently calved. The onset may be marked by tonic muscular spasms and twitching that are soon replaced by the dominant clinical signs of paresis and depressed consciousness, which are seen in the majority of cases. It is caused by a sudden drop in blood calcium (hypocalcemia) associated with the onset of lactation, and is most common in high-producing dairy cows.

Canine puerpenal tetany (eclampsia)

Puerpenal tetany is an acute condition usually seen at peak lactation 2–3 weeks after whelping and, like parturient paresis, is associated with hypocalcemia. Small-breed bitches with large litters are most often affected. Early clinical signs are restlessness. Subsequent changes include mild tremors, twitching, muscle spasms, stiffness, and ataxia. Severe tremors, tetany, and generalized seizure activity may be seen. The functional disturbances associated with hypocalcemia in the bitch are primarily the result of neuromuscular tetany, whereas in cows the clinical signs are related to paresis. The contrast is related to differences in function of the neuromuscular junction between the cow and the bitch. In cows, release of acetylcholine and transmission of nerve impulses across the neuromuscular junction is blocked by hypocalcemia, leading to muscle paresis. In the bitch, excitation–contraction coupling is maintained at the neuromuscular junction. The low concentration of calcium in the extracellular fluid has an excitatory effect on nerve and muscle cells, because it lowers the threshold potential and requires a stimulus of lesser magnitude to depolarize. Tetany occurs as a result of spontaneous repetitive firing of motor nerve fibers.

Dark cutting beef (dark cutters)

Dark cutting beef is a description for cuts of beef that do not "bloom" or brighten when they are exposed to air when marketed in a display case. Accordingly, it represents a financial loss to the meat industry. The retail products are referred to as "dark cutters."

The causes are linked to pre-harvest stress of live animals prior to slaughter and the depletion of muscle glycogen. The loss of muscle glycogen causes the pH to become more alkaline because glycogen content would ordinarily determine the concentration of lactic acid and acidity. Bacterial growth in meat is inhibited by low pH, and the higher pH of meat from glycogen-depleted animals spoils more easily. The meat has a firm texture and a dark appearance. Stress factors identified as contributing to dark cutting beef and that decrease the levels of muscle glycogen in the live animal include low energy intake by livestock, poor livestock handling, mixing groups of animals, and severe weather conditions during transport.

Self-evaluation

Answers can be found at the end of the chapter.

1 As compared to skeletal muscle fibers, the diameter and length of cardiac muscle fibers are:
   A Smaller
   B About the same
   C Larger
   D Larger in diameter but shorter in length

2 As compared to skeletal muscle fibers, the duration of action potentials in cardiac muscle fibers is:
   A Shorter
   B About the same
   C Longer
   D Too close to call

3 The predominant energy source for cardiac muscle fibers when engaged in aerobic metabolism is:
   A Glucose
   B Fatty acids
   C Amino acids
   D Triglycerides

4 Full contraction strength in cardiac muscle is related to release of Ca^{2+} into the sarcoplasm from:
   A Sarcoplasmic reticulum only
   B Sarcoplasmic reticulum and the T tubules
   C Sarcoplasmic reticulum, T tubules, and the extracellular fluid
   D Gap junctions

5 An increase in cardiac muscle size is associated with:
   A Atrophy
   B Hypertrophy and hyperplasia
   C Satellite cells
   D Hypertrophy

6 If myocardial fibers die:
   A Regeneration occurs from satellite cells
   B They are replaced by fibrous noncontractile scar tissue
   C There is replacement of cells followed by hypertrophy and hyperplasia
   D There is replacement of cells followed only by hypertrophy

7 Could the inability to swallow, causing difficulty in prehension and mastication and drooling of saliva, be the only clinical sign of tetanus (caused by a bacterial neurotoxin) in horses and/or cattle?
   A True
   B False

8 Which of the following clinical signs or characteristics are associated with exertional rhabdomyolysis in horses?
   A A suddenly developing muscle pain or cramping of the hindlimbs
   B Occurs in well-nourished animals and appears during exercise after a period of idleness
   C Exercise-induced muscle necrosis and release of myoglobin into the circulation
   D Acute episodes may be sporadic or recurring
   E All of the above

9 As compared to bovine parturient paresis, which of the following is not characteristic of canine puerperal tetany?
   A Both are associated with hypocalcemia
   B Both are associated with the onset of lactation
   C The transmission of nerve impulses across the neuromuscular junction is blocked

D The hypocalcemia lowers the threshold potential at the neuromuscular junction that results in spontaneous repetitive firing of motor nerve fibers

E Both **B** and **C**

10 Which one of the following statements relates to retail products known as "dark cutters"?

A They give a nice brightness when displayed at the meat counter

B Pre-harvest stress is not a factor because muscle glycogen is normal at the time of slaughter

C The causes are linked to pre-harvest stress (e.g., low energy intake, poor livestock handling) that decrease the levels of muscle glycogen in the live animal

D It is a preferred cut of beef by the meat industry

Suggested reading

Bailey, J.G. (2004) Muscle physiology. In: *Dukes' Physiology of Domestic Animals*, 12th edn (ed. W.O. Reece), pp. 885–887. Cornell University Press, Ithaca, NY.

Hall, J.E. (2011) Cardiac muscle: the heart as a pump and function of the heart valves. In: *Guyton and Hall Textbook of Medical Physiology*, 12th edn, pp. 101–104. Saunders Elsevier, Philadelphia.

Reece, W.O. (2009) Muscle. In: *Functional Anatomy and Physiology of Domestic Animals*, 4th edn, pp. 222–224. Wiley-Blackwell, Ames, IA.

Answers

1	A	6	B
2	C	7	A
3	B	8	E
4	C	9	E
5	D	10	C

Section V: Muscle Physiology

SECTION VI

The Cardiovascular System

Section Editor: Howard H. Erickson

30 The Heart and Vasculature: Gross Structure and Basic Properties

Dean H. Riedesel and Richard L. Engen
Iowa State University, Ames, IA, USA

The heart and a vast array of blood vessels that vary in size and tissue composition form the cardiovascular system. The function of the cardiovascular system can be simplified to that of a transportation system which distributes oxygen and nutrients to the tissues and removes carbon dioxide and other metabolic byproducts. The interstitial fluid environment surrounding the cells of an animal's body must remain relatively "constant" and maintaining this consistency is known as **homeostasis**. The role of the cardiovascular system in homeostasis cannot be overlooked. In addition to oxygen and nutrients, hormones, white blood cells, platelets, electrolytes, and heat are also transported by the cardiovascular system and closely controlled for maintaining homeostasis. Although the cardiovascular system does not control these variables, it is used for the transportation and distribution of essential substances and byproducts that diffuse between the dense capillary networks and the interstitial fluid of tissues.

William Harvey described the mammalian circulatory system in 1628. Since that time much work has been done to study the system and research continues to this day. Although simple in principle, the cardiovascular system must have the ability to alter organ perfusion rapidly. For example, a resting skeletal muscle does not require much blood flow but as soon as it starts to exercise the need for oxygen and glucose increases rapidly. Thus, changes in the total flow of blood (**cardiac output**) and its distribution within the body will have to change to meet those demands. The mechanical and physiologic factors which cause and control the flow of blood in the body are better understood when basic principles of hemodynamics are reviewed. Although the direct application of physics concerning fluid flow in rigid tubes is not appropriate, the concepts are useful in understanding blood flow.

Gross structure

1 Describe the location of the heart in the chest cavity.
2 Is the heart free to move or is it held in a fixed position?

The heart is in the thoracic cavity within the mediastinum between the left and right pleural cavities and protected by the ribs from about the third to the sixth intercostal spaces. The dorsal aspect is horizontally in line with the middle of the first rib and the ventral aspect is on the sternum. The long axis of the cardiac silhouette is oriented vertically in the horse, almost vertically in ruminants, and progressively more obliquely in the pig, dog, and cat. The dorsal part of the heart is known as the base and is formed by the atria and the major vessels entering (veins) and leaving (arteries) the heart. The major vessels tend to hold the heart in a relatively fixed position dorsally while ventrally it is free within the pericardial sac.

Dukes' Physiology of Domestic Animals, Thirteenth Edition. Edited by William O. Reece, Howard H. Erickson, Jesse P. Goff and Etsuro E. Uemura.
© 2015 John Wiley & Sons, Inc. Published 2015 by John Wiley & Sons, Inc.
Companion website: www.wiley.com/go/reece/physiology

Section VI: The Cardiovascular System

Cardiovascular system

> 1 Describe the arterial and venous systems as being high resistance or high capacitance and explain why.
>
> 2 Which organ receives more blood flow, the kidney or the myocardium?
>
> 3 What percent of a dog's body weight is blood?

The cardiovascular system has two circulations in series: (i) the **pulmonary circulation** composed of the right atrium (RA), right ventricle (RV) and lungs; and (ii) the **systemic circulation** composed of the left atrium (LA), left ventricle (LV), and the systemic organs. Each circulation has three major divisions: (i) the distribution system (ventricles, arteries, and arterioles), (ii) the perfusion/exchange system (capillaries), and (iii) the collecting system (venules, veins, and atria). The major components of the cardiovascular system are shown in Figure 30.1, with the **arterial** (high-pressure) system on the right and **venous** (low-pressure) system on the left. The areas shaded blue represent the venous and the pulmonary arterial systems that carry blood with reduced oxygen content. The areas shaded red include the arterial and pulmonary venous systems that carry oxygenated blood. The pulmonary and systemic systems are in series such that blood flow to the lungs from the right ventricle equals blood flow in the aorta coming from the left ventricle. The amount of blood pumped by the right or left ventricle is called the cardiac output ($\dot{Q}$) and is measured in liters per minute. The distribution of blood flow is indicated (see Figure 30.1) by percentages on the arteries supplying the various organs (e.g., 15% of the cardiac output goes to the head and endocrine glands). The intravascular pressures are measured in millimeters of mercury (mmHg) and are shown (see Figure 30.1) as mean values in parentheses on both the arterial and venous systems (e.g., the mean blood pressure in the aorta is 100 mmHg).

Figure 30.1 can be used to illustrate the following.

1 The arterial system (right side of diagram) is the high-**resistance**, low-compliance system and distributes blood from the left ventricle. Resistance (R) = pressure (ΔP)/flow ($\dot{Q}$).

2 The venous system (left side of diagram) is the low-pressure, high-**capacitance** system that stores and returns blood to the atria. Capacitance (C) = volume (ΔV)/pressure (ΔP).

3 Capillaries connect the arteries and veins and exchange gases and small molecules by diffusion with the tissues.

4 The cardiac output distribution ($\dot{Q}$) is indicated by numbers in parentheses on the arterial side of the diagram. The organs involved with the transport of heat and waste products out of the body and those that provide oxygen and nutrients receive a higher percentage of cardiac output than they need for their metabolism.

5 The major resistance sites on the arterial side occur at the precapillary beds (solid black circles).

6 Blood usually flows through only one capillary bed between an artery and vein. Unique portal systems occur in the renal and the digestive organ circulations. A **portal system** is defined as two capillary beds connected in series between an artery and a vein. In the renal circulation, there is a glomerular capillary bed between two arterioles and another normal capillary bed between an arteriole and a venule. Another portal system is shown in the digestive venous circulation as it drains into the liver via the portal vein. Additionally, the liver has an arterial supply for delivery of oxygen and nutrients. A third portal system occurs in the hypothalamus/pituitary area of the cranial blood flow.

7 The lungs receive 100% of the cardiac output from the right heart. This is a system with a greatly reduced blood pressure. The pulmonary artery pressure is approximately one-fifth that of the aorta on the arterial systemic side. Therefore, the vascular resistance is low ($\downarrow R = \downarrow P/\dot{Q}$) and the cross-sectional area of the pulmonary capillaries is large compared with the areas within the other organ systems.

8 The **preload** to the right ventricle (volume of blood in the ventricle prior to contraction) is blood returning to the heart from the high-capacitance, low-pressure venous system. The pressures in the right and left ventricle shown in Figure 30.1 approximate the mean diastolic pressures. The **afterload** (load on the ventricle during contraction, usually considered to be the pressure in the aorta) for the left ventricle is created by the high-resistance, low-capacitance arterial system or, more simply stated, the high-pressure arterial compartment.

9 The blood flow resistance of each organ can be calculated from the flow (percentage of cardiac output) and the blood pressure drop (ΔP) across the organ ($R = \Delta P/\dot{Q}$).

10 The mean blood pressure will vary somewhat depending on the effects of gravity on the vascular beds. A good example of this is the mean aortic blood pressure of the giraffe (mean, 190 mmHg) or other long-necked animals. In this example, the vascular pressure at the level of the heart must be increased to overcome the hydrostatic pressure created by the column of blood from the giraffe's head to the level of the heart in order to adequately perfuse the brain.

11 The circulatory system is a closed circuit and the flow (L/min) of venous blood returning to the heart or **venous return** must equal the flow of blood pumped by the left ventricle into the aorta. The heart cannot pump more blood than is supplied by the venous return. The exact amount of flow around the circuit depends on the number and strength of the heart contractions, total volume of blood, and the characteristics of the vessels.

The fluid and nutritive balance of the total organism depends on maintaining the distribution, perfusion, and collecting systems in balance (pressure and volume) at all times. This balance requires a synchronized concert of adequate hydrostatic pressure, normal osmotic and oncotic pressures, balanced distribution of blood flow, appropriate vessel diameters, and functional tissue capillaries.

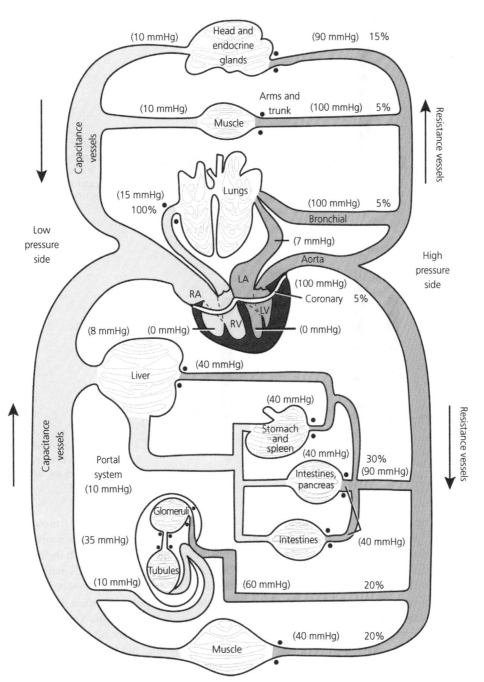

Figure 30.1 Overview of the cardiovascular system. The blue areas represent the venous blood with reduced oxygen content; the red vessels represent the arterial system with oxygenated blood. The solid black circles indicate areas of resistance, and the percentages indicate the proportion of cardiac output delivered to the organ system at rest. The size of the capillary bed varies with organ systems. From Reece, W.O. (2004) *Dukes' Physiology of Domestic Animals*, 12th edn. Cornell University Press, Ithaca, NY. Reproduced with permission from Cornell University Press.

Section VI: The Cardiovascular System

Blood volume versus body weight

In mammals, there is a relationship of heart weight and **blood volume** to body weight. The heart weight and the blood volume are approximately 0.6 and 8.0% of body weight, respectively. The distribution of blood volume within the vascular system (Figure 30.2) is very important for establishing the pressure gradients throughout the circulatory system. Comparison of the distribution of blood and the cross-sectional areas (Figure 30.3) within the vascular system segments clearly defines the arterial system as the resistance system (low volume, high pressure) and the venous system as the capacitance system (high volume, low pressure). The molecular structure of the arterial system resists

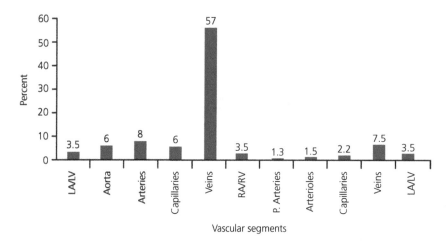

Figure 30.2 Distribution of blood in the vascular system (percentage). LA/LV, left atrium/left ventricle; RA/RV, right atrium/right ventricle; P, pulmonary. From Reece, W.O. (2004) *Dukes' Physiology of Domestic Animals*, 12th edn. Cornell University Press, Ithaca, NY. Reproduced with permission from Cornell University Press.

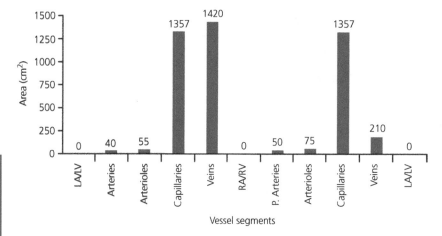

Figure 30.3 Cross-sectional area (cm²) of the cardiovascular system for a 20-kg dog. Data adapted from Berne, R.M. and Levy, M.N. (1998) *Physiology*, 4th edn, p. 327. Mosby, St Louis, MO.

expansion and therefore contains a small percentage of total blood volume at any time period. This physiologic condition allows the development of an elevated pressure. Because the expansion of the arteries is primarily due to stretch of the collagen and elastin fibers, no energy is required to return the vessel diameter to the normal state (diastolic phase). Thus, the arterial system becomes an additional pump sustaining the blood flowing away from the heart. This elastic recoil to the diastolic distension diameter has been called the Windkessel effect.

The arterial divergence aids in reducing the distal blood pressure and allows the distribution of blood to the organ tissues. The venous system can increase significantly in volume with an insignificant change in the internal pressure (i.e., high capacitance or $\Delta V/\Delta P$). Although small in magnitude, the pressure gradients are sufficient to allow the continuous flow of blood from the capillaries to the right heart.

Vascular tone

Organ blood flow is largely determined by its vascular resistance which, in turn, is determined by the tone or constriction of the smooth muscles in the walls of the arterioles which control the vessel radius. Arterioles are normally partially constricted even when all external influences are removed. This is known as basal

tone and may be due to the smooth muscles resisting the stretch caused by the internal vascular pressure or the production of a constrictor substance by the endothelium. In the smaller precapillary vessels, **vascular tone** is maintained by rhythmic contractions of the arteriolar smooth muscle, the frequency, duration, and amplitude of which determine resistance to blood flow through those vessels. The underlying smooth muscle contractile activity may be modulated by vasomotor nerves, vasoactive agents, and the local ionic and metabolic environment. The vascular tone varies in different segments of a given vascular bed, for example the tone of precapillary resistance vessels is high, while it is less so in the venous capacitance vessels. The degree of basal tone varies in different tissues, for example there is high resistance in vessels of the brain, myocardium, skeletal muscle, and splanchnic organs but resistance is practically absent in the open arteriovenous anastomoses of the skin. Variations in vascular tone are determinants of vascular resistance, capillary blood flow and exchange, arteriovenous shunting, and vascular capacitance. When an organ system requires maximal blood flow there may be limitations on how low vascular resistance will become because if all the circulatory beds dilated maximally at once, cardiac output could not equal the total flow rate required and systemic blood pressure would fall. Thus overall vascular resistance must be maintained at some minimal level by appropriate adjustments when maximal blood flow is required in some organs.

Blood volume distribution

The blood volume distribution (see Figure 30.2) does not parallel the total cross-sectional area (see Figure 30.3) of the vascular segments, as exemplified by the largest cross-sectional area (systemic plus pulmonary capillaries) containing only a small fraction (8.2%) of blood volume. The length of a typical capillary is very short, making the volume very small even though the cross-sectional area is large. The capillaries need the large surface area to distribute the blood efficiently because blood remains in the capillaries only a very short time, usually less than 750 ms. The time in the capillary is shortened to 250 ms during exercise.

Dynamic parameters

> 1 Define the systolic, diastolic, and mean blood pressures.
> 2 How would you measure the blood pressure of a dog noninvasively?
> 3 What effect does decreasing the radius of an artery have on blood flow through that vessel?
> 4 Is laminar blood flow more or less likely to occur in areas of high flow velocity?

Hemodynamics is the study of the physical laws of blood circulation and understanding some basics helps to understand the relationships between blood flow, pressure, and dimensions of the vascular beds. The major dynamic parameters of the cardiovascular system are blood pressure, volume, flow, and resistance.

Pressure

Bernoulli, in the eighteenth century, developed many of the basic concepts of energy and its relationship to fluid flowing through a straight tube. Bernoulli's concept of pressure in a tube (blood vessel) can be simplified to three components: lateral pressure, kinetic energy, and gravitational force. The lateral force is a form of potential energy produced by the stretching or expansion of a blood vessel. The kinetic energy is the flow of blood initiated by the ventricles as they contract and force blood into the pulmonary artery and aorta. The gravitational forces are greatest in the standing animal and are exemplified by the pressure in the arteries of the distance limbs, which is much higher than the pressure in the aorta due to gravity, and the pressure in the erect head (e.g., horse or giraffe) being much lower than the pressure in the aorta for gravitational reasons as well. The quantitative gravitational effect can be calculated by measuring the distance (e.g., millimeters of height the head is above the heart) and dividing by 13 (mercury is 13 times denser than water) to determine the mmHg pressure effect of gravity.

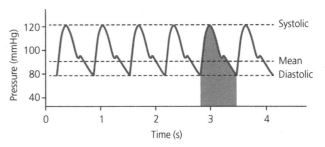

Figure 30.4 Direct pressure measurement from the dorsal metatarsal artery of a canine showing the systolic, diastolic, and mean pressures. The mean pressure is the average pressure of one pressure cycle shown by the shaded area. If the mean pressure cannot be measured, an estimate is calculated: mean = ⅓ (systolic − diastolic) + diastolic pressure.

The arterial blood pressure can be further defined as **systolic** pressure (highest), **diastolic** pressure (lowest pressure whether in the arteries or ventricles), **pulse** pressure (difference between the systolic and diastolic pressure), and **mean** pressure (approximately one-third pulse pressure + diastolic pressure) (Figure 30.4). Cardiovascular pressure is usually measured in units of millimeters of mercury (mmHg) but kilopascals (kPa) are used internationally (1 kPa = 7.5 mmHg). The systemic blood pressure is monitored by the central nervous system and controlled by several mechanisms: (i) the heart rate (beats per minute) and **stroke volume** (amount of blood pumped by each heartbeat) are regulated by both intrinsic and extrinsic factors; and (ii) the blood volume and vascular tone are controlled by the endocrine, neural, and renal systems. The importance of the heart rate and stroke volume in regulating the cardiac output cannot be understated. It is essential that the control of these two parameters be maintained to assure the cardiac output necessary to deliver the oxygen required by the tissues. The cardiac output is the primary parameter responsible for assuring the tissue oxygen requirements. Figure 30.5 summarizes the pressure changes that occur within the vascular system and Tables 30.1 and 30.2 list the systemic and pulmonary arterial blood pressures of several different species. The pressures in these tables were recorded using **invasive or direct** methods, which involve placing a catheter (hollow, stiff-walled but pliable tube) in the lumen of a vessel and advancing it so the tip is at the desired location for recording. For example, to record systemic arterial blood pressure a catheter would be placed in a peripheral artery (e.g., femoral or dorsal metatarsal artery) and attached by saline-primed low-compliance tubing to an **electronic transducer**. The transducer contains a pressure-sensitive membrane that converts the mechanical pressure into an electrical signal that can be viewed on, and measured by, a monitoring device (see Figure 30.4). When properly calibrated this system provides accurate systolic, diastolic, and mean blood pressures from the cannulated vessel. It is important that the transducer or catheter tip be zeroed at the same horizontal level as the heart or mathematical correction

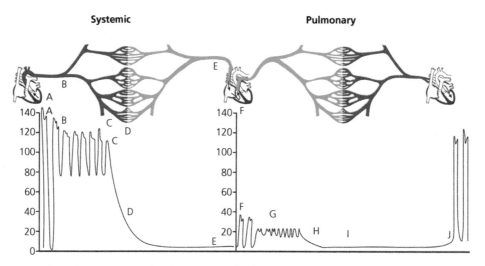

Figure 30.5 Pressure waveform characteristics within the systemic and pulmonary vascular systems (mmHg). (A) Left ventricle; (B) aorta; (C) small arteries and arterioles; (D) capillaries; (E) vena cava; (F) right ventricle; (G) pulmonary artery; (H) small pulmonary arteries and arterioles; (I) pulmonary capillaries; (J) left ventricle. From Reece, W.O. (2004) *Dukes' Physiology of Domestic Animals*, 12th edn. Cornell University Press, Ithaca, NY. Reproduced with permission from Cornell University Press.

Table 30.1 Comparison of the systemic arterial blood pressure (mmHg) of different species.

Species	Systolic	Diastolic	Mean	Pulse
Equine	130	95	107	35
Bovine	140	95	110	45
Ovine	140	90	107	50
Porcine	140	80	100	60
Canine	120	70	87	50
Feline	140	90	106	50
Giraffe	260	160	193	100

Table 30.2 Comparison of the pulmonary arterial blood pressure (mmHg) of different species.

Species	Systolic	Diastolic	Mean	Pulse
Equine	36	21	26	15
Bovine	39	20	26	19
Ovine	32	10	18	22
Porcine	40	24	32	16
Canine	21	10	14	11
Feline	31	16	21	15

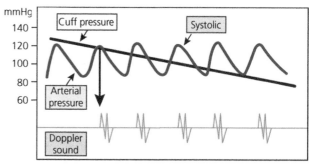

Figure 30.6 Noninvasive blood pressure measurement using a Doppler ultrasound flow probe. The flow probe is positioned over a distal artery (e.g., cranial tibial artery) and an inflatable cuff is wrapped around the extremity proximally (e.g., around the distal tibia just proximal to the hock joint). The diagram shows the mechanics of obtaining a systolic blood pressure value. The arterial blood pressure wave (red line) is shown along with a slowly decreasing cuff pressure. The Doppler ultrasound audible signal is shown at the bottom and an audible sound is produced as soon as the cuff pressure declines below the systolic blood pressure. The cuff pressure is read visually when the blood flow is audible and this is an estimate of the systolic arterial pressure.

for gravitational forces be made for the distance the transducer is above or below heart level. An aneroid manometer may also be used for direct pressure measurement but will only provide an accurate mean pressure. Aneroid devices measure air pressure and have a column of air between the manometer and the saline-primed low-compliance tubing connected to the intravascular catheter. **Noninvasive** methods of measuring systemic blood pressure in animals involve a Doppler ultrasound flow detector or oscillometer. Both of these techniques

require placement of an inflatable cuff around the base of the tail or a short segment of an extremity. A Doppler flow probe is then placed over an artery distal to the cuff, providing an indicator of blood flow. The cuff and Doppler flow provide a systolic blood pressure measurement by inflating the cuff to a pressure that occludes blood flow distally and then slowly deflating the cuff while visually monitoring the pressure with an aneroid manometer (Figure 30.6). The pressure at the exact moment when blood flow is audible is an estimate of systolic blood pressure. The Doppler technique is very similar to the auscultation of Korotkoff sounds over an artery distal to a deflating cuff around the upper arm of a human, except that blood flow is detected by the Doppler ultrasound flow transducer instead of a stethoscope.

The oscillometric technique also involves an inflatable cuff but an electronic device automatically inflates and deflates the cuff while monitoring the cuff pressure. The pulsations (oscillations) of the cuff pressure during deflation or inflation are used by the electronic device to estimate the systolic, diastolic, and mean systemic blood pressure of the animal.

The measurement of venous pressures requires a catheter in the lumen of the vessel. An electronic transducer may be used to measure venous pressures but frequently a saline-filled manometer will suffice.

Velocity and flow

Blood flows from areas of high pressure (e.g., left ventricle) to areas of low pressure (e.g., right atrium) and the cardiac output is the volume of blood pumped by a ventricle per minute. The term **blood velocity** refers to the distance a blood bolus travels per unit of time (e.g., mm/s) and describes how fast the blood from each contraction of the heart travels in the arterial system. The values for blood velocity are very high in the major arteries and decreases as the vessels arborize (divide and branch) and the cross-sectional area increases. **Blood flow** is measured as volume per unit time (e.g., L/min) and is called cardiac output (CO or $\dot{Q}$) when the total flow from the right or left ventricle is measured. Figure 30.7 shows a tube that might represent a portion of a blood vessel in an animal body, where $\dot{Q}$ represents the flow that develops from the pressure difference ΔP ($P_1 - P_2$).

The blood velocity, when measured in the aorta, usually peaks very quickly during the ejection phase (systolic phase) of ventricular contraction and reduces to nearly zero at the end of diastole. The velocity in the aorta actually reverses slightly, which aids in closure of the semilunar valves.

Cardiac output (designated as either CO or $\dot{Q}$) depends on several major factors that are taken into account by the **Poiseuille–Hagen equation**. The equation was originally used to describe the physics of liquid flow through rigid tubes but also applies for short segments of the vascular system where the radius stays relatively constant (see Figure 30.7). Besides the taper, another important difference between the rigid tube concept and the vascular system is the dynamic state of the vascular system, where radius changes with each ejection cycle of the heart. However, the equation can be used to describe the flow in large arteries but the values obtained are relative and should be considered as such. The derivation of the equation can be found in physics textbooks or the original manuscript publication. The Poiseuille–Hagen equation can be applied to describe the factors involved in total aorta blood flow or that to individual organs ($\dot{Q}$ = volume/time):

$$\dot{Q} = \text{flow} = \left(P_A - P_B\right) \times \frac{\pi}{8} \times \frac{1}{\eta} \times \frac{r^4}{L}$$

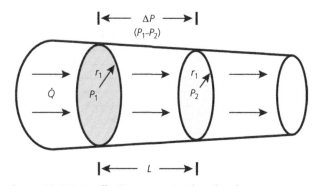

Figure 30.7 Poiseuille–Hagen equation describes the parameters that control flow: $\dot{Q}$, flow; ΔP, pressure drop $P_1 - P_2$; r, radius of vessel; L, length of vessel; η, viscosity. From Reece, W.O. (2004) *Dukes' Physiology of Domestic Animals*, 12th edn. Cornell University Press, Ithaca, NY. Reproduced with permission from Cornell University Press.

where $\dot{Q}$ represents flow (volume/time), $P_A - P_B$ change in pressure (mmHg, where 1 mmHg = 133 Pa) over the measured length, π = 3.14, r is vessel radius (cm), L vessel length (cm), η blood **viscosity** [Pascal second (Pa·s), equivalent to kg/(m·s)] and 8 is a predetermined constant for rigid tube measurements. The major factors affecting the flow of blood in the vascular system are blood pressure, vessel length and radius, and the viscosity of the blood. From the equation, flow is directly proportional to the difference in the inflow and outflow pressure, inversely proportional to the length of the vessel, and directly proportional to the radius raised to the fourth power. Note that if the vessel radius is decreased slightly, the flow decreases tremendously. Viscosity inversely affects flow and viscosity is increased by cellular components, as exemplified by what happens in greyhounds and horses when the hematocrit increases from about 40% to 55 or 60% during a race. Blood with a normal hematocrit has a viscosity about two to three times that of water or saline. From the above equation, one notes that when flow is decreased by the increased blood viscosity, a greater driving pressure (ΔP) is required to return the flow to normal.

Laminar or turbulent blood flow

Laminar (streamlined) flow is characterized by layers of fluid moving in series, with each layer having a different velocity of flow (Figure 30.8). The laminar flow profile within a vessel is parabolic, with the maximum (V_m) near the center of the vessel and a progressive decrease toward the vessel walls where it falls to zero (V_0). Plasma skimming is another term used to describe laminar flow. Components of a fluid layer remain in that lamina as the fluid progresses along the tube. When the laminar or streamline flow pattern is disrupted and develops irregular motion within a tube, the flow is termed **turbulent** and is usually accompanied by audible vibrations. Sound due to turbulence is associated with high blood velocity and is more prominent around arterial bifurcations, stenotic vessels and near valves, where there are major changes in diameter of the conducting vessel.

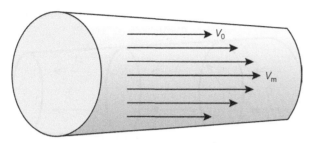

Figure 30.8 Demonstration of laminar blood flow within a vessel: V_0 is the minimum blood velocity (near zero), near the vessel walls; V_m is the maximum blood velocity, near the center of the vessel. From Reece, W.O. (2004) *Dukes' Physiology of Domestic Animals*, 12th edn. Cornell University Press, Ithaca, NY. Reproduced with permission from Cornell University Press.

Reynolds number (Re) is a dimensionless value used to predict turbulent areas:

$$Re = \frac{V \rho d}{\eta}$$

where V represents velocity (cm/s), ρ density (g/mL), d diameter (cm), and η viscosity. The viscosity of blood is usually equal to $3-4 \times 10^{-3}$ Pa.s (3–4 centipoise).

When Re is greater than 3000, turbulence will usually produce a sound sufficient to hear. One only needs to understand that the magnitude of the number predicts whether turbulence or sound will be heard from the vessel. The viscosity will usually remain relatively constant under normal conditions. However, during excitement, especially in greyhounds, the viscosity may increase to 1.5 times the normal value and because of the inverse relationship of viscosity to Re, the number will decrease.

Vascular resistance

> 1 What are the effects of vessel length, vessel radius, and blood viscosity on resistance to blood flow?
>
> 2 If you know the pressure difference between the renal artery and vein and the blood flow through the kidney, can you calculate the renal vascular resistance?

Another major factor that controls organ blood flow is the diameter of the distributing vessels. The major components of a blood vessel are collagen and elastin, which expand and contract during each beat of the heart. The primary control of the systemic vascular resistance and ultimately the systemic blood pressure is the responsibility of the smaller muscular arteries and arterioles. These vessels contain more smooth muscle and are controlled by the organ's metabolic needs, autonomic nervous system, and the endocrine system. The smaller arterioles can be controlled by local metabolites such as adenosine, pH, K^+, Ca^{2+}, O_2, CO_2, nitric oxide, and local cytokines.

The vascular resistance can be evaluated with reference to Ohm's law of electricity. Ohm's law states that volts (V) are equal to the current (I) times the resistance (R) or $V = IR$. When solved for R the equation becomes V/I. To relate this to the biological system, volts (V) will equal the hydrostatic pressure (ΔP), current (I) will equal flow ($\dot{Q}$), and vascular resistance will equal the hydrostatic pressure ($P_A - P_B$) divided by flow ($\dot{Q}$). Hence the Poiseuille–Hagen equation becomes:

$$R = \frac{8 L \eta}{\pi r^4} = \frac{\left(P_A - P_B\right)}{\dot{Q}}$$

From this equation, the major controlling factor is the vessel radius to the fourth power. If the vessel radius is doubled, the resistance is decreased by 16 times; similarly, if the vessel radius is halved, the resistance is increased by 16 times. An increase in vessel radius occurs in the venous system where small vessels converge into larger vessels, thus causing a decrease in the resistance. The diverging effect of the arterial system (larger to smaller vessels) causes the resistance to increase. However, there is a decrease in blood pressure because of the great increase in the blood distribution area. The vascular smooth muscle cells control the radius of the smaller vessels. In the larger arterial vessels the radius is controlled primarily by the amount of collagen and elastin. Collagen and elastin can maintain vessel structure without an energy requirement and can actually act as a support pump to move blood into the vessels during diastole.

The vascular resistance can vary considerably and can be difficult to evaluate from organ to organ. For example, the cardiovascular anatomy of the nephron allows instantaneous control of the blood flow through the glomerulus. The fluid dynamics within the capillary bed between the afferent and efferent arteriole is controlled by the vascular smooth muscle located in the arterioles. Therefore, the capillary bed between the arterioles is pressure regulated to ensure adequate filtration pressure.

Vascular compliance

> 1 Which has more compliance, the aorta or the vena cava? Why?
>
> 2 Which has more blood volume, the systemic arteries or veins?

The term **compliance** (C) is used to describe the elastic nature of blood vessels and is the change in vascular volume (ΔV) with a given change in internal pressure (ΔP), thus $C = \Delta V / \Delta P$. The compliance of the vascular system varies considerably. The arterial system, which structurally contains mostly collagen and elastin, has little compliance. The vessels will not expand easily and thus resist the flow of blood producing the systemic blood pressure required for tissue perfusion. However, the venous system is structurally different, because the vessel walls contain less collagen and elastin than the arteries. The venous system is

Table 30.3 Estimation of compliance of segments of the vascular system (20-kg dog).

Segment	Percent blood volume	Blood volume (mL)	Blood pressure (mmHg)	Compliance (mL/mmHg per kg)
LA/LV	3.5	56	75	0.037
Aorta	6	96	100	0.048
Arteries	8	128	75	0.085
Capillaries	6	96	35	0.137
Veins	60	960	10	4.800
RA/RV	3.5	56	15	0.186
Pulmonary artery	1.3	21	17	0.061
Arteries	1.5	24	12	0.100
Capillaries	2.2	35	12	0.145
Veins	4	64	10	0.320
LA/LV	3.5	56	75	0.037

LA/LV, left atria and left ventricle; RA/RV, right atria and right ventricle.

able to expand easily and hold larger volumes of blood. Thus, the arterial system has been defined as the resistance system and the venous system as the compliance system of the vascular system. If vessel walls are more compliant, they can hold more blood per increment of distending pressure (i.e., $\Delta V/\Delta P$).

Table 30.3 compares the compliance within the vascular system, including the systemic and the pulmonary circulations, for a 20-kg dog with an 8% blood volume.

The heart

> 1 List the three functions of the atria.
>
> 2 What are the four cardiac valves and where are they located?
>
> 3 What is found between the epicardium and the fibrous pericardium?
>
> 4 What is the difference between a morphologic and functional syncytium?
>
> 5 What is the function of gap junctions of the intercalated disks?

Gross structure

The four-chambered mammalian heart consists of the right and left **atria** and the right and left **ventricles** (Figure 30.9). This muscular pump circulates the blood throughout the body. The size of the mammalian heart (0.3–1.0% of body weight) correlates with the degree of physical activity characteristic of the species or breed. For example, the relatively sedentary pig's heart is approximately 0.3% of body weight while the athletic greyhound dog and thoroughbred horse heart is 1.2% of body weight.

Atria

The thin-walled, low-pressure atria serve three functions: (i) as an elastic reservoir and conduit from the venous bed to the ventricle; (ii) as a booster pump, enhancing ventricular filling; and (iii) assisting atrioventricular (AV) valve closure before ventricular systole.

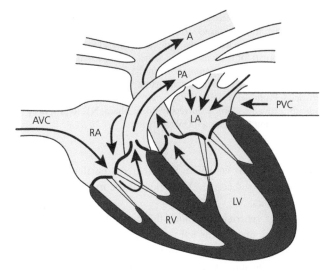

Figure 30.9 The four chambers of the mammalian heart, the great veins, the great arteries, and the direction of blood flow. AVC, anterior vena cava; PVC, posterior vena cava; RA, right atrium; RV, right ventricle; LA, left atrium; LV, left ventricle; PA, pulmonary artery; A, aorta. From Reece, W.O. (2004) *Dukes' Physiology of Domestic Animals*, 12th edn. Cornell University Press, Ithaca, NY. Reproduced with permission from Cornell University Press.

Cardiac valves

The four sets of fibrous cardiac valves are oriented to maintain a unidirectional flow of blood through the heart (Figure 30.10). The passive opening and closing of these valves occurs in response to pressure changes produced by contraction and relaxation of the four muscular chambers. The **atrioventricular** (AV) valves separate the atria from the ventricles and the **semilunar** valves are positioned between the ventricles and the great arteries (pulmonary artery and aorta).

Ventricles

The ventricular myocardial mass comprises most of the heart's weight. During contraction a decrease in transverse diameter and some shortening in the base–apex direction reduce the

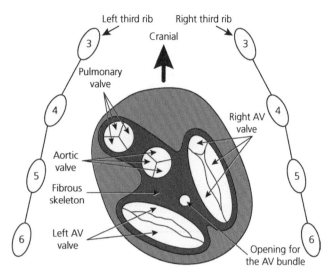

Figure 30.10 Simplified dorsal view of the heart illustrating the fibrous skeleton. This fibrous structure electrically insulates the atria from the ventricles and physically forms the attachment rings (annulus fibrosi) for the four cardiac valves and muscle fibers of the atria and ventricles. An opening exists in the fibrous plate for the atrioventricular (AV) bundle to conduct impulses from the atria to the ventricles. From Reece, W.O. (2004) *Dukes' Physiology of Domestic Animals*, 12th edn. Cornell University Press, Ithaca, NY. Reproduced with permission from Cornell University Press.

volume of the left ventricle. The former is particularly effective, owing to the constrictor action of the mid-wall circumferential fibers.

The right ventricle has much thinner walls and only about one-third the mass of the left ventricle. During systole, its free wall moves toward the interventricular septum due to the contraction of the spiral muscles. Systole in the left ventricle also functions to assist ejection from the right ventricle by the curvature of the septum, pulling the right ventricular free wall toward the septum (called left ventricular aid).

Pericardium

The heart is surrounded by two layers of **pericardium**, with the relationship between the two being compared to pushing a clenched fist (representing the heart) into the middle of a partly inflated balloon (representing the pericardium). The clenched fist (heart) would then be surrounded by two layers (pericardium) but would not be within the lumen of the balloon (pericardial cavity). The inner layer or visceral pericardium is firmly attached to the external surface of the heart forming the **epicardium**. Between the visceral and parietal pericardium is a small amount of serous fluid that gives a lubricated surface for the heart movements. The outer layer or **parietal** pericardium is slightly larger than the heart in diastole (relaxation) and is reinforced by an external layer of inelastic collagen-rich fibrous connective tissue. The surface of the fibrous pericardium is covered by the parietal pleura of the mediastinum.

The pericardium is relatively inelastic and thus protects against acute expansion of the heart. Because of this inelasticity, the acute accumulation of intrapericardial fluid under pressure will tend to collapse the veins that enter the atria and impede or halt cardiac filling (cardiac tamponade). When cardiac enlargement develops gradually, as in hypertrophy, or when there is slow accumulation of fluid (pericardial effusion), the pericardium will enlarge to accommodate the increased contents. Congenital absence or surgical removal of the pericardium ordinarily does not disturb cardiac function. The restraining effect of the pericardium promotes mechanical interplay between the cardiac chambers, so that the volume and pressure effect of distension of one chamber will be transmitted to the other chambers. For example, enlargement of the right ventricle due to obstructed blood flow through the lungs will lead to displacement of the interventricular septum and reduction in volume of the left ventricular chamber.

Myocardial cell

Although the pacemaker, conduction, and working cells account for the majority (>70%) of the heart's mass, they only constitute one-third of the total number of cells in the heart. The remaining cells are fibroblasts, endocardial cells, endothelial cells, and vascular smooth muscle cells.

The working myocardial cells or **myocardium** are striated muscle surrounded by a plasma membrane (sarcolemma) and do not form a **morphological syncytium**. They do, however, form a **functional syncytium** because of the presence of tight (gap) junctions that have low electrical resistance and allow passage of ions and small molecules between adjacent cells. The atrial functional syncytium is separated (insulated) from the ventricular functional syncytium by the annulus fibrosi.

The working myocardial cells are specialized for contraction and impulse conduction, but most cells do not initiate impulses. The contractile cells of smaller mammals (rat, guinea pig) are somewhat thinner than those of larger mammals. Each myocardial cell has a centrally located nucleus, is packed with contractile **myofibrils**, and contains numerous mitochondria. The working myocardial cells are organized in series and connected end to end by intercalated disks to form myocardial fibers. The term "fiber" is applied to individual cells as well as to a chain of cells connected by intercalated disks. Parallel groups of fibers are separated into bundles that are surrounded by connective tissue sheaths. The heart wall contains layers of muscle fibers that characteristically show a smooth change in orientation across the wall. The superficial layers of fibers spiral around the heart after arising from the annulus fibrosi. They seem to spiral toward the apex just beneath the epicardium. At the apex these fibers traverse the myocardial wall and spiral back to the heart's base just beneath the endocardium and form the papillary muscles.

Within each cell or fiber are myofibrils consisting of **sarcomeres** joined end to end at their Z lines. Each myofibril extends the entire length of the cell and is anchored at each end to the intercalated disk. The sarcomere is the fundamental contractile

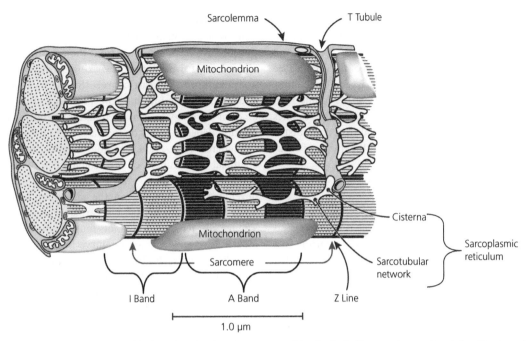

Figure 30.11 The working myocardial cell. The A band is the region occupied by the thick filaments (myosin) and thin filaments (actin); the I band is the region occupied by thin filaments only. These thin filaments attach at the Z line (the line bisecting each I band) and extend toward the center of the sarcomere, which is the shaded area between two lines and is the functional contractile unit. The sarcoplasmic reticulum is a tubular structure that surrounds the contractile proteins, forming the sarcotubular network at the center of the sarcomere and the cisternae that contact the T tubules and sarcolemma, which is a thin enveloping sheath. The transverse tubules are continuous with the sarcolemma and thus extend the cell surface into the depths of the cell. From Reece, W.O. (2004) *Dukes' Physiology of Domestic Animals*, 12th edn. Cornell University Press, Ithaca, NY. Reproduced with permission from Cornell University Press.

unit between two cross-striations (Z lines) (Figure 30.11). The sarcomeres of parallel myofibrils are aligned in transverse register across the cell, giving the cross-banded appearance.

The sarcomeres, in turn, are composed of still finer structures, the myofilaments, which are strands of the contractile proteins **myosin** and **actin**. Dark transverse bands called Z lines form the boundaries of each sarcomere. Light (I band) and dark (A band) zones exist within the sarcomere because of the overlapping arrangement of actin and myosin. At least two other proteins, **tropomyosin** and **troponin**, modulate the contractile process.

Intercalated disks

Intercalated disks are specialized paired membrane junctions that interdigitate and connect the ends of adjacent cells in series. The transverse portions of these disks are at right angles to the fibers. They are always located at the level of a Z line but frequently run longitudinally the length of a sarcomere to the next Z line, forming a zig-zag or step-like pattern. The intercalated disks have three types of functional specializations.

1 The fascia adherens occupies the major part of the transverse segment of the disk and forms a strong connection between adjacent fibers and a locus for insertion of actin myofilaments.

2 Desmosomes are round bodies in the transverse segment of the disk that appear to weld the sarcolemma of adjacent fibers

together, allowing transmission of the force of contraction and producing the mechanical syncytium.

3 Gap junctions are found in the longitudinal segments of the disk. The gap junctions contain channels for the free diffusion of ions between cells and have low electrical impedance, which together result in the electrical syncytium of the myocardium. Gap junctions are sparse and small in sinoatrial (SA) and AV nodal cells, where conduction is slow, whereas gap junctions are plentiful and elongated in Purkinje cells, where conduction is rapid.

Mitochondria

The mitochondria are numerous (see Figure 30.11), making up 25–30% of cell volume. In some myocardial cells the mass of the mitochondria equals that of the myofibrils. The mitochondria are the major sites of oxidative phosphorylation, in which energy provided from substrate oxidation is converted to adenosine triphosphate, the source of energy for cell function.

Glycogen granules and lipid droplets

Glycogen granules are found in large numbers and are evenly dispersed in cardiac muscle. Lipid droplets are frequently encountered and are commonly located adjacent to mitochondria.

Transverse tubular system or interior sarcolemma

The **transverse tubular or T system** consists of relatively thick-walled tubules formed by invaginations of the sarcolemma and extends into the myocardial fiber at the level of the Z lines (see Figure 30.11). The membrane forming the T tubule is continuous with the sarcolemma and the lumen of the tubule is in direct connection with the extracellular space. These tubules are believed to transmit the action potential from the outside surface of the sarcolemma to the interior of the fiber and accumulate calcium.

Sarcoplasmic reticulum

The **sarcoplasmic reticulum** consists of a series of anastomosing thin-walled tubules that invest the sarcomere and which have no direct contact with the cell exterior (see Figure 30.11). The sarcoplasmic reticulum can be subdivided into two parts: (i) the longitudinal (L) system located adjacent to the myofilaments, and (ii) the terminal portion (cisternae) found adjacent to the T tubules. The L system functions in the uptake and storage of calcium ions. The juxtaposition of the T system with the sarcoplasmic cisternae has led to the hypothesis that the depolarizing impulse travels along the transverse tubule from the outer cell membrane, triggering release of calcium from the stores within the terminal ends (cisterna) of the sarcoplasmic reticulum. The released calcium diffuses over to the myofilaments activating contraction. Subsequently, the L system accumulates the released calcium leading to myofilament relaxation.

Properties of myocardial cells

> 1 What are the three major properties of myocardial cells?
> 2 Is the myocardium primarily equipped for aerobic or anaerobic metabolism?
> 3 Is the myocardium more like red or white skeletal muscle? Why?

Spontaneous depolarization

The normal pacemaker of the heart is the SA node located in the right atrium. The spontaneous phase 4 depolarization of these cells initiates an action potential that is conducted throughout the heart. Several ion currents are responsible for the spontaneous depolarization. Other slower pacemakers are located in the AV node and the His–Purkinje system. The slower pacemakers may capture the heart's rhythm when they fire more rapidly than normal, when the SA node pacemaker is slowed, or when impulses generated in the SA node are blocked.

Conduction

Myocardial cells are capable of transmitting action potentials. Although individual cells are separated by plasma membranes, the impulse can pass from cell to cell through the specialized gap junctions in the intercalated disks.

Contraction

Four major proteins (actin, myosin, tropomyosin, and troponin) have been extracted from the myofibrils and make up about half of the volume of working cardiac myocytes. Actin and myosin of the heart convert the chemical energy of substrate metabolism into mechanical energy of contraction. The amount of energy so converted and the resulting force of contraction depend mainly on two factors: (i) the resting length of sarcomeres (the Frank–Starling mechanism) and (ii) the chemical environment of the proteins before and during the activation–contraction reaction. The relationship of force developed by a muscle and the sarcomere length has been described in both skeletal and cardiac muscle (Figure 30.12). The **length–tension curve** plots muscle tension (force) against muscle length. The resulting curve is examined left to right, with the ascending limb produced by the increase in developed muscle tension on contraction as the muscle is stretched to a greater length. The descending limb (right side of the curve) is where muscle tension decreases as sarcomere length is increased further by muscle stretch. Cardiac muscle only functions on the ascending limb of the length–tension curve because the fibers begin to tear when stretched further. The cross-bridge

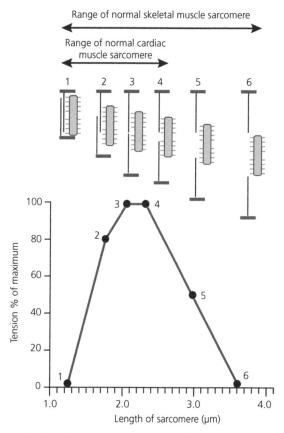

Figure 30.12 Relationship of the myocardial resting sarcomere length prior to contraction and the isometric force developed during contraction. From Reece, W.O. (2004) *Dukes' Physiology of Domestic Animals*, 12th edn. Cornell University Press, Ithaca, NY. Reproduced with permission from Cornell University Press.

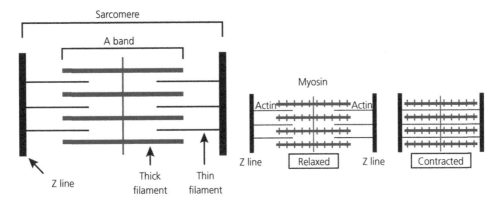

Figure 30.13 Diagram of the thick and thin myofilaments in a sarcomere and how the Z lines move closer together during contraction (systole). From Reece, W.O. (2004) *Dukes' Physiology of Domestic Animals*, 12th edn. Cornell University Press, Ithaca, NY. Reproduced with permission from Cornell University Press.

Table 30.4 Mechanisms regulating the contractile performance of skeletal and cardiac muscle.

Mechanism	Role in cardiac muscle	Role in skeletal muscle
Ability to summate responses to rapidly delivered stimuli	None	Minor
Ability to vary the number of active muscle fibers	None	Major
Ability to alter contractility	Major in sustained responses Minor in beat-to-beat regulation	Minor
Ability to alter contractile response by changing initial fiber length	Major in beat-to-beat regulation Minor in sustained responses	Usually minor

Source: adapted from Katz, A.M. (2011) *Physiology of the Heart*, 5th edn. Lippincott Williams & Wilkins, Philadelphia. Reproduced with permission from Lippincott Williams & Wilkins.

Section VI: The Cardiovascular System

hypothesis suggests that in striated skeletal muscle the reduction in force seen on the descending limb is due to the reduction in the overlap of thin and thick filaments and force approaches zero when this overlap is totally eliminated. The lengths of the thick and thin filaments remain constant during contraction and relaxation (Figure 30.13).

There is experimental evidence that the increased force seen with stretch of the myocardial fibers in the ascending limb of the length–tension curve may be due to factors other than cross-bridge formation. Another hypothesis is that the distance between the thin and thick myofilaments decreases as the muscle fiber is stretched. The closer proximity of the myofilaments increases the probability and number of actin–myosin interactions resulting in increased muscle strength.

Working myocardial cells have many features and properties resembling red skeletal muscle. However, contraction of the myocardium differs from that of skeletal muscle in several respects:

1 the individual myocardial cells, while anatomically discrete, rapidly transmit impulses across the cell boundaries and thus behave as a functional syncytium;
2 the duration of contraction is longer;
3 the refractory period is longer;
4 the rate of force development during contraction is slower and velocity of shortening is slower;

5 the maximum tension developed per unit of cross-section of cardiac muscle is only one-third to one-half that of skeletal muscle.

The physiologic features that distinguish cardiac from red and white skeletal muscle are summarized in Table 30.4. Tension development in skeletal muscle is regulated by the frequency of motor nerve impulses (temporal summation, tetanus) and by variations in the number of muscle units activated during a single contraction. Cardiac muscle is not organized on a muscle unit basis, does not have myoneural junctions, and behaves as a physiologic syncytium so that all myocardial cells are activated during each contraction in an all-or-none fashion. Under physiologic conditions, myocardial cells cannot be summated temporally; nor can they develop tetanic contraction because of their long refractory period.

There are other differences between cardiac and skeletal muscle. First, cardiac muscle has more mitochondria than skeletal muscle, probably because of its continual need for oxidative phosphorylation to supply high-energy phosphates for contraction. Skeletal muscle does not need this capability because it can develop an oxygen debt, with a far greater lowering of pH and high-energy phosphate levels during activity since, unlike the myocardium which does not fatigue, skeletal muscle can go through a rest period during which it restores metabolites and pH. Second, skeletal muscle fibers can run the length of the muscle whereas in cardiac muscle intercalated disks longitudinally connect cells into chains. Finally, skeletal muscle has multiple peripheral nuclei while cardiac muscle cells have a single centrally placed nucleus. Compared with red and white skeletal muscle, myocardial cells have structural and functional features that are more closely allied with those of red than with white skeletal muscle.

Metabolism and energetics

Under normal circumstances, myocardial cells operate almost exclusively on an aerobic metabolic system that provides a constant supply of high-energy phosphate bonds for mechanical and chemical work. Usually the major fuel for red muscle or cardiac metabolism is free fatty acids (Table 30.5). Glucose and lactate are also important contributors, whereas amino acids, ketones, and pyruvate make lesser contributions. The mitochondria are the sites of the major aerobic and oxidative processes on which the heart depends for its energy supply. The heart, like red skeletal muscle, is organized to maintain its work over long periods of time without rest; both types of muscle rely on oxidative metabolism for ATP regeneration and have little ability to function anaerobically or to incur oxygen debt. This is in contrast to white skeletal muscle, which is organized for brief bursts of intense activity followed by periods of relaxation. Cardiac muscle contains large numbers of mitochondria and the myoglobin content is large, favoring oxygen diffusion into the fiber. In white skeletal muscle the enzymes responsible for anaerobic glycolysis are more abundant, whereas cardiac muscle is richer in enzymes providing for oxidative metabolism. Under anaerobic conditions the heart has a very limited capacity to use glycolysis for energy release, and its slender reserve of phosphocreatine is quickly depleted.

The energy-utilization phase of cardiac and red skeletal muscle also differs characteristically from that of white skeletal muscle. The ATPase activity of myosin from the former is less active than that of white skeletal muscle myosin. The maximal shortening velocities of both red skeletal and cardiac muscles

Table 30.5 Biochemical differences between myocardial/red and white muscle.

Biochemical characteristic	Myocardial/red muscle	White muscle
Pathways of energy production	Aerobic	Anaerobic
Major substrates	Lipid, carbohydrates	Carbohydrates
Major metabolites	CO_2 and H_2O	Lactic acid
Dependence on oxygen	Marked	Little
Mitochondria	Abundant	Sparse
Reserve of phosphocreatine	Minor	Significant

Source: adapted from Katz, A.M. (2011) *Physiology of the Heart*, 5th edn. Lippincott Williams & Wilkins, Philadelphia. Reproduced with permission from Lippincott Williams & Wilkins.

are slower than those of white skeletal muscle, presumably because of the slow rate of ATP hydrolysis by the contractile proteins. The lower tensions developed per cross-sectional area by cardiac muscle, as contrasted with white skeletal muscle, may be attributed in part to the larger number of mitochondria and the space they occupy within myocardial cells rather than a difference in the strength of the contractile elements.

Regeneration

In the embryogenesis of skeletal muscle, once the cells have differentiated to the point where they are capable of contraction, there is no further cell division or increase in DNA content. In the developing heart, on the other hand, the cells multiply – they undergo hyperplasia. At just what stage of development the heart loses its capacity for hyperplasia is not known for certain. However, the consensus is that an increase in myocardial mass, particularly in an adult animal, can be accomplished only through the enlargement or hypertrophy of cardiac cells already differentiated, leading to the enlargement and multiplication of intracellular structures such as myofilaments and mitochondria.

Dilatation

The term cardiac **dilation** refers to an increase in the volume or capacity of the heart chambers. Alterations in cardiac volume occur normally whenever there is a change in cardiac output, especially stroke volume. In various abnormal states, however, enlargement beyond usual physiologic limits may occur either acutely or as a chronic condition.

The three factors involved in acute dilation are (i) sarcomere lengthening, which leads to (ii) fiber slippage and (iii) fiber stratification. Fiber slippage occurs as the sarcomeres are lengthened and individual fibers slide past one another longitudinally. This can produce dilation (lengthening of the dimensions of the wall of the heart) in any direction because of the disparate fiber orientation and branching. Different from this is the process of change in stratification of fibers, where the heart chamber dilates at right angles to the direction of myocardial fibers. As the myocardium is stretched longitudinally, the individual fibers become thinner and adjacent layers slide between one another. This increases the number of fibers within a single layer and decreases the number of layers in the myocardial wall. The wall thickness is reduced and the chamber diameter increased.

Dilation has two functional implications: (i) increasing sarcomere length, which increases the contractile strength of myocardial fibers (Frank–Starling relationship); and (ii) increasing chamber diameter, which increases the wall stress for a given intracardiac pressure in accordance with the Laplace law (Figure 30.14). Physiologically, increased stretch results in increased **wall stress**, but at the same time the force of contraction is increased. In theory, if the sarcomeres are stretched excessively, contractile strength decreases. However, studies on experimental animals in which acute cardiac dilatation has been induced (e.g., acute asphyxia) indicate that sarcomere stretch

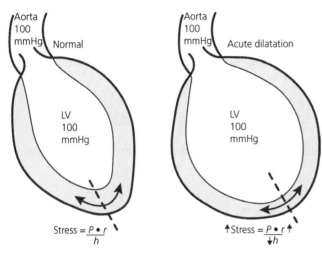

Figure 30.14 Wall stress in the ventricles is a force per unit area (e.g., mmHg/cm²). The law of Laplace is applied to thick-walled ventricles to calculate the stress developed during contraction. By examining the components of the formula, one can estimate how stress would change with ventricular dilation if the pressure remained unchanged. *P*, pressure inside the ventricular lumen; *r*, radius of the ventricle; *h*, wall thickness of the ventricle. From Reece, W.O. (2004) *Dukes' Physiology of Domestic Animals*, 12th edn. Cornell University Press, Ithaca, NY. Reproduced with permission from Cornell University Press.

beyond physiologic limits does not ordinarily occur (see Figure 30.12). However, sarcomere length can be increased to the point that there is little reserve to further increase contractile strength through the Frank–Starling mechanism. The increase in sarcomere length that does take place cannot fully account for the degree of observed dilatation, so that fiber slippage and stratification change must play a significant role.

The wall stress during ventricular contraction (systole) is a function of the intraventricular pressure, radius of the ventricular cavity, and the thickness of the myocardial wall. Assuming that the ventricle has a spherical cavity, its wall stress can be specified by **Laplace's law** (see Figure 30.14):

$$T = (P \cdot r)/h$$

where *T* is mean stress (i.e., mean force per unit cross-sectional area of the wall during systole) which, for practical purposes, is tension circumferentially directed; *P* is mean transmural pressure per unit endocardial area (again during systole), which is radially directed; *r* is mean radius of the chamber; and *h* is mean thickness of the wall. If intraluminal pressure is increased and the wall becomes thinner or the mean radius becomes greater, the ventricle will have to develop a greater circumferential tension to shorten during systole.

The Laplace relationship shows the disadvantage of an excessively dilated ventricle. In the normal ventricle the radius of the chamber during systole decreases as the blood is ejected. Normally, the wall tension begins to decrease after the beginning

of ejection, and at the time of peak systolic pressure may actually be less than at the onset of systole. When the ventricle is markedly dilated (see Figure 30.14), however, the wall tension is greater than normal and the magnitude of fiber shortening may be so compromised that reduction in chamber radius is minimal. In such instances, the tension produced by myocardial fibers may continue to increase from the beginning of ejection to the peak of systolic pressure. These factors diminish the ability of the ventricles to eject blood. It is the increased tension in dilated hearts that is believed to be the stimulus for myocardial **hypertrophy**. Similarly, it may account for hypertrophy in conditions in which there is volume overload, even though intraluminal pressure is not increased (e.g., right ventricular hypertrophy in atrial septal defects). The relation also applies, of course, to an atrium.

Hypertrophy and atrophy

Myocardial hypertrophy is an increase in muscle mass beyond its usual limits. At present the molecular biology of myocardial hypertrophy is speculative. In most types of cells, the predominant extracellular signals for hypertrophy involve the induced synthesis and secretion of potent growth factors. Mechanical stretch affecting ion channels in the cell membrane has also been hypothesized as a signal for hypertrophy. Physiologic hypertrophy, as seen in exercise training, is accompanied by a normal or enhanced contractile state, proportional growth of cellular constituents, and normal myosin ATPase activity. Pathologic hypertrophy, seen in diseased hearts, is accompanied by a decrease in contractile state, decreased myosin ATPase activity, diminished cyclic AMP, and disproportionate biosynthesis of subcellular structures (e.g., mitochondria). There is no convincing evidence of hyperplasia in myocardial hypertrophy. Rather, the myocardial fibers increase in diameter by the addition of more myofibrils and in length by the addition of more sarcomeres.

Concentric hypertrophy (Figure 30.15) consists of an increased thickness of the ventricular wall without an increase in size of the ventricular chamber. This adaptation occurs in response to a long-standing pressure overload (e.g., aortic valve or aortic outflow obstruction) and the myocardial cells respond by adding more myofibrils in parallel. **Eccentric hypertrophy** consists of an enlarged ventricular chamber with a relatively small increase in wall thickness. This adaptation is due to a long-standing volume overload (e.g., patent ductus arteriosus or atrioventricular valve insufficiency) and the myocardial cells respond by adding more sarcomeres in series. The hypertrophied myocardium in cardiac disease frequently exhibits abnormal systolic or diastolic function and electrical instability leading to arrhythmias of various kinds. Myocardial cells adjust their size to their workload: mechanical overload induces hypertrophy, the cells return to control size when the workload returns to normal, and reduction in workload below normal causes atrophy. Examples of the latter are the reduction in left ventricular mass when right ventricular output is reduced in

Section VI: The Cardiovascular System

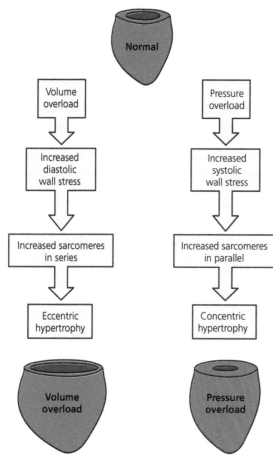

Figure 30.15 The development of eccentric and concentric hypertrophy as a result of volume and pressure overload of the left ventricle. Modified from Kittleson, M.D. and Kienle, R.D. (1998) *Small Animal Cardiovascular Medicine*. Mosby, St Louis, MO. With permission from Elsevier.

pulmonary hypertension, the small subepicardial myocardial cells seen in long-standing pericardial effusion that decreases cardiac output, and the reduction in heart and fiber size in starvation. Normalization of the myocardial wall stress is considered the feedback signal that governs the rate and degree of ventricular hypertrophy.

Self-evaluation

Answers can be found at the end of the chapter.

1 Which one of the following statements is true?
  A The arterial system is a high-resistance, high-compliance system
  B The venous system is a low-resistance, low-compliance system
  C The arterial system is a low-resistance, low-compliance system
  D The venous system is a low-resistance, high-compliance system

2 Which one of the following organs has a portal system?
  A Adrenal gland
  B Heart
  C Kidney
  D Eye

3 Which animal has the highest aortic systolic pressure?
  A Horse
  B Dog
  C Sheep
  D Giraffe

4 Where does the heart normally function on the length–tension diagram?
  A Ascending limb
  B Descending limb
  C At the peak
  D All of the above, depending on the preload, afterload, and contractility

5 Which one of the following is a major mechanism of increased muscle performance in skeletal but not cardiac muscle?
  A Ability to vary the number of active muscle fibers during contraction
  B Ability to alter contractility
  C Ability to respond to an increased initial fiber length

6 What structure in the intercalated disk allows the free diffusion of ions between cells and has low electrical impedance?
  A Gap junctions
  B Desmosomes
  C Fascia adherens
  D T tubules

7 What is the difference between the aortic and pulmonary artery systolic pressure?
  A Aortic pressure is twice the pulmonary artery systolic pressure
  B They have the same flow and systolic pressure
  C Pulmonary artery pressure is three times higher than aortic systolic pressure
  D Aortic systolic pressure is five times higher than pulmonary pressure

8 Which of these vessel groups has the highest cross-sectional area?
  A Systemic arteries
  B Systemic arterioles
  C Systemic capillaries
  D Pulmonary arteries

9 Which vessel group contains the most blood volume?
  A Systemic arteries
  B Systemic capillaries
  C Systemic veins
  D Pulmonary capillaries

10 Under normal circumstances, which of the following is the major fuel for cardiac metabolism?
  A Glucose
  B Protein
  C Free fatty acids
  D Ketones

Suggested reading

Boulpaep, E.L. (2009) Organization of the cardiovascular system. In: *Medical Physiology*, 2nd edn (eds W.F. Boron and E.L. Boulpaep). Saunders Elsevier, Philadelphia.

Hill, J.A. and Olson, E.N. (2008) Cardiac plasticity. *New England Journal of Medicine* 358:1370–1380.

Katz, A.M. (2011) *Physiology of the Heart*, 5th edn. Lipppincott Williams & Wilkins, Philadelphia.

King, A.S. (1999) *The Cardiorespiratory System*. Blackwell Science, Oxford.

Kittleson, M.D. and Kienle, R.D. (1998) *Small Animal Cardiovascular Medicine Textbook*. Elsevier, Philadelphia.

Mohrman, D.E. (2010) *Cardiovascular Physiology*, 7th edn. McGraw-Hill, New York.

Pappano, A.J. and Wier, W.G. (2013) *Cardiovascular Physiology*, 10th edn. Mosby, Philadelphia.

Answers

1	D	6	A
2	C	7	D
3	D	8	C
4	A	9	C
5	A	10	C

Section VI: The Cardiovascular System

31 Electrophysiology of the Heart

Robert F. Gilmour, Jr
University of Prince Edward Island, Charlottetown, Prince Edward Island, Canada

Structural basis for electrical activation of the heart

> 1 What is the normal sequence of electrical activation in the heart?
>
> 2 Why does a highly structured activation sequence promote efficient cardiac performance?

The primary function of the heart is to pump blood, which requires that the heart generate contractile force. Because the cardiac **action potential** is the trigger for cardiac contraction, the mechanical activity of the heart is dependent on the electrical activity of the heart. For the heart to beat efficiently and continuously over the lifespan of an animal, which may encompass many millions of heartbeats, electrical activation of the heart must occur repetitively in the proper sequence.

Orderly electrical activation of the heart is accomplished by the sequential **propagation** of action potentials along the anatomically defined structures shown in Figure 31.1. The heartbeat begins in the sinoatrial (SA) node with a spontaneously generated action potential. Electrical activation subsequently spreads outward from the SA node to surrounding right atrial myocardium and across Bachmann's bundle to the left atrium. Activation wavefronts traversing atrial myocardium eventually converge on the only electrical connection between the atria and the ventricles, the atrioventricular (AV) node. On exit from the AV node, these wavefronts enter a specialized conducting system consisting of the bundle of His and the left and right bundle branches, which are arborizing networks of cardiac Purkinje cells. The His–Purkinje system distributes activation rapidly and widely to ventricular myocardium.

Some fundamental electrophysiological principles

> 1 What is the general process by which cardiac action potentials propagate?
>
> 2 What are the two major factors that influence action potential propagation?
>
> 3 What types of driving forces are present in heart cells and how are they maintained?

Propagation of action potentials throughout the heart requires **depolarization** of a cardiac cell from a resting state to an excited state, during which the cell generates an action potential. Ionic current flowing into the cell during the action potential is transferred from an excited cell to its unexcited neighbors, until they in turn are excited and propagate action potentials to their neighbors. Thus, propagation of cardiac action potentials requires the flow of electrical charge (current) both across the cell membrane of an individual myocyte, to cause an action potential, and across the cell membranes that interconnect myocytes, to raise cell membrane potential to threshold for an action potential. The charge is carried primarily by cations (Na^+, K^+ and Ca^{2+}), because anions (Cl^- excepted) are generally large charged proteins that cannot easily diffuse across cell membranes.

For current to flow across a cell membrane, two conditions are required: a driving force and a path for current flow (such as an ion channel or gap junction). The relationship between current, driving force and presence of a path can be expressed by Ohm's law:

$$V = IR$$

Dukes' Physiology of Domestic Animals, Thirteenth Edition. Edited by William O. Reece, Howard H. Erickson, Jesse P. Goff and Etsuro E. Uemura.
© 2015 John Wiley & Sons, Inc. Published 2015 by John Wiley & Sons, Inc.
Companion website: www.wiley.com/go/reece/physiology

Section VI: The Cardiovascular System

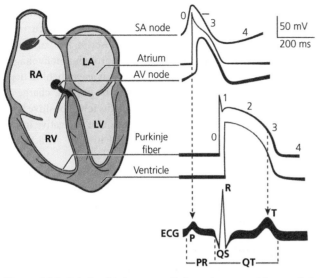

Figure 31.1 Relationship between cellular action potentials recorded from different regions of the heart and the surface electrocardiogram. RA, right atrium; RV, right ventricle; LA, left atrium; LV, left ventricle. From Reece, W.O. (2004) *Dukes' Physiology of Domestic Animals*, 12th edn. Cornell University Press, Ithaca, NY. Reproduced with permission from Cornell University Press.

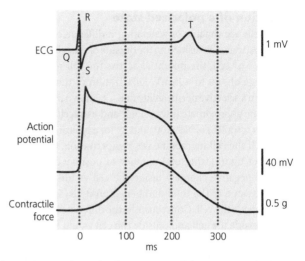

Figure 31.2 Relationship between the cellular action potential (middle trace) and the surface electrocardiogram (upper trace) and developed tension (bottom trace). From Reece, W.O. (2004) *Dukes' Physiology of Domestic Animals*, 12th edn. Cornell University Press, Ithaca, NY. Reproduced with permission from Cornell University Press.

where V is voltage (driving force), I current and R resistance (of the path). Another way to express resistance is as its reciprocal ($1/R$) or conductance (g). Thus:

$$I = Vg$$

From this expression it is apparent that current flow is promoted by a high path conductance (open channel) and by a high driving force. Conversely, current flow is inhibited by a low path conductance (closed channel) and by a low driving force. Thus, transmembrane current flow requires both a driving force and an open channel.

The total driving force for transmembrane current flow typically is the sum of two individual driving forces, the force resulting from the difference in membrane potential between the inside and the outside of the cell (the electrical driving force) and the force resulting from the difference in the concentration of a given cation between the inside and the outside of the cell (the chemical driving force). Under certain circumstances, discussed in more detail later in the chapter, the electrical and chemical driving forces may reinforce one another, whereas in other situations they may oppose one another.

The paths for current flow across cell membranes comprise several types of ion channels, some of which are open continuously and some of which open only in response to changes in transmembrane potential. The latter are known as voltage-dependent ion channels, the opening and closing of which typically occur as a function of time. In addition to being voltage-dependent and time-dependent, some channels are also regulated by changes in channel phosphorylation state. The rather complex regulation of ion channels provides a

variety of mechanisms to alter channel behavior in response to changes in an animal's cardiovascular requirements. Alterations of ion channel behavior, in turn, mediate adaptations of cardiac action potentials to a changing environment. The nature of cardiac action potentials and their response to certain changes in the environment are discussed in the next section.

Cardiac action potentials

1 In the resting state the myocardial cell is selectively permeable to what ion? How does this selective permeability account for generation of the resting membrane potential?

2 What ionic currents are primarily responsible for phases 0, 2 and 3 of fast-response and slow-response action potentials?

3 How does the cell maintain its sodium and potassium gradients?

4 What steps are involved in the opening and closing of sodium and calcium channels?

5 Why are calcium channels sensitive to changes in intracellular concentrations of cyclic AMP? How are the effects of β-receptor agonists, β-receptor antagonists and acetylcholine on calcium channels related to cyclic AMP?

6 What is a **refractory** period? What is the relationship between action potential duration and the refractory period?

The generation of an action potential by a cardiac cell involves a specific series of events, which can be summarized as follows: (i) generation of a polarized state; (ii) depolarization; (iii) **repolarization**. In the next two sections we will examine the general features of the cardiac action potential, as shown in Figure 31.2, and then discuss two specific types of cardiac action potentials, **fast responses** and **slow responses**.

Generation of a polarized state

Cardiac cells are capable of generating a difference in electrical potential between the inside and the outside of the cell. Depending on the type of cell, the potential across the cell membrane is in the range of –60 to –95 mV. Polarization of the cardiac cell results from a selective permeability to K+, as shown in Figure 31.3, in which the approximate intracellular and extracellular concentrations (in mmol/L) of Na+, Ca2+ and K+ for a typical excitable cell are given. If the cell membrane were impermeable to all cations (left side of figure), the total number of positive charges (and associated negative charges) inside the cell would be approximately the same as the total number of positive (and negative) charges outside the cell. Consequently, the difference between the potential inside the cell and outside the cell would be near zero.

However, the normal cardiac cell membrane is selectively permeable to K+ (increased g_K), which allows K+ to flow out of

the cell down its concentration gradient. K+ efflux generates a specific current, the **inward rectifier** (I_{K1}, where I is current, subscript K represents potassium and subscript 1 a particular type of potassium current), which flows through a nonvoltage-gated channel. As K+ moves out of the cell, it leaves behind negative charge. Consequently, the balance in positive charge is altered, so that the inside of the cell contains fewer positive ions than the outside, resulting in the generation of a negative intracellular potential. The negative potential in turn attracts K+, thereby reducing its efflux.

At equilibrium, the chemical force driving K+ out of the cell is offset by the electrical force attracting K+ into the cell. This membrane potential, called the K+ equilibrium potential (E_K), can be calculated using the Nernst equation, a simplified version of which is shown in Figure 31.3.

Thus, the resting cardiac cell is **polarized**, in that the interior of the cell represents a negative pole, whereas the exterior represents a positive pole. If positive charge is added to the inside of the cell, the cell becomes less polarized, or **depolarized**. Conversely, if positive charge is removed from the cell, it becomes more polarized, or **hyperpolarized**. Finally, if a cell has been depolarized (by adding positive charge), removal of that positive charge will cause the cell to **repolarize**.

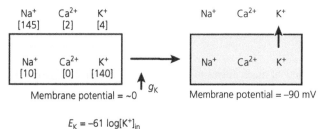

$$E_K = -61 \ \frac{\log[K^+]_{in}}{[K^+]_{out}}$$

$$= -61 \ \log(35)$$

$$= -61(1.54)$$

$$= -94.2 \ \text{mV}$$

Figure 31.3 Generation of the resting membrane potential in a cardiac cell. From Reece, W.O. (2004) *Dukes' Physiology of Domestic Animals*, 12th edn. Cornell University Press, Ithaca, NY. Reproduced with permission from Cornell University Press.

Depolarization

During the depolarization phase of an action potential, the cell membrane potential moves from the resting membrane potential to a depolarized potential (in the range of 0 to +40 mV) over a time course of 1–10 ms. This phase is called the action potential upstroke or phase 0 (see Figure 31.1). In atrial and ventricular muscle cells and in cells of the His–Purkinje system, depolarization is mediated by the opening of voltage-gated Na+ channels and the resulting influx of Na+ via the fast inward **sodium current** (I_{Na}). A simple conceptual framework for operation of the Na+ channel is shown in Figure 31.4 (discussion

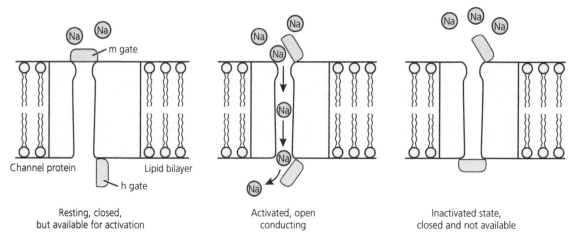

Figure 31.4 Scheme for opening and closing of the cardiac sodium channel, where m and h represent the activation and inactivation gates, respectively. From Reece, W.O. (2004) *Dukes' Physiology of Domestic Animals*, 12th edn. Cornell University Press, Ithaca, NY. Reproduced with permission from Cornell University Press.

of a more complex and contemporary theory is available at http://www.scholarpedia.org/article/Gating_currents). The channel is a protein that spans the lipid bilayer of the cell membrane. The conductance (*g*) of the channel is controlled by sets of voltage- and time-dependent "gates" that are subunits of the channel protein and which move into or out of the channel pore in response to changes in the transmembrane potential.

In the channel's resting state, which occurs only at or near the resting membrane potential, one type of gate, the inactivation (or "h") gate, is in the open position, whereas the other type, the activation (or "m") gate, is in the closed position. Because the activation gate occludes the channel pore, no Na^+ enters the cell, despite the presence of two driving forces for Na^+ influx: a concentration gradient (higher Na^+ concentration outside the cell than inside) and an electrical gradient (the negative interior of the cell attracts positively charged Na^+ ions).

When the transmembrane potential is reduced from the resting membrane potential to $-65\,mV$ (by a process described later), the activation gate opens almost instantaneously, thereby creating an open channel state and allowing Na^+ ions to flow into the cell down their electrochemical gradient. Depolarization also induces the voltage-dependent inactivation gate to close. However, closure requires $1–2\,ms$. Thus, for a brief time the channel is open. Once the inactivation gate closes, the channel pore is occluded (inactivated) and no further entry of Na^+ occurs.

The Na^+ channel remains inactivated unless and until the membrane potential returns to the vicinity of the resting membrane potential. As long as the membrane potential remains depolarized, no amount of additional stimulation can induce the channel to reopen. Consequently, the channel, and the cell in which it resides, are **absolutely refractory**. As the membrane potential returns to voltages near the resting membrane potential, channels begin to revert to the rest state, where the activation gate once again is closed and the inactivation gate is open. The closer the membrane potential is to the resting membrane potential, the larger the number of channels that have reverted to the resting state. If a sufficiently large stimulus is delivered to the cell after the end of the absolute refractory period but before complete repolarization, another action potential can be induced. However, the amplitude of such an action potential is lower than normal because only a fraction of the Na^+ channels have returned to the resting state and are available for activation. Thus, the cell is **relatively refractory**. As repolarization proceeds to the **resting potential** of $-90\,mV$, all the Na^+ channels return to the resting state and are available for reopening.

The prolonged refractory period is a very useful feature of the heart, in that the duration of the cardiac action potential encompasses the contractile event (see Figure 31.2). Because cardiac cells do not repolarize until after the contractile event has subsided, no new action potential and therefore no new contractile event can be induced until the muscle has nearly completed relaxation. Consequently, heart muscle, in contrast to skeletal muscle, cannot be rapidly stimulated into tetany, which is highly desirable – skeletal muscle tetany may be inconvenient (and painful) for an animal, but heart muscle tetany would be lethal.

In some cells, particularly those of the SA and AV nodes, the depolarization phase of the action potential is mediated by the opening of Ca^{2+} channels. Ca^{2+} channels operate in much the same way as Na^+ channels, with one important difference: in addition to the voltage- and time-dependent activation and inactivation gates, Ca^{2+} channels contain phosphorylation-dependent gates. In the resting state, a certain fraction of the phosphorylation-dependent gates are phosphorylated and are therefore open. However, no current can flow through the channel because the voltage-dependent activation gate is closed. As the cell is depolarized past the threshold for opening of the activation gate ($-40\,mV$), the channel opens and Ca^{2+} flows into the cell down its electrochemical gradient. With time, the inactivation gate closes and the channel once again is blocked. Ca^{2+} channels, as a group, take longer to open than Na^+ channels and remain open longer. For that reason, the Ca^{2+} current has been referred to as the slow inward Ca^{2+} current, in contrast to the fast inward Na^+ current.

The primary physiologic mechanism for increasing I_{Ca} is augmentation of Ca^{2+} channel phosphorylation by activation of β-adrenergic receptors. The β-adrenergic receptor agonists include the predominant neurotransmitter of the sympathetic nervous system, norepinephrine, the circulating catecholamine epinephrine and synthetic compounds such as isoproterenol. As shown in Figure 31.5, occupancy of the β-adrenergic receptor promotes binding of the agonist–receptor complex to a stimulatory guanine nucleotide-binding protein (G_s), resulting in G_s activation. Activated G_s subsequently stimulates the catalytic activity of adenylyl cyclase, thereby increasing cyclic AMP production and the subsequent activation of cyclic AMP-dependent protein kinase (PKA). The latter enzyme phosphorylates a regulatory component (or "gate") of the Ca^{2+} channel, increasing the probability that the channel will open during depolarization of the membrane.

Stimulation of I_{Ca} by activation of β-adrenergic receptors is antagonized by activation of muscarinic cholinergic receptors (MCRs), such as occurs during stimulation of parasympathetic nerves (e.g., vagus nerve) (see Figure 31.5). Binding of the parasympathetic neurotransmitter acetylcholine to MCRs activates a G protein (G_i) that inhibits adenylyl cyclase. Consequently, cyclic AMP production is reduced, as is the activation of cyclic AMP-dependent protein kinase. Reduced activity of the kinase is associated with less phosphorylation of Ca^{2+} channels and a reduction in the magnitude of I_{Ca}.

In addition to causing the activation of I_{Na} and I_{Ca}, depolarization during the upstroke of the action potential results in the blockade of I_{K1}. As discussed above, the I_{K1} channel is not a gated channel. One would expect that as the membrane is depolarized the chemical driving force would exceed the electrical driving force, resulting in efflux of K^+. However, with progressive depolarization, not only does the outward K^+ current not increase linearly (according to $V = IR$), it actually turns off.

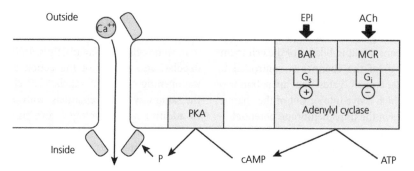

Figure 31.5 Regulation of the L-type calcium channel by the autonomic nervous system, where current flow through the channel requires not only the opening of activation and inactivation gates, as for Na channels (see Figure 31.4), but also the opening of a phosphorylation (P)-dependent gate. BAR, β-adrenergic receptor; PKA, cyclic AMP-dependent protein kinase; MCR, muscarinic cholinergic receptor; EPI, epinephrine; ACh, acetylcholine. From Reece, W.O. (2004) *Dukes' Physiology of Domestic Animals*, 12th edn. Cornell University Press, Ithaca, NY. Reproduced with permission from Cornell University Press.

This unexpected (or anomalous) behavior is known as inward rectification, i.e., current passing through the channel at depolarized membrane potentials is less outward than expected. In fact, depolarization induces rapid blockade of the channel by magnesium and certain polyamines. The larger the degree of depolarization, the larger the degree of block (rectification) by these positively charged molecules. Depolarization-dependent blockade is a useful feature of I_{K1}, in that the objective during the upstroke phase of the action potential is to depolarize the cell. Were I_{K1} not blocked during this phase, K$^+$ efflux down its electrochemical gradient might partially offset the depolarizing influence of Na$^+$ influx.

Repolarization

In some species (e.g., dog, cat, monkey), but not all (e.g., guinea pig), phase 0 of the action potential is followed by a rapid repolarization phase (phase 1, see Figure 31.1). The transient repolarization during this phase is caused by activation of a calcium-independent outward current carried by K$^+$ (I_{to1}) and by a calcium-dependent current carried by Cl$^-$ (I_{to2}). Following phase 1, the membrane potential becomes progressively more negative over a time course ranging from 20 to 500 ms, eventually returning to the resting membrane potential. This process is mediated primarily by a gradual reduction of Ca^{2+} influx coupled with an increase in K$^+$ efflux.

As discussed above, depolarization of the cell membrane during phase 0 exceeds the threshold for the opening of Ca^{2+} channels. Threshold is also exceeded for the opening of a second type of potassium channel, the **delayed rectifier**. In most species, two types of delayed rectifier channels exist. One opens (activates) slowly on depolarization and closes (deactivates) slowly on repolarization. The second activates rapidly on depolarization, but inactivates rapidly as well and remains largely inactivated until the membrane potential begins to repolarize, at which time it reverts to the activated state before deactivating. The currents that flow through these two types of channels are called the slow (I_{Ks}) and rapid (I_{Kr}) components of the delayed rectifier, respectively. The slow activation of I_{Ks} and

rapid inactivation of I_{Kr} ensure that appreciable K$^+$ efflux does not begin until after the depolarization phase has peaked.

Immediately following phase 1 the efflux of K$^+$ via I_{Kr} and I_{Ks} is more or less balanced by the influx of Ca^{2+} via I_{Ca}, resulting in the plateau phase of the action potential (phase 2). With time, I_{Ca} inactivates, leaving K$^+$ efflux unopposed and terminal repolarization (phase 3) proceeds. As the membrane potential repolarizes to potentials more negative than –60 mV, the voltage-dependent delayed rectifiers begin to decline (deactivate). However, unblocking of I_{K1} also occurs within this range of membrane potentials, resulting in efflux of K$^+$ via this current and a return to the resting membrane potential.

Regulation of action potential duration via alterations of plateau currents is an important adaptive mechanism for the heart, particularly with respect to modulation by sympathetic neurotransmitters. During activities that require greater cardiac output, such as exercise, sympathetic tone increases. Increased release of norepinephrine and epinephrine results in increased heart rate, by a mechanism described below. In addition, the contractile force of the heart increases, secondary to increased I_{Ca} (see Chapter 33 for a more complete description of this effect). The combination of increased heart rate and increased force of contraction yields an increase in cardiac output, which is desirable during exercise.

From an electrophysiological standpoint, increased I_{Ca} would be expected to increase the influx of positively charged ions during the plateau phase of the action potential, which would prolong the duration of the action potential. If action potential duration were prolonged at the same time that heart rate was increased, the diastolic interval between action potentials would be shortened. Given the correspondence between electrical and mechanical diastole (see Figure 31.2), a shorter electrical diastole would create a shorter mechanical diastole. The latter, in turn, would result in less filling time for the ventricle, which would result in a decreased cardiac output, the opposite of what activation of the sympathetic stimulation is attempting to achieve during exercise. However, concomitant phosphorylation of I_{Ks} by sympathetic neurotransmitters increases outward repolarizing current, shortens action potential duration and helps to preserve, insofar as possible, adequate filling time.

Redistribution of ions

Although the number of cations flowing across the cell membrane during any given action potential is exceedingly small compared with the total number of cations, repetitive generation of action potentials would eventually dissipate the concentration gradients that make up one of the driving forces for ion flow. Consequently, some means of redistributing cations must exist. In the case of Na^+ and K^+, Na^+ is extruded from the cell interior and K^+ is restored to the cell interior by the Na^+/K^+-ATPase pump (the sodium pump). A pump is required for the movement of these ions because they are being transported against their concentration gradients.

The sodium pump exchanges three Na^+ ions for two K^+ ions. Thus, each cycle of the pump results in the net loss of one positive charge from the interior of the cell. However, under most circumstances the current generated by the pump is quite small and is offset by other pump or exchange currents.

Calcium ions entering the cell during the action potential are restored to the extracellular space primarily by an exchange mechanism that exploits the driving force for Na^+ influx to drive Ca^{2+} out of the cell against its concentration gradient. The operation of the Na^+/Ca^{2+} exchanger is analogous to that of a revolving door, where extracellular Na^+ ions enter the cell via the exchanger, driven by their concentration gradient, and intracellular Ca^{2+} ions caught in the "door" are propelled out of the cell against their concentration gradient. Although no ATP is consumed in this process, the exchange requires an intact Na^+ gradient, which in turn is maintained by the ATPase-driven sodium pump as discussed.

Fast- and slow-response action potentials

> 1 Which regions of the heart generate fast-response action potentials?
>
> 2 Which regions generate slow-response action potentials?

Although the morphology and ionic bases for cardiac action potentials differ significantly between different regions of the heart in a given species and within a single region of the heart across species, it is useful to generalize action potential characteristics into two types: fast responses and slow responses (Figure 31.6). The descriptors "fast" and "slow" refer to the speed with which the depolarization phases of these action potentials occur. As will be discussed subsequently, fast and slow upstroke velocities translate into fast and slow conduction, respectively. Because conduction through different regions of the heart is mediated either by fast responses (in atrial and ventricular myocardium and in the His–Purkinje system)

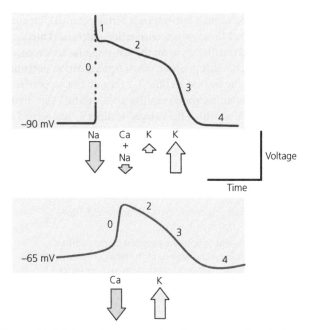

Figure 31.6 Schematic representation of ionic current flow during fast- and slow-response action potentials (inward currents represented by downward arrows and outward currents by upward arrows). From Reece, W.O. (2004) *Dukes' Physiology of Domestic Animals*, 12th edn. Cornell University Press, Ithaca, NY. Reproduced with permission from Cornell University Press.

or by slow responses (in the SA and AV nodes), and because the upstroke of each type of response is generated by a different ionic current, it is possible to preferentially alter conduction in a given region of the heart using selective ion channel-blocking drugs or other interventions. Regional depression or enhancement of conduction is useful for the treatment of a number of clinical conditions (discussed in Chapter 32).

The distinguishing features of a fast-response action potential are a resting membrane potential near $-90\,mV$, a rapidly rising upstroke mediated by the fast inward Na^+ current and a prolonged plateau phase, sustained by a relative balance between I_{Ca} and I_K (Figure 31.6). The membrane potential during phase 4 is constant in atrial and ventricular myocardium and slowly depolarizing in His–Purkinje cells.

Strictly speaking, slow-response cells do not exhibit a "resting" membrane potential, in that phase 4 in these cells is characterized by progressive depolarization. The ionic basis for phase 4, or diastolic, depolarization is discussed in the section on the spontaneous initiation of action potentials. The upstroke of the slow-response action potential is mediated primarily by influx of Ca^{2+} via I_{Ca}, the same Ca^{2+} current responsible for Ca^{2+} influx during the plateau phase of the fast-response action potential. Na^+ channels are generally not found in cells that generate slow-response action potentials.

The early repolarization and plateau phases are largely absent from slow-response action potentials, giving the slow-response action potential a somewhat triangular appearance, in contrast to the more rectangular fast-response action potential. Terminal repolarization of the slow-response action potential is mediated by the delayed rectifier, I_K, as for the fast-response action potential. Because cells that generate slow-response action potentials typically lack the inward rectifier I_{K1}, they do not repolarize to membrane potentials more negative than –65 mV (the membrane potential at which the delayed rectifier I_K has turned off completely).

Propagation of action potentials

> 1 Why do "fast responses" conduct rapidly and "slow responses" conduct slowly?
>
> 2 What treatment options are provided by the fact that conduction in certain regions of the heart is dependent on "fast responses" whereas conduction in other regions is dependent on "slow responses"?

The propagation of action potentials from cell to cell is governed by the same general principles as the generation of an action potential within a single cell. For an action potential to move from one cell to another, there must be a driving force for such movement and a connection between the two cells. The driving force is the difference in voltage between the cell that has generated an action potential, which is depolarized, and the cell that has not yet generated an action potential, which is at the resting membrane potential. Intercellular connections between cardiac cells are composed of honeycomb structures called connexons, which are not present along the entire cell membrane but are concentrated at gap junctions in the region of the intercalated disks. Although the permeability of the connexons can be regulated by Ca^{2+} and H^+ and certain second messengers, connexons typically function as permanently open, low-resistance channels in the normal heart.

When two interconnected cardiac cells are at rest, there is no voltage gradient between them (Figure 31.7). Consequently, no current flows, despite the presence of an open connection. If one cell develops an action potential, the resultant depolarization creates a voltage gradient between that cell and its unexcited neighbor. As a result, positive charge flows. If sufficient positive charge flows into the resting cell, the membrane potential of that cell reaches threshold for the opening of Na^+ or Ca^{2+} channels and generates an action potential. Charge is prevented from moving back into the previously excited cell by the lack of a voltage gradient (i.e., both cells are now fully activated and their voltages are nearly identical).

From this series of events, it follows that the larger the voltage gradient between cells, the more likely current is to flow from one cell to another and sustain propagation. In addition, the more rapidly a cell depolarizes, the more rapidly the voltage gradient is established. Thus, large amplitude, rapidly rising action

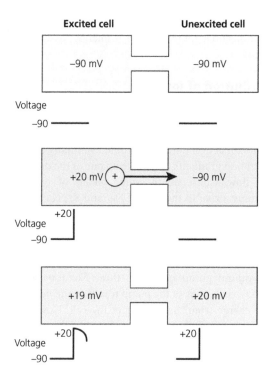

Figure 31.7 Sequence of events leading to conduction of an action potential from an excited cell (left) to an unexcited cell (right). From Reece, W.O. (2004) *Dukes' Physiology of Domestic Animals*, 12th edn. Cornell University Press, Ithaca, NY. Reproduced with permission from Cornell University Press.

potentials conduct more rapidly than lower amplitude, slowly rising action potentials.

In addition to its dependence on the driving force (voltage gradient), conduction through either fast- or slow-response tissue is dependent on the resistance of the path between cells, in this case the intercellular connections (the cytoplasm of the cells also contributes to path resistance but cytoplasmic resistance is much less than intercellular resistance). The density of gap junctions between fast-response cells is greater than between slow-response cells, a feature that further contributes to the disparity in conduction velocity between these two cell types.

Rapid conduction of fast-response action potentials is a necessity if synchronous activation is to occur over a large area of myocardium, particularly in a large mammalian heart. The usefulness of slow conduction may be less obvious. Yet, slow conduction performs an important function in the AV node, where a step delay in transmission of the cardiac impulse from the atria to the ventricles is necessary to allow blood to flow from the atria to the ventricles before the ventricles are electrically activated and contract. Furthermore, slow conduction in the AV node contributes to the "filter" function of the node, in that the AV node simply will not conduct rapidly. Consequently, if an abnormally rapid rhythm should develop in the atria, that rhythm will not be transferred intact to the ventricles. In this way, the ventricles are protected from rapid supraventricular rhythms that might compromise ventricular filling time and reduce cardiac output.

The reliance of slow-response conduction on I_{Ca} provides an opportunity for regulation of conduction through slow-response tissues by the autonomic nervous system. Such regulation is particularly important for conduction through the AV node. Activation of the sympathetic nervous system and the resultant increase in I_{Ca} promote conduction through the AV node. Conversely, activation of the parasympathetic nervous system reduces I_{Ca} and slows conduction through the node. In addition, activation of $I_{K,Ach}$ by acetylcholine may hyperpolarize AV nodal cells, moving their resting membrane potential further from threshold for I_{Ca}. As a result, more time and depolarizing current may be required to bring the AV nodal cell to threshold, further slowing conduction through the node. These actions of acetylcholine contribute importantly to the induction of AV conduction delay and block by intense vagal stimulation.

Spontaneous initiation of action potentials

> 1 What is automaticity?
>
> 2 What is the normal hierarchy of pacemaker activity in the heart?
>
> 3 How do β-receptor agonists and acetylcholine alter automaticity?

As discussed previously, generation of a cardiac action potential requires that the membrane potential reach threshold for the opening of Na^+ or Ca^{2+} channels. Depolarization to threshold is caused by transfer of current from an excited cell to an unexcited cell. The latter, once excited, subsequently provides current to its neighbors. But how does this chain of events begin, i.e., what is the original source of depolarizing current? The answer to that question lies in the ability of certain cardiac cells to self-stimulate by a process known as **automaticity**. Automaticity typically involves slow progressive depolarization of the membrane potential (spontaneous diastolic depolarization or phase 4 depolarization) until a threshold potential is reached, at which point an action potential is initiated. Hypothetically, the net gain in positive charge during phase 4 depolarization could result from slowly increasing inward current with outward current being constant, or slowly decreasing outward current with inward current being constant. As discussed in more detail below, there is experimental support for both hypotheses.

Although all myocardial cells are capable of spontaneously generating action potentials under the appropriate circumstances, their intrinsic discharge rates differ. Consequently, a hierarchy of spontaneous discharge rates exists, in which the discharge frequency of the SA node is higher than that of subsidiary pacemakers in the atrium and AV junction. Similarly, the discharge rates of the junctional pacemakers are more rapid

than those of the His–Purkinje system. In the normal heart wavefronts of action potentials initiated in the SA node activate subsidiary pacemaking sites before they can spontaneously depolarize to threshold. If, however, the SA node pacemaker becomes quiescent or impulses generated by the SA node are unable to activate surrounding atrial myocardium, more slowly depolarizing latent pacemakers may assume control of the cardiac rhythm, albeit at a slower rate. The emergence of these subsidiary pacemakers provides a fail-safe mechanism, assuring that ventricular activation is maintained.

SA node

Automaticity in the SA node is associated with progressive depolarization during phase 4, until the threshold for I_{Ca} is reached and a slow-response action potential is generated. Hypotheses regarding the cellular mechanism for automaticity are complex and still evolving, as they have for decades. Currently, the spontaneous generation of action potentials in the SA node is believed to involve the coordinated interactions of two "clocks," one generated by cyclical changes in transmembrane ionic currents (the "membrane clock") and one generated by cycling of intracellular calcium stores (the "calcium clock") (Figure 31.8).

The membrane clock produces a net influx of positive charge during diastolic (phase 4) depolarization, which depolarizes the cell to threshold for activation of L-type calcium channels. The resulting slow inward **calcium current** mediates the upstroke of a slow-response action potential that subsequently is conducted to neighboring cells in the perinodal region and eventually to atrial myocardium.

The net influx of positive charge during phase 4 depolarization results from the activation of several inward currents and the deactivation of outward current. The inward currents include I_f (the "funny" current, in the sense of unusual, in that I_f is activated by hyperpolarization, in contrast to most cardiac ion channels which are activated by depolarization). I_f conducts a slowly developing inward sodium current during phase 4. Other inward currents include inward Na^+/Ca^{2+} exchange current (three Na^+ ions enter the cell for each Ca^{2+} ion that is extruded, resulting in a net gain of one positive charge) and T-type calcium current, which is activated at more negative membrane potentials than L-type calcium current. Changes in outward currents include the time-dependent deactivation of both components of the delayed rectifier, I_{Kr} and I_{Ks}.

The calcium clock is set by intracellular cycling of calcium. During phase 4 depolarization, spontaneous local Ca^{2+} release from the sarcoplasmic reticulum (SR) leads to accumulation of calcium in the cytosol and an increase in cytosolic calcium concentration. The latter increases the driving force for Na^+/Ca^{2+} exchange, where extrusion of a single calcium ion in exchange for the influx of three sodium ions creates an electrogenic (i.e., positive) current that contributes to diastolic depolarization. Following sufficient depolarization, L-type Ca^{2+} channels are activated, which causes Ca^{2+}-induced Ca^{2+} release from the SR via ryanodine receptors, resulting in the whole-cell

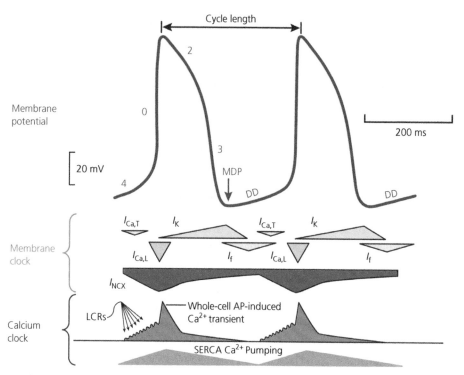

Figure 31.8 Cellular mechanism for automaticity in the SA node. The red trace (top) shows an example of a typical action potential of a spontaneously beating rabbit SA node. A schematic representation of the timing and magnitude of the different components of the "membrane clock" is shown in the middle, whereas the timing and magnitude of the different components of the "calcium clock" are shown at the bottom. MDP, maximum diastolic potential; DD, diastolic depolarization; AP, action potential; $I_{Ca,T}$, T-type voltage-dependent Ca^{2+} current; $I_{Ca,L}$, L-type voltage-dependent Ca^{2+} current; I_{NCX}, sodium calcium exchange current; I_K, delayed rectifier potassium current; I_f, funny current; SERCA, sarco-endoplasmic reticulum ATPase; LCRs, local calcium releases. Reproduced from Monfredi, O., Maltsev, V.A. and Lakatta, E.G. (2013) Modern concepts concerning the origin of the heartbeat. *Physiology* **28**:74–92; doi:10.1152/physiol.00054.2012 with permission.

Ca^{2+} transient. Cytoplasmic Ca^{2+} is then pumped back into the SR by the SR Ca^{2+} pump, SERCA, and extruded from the cell by the sarcolemmal Na^+/Ca^{2+} exchanger.

The exact ionic mechanisms for spontaneous impulse generation in the sinus node vary across species in order to account for the wide variety of resting heart rates (e.g., about 600 beats per minute for a mouse compared with about 30 beats per minute for a horse) as well as for the species-dependent differences in the response of heart rate to changes in autonomic nervous system tone and other chronotropic (rate-changing) influences.

As discussed previously, drugs and neurotransmitters that bind to the β-adrenergic receptor increase I_{Ca} secondary to phosphorylation of a protein that modulates the opening of Ca^{2+} channels (Figure 31.9). The larger influx of Ca^{2+} via augmented I_{Ca} may accelerate the rate of diastolic depolarization and thereby account for the positive chronotropic effect (increase in heart rate) of sympathetic stimulation (Figure 31.10). Acceleration of SA node automaticity by β-adrenergic agonists has also been proposed to result from an increase in the pacemaker current I_f, a process that may be mediated by a direct effect of cyclic AMP on channel conductance. Activation of both I_{Ca} and I_f have also been proposed to result from a direct stimulatory effect of G proteins (specifically G_s) on the respective channels, independent of phosphorylation.

SA node automaticity is also regulated importantly by the parasympathetic nervous system (Figure 31.9). In general, stimulation of the parasympathetic nervous system decreases heart rate. The negative chronotropic effects of acetylcholine have been attributed to increased K^+ conductance, secondary to induction of the potassium current $I_{K,ACh}$. Efflux of K^+ via $I_{K,ACh}$ hyperpolarizes the membrane potential, which lengthens the time required to depolarize to threshold. In addition, acetylcholine may inhibit I_{Ca} or the pacemaker current I_f. A reduction of either of these currents would be expected to decrease the rate of phase 4 depolarization (as shown in Figure 31.10).

Subsidiary supraventricular pacemakers

Latent supraventricular pacemakers have been identified in the AV node, as well as in various regions of the atria, including the coronary sinus, Bachmann's bundle, the AV valves, atrial plateau fibers and the inferior right atrium near its junction with the inferior vena cava. Automaticity of the AV node appears to arise from a mechanism similar to that occurring in the SA node. Diastolic depolarization is caused by decay of I_K concomitant with activation of I_{Ca}, culminating in full activation of I_{Ca} and a slow-response action potential. I_f is also present in the AV node but, as in the SA node, its role with respect to generating the pacemaker potential has not been fully defined. Acceleration of

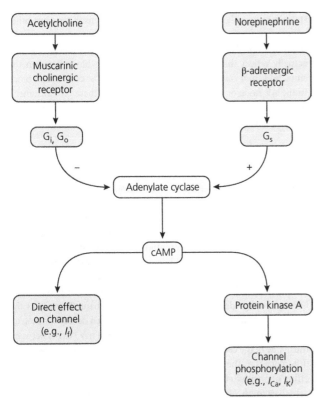

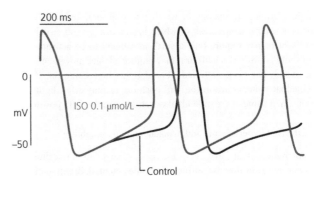

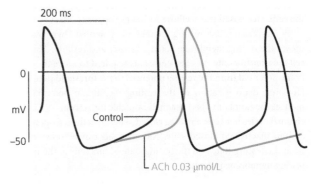

Figure 31.9 Influence of parasympathetic (acetylcholine) and sympathetic (norepinephrine) neurotransmitters on ionic currents involved in automaticity. From Reece, W.O. (2004) *Dukes' Physiology of Domestic Animals*, 12th edn. Cornell University Press, Ithaca, NY. Reproduced with permission from Cornell University Press.

Figure 31.10 Effects of a β-adrenergic agonist (isoproterenol, ISO; upper traces) and a muscarinic cholinergic agonist (acetylcholine, ACh; lower traces) on spontaneous impulse generation (automaticity) in the sinoatrial node. Reproduced from Difrancesco, D., Mangoni, M. and Maccaferri, G. (1995) The pacemaker current in cardiac cells. In: *Cardiac Electrophysiology. From Cell to Bedside*, 2nd edn (eds D.P. Zipes and J. Jalife), pp. 96–103. W.B. Saunders, Philadelphia, with permission.

AV nodal automaticity by β-adrenergic agonists is believed to result from activation of I_{Ca} via the second messenger system described above.

Ventricular pacemakers

Isolated cells of the His–Purkinje system discharge spontaneously, whereas ventricular myocardial cells usually do not exhibit spontaneous diastolic depolarization or automaticity. Diastolic depolarization in Purkinje cells is believed to result from activation of I_p, although a time-dependent reduction of an outward current may also play a role. Na$^+$ influx via I_f slowly depolarizes the membrane potential until the threshold potential for I_{Na} is reached, at which point a fast-response action potential is elicited. The relatively slow spontaneous discharge rate of Purkinje fibers ensures that pacemaker activity in the His–Purkinje system will be suppressed on a beat-to-beat basis by the more rapid discharge rate of the SA node.

Self-evaluation

Answers can be found at the end of the chapter.

1 Define and explain the effects of hyperkalemia and hypokalemia on the excitability of ventricular myocardium and on heart rate.

2 Define and explain the effects of hypercalcemia and hypocalcemia on the excitability of ventricular myocardium.

Suggested reading

Berne, R.M. and Levy, M.N. (2000) *Cardiovascular Physiology*, 8th edn, pp. 5–52. Mosby Year Book, St Louis, MO.

Dobrzynski, H., Boyett, M.R. and Anderson, R.H. (2007) New insights into pacemaker activity: promoting understanding of sick sinus syndrome. *Circulation* **115**:1921–1932.

Grant, A.O. (2009) Cardiac ion channels. *Circulation: Arrhythmias and Electrophysiology* **2**:185–194.

Monfredi, O., Maltsev, V.A. and Lakatta, E.G. (2013) Modern concepts concerning the origin of the heartbeat. *Physiology* **28**:74–92.

Answers

The effects of changes in serum concentrations of Ca^{2+} and K$^+$ on excitation in cardiac muscle are complex. Accordingly, it is useful to separate the effects of these ions on the threshold potential (the potential at which fast Na$^+$ channels open) from their effects on conductance (roughly, the number of Na$^+$ channels that are available for opening once the threshold potential has been reached). In this context, you might consider an analogy in which one wall-mounted light switch controls several lamps, each of which has its own on–off switch. The wall switch may require only a small movement to be activated (i.e., threshold is easily reached) or it may require a larger movement. Once the switch has been activated, several lights may come on, if their individual switches are in the "on" position, or only a few lights may come on, if some of the individual switches are in the "off" position.

1 Effects of hyperkalemia and hypokalemia on excitability

For reasons that have been discussed, changes in extracellular K^+ concentration alter the resting membrane potential. Briefly, increased extracellular K^+ reduces the driving force for K^+ efflux via the inward rectifier K^+ current and thereby reduces (makes less negative) the resting membrane potential (fewer positively charged K^+ ions leave the cell). Decreased extracellular K^+ has the opposite effect.

By decreasing the resting membrane potential, hyperkalemia moves the resting membrane potential closer to threshold. Thus, the cell is easier to excite (i.e., less current is required to move the membrane potential from the resting potential to the threshold potential). However, depolarization of the resting membrane potential also reduces the number of Na^+ channels available for activation. The Na^+ channel cycles between a resting closed state, an activated open state, and an inactivated closed state. Na^+ channels can be opened only from the resting state and the resting state occurs only at the normal resting membrane potential.

Depolarization of the resting membrane potential "locks" Na^+ channels in the inactivated state (the greater the depolarization, the greater the number that are inactivated). With moderate hyperkalemia ($[K^+]_o$ 5–8 mmol/L), cardiac muscle cells may be "hyperexcitable", whereas with more severe hyperkalemia depression of conduction secondary to inactivation of a large fraction of Na^+ channels occurs, as reflected by cardiac muscle weakness and conduction disturbances, including asystole.

During hypokalemia, the resting membrane potential is more negative than normal. Consequently, there is a greater difference between the resting potential and the threshold potential, rendering the cell less excitable. However, all the Na^+ channels are in the resting state and are therefore available once the threshold potential has been reached. With sufficiently severe hypokalemia, however, threshold is reached rarely, resulting in cardiac conduction disturbances.

Thus, during hyperkalemia, the wall switch is easier to flip, but fewer lights come on. If the hyperkalemia is sufficiently severe, no lights come on and therefore no excitation (or contraction) occurs. During hypokalemia, the wall switch is harder to flip, but once flipped produces a very bright room.

With respect to the effects of hyperkalemia and hypokalemia on heart rate, it is important to remember that heart rate is normally controlled by the rate of spontaneous discharges in the sinus node, via the process of automaticity. Impulses generated in the sinus node subsequently are conducted to the rest of the heart, a process that is affected by the changes in excitability discussed above. The process of automaticity is very resistant to changes in extracellular K^+ concentration, in part because the sinus node lacks the inward rectifier. Consequently, its resting membrane potential is much less affected by hyperkalemia or hypokalemia than is the resting potential of other cardiac cells. Changes in heart rate that accompany hyperkalemic or hypokalemic

states are more likely to result from the primary insult, or some other consequence of that insult, than from changes in serum K^+ concentration, the exception being apparent changes in heart rate that actually reflect the development of conduction block between the sinus node and surrounding atrial myocardium or conduction block in the AV node or His–Purkinje system. Under these circumstances, the sinus node may be discharging at its normal rate, but not all impulses are conducted to the ventricles.

2 Effects of hypercalcemia and hypocalcemia on excitability (sometimes referred to as "irritability")

Changes in the extracellular concentration of Ca^{2+} alter excitation primarily by altering the threshold potential for activation of Na^+ channels, without affecting the number of Na^+ channels available for activation. Increased extracellular Ca^{2+} concentration (hypercalcemia) shifts the threshold potential for Na^+ channels to less negative membrane potentials, whereas decreased extracellular Ca^{2+} concentration (hypocalcemia) has the opposite effect.

One potential mechanism to explain the effects of extracellular Ca^{2+} on voltage-dependent activation of Na^+ channels involves the concept of surface charge. In a normally polarized cardiac or skeletal muscle cell, a difference in potential (of about 90 mV) exists between the inside of the cell and the extracellular environment. The potential difference (i.e., the resting membrane potential) is created by the net efflux of positive charge from the interior of the cell via K^+ ions. The actual strength of the electric field within the sarcolemmal membrane is determined by the potential difference between the inside and outside surfaces of the membrane. This potential need not be the same as the difference between the potentials existing in the cytoplasm and the bulk extracellular fluid. In this regard, the outer surface of the membrane contains a number of fixed, predominantly negative surface charges, provided by amino acid side chains on ion channels and sialic acid residues.

Assuming that negative intracellular charge congregates on the inside surface of the membrane, negative charge on the outside surface of the membrane would reduce the potential difference sensed by molecules within the membrane, ion channels in particular. Conversely, neutralization of the negative surface charges by cations such as Ca^{2+} would increase the potential difference across the inner and outer membrane surfaces.

In the case of the Na^+ channel, depolarization is needed to open the channel, presumably because some component of the channel senses voltage and induces some other part (or parts) of the channel to move in response to a sufficiently large change in voltage. If during rest the potential (voltage) gradient across the membrane itself is small, as it would be in the absence of extracellular Ca^{2+}, a smaller change in the total transmembrane potential would be required to overcome the resting voltage gradient and open the channel. On the other hand, if a large potential difference across the membrane exists at the resting membrane potential, as it would in the presence of elevated extracellular Ca^{2+}, a larger additional voltage change would be required to open the channel.

Thus, Na^+ channels are more easily opened during hypocalcemia, which increases excitability. Conversely, hypercalcemia reduces the probability that sodium channels will open during a normal depolarization, which decreases excitability.

32 The Electrocardiogram and Cardiac Arrhythmias

Robert F. Gilmour, Jr[1] and N. Sydney Moïse[2]

[1] University of Prince Edward Island, Charlottetown, Prince Edward Island, Canada
[2] Cornell University, Ithaca, NY, USA

Surface representation of cardiac electrical activity (electrocardiogram)

1 How can cardiac electrical activity be assessed in patients?

2 What is the theoretical basis for bipolar recordings and how are they used to record the electrocardiogram?

3 What are summed vectors and what information do they convey?

ECG and cellular electrical activity

The discussion of cardiac electrical activity in Chapter 31 relied heavily on the analysis of recordings of action potentials and ionic currents, recordings that require direct contact between an electrode and a cardiac cell. Such recordings obviously are not feasible in clinical cases. Consequently, the clinician typically must rely on recordings made from the body surface, in the form of an electrocardiogram (ECG).

The correspondence between cellular electrical activity and the ECG is illustrated in Figure 31.1. Note that there is no ECG deflection corresponding to the discharge of the SA node. The voltage generated by the relatively small number of cells in the SA node is too small to be detected on the body surface. Consequently, discharge of the SA node is assumed to have occurred just prior to the initial wave on the ECG, the P wave, representing depolarization of atrial muscle. The P wave is followed by a return to baseline (the isoelectric line) and the apparent absence of electrical activity. However, during this segment of the ECG the cardiac impulse is traversing the atrioventricular node which, like the SA node, is too small to

generate sufficient voltage to be recorded on the body surface. As the impulse emerges from the AV node and activates the His–Purkinje system and ventricular muscle, a QRS complex is generated (Figure 32.1). Depolarization of the ventricles, as represented by the QRS complex, is followed by repolarization of the ventricles, represented by the T wave. Repolarization of atrial muscle typically occurs simultaneously with depolarization of the ventricles and is therefore masked by the QRS complex.

The most clinically useful ECG intervals are as follows.

1 The P–R interval, measured from the beginning of the P wave to the beginning of the QRS complex, represents the time required for the wave of excitation to travel from the SA node to the ramifications of the His–Purkinje system.

2 The duration of the QRS complex represents the spread of impulses throughout ventricular muscle and is a measure of the intraventricular conduction time.

3 The Q–T interval, measured from the beginning of the Q to the end of the T wave, reflects the approximate duration of ventricular systole and the ventricular refractory period.

Principles of surface recordings

The ECG is recorded using a set of bipolar and unipolar leads. In bipolar electrocardiography a lead is the connection of two parts of the body by electrodes and wires with the electrocardiograph. For the standard limb leads, the potential difference between two electrodes is recorded (Figure 32.2). For the augmented leads, the recordings from two electrodes are summed

Section VI: The Cardiovascular System

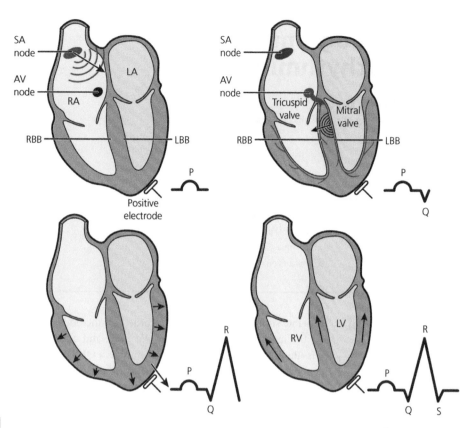

Figure 32.1 Sequence of electrical activation of the heart and its relationship to the electrocardiogram. RA, right atrium; RV, right ventricle; LA, left atrium; LV, left ventricle; RBB, right bundle branch; LBB, left bundle branch. From Reece, W.O. (2004) *Dukes' Physiology of Domestic Animals*, 12th edn. Cornell University Press, Ithaca, NY. Reproduced with permission from Cornell University Press.

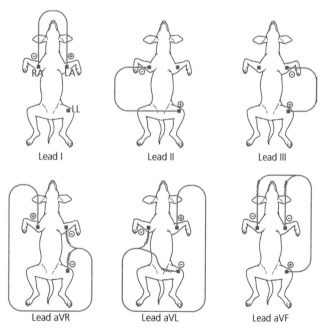

Figure 32.2 (*Top*) Standard bipolar limb leads (leads I, II and III) and (*bottom*) the augmented leads (leads aVR, aVL, aVF). The connections between the recording electrodes are made internally in the ECG machine by turning a switch. From Reece, W.O. (2004) *Dukes' Physiology of Domestic Animals*, 12th edn. Cornell University Press, Ithaca, NY. Reproduced with permission from Cornell University Press.

and compared with the recording from the third electrode. The resulting recording is equivalent to comparing the potential recorded by one electrode with the potential recorded by an imaginary (virtual) lead located midway between the summed electrodes. Recordings can also be obtained using unipolar leads, known as precordial leads. Such recordings are used to interrogate specific areas of the chest wall.

Recordings from each of the bipolar ECG leads represent the difference in voltage between a given pair of electrodes. Because the ECG signal is generated by the difference in potential between two electrodes, the position of the electrode pair with respect to the activation wavefront significantly affects the recording, as illustrated in Figure 32.3. In this figure depolarization is represented by a reversal of polarity from inside negative to inside positive (with reciprocal changes on the outer surface of the fiber). The output from the recorder is the difference between the potential sensed by the two poles of the electrode. The fiber is stimulated initially on the left end and a wavefront propagates from left to right. With a parallel lead orientation, a biphasic potential (not unlike a QRS complex), recorded as a potential difference between the two electrodes, develops and then subsides. In contrast, with a perpendicular lead orientation, the difference in potential remains constant during the same left-to-right sequence of activation. Consequently, no deflection is seen on the recorder output.

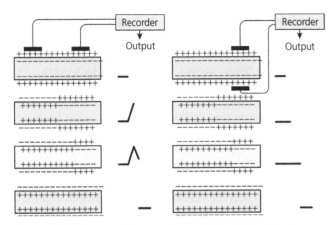

Figure 32.3 Diagram of the recordings obtained using a bipolar electrode oriented parallel (left panels) or perpendicular (right panels) to a depolarizing wavefront traveling along a piece of cardiac tissue. From Reece, W.O. (2004) *Dukes' Physiology of Domestic Animals*, 12th edn. Cornell University Press, Ithaca, NY. Reproduced with permission from Cornell University Press.

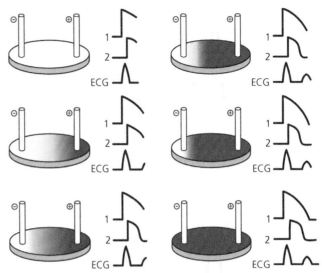

Figure 32.5 Schematic representation of the electrical signals produced by a repolarizing wavefront. Same format as in Figure 32.4. From Reece, W.O. (2004) *Dukes' Physiology of Domestic Animals*, 12th edn. Cornell University Press, Ithaca, NY. Reproduced with permission from Cornell University Press.

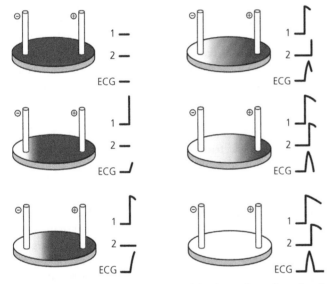

Figure 32.4 Schematic representation of the electrical signals produced by a depolarizing wavefront as assessed using two recording sites. Signals from each of the sites (1, corresponding to the negative electrode; 2, corresponding to the positive electrode) are shown, as is the difference between the two sites (ECG). From Reece, W.O. (2004) *Dukes' Physiology of Domestic Animals*, 12th edn. Cornell University Press, Ithaca, NY. Reproduced with permission from Cornell University Press.

The difference in potential recorded by a bipolar lead corresponds to a difference in cellular electrophysiological properties. For example, a lead II recording of the QRS–T complex can be thought of as representing the difference between action potentials generated by two regions of the heart, as shown in Figure 32.4. As depolarization (lighter areas in the figure) proceeds from left to right across a piece of cardiac tissue, site 1 is activated. Activation of site 1 while site 2 is still at rest results in a difference in potential between the two sites,

represented by the initial upward deflection of the ECG (middle left). Further depolarization of site 1 results in a larger ECG deflection (lower left). As site 2 becomes progressively more depolarized (right panels), the difference between the two sites declines and the ECG returns to baseline. Note the similarity between the ECG signal and the QRS complex of Figure 32.1.

Thus, during the normal spread of activation throughout the ventricles, a difference in activation times results in the QRS complex. If the two regions have different action potential durations, then the resulting difference in repolarization times produces a T wave, as shown in Figure 32.5. In contrast to the sequence of depolarization, where site 1 was activated before site 2, during repolarization the site with the shorter action potential duration (site 2) repolarizes before the site with the longer action potential duration (site 1). Thus, repolarization (shaded area) proceeds from right to left. Because site 2 repolarizes before site 1, a difference in membrane potential develops, represented by the upward deflection of the ECG (left panels). As repolarization proceeds, the difference between the two sites declines and the ECG returns to baseline. The resulting waveform is similar to that of the T wave .

Variations in the duration and polarity of the T wave are associated with differences in action potential duration, such as those that normally exist between the epicardium and endocardium, where action potential duration is shorter in the epicardium, and between the base and the apex of the ventricles, where action potential duration is shorter at the apex. The relationship between action potentials from these regions in canine myocardium is shown in the top panel of Figure 32.6. The differences in action potential duration

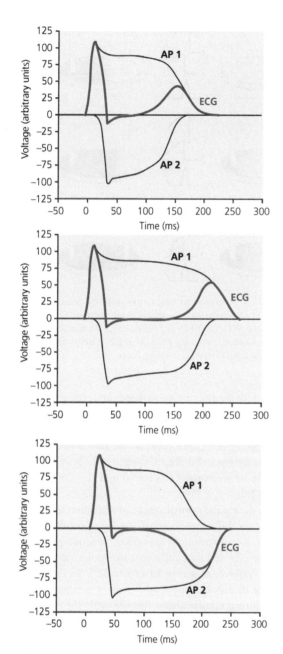

Figure 32.6 Generation of the ECG as the difference in potential between two regions of the heart. The difference in membrane potential is calculated by adding the negative of one action potential (AP) to the other. From Reece, W.O. (2004) *Dukes' Physiology of Domestic Animals*, 12th edn. Cornell University Press, Ithaca, NY. Reproduced with permission from Cornell University Press.

result in a T wave with normal duration and upright polarity. In the middle panel, the duration of both action potentials is prolonged, as might occur in response to a drug that blocks K⁺ channels, resulting in upright T-wave polarity but prolongation of the QT interval. In the bottom panel, only one of the action potentials is prolonged, resulting in inversion of the T wave.

Summed vectors

Electrical activation of the heart is a complex process that proceeds in three spatial dimensions (vertical, horizontal and front-to-back) simultaneously. The sequence of activation – SA node, atria, AV node, His–Purkinje system, ventricles – is uniform across species, but the specific patterns of activation may differ. For example, the His–Purkinje system is largely restricted to the subendocardium in species such as dogs, cats, rodents and primates, whereas it penetrates more deeply in horses, ruminants, swine and birds. As a result, activation of dog ventricle, for example, occurs from endocardium to epicardium compared with activation of horse ventricle, where the sequence of activation is largely reversed.

Activation of the heart can be represented by a series of **vectors** in three-dimensional space, each of which displays a direction and a magnitude. The ECG samples these vectors as they project onto a two-dimensional surface, represented in the frontal plane by Einthoven's triangle. Any given ECG lead, by recording the difference in potential between two sites on the torso, captures the magnitude of a given vector, but not its direction. Consequently, the measurements provided by ECG leads are scalar, rather than vector, quantities. However, the cardiac vector, represented by the mean electrical axis, can be reconstructed using recordings from at least three ECG leads. There are several procedures that can be used for this reconstruction, two of which are described here: the first is more accurate but the second is quicker, easier and more likely to be used clinically.

In the first method, the Einthoven triangle is used. The theoretical "center of electrical activity" is obtained by dropping perpendiculars from the midpoints of the sides of the equilateral triangle, the sides of which represent the three standard bipolar limb leads (Figure 32.7). To find the mean QRS vector, the amplitude of the R wave for each lead is plotted along one side of the triangle in the positive direction from the midzero point. After plotting the vectors for all three leads, perpendiculars are drawn from these points. The mean electrical axis is found by connecting the two points at which all three perpendiculars intersect with a straight line.

In the second method all six leads are used (Figure 32.7). The initial step is to find the lead with a net amplitude of near zero for the QRS complex (where a net amplitude of zero means that the magnitude of the positive QRS deflection is the same as the magnitude of the negative QRS deflection). For the reasons discussed above (Figure 32.3), the mean electrical axis must have been perpendicular to this lead. Once the perpendicular lead has been identified, the polarity of the QRS complex in the perpendicular lead is determined. The axis can then be read from the corresponding pole of the lead (Figure 32.7).

As an example, if the net amplitude of the QRS complex is nearly zero in lead aVL, then the electrical axis is parallel to lead II. If the QRS complex is positive in lead II, then the axis is +60°, which is within the normal range for most species. Should the vector point to between 0 and –90°, there is left-axis deviation,

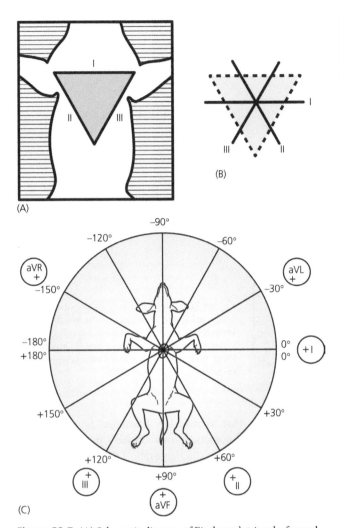

Figure 32.7 (A) Schematic diagram of Einthoven's triangle, formed by leads I, II and III. (B) Transposition of the three sides of Einthoven's triangle to a common central point of zero potential. Diagram of the hexaxial lead system, formed by superimposing the three limb leads and the three augmented leads so that the midpoints of the lead axes coincide. (C) The hexaxial lead system can be enclosed in a circle and used to determine the magnitude and direction of the mean electrical axis. From Reece, W.O. (2004) *Dukes' Physiology of Domestic Animals*, 12th edn. Cornell University Press, Ithaca, NY. Reproduced with permission from Cornell University Press.

which may occur for example with left ventricular hypertrophy. If the vector is between +90 and +180°, there is right-axis deviation (depending on the species), which may accompany right ventricular hypertrophy.

Mechanisms of cardiac arrhythmias

1 What are the major classes of cellular mechanisms for the development of cardiac arrhythmias?

2 Why do cardiac arrhythmias disrupt cardiovascular function?

3 What are the different classes of abnormal impulse formation?

4 How does enhanced normal automaticity differ from abnormal automaticity?

5 How does automaticity differ from triggered activity?

6 What are the different types of triggered activity and how are they generated?

7 How is conduction block characterized?

8 What are the primary determinants of conduction block?

9 How does conduction block precipitate reentry?

10 What are the prerequisites for reentry?

Cardiac **arrhythmias** (or dysrhythmias) are defined as variations of the cardiac rhythm from normal sinus rhythm. Such variations may be appropriate responses to changes in an animal's state, such as increased heart rate during exercise or decreased heart rate during sleep. Others may be undesirable (e.g., ventricular **fibrillation**) and require treatment. The underlying mechanisms for cardiac arrhythmias can be grouped into two general classes: abnormalities of impulse formation and abnormalities of impulse propagation. Abnormalities of impulse formation encompass changes in normal pacemaker activity and the emergence of abnormal pacemakers, which may compete with the SA node for control of cardiac rhythm. Abnormalities of impulse propagation include block of impulses into or out of various regions of the heart and **reentrant excitation**, where activation circles an anatomical or functional object.

The development of additional pacemakers, conduction block or reentrant excitation disrupts the normally synchronous activation of the heart. Consequently, cardiac output may be adversely affected. If cardiac output is reduced sufficiently, blood pressure falls, which initially may cause symptoms such as dizziness (presyncope) and passing out (syncope) and in more severe cases may cause death. Treatment of certain cardiac arrhythmias is therefore indicated. Although in many cases the exact mechanism of a given arrhythmia cannot be determined with certainty, knowing the mechanism permits a more rational therapeutic approach.

In addition to the textual description of cardiac arrhythmias provided in the following sections and the examples of arrhythmias given in Figures 32.8 to 32.15, an excellent visual representation of common cardiac arrhythmias can be viewed in the video *Living Arrhythmias* (available at https://www.youtube.com/watch?v=TJR2AfxVHsM).

Abnormalities of impulse formation
Altered normal automaticity
Altered normal automaticity is a physiological feature of the SA node that permits the heart to match its output to demand. Under circumstances of increased demand, such as during exercise, automaticity is enhanced. Enhanced normal automaticity, manifest as sinus **tachycardia** (Figure 32.8), is typically associated with physiological stimuli that increase sympathetic tone and/or decrease parasympathetic tone. As discussed in Chapter 31, both enhanced sympathetic tone and reduced

Normal sinus rhythm

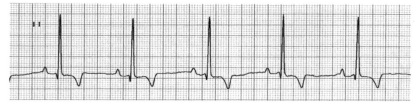

Sinus bradycardia

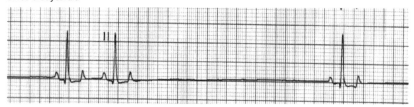

Sinus tachycardia

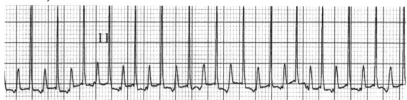

Figure 32.8 Normal sinus rhythm, sinus bradycardia, and sinus tachycardia in a dog. From Reece, W.O. (2004) *Dukes' Physiology of Domestic Animals*, 12th edn. Cornell University Press, Ithaca, NY. Reproduced with permission from Cornell University Press.

parasympathetic tone increase pacemaker current in the SA node. Decreased demand, as typically occurs during sleep, is associated with a reduction in the spontaneous discharge rate of the SA node, manifest as sinus **bradycardia** (Figure 32.8). The slowing of the SA node discharge rate is caused by increased parasympathetic and/or reduced sympathetic tone. Changes in the SA node discharge rate may also result from shifts of the primary pacemaker region within the right atrial pacemaker complex, secondary to differential distribution of sympathetic and parasympathetic innervation within different regions of the pacemaker complex and/or different sensitivities to autonomic neurotransmitters.

Modulation of normal SA node automaticity by the autonomic nervous system can also contribute to variations in sinus rate during respiration. Respiratory sinus arrhythmia is caused primarily by decreased vagal tone during inspiration, leading to acceleration of the heart rate, and by increased vagal tone during expiration, leading to slowing of the heart rate. The alterations of vagal tone are determined by inputs from the central nervous system, where central inspiratory drive inhibits vagal nerve traffic to the SA node, and from peripheral sensors linked to arterial chemoreceptors and baroreceptors, intracardiac reflexes, and pulmonary stretch receptors.

If the SA node pacemaker becomes quiescent or impulses generated by the SA node are unable to activate surrounding atrial myocardium, more slowly depolarizing latent pacemakers in the atrium, atrioventricular (AV) node or ventricle may assume control of the cardiac rhythm. The back-up function provided by subsidiary pacemakers is desirable, in that it assures that ventricular activation is maintained. Enhancement of automaticity in subsidiary pacemakers may increase the spontaneous discharge rate of these pacemakers so that it more closely approximates the normal discharge rate of the SA node.

However, enhanced automaticity of subsidiary pacemakers in the continued presence of normal SA node automaticity may not be desirable. For example, acceleration of the spontaneous discharge rate of subsidiary pacemakers can be precipitated by various drugs, certain forms of cardiac disease, or alterations in autonomic nervous system tone. Under these circumstances, the emergence of subsidiary pacemaker activity is not warranted and the competition between normal pacemaker activity in the SA node and accelerated pacemaker activity arising from a subsidiary pacemaker may create an irregular cardiac rhythm (Figure 32.9).

Abnormal automaticity

Cardiac Purkinje fibers usually have relatively slow spontaneous discharge rates, whereas atrial and ventricular muscle are quiescent. Depolarization of these tissues secondary to certain forms of cardiac disease induces spontaneous activity (Figure 32.10), the rate of which increases with increasing depolarization. Depolarization-induced automaticity is more easily suppressed by calcium channel blockade than by sodium channel blockade and is accelerated by β-adrenergic agonists. In this respect, **abnormal automaticity** in Purkinje fibers and atrial and ventricular myocardium resembles normal automaticity in the SA node.

Premature atrial complexes

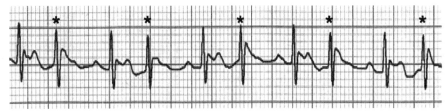

Premature ventricular complex

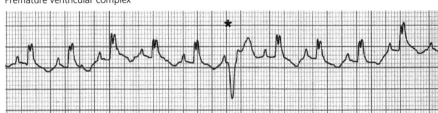

Figure 32.9 Premature atrial complexes and a ventricular complex (indicated by asterisks) in a cat. From Reece, W.O. (2004) *Dukes' Physiology of Domestic Animals*, 12th edn. Cornell University Press, Ithaca, NY. Reproduced with permission from Cornell University Press.

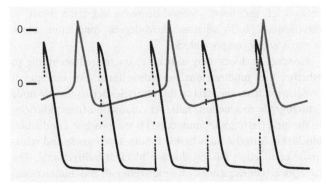

Figure 32.10 Abnormal automaticity in diseased ventricle. The lower recording is from normal myocardium bordering a region of diseased myocardium. The upper recording is from the diseased region. During pacing at a constant cycle length, the normal region generates normally appearing fast-response action potentials. In contrast, the abnormal region exhibits slow diastolic depolarization leading to automatic slow-response action potentials. Reproduced from Gilmour, R.F. Jr and Zipes, D.P. (1986) Abnormal automaticity and related phenomena. In: *The Heart and Cardiovascular System*, 2nd edn (eds H.A. Fozzard, E. Haber, R.B. Jennings, A.M. Katz and H.E. Morgan), pp. 1239–1257. Raven Press, New York.

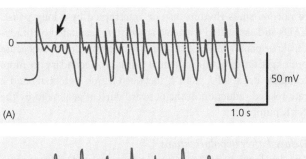

(A)

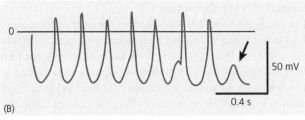

(B)

Figure 32.11 Examples of (A) early and (B) delayed after depolarizations (at the arrows) in diseased rat myocardium. From Reece, W.O. (2004) *Dukes' Physiology of Domestic Animals*, 12th edn. Cornell University Press, Ithaca, NY. Reproduced with permission from Cornell University Press.

Triggered activity

In certain forms of cardiac disease, the repolarization phase of a cardiac action potential may be interrupted, or followed, by another depolarization phase, or **afterdepolarization** (Figure 32.11). Afterdepolarizations that interrupt repolarization are called **early afterdepolarizations** (EADs), whereas afterdepolarizations that follow repolarization are called **delayed afterdepolarizations** (DADs). If the magnitude of the afterdepolarization is sufficiently large, threshold for activation of Na^+ or Ca^{2+} channels may be exceeded, resulting in the generation of an action potential. Such an action potential is known as a triggered response, in that it did not occur spontaneously but was triggered by the afterdepolarization.

Early after depolarizations

EADs may result either from enhanced inward current or from reduced outward current during the action potential plateau. Enhancement of inward current can be mediated by augmented calcium (I_{Ca}), sodium (I_{Na}), or Na/Ca exchange ($I_{Na/Ca}$) currents. Although Na^+ and Ca^{2+} channels are expected to be inactivated at the end of the plateau phase, when EADs most commonly develop, a small fraction of channels does not inactivate. As a result, an inward current persists during the plateau. The magnitude of the current is small, yet even a small current (I, where $V = IR$) may produce significant changes in membrane potential (V) during the plateau because membrane resistance (R) during this phase of the action potential is high (not many channels are open). If the depolarization caused by the inward plateau current is sufficient, activation of I_{Ca} or I_{Na} may occur and initiate triggered responses.

EADs may also result, indirectly, from a reduction in outward current. If the reduction of outward current is nonuniform throughout the action potential or coincides with activation of a particular inward current, net current may become inward and produce a discrete depolarization. Alternatively, reduction of outward current may simply prolong action potential duration and thereby provide sufficient time for the recovery and subsequent reopening of inward currents. The induction of EADs secondary to reduced outward current occurs during exposure to certain drugs (e.g., quinidine and type III antiarrhythmic drugs) and abnormal extracellular ionic milieu, including hypokalemia, hypocalcemia and acidosis. In addition, a reduction of outward current in certain disease states, such as hypertrophy and some variants of the long QT syndrome, may predispose to the development of EADs.

The development of EADs usually occurs in the setting of a slow heart rate or pronounced sinus arrhythmia, where a period of normal sinus rhythm may be interrupted by a long pause. EADs and associated triggered activity are facilitated by bradycardia or pauses in sinus rhythm because slow heart rates cause prolongation of action potential duration, secondary to more complete decay of I_{Kr} and I_{Ks} between action potentials and a rate-related reduction of the outward current generated by the Na/K pump.

Delayed after depolarizations

The development of DADs is typically associated with exposure of a cardiac myocyte to higher than normal intracellular calcium concentrations ($[Ca^{2+}]_i$), as may occur in environments that promote calcium influx (e.g., toxic levels of digitalis, hypercalcemia, and intense sympathetic stimulation). If the rate of calcium influx is more rapid than its rate of efflux, the calcium sequestration reserve of the sarcoplasmic reticulum becomes saturated. As a result, cytosolic $[Ca^{2+}]_i$ increases, which in turn either activates a calcium-dependent transient inward current (I_{ti}), carried primarily by sodium ions, or increases the exchange of intracellular calcium for extracellular sodium via the Na/Ca exchanger. In either case, sodium entry depolarizes the cell, which may lead to the generation of a triggered response (Figure 32.11).

In contrast to the induction of EADs, initiation of DADs is facilitated by rapid pacing. Increasing the number of action potentials increases calcium entry via I_{Ca} and decreases the time available for calcium extrusion. Both effects promote an increase in $[Ca^{2+}]_i$. Such a process may become self-sustaining, where a DAD leads to a triggered response and calcium entry during the plateau of the triggered response leads to another DAD.

Abnormalities of impulse propagation
Conduction block

The orderly spread of activation throughout the heart is predicated on each cell being in the rest state at the moment it is activated. Cells that are still refractory from a previous activation will not respond to another input. Consequently, action potential propagation fails in refractory tissue, producing conduction block. In cells with a normal resting membrane potential, the duration of the refractory period is determined by the duration of the action potential, for the reasons given in Chapter 31. In cells that have been depolarized by a disease process, however, the refractory period may outlast repolarization, leading to "post-repolarization" refractoriness. The latter is caused by persistent inactivation of sodium channels at membrane potentials less negative than the normal resting membrane potential.

Block of impulses is generally an abnormal phenomenon in the heart, with the exception of the AV node, where partial block of rapid atrial rhythms may be protective. For clinical characterization of the severity of conduction block, it is useful to describe the degree to which conduction is impaired. An illustration of the different degrees of conduction block as they occur in the AV node is given in Figure 32.12. First-degree conduction block is actually not block at all, but prolongation of activation times, reflecting slow conduction between two regions of the heart. Second-degree conduction block is intermittent block, whereas third-degree conduction block is persistent or complete block.

Conduction block may also be characterized according to whether it is unidirectional or bidirectional. For example, if conduction from the atria to the ventricles across the AV node (anterograde conduction) fails, yet conduction from ventricles to the atria (retrograde conduction) is still possible, conduction block is unidirectional, whereas if both anterograde and retrograde conduction fail, conduction block is bidirectional. The functional consequences of unidirectional and bidirectional conduction block for the development of certain forms of reentry are discussed in the next section.

Reentry

Reentry is probably responsible for the majority of the life-threatening tachyarrhythmias that occur clinically. As such, reentry has been studied extensively and several forms have been identified. The most venerable concept of reentry is that of circus movement reentry. The hallmarks of this type of reentry are unidirectional conduction block in one limb of a branching conduction network, slow conduction around a large anatomical obstacle, and reexcitation of the previously blocked region of tissue. In the example shown in Figure 32.13, an impulse emerging from the top of the diagram conducts along the right pathway but blocks in the left pathway, which has a longer refractory period, perhaps secondary to some form of cardiac disease. The impulse in the right pathway conducts around an anatomical obstacle, which may be formed by a region of necrotic tissue or a valve orifice for example. If the time taken to circumnavigate the obstacle is sufficiently long, the refractory period of the previously blocked region will have expired before the impulse arrives. As a result, the impulse may then conduct retrogradely through that region and initiate a self-sustaining circular excitation of the circuit.

First-degree AV block

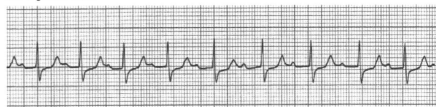

Second-degree AV block

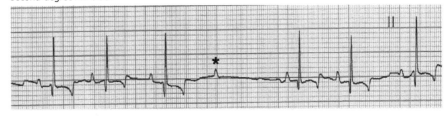

Third-degree AV block

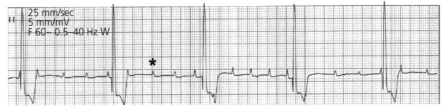

Figure 32.12 First-degree, second-degree and third-degree AV block in a dog. Note prolongation of the PR interval during first-degree block. During second-degree block, one of the P waves blocks (asterisk), whereas in third-degree block all of the P waves block (one of which is indicated by the asterisk). Activation of the ventricle was maintained in this animal with a ventricular pacemaker (note the stimulus artifact preceding each QRS complex). From Reece, W.O. (2004) *Dukes' Physiology of Domestic Animals*, 12th edn. Cornell University Press, Ithaca, NY. Reproduced with permission from Cornell University Press.

Fixed obstacle   Spiral wave

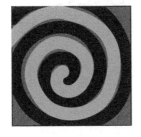

Figure 32.13 Schematic diagrams of circus movement reentry around a fixed obstacle (*left*) and spiral wave reentry (*right*). From Reece, W.O. (2004) *Dukes' Physiology of Domestic Animals*, 12th edn. Cornell University Press, Ithaca, NY. Reproduced with permission from Cornell University Press.

Once initiated, the reentrant pattern of excitation may become self-sustaining if the impulse continues to revolve around the circuit. Under these circumstances, the reentrant circuit generates pinwheel-like waves of activation that compete for activation of the ventricle with wavefronts initiated by the SA node. The result is often a rapid irregular rhythm that reduces filling time and disrupts normal synchronous activation, thereby impairing cardiac output.

A large obstacle and slow conduction around the circuit are necessary for maintenance of reentry, otherwise the activation wavefront may impinge on refractory tissue and stop (the "head" catches the "tail"). In the normal heart, few if any obstacles exist

that are sufficiently large to support a reentrant circuit, nor is conduction normally very slow anywhere in the heart except in the AV node. Thus, reentry typically occurs only in hearts that have been damaged. Under such circumstances, regions of the heart that are necrotic or permanently inexcitable may contribute to the formation of an obstacle. In addition, myocardial injury may cause cells to become partially depolarized, in which case Na⁺ channels are permanently inactivated and cells must then rely on slow Ca²⁺ current for excitation. Injury may also impair gap junction conductance and slow conduction by that mechanism.

More recent additions to the potential mechanisms for reentrant excitation in the heart are leading circle reentry and spiral wave reentry. A spiral wave is a curved wavefront of excitation that revolves around a core of inexcitable cells (see Figure 32.13). However, the core need not be damaged tissue. Instead, it may be a region of normally excitable cells that has been rendered temporarily inexcitable, secondary to extreme wavefront curvature. This phenomenon reflects the process discussed in Chapter 31, where an excited cell delivers current to its unexcited neighbor and raises that cell to threshold, which is typical of a normal planar wave. If the wavefront has curvature, however, the cell at the tip of the wavefront disperses current to several cells, with the result that there may be insufficient current delivered to any cell to raise it to threshold. Sustained depolarization of the core and the resultant inactivation of Na⁺ channels may also contribute to inexcitability.

Supraventricular tachycardia

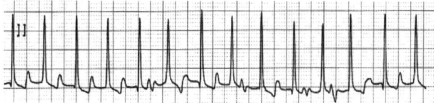

Ventricular tachycardia

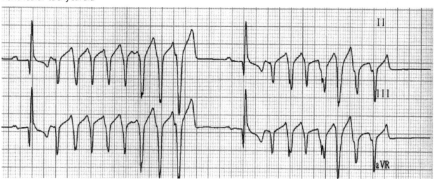

Figure 32.14 Supraventricular and ventricular tachycardia in a dog. During supraventricular tachycardia, the QRS complexes remain upright and narrow, indicating that the ventricular activation sequence is normal. During ventricular tachycardia, the QRS complexes are inverted in polarity and prolonged in duration, reflecting an abnormal sequence of ventricular activation. From Reece, W.O. (2004) *Dukes' Physiology of Domestic Animals*, 12th edn. Cornell University Press, Ithaca, NY. Reproduced with permission from Cornell University Press.

Atrial fibrillation

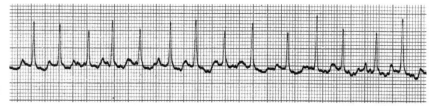

Ventricular fibrillation

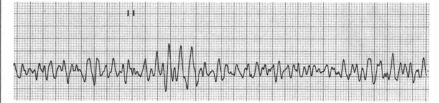

Figure 32.15 Atrial fibrillation in a cat and ventricular fibrillation in a dog. During atrial fibrillation, the intervals between QRS complexes show no discernible pattern. From Reece, W.O. (2004) *Dukes' Physiology of Domestic Animals*, 12th edn. Cornell University Press, Ithaca, NY. Reproduced with permission from Cornell University Press.

Just as a cyclone may move erratically along the ground, spiral waves may meander through the heart, creating the irregular activation patterns that typify certain tachyarrhythmias, such as atrial and ventricular tachycardia and fibrillation (Figures 32.14 and 32.15) (see also movies section at http://thevirtualheart.org). In addition, a single spiral wave may, under the appropriate circumstances, disintegrate into many wavelets. Similarly, a single circus movement reentry circuit may break up and spawn multiple wavelets. The transformation of a single spiral wave or reentry circuit into many smaller waves or circuits has been proposed to underlie the transition from ventricular tachycardia to ventricular fibrillation.

Self-evaluation

Answers can be found at the end of the chapter.

1 Define and explain the effects of hyperkalemia and hypokalemia on the QT interval of the ECG.

2 Define and explain the effects of hypercalcemia and hypocalcemia on the QT interval of the ECG.

For questions 1 and 2, remember that the duration of the QT interval is determined by the duration of the ventricular action potential. Accordingly, changes in the QT interval can be largely predicted on the basis of changes in action potential duration.

3 Your patient is an elderly Great Dane that has displayed chronic atrial fibrillation of unknown etiology for the last 6 months. At rest, the ventricular rate is fairly regular at approximately 160 beats per minute. The owner is concerned because recently the animal seems to get dizzy when it runs or gets excited.

  A How can the ventricular rate be fairly regular when the atria are fibrillating?

  B What is the most likely reason for the animal's presyncope (dizziness)?

4 You have been asked to evaluate a new drug that may (or may not) block both calcium and sodium channels. Following administration of the drug to an animal, what changes in ECG parameters (e.g., P–P interval, PR interval, QRS duration, QT interval) would be expected if the drug blocked:

  A Calcium channels

  B Sodium channels

5 Addison's disease may be accompanied by excessive retention of potassium. Consequently, blood levels of potassium may be elevated (hyperkalemia). Describe and give mechanisms for the potential effects of hyperkalemia on the following aspects of the electrical activity of ventricular muscle.

  A Resting membrane potential

  B The amplitude of phase 0 of the action potential

  C Conduction velocity

Suggested reading

Cherry, E.M., Fenton, F.H. and Gilmour, R.F. Jr (2012) Mechanisms of ventricular arrhythmias: a dynamical systems-based perspective. *American Journal of Physiology* 302:H2451–H2463.

Fox, P.R., Sisson, D. and Moïse, N.S. (1999) *Textbook of Canine and Feline Cardiology*, 2nd edn, pp. 67–106, 291–306. W.B. Saunders, Philadelphia.

Tilley, L.P. (1992) *Essentials of Canine and Feline Electrocardiography*, 3rd edn. Lea & Febiger, Philadelphia.

Zipes, D.P. (2011) Genesis of cardiac arrhythmias. In: *Braunwald's Heart Disease*, 9th edn (eds R.O. Bonow, D.L. Mann, D.P. Zipes and P. Libby), pp. 548–592. W.B. Saunders, Philadelphia.

Answers

1 A seemingly anomalous (and frequently confusing) observation is that as extracellular K^+ is increased, action potential duration decreases, and as extracellular K^+ concentration is decreased, action potential duration increases. One might expect that the augmented driving force for K^+ efflux created by hypokalemia would increase outward K^+ current and thereby shorten action potential duration. The opposite effects might be expected to accompany hyperkalemia. In fact, increased outward current during hypokalemia and decreased outward current during hyperkalemia does apply to current flowing via the delayed rectifier. However, action potential duration is also determined by the inward rectifier and, as discussed in the text, the inward rectifier channel is regulated by extracellular K^+ concentration. Thus, during hypokalemia, K^+ efflux via the inward

rectifier is reduced, leading to a prolongation of action potential duration, whereas K^+ efflux during hyperkalemia is increased (despite the reduced driving force) and action potential duration is shortened. Prolongation or abbreviation of action potential duration is reflected by a lengthening or shortening, respectively, of the QT interval on the surface ECG.

2 Another seemingly anomalous (and frequently confusing) observation is that as extracellular Ca^{2+} concentration is increased, action potential duration decreases, whereas as extracellular Ca^{2+} is decreased, action potential duration increases. Again, one might expect that the increased driving force for Ca^{2+} influx created by hypercalcemia would increase inward Ca^{2+} current and thereby prolong action potential duration (more depolarizing current during the action potential plateau). Conversely, the decrease in driving force created by hypocalcemia should shorten action potential duration. However, extracellular Ca^{2+}, in addition to serving as the charge carrier for the Ca^{2+} current, also regulates the conductance of the delayed rectifier. Hypercalcemia increases the delayed rectifier (via an unknown mechanism), which shortens action potential duration, whereas hypocalcemia has the opposite effects. Thus, hyperkalemia is accompanied by shortening of the QT interval and hypocalcemia by prolongation of the QT interval.

Although the relationship between serum Ca^{2+} concentration and action potential duration may seem somewhat convoluted, one can rationalize the usefulness of such a relationship from a physiological standpoint, in that during hypocalcemia contractile force generation would tend to decrease, secondary to a reduction of Ca^{2+} current and the resultant reduction in intracellular Ca^{2+} concentration. Prolongation of action potential duration during hypocalcemia increases the period of time during which the calcium current flows, thereby partially compensating for the reduced magnitude of Ca^{2+} current at any given point in time. On the other hand, during hypercalcemia, the danger of excessive Ca^{2+} influx and the generation of arrhythmias secondary to "Ca^{2+} overload" exists (by rather complex mechanisms that are not covered here). Shortening of action potential duration and the time during which the Ca^{2+} current flows would tend to offset the potential for Ca^{2+} overload.

3 A. The ventricle is protected from rapid activation during atrial fibrillation because the slow response-dependent AV node cannot conduct rapidly enough to transmit the atrial activation to the ventricle.

B. Excitement is typically accompanied by an increase in sympathetic tone and a decrease in parasympathetic tone. Both would tend to increase calcium current in AV nodal cells and thereby increase conduction velocity through the AV node. If more impulses are allowed to pass from the atria to the ventricles, the ventricular rate will become more rapid and irregular, which would decrease filling time. The reduction in preload might reduce cardiac output and blood pressure to the point where blood supply to the brain is impaired.

4A *P–P interval*: increase. The P–P interval is determined by the discharge rate of the sinus node, which is a slow-response (calcium channel-dependent) tissue. Decreased calcium current reduces the slope of phase 4 depolarization. As a result, more time is required to reach threshold.

PR interval: increase. The PR interval is determined by conduction velocity through the AV node, a slow-response tissue. Blocking calcium channels reduces upstroke velocity and action potential amplitude and thereby slows conduction velocity.

QRS duration: no change. QRS duration is determined by conduction velocity through ventricular muscle, which is fast-response (sodium channel-dependent) tissue.

QT interval: decrease. The QT interval is determined by the duration of action potentials in ventricular muscle. The latter is determined largely by a balance between calcium and potassium currents. Decreased inward calcium current tips the balance between inward and outward current to net outward, which accelerates repolarization. However, the expected decrease in the QT interval is typically offset by the increase in QT interval that accompanies a slowing of the heart rate (see changes in P–P interval above).

4B *P–P interval*: no change. The P–P interval is determined by the discharge rate of the sinus node, which is a slow-response (calcium channel-dependent) tissue.

PR interval: no change. The PR interval is determined by conduction velocity through the AV node, a slow-response tissue.

QRS duration: increase. QRS duration is determined by conduction velocity through ventricular muscle, which is a fast-response (sodium channel-dependent) tissue. Blocking sodium channels will reduce upstroke velocity and action potential amplitude and thereby slow conduction velocity.

QT interval: no change. The QT interval is determined by the duration of action potentials in ventricular muscle. The latter is determined largely by a balance between calcium and potassium currents.

5 A. Hyperkalemia reduces (makes less negative) resting membrane potential by decreasing the chemical gradient for potassium efflux. Less efflux of positive charge equals retention of positive charge by the cell.

B. Reduction of the resting membrane potential produces persistent inactivation of sodium channels. If less sodium channels are available to carry current, the membrane potential will not become as depolarized during phase 0. Also, because action potential amplitude is defined as the difference between the resting membrane potential and the peak voltage attained during the upstroke, reduction of the resting membrane potential necessarily reduces action potential amplitude.

C. If sodium current is reduced, action potential amplitude and the upstroke velocity of phase 0 will be reduced. Accordingly, the action potential will propagate more slowly to offset the potential for Ca^{2+} overload.

33 Mechanical Activity of the Heart

Dean H. Riedesel

Iowa State University, Ames, IA, USA

Heart as a pump

1 If the stroke volume of a healthy dog was 20 mL and the heart rate was 100 beats per minute, what would the cardiac output be in liters per minute?

2 Where does the calcium come from to initiate contraction of myocardial muscle?

3 If the volume of a dog's right ventricle at the end of diastole was 45 mL and the volume at the end of systole was 18 mL, what is the dog's stroke volume?

4 What would be the ejection fraction of the dog described above?

5 Draw a cross-section of the mammalian ventricles in the frontal plane and label the septum, right and left ventricular free walls, and right and left ventricular chambers.

The heart is an amazing pump that over the lifetime of an animal performs a huge amount of work in extremely variable conditions. Although the heart is independent functionally, humoral and neural factors influence its performance tremendously. All the myocardial cells contract with each heartbeat but the strength of each cell contraction depends on **excitation–contraction coupling** and **sarcomere length**. This chapter describes the intrinsic mechanisms that affect myocardial cell activity, the cardiac cycle (contraction and relaxation) of the heart using the classical Wiggers diagram to plot various events and pressures over time, and the pressure–volume loop. Although most of the examples utilize the left atrium, ventricle, and aorta, the same principles apply to the right atrium, ventricle, and pulmonary artery.

Excitation–contraction and the membrane system of cardiac cells

As in all excitable cells, excitation is mediated in myocardial cells by depolarization of cell membranes (sarcolemma). From the sarcolemma, the excitatory process is distributed via intercalated disks to adjacent cells and by the transverse tubular system throughout the entire thickness of the cell. The intercalated disks, along with the gap junctions of low electrical resistance, permit rapid transmission of depolarizing impulses from cell to adjacent cell. The transverse tubular network extends the extracellular compartment to all levels of the myocardial cell, shortening diffusion distance from the cell exterior to structures in the cell interior. Depolarization and repolarization of the sarcolemma occurs in intimate association with intracellular structures.

Excitation–contraction coupling

Ionic calcium is the link between excitation and contraction. Calcium enters the cell from the extracellular fluid and is also released from intracellular sites during the plateau of the action potential (Figure 33.1). The sarcolemma membrane regulates inward diffusion of calcium by opening and closing voltage-dependent Ca^{2+} channels (L-Ca^{2+}) as depolarization alters the transmembrane electrical potential.

There is evidence of the existence of two different Ca^{2+} pools within the myocardial cell: (i) a calcium-binding site in the longitudinal tubules of the **sarcoplasmic reticulum** and (ii) a calcium-storage site in the terminal cisternae of the sarcoplasmic reticulum. In response to the action potential, Ca^{2+} enters the cell across the sarcolemma from the extracellular space. This

Dukes' Physiology of Domestic Animals, Thirteenth Edition. Edited by William O. Reece, Howard H. Erickson, Jesse P. Goff and Etsuro E. Uemura.

© 2015 John Wiley & Sons, Inc. Published 2015 by John Wiley & Sons, Inc.

Companion website: www.wiley.com/go/reece/physiology

Section VI: The Cardiovascular System

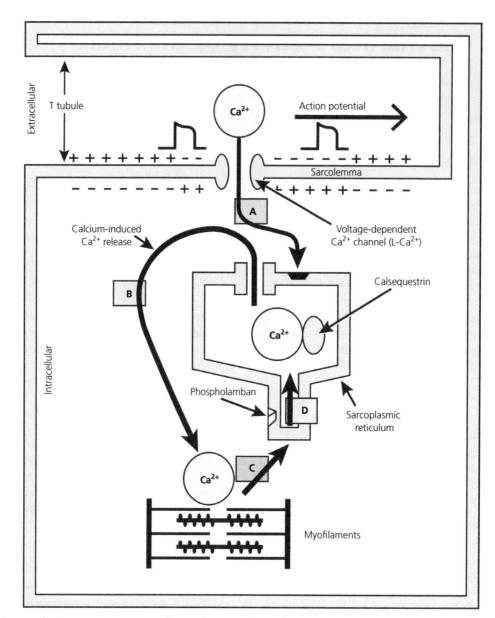

Figure 33.1 Diagram of excitation–contraction coupling in the myocardium. The action potential spreads into the cell via T tubules. During the plateau phase of the action potential, voltage-dependent calcium channels open and extracellular calcium enters the cell (A). This small amount of calcium triggers the release of a large amount of calcium from the sarcoplasmic reticulum (B). The released calcium diffuses within the cytosol and binds to troponin and leads to myocardial contraction (C). When the action potential-induced calcium release ceases, the cytosolic calcium levels decrease owing to uptake by the sarcoplasmic reticulum (D). Sarcolemma ion pumps are activated and remove cytosolic calcium into the extracellular space. Phospholamban is a small protein that accelerates calcium uptake by the sarcolemma cisternae. From Reece, W.O. (2004) *Dukes' Physiology of Domestic Animals*, 12th edn. Cornell University Press, Ithaca, NY. Reproduced with permission from Cornell University Press.

calcium binds to a receptor on the cisternae of the sarcoplasmic reticulum and results in the massive release of calcium from storage and contraction of the myofilaments (systole). Contraction is terminated when the longitudinal tubules of the sarcoplasmic reticulum accumulate the Ca²⁺, removing it from the site of interaction with contractile proteins.

As the contractile event depends on the presence of Ca²⁺ ions, so relaxation depends on its removal. When Ca²⁺ ions are removed from the area of the myofilaments, cross-bridge formation between actin and myosin ceases and the sarcomere returns to its resting length. Thus, the sarcoplasmic reticulum, with its ability to bind, transport, and sequester calcium in an inactive site, is considered the subcellular system initiating contraction, regulating tension, and achieving relaxation.

Muscle mechanics

Studying an isolated piece of cardiac muscle may help one understand the response of the whole heart to changes in blood pressure (**afterload**), return of venous blood (**preload**), and myocardial contractility (**inotropic state**). The concepts and

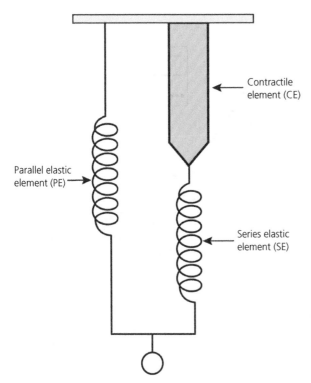

Figure 33.2 A.V. Hill's model for muscle. The series elastic element (SE) lies between the contractile element (CE) and the muscle ends. Stretching of the SE at the initiation of a muscle (CE) contraction delays the development of tension at the ends of the muscle. From Reece, W.O. (2004) *Dukes' Physiology of Domestic Animals*, 12th edn. Cornell University Press, Ithaca, NY. Reproduced with permission from Cornell University Press.

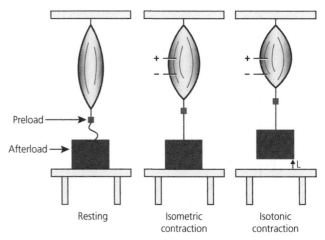

Figure 33.3 Experimental arrangement used to study the mechanics of an isolated muscle (e.g., papillary heart muscle). Preload stretches the muscle fiber and consequently the sarcomeres to some pre-contraction length. The muscle is then electrically stimulated to contract. Isometric contractions occur when the muscle cannot lift the afterload. The relationship between the preload and the amount of isometric force is used to develop the length–tension diagram. The relationship between preload, afterload, and velocity of lifting ($\Delta l/\Delta t$) the afterload during isotonic contractions is used to develop the force–velocity curve. From Reece, W.O. (2004) *Dukes' Physiology of Domestic Animals*, 12th edn. Cornell University Press, Ithaca, NY. Reproduced with permission from Cornell University Press.

techniques are those of A.V. Hill, which were developed to analyze skeletal muscle. Two types of muscle contraction are used: **isometric** (*iso*, constant or equal; *metric*, length) and **isotonic** (at constant force or load). The force of contraction and the velocity of shortening are measured under variable loading conditions of the isolated muscle. Force and velocity are inversely related; thus, with no load, force is negligible and velocity is maximal. At the other extreme, isometric contractions develop maximal force and zero velocity of contraction.

Three-component model of muscle

The original skeletal muscle model proposed by Hill (Figure 33.2) consists of a **contractile element** (CE), a series elastic element (SE), and a parallel elastic element (PE). The elastic elements have no anatomical counterpart. The muscle functions as if the elastic elements existed as shown in the model. Since the PE has no role in muscle contraction, it is not considered further in this discussion.

Figure 33.3 shows the arrangement employed for studying muscle mechanics in the isolated papillary muscle from the right ventricle of a cat. The mechanical energy produced by the contraction of cardiac or skeletal muscle is a function of its sarcomere length just before contraction. Preload is the term given to the weight attached to stretch the muscle to its pre-contraction

length and tension. In the intact ventricle, preload is analogous to factors that determine end-diastolic volume. Additional weight is then added to the preload; in the system as diagrammed, this added weight, the afterload, has no effect on the muscle until it has been stimulated and begins to shorten. In the heart, the aortic pressure against which the left ventricle contracts to raise pressure and eject blood approximates afterload. Together the preload and afterload make up the total load or total weight against which the muscle contracts when stimulated.

When the muscle is stimulated, excitation–contraction coupling takes place, and the CE becomes capable of shortening and developing force. The SE element (see Figure 33.2) is given properties of a spring against which CE contracts. Consequently, the active state of CE is translated into mechanical force development or shortening only after some delay. The time course of the contraction depends on the contractile properties of the CE, the duration of the active state, and the elastic properties of the SE element. During an isometric contraction (see Figure 33.3) the muscle cannot shorten and the afterload is not lifted. Figure 33.3 also illustrates an isotonic contraction in which the contractile force stretches the SE element to the point that its elastic tension equals the load and the afterload is lifted by the distance L.

Length–tension diagram

In both cardiac and skeletal muscle the force of an isometric contraction depends on initial muscle length (see Figure 30.12, Chapter 30). Normally, the ventricles operate on the ascending

Section VI: The Cardiovascular System

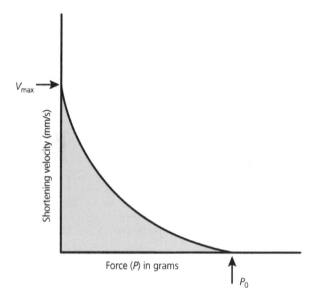

Figure 33.4 Force–velocity curve from an isolated papillary muscle at a constant preload and varying afterloads. The velocity (mm/s) of shortening is determined by measuring how fast the muscle lifts the afterload during the initial stage of contraction. P_0, the maximum load the muscle can lift; V_{max}, the theoretical maximum velocity determined by extrapolation of the experimental points to a zero load. From Reece, W.O. (2004) *Dukes' Physiology of Domestic Animals*, 12th edn. Cornell University Press, Ithaca, NY. Reproduced with permission from Cornell University Press.

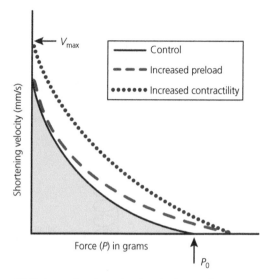

Figure 33.5 Increasing the preload on the force–velocity curve does not alter V_{max} but increases P_0. Increasing the contractility or inotropic state of the muscle increases both V_{max} and P_0. From Reece, W.O. (2004) *Dukes' Physiology of Domestic Animals*, 12th edn. Cornell University Press, Ithaca, NY. Reproduced with permission from Cornell University Press.

limb of the length–tension curve so that any increase in filling of the ventricle increases the force of contraction and thus the volume of the blood pumped out per beat. This relationship in the heart was first described by Otto Frank in 1895 and later elaborated by Ernest Starling in 1918, hence it is known as the Frank–Starling relationship (mechanism) or **Starling's law** of the heart.

Force–velocity curve

If an isolated muscle is allowed to contract isotonically against various total loads (preload and afterload), and the beginning or initial velocity of contraction ($\Delta l/\Delta t$) is plotted as a function of load (P) the force–velocity curve can be developed (Figure 33.4). When preload and therefore initial muscle length is kept constant, an inverse relation is found between velocity and force. The load at which the muscle cannot shorten and where its velocity is zero is denoted as P_0 on the abscissa; this represents maximum isometric force. If the curve is extrapolated to its intersection with the ordinate (i.e., the velocity at zero load) the maximum velocity of shortening (V_{max}) is obtained. Force and velocity are inversely related. When the load is zero the velocity is maximal and when the load is maximal (isometric contraction) velocity is zero (see Figure 33.4). The relationship is altered when preload and consequently initial muscle length changes. When initial muscle length (preload) is increased, there is a change in maximal force developed (P_0) without a change in maximal velocity of shortening (Figure 33.5). In the

intact heart this changing relationship is synonymous with the Frank–Starling mechanism in which the stroke volume (i.e., force of contraction) is found to increase with larger ventricular end-diastolic volumes.

The force (i.e., load) and velocity relationship of cardiac muscle varies with changes inherent in the contractile mechanism, including the property known as contractility or the inotropic state. Inotropic agents such as norepinephrine, calcium, and certain drugs (e.g., pimobendan) increase contractility of the heart. These agents cause the heart muscle to contract faster at any given load and to contract more strongly with an isometric load (see Figure 33.5). The fact that V_{max} does not change with stretching of the muscle but does change during inotropism led to the use of V_{max} as an index of myocardial contractility.

In summary, the application of these papillary muscle experiments to the functioning heart is important. For example, the length–tension response of the papillary muscle is the same as the relationship between the volume of the heart prior to contraction (end-diastolic volume) and the strength of that contraction, i.e., Starling's law of the heart. The afterload used in the papillary muscle experiments affects the length of muscle shortening. A papillary muscle under a constant preload will progressively shorten less length as the afterload is increased. This observation can be applied to the heart because afterload can be considered similar to the pressure in the aorta that the left ventricle has to eject blood against. The heart will eject less blood when the aortic pressure increases just as the papillary muscle shortens less with increasing afterload. Decreasing the afterload of the left ventricle is one possible treatment option to increase the volume of blood ejected by each contraction of the ventricle (stroke volume).

Definitions and general considerations

The output of the right and left ventricle per beat is approximately equal and termed the **stroke volume** (SV). The SV from either ventricle multiplied by the heart rate equals the **cardiac output** (CO). For example, the quantity of blood ejected by each beat (SV) of the left ventricle in a 20-kg mongrel dog is about 20 mL, giving a CO of 2.0 L/min when the heart rate is 100 beats per minute. An equal volume of blood is ejected at the same time by the right ventricle. The stroke volumes and cardiac output are always expressed in terms of one ventricle and thus represent the quantity of blood flowing consecutively through the lungs and into the systemic vessels during the same period. If the heart rate in our hypothetical dog averaged 100 beats per minute over 24 hours, the amount of blood circulated during that period would be 2880 L (approximately 720 gallons).

To compare the cardiac output in animals of different size, the value is generally expressed in terms of body weight (kg), surface area (m²), or metabolic weight (kg$^{0.75}$) and is referred to as the cardiac index. For example, the cardiac index for a resting 450-kg horse is about 72–88 mL/min per kg, whereas for a 20-kg dog it is 155–175 mL/min per kg. In the dog, one formula for surface area is:

$$\text{Surface area}\left(m^2\right)=\left[10.1\times\text{weight}\left(g\right)^{0.67}\right]\times10^{-4}$$

where 10.1 is a constant. Using this equation for a 20-kg dog, the surface area would be 0.77 m² and the cardiac index 4000–4500 mL/min per m² or 4.0–4.5 L/min per m².

Mathematical scaling has been used to estimate the cardiac output for animals of various body weights. Like many biologic variables, cardiac output does not change linearly with body weight but is logarithmic. There is some disagreement on which power function is more appropriate for scaling cardiac output as a function of body mass. However, it has been shown that for dogs, horses, cows, humans, and other species the cardiac output is linearly related to body weight raised to the power 0.78–0.81, for example:

$$CO\left(L/min\right)=0.187\times\text{body weight}\left(kg\right)^{0.81}$$

In this regard, the relationship between body mass and cardiovascular function in birds differs from mammals of similar size. Birds have relatively larger hearts and lower heart rates.

It turns out that cardiac output and metabolism are correlated and have similar logarithmic exponents. In fact, the total oxygen requirement of the tissues, which reflects the overall metabolism or energy exchange, is the primary determinant of cardiac output in all animals. Since the oxygen requirement of the tissues is the basic determinant of cardiac output, the volume (content) of oxygen carried per unit of blood and the percent extraction by the tissues (arteriovenous oxygen difference) governs the actual cardiac output required to meet the tissue needs. The oxygen content of blood depends on the

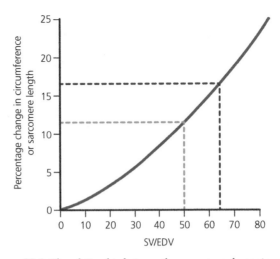

Figure 33.6 The relationship between the percentage change in mid-wall circumference or sarcomere length and ventricular ejection fraction (SV/EDV) for the left ventricle. From Reece, W.O. (2004) *Dukes' Physiology of Domestic Animals*, 12th edn. Cornell University Press, Ithaca, NY. Reproduced with permission from Cornell University Press.

concentration of hemoglobin and its oxygen saturation. The tissue extraction of oxygen depends on the gradient in the partial pressure of oxygen between plasma and tissue, the capillary surface area available for exchange, and the time the blood is exposed to this surface. In species other than mammals, these factors become increasingly significant in determining cardiac output. Thus, in fish or crustaceans that have blood with low oxygen-carrying capacity, a higher flow rate must be maintained. Similarly, in mammals, when the oxygen-carrying capacity is reduced (as in severe anemia) cardiac output must increase. In humans and other mammals the ratio of cardiac output ($\dot{Q}$) to oxygen uptake ($\dot{V}O_2$) is approximately 20 : 1 (e.g., for a 20-kg dog, $\dot{Q}/\dot{V}O_2 = 2000$ mL/100 mL). In anemia this ratio increases as blood flow (cardiac output) is elevated to carry the required amount of oxygen.

Stroke volume, the output per beat, is the difference between ventricular **end-diastolic volume** (EDV) and **end-systolic volume** (ESV). The ratio SV/EDV (**ejection fraction**) has been shown to be quite constant in mammals that vary in size from rat to horse. This constancy in heart function over vastly different sizes is explained on the basis of sarcomere characteristics. In Figure 33.6, percentage change in ventricular mid-wall circumference (i.e., sarcomere length) is plotted against ejection fraction (SV/EDV). The dashed lines represent normal ejection fractions within the reported range of 50–65%, indicating that the ventricle is not completely emptied of blood during systole. This would require sarcomere shortening of 12–17%, which corresponds well with predictions. Thus, the characteristics of sarcomeres, which are uniform in different-sized hearts, would explain ventricular ejection and apply to hearts of any size.

Patterns of ventricular emptying

Direct measurements of changing ventricular dimensions in unanesthetized dogs indicate that the left ventricle resembles a cylinder with a cone-shaped apex. Left ventricular systole primarily involves thickening of the walls and reduction in transverse lumen diameter. There is relatively little rotation or shortening of the longitudinal axis. All this would be expected since the bulk of the fibers are circularly arranged.

In contrast, right ventricular ejection of blood can be effected by three means.

1 Longitudinal shortening of the chamber (i.e., apex moving toward the base) is the most obvious gross movement. This might be expected since the inner and outer layers of spiral muscle making up the right ventricle are oriented about 90° to each other. Simultaneous contraction of these two layers of spiral muscle produces a shortening movement along the longitudinal axis.

2 A bellows-like action as a result of the right ventricular chamber being crescent shaped (Figure 33.7), with a convex septal wall and a concave free or lateral wall. During contraction the lateral wall moves toward the convex surface of the septum operating like a bellows; since the sides of the ventricle or bellows are large compared to the enclosed space, slight movement of the lateral wall toward the septum should cause displacement of a large volume of blood.

3 Contraction of the left ventricle increases the curvature of the septum, pulling the attached right ventricular lateral wall toward the septum and adding to the bellows action. That this can be a potent mechanism is borne out by the observation that right ventricular ejection can be maintained when the free wall of the right ventricle has been almost completely destroyed by cautery in the dog or by coronary occlusion in humans.

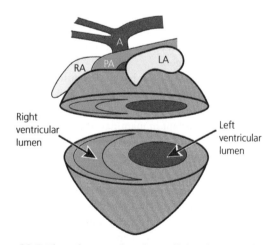

Figure 33.7 The right ventricle is thin-walled and crescent shaped. The left ventricle is thick-walled and circular. RA, right atrium; LA, left atrium; PA, pulmonary artery; A, aorta. From Reece, W.O. (2004) *Dukes' Physiology of Domestic Animals*, 12th edn. Cornell University Press, Ithaca, NY. Reproduced with permission from Cornell University Press.

Pressure and volume events of a cardiac cycle

1 Draw a ventricular pressure wave so it corresponds with the timing of the ECG.
2 Put units (mmHg) of pressure on the ventricular curve.
3 What is the difference between a right and left ventricular pressure curve?
4 Draw a pressure wave from the artery that receives blood from the left ventricle.
5 Put units (mmHg) on the arterial pressure wave.
6 What valve(s) is leaking if a systolic murmur is auscultated?

Overview of the cardiac cycle

Contraction (**systole**) and relaxation (**diastole**) of various chambers of the heart result in the characteristic pressure changes and valve movements comprising the **cardiac cycle**. The cycle repeats with every heartbeat and includes systole (isovolumetric contraction, ejection), diastole (isovolumetric relaxation and filling), and then back to systole. The right and left ventricular cycles are basically identical except for the peak pressures. The right ventricle usually only achieves peak systolic pressures of 20–40 mmHg while the left ventricle develops pressures of 100–160 mmHg in the resting animal.

As a pump the heart ejects blood with kinetic energy due to the potential energy developed (pressure) within its chambers. The repeated contraction and relaxation of the heart is known as the cardiac cycle and can be divided into phases or stages (see Figure 33.8). The reference point for the cycle is the electrocardiogram (ECG). The **P wave** corresponds with atrial depolarization, **QRS complex** with ventricular depolarization, and **T wave** with ventricular repolarization.

The pressure in the left ventricle (LV) during diastole (relaxation) is quite low and basically the left atrium (LA) and LV will have the same pressure at this point in the cardiac cycle (Figure 33.9). After the P wave of the ECG the atria will contract and the resulting increase in blood volume added to the LV will raise the pressure slightly. After the QRS complex the ventricles contract and the pressure in the lumen of the LV increases rapidly. As soon as LV pressure exceeds LA pressure the left **AV valve** closes and the **first heart sound** (S$_1$) or "lub" (of the "lub-dub") is produced. When the pressure in the LV exceeds that in the aorta, the **semilunar valve** (aortic valve) opens and blood is ejected from the ventricle. The ejected volume of blood expands the aorta causing the pressure to increase. In Figure 33.9, pressures in the LV and aorta are plotted simultaneously using the same scale. Notice the virtually identical pressures in the LV and aorta during systole. Toward the end of systole the ventricular muscle repolarizes producing the T wave on the ECG. As the ventricle relaxes (diastole), LV pressure decreases below aortic pressure and the blood in the aorta flows backwards for a short period of time until the semilunar valve closes, producing a small oscillation or notch (**dicrotic notch**) in the aortic pressure trace. The semilunar

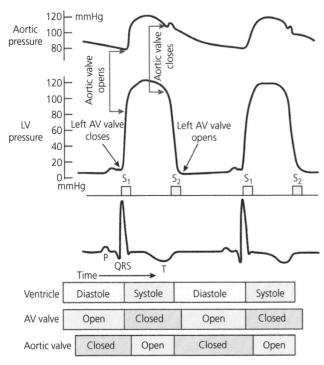

Figure 33.8 Diagram of an ECG and pressure in the left ventricle (LV) and aorta. The pressure scales for the aorta and left ventricle are identical. The diastolic pressure in the ventricle is almost zero while it fills. After the aortic valve opens, the pressure in the aorta and left ventricle are almost identical. After the aortic valve closes, the pressure in the aorta slowly decreases as blood drains through the tissues of the body. S_1, first heart sound; S_2, second heart sound; AV, atrioventricular. From Reece, W.O. (2004) *Dukes' Physiology of Domestic Animals*, 12th edn. Cornell University Press, Ithaca, NY. Reproduced with permission from Cornell University Press.

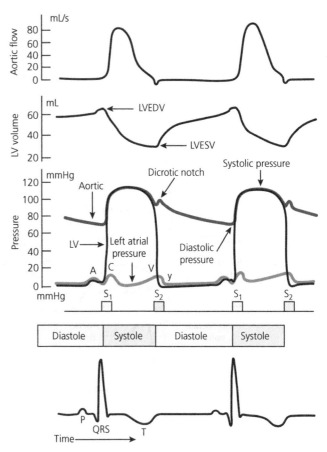

Figure 33.9 The aortic and left ventricular pressures have been superimposed, and the pressure from the left atrium is shown, as is the volume plot of the left ventricle (LV). The ventricular volume changes rapidly early in systole (rapid ejection phase) and early in diastole (rapid filling phase). LVEDV, left ventricular end-diastolic volume; LVESV, left ventricular end-systolic volume; A, C, V, pressure waves in the atrium. From Reece, W.O. (2004) *Dukes' Physiology of Domestic Animals*, 12th edn. Cornell University Press, Ithaca, NY. Reproduced with permission from Cornell University Press.

valve closing produces audible vibrations of the **second heart sound** (S_2) or "dub" (of the "lub-dub"). With the closure of the semilunar valve the blood ejected into the aorta is trapped and can only flow from the high-pressure aorta through the peripheral tissues. Thus, aortic pressure decreases slowly during diastole and never reaches the low values found in the ventricles. The peak pressure in the aorta is called systolic and the lowest pressure is the diastolic pressure. When pressure in the LV decreases to a level below that in the LA, the left AV valve opens and the ventricles begin to fill and a new cardiac cycle begins.

Wiggers diagram

In 1949 Carl Wiggers described the cardiac cycle in phases, and understanding the Wiggers diagram is essential by all who need to appreciate the pumping action of the heart. The phases and events occurring in the chambers are correlated with the opening and closing of the semilunar and AV valves, left ventricular and aortic pressures, and the ECG (Figure 33.10 and Table 33.1). The phases of the cardiac cycle are as follows.

1. *Isovolumetric contraction.* At the onset of ventricular contraction the pressure in the lumen is essentially equal to that in the atria and the AV valves have floated almost into apposition.

The QRS complex signifies ventricular depolarization and follows the P wave by a time interval (PR interval) necessary for the impulse to traverse the conduction system and reach the ventricular muscle cells. At the time of the peak of the R wave in the ECG, ventricular contraction begins. As soon as ventricular pressure exceeds atrial pressure the AV valves close. This marks the end of diastole and the beginning of systole. Both AV and semilunar valves are now closed, and the ventricles are contracting around the contained blood, which is incompressible. During this phase of the cardiac cycle the volume of the ventricles does not change and pressure increases rapidly. This phase terminates and the next begins at the moment the ventricular pressure exceeds aortic or pulmonic pressure. The semilunar valves then open and blood is accelerated into the great arteries (aorta and pulmonary).

2. *Maximum ejection.* The period of maximum ejection begins with the opening of the semilunar valves and lasts until

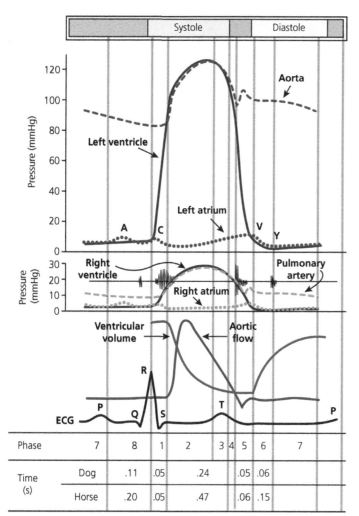

Figure 33.10 Wiggers diagram showing the eight phases of the cardiac cycle for the right and left ventricles. Time indicates the approximate length of the phases in a normal resting dog and horse. The length of phase 7 is not shown because it varies with heart rate. The phonocardiogram, shown in the middle of the diagram with the pressure waves from the right side of the heart, displays four heart sounds from left to right: fourth (S_4), first (S_1), second (S_2), third (S_3). From Reece, W.O. (2004) *Dukes' Physiology of Domestic Animals*, 12th edn. Cornell University Press, Ithaca, NY. Reproduced with permission from Cornell University Press.

Phase		7	8	1	2	3	4	5	6	7
Time (s)	Dog	.11	.05		.24		.05	.06		
	Horse	.20	.05		.47		.06	.15		

Table 33.1 Phases of the cardiac cycle.

Phase	Number*	Events at onset	Main events during	Events at close
Isovolumetric contraction	1	Onset of ventricular contraction	Closure of atrioventricular (AV) valves, rapid rise of intraventricular pressure with no volume change	Opening of semilunar valves
Maximum ejection	2	Opening of semilunar valves	Rapid outflow of blood from ventricles	Peak of intraventricular pressure
Reduced ejection	3	Peak of intraventricular pressure	Declining outflow of blood from ventricles	Onset of ventricular relaxation
Protodiastole	4	Onset of ventricular relaxation	Rapid decrease in intraventricular pressure	Closure of semilunar valves
Isovolumetric relaxation	5	Closure of semilunar valves	Continued ventricular relaxation, rapid decrease in intraventricular pressure with no volume change	Opening of AV valves
Rapid filling	6	Opening of AV valves	Rapid flow of blood from atria to ventricles	Decreased rate of filling
Diastasis	7	Slow rate of flow from atria to ventricles	Continued slow filling of ventricles	Onset of atrial contraction
Atrial systole	8	Onset of atrial contraction	Increased flow from atria to ventricles	Termination of atrial and onset of ventricular contraction

*The numbers correspond to those in Figure 33.10.
Source: Reece, W.O. (2004) *Dukes' Physiology of Domestic Animals*, 12th edn. Cornell University Press, Ithaca, NY. Reproduced with permission from Cornell University Press.

the peak of the arterial pressure curve. About 75% of the blood ejected during systole flows during this period and flow into the aorta (and pulmonary artery) exceeds runoff into the peripheral arteries, causing the pressure to rise. During this period of systole, aortic pressure is exceeded by left ventricular pressure and the blood is accelerated to a peak velocity of 1–2 m/s.

3. *Reduced ejection.* As peripheral runoff reaches equilibrium with ventricular ejection into the great arteries, the pressure curve reaches a maximum. This is the beginning of the reduced ejection phase and blood runoff begins to exceed the ejection rate, causing the pressures to decrease. It would make sense that the pressure in the ventricles exceeds that in the great vessels throughout systole. However, the pressure within the ventricle only exceeds that in the great vessels during the first half of systole when most of the blood is ejected. During the last half of systole pressure in the great vessels exceeds that in the ventricle even though blood is still flowing out of the ventricle. This paradox occurs because of the reduced momentum and kinetic energy of the blood as it leaves the ventricle. The low momentum of the blood during this slow ejection phase of the ventricle and the conversion of the blood's kinetic energy to potential energy in the aorta produces the reversal of the pressure gradient.

4. *Protodiastole.* This marks the beginning of ventricular relaxation and is a point on the ventricular pressure curve that is often difficult to identify. The pressure in the ventricle continues to fall below that in the aorta and pulmonary artery. A brief retrograde flow occurs, closing the semilunar valves. This marks the end of protodiastole and the beginning of the next phase. The volume of blood remaining in the ventricle at the end of a contraction is the ESV (Figure 33.11, see also point 6 further on). Each ventricle has an ESV, i.e., left ventricular ESV (LVESV) and right ventricular ESV (RVESV). The difference between the EDV and the ESV is the SV:

$$\text{Left ventricular stroke volume (LVSV)} = \text{LVEDV} - \text{LVESV}$$

The ESV is not zero and the normal amount of blood ejected (pumped) by each heartbeat is about 50–65%.

5. *Isovolumetric relaxation.* The T wave signifies ventricular repolarization and muscle relaxation. This marks the end of ventricular systole and the beginning of diastole. The short period of reversal of blood flow in the great vessels as the ventricles relax closes the semilunar valves and produces the incisura or dicrotic notch on the pressure wave in the great vessels. The semilunar valves keep blood from leaking back into the ventricles as the ventricular pressure drops to very low values. Since the ventricles are closed chambers, myocardial relaxation results in a steep fall in intraventricular pressure but no alteration in ventricular volume. This phase, with a rapid decrease in ventricular pressure and no blood flowing into or out of the ventricles, is isovolumetric relaxation. The aortic and pulmonary artery pressures decline during diastole as blood flows through the tissues.

6. *Rapid filling.* Beginning with the opening of the AV valves, ventricular volume increases as blood that has accumulated in the

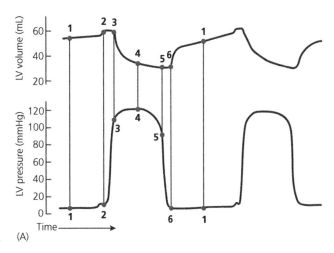

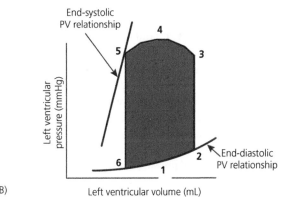

Figure 33.11 (A) The tracing of left ventricular (LV) volume and pressure are taken from the Wiggers diagram. Points 1–6 are values taken simultaneously during the cardiac cycle to develop panel B. (B) The pressure–volume (PV) loop is developed from the Wiggers diagram and each counterclockwise revolution is one cardiac cycle. Points 1–6 occur in sequence as the phases develop. Point 1, during ventricular filling; 2, when the mitral valve closes and pressure starts to rise in the LV; 3, aortic valve opens at the end of the isovolumetric phase; 4, peak or systolic pressure of the ventricle; 5, closure of the aortic valve, end of ejection, and beginning of ventricular relaxation; 6, end of isovolumetric relaxation, opening of the mitral valve, and beginning of ventricular filling. The curve created by points 6, 1, and 2 is called the end-diastolic PV relationship. The slope of this line indicates the compliance of the ventricle. Changes in compliance due to disease can have profound effects on the filling of the ventricle. The end-systolic PV relationship line is determined by the contractility of the heart. Stroke volume can be calculated from the diagram by subtracting the end-systolic volume (points 5–6) from the end-diastolic volume (points 2–3). From Reece, W.O. (2004) *Dukes' Physiology of Domestic Animals*, 12th edn. Cornell University Press, Ithaca, NY. Reproduced with permission from Cornell University Press.

atria under increasing pressure flows quickly into the relaxed ventricle. The blood volume in each atrium is slightly greater than that of the corresponding ventricle, thus providing a reservoir of blood sufficient to fill the ventricle completely for each beat. The end of this phase is not clear-cut as it merges with the next. At the transition between this and the following phase the usually inaudible third heart sound (S_3) may be recorded on a phonocardiogram.

7. *Reduced filling (diastasis).* This is a period of slower filling during which blood continues to flow into both atria and ventricles as into a common chamber. It is terminated by onset of atrial systole.

8. *Atrial systole.* In the normal heart the initial impulse for a heartbeat arises within the SA node and quickly spreads to the two atria. The atria depolarize, producing the P wave on the ECG, and begin to contract shortly after depolarization. The muscle in the atrial wall is basically arranged in a circular fashion such that the volume of blood within the atria decreases with each contraction. The ventricles are relaxed when the atria contract and blood enters the ventricle due to the pressure gradient. Atrial contraction produces only a small increase in ventricular volume and pressure. This phase ends at the onset of ventricular isovolumetric contraction, completing the cardiac cycle.

Atrial pressure waves (A, C, and V waves)

The pressures in the atria (see Figure 33.9) are low compared with those in the arteries but there are several characteristic waves present. At the end of phase 7 the ventricles are usually well filled with blood and atrial contraction raises the pressure (A wave) to add yet a little more volume to the ventricle just prior to its contraction. The C wave of atrial pressure is due to the bulging of the AV valves into the atrium as each ventricle increases the intraluminal pressure during phase 1 of the cardiac cycle. While the ventricles contract blood is returning to the atria from the veins and the atrial pressure rises continuously to the end of the isovolumetric relaxation period of the ventricles, forming the V wave. When the ventricular pressure drops below the atrial pressure and the AV valves open, the accumulated blood flows rapidly into the ventricle. The period of rapid ventricular filling (i.e., phase 6 or early diastolic filling) is marked by a continuous decline in atrial pressure, producing the descent of the V wave (labeled "y" on Figures 33.9 and 33.10).

Atrial contraction

The dynamic importance of atrial contraction on ventricular filling has been much debated. It has been observed that animals with atrial fibrillation, which do not exhibit functional coordinated contraction of the atria, maintain a reasonable cardiac output unless the ventricular contraction rate per minute exceeds normal values. However, the atria are not totally without benefit to animals, because dogs with rapid heart rates may attribute 20–30% of ventricular filling to atrial contraction. Also, atrial contraction and relaxation are instrumental in bringing about normal closure of the AV valves.

Aorta and pulmonary artery pressures

Aortic pressure throughout the cardiac cycle is uniformly higher than pulmonary artery pressure. For dogs, the peak systolic pressure in the aorta is about 100–125 mmHg, approximately five times higher than the corresponding pressure of 20–25 mmHg in the pulmonary artery. The relative end-diastolic pressures are 80 mmHg in the aorta and 10 mmHg in the pulmonary artery; the relative pulse pressures (pulse pressure = systolic pressure – diastolic pressure) are 40 mmHg and 15 mmHg, respectively. The diastolic pressure in both ventricular cavities is quite low, with a small pressure gradient from the left ventricle (0–5 mmHg mean diastolic, 5–12 mmHg end-diastolic) to the right ventricle (0–3 mmHg mean diastolic, 0–5 mmHg end-diastolic). The atrial pressure values are only a few millimeters of mercury and are uniformly somewhat higher in the left atrium (mean 0–5 mmHg).

Although dynamic events on the two sides of the heart are generally similar, there is minor asynchrony and difference in duration of parts of the cardiac cycle. For example, the onset of contraction of the right atrium precedes that of the left atrium, whereas the onset of contraction of the right ventricle follows that of the left ventricle. Nevertheless, right ventricular ejection begins earlier and is completed later than left ventricular ejection.

ECG versus onset of pressure events

In the dog the interval between the onset of electrical and mechanical activity in the left atrium (rise of P wave versus onset of rise of atrial A wave) is on the order of 0.04 s. For the left ventricle, the interval between the onset of ventricular depolarization (Q wave) and the onset of left ventricular contraction (onset of pressure rise) approximates 0.02 s. The T wave has a variable relation to the end of systole but terminates usually before the incisura of the aortic pressure curve.

Aortic flow

The blood flow rate in the root of the aorta (see Figure 33.10) increases rapidly during the phase of **maximum ejection** when most of the stroke volume of the heart is expelled. The flow rate then decreases during the phase of **reduced ejection** and actually reverses at the end of ejection. During diastole aortic flow remains at about zero, but forward flow continues in the peripheral arteries under the impetus of its initial momentum and the elastic recoil of the larger arteries.

Ventricular pressure–volume diagram

These diagrams combine two key ventricular functions (i.e. developing pressure and ejecting volume) into one graph. In Figure 33.11A, the pressure and volume in the left ventricle are plotted against time. The **pressure–volume loop** (PV) combines these two key components into a single diagram (Figure 33.11B). The normal PV loop of an ejecting ventricle progresses counterclockwise and begins at point 2, which is the end of diastole, time of mitral valve closure, and onset of isovolumetric contraction. The ventricular pressure rises without ejection to point 3 (period of isovolumetric contraction), where the aortic valve opens and ventricular ejection begins. The ventricular volume then decreases as the myocardial fibers shorten and blood is ejected into the aorta (point 4). At point 5 systole ends and the aortic valve closes. From point 5 to point 6 the

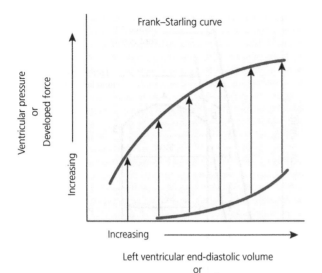

Figure 33.12 The relationship between systolic pressure developed during isovolumetric contraction of the heart at various end-diastolic volumes (Starling's law of the heart). Increasing the end-diastolic volume produces a stronger contraction of the ventricle (heterometric autoregulation). From Reece, W.O. (2004) *Dukes' Physiology of Domestic Animals*, 12th edn. Cornell University Press, Ithaca, NY. Reproduced with permission from Cornell University Press.

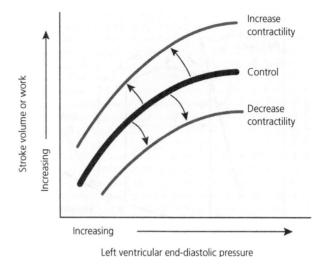

Figure 33.13 Ventricular function curves of the heart. A curve can be altered by changes in autonomic nervous system activity. A change in contractility will alter the amount of work performed by the heart at each end-systolic pressure point. From Reece, W.O. (2004) *Dukes' Physiology of Domestic Animals*, 12th edn. Cornell University Press, Ithaca, NY. Reproduced with permission from Cornell University Press.

ventricle relaxes isovolumetrically, and from point 6 to point 2 it fills again, with the mitral valve opening at point 6. Note that the point on the loop corresponding to the end of systole (point 5) lies on a sloped line. This line is called the end-systolic pressure–volume relationship (ESPVR). This line will predict the end-systolic point for a ventricle if preload or afterload is varied. The position and slope of the line will change if contractility of the myocardium changes.

Ventricular function curves

The **Starling curve** resulted from experiments on isolated dog heart–lung preparations. This curve, shown in Figure 33.12, describes the relationship between energy output (developed force or pressure) and ventricular diastolic size (initial myocardial fiber length). In essence, the energy output is related to the presystolic length of individual fibers. **Heterometric** (*hetero*, different; *metric*, length) **autoregulation** is the name given to the heart's ability to alter its output in response to altered myocardial fiber length.

Since these early experiments, ventricular function curves have been developed which plot various indices of ventricular performance along the ordinate and some index of fiber length along the abscissa (Figure 33.13). A ventricle may move from one curve to another, depending on the level and balance of autonomic input into the heart. **Homeometric** (*homeo*, same; *metric*, length) **autoregulation** refers to the ability of the ventricle to alter its vigor of contraction without altering the initial myocardial length.

Five major factors that influence ventricular performance

Preload (Frank–Starling mechanism)

Preload in the isolated muscle stretches the muscle and determines the resting fiber length. Increasing the preload of an isolated muscle causes an increased force on contraction (Starling's law of the heart). In the mammalian heart, preload occurs by diastolic filling of the ventricle. The resting muscle fiber length is determined for practical purposes by ventricular end-diastolic pressure or volume. The normal left ventricular end-diastolic pressure is about 5 mmHg and that for the right ventricle is 3 mmHg. On the Starling curve (see Figure 33.13) increasing the preload (end-diastolic pressure) results in an increased stroke volume or work. The physiologic reason for this increased strength of contraction is complex and involves a change in the geometry of the contractile elements and an increased quantity of calcium released by the sarcoplasmic reticulum. This relationship is very important for maintaining an equal output by both ventricles. If one ventricle pumps more volume than the other for a long period of time, blood would accumulate either in the lung or in the body's peripheral veins leading to edema formation. However, an increase in output of one ventricle will lead to an increase in venous return to the other ventricle. The increased return will result in a stronger contraction and increased output of the other ventricle (Figure 33.14). Thus, left and right ventricular outputs balance.

Afterload

The major component of afterload for the left ventricle is systolic aortic pressure; for the right ventricle, it is the systolic pulmonary artery pressure. The arterial pressures determine the

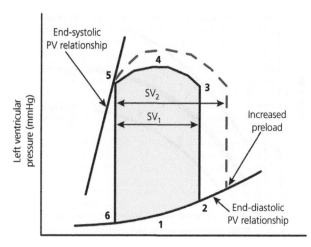

Figure 33.14 Left ventricular pressure–volume (PV) diagram showing the effect of increasing the end-diastolic pressure (preload). The normal stroke volume (SV_1) increased to SV_2 after the end-diastolic volume is increased. The afterload (point 3) has remained the same. From Reece, W.O. (2004) *Dukes' Physiology of Domestic Animals*, 12th edn. Cornell University Press, Ithaca, NY. Reproduced with permission from Cornell University Press.

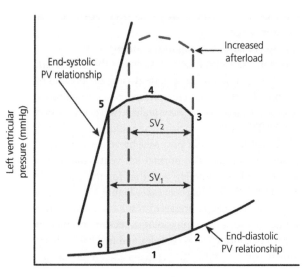

Figure 33.15 Left ventricular pressure–volume (PV) diagram showing the effect of increasing the end-systolic pressure (afterload). The normal stroke volume (SV_1) is decreased to SV_2 after the increase. The preload has remained the same (point 2). From Reece, W.O. (2004) *Dukes' Physiology of Domestic Animals*, 12th edn. Cornell University Press, Ithaca, NY. Reproduced with permission from Cornell University Press.

tension that must be developed by the ventricular wall. If aortic pressure is increased, the ensuing contractions of the ventricle will encounter more afterload and the ejected stroke volume will transiently decrease (Figure 33.15), just as the isolated muscle experiments showed that increasing the afterload decreased the velocity of shortening (see Figure 33.4). Conversely, decreasing

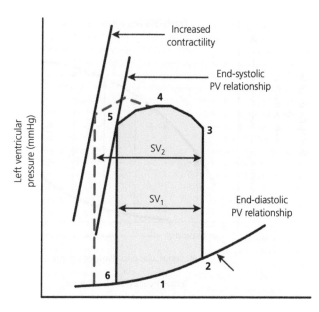

Figure 33.16 Left ventricular pressure–volume (PV) diagram showing the effect of increasing contractility (end-systolic PV relationship). The normal stroke volume (SV_1) has increased to SV_2 because point 5 lies on a different relationship line. The preload and afterload have remained the same. From Reece, W.O. (2004) *Dukes' Physiology of Domestic Animals*, 12th edn. Cornell University Press, Ithaca, NY. Reproduced with permission from Cornell University Press.

the afterload increases the velocity and length by which a muscle will contract. Preload determines the amount of muscle stretch before contraction. Afterload sets the amount of work needed to eject blood.

Inotropic state: contractility

The inotropic state affects muscle performance independent of preload and afterload. Increasing the inotropic state increases the peak (isometric) tension developed at each preload and the velocity of fiber shortening (see P_0 and V_{max} in Figure 33.5). The heart *in vivo* exhibits the same characteristics. The PV diagram (Figure 33.16) illustrates that altering the inotropic state leads to changes in stroke volume (fiber shortening). The sympathetic nervous system is an important determinant of inotropic state. Increasing the contractility but keeping preload and afterload constant results in an increased stoke volume and decreased LVESV (see point 6 of Figure 33.16).

Heart rate

In the isolated muscle, an increase in stimulation frequency leads to an increase in developed tension. This effect is known as the staircase, Bowditch, or treppe phenomenon. Although the inotropic state is increased slightly by an increase in heart rate, the effect that overshadows is the potential increase in cardiac output. Since cardiac output is the product of heart rate (HR) and stroke volume ($CO = HR \times SV$), the cardiac output of a slowly beating heart can be potentially doubled by doubling the heart rate.

Lusitropic reserve: ability to relax

Lusitropy is the inactivation of the myocardial contractile process and the return of the muscle to a relaxed state. The end-diastolic pressure–volume relationship (see Figure 33.16) reflects the lusitropic state of the myocardium, which is important for adequate ventricular filling before the next cardiac contraction. For example, during exercise the heart is required to beat faster and pump a larger stroke volume. The time interval for ventricular filling is reduced and the heart's ability to increase cardiac output depends partly on rapid relaxation. An increased inotropic state and heart rate normally initiate lusitropic reserve, shortening the process of myocardial muscle relaxation.

Measurement of cardiac output

> 1 Define cardiac output.
> 2 What is the difference in cardiac output between the right and the left ventricle?
> 3 How could you measure the cardiac output of a dog without injecting anything or removing any blood?

Four methods are currently in use for measuring an animal's cardiac output. Transthoracic or esophageal **echocardiography** utilizes high-frequency sound waves (ultrasound) aimed at the heart or aorta and records the echoes reflected from the various structures. A shift in the sound wave frequency occurs when the waves are reflected from a moving object and the magnitude of shift can be used to calculate blood flow velocity. Multiplying the integration of a velocity–time curve from the ascending aorta by the cross-sectional area of the aorta and the heart rate gives an estimate of cardiac output. A second method is the **indicator dilution technique,** used frequently in animal research laboratories and in a few clinical situations. A known quantity of indicator is injected into a large vein close to the right atrium and detected "downstream" in a pulmonary or systemic artery. The indicator may be a dye (e.g., indocyanine green), radioisotope, ion (e.g., lithium), or a thermal mass (e.g., cold saline). When a known quantity of the indicator is injected into an unknown volume and the diluted indicator's concentration measured by a detector situated in the flow of blood, the cardiac output can be calculated. The ultrasound velocity dilution method is an adaptation of the indicator dilution technique just described but requires an arteriovenous loop, which is only practical in anesthetized animals. However, it is a relatively noninvasive technique that has been described and adaptable to mammals under 250 kg. The third method (Fick principle) is also the oldest, being first described by Adolph Fick in 1870, and involves the application of the law of conservation of mass. For the Fick method of determining cardiac output the animal's oxygen consumption is measured as well as the oxygen content of arterial and venous blood:

$$CO = O_2 \text{ consumption} / (\text{arterial} - \text{venous } O_2 \text{ content})$$

The fourth method is analysis of the arterial pressure wave contour by a dedicated monitor. This is an old method that has recently been commercialized but its accuracy in animals has yet to be determined.

Clinically, in the awake animal the transthoracic ultrasound method is the most feasible, while the lithium dilution and pulmonary artery thermodilution techniques are being utilized in anesthetized patients.

Self-evaluation

Answers can be found at the end of the chapter.

1 Where is most of the calcium stored during diastole in the working myocardium?
   A Extracellular fluid
   B Intracellular fluid
   C Intracellular sarcoplasmic reticulum
   D T tubules

2 What is the force stretching the myocardium to its pre-contraction length?
   A Isometric force
   B Isotonic force
   C Preload
   D Afterload

3 If the stroke volume of a horse was 500 mL, the ejection fraction was 60%, and the heart rate was 40 beats per minute, what would the cardiac output be?
   A 8 L/min
   B 12 L/min
   C 20 L/min

4 Which cardiac valves close with the first heart sound?
   A Atrioventricular valves
   B Semilunar valves
   C Both
   D Neither, both valves open with the first heart sound

5 Which cardiac event occurs shortly after the QRS complex of the ECG?
   A Atrial contraction
   B Ventricular contraction
   C Ventricular relaxation
   D Rapid filling of the ventricles

6 What cardiac event is associated with lusitropy?
   A Atrial contraction
   B SA node spontaneous depolarization
   C Ventricular relaxation
   D Impulse conduction through the AV node and Purkinje system

Section VI: The Cardiovascular System

7 What cardiac event is associated with the A wave in the right atrium?
  A Atrial contraction
  B Ventricular contration
  C Atrial relaxation and rapid filling
  D Ventricular relaxation and rapid filling

8 Based on Starling's law of the heart, what cardiac response would you predict to occur with the rapid infusion of intravenous fluids to a dog with a normal heart?
  A The heart would not alter its function because the extra fluids would be stored in the veins
  B The stroke volume of the heart would decrease due to the decreased preload
  C The stroke volume of the heart would increase due to the increased preload
  D The stroke volume of the heart would decrease due to the increased afterload

9 If the preload and afterload of the heart were unchanged but the contractility was increased by the infusion of dobutamine, which one of the following responses would be most likely to occur?
  A The stroke volume and ejection fraction would increase
  B The stroke volume would be unchanged but the ejection fraction would increase
  C The stroke volume and ejection fraction would decrease
  D The stroke volume would increase but the ejection fraction would decrease

10 Which one of the following correctly describes the events occurring during isovolumetric contraction of the left ventricle?
  A The AV valve is closed, the semilunar valve is open and the ventricle is rapidly ejecting blood into the aorta
  B The AV valve is open, the semilunar valve is closed and the ventricle is rapidly filling with blood from the left atrium

  C The AV and semilunar valves are both open and the ventricle is rapidly ejecting blood into the aorta
  D The AV and semilunar valves are both closed and the intraventricular pressure is rapidly increasing but no blood is being ejected yet

Suggested reading

Haskins, S., Pascoe, P.J., Ilkiw, J.E., Fudge, J., Hopper, K. and Aldrich, J. (2006) Reference cardiopulmonary values in normal dogs. *Comparative Medicine* **55**:156–161.

Katz, A.M. (2011) *Physiology of the Heart*, 5th edn. Wolters Kluwer Lippincott Williams & Wilkins, Philadelphia.

King, A.S. (1999) *The Cardiorespiratory System*. Blackwell Science, Oxford.

Mohrman, D.E. and Heller, L.J. (2010) *Cardiovascular Physiology*, 7th edn. McGraw-Hill, New York.

Pappano, A.J. and Wier, W.G. (2013) *Cardiovascular Physiology*, 10th edn. Elsevier Mosby, Philadelphia.

Shih, A. (2013) Cardiac output monitoring in horses. *Veterinary Clinics of North America Equine Practice* **29**:155–167.

Answers

1	C	6	C
2	C	7	A
3	C	8	C
4	A	9	A
5	B	10	D

34 Regulation of the Heart

David D. Kline, Eileen M. Hasser and Cheryl M. Heesch

University of Missouri, Columbia, MO, USA

Cardiac output (CO, the amount of blood ejected per minute) may be altered by changing the rate at which the heart beats (heart rate, HR) or by changing stroke volume (SV), the amount of blood ejected by each beat, that is $CO = HR \times SV$. These parameters are controlled by local intrinsic mechanisms within the myocardium and by extrinsic regulation through the autonomic nervous system. Such intrinsic and extrinsic factors adjust HR and SV by changing the force, velocity, duration, and extent of contraction. Electrical conduction through the heart is adjusted to maintain proper timing of atrial and ventricular systole and the temporal sequence of ventricular activation.

Intrinsic regulation of cardiac function

> 1 What is the difference between heterometric and homeometric regulation?
>
> 2 Define preload and afterload.

Local mechanisms within the heart make it possible for the myocardium to adapt to changes in workload. For example, in an experimental animal with a denervated heart, local mechanisms contribute to the ability to appropriately adjust cardiac output during exercise and rest. In the following section, we discuss the two types of mechanisms that mediate intrinsic regulation, their similarities and their differences. The best known of these is the Frank–Starling mechanism, which is the response to changes in resting myocardial fiber length, or heterometric autoregulation. This is in contrast to homeometric autoregulation of the heart which does not involve changes in cardiac fiber length but rather uses intrinsic molecular mechanisms.

Heterometric, or Frank–Starling, mechanism for regulation of cardiac function

The mechanical basis for the Frank–Starling mechanism has been described for isolated papillary muscle and heart. This effect, also called the length–tension relationship or Starling's law of the heart, results in an increase in the force of muscle contraction as fiber length is increased to its optimal length, thus allowing maximal cross-bridge formation. Increasing the volume of the heart at the end of diastole, which enhances cardiac muscle fiber length, thereby augments contractile force and ventricular stroke volume. End-diastolic volume, and thus filling pressure, constitutes preload. Assuming that ventricular compliance remains unchanged, ventricular end-diastolic pressure or preload can be used as a measure of the volume change or stretch of the myocardial fibers. An increase in preload subsequently enhances ventricular contraction and as a result increases stroke volume. At very large end-diastolic volumes, maximum contraction is decreased because the muscle fibers are stretched beyond optimal myofilament cross-bridge interactions. However, such excessive stretching is rarely observed in the normal heart.

An increase in diastolic volume/pressure and fiber length permits the heart to compensate for increases in arterial resistance. Increases in arterial resistance, or afterload, can impede the ability of the heart to eject blood. Aortic pressure (which rises and falls during ejection), blood viscosity, viscoelastic properties of the arterial system, and vascular resistance all contribute to

Dukes' Physiology of Domestic Animals, Thirteenth Edition. Edited by William O. Reece, Howard H. Erickson, Jesse P. Goff and Etsuro E. Uemura.

© 2015 John Wiley & Sons, Inc. Published 2015 by John Wiley & Sons, Inc.

Companion website: www.wiley.com/go/reece/physiology

afterload. When afterload is initially increased, there is a decrease in stroke volume and ventricular emptying. Venous return following the elevated end-systolic volume increases preload and cardiac fiber length, augmenting the subsequent contraction to maintain stroke volume despite the enhanced afterload.

Homeometric regulation

Contractile strength of cardiac muscle for any given fiber length can be modulated by its frequency of contraction, as well as temperature.

Rate and rhythm effects

The strength of myocardial contraction is markedly influenced by heart rate. This was first described as the **staircase** or **treppe phenomenon** in the frog ventricle: after a period where rate and tension of contractions have been regular, an abrupt increase in rate results in progressive augmentation in the strength of contractions until a plateau or steady state is reached (Figure 34.1A). The staircase phenomenon is an example of the interval and force relationship of the heart. That is, as the rate (frequency) of contractions increases, there is an increase in the peak tension and maximum shortening that develops over the physiological range. This frequency potentiation requires many beats to attain a steady state (Figure 34.1B). However, a brief increase in heart rate for one or two beats may substantially alter subsequent force development. Specifically, in mammalian ventricular muscles, a premature contraction (extrasystole) is weaker than the preceding beats, but then for several regular beats following the premature beat the contractions are stronger than normal. This phenomenon in heart muscle is termed **post-extrasystolic potentiation** (Figure 34.1C) and seems to be almost complete in the first potentiated contraction. However, if the premature contractions are repeated in series, the magnitude of potentiation increases.

Changes in intracellular calcium appear to account for these interval–strength phenomena of the heart. Calcium is vital to cardiac muscle contraction. Calcium enters the cell during each contraction during the plateau phase of the cardiac action potential. As heart rate is elevated, there is a resulting increase in the number of action potential plateaus. In addition, elevated frequency enhances the amount of calcium that enters through L-type calcium channels as well as slowing channel inactivation. As a result of these processes, there is an increase in the amount of intracellular calcium in the myocardium. At excitation, sarcoplasmic reticulum (SR) calcium is released from the terminal cisternae of the SR as a result of the increase in intracellular calcium via the L-type membrane channels. The greater increase in intracellular calcium from the SR results in augmented force of contraction. Relaxation is caused by pumping this calcium back into the longitudinal SR by the Ca-ATPase. Post-extrasystolic potentiation has also been suggested to result from increases in intracellular calcium taken up by SR stores in the pause following the weak extrasystole. The subsequent beat results in more calcium release and greater tension. In addition,

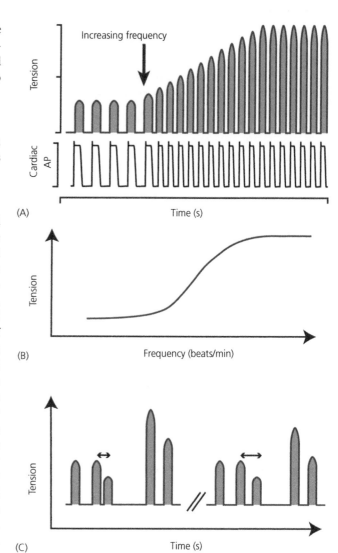

Figure 34.1 The effect of interval changes in heart rate on cardiac muscle tension. (A) Treppe phenomenon: as heart rate frequency suddenly increases, there is a gradual increase in force or tension development. (B) As heart rate increases, there is a subsequent rise in tension (i.e., force–interval relationship). (C) Extrasystolic potentiation is observed when the interval between beats is reduced. The premature beat results in weak force development, but the subsequent beat is strong. If the premature beat is later, the potentiation is reduced.

Starling's law mechanisms due to changes in filling time contribute to increased force of contraction.

The force–interval relationships may differ in detail among mammals (e.g., rat vs. other mammals); they are present in the heart muscle of birds, reptiles, and fish but absent in amphibia.

Temperature

A rise in body temperature, such as during fever, increases heart rate. Conversely, a decrease in body temperature, such as during hypothermia, dramatically suppresses heart rate. In isolated mammalian heart preparations, hypothermia augments contractile strength. However, in intact dogs either moderate hypothermia (body temperature of 25–30 °C) or pyrexia (body temperature of 41–43 °C) decreases ventricular contractile capacity. A possible explanation of this apparent discrepancy is that, in the intact heart, cooling depresses cardiac sympathetic tone. The thermal limits of both human and dog hearts are between 26 and 44 °C; as the heart approaches either of these limits, myocardial conduction and contractility are both depressed.

Extrinsic regulation of cardiac function

1 What are the heart rates for different animals?

2 How is heart rate related to body size, metabolic rate, and autonomic balance?

3 Explain the innervation of the heart.

4 Define the following: chronotropic action (chronotropy), inotropic action (inotropy), dromotropic action (dromotropy), and bathmotropic action (bathmotropy).

5 Explain chemical and hormonal control of the heart.

From the previous section it can be seen that the three intrinsic factors that affect the contractile force of the myocardium and thus cardiac performance are preload, afterload, and heart rate and rhythm. In this section, various extrinsic factors that govern regulation of the inotropic state as well as heart rate will be elaborated.

Resting heart rate and its influence on cardiac output

The resting heart rate of an animal is related to its body size, metabolic rate, and the autonomic balance characteristics of the species. In the scientific literature, data on heart rates is often disparate because of differing environmental conditions. For domestic animals, values found in the clinical literature may be more representative. Table 34.1 lists representative heart rates for various species.

In most cases, body mass and heart rate are inversely related. A logarithmic equation has been proposed to represent the relation between heart rate (HR) and body weight (BW, kg) in mammals: $HR = 241 \times BW^{-0.25}$. However, certain species depart from this relationship. The heart rate of the domestic rabbit ranges from 180 to 350 beats per minute (bpm), while that of the hare is much slower at 60–70 bpm. The heart rate range for dairy cattle is 48–84 bpm, while that for horses is lower at 28–40 bpm. In short, more athletic animals like the hare and horse have lower resting heart rates than sedentary species of similar size. Higher parasympathetic tone is responsible for lower heart rates in these species.

Avian heart rates also vary greatly depending on the age of the subject and conditions of recording. In general, restraint tends to induce marked tachycardia. Some reported rates for adult birds are as follows: chicken, 191–354; turkey, 160–219; duck, 175–194; and geese, 80–144 bpm.

Table 34.1 Representative heart rate ranges (bpm).

Animal	Rest	Exercise	Newborn/young
Elephant	25–35		60–70
Horse	28–40	180–240	60–80
Ox	36–60	180–200	105–150
Dairy cow	48–84	180–200	140–160
Swine	70–120	200–280	230
Human	60–80	100–200	100–160
Sheep	70–80	290	
Goat	70–80		
Dog	70–120	220–325	140–275
Cat	120–140		170–300
Rhesus monkey	160–330		
Rabbit	180–350		120–240
Hare	60–70		
Guinea pig	200–300		
Rat	250– 400	500–600	
Mouse	450–750		

More rapid resting rates are often reported for nonhuman species owing to excitement during restraint.
Source: revised from Table 9.1, Detweiler, D.K. (1993), in *Dukes' Physiology of Domestic Animals*, 11th edn (eds M.J. Swenson and W.O. Reece). Cornell University Press, Ithaca, NY. With permission from Cornell University Press.

At lower physiological heart rates and up to a certain level, cardiac output increases with elevated heart rate. This is especially true in an isolated experimentally paced heart. However, depending on the physiological state of the circulatory system, as rate accelerates a point is reached where further increases in heart rate result in a progressive decrease in stroke volume due to decreased ventricular filling time and end-diastolic volume. The result is a reduction in cardiac output. For a physiological rate range, the relationship is such that the larger the stroke volume at the lowest rate, the higher the heart rates at which peak outputs occur. Thus if the stroke volume is small at the resting or control heart rate, rate acceleration will increase output very little initially and output will begin to decline at relatively low frequencies. The smaller the initial stroke volume, the greater the fractional decrease of stroke volume as heart rate increases. Excessive rates result in lowered cardiac output; in dogs, for example, pacing the heart at 280 bpm for 11–29 days results in low-output congestive heart failure.

Innervation of the heart by the autonomic nervous system

Innervation of the heart arises primarily from the autonomic nervous system via bilateral sympathetic and parasympathetic (vagal) nerves. In mammals, the general anatomic pattern is similar across species but differs in detail among the various species. The autonomic nervous system innervates the atria and ventricles to modulate their function and coordination.

The **atria** are extensively innervated by sympathetic and parasympathetic fibers, as well as afferent fibers, especially on

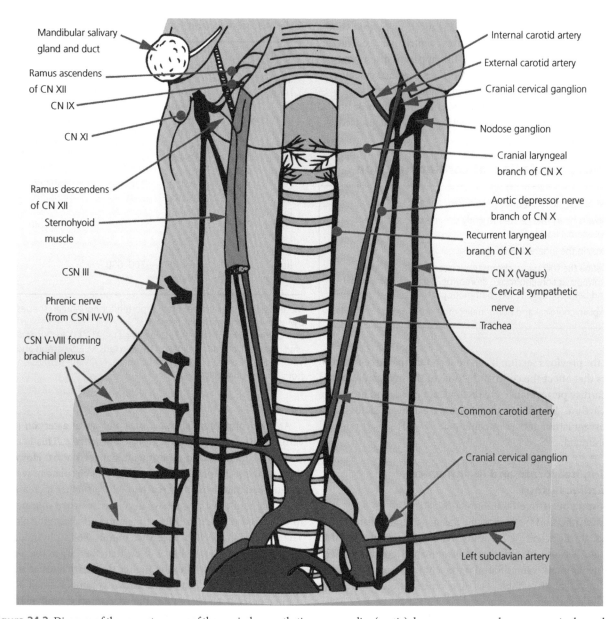

Figure 34.2 Diagram of the separate course of the cervical sympathetic nerve, cardiac (aortic) depressor nerve, and vagus nerve in the neck of the rabbit. Jugular veins are not shown. Spinal and cranial nerves shown unilaterally only. CN, cranial nerve; CSN, cervical spinal nerve. Modified from Wells, T.A.G. (1964) *The Rabbit: A Practical Guide.* Heinemann, London.

their posterior surfaces. The sinoatrial (SA) and atrioventricular (AV) nodes are richly innervated; the SA node receives fibers primarily from the right side of the body and the AV node from both sides. **Ventricular** innervation, with the exception of the bundle of His, is much less profuse than atrial innervation (in mammals, not birds), and most species have only moderate parasympathetic innervation, primarily following the course of the coronary arteries. Diving mammals may be the exception since they can slow their hearts well below the AV rate as part of the diving reflex. In ungulates, the AV bundle of His is richly innervated. The ventricular myocardium receives its modest innervation from the coronary plexuses that follow these arteries. They are predominantly composed of sympathetic

fibers. In many species, the vagus and cervical sympathetic nerve fibers are closely associated and enclosed in the same epineural sheath, the vagosympathetic trunk.

Sympathetic nervous system control of the heart

The **sympathetic** fibers arise from the thoracic lumbar spinal cord (Figure 34.2). Myelinated preganglionic sympathetic fibers originate from the central nervous system in the intermediolateral (IML) column of the spinal cord. The IML is under the control of pre-sympathetic regions, including the rostral ventrolateral medulla (RVLM) of the brainstem and paraventricular nucleus (PVN) of the hypothalamus. Preganglionic fibers leave the thoracic and lumbar spinal cord between T1 and L3 via the

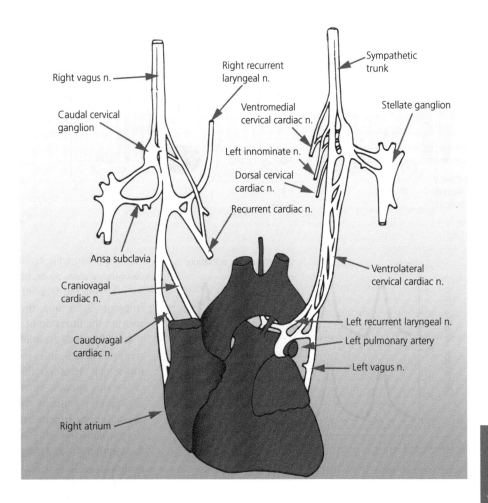

Right vagus n.

Caudal cervical ganglion

Right recurrent laryngeal n.

Ventromedial cervical cardiac n.

Left innominate n.

Dorsal cervical cardiac n.

Recurrent cardiac n.

Sympathetic trunk

Stellate ganglion

Ventrolateral cervical cardiac n.

Left recurrent laryngeal n.

Left pulmonary artery

Left vagus n.

Ansa subclavia

Craniovagal cardiac n.

Caudovagal cardiac n.

Right atrium

Figure 34.3 Diagram of the vagosympathetic trunks and their relations to the stellate ganglia, ansa subclavia, and caudal cervical ganglia of the dog. From Mizeres, N.J. (1957) The course of the left cardioinhibitory fibers in the dog. *Anatomical Record* 127:109–115. Reproduced with permission from Wiley.

ventral roots. Cardiac preganglionic fibers pass into peripheral ganglia of the sympathetic chain located adjacent to the vertebral column. Unmyelinated postganglionic fibers leave the ganglia to innervate the heart. Such innervation of the myocardium arises from postganglionic fibers exiting the cranial, middle, and caudal cervical ganglia and from the first four or five thoracic ganglia. The stellate ganglia or cervicothoracic ganglia, right and left, result from fusion of vertebral sympathetic ganglia in the anterior thoracic and caudal cervical regions (Figure 34.2). The majority of sympathetic nerve impulses reach the heart through the **stellate ganglia** (Figure 34.3). Postganglionic fibers subsequently innervate the base of the heart and innervate cardiac tissue. In addition, a substantial proportion of afferent fibers, probably mediating pain sensation, course with the sympathetic nerves.

Stimulation of the right stellate ganglion has a relatively greater effect on heart rate, and stimulation of the left stellate ganglion has a relatively greater effect on left ventricular contractility. This asymmetry occurs in humans and dogs, but may vary among other species. Overall, the sympathetic nerves have positive **chronotropic** (rate of contraction), **inotropic** (force of contraction), **bathmotropic** (increase in excitability) and **dromotropic** (rate of conductivity) actions on the heart. Sympathetic stimulation increases the discharge rate of the SA

node, increases AV conduction, and powerfully increases atrial and ventricular contractility.

Activation of the sympathetic nervous system results in the release of **acetylcholine** (ACh) from the preganglionic nerve terminals located in peripheral ganglia. ACh activates nicotinic ganglionic acetylcholine receptors on the postganglionic cell. The catecholamine **norepinephrine** is subsequently released from the postganglionic nerve terminal (Figure 34.4). Norepinephrine binds to **adrenergic receptors** on the heart. There are two major types of adrenergic receptors, **alpha (α)** and **beta (β)**. In cardiac tissue, β receptors predominate.

There are two major types of β receptors. In general, β_1-adrenergic receptors are responsible for inotropic and chronotropic myocardial responses, while β_2-adrenergic receptors mediate glycogenolysis and vasodilatation. Sympathetic activation of the SA node in the right atrium via release of norepinephrine and binding to β_1 receptors activates the G_s α-subunit, adenylyl cyclase, cyclic AMP, and protein kinase A (PKA) second messenger system (Figure 34.4). As a result, there is enhancement of SA node ion channels responsible for its rhythmicity, specifically the depolarizing I_f, L-type calcium (I_{Ca}) and hyperpolarizing potassium (I_K). The former effects predominate and increase the rate of diastolic depolarization, reduce action potential threshold, and overall shorten diastole

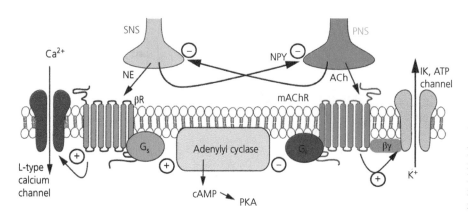

Figure 34.4 Cellular mechanisms for sympathetic (SNS) and parasympathetic (PNS) nervous system actions at the heart. ACh, acetylcholine; NE, norepinephrine; cAMP, cyclic AMP; PKA, protein kinase A; βR, β-adrenergic receptor; mAChR, muscarinic acetylcholine receptor; NPY, neuropeptide Y.

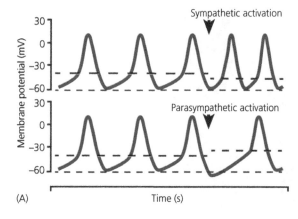

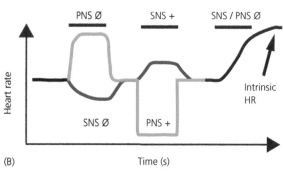

Figure 34.5 Relative effect of sympathetic (SNS) and parasympathetic (PNS) nervous system on heart rate. (A) SNS stimulation increases the rate of SA node action potential discharge, whereas PNS stimulation reduces its discharge rate. Blue dashed line denotes membrane potential, black dashed line action potential threshold. (B) Individually, SNS and PNS blockade (Ø) or stimulation (+) alter heart rate. Blockade of both SNS and PNS (SNS/PNS Ø), or ganglionic blockade, elevates heart rate to its intrinsic rate. Denervation would produce similar responses.

calcium channels, ryanodine receptors on SR to enhance calcium release, phospholamban to increase calcium reuptake into the SR, and troponin I to enhance Ca^{2+} dissociation from troponin C. In total, these effects enhance contractility and shorten the duration of contraction.

Initially it was generally accepted that myocardial adrenergic receptors were β_1 and vascular smooth muscle adrenergic receptors were β_2. However, there are exceptions to this generalization in various species. In most mammals tested the ventricular myocardium contains chiefly β_1 receptors, whereas β_2 receptors abound in the frog heart. In the human ventricle the β_1/β_2 ratio is approximately 80 : 20 and an even higher percentage of β_2 receptors is found in the atria. Unlike the foregoing functional properties of β_1 and β_2 receptors, in the hearts of many mammals β_1 receptors apparently mediate glycogenolysis through their actions on phosphorylase b and a. It had been assumed that β_2 receptors mediated coronary vasodilation, but in the coronary artery of the pig the majority of receptors have been found to be β_1 subtype. In any case, β-adrenergic receptors enhance myocardial contractility, dilate coronary arteries, mediate positive chronotropic effects, speed AV conduction, and increase automaticity.

The α-adrenergic receptors are also separated into two subgroups: α_1 and α_2. α_1-Adrenergic receptors are present in the myocardium, but their density is low in the ventricles where their role, if any, is minor. α_1-Adrenergic receptors are more relevant in atrial tissue, where they may participate to a greater extent in the production of positive inotropic effects. Postsynaptic α receptors mediate vasoconstriction in vascular smooth muscle in many locations, including the coronary arteries. There is evidence that adrenergic receptors can mediate coronary vasoconstriction, which is more readily observed when β receptors are blocked, and negative chronotropy at the SA node and in ventricular pacemaker cells. However, β_1 positive chronotropic and ionotropic effects predominate in the heart.

Released norepinephrine and termination of its action is through slow removal by sodium-dependent **reuptake** transporters on nearby nerve terminals, as well as by **diffusion** into the bloodstream.

(Figure 34.5A). As a result, there is an increase in heart rate (Figure 34.5B). Activation of β_1 receptors on the atria and ventricular myocardium through PKA also enhances contractility. This effect is multifactorial and involves PKA-mediated phosphorylation and augmentation of plasma membrane L-type

Parasympathetic nervous system control of the heart

The **parasympathetic** preganglionic cell bodies originate in the brainstem primarily in the dorsal motor nucleus of the vagus (DMnX) and nucleus ambiguus (nA). Parasympathetic myelinated preganglionic fibers leave the central nervous system via the vagus nerve (cranial nerve X; Figure 34.2) and travel to terminal ganglia on or near the epicardial surface of the heart where they form a synapse with short postganglionic neurons. As in the sympathetic nervous system, ACh is released from preganglionic terminals and binds to and activates nicotinic acetylcholine receptors on postganglionic neurons. The preganglionic fibers pass to the heart along the great veins and arteries. In addition to these efferent fibers, a considerable proportion of the vagus nerve contains afferent fibers which participate in cardiovascular reflexes (see Chapter 35).

The right and left vagus nerves differentially innervate the SA node. Stimulation of the right vagus ordinarily has a greater effect in decreasing the firing rate of the SA node (located in the right atrium) and thus decreasing heart rate (negative chronotropy) than stimulation of the left vagus. The negative inotropic effects of the vagus are primarily exerted on the atria where the vagal innervation is relatively rich. However, effects from the vagi can also be demonstrated on the ventricles. Left vagus nerve stimulation inhibits AV conduction and can produce AV block. Thus, vagal fibers have negative chronotropic (rate of contraction), inotropic (force of contraction), and dromotropic (conduction rate) actions on the heart. Vagal stimulation slows the discharge rate of the SA node, slows or blocks AV conduction, and decreases atrial and to a small extent ventricular contractility.

At rest, the vagus nerves exert a continuous or tonic restraint on the heart. When the vagi are cut or cooled in experimental animals, heart rate becomes greatly accelerated. Various conditions, physiological and pathological, may alter the intensity of baseline vagal activity, or vagal tone. In addition, vagal tone is naturally higher in some species (e.g., horse) than in others (e.g., domestic rabbit).

ACh is released from postganglionic vagal efferent nerve terminals at the level of the heart SA and AV nodes, where it binds to muscarinic acetylcholine receptors (mAChR; Figure 34.4). These receptors are negatively coupled via $G_i\alpha$ to adenylyl cyclase and inhibit activation of I_f and L-type calcium channels (I_{Ca}), thus reducing the rate of diastolic depolarization and making action potential threshold more positive (Figure 34.5). Muscarinic receptors are also coupled to G protein $\beta\gamma$ subunits to directly open potassium (K^+, $I_{K,ACh}$) channels that hyperpolarize the cell and decrease the frequency of action potentials. The summation of these effects is a reduction in heart rate (Figures 34.4 and 34.5). ACh may also mildly reduce cardiac contractility via its action in myocardial cells. This effect occurs through activation of $G_i\alpha$ and subsequent decrease in adenylyl cyclase activation and cyclic AMP production, which counterbalances the effect of sympathetic β-receptor activation. Muscarinic receptors also activate the phospholipase C pathway to produce nitric oxide that inhibits I_{Ca}. ACh has a mild vasodilatory effect on the coronary vessels, especially near the SA node. Thus the net primary response to parasympathetic activation is a reduction in heart rate and contractility.

ACh is rapidly broken down by **cholinesterase** into choline and acetate. Choline is taken up by the synaptic terminal to be recycled in the production of more ACh.

Sympathetic versus parasympathetic stimulation

The heart is under the control of both the sympathetic and parasympathetic nervous systems. Sympathetic activation will increase (accelerate) heart rate, whereas parasympathetic activation will decrease (decelerate) heart rate (Figure 34.5B). However, the heart is under tonic control of the autonomic nervous system. For instance, blockade of sympathetic β_1 receptors slightly decreases heart rate whereas blockade of parasympathetic muscarinic acetylcholine receptors substantially increases heart rate (Figure 34.5B). Such data demonstrate the predominance of parasympathetic activity on heart rate. Blockade of both systems, or ganglionic blockade, eliminates autonomic control of the heart and elevates heart rate to its intrinsic rate (Figure 34.5B). While normally parasympathetic activation predominates, these two systems act in a reciprocal manner. For instance, an increase in heart rate typically results from both the removal of vagal drive and an increase in sympathetic drive.

The heart rate responses to sympathetic versus vagal nerve stimulation follow different latent and decay periods. During sympathetic nerve stimulation, the response is sluggish, with heart rate acceleration beginning in 1–2 s and reaching a plateau after 30–60 s. In contrast, with vagal stimulation, the latency to response is short (0.15–0.20 s) and a plateau is reached within a few heartbeats (Figure 34.5B). After cessation of vagal stimulation, heart rate increases within a few heartbeats, although the rate may oscillate somewhat for a few seconds. This rapid response to changes in vagal activity allows beat-by-beat regulation of cardiac cycle length or heart period (i.e., the interval between two consecutive beats).

The rapid on–off response of the vagal versus sympathetic activation of heart rate is due to the mechanisms involved. The rapid "on" response of vagal activation is due to the direct coupling of muscarinic receptors to potassium ($I_{K,ACh}$) channels that allow a rapid response (Figure 34.4), whereas sympathetic stimulation requires activation of the second messenger adenylyl cyclase and cyclic AMP system. The rapid "off" response to parasympathetic nervous system activation is due to the abundant cholinesterase in the SA and AV nodes of the heart, allowing the rapid breakdown of ACh. On the other hand, sympathetic deactivation requires the slower reuptake and diffusion of norepinephrine. Accordingly, it is the sudden removal and reinstatement of vagal tone that accounts for the brief increase and decrease of heart rate in an animal with high vagal tone, such as the horse. For example, when a horse is briefly startled (e.g., response to a loud noise), a rapid change in heart rate occurs due to the release of parasympathetic tone and continued sympathetic effects on the heart. This tachycardia is short-lived.

Sympathetic and parasympathetic interactions

Since the postganglionic sympathetic and parasympathetic nerve terminals intermingle, their respective neurotransmitters are capable of affecting the other division of the autonomic nervous system. ACh released from vagal endings reacts with presynaptic muscarinic receptors on sympathetic nerve endings to reduce the amount of norepinephrine released from sympathetic efferent terminals (Figure 34.4). In addition to norepinephrine released from sympathetic terminals, transmitters such as neuropeptide Y are also released which inhibits the release of ACh from vagal nerve endings. At the level of the effector muscle cells, the two antagonistic transmitters oppose one another's effects via activation of their respective receptors and activation of second messenger systems.

The term **accentuated antagonism** has been given to the inhibitory effect of a given level of vagal stimulation that becomes more pronounced as the level of sympathetic activity increases. The inhibiting effect of vagal activity in the ventricles, where vagal fibers are sparse, appears to be achieved mainly by opposing the existing level of sympathetic activity. In the AV node, most evidence indicates that the left vagus and left sympathetic nerves dominate over the right-sided innervation. As discussed above, left vagus nerve stimulation inhibits AV conduction and can produce AV block. Negative dromotropic, chronotropic and inotropic vagal effects become more potent as the level of cardiac sympathetic activity becomes greater.

Denervated heart

Experimentally, elimination of the extrinsic cardiac nervous supply by sectioning or destruction of the nerves or by excision and reimplantation (autotransplantation) of the heart permits evaluation of the role of the nervous system in regulation of the heart. After autonomic denervation surgery in dogs, the resting heart rate stabilizes at 90–120 bpm, the **intrinsic heart rate** (Figure 34.5) of the denervated SA node. Respiratory sinus arrhythmia (see below) is abolished. The prompt acceleration of heart rate associated with a startle reaction or onset of exercise does not occur, rather a slower increase in heart rate to values about one-third lower than those in control dogs occurs. Thus the innervated heart satisfies the need for increased cardiac output largely by increasing heart rate and contraction while the denervated heart responds with a lesser heart rate increase but a large increase in stroke volume via the Frank–Starling (length–tension) mechanism. The denervated heart is supersensitive to circulating catecholamines, which support the needed augmentation of ventricular performance and heart rate in exercise. There is depletion of catecholamine stores, but apparently there are no major alterations in myocardial metabolism in denervated hearts. Parasympathectomy alone results in persistent sinus tachycardia at rest with rates of 140–160 bpm; this reveals the high vagal

resting tone of normal dogs and the effect of unopposed sympathetic tone on heart rate. Reinnervation becomes evident 1–2 months after denervation and is functionally complete in the dog in about 9 months; unfortunately this level of recovery does not occur following human cardiac transplantation.

Cardiac reflexes

A variety of reflexes affect both cardiac activity and vascular tone simultaneously and are discussed in Chapter 35. Under natural conditions, the rate of the heartbeat and physiological variations in this rate are controlled by the interaction of the regions responsible for vagal (i.e., nA, DMnX) and sympathetic (i.e., RVLM, PVN) outflow. These regions, in turn, are under the influence of other parts of the central nervous system, including the hypothalamus and the limbic system. They also receive input or information that enters the brainstem from all parts of the body, including the heart itself. Under these influences, the level of activity of either region may be elevated or depressed, with corresponding changes in heart rate.

There are certain reflex changes that primarily affect heart rate and these are discussed here. For example, pressure on the eyeball at the outer canthus usually slows the heart (oculocardiac reflex). In addition, increased pressure at the carotid sinus or aortic arch also reduces heart rate (baroreflex). Stimulation of afferent fibers in the respiratory passages by the inhalation of irritating vapors (e.g., anesthetics) is particularly likely to cause reflex inhibition of the heart. Extrasystole and bradycardia have been demonstrated electrocardiographically during abdominal operations, the irregularities apparently being the consequence of stimulation of visceral reflexes. Changes in heart rate that accompany emotions or those that precede muscular exercise are believed to result from the influence of higher cerebral centers on central autonomic regions.

The pulse rate is generally inversely related to the arterial blood pressure, a rise or fall in pressure causing, respectively, a decrease or increase in heart rate (i.e., the baroreflex; see Chapter 35). These adjustments are subserved by activation of two afferent limbs of the baroreflex, one via afferent vagal fibers (aortic depressor nerve) originating from the aortic arch and the other through the carotid sinus nerve originating from the carotid sinus. Activation of either set of afferent nerves via elevation of blood pressure increases activity of the brainstem nucleus tractus solitarius (nTS). Increases in nTS activity augment discharge of inhibitory neurons in the caudal ventrolateral medulla (CVLM) to reduce activation of the RVLM and IML, and result in a reduction in sympathetic nervous system activity, blood pressure, and heart rate. Activation of the nTS to nA or DMnX pathways (depending on the species) increases vagal tone to also reduce heart rate. Thus, changes in heart rate are brought about not simply by an increase or decrease in activity of one region or the other but by reciprocal variations in the tone of both.

Heart rate can also be altered by arterial blood gases (i.e., the chemoreflex). A decrease in arterial oxygen or increase in carbon dioxide activates carotid body chemoreceptors located

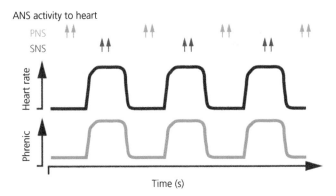

ANS activity to heart

Figure 34.6 Heart rate is elevated during inspiration and decreases during expiration (respiratory sinus arrhythmia). Phrenic nerve discharge represents neural respiration. Such arrhythmia is due to reciprocal activation and deactivation of the sympathetic (SNS) and parasympathetic (PNS) nervous systems. ANS, autonomic nervous system.

in the bifurcation of the common carotid artery and adjacent to baroreceptors. Such activation results in elevated discharge of chemoafferent nerves in the glossopharyngeal cranial nerve that project to the central nervous system. The subsequent elevation of nTS and nA and/or DMnX activity will decrease heart rate. Chemoreflex activation also elevates respiratory rate and depth. Not surprisingly, these reflexes as well as many others may interact with each other.

Respiratory sinus arrhythmia

An increase in heart rate during inspiration and a decrease during expiration is known as **respiratory sinus arrhythmia** (Figure 34.6). Such variations in heart rate maintain pulmonary blood flow during lung inflation. A number of different factors appear to interact in producing the phasic variation in vagal tone that causes this type of sinus arrhythmia, which has no pathological implications and is believed to be healthy. These factors include sensory and central influences. Sensory-related input is thought to be due to the cardiac component of several reflexes, including the respiratory **Hering–Breuer reflex** (tachycardia during lung inflation), the **Bainbridge reflex** (tachycardia in response to filling of the right atrium and great veins during inspiration), and the baroreceptor reflex (bradycardia when blood pressure increases). However, it is generally believed that the central nervous system is responsible for respiratory sinus arrhythmia since respiratory sinus arrhythmia persists when lung inflation is maintained. Also, respiratory sinus arrhythmia is sustained during sympathetic block, but eliminated when the parasympathetic (vagal) system is disrupted. In addition to the effect on heart rate, a positive inotropic action on left ventricular contraction during the acceleratory phase has been demonstrated.

Autonomic effects on contractility

Sympathetic effects, as already indicated, markedly increase both atrial and ventricular contractility. Parasympathetic effects profoundly inhibit the atria, decreasing heart rate and atrial

contractility and, paradoxically, shortening the action potential and refractory period of atrial cells. The inhibitory effects of parasympathetic stimulation on the ventricles are negligible compared with those on the atria, although a definite depression of ventricular contractility occurs with vagal stimulation, especially in the presence of high concurrent sympathetic activity. The reason for this latter characteristic is that the ACh liberated by vagal stimulation acts to inhibit norepinephrine release from the postganglionic sympathetic nerve terminals. This dependency of the vagal effect on contractility on the background sympathetic activity has been termed "accentuated antagonism."

Atrioventricular conduction

AV conduction is also regulated by the autonomic nervous system and its transmitters. Sympathetic neural activity and catecholamines decrease AV conduction time, acting especially in the upper (i.e., atrionodal and nodal) regions of the AV junctional area. Conduction in the lower (i.e., nodal–His) region is little affected. Blockade of β-adrenergic receptors decreases the SA node rate of discharge, prolongs AV conduction, and prolongs the refractory period of the AV junction. Vagal stimulation and cholinergic drugs slow conduction through the AV junction and increase the refractory period, acting primarily at the atrionodal and nodal regions rather than at the nodal–His region.

Hormonal control of the heart

Several hormones have a direct influence on the heart. Table 34.2 lists the effects of various humoral agents on cardiac function. In addition to sympathetic nervous release of norepinephrine from sympathetic nerve terminals, the catecholamines epinephrine and norepinephrine are also released from the adrenal medulla. While the ratio of epinephrine to norepinephrine released from the adrenal medulla may differ across species, these hormones both have profound effects on the heart, especially under stressful conditions. Glucagon causes a similar effect to catecholamines, possibly by a similar mechanism. It does not act as a β-receptor agonist but appears to stimulate cardiac adenylyl cyclase via a mechanism distinct from β-receptor activation. In addition to these hormones, a role for insulin, adrenocortical and thyroid hormones, angiotensin II, and others have been established (Table 34.2).

Although a physiological role for histamine in cardiac regulation has not been established, a histamine receptor system analogous to the adrenergic receptor system is present in the heart. Like β_1-adrenergic receptors, histamine H_2 receptors mediate positive chronotropy and inotropy, stimulate adenylyl cyclase, and cause coronary vasodilatation. H_1 receptors, like α-adrenergic receptors, mediate coronary vasoconstriction. Better known are the pathological effects of massive histamine release in anaphylactic shock, which cause hypotension, venodilatation, tachycardia, increased myocardial oxygen demand and, ultimately, cardiovascular

Table 34.2 Cardiac effects of humoral agents.

Hormone	Inotropic effect	Chronotropic effect	Coronary vasoactive effect	Remarks
Epinephrine	Positive, β_1	Positive, β_1	Constriction, α Dilation, β_1,β_2	Increased myocardial metabolism with β_1, stimulation causes coronary dilation by autoregulation
Norepinephrine	Positive, β_1	Positive, β_1	Constriction, α Dilation, β_2	
Acetylcholine	Negative	Negative	Dilation	
Glucagon	Positive	Positive	Dilation	No β-receptor effect; stimulates cyclase at another receptor site
Insulin	Positive	None	Dilation	
Mineralocorticoids	Positive	None	None	
ACTH	Little or none	Positive	None	May release corticosteroids
Vasopressin	Negative	Positive	Constriction, marked	Inotropic effect secondary to coronary constriction
Oxytocin	Little or none	Positive	Constriction, slight	
Angiotensin I	Positive, moderate	Positive, moderate	Constriction, weak	
Angiotensin II	Positive	Variable	Constriction	Strong inotropic and vasoconstrictor effect
Angiotensin III	Positive	Unknown	Constriction	Strong vasoconstrictor effect
Thyroxine	Positive	Positive	Increased flow	Inotropic effect chiefly on V_{max}; coronary effect chiefly secondary to increased myocardial O_2 consumption
Prostaglandins	Positive	Variable	Dilation	Reflex tachycardia; central nervous system stimulation tachycardia

ACTH, adrenocorticotropic hormone.
Source: data from Bourne, G.H. (ed.) (1980) *Hearts and Heart-like Organs*, Vols 1, 2 and 3. Academic Press, New York; Berne, R.M., Sperelakis, N. and Geiger, S.R. (eds) (1979) Handbook of Physiology, Section 2, Vol. 1, The Heart. American Physiological Society, Bethesda, MD.

collapse. Although histamine may play a role in local vascular autoregulation, it does not appear to be a likely candidate as a physiologic regulator of cardiac function under ordinary circumstances.

Finally, although oxygen, carbon dioxide, and pH have profound effects on the cardiorespiratory system via actions on the carotid body and central chemoreceptors, they may also directly influence cardiac function. Hypoxia and hypercapnia may depress cardiac contractility and performance through reduction in calcium sensitivity of contractile proteins. Hypercapnic effects likely occur through decreases in intracellular pH (acidosis). While changes in arterial blood gas composition may directly affect the heart, the reflex responses are likely to predominate.

Self-evaluation

Answers can be found at the end of the chapter.

1 What are the intrinsic factors that affect cardiac performance?

2 The resting heart rate of a horse is 30 bpm and the stroke volume is 1 L. The heart rate is increased by pacing to 200 bpm and the stroke volume decreases to 0.7 L. During exercise, the heart rate increases to 200 bpm and the stroke volume increases to 1.3 L. What is the cardiac output at rest, during pacing, and during exercise?

3 Increasing cardiac contractility by activation of sympathetic nerves is likely caused by which neurotransmitter and receptor?

4 What mechanism is most important in causing the staircase or treppe phenomenon?

5 What are three primary effects of activating parasympathetic efferent nerves to the heart?

Suggested reading

Berne, R.M., Sperelakis, N. and Geiger, S.R. (eds) (1979) *Handbook of Physiology, Section 2, Vol. 1, The Heart*. American Physiological Society, Bethesda, MD.

Boron, W.F. and Boulpaep, E.L. (eds) (2008) *Medical Physiology*, 2nd edn. Saunders Elsevier, Philadelphia.

Braunwald, E., Ross, J. Jr and Sonnenblick, E.J. (1968) *Mechanisms of Contraction of the Normal and Failing Heart*. Little, Brown, Boston.

Cohen, P.F. (1985) Cardiac pumping action and its regulation. In: *Clinical Cardiovascular Physiology* (eds P.F. Cohen, E.J. Brown Jr and S.C. Vlay). W.B. Saunders, Philadelphia.

Hall, J.E. (2011) *Guyton and Hall Textbook of Medical Physiology*, 12th edn. Saunders Elsevier, Philadelphia.

Katz, A.M. (2011) *Physiology of the Heart*, 5th edn. Lippincott, Philadelphia.

King, A.S. (1999) *The Cardiorespiratory System*. Blackwell Science, Oxford.

Levy, M.N. (1990) Neural and reflex control of the circulation. In: *Current Concepts in Cardiovascular Physiology* (ed. O.B. Garfein), pp. 133–207. Academic Press, New York.

Milnor, W.R. (1990) The heart as a pump. In: *Cardiovascular Physiology* (ed. W.R. Milnor). Oxford University Press, New York.

Pappano, A.J. and Wier, W.G. (eds) (2012) *Cardiovascular Physiology*, 10th edn. Mosby-Year Book, St Louis, MO.

Richardson, D.R., Randall, D.C. and Speck, D.F. (1998) *The Cardiopulmonary System*. Fence Creek Publishing, Madison, CT; Blackwell Science, Malden, MA.

Answers

1. (A) Preload, (B) afterload, (C) inotropic state (contractility), and (D) heart rate and rhythm.
2. At rest the cardiac output is 30 bpm × 1 L = 30 L/min. During pacing, the cardiac output is 200 bpm × 0.7 L = 140 L/min. During exercise, the cardiac output is 200 bpm × 1.3 L = 260 L/min.
3. Norepinephrine, β1 receptors.
4. Increased intracellular calcium.
5. Decreased (A) chronotropy, (B) dromotropy and (C) inotropy (mild effect).

Section VI: The
Cardiovascular System

35 Control Mechanisms of the Circulatory System

Cheryl M. Heesch, David D. Kline and Eileen M. Hasser
University of Missouri, Columbia, MO, USA

Introduction: systemic pressure and flow

1 What are some of the factors that determine arterial blood pressure?

2 What are normal values for arterial blood pressure?

3 Which species have much higher blood pressures and why might this occur?

Baseline arterial blood pressure

Arterial blood pressure is determined by (i) the pumping action of the heart (cardiac output), (ii) the peripheral resistance, (iii) the quantity of blood in the arterial system, and (iv) the elasticity of the arterial walls (see Chapter 30). These factors are controlled by complex regulatory systems that maintain the arterial pressure within narrow limits. Normal values for arterial pressure in various species are given in Table 35.1. Unlike heart rate (see Table 34.1, Chapter 34), blood pressure does not differ among species based on body weight; most mammals fall within the same ranges. However, there is a positive relationship between blood pressure and the height of the head above the heart level. Resting blood pressure at heart level increases with neck length from dog to cow to giraffe, while the differences in blood pressure at brain level among these species are much less. Birds have blood pressure ranges higher than those of mammals, possibly to buffer gravitational forces in flying. Blood pressure of newborn animals is significantly lower than that of adults in both birds and mammals.

Local regulation of blood flow

Regulation of blood flow plays a critical role in meeting the metabolic needs of tissues throughout the body. Numerous mechanisms involving the vascular endothelium, locally produced vasoactive substances, and intrinsic properties of vascular smooth muscle participate in regulation of blood flow in response to varying tissue demands. These mechanisms occur predominantly at the level of the microcirculation and are discussed in Chapter 36. Autoregulation of blood flow is especially important in maintaining blood flow to the heart, kidney, and brain (see Chapter 38). In addition to local control

Dukes' Physiology of Domestic Animals, Thirteenth Edition. Edited by William O. Reece, Howard H. Erickson, Jesse P. Goff and Etsuro E. Uemura.
© 2015 John Wiley & Sons, Inc. Published 2015 by John Wiley & Sons, Inc.
Companion website: www.wiley.com/go/reece/physiology

Section VI: The Cardiovascular System

Table 35.1 Representative adult arterial blood pressures.

Species	Systolic/diastolic (mmHg)*	Mean (mmHg)
Giraffe	211/151	185
Horse	130/95	115
Cow	140/95	120
Swine	140/80	110
Sheep	140/90	114
Human	120/70	100
Dog	150/87	107
Cat	125/89	105
Rabbit	120/80	100
Guinea pig	100/60	80
Rat	110/70	90
Mouse	111/80	100
Turkey	250/170	190
Chicken	175/145	160
Canary	220/150	185

* Published values are extremely variable because of the lability of blood pressure in response to environmental factors. These values were selected from various sources as reasonable for resting animals. *Source:* data from Mitchell, G., Maloney, S.K., Mitchell, D. and Keegan, D.J. (2006) The origin of mean arterial and jugular venous blood pressures in giraffes. *Journal of Experimental Biology* 209: 2515–2524; Brown, S., Atkins, C., Bagley, R. *et al.* (2007) Guidelines for the identification, evaluation, and management of systemic hypertension in dogs and cats. *Journal of Veterinary Internal Medicine* 21:542–558. Revised from Table 17.1, Erickson, H.H. and Detweiler, D.K. (2004), in *Dukes' Physiology of Domestic Animals*, 12th edn (ed. W.O. Reece). Cornell University Press, Ithaca, NY. Reproduced with permission from Cornell University Press.

mechanisms, the cardiovascular system is richly innervated by the parasympathetic (predominantly to the heart) and sympathetic (to heart and blood vessels) branches of the autonomic nervous system. Important neural reflexes provide the brain with constant sensory information from the periphery and initiate adjustments in autonomic outflow to maintain homeostasis and regulate arterial blood pressure, heart rate, cardiac output, and regional blood flow under a variety of physiological conditions.

Nervous control

1 Describe the autonomic innervation of the cardiovascular system, the transmitters, cotransmitters, and receptors involved.

2 Is sympathetic innervation greatest in arterioles or conduit vessels?

3 Explain various mechanisms for active vasodilation.

Overview: autonomic nervous system innervation of the cardiovascular system

Figure 35.1 provides an overview of the autonomic innervation of the cardiovascular system. **Parasympathetic innervation** of the heart originates from cell bodies within the dorsal motor nucleus of the vagus and the nucleus ambiguus in the medulla oblongata of the brainstem (see Figure 35.6), although the contribution of a given region is species-dependent. **Preganglionic fibers** to the heart course through the **vagus nerves** and release **acetylcholine (ACh)** onto postganglionic cell bodies. Although M_1-type muscarinic cholinergic receptors have been identified in autonomic ganglia, the major receptor type mediating activation of postganglionic cell bodies are **nicotinic ganglionic cholinergic receptors (N_2 type)**. For clarity parasympathetic ganglia are shown some distance from the heart in Figure 35.1, but actually the parasympathetic ganglia are located very near to, or on, the heart. The major postganglionic parasympathetic innervation of the heart is to the atria and the conduction system, including the sinoatrial (SA) and atrioventricular (AV) nodes. Postganglionic nerve terminals release ACh which activates **M_2-type muscarinic cholinergic receptors** and decreases heart rate and atrial contractile force. In the ventricles, parasympathetic innervation can mediate modest decreases in cardiac contractility through a presynaptic action to decrease ongoing **norepinephrine (NE)** release from sympathetic postganglionic nerve terminals. Most blood vessels are devoid of parasympathetic innervation, with a few notable exceptions. **Parasympathetic vasodilator fibers** innervate restricted cranial and sacral areas such as blood vessels in the brain, tongue, salivary glands, bladder, rectum, and external genitalia (shown in Figure 35.1). These fibers are probably not concerned with cardiovascular homeostasis or reflex control of blood vessels, nor are they tonically active. It is generally believed that they are cholinergic. The vasodilation caused by ACh is caused by interaction with muscarinic cholinergic receptors on (i) vascular endothelial cells, which mediate release of the gaseous vasodilator nitric oxide (also known as endothelium-derived relaxing factor, EDRF) (see Chapter 36); and (ii) sympathetic nerve terminals, where their activation inhibits NE release. Table 35.2 summarizes the transduction pathways and cardiovascular effects of activation of M_2-type muscarinic receptors.

The heart and most vascular beds receive innervation from the sympathetic branch of the autonomic nervous system. Preganglionic cell bodies in the **sympathetic nervous system** are located in the intermediolateral cell column of the thoracic and lumbar regions of the spinal cord and send projections to postganglionic cell bodies in the paravertebral (or prevertebral, not shown) ganglia (see Chapter 10). Similar to the parasympathetic ganglia, ACh released from preganglionic nerve terminals activates nicotinic ganglionic receptors on postganglionic cell bodies. Postganglionic sympathetic innervation to the atria, conduction system, and ventricles of the heart arise from the stellate ganglia. Sympathetically mediated increases in heart rate and cardiac contractility are due to release of NE from nerve terminals and activation of β_1-adrenergic receptors in the heart (see Chapter 34). Most blood vessels throughout the body receive sympathetic postganglionic innervation and, in general, release of NE results in vasoconstriction via activation of postsynaptic vascular α_1 receptors. However, α_2-adrenergic

Parasympathetic   Sympathetic

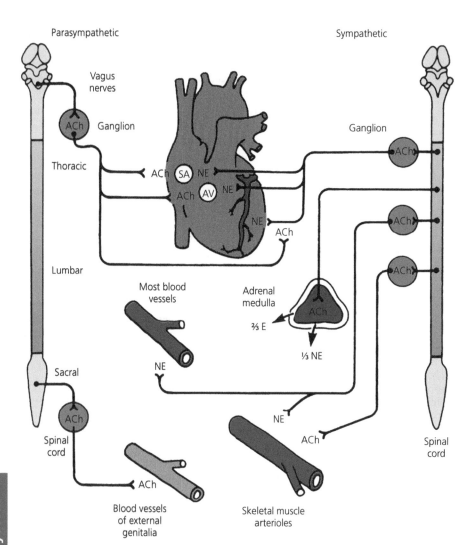

Figure 35.1 Autonomic innervation of the cardiovascular system. ACh, acetylcholine; NE, norepinephrine; E, epinephrine; SA, sinoatrial node; AV, atrioventricular node. See text for details. Adapted from Sparks, H.V. and Rooke, T.W. (1987) *Essentials of Cardiovascular Physiology.* University of Minnesota Press, Minneapolis, MN. Reproduced with permission from University of Minnesota Press.

Table 35.2 Muscarinic effects on the cardiovascular system.

Receptor subtype	Location	Transduction pathway	Second messenger	Functional response
Muscarinic M_1	Autonomic ganglia	Coupled by $G\alpha_q$ Activation of PLC	IP_3 and DAG	Depolarization (minor role compared with nicotinic N_2 receptors)
Muscarinic M_2	Heart	Coupled by $G\alpha_i/G\alpha_o$ and inhibition of AC	Decreased cyclic AMP	*SA node*: decreased spontaneous depolarization, hyperpolarization, decreased heart rate
		Activation: inwardly rectifying K^+ Inhibition of voltage-gated Ca^{2+} channels		*AV node*: decreased conduction velocity *Atrial myocardium*: decreased refractory period, decreased contractility *Ventricular myocardium*: slight decreased contractility
	Peripheral nerve terminals			Inhibition of transmitter release
	Blood vessels (arterioles in skeletal muscle)	Activation of guanylate cyclase	Increased cyclic GMP: nitric oxide released from endothelium	Vasodilation (in some species)

$G\alpha_q$, G-protein subunit that activates PLC; $G\alpha_i/G\alpha_o$, G-protein subunit that inhibits production of cyclic AMP from ATP; PLC, phospholipase C; IP_3, inositol trisphosphate; DAG, diacylglycerol; AC, adenylate cyclase.
Source: data from Table 8.3, Westfall, T.C. and Westfall, D.P. (2011) Neurotransmission: the autonomic and somatic motor nervous systems. In: *Goodman & Gilman's Pharmacological Basis of Therapeutics*, 12th edn (eds L.L. Brunton, B.A. Chabner and B.C. Knollmann). McGraw-Hill, New York; and Table 14.2, Richerson, G.B. (2009), in *Medical Physiology*, 2nd edn (eds W.F. Boron and E.L. Boulpaep). Saunders Elsevier, Philadelphia.

Table 35.3 Adrenergic effects on the cardiovascular system.

Receptor subtype	Primary location	Transduction pathway	Second messenger	Functional response
Adrenergic α_1	Arterioles and veins	Coupled by $G\alpha_q$ Activation of PLC	IP_3 and DAG	Depolarization Vasoconstriction
Adrenergic α_{2B}	Arterioles	Coupled by $G\alpha_i/G\alpha_o$ Inhibition of AC Decreased PKA activity	Decreased cyclic AMP	Vasoconstriction
Adrenergic α_{2A}	Sympathetic nerve terminals			Inhibition of NE release
Adrenergic β_1	Heart	Coupled by $G\alpha_s$ Activation of AC Activation of PKA Activation of L-type Ca^{2+} channels	Increased cyclic AMP	Increased heart rate Increased contractility
Adrenergic β_2	Blood vessels	Coupled by $G\alpha_s$ Activation of AC Activation of PKA Activation of Ca^{2+} channels	Increased cyclic AMP	Smooth muscle relaxation Vasodilation

$G\alpha_q$, G-protein subunit that activates PLC; $G\alpha_i/G\alpha_o$, G-protein subunit that inhibits production of cAMP from ATP; $G\alpha_s$, G-protein subunit that activates adenylate cyclase; PLC, phospholipase C; PKA, protein kinase A; IP_3, inositol trisphosphate; DAG, diacylglycerol; AC, adenylate cyclase. *Source*: data from Table 8.6, Westfall, T.C. and Westfall, D.P. (2011) Neurotransmission: the autonomic and somatic motor nervous systems. In: *Goodman & Gilman's Pharmacological Basis of Therapeutics*, 12th edn (eds L.L. Brunton, B.A. Chabner and B.C. Knollmann). McGraw-Hill, New York; and Table 14.2, Richerson, G.B. (2009), in *Medical Physiology*, 2nd edn (eds W.F. Boron and E.L. Boulpaep). Saunders Elsevier, Philadelphia.

receptors are present in certain arterioles and their activation also mediates vasoconstriction. In addition, α_2 receptors located on efferent presynaptic adrenergic terminals provide a local negative feedback mechanism, by inhibiting NE release during periods of high sympathetic activation. Table 35.3 provides a summary of the major adrenergic receptor subtypes, transduction pathways, and effects on the cardiovascular system.

In some species arterioles in skeletal muscle also receive specialized sympathetic innervation in which ACh is released from the postganglionic nerve terminals and mediates vasodilation. The functional significance of these **sympathetic cholinergic vasodilator fibers** is not entirely clear, but it has been proposed that they participate in the initial increase in skeletal muscle blood flow that originates from activation of the motor cortex in anticipation of skeletal muscle exercise.

In addition to these neural pathways, the **adrenal medullae** are also considered a part of the sympathetic nervous system. Chromaffin cells in the adrenal medulla function like postganglionic sympathetic neurons, with the exception that the catecholamines **epinephrine (adrenaline)** and **norepinephrine (noradrenaline)** are released directly into the bloodstream. Epinephrine is the predominant catecholamine secreted by the adrenal medulla, but the ratio of epinephrine to norepinephrine differs among species. Circulating catecholamines function in an endocrine fashion to mediate effects on both the heart and blood vessels.

Sympathetic vasoconstrictor fibers
Distribution
Sympathetic vasoconstrictor fibers were discovered in 1852 by Claude Bernard, who stimulated the cervical sympathetic nerve in the rabbit and observed constriction of the vessels of the ear.

These fibers belong to the thoracolumbar (sympathetic) division of the autonomic nervous system (see Chapter 10).

Adrenergic nerve endings (containing NE) have been identified in all types of blood vessels except the true capillaries. In general, precapillary resistance vessels (small arteries and arterioles) have a rich innervation, although the number of fibers is lower in the smallest precapillary vessels. The venules have fewer adrenergic fibers than the larger veins, which themselves are less richly innervated than the precapillary vessels. It is solely through such sympathetic fibers traveling with somatic nerve trunks that constrictor impulses are conveyed to the small vessels of the limbs. Sectioning of a peripheral nerve therefore causes complete degeneration of vasoconstrictor fibers in the area of its distribution.

Site and mode of action
The sympathetic nerve fibers constitute a powerful source of vasoconstrictor drive. Low levels of discharge of the vasoconstrictor fibers maintain normal vessel tone at rest, and maximal physiological excitation of sympathetic outflow to the vasculature causes profound vasoconstriction. Although NE is the major chemical transmitter released at the smooth muscle cell, neuropeptide Y (see next section) and **ATP** can be coreleased with NE from many sympathetic fibers. ATP released from perivascular nerves is capable of producing vasoconstriction by activating P_2 purinergic receptors on vascular smooth muscle cells, but the dominant effect of ATP is vasodilation due to activation of P_2 receptors on endothelial cells, promoting release of the potent vasodilator nitric oxide.

The overall effect of sympathetic innervation to resistance vessels is vasoconstriction, since a marked increase in blood flow in a vasoconstricted limb occurs immediately following sympathetic blockade or denervation. During prolonged constriction, accumulation of vasodilator metabolites in the tissue can oppose neurogenic influences, relaxing precapillary resistance vessels.

Excitation of sympathetic vasoconstrictor fibers to the aorta and largest arteries has only a moderate effect on these vessels. There is little or no rise in pressure as a direct effect of contraction or vasoconstriction of these large vessels; presumably, the most significant change is in their distensibility. In conduit arteries with diameters of 1 mm or greater, vasoconstriction or vasodilation related to changes in sympathetic nerve activity does not alter diameter of the vessels by more than 10%.

The postganglionic sympathetic neurons to blood vessels usually form two plexuses in the vascular adventitia. The innermost plexus is composed of unmyelinated fibers located in the boundary between the adventitia and the media. Small varicosities (2 μm in diameter) along each axon contain storage granules that release their contents upon depolarization. As discussed already, the chief neurotransmitter released from sympathetic nerve terminals is NE, but other transmitters or modulators are also present and may contribute to the response to activation of sympathetic nerves.

In addition to vasoconstrictor activity, sympathetic innervation exerts strong control over cardiac contractility and the capacity of vessels, mainly the veins. Augmented venous return and force of ventricular contraction contribute to increased cardiac output due to sympathetic nerve activation.

Neuropeptide Y

Neuropeptide Y (NPY) is one of the important cotransmitters released along with NE from sympathetic nerve terminals and, since it is a strong vasoconstrictor, contributes to the vasoconstrictor response especially during intense sympathetic activation. This 36-amino acid peptide is widely distributed together with NE in peripheral sympathetic nerve endings. Similar to previously discussed effects on NE release, activation of presynaptic α_2-adrenergic receptors also inhibits release of NPY from sympathetic nerve endings.

Functional significance

Vasoconstrictor fibers are of major importance in homeostasis of blood pressure and blood flow, including those reflex adjustments that arise from baroreceptors, cardiopulmonary receptors, and chemoreceptors. They also control blood flow through the skin and thus influence peripheral heat exchange. Vasodilation, particularly of a reflex nature, is predominantly due to removal of existing vasoconstrictor tone. Figure 35.2 graphically illustrates that at rest (baseline conditions) there is tonic vasoconstrictor sympathetic nerve discharge, so that the vessels are partially constricted. A decrease in sympathetic nerve discharge will result in an increase in arteriole diameter (vasodilation), while an increase in sympathetic drive above the baseline level will further constrict arterioles. In fulfilling its role as the main

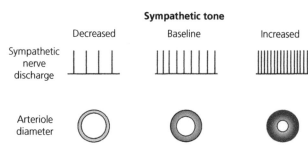

Figure 35.2 Sympathetic nerve discharge and arteriole diameter. Under baseline conditions (*middle*) there is tonic sympathetic nerve activity to the vasculature and arterioles are partially constricted. When sympathetic nerve activity is increased (*right*), arterioles constrict further. When sympathetic nerve activity decreases (*left*), arterioles dilate. Adapted from Heesch, C.M. (1999) Reflexes that control cardiovascular function. *American Journal of Physiology* 277:S234–S243. American Physiological Society with permission.

neural control for the peripheral circulation, the sympathetic vasoconstrictor system may exhibit generalized, segmental, or regional function, depending on the type of stimulus.

Active vasodilation

With abolition of sympathetic vasoconstrictor effects, there remains a residual contractile state in blood vessels, sometimes referred to as myogenic or intrinsic tone. **Active dilation** refers to a further reduction in vascular contractile tone below the level of tone present in the absence of sympathetic vasoconstrictor activity. Interestingly, increased sympathetic activity can actually contribute to active dilation in three ways: (i) indirectly by increasing tissue metabolic rate (e.g., through autoregulation and locally released metabolites, coronary dilation occurs when cardiac work increases in response to sympathetic stimulation); (ii) by action on **vascular β_2-adrenergic receptors** that cause vasodilation in certain vascular beds (e.g., skeletal muscle); and (iii) in special circumstances, through sympathetic cholinergic fibers (see Figure 35.1).

Sympathetic cholinergic vasodilator fibers

In addition to the vasodilation that occurs due to inhibition of vasoconstriction, there also exists a system of efferent dilator nerves emanating from the central nervous system, but they seem to be distributed primarily to skeletal muscle. Vasodilator nerves can be activated by stimulation of the motor cortex and certain regions of the hypothalamus (Figure 35.3) in some species (dog and cat). These vasodilatory pathways are distinct from pathways involving the rostral ventrolateral medulla which provides excitatory drive to preganglionic sympathetic neurons in the spinal cord to promote vasoconstriction (see section Central nervous system sites for cardiovascular control). The active dilator response is mediated by ACh released from postganglionic sympathetic nerve terminals and seems to be limited to arterioles, since the smallest precapillary resistance vessels and capacitance vessels of the venous side have no known cholinergic innervation.

It has been proposed that a pathway involving the motor cortex activates these fibers to dilate vessels in skeletal muscle and increase blood flow in anticipation of exercise. However, the dilation that accompanies physical exercise is not entirely cholinergic or adrenergic because it is not completely blocked by atropine or sympathectomy. Local control mechanisms contribute importantly to vasodilation in exercising muscle and it is believed that the sympathetic cholinergic vasodilator fibers to skeletal muscle play a limited role in the overall integrated response to exercise, likely by causing an initial increase in blood flow just before exertion.

Other vasodilator fibers

Although their exact neural pathways and physiological roles are not as well defined as those related to the autonomic nervous system and traditional transmitters/modulators, other neural vasodilator responses have been identified. Vasodilator fibers that liberate histamine have been demonstrated in the hindlimb of the dog. Independent of the sympathetic innervation, purinergic vasodilator fibers that liberate adenosine triphosphate (ATP) or adenosine have also been identified. In many blood vessels the powerful dilator actions of extracellular ATP and ADP are mediated through the release of nitric oxide by the endothelial cells. ATP and ADP also promote the release of prostacyclin (a vasodilator in some blood vessels and a potent inhibitor of platelet aggregation).

Summary of efferent cardiovascular innervation

In summary, most vasomotor nerves that supply arteries are sympathetic adrenergic fibers which mediate vasoconstriction primarily by activation of postsynaptic α_1-adrenergic receptors.

Parasympathetic and sympathetic cholinergic vasodilator nerves exist and likely mediate functionally specific vasodilation in certain restricted vascular beds in some species. Nonadrenergic and noncholinergic innervation has also been demonstrated in blood vessels. Many transmitters appear to be purinergic, but other possible vasodilator transmitters/modulators have been identified, including prostaglandins, serotonin, dopamine, bradykinin, vasoactive intestinal peptide (VIP), and ATP. The largest elastic arteries that have relatively little smooth muscle are sparsely innervated. As arteries get smaller and smooth muscle content increases, innervation density increases. Veins are less densely innervated than arteries.

Central nervous system sites for cardiovascular control

Multiple levels of the central nervous system contribute to cardiovascular control. Stimulation of discrete central nervous system areas and ablation experiments have identified a hierarchical array of control levels in the spinal cord, medulla, pons, hypothalamus, thalamus, cerebellum, and cerebral hemispheres (see Figure 35.3). Although such experiments demonstrate a certain autonomy and dominance in blood pressure control for centers in the bulbar region (primarily the medulla), they should not necessarily be considered the chief integrators for a given autonomic response when the various other control loops are intact. The other areas may play an important complementary and modifying role in neural regulation in the intact animal. Also, the contribution of various central pathways likely changes during physiological challenges and in pathophysiological states.

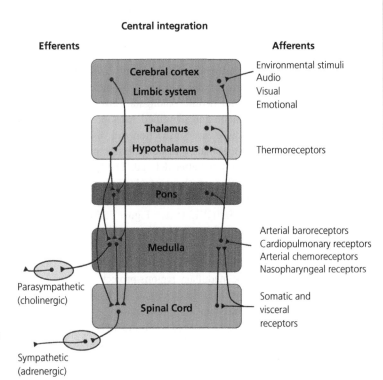

Figure 35.3 Central integration in cardiovascular regulation. The schematic is a simplified summary of central nervous systems sites involved in cardiovascular regulation. Projections are bilateral, but for presentation purposes afferent and ascending inputs are shown on the right, and efferent and descending inputs are shown on the left. This diagram emphasizes that the medulla in the brainstem is an important center for integration of sensory input. However, various levels of the central nervous system are reciprocally innervated and are capable of contributing to the integrated output of the parasympathetic and sympathetic branches of the autonomic nervous system.

It was once believed that discrete centers provided unitary control of preganglionic sympathetic spinal neurons. It is now well accepted that the inputs to the spinal neurons originate from, and are integrated at, several levels of the central nervous system, such as the pontomedullary region, midbrain, hypothalamus, and cerebral cortex (see Figure 35.3). Thus complicated responses, such as adjustments during blood loss, the defense reaction, temperature regulation, and adaptations during exercise, are the result of integration longitudinally along the neuraxis.

Spinal cord

Neurons of nearby spinal cord segments, as well as descending axons from several higher centers, synapse with soma of preganglionic sympathetic neurons in the **intermediolateral cell column (IML) of the spinal cord**. Therefore integration of neural activity from various central nervous system levels can occur at these spinal synapses.

The preganglionic sympathetic neurons may, under some circumstances, exhibit spontaneous activity that is independent of descending excitatory drive from higher levels of the nervous system. This phenomenon has been observed in spinal animals (e.g., following spinal cord injury) where spinal interneurons and possibly altered tensions of oxygen or carbon dioxide are believed to contribute to the "spontaneous" activity.

Various types of afferent stimulation can initiate vasoconstriction via reflexes at the level of the spinal cord. For example, pain or cold stimulation of the skin induces a segmentally arranged constriction of splanchnic (relating to the viscera) vessels in animals lacking descending input from supraspinal brain regions (spinal animals). Cutaneous vasodilation occurs in these animals when the skin is moderately warmed.

Medulla oblongata

In intact animals, spinal cord neurons subserving vasomotor function are under the control of higher-order neurons located particularly in the ventrolateral medulla oblongata. Early studies used local electrical stimulation and identified "pressor areas" and "depressor areas" that cause vasoconstriction and vasodilation, respectively. The sites primarily responsible for pressor and depressor responses are now better defined. The "pressor area" is located in the region of the **rostral ventrolateral medulla (RVLM)** and the "depressor area" is located in the **caudal ventrolateral medulla (CVLM)** (see Figure 35.5). The vasodilation due to activation of the CVLM is caused by inhibition of ongoing vasoconstrictor tone emanating from the RVLM, specific vasodilator fibers not being involved.

In the intact animal these medullary regions project to, and receive input from, still higher level neurons in the hypothalamus and the cerebral cortex. At rest, the contribution of inputs to the medulla from these higher centers is minimal. However, input from higher centers contributes importantly to integrated patterns of vasomotor activity in response to physiological challenges such as water deprivation and exercise.

The activity of the medullary neurons involved in control of sympathetic outflow is modulated by afferent nerve impulses which convey information from various organs and regions of the body, as well as from other central nervous system centers, such as respiratory centers.

Sectioning of the brainstem above the medulla does not affect baseline blood pressure, which indicates that upper levels do not dominate the medullary level, even though they can modify its state of activity. In addition, pre-sympathetic neurons that project to the spinal cord continue to discharge and maintain arterial blood pressure through vasoconstriction even after elimination of incoming afferent sensory input from the periphery, suggesting that networks within the brainstem are capable of generating sympathetic drive to the spinal cord.

Hypothalamus

Both increases and decreases in heart rate and arterial blood pressure may be elicited by stimulation of various areas in the hypothalamus. In the **paraventricular nucleus of the hypothalamus (PVN)**, pressor effects are mediated in part by activation of sympathetic adrenergic fibers via either direct or indirect (involving a synapse in the RVLM) projections from the PVN to preganglionic sympathetic neurons in the IML of the spinal cord. In several pathological states associated with increased sympathetic vasoconstrictor activity, including hypertension, heart failure and diabetes, increased activity of these **pre-sympathetic** neurons in the PVN have been implicated. The region of the dorsal medial hypothalamus, along with the periaqueductal gray region in the midbrain (PAG), is involved in eliciting the classical defense reaction and sympathoexcitation in response to stressful stimuli. In general, depressor effects mediated via the hypothalamus result from inhibition of ongoing sympathetic adrenergic drive. However, in certain species and vascular beds stimulation of sympathetic cholinergic vasodilator fibers (cat and dog) may contribute to depressor responses due to activation of the hypothalamus.

An important function of the hypothalamus is control of body temperature. The rostral hypothalamus and preoptic area contain neurons that protect the body against overheating; they also control the discharge to the vasoconstrictor fibers of the cutaneous blood vessels. Electrical stimulation or local cooling of this area brings about a rise in blood pressure (vasoconstriction), and direct warming of this region produces a fall in blood pressure (vasodilation). The cutaneous arterioles and precapillary vessels, and especially the arteriovenous anastomoses (shunts) in the skin, are the vessels most sensitively engaged in control of heat loss.

Cerebral cortex

Stimulation of the motor and premotor cerebral cortex results in marked elevation of blood pressure with constriction of the cutaneous, splanchnic, and renal vessels and, at the same time, considerable vasodilation in the skeletal muscle. A generalized depressor response accompanied by somatic inhibition ("playing dead" reaction) can be produced by stimulation of the cingulate gyrus (and also regions of the PAG in the midbrain). It is believed that these higher centers play significant roles in the blood pressure response to pain and anxiety and also to the initial central command response in anticipation of exercise.

Cerebellum

Stimulation of various areas in the cerebellum can produce depressor and pressor effects and peripheral redistribution of blood supply (e.g., decreased renal blood flow and increased skin and muscle flow).

Neurohumoral regulating mechanisms

> **1** What determines classification of endogenous compounds as endocrines, paracrines, or autocrines?
>
> **2** Describe the renin–angiotensin–aldosterone system and its role in control of the circulation.
>
> **3** Under normal conditions, what is the major role of vasopressin (antidiuretic hormone, ADH) in the body and what regulates its release?
>
> **4** Describe the major eicosanoid pathways.

In addition to cardiovascular control by autonomic nerves and their chemical mediators, there are blood-borne endocrine secretions that act on the heart and blood vessels and paracrine substances made by cells in many tissues that diffuse in the extracellular spaces to affect nearby blood vessels. Some of these endocrine and paracrine substances are also neurally released, so that a clear distinction between endocrines, paracrines, and neurotransmitters cannot always be made (e.g., norepinephrine, NPY, VIP, substance P).

Vasoactive substances that are synthesized and released by non-neural cells have been variously classified as autocoids, local hormones, autocrines, or paracrines. In general, **endocrines** are substances carried in the bloodstream and act on distant cells; **paracrines** act on target cells close to the releasing cell; and **autocrines** act on the cells that release them (e.g., growth factors from tumor cells that stimulate their own growth).

Endocrine control
Adrenal medulla

One of the oldest known neurohumoral relationships is the secretion of epinephrine (and smaller quantities of norepinephrine) from the adrenal medullae after stimulation of (i) the splanchnic nerves, (ii) the lateral columns of the spinal cord, (iii) the RVLM, or (iv) the hypothalamus. These catecholamines are released directly into the bloodstream and are thus true endocrines, although norepinephrine, when released from postganglionic sympathetic fibers, serves also as a neurotransmitter. The α_1-, α_2-, β_1-, and β_2-adrenergic receptors which are activated

by catecholamines and their cardiovascular actions are outlined in Table 35.3.

Although the exact proportions vary based on species and physiological state, the main catecholamine released from the adrenal gland is epinephrine, with lesser amounts of norepinephrine released. Epinephrine has a high affinity for both α- and β-adrenergic receptors, and its effects in a particular vascular bed (and on the heart) are the result of the balance of each type of receptor in the tissue. Moderate levels of circulating epinephrine result in dilation of arterioles in skeletal muscle, cutaneous and renal vascular beds (due to activation of extrasynaptic vascular β_2 receptors) and enhanced cardiac output (due to activation of cardiac β_1 receptors). Peripheral resistance decreases, cardiac output increases, and there is usually a modest increase in arterial blood pressure due to the increased cardiac output. However, with high levels of circulating epinephrine, α_1 vasoconstriction predominates because there are more peripheral α_1 receptors than β_2 receptors in the vasculature, and an increase in peripheral resistance contributes to a further rise in blood pressure.

Norepinephrine has about the same affinity for α-adrenergic receptors as epinephrine but much less affinity for β-adrenergic receptors. Thus, compared with epinephrine, norepinephrine produces greater vasoconstriction and less cardiac stimulation. Most arterioles constrict, peripheral resistance increases, and there is a greater rise in blood pressure.

The physiological role of adrenal medullary hormones in vasomotor control has long been debated. In experimental comparisons of these hormones and vasomotor fibers on peripheral vascular beds, resistance in most blood vessels has been found to be dominated by vasomotor fibers. The exception is the peripheral resistance of skeletal muscle vessels, which are almost maximally dilated by moderate levels of epinephrine with a significant reduction in the ratio of precapillary to postcapillary resistance. Epinephrine secretion increases progressively with increased intensity and duration of exercise, and during the fight or flight response. In these states secreted epinephrine may contribute to vasodilation in the exercising skeletal muscle. If the amount of secreted catecholamines is large, as after hemorrhage, α_1-adrenergic effects predominate and reinforce neurally mediated α_1-receptor vasoconstrictor effects, especially in the renal vascular bed.

Renin–angiotensin-aldosterone system

The renin–angiotensin–aldosterone system functions as a neurohumoral regulating mechanism in the control of blood volume and blood pressure and is critically involved in the pathophysiology of such clinical states as arterial hypertension and congestive heart failure (see Chapter 40).

Renin is a proteolytic enzyme that is synthesized, stored, and secreted by a variety of organs, including the kidney, brain, adrenal gland, arterial wall, uterus, placenta, fetal membranes, and amniotic fluid. Traditionally, the role of the renin–angiotensin system as a modulator of cardiovascular function has emphasized renal renin in the generation of circulating angiotensin, but more recently it has become clear that angiotensin generated outside the kidney may contribute to blood pressure control by local as well as systemic effects.

Renin cleaves the α_2-globulin angiotensinogen (from the liver) to form a relatively vasoinactive decapeptide, **angiotensin I**. Angiotensin-converting enzyme (ACE), a dipeptidyl carboxypeptidase, then converts angiotensin I to an active vasopressor octapeptide, **angiotensin II**. This converting enzyme is derived mainly in the capillary endothelium of the lung but is also found in the circulating plasma, the kidney, and other organ beds. Next to vasopressin, angiotensin II is the second most potent vasoconstrictor produced in the body. However, in normal animals at rest its pressor action is limited by rapid destruction in peripheral capillary beds by various peptidases. Angiotensin II plays a pivotal role in body fluid balance by acting directly on the adrenal cortex to promote the secretion of **aldosterone**, which in turn promotes Na^+ and water reabsorption by the kidney (see Chapter 18). Under pathological conditions the release of aldosterone, stimulated by angiotensin II, may contribute to blood pressure elevation in hypertension and fluid retention in heart failure (see Chapter 40).

In mammals the direct vasoconstrictor effect of angiotensin II is due to activation of angiotensin receptors on the arterial smooth muscle. It also potentiates α-adrenergic effects through a presynaptic mechanism to increase NE release from sympathetic postganglionic nerve terminals. In nonmammalian vertebrates (e.g., chickens) the action of angiotensin II is largely indirect, mediated by catecholamine release, and it may exert an initial vasodilator action by acting directly on smooth muscle. Angiotensin II is not required for maintenance of blood pressure in the normal state. However, when the extracellular fluid volume is depleted, small reductions in renal perfusion pressure promote the release of enough renin to increase circulating angiotensin II, raise blood pressure and cause, within 20 min, a 65% compensation of the fall in renal pressure. Thus the system has enough gain and operates with sufficient speed to function in short-term blood pressure control. Angiotensin II plays a significant role in blood pressure maintenance under stress conditions (e.g., salt deficiency, adrenalectomy, diuretic administration, reduction in renal perfusion pressure) through its vasoconstrictor and aldosterone-stimulating actions.

Circulating angiotensin II also contributes to blood volume and pressure regulation by activating central neural structures devoid of a blood–brain barrier which then project to regions within the brain that participate in pathways that stimulate thirst, secretion of vasopressin (ADH) and adrenocorticotropic hormone (ACTH), and increase sympathetic nerve activity. In addition, the brain has its own renin–angiotensin system and locally produced angiotensin peptides have been shown to modulate neuronal function in pathways involved in control of fluid balance and sympathetic outflow. In pathological states such as hypertension and heart failure, central nervous system effects of angiotensin II have been shown to contribute to the increase in sympathetic nerve activity which occurs.

While angiotensin II is capable of activating the sympathetic nervous system, the converse is also true. Activation of renal sympathetic nerves is an important stimulus for renin release, as are adrenergic agonists (see Chapter 18).

Vasopressin system

Vasopressin (antidiuretic hormone, ADH) is synthesized in magnocellular neurons in the hypothalamus which project to the posterior pituitary gland where it is then released into the bloodstream. ADH has two major actions that are important in blood volume and blood pressure regulation: antidiuresis and vasoconstriction. While *in vitro* it is the most powerful vasoconstrictor known (even more potent than angiotensin II), the physiological concentrations required for its antidiuretic action in the kidney are 10 to 100 times less than those required to elevate blood pressure. The normal physiological role of vasopressin related to long-term regulation of blood pressure is through its influence on water reabsorption in the collecting ducts of the renal tubules. In hemorrhage, however, vasopressin can be released in large quantities and both its vasoconstrictor and fluid-retaining actions contribute importantly in restoring blood pressure toward normal levels. Independent of its endocrine function, there is evidence that vasopressin serves as a neurotransmitter in pre-sympathetic neurons that project from the hypothalamus to both the RVLM and the spinal cord, and control sympathetic outflow.

Atrial natriuretic peptide

Atrial natriuretic peptide (ANP) is synthesized in atrial cells and stored in membrane-bound secretory granules. Stretching of the atria, as may occur with an increase in blood volume, causes release of ANP into the circulation. ANP acts directly on the inner medullary collecting ducts to inhibit sodium reabsorption. In addition, an increase in this hormone can result in inhibition of sodium reabsorption in other segments of the renal tubule by indirect mechanisms, including the inhibition of several steps in the renin–angiotensin–aldosterone pathway: it inhibits the secretion of renin, and it acts directly on the adrenal cortex to inhibit angiotensin-induced aldosterone secretion. ANP, by its effects on the renal arterioles, can also cause an increase in glomerular filtration rate, and this contributes to the increased sodium excretion produced by this hormone.

Other endocrines

Thyroid hormones stimulate protein synthesis (including cardiac contractile proteins), increase heart rate, shorten the refractory period of myocytes, enhance myocardial contractility, and increase the heart's responsiveness to catecholamines. By increasing metabolic activity of most tissues, thyroid hormones increase demand for increased cardiac output and blood flow. Parathyroid hormone at physiological levels decreases the vasoconstrictor response to angiotensin II. **Estrogens** increase cardiac output, stroke volume and plasma volume and cause vasodilation. **Progesterone** has vasodilator and natriuretic properties. Androgens such as testosterone are associated with higher blood pressures in men than in premenopausal women and in male rats with hereditary hypertension and are therefore thought to influence blood pressure.

Paracrine control

As mentioned earlier, locally secreted agents may function purely as paracrine-control agents (e.g., bradykinin), may have paracrine and endocrine functions (e.g., renin and angiotensin II), or may serve as both paracrine and neurotransmitter substances (e.g., serotonin and various peptides that are neurally released, such as VIP and substance P).

Eicosanoids

Eicosanoids are signaling molecules that are widely distributed in the body and which have numerous cardiovascular effects. Eicosanoid synthesis begins with the liberation of the essential fatty acid arachidonic acid from cell membranes by the enzyme phospholipase A_2. Through the cyclooxygenase (COX) pathway arachidonic acid is converted into various prostanoids: thromboxanes, prostacyclin, and various other prostaglandins. COX is inhibited by nonsteroidal anti-inflammatory drugs such as indomethacin. The enzymes that produce different prostanoids are tissue-specific so that the particular prostanoid produced is characteristic of a tissue, for example thromboxane A_2 in platelets and prostacyclin (PGI_2) in blood vessels. PGI_2 is a powerful vasodilator and inhibitor of platelet aggregation, while thromboxane A_2 has the opposite effect, causing vasoconstriction and platelet aggregation. Prostaglandin E_2 (PGE_2) dilates vascular and bronchial smooth muscles; $PGF_{2\alpha}$ constricts blood vessels. The products of the COX pathway are important signaling molecules in normal physiology and they also participate in inflammatory responses. Under normal conditions, levels of the prostanoids in circulating blood are low because many of them are removed from the bloodstream by a single passage through the pulmonary circulation and they are also taken up by the liver and kidney.

Vasodilator prostaglandins are present in the fetal plasma in relatively high concentrations. Since one of these, PGI_2, is little metabolized in the lungs, it may act as a circulatory hormone in the fetus, maintaining patency of the ductus arteriosus *in utero*. This has led to the use of indomethacin to aid closure of the patent ductus arteriosus in premature infants (see Chapter 38 for information on the ductus arteriosus and the fetal circulation).

Leukotrienes

Leukotrienes, another subclass of eicosanoids, are produced from arachidonic acid by the lipoxygenase pathway and are not influenced by indomethacin or other nonsteroidal anti-inflammatory drugs which block COX. The term "leukotriene" was used because these compounds were first found in leukocytes. Leukotrienes are produced not only by nucleated cells in bone marrow but by many other tissues, including skin, brain,

liver, kidney, heart, and tracheal epithelium. They are powerful mediators of inflammation and bronchial smooth muscle contraction and are involved in asthma and immune-mediated disease. Leukotrienes are major contributors to anaphylactic responses, which are characterized by marked hypotension, myocardial depression, and leakage of blood plasma into the tissues (see Chapter 40).

Kallikrein–kinin system

Kinins are vasodilator peptides produced by proteases from precursor proteins (kininogens). The enzyme kallikrein is found in certain glands, in the brain, in plasma, and in many other tissues. Plasma kallikrein is responsible for the production of bradykinin from high-molecular-weight kininogen, while tissue kallikrein hydrolyzes low-molecular-weight kininogen to produce kallidin. Glandular kallikrein–kinin systems appear to regulate local vasodilation associated with secretion. Intrarenally released kinins cause natriuresis, diuresis, and the release of vasoactive prostaglandins.

The kallikrein–kinin system and the renin–angiotensin system have opposing effects, whereby bradykinin is a vasodilator which stimulates Na^+ excretion, and angiotensin II is a vasoconstrictor that promotes Na^+ retention by stimulating aldosterone secretion from the adrenal cortex. The enzyme responsible for degradation of bradykinin, kininase II, is the same enzyme responsible for converting angiotensin I to the active peptide angiotensin II (i.e., ACE). The effects of this enzyme's activity are prohypertensive, and the therapeutic benefits of the commonly used class of antihypertensive drugs called ACE inhibitors are likely due not only to decreases in angiotensin II, but also increases in vasodilator kinins.

Summary of nervous/neurohumoral circulatory control

The autonomic nervous system neurotransmitters effect rapid regulatory changes in both the vasculature and the heart through actions on specific adrenergic and cholinergic receptors. Catecholamines secreted into the bloodstream by the adrenal medulla act on adrenergic receptors throughout the body.

NPY is released together with catecholamines from nerve endings in the adrenal medulla and peripheral sympathetic nervous system. NPY has direct vasoconstrictor properties, potentiates the effects of NE and regulates the release of other vasoactive substances. In general, NPY effects, like those of NE and ACh, are short lived, permitting moment-by-moment regulation of blood pressure and blood flow.

The renin–angiotensin system can be activated rapidly by sympathetic stimulation, controlled by such mechanisms as arterial and cardiopulmonary baroreceptor and chemoreceptor reflexes (see next section). The resultant support or increase in arterial blood pressure is sustained for minutes to hours because of aldosterone release, which has a long half-life in the circulation and increases plasma volume by renal sodium and associated water retention.

Section VI: The Cardiovascular System

ANP release is stimulated by atrial stretch due to increased blood volume and serves as an important part of a negative feedback loop to regulate volume effects on blood pressure. ANP promotes natriuresis, diuresis, and vasodilation, thus opposing the accumulation of increased fluid in the extracellular fluid compartment.

Vasopressin, although a potent vasoconstrictor, functions in blood pressure control primarily through its antidiuretic properties in the maintenance of optimal blood volume.

The kallikrein–kinin system generates natriuretic and vasodilator peptides such as bradykinin which oppose the sodium-retaining and vasoconstrictor actions of angiotensin II.

Reflex control mechanisms

1 Describe the central nervous system pathways for the arterial baroreflex, cardiopulmonary reflexes, and the arterial chemoreflex.

2 Why are the carotid sinus and aortic nerves called buffer nerves?

3 What are the baroreflex responses to an increase and decrease in arterial pressure?

4 Where are the chemoreceptors located and what are the cardiovascular responses to chemoreceptor activation?

5 Which cardiovascular control systems are involved in compensatory responses to progressive hemorrhage and what are the neural and humoral responses?

The effects of activating vasomotor nerve fibers and neurohumoral systems on the heart and circulation have been discussed in the preceding sections. These systems represent the **efferent limb of reflexes** that mediate moment-to-moment adjustments in distribution of blood flow in response to variations in regional or organ function. The **afferent limb of cardiovascular reflexes** comprises sensory nerves that continuously provide the brain with information from the periphery, so that appropriate adjustments in efferent outflow and humoral secretions can be made to maintain homeostasis and meet tissue demands under a variety of physiological conditions.

Afferent nerves providing input to the brainstem

Figure 35.4 illustrates some of the important peripheral sensory afferent nerves that provide input to the medulla of the brainstem. Located in the region of the bifurcation of the internal and external carotid artery (**carotid sinus region**) a network of nerve endings in the adventitia of the vessel wall (**carotid sinus baroreceptors**) send afferent fibers through the **carotid sinus nerve** to join the glossopharyngeal nerve projecting to the brainstem. The carotid sinus is especially distensible, and when blood pressure increases these nerve endings are stretched, which increases discharge in the carotid sinus nerves. Although the actual stimulus that activates these receptors is stretch, because the stretch is produced by an increase in pressure they

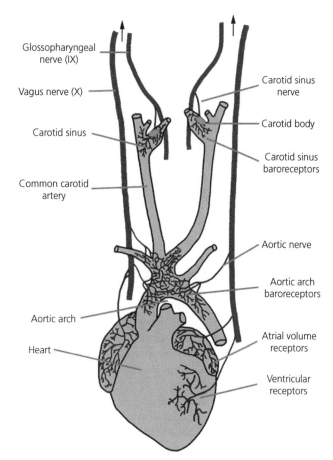

Figure 35.4 Afferent nerves for cardiovascular reflexes, showing the major sites for arterial baroreceptors, cardiopulmonary receptors, and arterial chemoreceptors and their afferent nerves. See text for details.

are referred to as **arterial baroreceptors** or **pressoreceptors**. Similar baroreceptors are present in the aortic arch region. **Aortic arch baroreceptors** send afferent fibers through the **aortic nerve**, or **aortic depressor nerve**, which in most species joins the vagus nerve before entering the central nervous system. The main function of arterial baroreceptors, which operate on the "high-pressure" side of the circulation, is to provide the brain with information regarding arterial blood pressure on a beat-by-beat basis.

Located in cardiopulmonary regions, including the atria, ventricles, and pulmonary vessels, there are receptors that respond to stretch and also to chemical activation. A major function of these **cardiopulmonary receptors**, in the "low-pressure" side of the circulation, is to provide information to the brain regarding blood volume.

In addition to arterial baroreceptors, there are specialized structures located near the bifurcation of the carotid arteries, the **carotid bodies**, which are exquisitely sensitive to changes in partial pressure of oxygen in the arterial blood (Pao_2). Decreased Pao_2 (and to a lesser extent increased $Paco_2$ or decreased blood pH) results in increased discharge of **carotid body chemoreceptors**, which send afferent fibers through the same carotid sinus–glossopharyngeal nerve pathway used by the carotid sinus baroreceptor afferent nerves. There are similar chemoreceptors in the aortic arch region (aortic bodies) of some species, although the carotid bodies appear to provide the predominant chemoreceptor input. Afferent signals from the aortic bodies are carried through the aortic nerves which then join the vagus.

Arterial baroreflex
Arterial baroreflex pathways

The importance of the carotid sinus in regulation of heart rate and arterial blood pressure was first demonstrated by Hering in 1923. Compression of the common carotid artery at its bifurcation (which would mimic elevated systemic arterial pressure by distorting afferent nerve endings in the carotid sinus) caused a marked slowing of heart rate, vasodilation, and a fall in blood pressure. Pressure on the common carotid artery some distance below the carotid sinus, which reduced blood pressure within the sinus (and decreased stretch of the nerve endings), caused cardiac acceleration, vasoconstriction, and a rise in arterial pressure. Current knowledge regarding the medullary arterial baroreflex pathways is summarized in Figures 35.5 and 35.6.

The arterial baroreflex pathway for control of sympathetic nerve activity is shown in Figure 35.5. A very important feature of this pathway is that at resting arterial blood pressure there is ongoing baseline activity in both the efferent and the afferent limbs. The mechanism for generating tonic activity in the RVLM is not fully understood, but as discussed previously, at rest the RVLM provides tonic excitatory input to preganglionic cell bodies in the IML of the spinal cord. Arterial baroreceptor afferent nerves enter the central nervous system and synapse on neurons in the nucleus tractus solitarius (nTS). When arterial blood pressure increases, afferent baroreceptor nerves increase their discharge rate resulting in increased release of the excitatory transmitter glutamate (Glu) from their nerve terminals, which activates second-order neurons in the nTS. Projections from activated nTS neurons then release Glu onto γ-aminobutyric acid (GABA)-containing neurons in the CVLM. Activation of these CVLM neurons results in the release of the inhibitory transmitter GABA from their nerve terminals which synapse on sympathoexcitatory neurons in the RVLM. Inhibition of the RVLM by GABA results in less descending excitatory input to the IML and efferent sympathetic nerve activity to blood vessels and the heart rate decreases. The pathway for arterial baroreflex control of parasympathetic innervation to the heart is depicted in Figure 35.6. An increase in arterial pressure will result in increased baroreceptor afferent nerve discharge and activation of second-order neurons in the nTS which project to the dorsal motor nucleus of the vagus (DMnX) and the nucleus ambiguus (nA). Activation of parasympathetic preganglionic cell bodies located in these medullary nuclei results in increased efferent discharge in the vagus nerve, release of ACh primarily on the conducting system of the heart (SA and AV nodes), and a decrease in heart rate.

Arterial baroreflex function

The arterial baroreflex is a negative feedback system that buffers changes in arterial blood pressure on a beat-to-beat basis. Figure 35.7 demonstrates the baroreflex-mediated adjustments in both sympathetic and parasympathetic branches of the

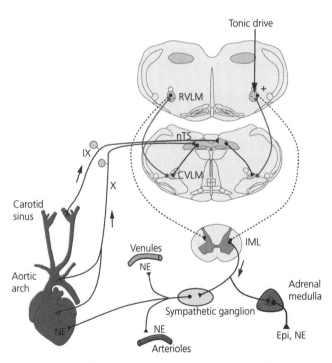

Figure 35.5 Medullary pathway for arterial and cardiopulmonary reflex control of the sympathetic nervous system. IX, glossopharyngeal nerve; X, vagus nerve; nTS, nucleus of the solitary tract; CVLM, caudal ventrolateral medulla; RVLM, rostral ventrolateral medulla; IML, intermediolateral cell column of the spinal cord; Epi, epinephrine; NE, norepinephrine. See text for details.

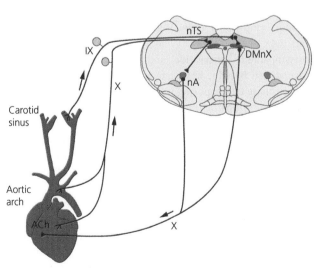

Figure 35.6 Medullary pathway for arterial and cardiopulmonary reflex control of the parasympathetic nervous system. DMnX, dorsal motor nucleus of the vagus; nA, nucleus ambiguus; nTS, nucleus of the solitary tract; ACh, acetylcholine. See text for details.

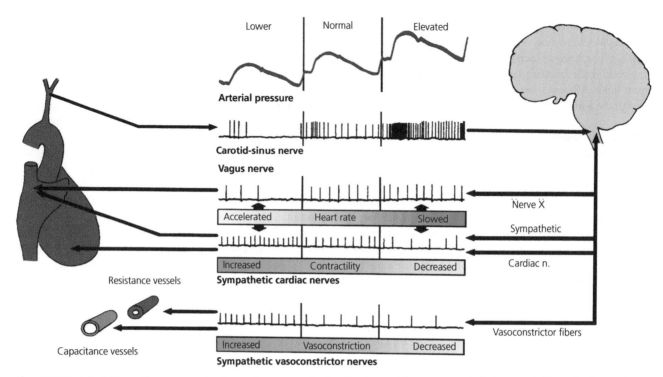

Figure 35.7 Arterial baroreflex responses to changes in pressure. An elevation in arterial pressure results in increased afferent discharge of the carotid sinus nerve, which reflexly decreases efferent sympathetic nerve activity to the heart and blood vessels and increases parasympathetic nerve activity to the heart. When arterial pressure is lowered, the opposite responses occur. In either case reflex responses return blood pressure toward normal levels. Adapted from Schmidt, R.F. and Thews, G. (eds) (1989) *Human Physiology*, 2nd edn. Springer-Verlag, Berlin. Reproduced with permission from Springer-Verlag.

autonomic nervous system in response to perturbations in baseline arterial pressure. Before considering baroreflex adjustments, note that at normal arterial pressure (Figure 35.7, middle panel) there is activity from all neural components of the arterial baroreflex including the afferent and efferent limbs. Both resistance and capacitance vessels are partially constricted due to ongoing sympathetic tone. With regard to determinants of heart rate, the SA and AV nodes receive sympathetic and parasympathetic innervation, and both efferent outflows are active at rest. Baseline heart rate is determined by the balance between these two opposing influences and the relative contribution of the sympathetic and parasympathetic nervous systems varies among species. Stroke volume is influenced by venous return and cardiac contractility. Increases or decreases in sympathetic nerve activity to the capacitance vessels and the ventricles will therefore affect stroke volume and cardiac output (see Chapter 33 for review).

Carotid sinus baroreflex responses to an increase in arterial pressure are shown on the right of Figure 35.7. Increased stretch of carotid sinus baroreceptors results in increased discharge in the carotid sinus nerves. Through the medullary pathways shown in Figures 35.5 and 35.6 this results in increased vagal output to the heart, and decreased sympathetic output to the SA node in the atria, cardiac ventricular muscle, and both capacitance vessels (veins) and resistance vessels (arterioles) in

the periphery. The overall response is a decrease in arterial blood pressure toward control levels due to decreased peripheral resistance and cardiac output. If arterial blood pressure falls below normal levels (Figure 35.7, left side), carotid sinus nerve discharge decreases, activation of the nTS barosensitive neurons decreases, vagal discharge decreases and through disinhibition of the RVLM (removal of inhibitory input from the CVLM), sympathetic nerve activity to the heart and vasculature increases. These adjustments act in concert to bring blood pressure back toward normal levels.

In addition to providing information about average arterial pressure, the rate of discharge in arterial baroreceptor afferent nerves increases if arterial pulse pressure or the rate of rise of pulse pressure increases, even if the mean arterial pressure does not change. In this way, the arterial baroreceptors provide the brain not only with information about blood pressure but also with information related to cardiac function.

The arterial baroreflex compensates for the effects of gravity on the circulation and is critical for the rapid adjustments which maintain circulation to the brain during postural changes. Figure 35.8 shows the predicted blood pressure change in a dog transitioning from a lying to a standing position. If the arterial baroreceptors are surgically denervated, recovery from the initial drop in blood pressure on standing is compromised. This is particularly important in large animals such as the giraffe and horse.

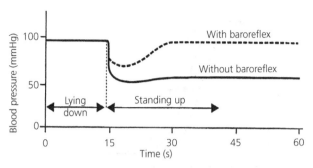

Figure 35.8 Arterial baroreflex maintains blood pressure during postural changes. Diagram shows the blood pressure response to standing in a dog with and without operational baroreflexes. From Figure 17.9, *Dukes' Physiology of Domestic Animals*, 12th edn (ed. W.O. Reece). Cornell University Press, Ithaca, NY. Reproduced with permission from Cornell University Press.

In normal animals there is a narrow range of blood pressure that is ideal for maintenance of adequate blood flow to the various vascular beds. Although the mechanism for determining the blood pressure **set point** is not fully understood, it appears to be independent of arterial baroreceptor input. This is illustrated in a classic study by Cowley *et al.* (Figure 35.9), which demonstrated that although complete surgical denervation of afferent arterial baroreceptor fibers in dogs resulted in an initial profound rise in arterial pressure (not shown), after several weeks mean arterial pressure was no different than in the pre-denervation state. However, in the absence of moment-to-moment buffering by arterial baroreflex input (after surgical denervation), the variability around mean arterial pressure was much greater.

It is generally accepted that mechanisms other than afferent neural input from arterial baroreceptors contribute to the determination of blood pressure set point. However, it is worth noting that other important negative feedback systems were intact in the experiment described in Figure 35.9, and there is evidence that afferent input from stretch receptors in the cardiopulmonary region may contribute to limiting increases in blood pressure set point in the absence of arterial baroreceptors, or in conditions such as exercise where baroreceptor set point is altered.

The approximate operating pressure range for carotid sinus baroreceptors is between 50 and 180 mmHg, although this range varies among species and is related to baseline arterial pressure (see Table 35.1). Even within species the "ideal" blood pressure can vary. For example, greyhounds characteristically maintain higher baseline blood pressure levels than other dogs and thus have a higher baroreceptor reflex set point.

The solid line in Figure 35.10A graphically depicts the typical sigmoidal relationship between mean arterial pressure and afferent baroreceptor nerve discharge at normal resting arterial pressure (**baroreceptor function curve**). Note that the steepest (most sensitive) portion of the curve occurs at pressures near baseline blood pressure, an ideal arrangement for limiting fluctuations in blood pressure. The resultant reciprocal reflex

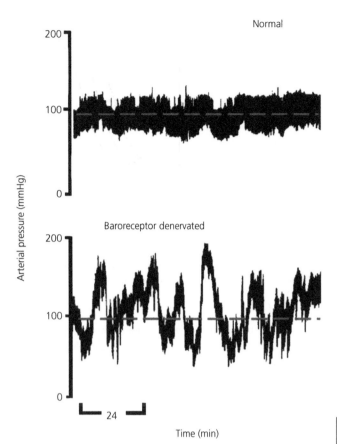

Figure 35.9 Recordings of pulsatile arterial pressure in a normal dog (*top*) and in the same dog (*bottom*) several weeks after baroreceptors were denervated. Arterial pressure was more variable after baroreceptor denervation, but the mean arterial pressure (dashed red lines) was similar with and without baroreceptors. Adapted from Cowley, A.W. Jr, Liard, J.F. and Guyton, A.C. (1973) Role of the baroreceptor reflex in daily control of arterial blood pressure and other variables in dogs. *Circulation Research* **32**:564–576. American Heart Association with permission.

changes in efferent sympathetic nerve discharge are depicted in Figure 35.10B (solid line). The **baroreflex function curve** for control of heart rate (not shown) is similar in directionality to the curve for overall control of efferent sympathetic nerve activity. However, remember that decreases in heart rate with increasing arterial pressure are not only due to decreasing cardiac sympathetic nerve activity, but that increases in efferent vagal discharge to the heart contribute importantly to baroreflex-mediated bradycardia. The responses of the aortic baroreceptors are similar.

Arterial baroreceptor and reflex resetting

As discussed, the arterial baroreceptors are very important for the beat-to-beat regulation of arterial pressure. They represent the most rapidly responding of the regulatory systems for buffering fluctuations in blood pressure, but do not determine the absolute level of blood pressure for long-term regulation. If, for whatever reason, arterial pressure is changed for a period of time, the arterial baroreceptors will reset to operate around the

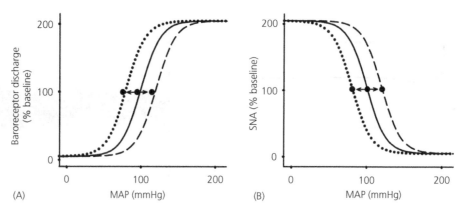

Figure 35.10 Short-term resetting of arterial baroreceptors and baroreflex. (A) Hypothetical curves showing sigmoidal relationship between mean arterial pressure (MAP) and baroreceptor afferent nerve discharge under control conditions (solid line) and after baseline arterial pressure (filled circles) is elevated (dashed line) or lowered (dotted line) for several days. (B) Hypothetical curves showing predicted baroreflex responses under the same conditions. Baroreceptor and baroreflex function curves shift in the direction of the prevailing pressure. Redrawn from Heesch, C.M. (1999) Reflexes that control cardiovascular function. *American Journal of Physiology* **277**:S234–S243. American Physiological Society with permission.

new pressure to which they are exposed. This process begins within a matter of minutes and is virtually complete within a couple of days to weeks. Figure 35.10 shows that exposure to an elevated arterial pressure will result in a rightward shift in the baroreceptor and baroreflex function curves toward higher operating blood pressures, while exposure to decreased blood pressure will result in a leftward shift in the baroreceptor and baroreflex function curves toward lower blood pressures. Although the arterial baroreceptors do not strictly maintain blood pressure around one set point, this rather acute baroreceptor and baroreflex resetting may be viewed as functionally advantageous. Should there be an overriding influence to increase or decrease baseline arterial pressure, the shift in the baroreceptor and baroreflex function curves in the direction of the prevailing pressure allows a wider range of pressures over which the baroreceptors maintain high sensitivity to immediate (beat-to-beat) fluctuations in pressure.

Chronic hypertension

During the initial development of hypertension, when arterial pressure is elevated above the normal level for that animal, the arterial baroreflex will shift to operate around the new elevated pressure, with maintained sensitivity to increments in pressure (Figure 35.10). However, with time, if blood pressure remains elevated, the sensitivity to increments in pressure will decrease. Decreased distensibility of the blood vessel wall (resulting in less stretch of baroreceptors for a given change in pressure) and various mechanisms within the central nervous system have been proposed to contribute to baroreflex resetting in chronic hypertension. The end result is that in established hypertension, the arterial baroreceptor reflex operates at higher pressures and is less able to correct for immediate fluctuations in blood pressure. Although unlikely to be the cause, this chronic baroreflex resetting may contribute to the maintenance of established hypertension.

Cardiopulmonary reflexes

There are stretch receptors located in the atria, ventricles, and pulmonary vessels that are tonically active under normal conditions, and participate in a negative feedback loop, similar to the arterial baroreceptors. Unlike the arterial baroreceptors, which are located on the high-pressure side of the circulation, these receptors are located on the low-pressure side of the circulation. Cardiopulmonary reflexes contribute to the overall regulation of arterial pressure and, in general, when activated or unloaded cause changes in sympathetic and parasympathetic nerve activity that are directionally similar to the reflex changes due to activation or unloading of the arterial baroreceptors. (An exception to this generalization is the tachycardic response that sometimes occurs when the atria are stretched, i.e., the Bainbridge reflex; see Chapter 34.) The effects of arterial and cardiopulmonary reflexes on control of arterial blood pressure are often the result of interactions between the two systems at the level of the central nervous system.

A major contribution of cardiopulmonary reflexes to circulatory control involves regulation of blood volume. The receptors are located in regions that will be stretched when blood volume is increased. Activation of these mechanically sensitive receptors results in a reflex decrease in renal sympathetic nerve activity, decreased renin secretion, and decreased angiotensin II. Vasopressin (ADH) secretion is inhibited through activation of a multisynaptic central nervous system pathway from the nTS to magnocellular neurons in the hypothalamus. Because of these reflex humoral changes, an increase in blood volume is compensated for by a loss of fluid into the urine.

In addition to mechanosensitive stretch receptors, afferent nerves in the heart also demonstrate chemosensitivity. Activation of afferent fibers that express serotonin receptors, primarily in the ventricles of the heart, produces a profound bradycardia and sympathoinhibition (Bezold–Jarisch reflex).

Arterial chemoreflex

The **arterial chemoreceptors** are collections of chemosensitive cells contained in the carotid and aortic bodies. They are located in the same general regions and their afferent nerves travel in the same nerve bundles as the arterial baroreceptors (see Figure 35.4). Per gram of tissue, the carotid bodies receive the highest blood flow of any region in the body. Direct flow measurements indicate a blood flow of approximately 2000 mL/100 g per min to the carotid bodies (for comparison, left ventricular flow at rest is about 80–100 mL/100 g per min). However, oxygen usage by the carotid bodies, about 9 mL/100 g per min, compares with that of the left ventricle. Thus the chemoreceptors are well positioned to sample Pa_{O_2} and provide the brain with information about oxygen delivery by arterial blood. Chemoreceptor reflexes buffer changes in arterial blood gases by controlling breathing. In general, when a decrease in Pa_{O_2} is sensed, increased discharge in the afferent chemoreceptor nerves promotes increased ventilation. This increase in ventilation occurs through medullary pathways from the nTS to respiratory-related cell groups in the medulla that control efferent discharge in motor nerves innervating the diaphragm and other respiratory muscles. Although arterial chemoreflexes are not a major mechanism for blood pressure regulation in normal states, their activation does lead to vasoconstriction mainly through a pathway involving excitation of nTS neurons with direct excitatory projections to the RVLM. In addition to the physiological role of the arterial chemoreflex to buffer changes in Pa_{O_2}, primarily through control of respiration, increased chemoreflex sensitivity has been implicated in overactivity of the sympathetic nervous system in heart failure and in pathological states associated with chronic hypoxia. In these conditions, higher centers, such as the PVN in the hypothalamus, are thought to contribute to increased sympathetic outflow.

Mayer waves, very slow oscillations in arterial pressure (2–3/min), are sometimes observed in hypotensive states. These are thought to be the result of periodic hypoxic stimulation of peripheral chemoreceptors during the nadir in arterial pressure, followed by chemoreflex activation of the sympathetic nervous system. This results in vasoconstriction and elevation of arterial pressure, until blood pressure again decreases and the cycle repeats. Other circumstances in which the respiratory and cardiovascular systems are coupled, such as respiratory sinus arrhythmia (increased heart rate during inspiration; see Chapter 34) and **Traube–Hering waves** (increases in blood pressure and sympathetic nerve activity synchronized with respiratory rate), are less dependent on afferent input and more likely the result of central nervous system interaction between brain regions responsible for controlling respiratory and cardiovascular function.

Heart rate responses to arterial chemoreceptor stimulation will vary depending on the respiratory effects. While chemoreceptor activation can increase vagal nerve activity and decrease heart rate, hypoxia also increases breathing and adrenal catecholamine secretion which can result in an increase in heart rate. With robust increases in ventilation, the overall effect of chemoreceptor stimulation will be an increase in heart rate.

In addition to input from peripheral chemoreceptors, which are activated primarily by decreased Pa_{O_2}, there are neurons within the central nervous system that are chemosensitive and are most responsive to an increase in Pa_{CO_2}. Activation of **central chemoreceptors** generally results in increased ventilation, increased sympathetic outflow, and increased blood pressure mediated by projections within the brainstem to respiratory and sympathetic outflow pathways.

Exercise pressor reflex

The **exercise pressor reflex**, also called the **somatic pressor reflex**, originates from sensory receptors located in exercising muscle and is characterized by an increase in arterial pressure and heart rate. Although this reflex can be demonstrated during both dynamic and static exercise, it is especially prominent during static exercise, where large increases in intramuscular pressure limit blood flow to active skeletal muscle. The afferent limb of this reflex is mediated by both mechanical and chemical stimuli acting on group III and IV muscle afferent nerves within the exercising muscle. Chemical activation of muscle sensory receptors is due to accumulation of byproducts of muscle metabolism, including lactic acid, H^+, K^+, adenosine, ATP analogs, and prostaglandins. Muscle afferent nerves from the muscle enter the dorsal horn of the spinal cord and project rostrally to, among other regions, the RVLM. When these muscle afferent fibers are activated, the efferent response is an increase in blood pressure and heart rate due to activation of sympathetic nerve activity and withdrawal of parasympathetic nerve activity. The overall effect is to increase blood pressure, which increases blood flow and oxygen delivery to the exercising muscle.

Reflex control of humoral systems

In addition to controlling the autonomic efferent outflow to blood vessels and the heart, cardiovascular reflexes modulate the secretion of vasoactive humoral agents. Decreased afferent discharge from arterial and cardiopulmonary receptors results in reflex increases in circulating levels of adrenal catecholamines, vasopressin, and angiotensin II. The effects on catecholamine secretion are mediated through efferent sympathetic nerves to the adrenal medulla. The effects on vasopressin secretion are via a central pathway to the hypothalamus. Sympathetic efferent nerves to the kidney control secretion of the enzyme renin and increases in renin secretion due to sympathetic stimulation increase circulating levels of angiotensin II. Hypoxic activation of carotid body chemoreceptors results in increased secretion of vasopressin, angiotensin II, and adrenal corticosteroids, including aldosterone. These humoral substances have vasoconstrictor properties and contribute to reflex adjustments in vascular resistance. However, the main peripheral effects of vasopressin (ADH) and angiotensin II are on the kidney and they influence arterial pressure primarily by regulating blood volume.

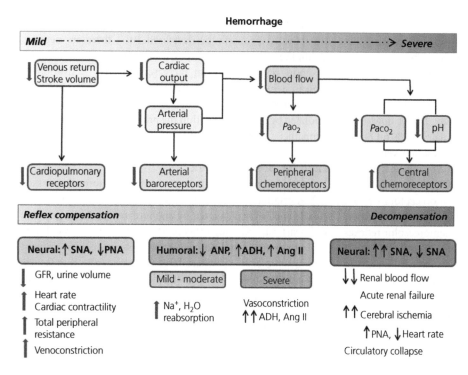

Figure 35.11 Cardiovascular reflex responses to progressive hemorrhage. Cardiopulmonary receptors, arterial baroreceptors, peripheral chemoreceptors, and central chemoreceptors contribute to neural and humoral compensatory responses to blood loss. See text for details. SNA, sympathetic nerve activity; PNA, parasympathetic nerve activity; GFR, glomerular filtration rate; Ang II, angiotensin II; ANP, atrial natriuretic peptide; ADH, antidiuretic hormone.

Integrated response to hemorrhage

In response to both physiological and pathophysiological challenges, the various reflexes seldom act in isolation. As an example, compensatory responses to progressive blood loss involve activation of multiple reflex systems involving both neural and humoral components, which work in concert to restore cardiac output and perfusion pressure (Figure 35.11). An initial loss of blood, up to 10% of total blood volume, results in little or no decrease in arterial blood pressure. The decrease in blood volume and venous return reduces stretch and thus "unloads" volume receptors on the low-pressure side of the circulation (cardiopulmonary receptors). As hemorrhage progresses, increased sympathetic nerve activity, especially to the kidney, results in vasoconstriction, decreased glomerular filtration rate, and decreased urine volume. Pulse pressure and blood pressure begin to fall and afferent discharge in arterial baroreceptors decreases and contributes to increased sympathetic nerve activity and decreased parasympathetic nerve activity. Heart rate, cardiac contractility, and total peripheral resistance increase and venoconstriction promotes venous return to the heart. The arteriolar constriction in response to hemorrhage is most pronounced in the cutaneous, skeletal muscle, and splanchnic beds, favoring maintenance of blood flow in the cerebral and coronary circulations. Although sympathetic outflow to the kidney increases, autoregulatory mechanisms in the kidney protect against ischemic damage until blood loss becomes severe.

Decreased stretch of the atrium due to reduced blood volume results in diminished secretion of ANP, while decreased renal perfusion pressure promotes secretion of renin and activation of the renin–angiotensin–aldosterone system. In addition, both cardiopulmonary and arterial baroreflex mechanisms promote increased circulating levels of ADH (vasopressin), angiotensin II, and aldosterone. These humoral changes promote sodium and water reabsorption in the kidney. As levels of ADH and angiotensin II continue to rise, direct vasoconstrictor effects of these peptides contribute to increased total peripheral resistance. If blood loss continues and mean arterial pressure falls to levels near the threshold for baroreceptor discharge (~60 mmHg in most species), baroreflex mechanisms are already maximally operational and no additional compensation due to baroreflex unloading is possible. With more severe hemorrhage, peripheral chemoreceptors sense hypoxia (decreased Pa_{O_2}) due to inadequate blood flow to the carotid body and contribute to further increases in sympathetic outflow. In addition, increased ventilation due to chemoreflex activation assists in promoting venous return. If cerebral ischemia occurs, elevated Pa_{CO_2} and decreased blood pH activate chemosensitive neurons in the brain, which results in a massive activation of the sympathoadrenal systems.

Although the compensatory mechanisms discussed here are able to restore arterial pressure and cardiac output following mild to moderate hemorrhage, it is important to realize that longer-term processes are critical for complete restoration of blood volume. These include Starling forces at the level of the microcirculation to move fluid and plasma proteins into the circulation (see Chapter 36), new synthesis of plasma proteins by the liver, and behavioral mechanisms regulating thirst and salt appetite (see Chapter 11) to restore the lost volume.

Pronounced renal and splanchnic vasoconstriction during severe hemorrhage help maintain adequate perfusion of the heart and brain. However, if prolonged, vasoconstriction in these circulations can result in irreversible damage. A patient may survive the initial blood loss, but die several days later due to acute renal failure. Prolonged intestinal ischemia may result in liver damage, an increase in intestinal blood loss, and the release of potent vasodilatory endotoxins into the general circulation.

Decompensation during hemorrhagic shock is the irreversible process whereby the hypotension induced by blood loss initiates processes which aggravate the hypotension and lead to circulatory failure and death. Acidosis, central nervous system depression, aberrations in blood clotting, cardiac failure, and increased circulating endotoxins are all factors which may participate in circulatory collapse in hemorrhagic shock (see Chapter 40). These processes are most likely to ensue with severe hemorrhage. The obvious therapeutic goal in treating a patient that has experienced hemorrhage is to treat rapidly and aggressively, preferably with infusion of whole blood, prior to the development of irreversible processes.

Centrally integrated patterns of circulatory responses

Stereotyped patterns of circulatory response characterized by specific changes in blood flow distribution and cardiac output occur in exercise, the defense reaction, diving, and thermoregulation. The hypothalamus is an important integrating center for many of these responses. In some cases influences from cortical and subcortical autonomic areas (especially the limbic system) and the premotor and motor cortex also contribute. Relay stations are found in mesencephalic structures and the medulla oblongata. Importantly, multiple afferent sensory inputs may interact within the central nervous system to produce the final integrated output.

Exercise

At the onset of exercise there is decreased vagal discharge and increased sympathetic adrenergic discharge to the heart and many vascular beds that results in increased cardiac output, vasoconstriction in nonexercising parts of the body, and vasodilation in the vascular beds of the exercising muscles. This results in alterations in regional peripheral resistance so that most of the increased blood flow goes to the exercising muscles. The cardiac and blood pressure adjustments that occur during exercise in fact begin before the exercise starts (**central command**). During dynamic exercise, both arterial blood pressure and heart rate increase. Arterial baroreflex function resets with an upward and rightward shift in the baroreflex function curve, so that, importantly, sensitivity to increments in pressure is maintained around the new set point (elevated arterial pressure and heart rate). Central nervous system modulation of baroreflex function by both central command and the exercise pressor reflex contribute to resetting of the baroreflex set point during exercise. Cardiopulmonary negative feedback reflexes are activated by increased venous return during exercise,

and the overall effect of cardiopulmonary reflex activation appears to be a restraint on the increase in sympathetic nerve activity, heart rate, and the degree of baroreflex resetting during exercise.

Defense response

The **defense reaction** in mammals (**fight or flight response**), extensively studied in cats, is classically defined by the combination of behavioral, somatic, and autonomic nervous system (primarily sympathetic) responses that accompany alerting, fear, or rage. Piloerection and pupillary dilation occur. Increased efferent sympathetic discharge to the heart accounts for tachycardia and increased cardiac contractility. Increased sympathetic nerve activity to the splanchnic, cutaneous, and renal circulations produces vasoconstriction in these vascular beds. However, blood flow to skeletal muscle is increased due to withdrawal of sympathetic outflow to skeletal muscle arterioles and, in some species (e.g., cats), activation of sympathetic cholinergic vasodilator fibers. This coordinated pattern of cardiovascular responses is integrated primarily at the level of the dorsal medial hypothalamus and prepares the animal for aggression or retreat in response to a threat.

Diving reflex

In diving mammals and birds, reflex bradycardia and vasoconstriction occur when the nostrils are submerged in water. The magnitude of the reflex response increases as water temperature decreases. The afferent limb of the reflex is in the trigeminal nerve (cranial nerve V) and the initial response to submersion is vagally mediated bradycardia, followed by increased sympathetic nerve activity and peripheral vasoconstriction. Blood flow to skeletal muscles and other tissues is thus restricted so that most of the blood flow is channeled to the heart and brain, conserving oxygen for these vital organs. Arteriovenous shunts in the skin remain patent, allowing a small venous return of blood that has not lost oxygen within the tissues. When the animal resurfaces, these changes are reversed; cardiac output and muscle blood flow promptly increase, the accumulated oxygen debt is repaid, and metabolites are removed from the muscles and other tissues that were poorly perfused.

Thermoregulatory responses

The skin is the largest organ of the body and regulation of cutaneous blood flow plays a critical role in control of core body temperature. Thermoregulatory responses are under control of the hypothalamus. With increased heat load, these responses include cutaneous vasodilation and opening of arteriovenous anastomoses by reduced sympathetic vasoconstrictor discharge. The result is redistribution of blood flow from other organs to increase cutaneous flow and favor heat loss. Local cooling of the hypothalamus or skin has the opposite effect. Thermoregulatory mechanisms and species differences are discussed in detail in Chapter 14.

Long-term regulation of blood pressure

> 1 Are arterial baroreflexes more important for short-term or long-term regulation of blood pressure?
>
> 2 What is the overall goal of integrated cardiovascular regulatory mechanisms?

As discussed throughout this chapter, important short-term neural reflexes and their interaction with humoral control systems contribute to the moment-to-moment regulation of arterial blood pressure. However, the mechanisms for long-term regulation of blood pressure, or whether there is one site or organ system which determines an ideal set point, remains controversial.

A widely accepted model proposed by Guyton and colleagues proposes that the blood pressure set point is dependent on the kidney, whereby arterial pressure is set at a level which will maintain sodium balance (Na^+ and water excretion equals Na^+ and water intake). By this model, increased sodium retention by the kidney would result in an initial increase in blood volume and increased cardiac output. The resultant increase in arterial pressure would promote excretion of the excess sodium. Hypertension would result if the renal pressure–natriuresis relationship reset, such that higher pressures were required to accomplish sodium balance. There is also convincing evidence that the brain, which receives input from sensory receptors throughout the body, is a major determinant of blood pressure set point. Various manipulations that modify central nervous system sites involved in regulation of sympathetic nerve activity can change set point, either promoting or attenuating the development of hypertension.

It is likely that mechanisms proposed in both of these models contribute to long-term regulation of blood pressure. Regardless, there is general agreement that the ultimate goal of cardiovascular regulation is to provide adequate perfusion (blood flow) and oxygen delivery to tissues throughout the body under a variety of physiological conditions. Regionally specific changes in flow, based on the needs of a particular tissue under a particular condition, are required and neural, humoral, and local control mechanisms acting in concert are critical to accomplish this goal.

Self-evaluation

Answers can be found at the end of the chapter.

1 Which of the following substances released from postganglionic sympathetic nerve terminals contribute in vasoconstriction?
   A Neuropeptide Y (NPY)
   B Acetylcholine (ACh)
   C Norepinephrine (NE)
   D Angiotensin II

2 The decrease in blood pressure that occurs in a hypertensive animal following blockade of the enzyme kininase II (angiotensin-converting enzyme, ACE) may be due to:

A Vasodilation as a result of decreased production of kinins
B Vasodilation as a result of decreased angiotensin II
C Vasodilation as a result of increased kinins
D Increased Na^+ reabsorption by the kidney

3 Which of the following is true regarding carotid body chemoreceptors.
   A Arterial chemoreceptors are primarily sensitive to changes in partial pressure of oxygen in the arterial blood (Pao_2) and increase their discharge rate when Pao_2 decreases
   B The arterial chemoreflex is critical for beat-to-beat regulation of arterial blood pressure
   C When afferent nerves from the carotid chemoreceptors are activated, they initiate a negative feedback loop which results in inhibition of efferent sympathetic nerve activity
   D Input from arterial chemoreceptors is critical for producing respiratory sinus arrhythmia

4 The arterial baroreflex response to a decrease in arterial blood pressure is:
   A Increased discharge in sympathetic nerves to the heart and blood vessels
   B Decreased discharge in arterial baroreceptor afferent nerves
   C Decreased discharge in the vagus nerve to the heart
   D An increase in heart rate, cardiac contractility, vasoconstriction, and increased venous return

5 In response to progressive hemorrhage:
   A Early activation of central chemoreceptors, which sense decreased Pao_2 in the cerebral circulation, limits the secretion of vasoconstrictor humoral substances such as vasopressin and angiotensin II
   B ANP secretion from the atria is increased and contributes to maintenance of renal function in response to decreased blood volume and the resultant decrease in renal blood flow
   C Early in hemorrhage, vasoconstriction in the renal and coronary circulation limits fluid loss and decreases the workload on the heart
   D Cardiopulmonary reflexes act in concert with the arterial baroreflex to maintain arterial pressure by increasing sympathetic nerve activity and the secretion of vasopressin and angiotensin II

Suggested reading

Barrett, K.E., Barman, S.M., Boitano, S. and Brooks, H.L. (2012) Cardiovascular regulatory mechanisms. In: *Ganong's Review of Medical Physiology*, 24th edn. McGraw-Hill Companies, Inc., New York.

Berne, R.M. and Levy, M.N. (2008) *Cardiovascular Physiology*, 8th edn. Mosby, St Louis, MO.

Boulpaep, E.L. (2009) Regulation of arterial pressure and cardiac output. In: *Medical Physiology*, 2nd edn (eds W.F. Boron and E.L. Boulpaep), pp. 554–576. Saunders Elsevier, Philadelphia.

Erickson, H.H. and Detweiler, D.K. (2004) Control mechanisms of the circulatory system. In: *Dukes' Physiology of Domestic Animals*, 12th edn (ed. W.O. Reece), pp. 275–302. Cornell University Press, Ithaca, NY.

Fadel, P.J. and Raven, P.B. (2012) Human investigations into the arterial and cardiopulmonary baroreflexes during exercise. *Experimental Physiology* **97**:39–50.

Hall, J.E. (2010) Nervous regulation of the circulation, and rapid control of arterial pressure. In: *Guyton and Hall Textbook of Medical Physiology*, 12th edn. Saunders Elsevier, Philadelphia.

Heesch, C.M. (1999) Reflexes that control cardiovascular function. *American Journal of Physiology* **277**:S234–S243.

Llewellyn-Smith, I.J. and Verberne, A.J.M. (2011) *Central Regulation of Autonomic Functions*, 2nd edn. Oxford University Press, New York.

Smith, S.A., Mitchell, J.H. and Garry, M.G. (2006) The mammalian exercise pressor reflex in health and disease. *Experimental Physiology* **91**:89–102.

Westfall, T.C. and Westfall, D.P. (2011) Neurotransmission: the autonomic and somatic motor nervous systems. In: *Goodman and Gilman's Pharmacological Basis of Therapeutics*, 12th edn (eds L.L. Brunton, B.A. Chabner and B.C. Knollmann). McGraw-Hill Companies, Inc., New York.

Answers

1 A, C. NE, the primary transmitter released from adrenergic nerve terminals, and NPY, an important cotransmitter often released with NE, are both potent vasoconstrictors. ACh is released primarily from postganglionic parasympathetic nerves. Although in certain species sympathetic cholinergic fibers innervate the skeletal muscle vascular bed, the effect of ACh released from these terminals is vasodilation. Angiotensin II is not released from postganglionic sympathetic nerve terminals, although angiotensin II present in the tissue can have a presynaptic effect to increase NE release from sympathetic nerve terminals.

2 B, C. In the renin–angiotensin–aldosterone pathway, kininase II (ACE) converts angiotensin I to the active peptide angiotensin II. In the kallikrein–kinin pathway, this enzyme degrades vasodilator kinins to inactive metabolites. Since angiotensin II is a vasoconstrictor that promotes Na^+ retention, and the kinins are vasodilators that promote Na+ excretion, blockade of the enzyme kininase II will decrease angiotensin II and increase kinins. Both actions will have an antihypertensive effect.

3 A. Carotid body chemoreceptors are most sensitive to changes in PaO_2, although increased $PaCO_2$ and decreased pH of arterial blood can also activate them. The response to arterial chemoreflex activation is an increase in sympathetic nerve activity and blood pressure increases; however, their major function in a normal animal is related to control of breathing. Respiratory sinus arrhythmia does not involve arterial chemoreflex activation.

4 All the choices are correct. A decrease in arterial pressure "unloads" arterial baroreceptors and decreases discharge in the baroreceptor afferent nerves. This results in a reflex decrease in vagal activity to the heart and increased sympathetic nerve activity to the heart and blood vessels (resistance and capacitance vessels). Peripheral resistance and cardiac output (heart rate × stroke volume) will increase and correct for the initial drop in arterial pressure.

5 D. Mild to moderate hemorrhage engages cardiopulmonary and arterial baroreflex mechanisms to maintain arterial pressure and limit loss of Na^+ and water through both neural (increased sympathetic, decreased vagal tone) and humoral (increased ADH and angiotensin II) mechanisms. Central chemoreceptors are activated by increased PaCO2 when blood loss is severe. Decreased blood volume results in less stretch of the atria and ANP secretion will decrease. Blood flow is redistributed to favor the cerebral and coronary circulations. In addition, local autoregulatory mechanisms in these regions, as well as in the kidney, contribute to maintenance of blood flow to these organ systems until blood loss is severe.

Section VI: The Cardiovascular System

36 Microcirculation, Lymph, and Edema

Luis A. Martinez-Lemus and M. Harold Laughlin
University of Missouri, Columbia, MO, USA

Functional organization of the vascular bed

1 How are the blood vessels classified according to function?
2 Which vessels are the major site of resistance?
3 Which vessels contain most of the blood volume?
4 Which vascular beds are encompassed in the microcirculation?
5 What kind of cells are the capillaries composed of?
6 What are the three general types of capillaries and where are they found?
7 What is the mean pressure in the systemic capillaries?
8 What is the mechanism for control of flow through and between individual capillaries?
9 Are there more erythrocytes in 100 mL of blood in the capillaries than in the larger vessels?

As blood circulates through the body, it passes in series through the parts of the circulatory system that have the functions designated in Figure 36.1. Each part of the body receives blood through a series of vessels. For the body as a whole, however, the circulation consists of multiple series like this, arranged in parallel channels.

Vascular classification by function

Vessels may be classified in accordance with their function as follows.
1 Conduit elastic vessels convert pulsatile inflow to a somewhat smoothed outflow.
2 Resistance vessels are the small arteries, the arterioles, and to a lesser extent the capillaries and smallest veins. Precapillary resistance resides primarily in the small arteries and arterioles. Postcapillary resistance is determined by the venules and veins. Capillary hydrostatic pressure and filtration–absorption exchange are determined by the ratio of precapillary to postcapillary resistance.
3 Terminal arterioles are the end segments of precapillary arterioles that control capillary flow. They determine the functioning area of capillary exchange surface.
4 Exchange vessels are the capillaries, which are not contractile but respond passively to changes in resistance and terminal arterioles.
5 Capacitance vessels are the veins that, through diameter changes that have little influence on resistance, can effect marked shifts of blood volume and dramatically affect venous return and volume flow. They contain about 80% of the regional blood volume.
6 Shunt vessels are arteriovenous anastomoses found in some tissues; these vessels allow the blood to bypass exchange vessels.

Resistance and capacitance vessels may react in accordance with their functions. Epinephrine dilates some resistance vessels while constricting capacitance vessels; norepinephrine constricts both but affects capacitance vessels more.

The microcirculation

The **microcirculation** is that portion of the circulatory system that is indistinguishable to the naked eye. It is composed of arterioles, capillaries, venules, and small lymphatics. Its major function is the transport of oxygen and nutrients to the tissues and the removal of waste products from the tissues.

Dukes' Physiology of Domestic Animals, Thirteenth Edition. Edited by William O. Reece, Howard H. Erickson, Jesse P. Goff and Etsuro E. Uemura.
© 2015 John Wiley & Sons, Inc. Published 2015 by John Wiley & Sons, Inc.
Companion website: www.wiley.com/go/reece/physiology

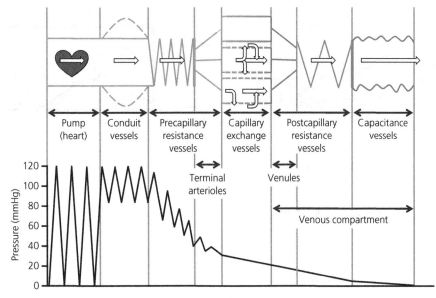

Figure 36.1 Functionally differentiated segments of the vascular bed. Adapted from Mellander, S. and Johansson, B. (1968) Control of resistance, exchange, and capacitance functions in the peripheral circulation. *Pharmacological Reviews* **20**:117–196. American Society for Pharmacology and Experimental Therapeutics.

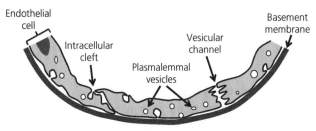

Figure 36.2 Structure of the capillary wall showing single layer of endothelial cells and an intercellular cleft at the junction between adjacent endothelial cells. Adapted from Fig. 16.1, Hall, J.E. and Guyton, A.C. (2001) *Textbook of Medical Physiology*, 10th edn. W.B. Saunders, Philadelphia. With permission from Elsevier.

Capillaries

The capillary bed is the main portion of the microcirculation where the exchange or transport of nutrients and waste occurs. As cells within tissues change their metabolic rate, adjustments in exchange or transport of nutrients and waste products are required. These adjustments take place through variations in the numbers of capillaries that are perfused with blood, which causes a change in diffusion surface, capillary blood volume, and the rate of blood movement through the capillaries.

The capillary is a small tube of internal diameter slightly smaller than the size of a nondeformed erythrocyte of the same animal species. Its wall is composed of a single layer of endothelial cells that does not exceed 0.5 μm in thickness except at the location of the cellular nucleus (Figure 36.2). Additional commonly found components of the capillary wall are a basement membrane, composed mainly of collagen IV, and a scarce

number of pericytes. Three general types of capillaries are distinguished on the basis of the completeness of their endothelial walls (Figure 36.3).

1 Continuous capillaries with complete endothelial walls and basement membranes are found in adipose tissue; smooth, skeletal, and cardiac muscle; the placenta; the lungs; and the central nervous system. They have pinocytic vesicles (60–70 nm in diameter) along their luminal and basal borders, form tight junctions with adjacent cells, and have pores or intercellular clefts between cells that allow the passage of water-soluble ions and molecules across the capillary wall. Many of these capillaries also possess gap junctions that allow for cell-to-cell communication along the capillary wall.

2 Discontinuous capillaries or sinusoids have gaps between the endothelial cells and incomplete or absent basement membranes. They are found in the liver, spleen, and bone marrow and allow passage of whole cells, macromolecules, and particles across the capillary wall. Although capillaries are generally considered passive, contractile properties of endothelial cells have been observed in liver sinusoids.

3 Fenestrated capillaries contain small openings of 0.1 μm or less in diameter that are closed (except for glomerular capillaries) by a thin diaphragm. These holes or fenestrae allow the rapid diffusion of solutes and water across the capillary wall. Fenestrated capillaries are found in endocrine and exocrine glands, gallbladder, synovial membrane, ciliary body, and choroid plexus and in countercurrent flow systems as found in the renal medulla.

Functionally, blood flows from an artery into arterioles that become smaller in internal diameter as they branch. The

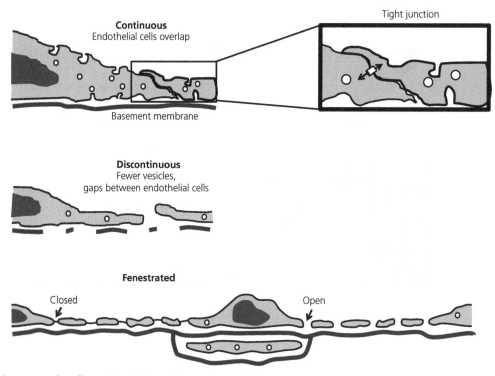

Figure 36.3 Three types of capillaries classified according to the completeness of the endothelium. Adapted from Majno, G. (1965) Ultrastructure of the vascular membrane. In: Hamilton, W.F. and Dow, P. (eds) *Handbook of Physiology*. Section 2: Circulation, Vol. **3**. American Physiological Society, Washington, DC.

terminal arterioles then lead into capillaries and capillary-like channels that connect directly with venules. In some vascular beds, such as portions of the rat mesentery, at the ostia of each capillary there is a small precapillary sphincter of smooth muscle. Sympathetic vasoconstrictor fibers innervate the arterioles and occasionally extend as far downstream as the terminal arterioles. However, the terminal arterioles are not usually innervated and are chiefly under the control of local conditions in the tissues. Under natural conditions the terminal arterioles undergo vasomotion with periodic contractions that last from seconds to a few minutes. When the tissue is in a resting state, the constrictor phase of this rhythm predominates and blood flow may be completely interrupted. When the tissue becomes active, terminal arterioles dilate allowing blood flow to the tissue. In contrast to this active vasomotion is the passive opening or closing of the capillaries. Their open or closed state depends on the hydrostatic pressure relationships within and without the capillary tube. The intracapillary pressure is controlled by the diameter of the upstream terminal arteriole, while the external capillary pressure depends on mechanical forces applied to the tissue in question. In skeletal muscle, the increase in blood flow produced during exercise is the result of dilation of arterioles decreasing vascular resistance and this is associated with recruitment of additional capillary exchange area (discussed later) through increased perfusion of capillaries as upstream arterioles dilate.

Capillary blood pressure

The mean hydrostatic blood pressure for systemic capillaries is about 25 mmHg. However, capillary pressure is normally quite variable both among and within tissues. Blood pressure decreases from the arterial to the venous end of the capillary, while capillary diameter usually increases. In systemic capillaries, pressures are 35 and 15 mmHg, respectively. This pressure gradient is higher per unit length than in any other segment of the vascular system except for the arterioles. Capillary pressure is an important determinant not only for capillary flow but also for exchange of fluid between the capillaries and the interstitial fluid. Pulse pressures are damped out in the arterioles and in the proximal segments of the capillaries.

Mean capillary pressure is determined by venous pressures downstream of the capillary, by blood pressure, and the interaction of vascular resistance in the arteriolar tree (precapillary pressure) and postcapillary resistance (resistance in the venous circulation). The capillary walls have no smooth muscle and are relatively inelastic. Changes in the relationship between the resistance to flow in vessels upstream and downstream from the capillary, specifically the ratio of postcapillary to precapillary resistance, determine capillary pressures if arterial and venous pressures are normal. Although precapillary resistance is relatively large due to the difference between mean arterial pressure (100 mmHg) and mean capillary pressure (25 mmHg), postcapillary resistance is relatively small because the difference between normal mean capillary pressure (25 mmHg) and mean peripheral venous pressure (6 mmHg) is small (19 mmHg). Thus a change in postcapillary resistance has a much larger effect on capillary pressure than the same change in precapillary resistance (five to ten times).

Normally an autoregulatory mechanism stabilizes capillary blood pressure and flow by altering postcapillary and precapillary resistance simultaneously, thus maintaining a normal ratio. When venous resistance to capillary outflow increases, capillary pressure increases. The smooth muscle in terminal arterioles responds by contracting the inflow vessels, and as a result capillary pressure returns to normal. This mechanism may be interrupted by potent vasoactive substances such as histamine and bradykinin.

Capillary blood flow

The total volume of blood flowing through the systemic capillaries is equal to the cardiac output. Compared with the systemic circulation, capillary blood flow is slow and remarkably nonuniform. The primary control of flow through and between individual capillaries occurs at the terminal arteriole. Terminal arterioles guard the entrances into capillary networks and serve as gates, with contractions that vary in frequency and duration. After blood enters the capillaries, the resistance to flow is determined by the complex anastomotic network of capillary tubes, the internal diameter of the tubes, which is usually greater at the venular than the arteriolar end, and the venular pressure. Pressure changes in the venules draining the capillaries and variations in arterial pressure due to the activity of the terminal arterioles cause the flow in capillaries to change intensity, reverse direction, or bypass some routes.

Additional factors that contribute to capillary flow include the presence of intermittent flow due to variations in extramural pressure on thin-walled vessels during muscular contraction (e.g., in the heart and skeletal muscle). In addition, obstruction by leukocytes may occur due to the ratio of capillary to leukocyte diameter. As mentioned earlier, capillary lumens are usually smaller than the erythrocytes. These cells are deformed as they pass through the small capillary lumen. They can pass through artificial pores less than half the size of their own diameters without incurring injury. Consequently, the rigidity of erythrocytes has been associated with conditions that affect flow through capillary beds such as pulmonary arterial hypertension in broiler chickens.

There are fewer erythrocytes per 100 mL of blood in the capillaries and other small vessels than in the larger vessels feeding and draining them. Consequently, the packed cell volume or hematocrit is lower relative to the amount of plasma. This is caused by the axial streaming of blood cells in blood vessels. In the very small vessels, such as the small arterioles, capillaries, and small venules, the red blood cells cannot flow near the vascular wall while plasma does. Therefore, the ratio of plasma to red blood cells is much greater in the small vessels such as the capillaries than in the large vessels.

The microcirculation is particularly susceptible to blood cell aggregation as occurs during inflammation, infections, shock, and the extracorporeal circulation of blood. Aggregation leads to the trapping of cells (a kind of anemia), stasis of flow in capillaries, and shunting of flow through arteriovenous anastomoses. Therapeutically it is reversed by the infusion of saline solutions or solutions of low-molecular-weight dextrans.

The pressure in the aorta and large arteries supplying the peripheral circulation is maintained at a relatively constant level through a series of reflexes that maintain perfusion pressure homeostasis (see Chapter 35). In addition, peripheral vascular beds possess intrinsic or local mechanisms that control vascular resistance and blood flow to the tissues. For example, exercise results in **vasodilation** within the exercising muscles, and digestion is accompanied by an increase in blood flow to the splanchnic circulation. When functional activity subsides, flow is diminished. If pressure in the large arteries transiently increases or decreases, local mechanisms preserve the normal rate of flow. Therefore, blood flow in many peripheral vascular beds is maintained relatively constant and, accordingly, is largely autoregulated.

Tone

Microvascular **tone** refers to the level of active constriction observed in the vessels comprising the microcirculation. Arterioles and venules are capable of developing active constriction, while capillaries are usually not. However, some capillary tubes are able to constrict in response to adrenergic stimulation. Based on their capacity to reduce their diameter from maximal dilation, terminal arterioles are the microvessels with greatest tone capabilities. A terminal arteriole is considered to have tone when contracting in a regular rhythmic fashion or even maximally to occlude blood flow. The tone of peripheral vessels is variable not only within the same vascular bed but also from bed to bed. *In vivo*, the degree of tone can be estimated by comparing the average blood flow through a tissue to that occurring when the vessels are maximally dilated. The latter condition is usually achieved with the use of potent vasodilators or disruptors of the vascular smooth muscle contractile machinery. The degree of tone in the microcirculation of a tissue at rest is a measure of its circulatory reserve. The reduction in vascular tone or vasodilation that occurs as a tissue changes from a resting state to increased activity (e.g., exercise) is important for balancing variations in the tissue demands for metabolic exchange and the amount of blood flow.

Vascular tone can be **myogenic** (intrinsic) or neural/humoral in origin, or both. This is due to the inherent property of automaticity found in vascular and other smooth muscle, and because microvessels may be innervated by vasoconstrictor nerve fibers. Intrinsic vascular tone persists after surgical or chemical interruption of all efferent vasomotor fibers and in the absence of circulating vasoactive compounds. The tone of blood vessels due to myogenic automatic contractility is called **basal tone**. The magnitude of basal tone is usually inversely related to the density of vasoconstrictor innervation and passive arteriolar diameter. Basal tone is relatively high in the vascular beds of the brain and myocardium; more moderate in skeletal muscle, splanchnic viscera, and kidneys; and very low or absent in the skin. Basal tone, however, may be quite variable among different vascular beds of similar types of tissue, and is subject to modulation by both extrinsic neural and local mechanisms.

The level of vascular tone varies depending on the nature and intensity of the stimuli that cause it and on the sensitivity of specific vascular beds to those stimuli. The stimuli for tone include impulses conducted over autonomic vasomotor nerves, vasoactive hormones originating in remote organs, autocrine or paracrine noncirculating vasoactive chemicals released locally, and local physical stimuli. The main physical stimuli originate from changes in hemodynamics including variations in shear rate, produced by changes in flow velocity and transmural pressure in the arterioles. Because changes in transmural pressure initially result in stretching force, stretch is considered the predominant physical stimulus. However, experimental data indicate that wall tension is the parameter normalized by intrinsic myogenic tone. Consequently, myogenically active vessels exposed to step changes in transmural pressure are able to constrict or dilate to diameters smaller or larger than those observed before the change in pressure. This suggests that stimuli other than stretching and sensors other than those activated by stretch participate in myogenic phenomena. The precise stimuli or sensors controlling basal tone are therefore not yet fully elucidated. Transmural pressure varies with the level of hydrostatic blood pressure, the pressure of the tissue fluid, and the contractions of skeletal muscles or surrounding tissue.

Autoregulation

Autoregulation refers to the process of local intrinsic regulation of blood flow whereby blood flow is maintained relatively unchanged despite changes in perfusion pressure. This process assures that the concentration of cell nutrients and waste products is maintained in a normal range despite variations in perfusion pressure, metabolic rate, or the influence of extrinsic vasomotor nerves. Autoregulation occurs at the level of the microcirculation through mechanisms that adjust vascular resistance. Consequently, arterioles are the main effectors of the autoregulation process as they are responsible for 65–80% of total vascular resistance in most vascular beds such the intestine and skeletal muscle. Autoregulation is important for the adjustment of the volumetric flow rate to the metabolic rate in individual tissues, and for the selective distribution of total blood flow among all the body tissues. In general, all vascular beds, except the pulmonary circulation, possess variable levels of autoregulation that occur over the physiological range of vascular pressures. The process of autoregulation interacts with other mechanisms that control blood flow and may be fully surmounted by them.

It is generally believed that two mechanisms are responsible for the autoregulation of blood flow: myogenic and metabolic. The myogenic mechanism, discovered by Sir William Maddock Bayliss, indicates that vascular smooth muscle responds by contracting when the transmural pressure increases and relaxing when it decreases. The metabolic hypothesis proposes a mechanism capable of acting on detected differences in the concentration of some chemical(s) (metabolites) so that tissue metabolism and vascular smooth muscle constitute a local control system.

Evidence of myogenic autoregulation has been obtained by perfusing denervated isolated vascular preparations *in vivo*, which eliminates neural and hormonal vasoactive factors. In this experimental scenario, the perfusion pressure in the arterial supply vessels may be adjusted. As pressure in these vessels is either increased or decreased, flow in resting tissue remains relatively constant. A reduction in pressure is followed by vasodilation, and a rise in pressure by **vasoconstriction**. Myogenic autoregulation is therefore a perfusion pressure-initiated autoregulation and the mechanisms that control it are for the most part the same as those inducing basal myogenic tone. An important consequence of myogenic autoregulation is preservation of normal capillary pressure and flow despite moderate changes in arterial pressure.

The metabolic hypothesis of autoregulation indicates that the concentration of some local chemical(s) (metabolites) alters the degree of contraction of vascular smooth muscle. The muscle may possess receptor sites on which metabolic vasodilators act.

Another example of local control of blood flow is reactive hyperemia. Reactive hyperemia is a local response of the microcirculation to the occlusion of the blood supply to a muscle for a brief interval (Figure 36.4). The increase in blood flow during the postocclusion period is called **reactive hyperemia** and depends on events occurring during both the occlusion and the release of occlusion. Reactive hyperemia is a classic example of local regulation of blood flow in which both myogenic and metabolic pathways are believed to contribute to an increase in blood flow. The myogenic portion of the response is a result of changes in transmural pressure that occur during occlusion of the supply artery and during release of the vascular occlusion. Metabolic responses are primarily due to accumulation of vasodilatory factors, or the depletion of the oxygen necessary for normal smooth muscle contractility that occurs during the occlusion. It is likely that the myogenic portion of the response, as well as the response to different metabolic factors accumulated during the occlusion, have different temporal effects on the vasculature. The evidence that both the intensity and duration of reactive hyperemia are directly related to the duration of occlusion strongly supports a greater role for metabolic factors in reactive hyperemia as occlusion duration increases.

Exercise or functional or active hyperemia is another example of regulation of blood flow (Figure 36.4). Venous blood draining from exercising muscle causes vasodilation when it is collected

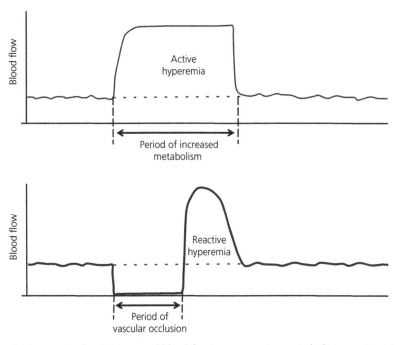

Figure 36.4 Active and reactive hyperemia showing increased blood flow in response to a period of increased metabolism (active hyperemia) or a period of vascular occlusion (reactive hyperemia). Adapted from Fig. 23.2, Cunningham, J.G. (2002) *Textbook of Veterinary Physiology*, 3rd edn. W.B. Saunders, Philadelphia. With permission from Elsevier.

and perfused through resting muscle. However, the magnitude of increased blood flow cannot be produced by this method. The principal metabolic factors shown to have a vasodilator effect in exercise hyperemia are lack of oxygen, and increased H^+, K^+, hyperosmolarity, adenine nucleotides, and adenosine. None of the substances by themselves account for all the phases of exercise hyperemia. They probably act in additive, synergistic and sequential patterns, with some being more important in the initiation (K^+ and hyperosmolarity) and others in the maintenance (oxygen tension and pH) of the response. The duration and intensity of exercise influence the extent of increased skeletal muscle blood flow during exercise and may affect the rate and kind of vasodilator metabolites generated.

It is now well established that local application of acetylcholine to a small arteriole in an arteriolar network initiates a local vasodilation that is conducted along the arteriolar wall to larger upstream vessels. This phenomenon is referred to as **conducted vasodilation**. The onset of vasodilation is rapid (<1 s), conducted rapidly (>2 mm/s), and decays with distance in a manner consistent with passive electrical decay. The initial vasodilation is followed by a slower component that appears to be related to a traveling calcium wave. Collectively, these mechanisms may lead to dilation of larger upstream arterioles and feed arteries that precede changes in wall shear rate. The major component of conducted dilation is independent of flow and thus distinguished from "flow-induced vasodilation." It has been proposed that acetylcholine release from alpha motor neurons thus assists in exercise hyperemia, working with metabolic control to increase blood flow to active skeletal muscle.

Oxygen plays a central role in most schemes of metabolic autoregulation and local control of blood flow. In the systemic circulation, a rise in oxygen tension above normal produces vasoconstriction whereas a fall produces vasodilation. Oxygen may act directly on smooth muscle. However, evidence points to a predominant indirect action of oxygen or the lack of it causing the release of vasoactive substances from parenchymal or other cells that in turn modulate vascular diameter. Oxygen tension may produce different reactions in smooth muscle cells of different precapillary vessels. In any event, oxygen is important to the intrinsic regulation of all tissues in situations resembling reactive hyperemia and in normal circumstances in tissues with high metabolic rates (e.g., heart, brain, and exercising muscle).

Other substances responsible for intrinsic regulation of blood flow include locally produced reactive oxygen species, inorganic phosphate, **nitric oxide**, carbon dioxide, arachidonic acid derivatives, histamine, serotonin, and bradykinin, some of which are partly related to the five main factors previously mentioned. Bradykinin, one of the vasoactive peptides, is involved in the functional hyperemia of the salivary glands and the pancreas and its activity includes the stimulation of **nitric oxide synthase**.

The relative importance of myogenic or metabolic control processes depends on both the circumstances and the individual vascular bed, but in most cases both mechanisms appear to be involved. In reactive hyperemia the initial vasodilation appears to be mostly myogenic that later is augmented and dominated by metabolic mechanisms. Similarly, the initial vasodilation occurring at the onset of muscular contraction prior to the development of vasoactive metabolites is likely myogenic in

Section VI: The Cardiovascular System

Table 36.1 Relative potentials of vascular autoregulation (intrinsic) and neural (extrinsic) regulation.

Vascular bed	Potency of vasoconstrictor nerves	Potency of autoregulation
Brain	+	++++
Heart	±	+++
Skeletal muscle	++	+++
Intestinal tract	+++	++
Hepatic (arterial)	+++	++
Kidney	++++	++++
Skin	++++	–

Increased and decreased potency is indicated by + and –.
Source: Table 10.1, Smith, C.R. and Hamlin, R.L. (1977), in *Dukes' Physiology of Domestic Animals*, 9th edn (ed. M.J. Swenson). Cornell University Press, Ithaca, NY. With permission from Cornell University Press.

origin. In most instances the duration of the stimulus determines the preponderance of the mechanisms controlling vascular resistance and blood flow, with the myogenic type dominating after brief stimuli and metabolic over longer durations of stimulation.

In some vascular beds with sparse vasomotor innervation (e.g., brain and kidney) autoregulation is functionally very well developed. The cutaneous vessels exemplify the opposite situation. In other vascular beds, central neurogenic and local autoregulatory mechanisms exist side by side (Table 36.1). Extrinsic neural regulation is concerned with general overall hemodynamics, is more homogeneous, is widely distributed, and is rapid in onset, in contrast to the more diversified and more slowly responding autoregulatory/local control mechanisms. When both extrinsic and local mechanisms operate simultaneously, the response is determined by the characteristics of the vascular smooth muscle in the arteriolar network. Strong stimulation of vasoconstrictor nerves can transiently overcome metabolically induced vasodilation. Similarly, metabolic vasodilation can break through neurally induced vasoconstriction. Autoregulatory escape is an emergency mechanism for preserving the integrity and function of a tissue. However, autoregulation breaks down with shock, prolonged periods of ischemia, and inflammation.

Arterioles

The arterioles constitute the circulatory segment of the microcirculation where the greatest drop in blood pressure occurs. They are also the primary effectors of the control of blood flow to the capillary beds. Arterioles are the primary resistance vessels that penetrate an organ. Their diameter varies greatly between animal species, vascular beds, and state of contraction. Therefore, they are better defined by their structural characteristic of containing only one or two layers of smooth muscle. Nonetheless, it is customary to set a limit of 150 μm as the maximal internal passive diameter that defines an arteriole.

The arteriolar wall consists of three structurally distinct layers, starting on the luminal side with the intima, followed by the media, and ending with an adventitia.

The intima is made of endothelial cells that sit on a basement membrane composed predominantly of collagen type IV. It serves to provide a barrier that contains the blood constituents inside the vascular tube. Endothelial cells also participate in controlling tone through the production and release of vasoactive factors that modulate the activity of nearby smooth muscle cells present in the medial layer (Figure 36.5). These factors are produced and released in response to a variety of physical, neural, and humoral stimuli. The main physical stimulus affecting endothelial cells is the shear stress produced by blood flow, which causes an increase in intracellular calcium concentrations in endothelial cells and activates endothelial nitric oxide synthase. This enzyme uses L-arginine for the production of the potent vasodilator nitric oxide. In most vascular beds there is constitutive production of nitric oxide as evidenced by the vasoconstriction and increase in blood pressure observed after the experimental infusion of nitric oxide synthase inhibitors. Muscarinic stimulation of the endothelium also results in the production of nitric oxide and endothelium-derived hyperpolarizing factor, both of which induce vasodilation. The identity of the latter is controversial but substantial evidence suggests it may be current generated by changes in cellular permeability to K^+ ions. An additional vasodilator produced by the endothelium in response to shear stress is prostacyclin. This major product of arachidonic acid metabolism and the cyclooxygenase pathway is also produced in response to hypoxia and through receptor-operated mechanisms. Within the vascular wall, its production is largely confined to endothelial cells and catalyzed by the enzyme prostacyclin synthetase. Prostacyclin causes relaxation of smooth muscle through cyclic AMP (cAMP) and, infused intravenously, it causes a fall in blood pressure. Prostacyclin also inhibits platelet aggregation. Therefore there is also a negative feedback mechanism that causes increased prostacyclin production where platelet aggregation occurs.

Endothelial cells also produce a number of vasoconstrictor factors such as **endothelin (ET)**, which is one of the most potent mammalian vasoconstrictors known. ET is a 21-amino-acid polypeptide produced primarily by the vascular endothelium. Three isoforms of ET have been reported of which ET-1 is the most prominent member of the family. In addition to vasoconstriction, ET-1 promotes vascularization, induces the release of norepinephrine and serotonin during the regulation of vascular tone, and participates in the redistribution of blood flow during exercise. ET-1 functions in a paracrine and autocrine fashion in pulmonary and systemic arteries and veins. Hypoxic conditions, increased pressure, and increased shear stress induce the release of ET-1. The synthesis and secretion of ET-1 occurs within minutes, with 75% of it being released into the basolateral interstitial space where it acts on vascular smooth muscle cells or endothelial cells. ET-1 causes not only vasoconstriction but also positive inotropy and atrial natriuretic peptide release at concentrations

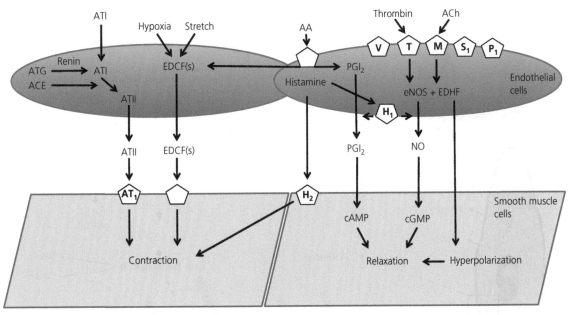

Figure 36.5 Vasoactive substances released from the vascular endothelium. AA, arachidonic acid; ACh, acetylcholine; V, vasopressinergic receptor; T, thrombin receptor; M, muscarinic receptor; S_1, serotonergic receptor; P_1, purinergic receptor; ATG, angiotensinogen; ATI, angiotensin I; ATII, angiotensin II; ACE, angiotensin-converting enzyme; eNOS, endothelium nitric oxide synthase; EDCF, endothelium-derived contracting factor; EDHF, endothelium-derived hyperpolarizing factor; NO, nitric oxide; PGI_2, prostacyclin; H_1/H_2, histaminergic receptors; AT_1, angiotensinergic receptor 1; cAMP, cyclic adenosine monophosphate; cGMP, cyclic guanosine monophosphate. Adapted from Luescher, T.F. (1988) *Endothelial Vasoactive Substances and Cardiovascular Disease.* Karger, Basel.

in the low nanomolar range. ET-2 does not have a known significant function, while ET-3 is found in high concentrations in the lung where it causes nitric oxide production by endothelial cells and vasodilation. There are four G protein-coupled receptor isotypes that bind ET: ET_A, ET_{B1}, ET_{B2} and ET_C. ET_A and ET_{B2} are mostly present in vascular smooth muscle cells and their activation induces vasoconstriction. ET_{B1} is localized in vascular endothelium where its ligation induces the production of nitric oxide and vasodilation. There is no well-defined role for the ET_C receptor. Responses subsequent to ET release vary depending on the affinity of the receptor for its ligand and the location of the release, but activation of any of the receptor isotypes results in an increase in intracellular free calcium concentration.

The medial layer of the arteriolar wall consists almost exclusively of smooth muscle cells and has an internal elastic lamina. The internal elastic lamina is not present at all levels of the arteriolar tree. In most vascular beds it tends to disappear as arterioles become smaller in diameter. Where present, the internal elastic lamina possesses holes or fenestrae that allow physical contact and communication between endothelial and smooth muscle cells via myoendothelial junctions. Smooth muscle is the most abundant component of the media in arterioles. The contraction and relaxation of smooth muscle cells control arteriolar diameter. These cells are spindle-shaped and arranged perpendicular to the long axis of the arteriole. Rapid changes in arteriolar diameter occur primarily as contractile activation or

deactivation of smooth muscle changes the interaction between actin fibers and myosin in the cytoskeleton. The principal event associated with vasoconstriction relies on the increase in intracellular free calcium and calcium–calmodulin interaction with the subsequent activation of **myosin light chain (MLC)** kinase. Phosphorylation of MLC causes the formation and cycling of actomyosin cross-bridges and vasoconstriction. Unlike skeletal and cardiac muscle, smooth muscle actin and myosin filaments are not organized into sarcomeric units. Instead, these contractile proteins are scattered throughout the cytoplasm of the smooth muscle cell. The smooth muscle also differs from sarcomeric muscle in that the regulation of contraction is based on the thick (myosin) filament rather than on the thin (**actin**) filament. Actin serves as a structural element. Smooth muscle myosin consists of a pair of heavy-molecular-weight chains and two pairs of light-molecular-weight chains. There are two types of MLC. One is required for myosin ATPase activity and is called essential, or alkali, MLC. The second type is called regulatory MLC and is the one that is phosphorylated by MLC kinase. The smooth muscle cell has a pair of each type of MLCs. Smooth muscle also contains tropomyosin.

In addition to the calcium-dependent activation of smooth muscle, it is now recognized that two additional processes participate in cell shortening and vasoconstriction (Figure 36.6). One consists of the activation of the small GTP-binding protein RhoA and the subsequent activation of Rho kinase, which results in the phosphorylation and deactivation of MLC

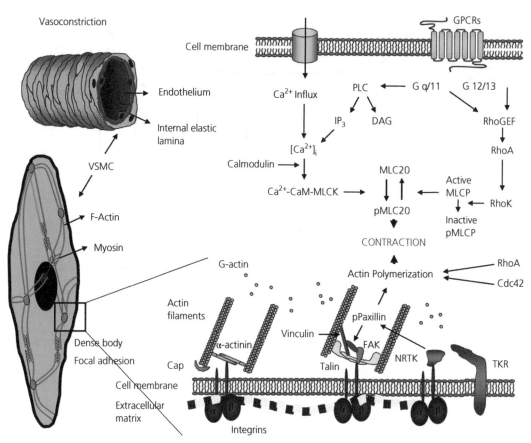

Figure 36.6 Vascular smooth muscle cells (VSMC) located in the medial layer of resistance arteries actively contract to reduce the internal diameter of resistance arteries via processes involving the phosphorylation state of myosin light chain (MLC20) and the remodeling of the actin cytoskeleton. Calcium-dependent pathways of MLC20 phosphorylation occur as intracellular calcium concentrations ($[Ca^{2+}]_i$) are elevated in response to extracellular calcium influx or the depletion of intracellular calcium stores in response to inositol trisphosphate (IP_3) and phospholipase C (PLC)-dependent signaling. Cytosolic calcium binds calmodulin (CaM) and activates myosin light chain kinase (MLCK), which in turn phosphorylates MLC20. Stimuli that activate G protein-coupled receptors (GPCRs) and elevate $[Ca^{2+}]_i$ are also capable of activating Rho guanine nucleotide exchange factors (RhoGEF), RhoA and Rho kinase (RhoK). This RhoK signaling cascade is a calcium-independent pathway that maintains pMLC20 via the phosphorylation and inactivation of myosin light chain phosphatase (MLCP). Actin polymerization participates in the acute phase of vasoconstriction as monomeric G-actin is incorporated into F-actin fibers and strengthens the cytoskeleton. This process requires the phosphorylation of paxillin and involves multiple focal adhesion-associated proteins with and without kinase activity such as integrins, talin, focal adhesion kinase (FAK), and possibly other nonreceptor tyrosine kinases (NRTK) as well as tyrosine kinase receptors (TKR), RhoA and Cdc42. Redrawn from Martinez-Lemus, L.A., Hill, M.A. and Meininger, G.A. (2009) The plastic nature of the vascular wall: a continuum of remodeling events contributing to control of arteriolar diameter and structure. *Physiology (Bethesda)* **24**:45–57.

phosphatase. This causes MLC phosphorylation to be sustained at relatively low levels of intracellular calcium, a process known as calcium sensitization. The second process encompasses the polymerization of actin and the strengthening of vascular smooth muscle actin fibers that in theory provides a rigid scaffold for the development of force. Evidence suggests that all these three processes (i.e., calcium-induced contraction, calcium sensitization, and actin polymerization) participate in all kinds of vasoconstriction, but their relative participation may vary depending on the stimuli (e.g., myogenic or humoral). For the most part, vasodilation results from mechanisms that oppose the vasoconstriction pathways and result in a reduction of intracellular free calcium concentration and MLC dephosphorylation in smooth muscle. Adenosine and prostacyclin

have their effect via the activation of adenylyl cyclase and production of cyclic AMP, while nitric oxide acts via the activation of guanylyl cyclase and production of cyclic GMP.

The outermost layer of arterioles is the adventitia. It is composed mostly of extracellular matrix components and a few fibroblasts and nerve ends. The most predominant extracellular matrix in the adventitia is collagen type I, but large arterioles also tend to have a well-defined external elastic lamina made of elastin fibrils. The presence and structural completeness of the external elastic lamina varies from vascular bed to vascular bed. The adventitia is considered mostly a structural support for the vascular wall, but it also provides functional signals that contribute to vascular function such as the production of reactive oxygen species by fibroblasts and the storage of vasoactive peptides that anchor to the extracellular matrix. In addition, adventitial fibroblasts play a preeminent role in vascular repair.

Inflammation

Inflammation is a local process associated with vascular changes, including hyperemia. The increase in blood flow becomes excessive and causes redness and an increase in temperature. In addition, the porosity of capillaries increases and promotes **edema** of the tissues. Analysis of the lymph draining sites of inflammation suggests that each substance associated with the inflammatory process has a definitive role at a certain stage in its course.

The inflammation site is relatively overperfused, as the redness and temperature indicate. Thus the hyperemia must have a somewhat different basis than does reactive or functional hyperemia. Among the vasodilators identified in inflammation are prostaglandins, bradykinin, and histamine. These also increase capillary permeability.

Microcirculatory exchange between blood and interstitial fluid

> 1 What is the primary mechanism for transcapillary exchange?
>
> 2 Name the four pressures or Starling forces that are involved in bulk flow.
>
> 3 What is pinocytosis?
>
> 4 Are the capillary hydrostatic pressures the same in all tissues?
>
> 5 How do hydrostatic pressures in the retinal capillaries differ from those of other capillaries?
>
> 6 How do hydrostatic pressures in the capillaries of the lungs differ from those in other capillaries?

The capillaries and postcapillary venules are the primary vessels in the microcirculation where the exchange between blood and the interstitium occurs. The walls of capillaries and venules form a semipermeable barrier that allows transport of fluid and solutes. This exchange is usually expressed in terms of permeability or flux and is responsible for the delivery of nutrients and removal of waste to and from the tissues. Diffusional flux represents the major spontaneous movement of molecules and particles that occurs across the capillary walls. Molecules move from regions of higher to lower concentration. The volume of water diffusion through the total capillary surface is about 15,000–18,000 times that of filtration. Lipid-soluble substances, including oxygen and carbon dioxide, diffuse freely through the capillary wall. Water molecules also diffuse through the capillary wall as well as through intercellular clefts or pores present in the wall. Water-soluble lipid-insoluble substances (e.g., electrolytes, glucose, urea) cannot pass through the lipid membrane of endothelial cells and must diffuse through capillary endothelial cell junctions and/or capillary pores.

Bulk fluid flux across the capillary wall, in contrast to diffusion, is the movement of fluid and solutes in bulk through capillary pores that occurs in response to hydrostatic or osmotic pressure differences across the capillary wall. The direction of this flux is into the capillary or out of the capillary depending on the balance of hydrostatic and osmotic pressures present inside and outside the capillary tube. Ernest Henry Starling first formulated the characteristics of these pressure forces in 1896. Later, Eugene M. Landis verified and amended those formulas with specific pressure measurements. Typical values for these pressure forces are given in Figure 36.7. There is a net filtration pressure of 8 mmHg at the arterial end of the capillary. The blood hydrostatic pressure falls toward the venous end while the other forces remain constant, resulting in an effective inward absorption pressure at the venous end of –7 mmHg. The net exchange over 24 hours is about 40 mL/100 g of tissue. Bulk flux of fluid across the capillary wall contributes little to the actual rate of exchange of other materials across capillary walls. Compared with bulk flux and total extracellular fluid volume, including plasma volume, the relatively enormous diffusional flux is the primary determinant of transcapillary exchange for most solutes, and for a given solute it may proceed along a concentration gradient in a direction opposite to that of net bulk flux.

An additional method for transcapillary exchange of solutes is transcellular transport. This occurs through the formation of plasmalemmal vesicles. Via pinocytotic processes, small particles are engulfed and brought into a cell through the invagination of plasma membrane structures. In the vasculature, and particularly in the capillary beds, it is the method endothelial cells use to ingest substances at their inner surface for transport to the outer cell surface, where they are discharged. Vesicular transport is believed to account for the absorption and transport of large molecules such as lipoproteins and polysaccharides across the endothelium.

Excess extracellular fluids and large molecules and particles that are not returned to the bloodstream through capillary absorption must be returned through the lymphatics.

The lymphatic system

> 1 What is the function of the lymphatic system?
>
> 2 What is the effect of gravity on lymph flow?

The blood vascular system transports compounds such as nutrients and metabolites to and from the blood–tissue exchange system at the capillary level. The interstitium is filled with a gel-like matrix (a water-filled network of fibers containing macromolecules) that can be considered "bounded" by two fluid compartments: the capillary network and the initial lymphatics. The interstitium and the lymphatics constitute an extravascular flow system on which the blood capillary–tissue exchanges

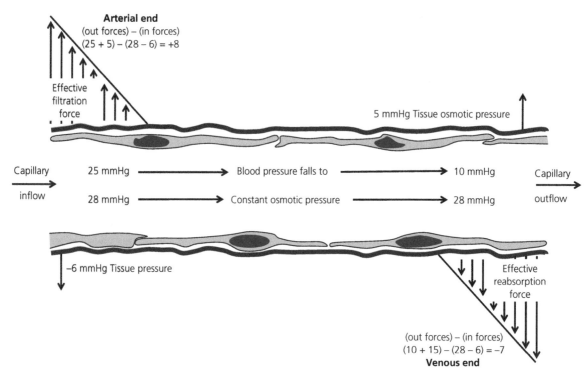

Figure 36.7 Hydrostatic and osmotic forces accounting for capillary filtration and reabsorption. Adapted from Fig. 10.4, Detweiler, D.K. (1993), in *Dukes' Physiology of Domestic Animals*, 11th edn (eds M.J. Swenson and W.O. Reece). Cornell University Press, Ithaca, NY. With permission from Cornell University Press.

depend. The steady state of the interstitium depends on the passage of materials in and out of the blood capillaries and the passage of materials into the lymph system and then back to the bloodstream. The excess of capillary filtration over reabsorption is normally balanced by lymph flow. Large molecules, such as plasma proteins, cannot be reabsorbed into the capillaries against their concentration gradients. Therefore, a primary function of the lymphatic system is to prevent accumulation of such large molecules in the interstitium. Failure to clear these large molecules will cause interstitial oncotic pressure to increase and lead to edema as outlined in the next section.

The lymphatic system originates in a network of initial lymphatics, also named capillary lymphatics, composed of blind-ended tubes, sacs or bulbs that move lymph centrally toward collecting lymphatic vessels (Figure 36.8). The tissue or interstitium pressure is subatmospheric, ranging from −0.2 to −8.0 mmHg. The blood capillary filtrate leaves the interstitium either by reabsorption through the Starling mechanism or via the lymphatic system. The latter is the only route for proteins and other macromolecules. This is aided by the pumping or suction action of the collecting lymphatic channels, which are spontaneously contractile, have one-way valves, and are massaged by mechanical movement of the tissue. The fluid flux across systemic capillaries (Starling mechanism) is substantially higher than the lymph flow, perhaps eight to ten times higher.

The lymphatic capillaries are composed of flat nonfenestrated endothelial cells that overlap and adhere to each other at sites more loosely connected than endothelial junctions in capillary beds. The cellular overlaps allow the collection and mostly unidirectional movement of lymph at the initial lymphatic. At sites of open intercellular junctions there are anchoring fibers attached to the outer membranes of endothelial cells that allow the formation of passages and the movement of fluid into the initial lymphatic. Initial lymphatics are larger than capillary tubes. As the lymphatic network is followed centrally toward the collecting vessels, specialized smooth muscle cells appear. These muscle cells provide tonic and phasic contractions that generate lymph flow. In this regard, lymph transport mechanisms in lymphatics are vastly different from blood transport in veins. Intravenous and intralymphatic pressures recorded from the limbs of sheep show that the venous pressure is steady at about 15–20 mmHg and fluctuates slightly with each heartbeat, whereas the intralymphatic pressure has a pressure pulse with an amplitude that reaches 25 mmHg and a frequency of about 5 cycles per minute. These lymphatic pressure pulses are generated by contractions of the lymphatics themselves that occur in response to pacemaker activity located within the smooth muscle layer of the wall. The lymphatics may be thought of as a series of contracting chambers or lymphangions, demarcated by the lymph unidirectional valves formed by endothelial cells. Thus it is better to describe their hydrodynamic function in

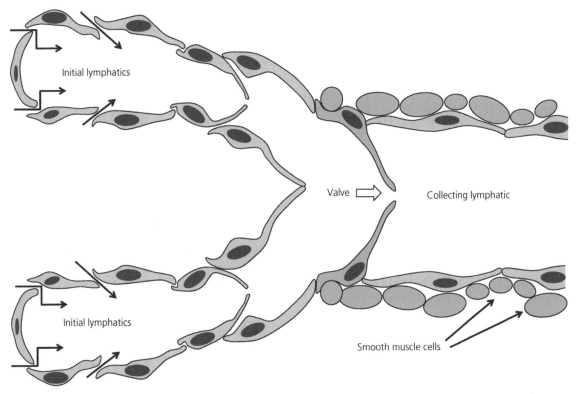

Figure 36.8 Initial lymphatics or lymphatic capillaries, valves, and collecting lymphatic. Adapted from Fig. 16.12, Hall, J.E. and Guyton, A.C. (2001) *Textbook of Medical Physiology*, 10th edn. W.B. Saunders, Philadelphia. With permission from Elsevier.

terms used for the heart, such as systole, diastole, preload (filling pressure), afterload (outflow resistance), stroke volume, and rate of beating. The main determinants of lymph flow are filling pressure (preload) and outflow resistance (afterload). When afterload, preload, or both are increased, the lymph vessel is stretched; it responds by increasing the rate and strength of contraction. Empty lymph vessels, as when preload is reduced to zero, do not contract. Complete obstruction increases the amplitude and frequency of contractions to raise peak lymphatic pressures to about 60 mmHg or even higher.

Hormones, vasoactive substances, and nerves affect the rate and strength of contraction in lymph vessels. Norepinephrine, epinephrine, and α-adrenergic sympathetic nerves stimulate motor activity and local lymph flow. Stimulation of β-adrenergic receptors results in the opposite effect. Similarly, a decrease in contractile activity is observed in response to stimulation with acetylcholine, which causes nitric oxide synthesis by endothelial cells. There is no evidence that motor effects cause negative pressure (or suction) at the lymph capillaries. Certain endotoxins can paralyze lymphatics.

Ordinarily, gravity has little effect on lymph flow because the column of fluid in the lymphatic is not continuous and a hydrostatic gradient (standpipe effect) is not present as it is in veins. If, however, lymphatics are markedly distended and their fluid column is continuous, then they behave like veins. Thus muscle or massage can propel lymph in the lymphatics as well as blood

in the veins centrally under conditions of lymph vessel distension. Also, movement of the limbs, manual massage, or both can induce lymphatic contractions as well as increase local production of lymph, causing an increase in lymph flow. When no lymph is present, its smooth muscle becomes quiescent and lymph pressure falls to zero. Stretching of the vessels by the lymph causes rhythmic contractions that increase in rate and strength, depending on the degree of stretch.

Edema

1 How would you define edema?

2 What are some causes of edema?

3 What is peripheral edema?

4 What causes overnight "stocking" or "ankle" edema in horses?

5 What are some causes of pulmonary edema?

Under normal physiological conditions, the volume of a tissue remains constant except for minor variations in capillary blood volume. The fluid and protein that escape from the blood capillaries return in equal amounts by absorption into either the blood or the lymph capillaries. Edema is an abnormal accumulation of interstitial fluid accompanied by swelling. Factors that result in edema are an increase in capillary pressure, increased capillary permeability, a decrease in the concentration of plasma proteins, and obstruction of the lymphatic vessels. An increase in capillary pressure due to increased venous pressure (because of obstruction of the veins) or due to excessive vasodilation of precapillary resistance vessels favors filtration and forces more fluid out through the capillary wall into the interstitium. An increase in capillary hydrostatic pressure may be caused by an increase in arterial blood pressure or venous pressure, or a decrease in arteriolar resistance. Heart failure often leads to increased capillary pressures and edema due to an increase in venous pressure.

An increase in capillary permeability may occur with severe burns, resulting in an increase in the permeability of the capillaries that allows protein to leak into the interstitium pulling water out and causing edema. A decrease in the plasma protein concentration also upsets the balance of forces across the capillary wall, resulting in increased filtration of fluid out of the capillary tubes. This may occur with the loss of protein in renal disease or with poor nutrition causing low production of plasma proteins by the liver.

Peripheral edema

Overnight "stocking" ("ankle"), or peripheral, edema in horses is caused by a deficiency of venous massage to aid in the return of venous blood from pendant blood capillaries and inability of the lymphatic system to remove this excessive interstitial fluid. With exercise, muscle massage decreases venous pressure and, insofar as the lymphatics are distended, exercise would aid lymph return. With exercise, stocking edema soon disappears. The lymphatics ordinarily handle minor increases in tissue flow, preventing the formation of edema. A cardinal reaction of tissue trauma is swelling caused by edema formation secondary to capillary damage. The edema that occurs in immunologically mediated tissue reactions (e.g., urticaria) and in various renal diseases is apparently caused by damage to the capillary basement membrane. After severe hemorrhage, capillary hydrostatic pressure falls and the resulting capillary uptake of tissue fluid immediately begins to dilute plasma proteins and red blood cell concentration, depending on the intensity of the hypotension. Spontaneous vasomotion of the lymphatic collecting vessels also occurs, further increasing fluid return to the bloodstream. Finally, excessive transcapillary fluid filtration in gastrointestinal or liver tissues can lead to ascites – excessive fluid in the abdominal space. This is often seen in cases of right-sided heart failure that increase central venous pressures.

Pulmonary edema

In the lungs, where edema is particularly dangerous, the rapid removal of capillary filtrate by the lymph system is especially important in preventing fluid accumulation in the alveoli when capillary hydrostatic pressure increases or when plasma protein concentration decreases. One of the most common causes of pulmonary edema is left-sided heart failure or mitral valvular disease. This results in a large increase in pulmonary venous pressure and pulmonary capillary pressure and the flooding of the interstitial spaces and alveoli with fluid. Another common cause of pulmonary edema is damage to the capillary membrane by infections such as pneumonia. This results in the rapid leakage of both plasma protein and fluid out of the capillaries into the interstitial spaces and the alveoli.

There is a safety factor to protect the lungs from pulmonary edema. The pulmonary capillary pressure must rise to a value equal to the colloid osmotic pressure or higher before significant pulmonary edema occurs. For example, in a dog with left-sided heart failure, left atrial pressure must rise above about 23–25 mmHg before fluid begins to accumulate in the lungs. When the pulmonary capillary pressure remains chronically elevated, the lungs become even more resistant to pulmonary edema because the lymph vessels expand, increasing their ability to carry fluid away from the interstitial spaces as much as tenfold. Thus, in chronic pulmonary edema, the safety factor can rise to 30–35 mmHg.

The accumulation of an excessive volume of extracellular fluid in congestive heart failure results in increased blood volume, edema, ascites, and (sometimes) hydrothorax. These increases are brought about mainly by renal retention of salt and water, aggravated by increased thirst and possibly by an increased appetite for salt. With the increase in blood volume, the blood vessels are more completely filled, whereas the swollen interstitial fluid volume compresses the blood vessels externally.

Self-evaluation

Answers can be found at the end of the chapter.

1 Which of the following vessels converts pulsatile inflow to a somewhat smoothed outflow?
   A Conduit vessels
   B Resistance vessels
   C Terminal arterioles
   D Exchange vessels
   E Capacitance vessels

2 What are the three general types of capillaries?

3 What is the mean hydrostatic pressure in the systemic capillaries?
   A 0 mmHg
   B 10 mmHg
   C 25 mmHg
   D 50 mmHg
   E 100 mmHg

4 What metabolic factors have a vasodilator effect?

5 Name the three main processes that participate in vasoconstriction.

6 Autoregulation is functionally very well developed in which vascular beds?

7 In which vascular bed is autoregulation very poorly developed?

8 What are the mechanisms for transcapillary exchange and what is the primary mechanism?

Suggested reading

Granger, D.N. (2010) *Inflammation and the Microcirculation*. Morgan & Claypool Life Sciences Publishers, San Rafael, CA.

Hall, J.E. (2011) *Guyton and Hall Textbook of Medical Physiology*, 12th edn. Saunders Elsevier, Philadelphia.

Moncada, S. and Higgs, A. (2006) *The Vascular Endothelium*. Springer, New York.

Tuma, R.F., Duran, W.N. and Ley, K. (2008) *Handbook of Physiology. Microcirculation*, 2nd edn. Academic Press, San Diego, CA.

Answers

1 A
2 Continuous capillaries, discontinuous capillaries, and fenestrated capillaries.
3 C
4 The principal metabolic factors shown to have a vasodilator effect are lack of oxygen, increased H^+, K^+, hyperosmolarity, adenine nucleosides, and adenosine.
5 The three main processes associated with vasoconstriction are intracellular calcium activation of vascular smooth muscle cells, calcium sensitization, and actin polymerization.
6 Brain and kidney.
7 Cutaneous vessels.
8 The three mechanisms for transcapillary exchange are diffusion, bulk flow, and pinocytosis. Diffusion flow is the major mechanism for transcapillary exchange.

Section VI: The Cardiovascular System

David C. Poole and Howard H. Erickson
Kansas State University, Manhattan, KS, USA

Section VI: The Cardiovascular System

Anatomy

1 Describe the anatomy of the pulmonary circulation.
2 How does the pulmonary circulation differ from the systemic circulation?

The pulmonary and systemic circulatory systems are considered two open circuits connected in series to form a single closed loop. The pulmonary circulation is interposed between the right and left sides of the heart and entirely located within the negative pressure confines of the thorax. The cardinal function of the pulmonary circulation is the **exchange of gases** in the lungs. Although the average volume flow through the two circuits is almost the same, there are marked structural and dynamic differences. The pulmonary circulation is a relatively short, **low-resistance, low-pressure system** (see Figure 37.1 for comparison with the systemic circulation) which conducts blood to and from a single but very dense capillary bed enveloping the **pulmonary alveoli**. It consists of the right ventricle, pulmonary arteries, pulmonary capillaries, pulmonary veins, and left atrium. Because the pulmonary vessels are very distensible, they serve not only as a channel but also as a reservoir between the right and left ventricles.

Right ventricle

The right ventricle functions as a "volume pump." It ejects almost the same volume per minute as the left ventricle but against a much lower pressure. The normal right ventricle can be identified by the right ventricular free wall, which is only about one-third as thick as the left ventricular free wall. When dissected from the rest of the heart, the free wall has a triangular shape. Its normal attachment to the cylindrical surface formed by the interventricular septum and the free wall of the left ventricle results in a crescent-shaped right ventricular lumen of relatively large dimensions. At rest, the right ventricle has a lower **fractional oxygen extraction** than the left ventricle (~0.5 vs. 0.8) which allows both increased oxygen extraction and blood flow to contribute to the elevated oxygen demands of the right ventricular muscle during the high heart rates found during exercise.

Pulmonary vessels

The pulmonary vascular system, like the systemic vascular system, consists of a series of tubes. However, the large pulmonary arteries are short and rapidly subdivide into peripheral branches, which have thinner walls and wider lumens than their systemic counterparts and which in general resemble systemic veins more than arteries. The wall of the pulmonary artery is less than

Dukes' Physiology of Domestic Animals, Thirteenth Edition. Edited by William O. Reece, Howard H. Erickson, Jesse P. Goff and Etsuro E. Uemura.
© 2015 John Wiley & Sons, Inc. Published 2015 by John Wiley & Sons, Inc.
Companion website: www.wiley.com/go/reece/physiology

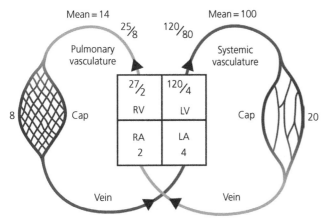

Figure 37.1 Comparison of pressures (mmHg) in the pulmonary and systemic circulations in the dog. These are altered by exercise (more pronounced in very athletic species such as the Thoroughbred horse) and also the vertical position of the lung region with respect to the heart. Such hydrostatic differences are particularly important in large animals where the vertical height of the lung may exceed 100 cm. Adapted from Fig. 4.1, West, J.B. (2000) *Respiratory Physiology: The Essentials*, 6th edn. Lippincott Williams & Wilkins, Baltimore. Reproduced with permission from Lippincott Williams & Wilkins.

one-third as thick as that of the aorta. Small arteries have only a thin media with relatively little smooth muscle. The small postcapillary venules are devoid of smooth muscle. Because the pressures throughout the pulmonary circuit are so low, even smaller amounts of vascular smooth muscle are capable of actively changing vessel radii.

Important features to consider in the dynamics of the pulmonary circulation are (i) the position within the negative (except for forced exhalations at rest and during exercise) but rhythmically variable pressure of the thorax; (ii) the position between the right ventricle and the left atrium; (iii) the relatively great distensibility and collapsibility of the vessels; (iv) the effect that the interaction of intravascular and extra-vascular pressures has on easily collapsible and distensible vessels, pulmonary vascular resistance (PVR), and flow distribution within the lung; (v) the relative paucity of vascular smooth muscle and vasomotor nerves; and (vi) the transport of venous blood in arteries and arterial blood (oxygenated) in veins in quantities per unit time equal to that of the systemic circulation.

There are species differences in the morphology of the pulmonary vessels. In the rabbit the small pulmonary arteries are relatively muscular. In the cow a distinct muscular media occurs in both arteries and veins down to vessels with diameters as small as 20 μm. Among the species studied, the bovine has the best developed muscular coat in the arterioles. Differences in pulmonary vasoactivity among species correlate well with the degree of development of the vasculature of the pulmonary vessels. These species differences become extremely important in the response to the inspired hypoxia found at altitude.

The pulmonary hypoxic vasoconstrictor response and consequent elevation of pulmonary arterial pressure that often leads to right heart failure is more extreme in the calf and the pig (very muscular pulmonary arterial systems) than in the dog and the sheep (relatively less well-developed pulmonary arterial musculature). In this respect, the horse is intermediate between the cow and the dog.

Bronchial vessels

In addition to the flow of venous blood delivered by the pulmonary artery to the alveoli for oxygenation, the lungs also receive a nutrient supply via the bronchial arteries. The blood supply to the bronchial connective tissue is part of the systemic circulation and consists of the broncho-esophageal artery and the right apical bronchial artery. The bronchial vessels supply oxygenated blood to the lung tissues at least to the level of the bronchioles. Normally the volume flow through the bronchial arteries amounts to no more than 1–2% of the cardiac output. Part of the venous drainage from the bronchial circulation is returned by systemic veins to the right atrium. The remainder drains into the pulmonary veins. There is free communication between the capillaries of the pulmonary and bronchial system. The communication of the two circulations at the capillary level provides a potential shunt which can serve to prevent elevation of capillary hydrostatic pressure if an increase should occur unilaterally in either right or left atrial pressure. Under such circumstances, capillary blood can drain through the venous system with the lower pressure. The bronchial vessels can also provide collateral circulation to the lungs when the pulmonary arterial supply is inadequate, such as in pulmonary artery atresia. In contrast to the pulmonary arterial system, hypoxia causes dilation of the bronchial arteries.

With lung transplantation, the bronchial arterial system is typically not reconnected and it appears that the nutritive role of this circulation can be effectively subserved by the pulmonary circulation.

Pressures

1 What are the pressures in the pulmonary circulation (see Figure 37.1)?
2 How do the pressures differ in the pulmonary and systemic circulations?
3 What are the effects of respiration on pressures in the pulmonary circulation?
4 How is pulmonary wedge pressure determined?

Right ventricular pressure

For the right ventricle the highest systolic pressures occur in the horse, cow, and pig, the lowest in the dog. Intermediate systolic pressures are found in the goat and sheep. The higher pressures

Table 37.1 Pressures in the pulmonary circulation (mmHg).

Species	Right ventricle pressures			Pulmonary artery pressures			
	Systolic	Diastolic	Source	Systolic	Diastolic	Mean	Source
Cow	42–56	0–1	Doyle *et al.* (1960)	33–46	19–21	24–31	Doyle *et al.* (1960)
Horse	49±11 (35–72)	14±6 (7–24)	Gall (1967)	36±9 (25–51)	21±5 (14–28)	28	Gall (1967)
Calf	55 (51–60)	0	McCrady *et al.* (1968)	45 (36–52)	16 (12–18)	26 (20–35)	McCrady *et al.* (1968)
Pig	51	0	Wachtel *et al.* (1963)	40	16 (9–20)	22.5	Maaske *et al.* (1965)
Dog	24	2	Moscovitz *et al.* (1956)	21	10	10	Moscovitz *et al.* (1956)
Human	25 (17–32)	4 (1–7)	Dittmer *et al.* (1959)	22 (11–29)	9 (4–13)	15 (9–19)	Dittmer *et al.* (1959)
Goat	24.5 (24–32)	−1.5 (−3 to 0)	Sporri (1962)				
Sheep	26.3 (18–37)	−3.1 (−6 to 0)	Sporri (1962)			9	Halmagi *et al.* (1961)
Cat	26	0	Tashjian *et al.* (1965)	26–36	15–17		Grauweiler (1965)

Source: data from Table 19.1, Reece, W.O. (ed.) *Dukes Physiology of Domestic Animals*, 12th edn. Cornell University Press, Ithaca, NY.

in larger animals are probably related in part to the higher resistances to flow encountered in larger lungs, especially in those with significant portions of the pulmonary vascular bed above the level of the heart. Diastolic pressures in the horse are also usually higher than those in the cow, dog and other smaller animals (Table 37.1). The higher diastolic pressures may be related to the weight of the column of blood (hydrostatic effect) between the ventricle and the head, i.e., contained within the right atrium and the jugular veins. The diastolic pressure in cows is increased when the head is elevated and decreased when the head is lowered.

The **pulse contour** of the right ventricle differs from the left: (i) it is smaller in amplitude, (ii) the rate of rise is smaller, (iii) the peak pressure occurs early rather than late in the ejection period, and (iv) the pressure falls rather rapidly following the early peak, in contrast to the plateau–peak sequence in the left ventricle pressure pulse (Figure 37.2). The lower rate of rise of pressure (i.e., **dP/dt**) is determined by the smaller myocardial mass of the right ventricle and the lower resistance and greater distensibility of the pulmonary circuit. The fall in pressure following the early peaking is due to the rapid passage of blood from the relatively short pulmonary arteries. When conditions in the pulmonic circuit become more like those in the systemic, the pulse contours become more alike. In **pulmonary hypertension**, for example, the PVR increases and the right ventricle hypertrophies.

Pulmonary artery pressure

The mean pressure in the pulmonary artery is approximately one-sixth that of the systemic arteries. Pressures in human, dog, cat, calf, and sheep tend to be lower than those in cow, pig, and horse (Table 37.1). The pressures vary with age as well as with species. *In utero*, the pulmonary and systemic pressures are nearly equal as a result of the **patent ductus arteriosus**. In newborn calves the pulmonary artery pressure decreases in three stages: it falls below systemic pressure during the first 2 hours after birth; it falls rapidly during the period between the second and twelfth hours; and it slowly decreases further until the animal is 14 days old.

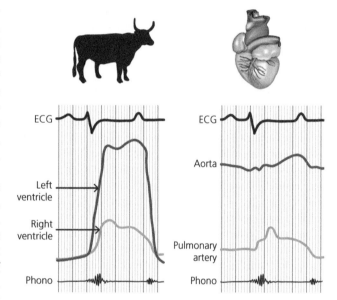

Figure 37.2 Contour of the pressure pulses in the right and left ventricles, aorta, and pulmonary artery in the ox. Adapted from Swenson, M.J and Reece, W.O. (eds) (1993) *Dukes' Physiology of Domestic Animals*, 11th edn. With permission from Cornell University Press.

In **Poiseuille's equation** ($\dot{Q} = P/R$), $\dot{Q}$, or volume of flow per unit time (i.e., per minute), is very nearly the same for both pulmonary and systemic circuits. On the other hand, the short lengths and large radii of the pulmonary arteries yield a small value for resistance, approximately one-fifth to one-tenth of the resistance to flow observed in the systemic arteries. The low resistance and therefore low pressures within the pulmonary versus the systemic circulation are explained by the different functions of the two circulations. The systemic circulation provides blood flow to many different organ systems some of which (i.e., the brain) may be considerably above the heart. In addition, in a resting animal the splanchnic bed, kidneys and skin may receive a substantial percentage of the cardiac output, whereas during intense running over 80% of the cardiac output is

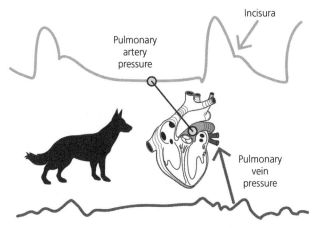

Figure 37.3 Record from an unanesthetized dog showing the pressure pulse contours in the pulmonary artery (upper curve) and pulmonary vein (lower curve). Pulmonary artery pressure, 42/11 mmHg (systolic/diastolic); mean pulmonary vein pressure, 2–12 mmHg in six dogs. A marked incisura occurs low in the dicrotic limb. Adapted from Hamilton, W.F., Woodbury, R.A. and Vogt, E. (1939) Differential pressures in the lesser circulation of the anesthetized dog. *American Journal of Physiology* **125**:130–141.

redirected to the active skeletal muscles. An arterial/arteriolar network with high vascular pressures and a powerful vasoconstrictor tone is thus essential for directing blood flow among the appropriate tissues dependent on their demands at rest and during exercise. By comparison, the lung must accept the entire cardiac output and its vascular pressures are consistent with the need to elevate blood to the top (i.e., apex or dorsum depending on body position and species) of the lung. This low-pressure system has two major advantages: (i) it minimizes work of the right heart, and (ii) allows a very **thin blood–gas barrier** suitable for high rates of gas exchange.

Contour of pressure pulse

The contour of the pulmonary arterial pressure pulse relative to that of the aorta is shown in Figure 37.2. Note the earlier systolic phase compared with that of the aorta. A marked incisura occurs low on the dicrotic limb (Figure 37.3). The low absolute value of the pulse pressure is a reflection of not only the marked distensibility of the pulmonary arterial vessels, which permits easy accommodation to the right ventricular stroke volume without a marked rise in the pressure, but also the low arteriolar resistance, which allows a larger fraction of the stroke volume to leave the arterial tree during each systole.

The ratio of pulse pressure to systolic pressure is higher than in the systemic circuit. Pulse pressure is half or more of systolic pressure due to the fact that the stroke volume represents a relatively larger fraction of the blood in the pulmonary arteries. For example, blood volume in the pulmonary arteries of a 20-kg dog is approximately 60 mL; stroke volume is 20–30 mL. Were it not for the marked distensibility of the pulmonary arterial tree, the pulse pressure would be still larger.

Effect of respiration

During inspiration the **intrapleural pressure** falls and the lungs expand. The reverse occurs during expiration. Pressures and flow in the pulmonary artery are both influenced by these events. Pulmonary artery pressure changes will parallel the intrapleural pressure fluctuations, i.e., fall during inspiration and rise during expiration. In contrast, **transmural pressures** will rise during inspiration and fall during expiration. The inspiratory rise is due to the increased flow that follows increased cardiac output occurring concomitantly with an increased venous return during the inspiratory fall in intrapleural pressure. In the dog at rest, an increase in cardiac output during inspiration is also aided by an increase in heart rate during **sinus arrhythmia**. During expiration the opposite takes place. With maximal expansion of the lungs (see section Pulmonary vascular resistance), or during a forced expiration with the glottis closed (**Valsalva maneuver**), the vessels are strongly compressed by the surrounding lung tissue and the pulmonary arterial pressure rises sharply.

Nonrespiratory pressure waves

Slow, noncardiac, and nonrespiratory rhythmic fluctuations in pulmonary arterial pressures are sometimes observed. They are most frequently found in association with systemic (**Traube–Hering–Mayer**) waves, with frequency and amplitude independent of the breathing pattern. They are passive effects of fluctuations in pulmonary blood flow due to rhythmic changes in systemic vascular resistance and flow.

Capillary and wedge pressures

If a small catheter is advanced along the pulmonary arterial tree until it wedges in a small branch artery, the mean pressure in the catheter reflects venous pressure and left atrial pressure (rather than mean capillary pressure). From a consideration of **wedge pressures** and the fact that mean capillary pressure is intermediate between mean pulmonary arterial and venous pressures, a value between 5 and 10 mmHg appears reasonable for the dog and between 20 and 30 mmHg for the horse. However, there is recent evidence that pulmonary capillary pressures may be quite close to pulmonary venous pressure, rather than midway between pulmonary arterial and pulmonary venous pressures as once thought.

Normally, the capillary pressure must be below the **oncotic pressure** of the plasma proteins (25–30 mmHg) or else bulk transfer of fluid from the capillaries to the alveoli of the lungs would occur. In the healthy animal, fluid does not accumulate in the alveoli but is rapidly absorbed and removed by the rich lymphatic system.

Pulmonary blood volume

1 What is the difference between central blood volume and pulmonary blood volume?

2 What are some of the causes of an increase in pulmonary blood volume?

The pulmonary blood volume is the volume of blood contained in the vessels of the lungs and should not be confused with the central blood volume, which includes the pulmonary blood volume plus the blood volumes in the heart and great vessels. One-third of the central blood volume is in the pulmonary blood vessels. Approximately 9% of total blood volume is contained in the pulmonary vessels. It is distributed about equally among the arteries, capillaries, and veins. Increases in pulmonary blood volume of 25–50% may occur when the pulmonary circulation serves a reservoir function to accommodate increases in total blood volume or when extensive systemic arterial and venous constriction causes a shift of blood volume from the systemic to the pulmonary circuit.

Pulmonary blood flow

---

1 What are some of the characteristics of phasic pulmonary blood flow?

2 Describe the sheet flow concept in the lung.

3 What are the determinants of PVR and how does it changes from rest to exercise and across lung volumes?

4 What effect does **hydrostatic pressure** have on capillary flow?

5 What is the **transit time** for blood in the pulmonary capillaries?

6 What are the hydrostatic and osmotic pressures across the capillary membrane?

Measurement

The **Fick principle** enables calculation of cardiac output (i.e., pulmonary blood flow, $\dot{Q}$) from straightforward measurements. The Fick principle states that whole-body oxygen uptake is the product of $\dot{Q}$ and the difference between systemic arterial oxygen content (Cao_2) and pulmonary arterial oxygen content (referred to as mixed venous, $C\bar{v}o_2$). Thus:

$$\dot{V}o_2 = \dot{Q}\left(Cao_2 - C\bar{v}o_2\right)$$

Rearranging to solve for $\dot{Q}$:

$$\dot{Q} = \dot{V}o_2/\left(Cao_2 - C\bar{v}o_2\right)$$

Typically, $\dot{V}o_2$ is measured by collecting expired gas, Cao_2 by sampling from any artery, and $C\bar{v}o_2$ from the pulmonary artery (or sometimes the right ventricle). This technique measures the average blood flow over multiple cardiac cycles. However, it is possible to measure the instantaneous uptake of a very soluble gas (e.g., nitrous oxide) from the lung and thereby follow the pulsatile nature of pulmonary blood flow.

Phasic flow

In the pulmonary artery the flow of blood rises and falls more slowly than in the aorta. A small backflow occurs at the end of systole, as in the aorta. Flow remains pulsatile throughout arteries and capillaries, and small oscillations persist into the left atrium. Depending on species and, in part, the vertical dimensions of the lung, the distribution of flow within the lung may be affected by gravitational hydrostatic forces that enhance blood flow to the base of the upright lung or the ventrum of the quadruped's lung. Measurements of regional pulmonary blood flow in the horse have determined that active vasomotor control may override gravitational effects.

Sheet flow concept

The alveolar microcirculation is organized into a vascular sheet in which two walls of endothelium are held apart by connective tissue and cellular posts enclose a sheet-like space, rather than the conventional model of a network of cylindrical tubes. The intra-alveolar capillary bed is visualized as an endothelium-lined, flat, vascular sinus with variable reservoir capacity through which blood advances as a moving sheet.

Capillary flow

In marked contrast to the systemic circuit, the resistance to outflow from the pulmonary arteries is low. Further, the volume of the pulmonary capillary network (dog, ~20 mL) and the right ventricular stroke volume (dog, ~20–30 mL) are much closer together than their systemic counterparts. Thus uneven or pulsatile capillary flow occurs. Pulsations of flow are accompanied by pressure pulsations of several mmHg. These may at times affect whether a pulmonary capillary is open, closed, or partially collapsed. They also provide rhythmic stimulation to the vascular smooth muscle in the small **precapillary arterioles**.

Effect of hydrostatic pressure

The pulmonary circulation is often considered to be a passive circuit in which blood flow distribution is determined by the hydrostatic gradient due to gravity. This concept is embodied in the traditional "zonal" model wherein distribution of regional blood flow is determined by local arterial, venous, and alveolar pressures within the lung. The weight of a column of fluid in a vessel exerts force as hydrostatic pressure. For blood this increases approximately 7.4 mmHg for each 10 cm of height. The development of high-resolution microsphere technology has advanced the study of regional blood flow distribution within the lung and other organs. The distribution of pulmonary blood flow, once believed to be primarily influenced by gravitational forces, when examined with these new techniques is found to be quite heterogeneous within isogravitational planes, at least in the horse. The branching pulmonary vascular tree is **fractal** by nature, and therefore fractal methods have emerged as an effective way to describe regional blood flow distribution. Gravity has been found to be a less important determinant of pulmonary perfusion in species such as the horse than originally supposed. In the lungs of resting unanesthetized horses – animals with a large vertical lung height – there is no consistent vertical gradient to pulmonary blood flow and there is a considerable degree of perfusion heterogeneity, indicating that gravity alone does not play the major role in determining blood flow distribution.

Pulmonary vascular resistance

As mentioned previously, PVR is extremely low in comparison to the systemic circulation. PVR may be calculated as:

$$PVR = \left(P_{pa} - P_{la}\right)/\dot{Q}$$

where P_{pa} is pulmonary artery pressure, P_{la} is left atrial pressure, and $\dot{Q}$ is pulmonary blood flow or cardiac output. For example, from Figure 37.1, if P_{pa} is 14 mmHg, P_{la} 4 mmHg, and cardiac output 30 L/min, then PVR is calculated as follows:

$$PVR = (14 - 4)/30 = 0.33 \text{ mmHg/L per min}$$

Despite this very low value at rest, PVR falls further during exercise due to the recruitment of vessels that are closed at rest and distension of vessels already open at rest. Because of the extremely thin walls of the pulmonary vasculature and the lack of external support, there is considerable room for expansion and this is seen clearly, for example, in the pulmonary capillaries which change their shape from elliptical to circular as pulmonary arterial (and also pulmonary capillary) pressures rise. Figure 37.4 demonstrates this reduction in PVR as pulmonary arterial pressure is elevated.

In addition to intravascular pressures, lung volume is an important determinant of PVR (Figure 37.5). This occurs for several reasons, the most important being that extra-alveolar vessels (primarily arterioles and venules) are pulled open by **torsional forces** imparted by the lung parenchyma as the lung expands. Thus, PVR decreases as lung volume increases from very low volumes as the thin smooth muscle and elastic tissue in the vessels walls allow the expanding parenchyma to pull them open thereby increasing their caliber. PVR reaches a minimum close to functional residual capacity. As lung volume is increased further, the vessel caliber reaches a maximum and additional lung volume increases PVR by increasing vessel length and, more importantly, by stretching and flattening the pulmonary capillaries. At very high lung volumes the resistance of the pulmonary capillaries can contribute substantially to PVR.

Transit time

The average time estimated for a red blood cell to traverse the pulmonary capillaries in the dog varies from 0.18 s (exercise) to 1 s (rest). The more capillaries open for a certain volume flow, the longer the average capillary transit time according to the relationship:

Red blood cell mean transit time
$$= \text{Pulmonary capillary volume}/\dot{Q}$$

Normally, blood does not accumulate in arteries, capillaries, or veins. With each heartbeat the stroke volume ejected replaces an equivalent volume in the pulmonary arteries, which is propelled onward to the succeeding segment. In a 15–20 kg dog the pulmonary capillary blood volume is about 20 mL, which

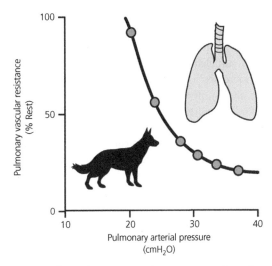

Figure 37.4 Fall in pulmonary vascular resistance as the pulmonary artery pressure is raised. When the arterial pressure was changed, the venous pressure was held constant at 12 cmH$_2$O. Data from an excised dog lung. Adapted from Fig. 4.4, West, J.B. (2000) *Respiratory Physiology: The Essentials*, 6th edn. Lippincott Williams & Wilkins, Baltimore. Reproduced with permission from Lippincott Williams and Wilkins.

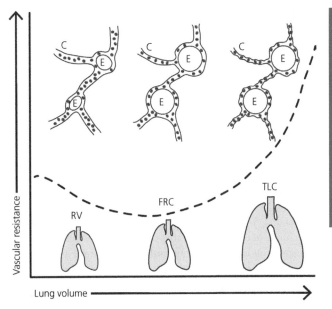

Figure 37.5 The change in vascular resistance incurred by increasing lung volume. The inset diagrams represent alveolar (C) and extra-alveolar (E) vessels. At residual volume (RV), the extra-alveolar vessels are narrowed but the walls of the alveolar vessels (capillaries) are not under longitudinal stress and thus the lumen is distended. At total lung capacity (TLC), the extra-alveolar vessels are distended but the alveolar vessels are flattened because of the tension in the alveolar septum. Minimal vascular resistance occurs close to functional residual capacity (FRC). Adapted from Fig. 45.5, Robinson, N.E. (1997) Pulmonary blood flow. In: *Textbook of Veterinary Physiology* (ed. J.G. Cunningham). W.B. Saunders, Philadelphia. With permission from Elsevier.

approaches the stroke volume. If these volumes were equal, the capillary transit time would equal the beat interval.

Normally, the time spent by the blood in the capillaries is more than sufficient for oxygenation. When the pulmonary flow rate increases, as during exercise, oxygenation is still near 100% (in healthy, nonelite or nonathletic animals) because (i) usually it only requires a fraction of the time spent in the capillaries under basal conditions, and (ii) when the beat-to-beat interval is decreased, as it is when cardiac output increases during exercise, the number of patent capillaries increases and they distend elevating the pulmonary capillary volume. The stroke volume thus becomes smaller compared with the capillary volume and transit time occupies more than one beat-to-beat interval. Only when blood flow and capillary volumes change disproportionately is there danger of reducing the time spent in the capillaries below that required for close to full oxygenation.

> In very athletic species, most notably the Thoroughbred horse and greyhound, from rest to maximal exercise, $\dot{Q}$ may increase as much as 5–16 times, whereas pulmonary capillary volume increases about twofold. This proportionality mandates that red blood cell transit time in the pulmonary capillary bed will decrease considerably to the extent that oxygen loading is compromised and arterial hypoxemia becomes manifest.

Hydrostatic and osmotic pressures across the capillary membrane

The extent of production and reabsorption of **interstitial fluid** in the lung ("lung water") in accordance with the **Starling principle** is somewhat controversial because of disagreements about the level of interstitial hydrostatic and oncotic pressures. Capillary pressures within the lung are low compared with those in the systemic circulation. Capillary hydrostatic pressure may be influenced by gravity, being lower at the apex and higher at the base; a mean value of 9 mmHg has been suggested. Because of the prevailing negative intrathoracic pressures, it is generally assumed that lung interstitial fluid pressure is subatmospheric (about −12 mmHg). If **colloid oncotic pressures** of 26 mmHg in the plasma and 5 mmHg in the interstitial fluid are assumed, then these forces at equilibrium across the capillary membrane would balance as follows: the total outward force of 26 mmHg is the sum of 9 mmHg of capillary hydrostatic pressure, 5 mmHg of interstitial colloid osmotic pressure, and 12 mmHg of negative interstitial fluid pressure. The total inward force of the plasma colloid osmotic pressure is 26 mmHg, and thus there is equilibrium.

However, in reality net outward forces slightly exceed the inward force, causing a very small excess of fluid to filter out of the capillaries. This is returned to the circulation through the lymphatics. In fact, it is the exceptionally rich lymphatic network that prevents pulmonary edema until capillary hydrostatic pressure exceeds 25 mmHg. The negative interstitial fluid pressure favors passage of fluid across the alveolar membranes into the interstitial fluid spaces, thus preventing accumulation of fluid in the alveoli.

Pulmonary edema

> 1 How is **pulmonary edema** prevented?
> 2 What are some of the causes of pulmonary edema?

The lymphatic vessels, which are contractile, serve as skimming pumps for maintaining the extravascular fluid volume. In mature normal unanesthetized sheep weighing 30–40 kg, lung lymph flow is estimated to be 10 mL/hour.

The alveolar epithelial membrane keeps fluid from entering the alveolar gas spaces. The uninjured membrane is normally impermeable to the common solutes of body fluids which pass freely over the capillary wall. Entrance of fluid into the alveoli only occurs as the final event in **lung edema**.

> Normally, the lung lymphatics can transport moderately increased fluid loads with only minimal increases in interstitial fluid volume and pressure. Only when they become overwhelmed does fluid accumulate and edema become evident.

For lung edema with alveolar flooding to occur, one or a combination of events must lead to an imbalance between the rate of formation of tissue fluid and the rate of its drainage. The rate of filtration of capillary fluid is determined by the capillary blood pressure, tissue oncotic pressure, permeability of the capillary wall, pressure of the environment surrounding the capillary, and oncotic pressure of the blood plasma. Increases in any of the first three or decreases in the last two favor more rapid filtration. The most frequent cause of pulmonary capillary hypertension and lung edema is a decrease in the pumping action of the left ventricle as occurs in chronic **congestive heart failure** or **acute myocardial infarction**. When the ventricle fails to empty, it accumulates blood, end-diastolic volume and pressure increase, and pressures more proximal to the lung in the left atrium and the pulmonary vessels rise. Obstruction to flow from the left atrium to the left ventricle (**mitral stenosis**) causes a similar chain of events. Noncardiac causes of pulmonary capillary hypertension include intravascular fluid overload, pulmonary veno-occlusive diseases, **exercise-induced pulmonary hemorrhage**, and congenital and acquired forms of venous narrowing or stenosis.

> Lymphatic obstruction or paralysis of lymphatic contractility decreases the rate of drainage and enhances the accumulation of fluid. In clinical situations, by far the most common cause of imbalance is increased capillary blood pressure.

Increases in the permeability of the pulmonary microvascular and alveolar membranes can be a primary factor in lung edema. Often permeability factors that are also mediators of inflammation, coagulation, or **embolism** are involved. Pulmonary edema due to increased permeability may be seen in pneumonia, following inhalation of irritating gases, in radiation sickness, in uremia, following aspiration of foreign material, as a result of poisoning with snake venoms or organophosphate insecticides, and with pulmonary microembolization which may accompany physical trauma, hemorrhagic and septic shock, hemodialysis, or cardiopulmonary bypass.

> **Neurogenic pulmonary edema** is the term given to acute pulmonary edema that may follow severe head injuries or experimental lesions of the medulla or hypothalamus. In some cases severe systemic hypertension leads to rising pulmonary capillary pressures that account for the pulmonary edema. In some instances increased pulmonary capillary pressure is not involved and an increase in capillary permeability occurs.

Regulation of vasomotor tone

> 1 What are the species differences in **vasomotion** in the pulmonary circulation?
> 2 Describe the causes of pulmonary arterial vasomotion.
> 3 Explain the concept of **autoregulation**.
> 4 What are some of the vasoactive substances that are synthesized, stored, or activated by cells in the lung?

Because pulmonary vessels are thin-walled and easily collapsible, passive mechanical forces, such as those associated with the consolidation of some pneumonias or with airless or **atelectic** areas, substantially increase resistance to flow. The structure of the pulmonary vessels is not particularly well suited for active vasoconstriction. Neither pulmonary arteries nor veins have much vascular smooth muscle. However, as already discussed, species differences exist; cattle and swine have relatively more, while sheep and dogs have relatively less muscle in arterial walls. Since pulmonary arterial pressure is so low, even mild contraction of vascular smooth muscle can cause constriction of vessels under normal circumstances.

The pressures of oxygen and carbon dioxide in the alveolar gas spaces are the most powerful stimuli for pulmonary arterial vasomotion. In health not all alveoli are equally well ventilated, but much more significant unevenness of ventilation develops in pneumonia, bronchitis, emphysema, or other diseases in which some regional airway is obstructed. Either a fall in Po_2 or a rise in Pco_2 in a lung region results in vasoconstriction of its arterial vessels. Extrinsic autonomic nerves are not required.

Autoregulation

Autoregulation is well developed in the pulmonary vascular system and helps match blood flow to ventilation. Experimental observations on isolated artificially perfused and ventilated lungs, as well as *in vivo* experiments employing drugs which block autonomic nerves, reveal that the major vasomotor activity of resistance vessels depends on local autoregulatory mechanisms rather than central neural reflex systems.

The action of **alveolar hypoxia** is limited to very short segments of arteries/arterioles less than 200 μm in diameter that are immediately adjacent to the alveolus. Carbon dioxide acts similarly but on somewhat longer segments. It is the effect that Pco_2 has on the local hydrogen ion concentration rather than the Pco_2 per se which stimulates the vasoconstriction. The site of action is important in that it renders autoregulation effective down to the level of the alveoli.

> The vasoconstrictor effect of alveolar hypoxia or hypercapnia diverts blood flow from underventilated to well-ventilated air spaces. Hypoxia is a more potent vasoconstrictor than hypercapnia.

Vasoactive substances

Because of the large surface area of the pulmonary vascular bed and the fact that practically the entire cardiac output passes through it during each circulatory cycle, there are multiple vasoactive substances which are synthesized, stored, or activated by cells of the lung. Although similar metabolic processes may take place elsewhere, in other organ beds, their access to blood is only in proportion to the percentage of cardiac output they receive. Cells of the **reticuloendothelial system**, blood platelets, white blood cells, and those of the alveolar epithelium participate in the local production and destruction of vasoactive chemicals. **Histamine**, widely distributed in mast cells, is a powerful but rapidly inactivated pulmonary vasoconstrictor, although it has been reported to have a vasodilator action on the neonatal bovine circulation. **Serotonin (5-hydroxytryptamine)** is found in mast cells and blood platelets and is also a potent vasoconstrictor. **Angiotensin II**, formed from **angiotensin I** by a lung converting enzyme, is also a vasoconstrictor. **Bradykinin**, a vasodilator, is both generated and destroyed in the lungs. The **prostaglandin vasodilators PGE$_1$ and PGE$_2$** can be synthesized and stored in the lungs, but the **vasoconstrictor PGF$_{2\alpha}$** is most abundant in lung parenchyma. **Nitric oxide (NO)** is a vascular smooth muscle relaxing factor that is produced by the action of nitric oxide synthase on L-arginine within vascular endothelial cells and elsewhere. Experiments using nitric oxide synthase inhibitors have revealed an important role for endogenous NO in setting the pulmonary vascular conductance in horses during exercise.

> These and other vasoactive compounds play important roles in a wide variety of pathological states, such as **endotoxic shock**, **hemorrhagic shock**, and **anaphylaxis**.

Vasomotor nerves

The small pulmonary vessels have muscular coats and are equipped with a dual nerve supply, sympathetic and parasympathetic; however, the predominant supply is via adrenergic sympathetic vasoconstriction. Stimulation of the sympathetic pulmonary nerves increases the PVR and hence pulmonary blood pressure. Stimulation of the baroreceptors results in increased pulmonary blood flow and decreased pulmonary arterial pressure. The capacious pulmonary vessels constitute one of the body's blood reservoirs, and the vasoconstrictor fibers function more in the reflex mobilization of blood (e.g., in hemorrhage) than in pressor or depressor pulmonary responses.

The presence of an adrenergic system within the lungs is confirmed by the actions of injected catecholamines in perfused isolated lungs. Small doses of epinephrine produce either minimal vasoconstriction or vasodilatation. Larger doses produce definite vasoconstriction. **Epinephrine** binds to both α-constrictor and β-dilator receptors, but has a stronger affinity for the latter. The β receptors are far fewer in number. Thus the larger the dose, the more conspicuous the vasoconstrictor effect. **Isoproterenol**, a pure β-stimulator, regularly produces vasodilatation. **Norepinephrine**, a pure α-stimulator, regularly produces vasoconstriction. Catecholamines are synthesized and stored in adrenergic nerve endings, but their release may be initiated not only by nerve impulses but also by local chemicals. For this reason the presence of adrenergic receptors is not absolute proof of neural reflex regulation. In the horse, endothelial cells mediate regional differences in pulmonary arterial relaxation to **methacholine**, which may favor the distribution of blood flow to dorsocaudal lung regions, the regions most affected by exercise-induced pulmonary hemorrhage.

Pulmonary hypertension

> 1 What are the factors involved in the setting and maintenance of pulmonary blood pressure?
>
> 2 How do the blood vessels in the lungs respond to high altitude and hypoxia?
>
> 3 Describe **brisket disease**. What species is primarily affected?
>
> 4 What is **emphysema** in horses?
>
> 5 Describe **heartworm disease** in dogs.
>
> 6 Describe exercise-induced pulmonary hemorrhage in horses.

The most important factors in the production and maintenance of pulmonary blood pressure are the rate of blood flow or the output of the right ventricle, the resistance to flow, the blood vessel volume, the expansiveness of the vascular system, and the blood viscosity. The pulmonary system is so extensive and capacious that increases in pulmonary blood flow and volume are often almost self-canceling due to the recruitment of additional pathways. Since the arterial resistance vessels are relatively thin-walled, pulmonary hypertension in the absence of lung or heart disease is less common than systemic hypertension in most species. When primary pulmonary hypertension occurs, it is often vaso-occlusive, i.e., there is curtailment of the pulmonary vascular bed or an impediment to flow through it. **Vaso-occlusive pulmonary hypertension** associated with a raised vascular resistance may be vasoconstrictive, a kind of functional vasospasm; obstructive, due to mechanical blockage of the vessel lumen by external pressure on vessel walls or plugging by thrombi or emboli; or obliterative, due to primary destructive or occlusive diseases of the walls of arteries and capillaries with a reduction in total functional cross-section. Often, several factors operate simultaneously or serially.

Often one mechanism recruits another. For example, the vaso-occlusion which accompanies obstruction by thrombi may be both mechanical and vasoactive because thrombi contain platelets, which are a source of the vasoconstrictor serotonin. Also, some chemicals that promote thrombosis and embolism, besides being vasospastic agents, may also be **vasculotoxic**, inducing inflammation and destruction of vessels. In animals, 30–50% of the vascular bed must be occluded to evoke pulmonary hypertension in the absence of increased pulmonary blood flow, volume, or viscosity.

High altitude

Unlike most other blood vessels, the vessels of the lungs constrict in response to hypoxia. This response may have evolved as part of the mechanism to divert blood away from the lungs and through the ductus arteriosus *in utero*. Thus as the arterial blood is hypoxemic *in utero*, PVR is high. At birth the first breath oxygenates the alveoli, raising oxygen pressures and relieving the vascular resistance. At high altitudes, airway or ventilatory hypoxia occurs in the absence of any **hypercapnic acidosis** or CO_2 retention. Ventilatory hypoxia elicits pulmonary arterial vasoconstriction and consequently an elevated pulmonary arterial pressure in mammals. Alveolar hypoxia, but not pulmonary arterial hypoxemia, causes this response. The hypertension is reversible when the hypoxia is relieved. The magnitude of the pressor response varies among species, being most pronounced in those having the most vascular smooth muscle. Calves and pigs, with relatively more vascular smooth muscle, are especially responsive (Figures 37.6 and 37.7). Hypoxia induced by breathing 12–13% oxygen in nitrogen considerably increases pulmonary arterial pressure, mildly increases cardiac output, and is without effect on left atrial pressure or central blood volume. Although generalized vasoconstriction of the pulmonary bed would seem to serve no useful purpose, a local hypoxia (e.g., as occurs when a bronchiole is partially or wholly occluded, decreasing or preventing ventilation to the dependent lung region) is helpful in regulating the distribution of blood flow by causing vasoconstriction, which would divert blood from the anoxic region to vessels in better-aerated parts of the lung.

> **Brisket disease** is a vasoconstrictive pulmonary hypertension due to alveolar hypoxia which is observed in some cattle at altitudes of 7000 feet (2133 m) or more above sea level. When pulmonary hypertension persists, it initiates responses in the right ventricle and systemic veins, capillaries, and tissues. The right ventricle hypertrophies, followed by right ventricular dilatation and failure, filling and distension of systemic veins, congestive edematous swelling of subcutaneous tissues, and **ascites**. Together, pulmonary hypertension, cardiac hypertrophy, and right heart dilation and failure constitute **cor pulmonale**, a heart disease secondary to pulmonary hypertension. The clinical signs in cattle are principally those associated with right heart failure, including

a dependent edematous swelling of the brisket region, a low exercise tolerance, **tachycardia**, distended and pulsating jugular veins, a loud pulmonic second heart sound, sometimes a systolic murmur due to incompetency of the tricuspid valve, ascites with congestion of the abdominal viscera, and profuse diarrhea. Pulmonary hypertension is the characteristic hemodynamic change that leads to right heart failure. The necropsy finds a hypertrophied and dilated right ventricle and hypertrophy of the vascular smooth muscle of pulmonary arteries. Bovine respiratory disease is the leading cause of mortality in cattle and altitude-induced pulmonary hypertension is associated with a substantially increased mortality despite improvements in antimicrobial and anti-inflammatory therapeutics.

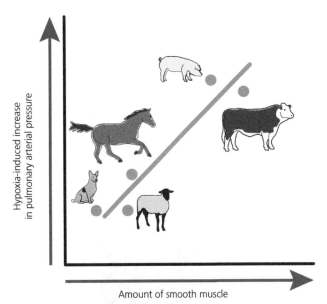

Figure 37.7 The relationship between the amount of muscle in the media of small pulmonary arteries and the change in pulmonary arterial pressure when animals are exposed to a hypoxic environment. Animals with thicker muscle layers, such as the cow and pig, have a greater vascular response to hypoxia than animals with far less muscle in the small pulmonary arteries, such as the dog and sheep. The horse has a low/intermediate response. Adapted from Fig. 45.6, Robinson, N.E. (1997) Pulmonary blood flow. In: *Textbook of Veterinary Physiology* (ed. J.G. Cunningham). W.B. Saunders, Philadelphia. With permission from Elsevier.

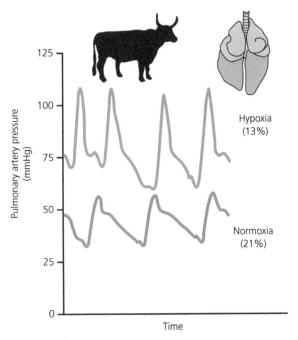

Figure 37.6 Effects of reduced oxygen in inspired air on pulmonary artery pressure in calves with unilateral (left) pulmonary artery ligation. Mean pulmonary artery pressure for control was 38 mmHg and for 13% oxygen mixture 84 mmHg. Adapted from Vogel, J.H.K., Averill, K.H., Pool, P.E. and Blount, S.G. (1963) Experimental pulmonary arterial hypertension in the newborn calf. *Circulation Research* **13**:557–571. Reproduced with permission from The American Heart Association, Inc.

> Hypertrophy and dilatation of the right ventricle secondary to the pulmonary hypertension of chronic obstructive lung disease have been reported in horses and cattle. PVR and pulmonary arterial pressure are also elevated in emphysematous horses.

Emphysema (heaves) in horses

Increased hindrance to airflow out of the lungs defines **chronic obstructive lung diseases,** such as COPD, chronic emphysema, and bronchitis. Increased PVR is particularly frequent in emphysema. The resulting pulmonary hypertension is vaso-occlusive. The primary lung disease results in destruction of vessels and thus a reduction in the overall radius of the pulmonary vascular system. Increased vascular resistance, pulmonary hypertension, and an apparent decrement in the density of capillaries occurs in emphysematous horses. In emphysema, airway hypoxia and hypercapnia result from ventilation–perfusion mismatch that favors pulmonary vasoconstriction.

Heartworm disease in dogs

Pulmonary hypertension is characteristic of heartworm disease in dogs (Figure 37.8). Pulmonary artery pressures as high as 158/59 mmHg have been observed. PVR is increased due to obstruction, narrowing, or closure of pulmonary vascular pathways. In large vessels this is the result of mature worms in their lumens. In the smaller vessels, mechanical obstruction is caused by thrombi containing fragments of disintegrating parasites, by emboli, and by fibroplasia involving the walls of arteries.

> Right heart failure is common in dogs infested with **Dirofilaria immitis**. Such failure is not always purely secondary to pulmonary hypertension. Both mature worms (up to 15 cm long) and microfilariae may be widely distributed in the chambers of the heart and the vessels of the systemic circulation. Mature worms may be found in the venae cavae, lumens of the right atrium and ventricle, and orifices of the tricuspid and pulmonary semilunar valves. They obstruct flow into and out of the right side of the heart and hinder normal function of cardiac valves.

Section VI: The Cardiovascular System

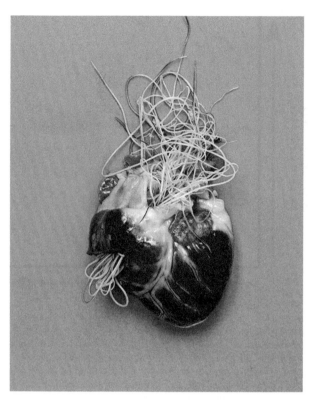

Figure 37.8 Severe *Dirofilaria immitis* infestation in the heart of a dog. This condition, in the extreme, leads to increased pulmonary vascular pressures, right heart failure, and death. Merial Ltd, Duluth, GA, USA, 2014. Reproduced with permission of Merial Ltd.

Exercise-induced pulmonary hemorrhage

Exercise-induced pulmonary hemorrhage (EIPH) occurs in racehorses during sprint racing and is characterized by pulmonary hypertension, edema in the gas exchange region of the lung, rupture of the pulmonary capillaries, intra-alveolar hemorrhage, and the presence of blood in the airways (Figure 37.9). Current evidence suggests that stress failure of the pulmonary capillaries results from pulmonary vascular hypertension combined with large negative intrapleural pressures or large changes in pressure which create a high capillary transmural pressure leading to hemorrhage. The cause of hypertension may also be related to the enormous cardiac output demanded by the racehorse associated with maximal recruitment and distension of the pulmonary capillaries. Experimental evidence indicates that there is significant EIPH above a mean pulmonary artery pressure of about 90 mmHg, and during maximal exercise pulmonary arterial pressures may exceed 120 mmHg in the Thoroughbred. **Diuresis** invoked by **furosemide** (Lasix or Salix) treatment lowers pulmonary vascular pressures and EIPH. **Laryngeal hemiplegia** narrows the respiratory passageways and elevates inspiratory resistance. This condition is detected initially by the distinct "**roaring**" heard on inspiration during exercise in affected horses and diagnosed by **endoscopy**. The elevated inspiratory resistance caused by laryngeal hemiplegia elevates negative alveolar pressures and worsens EIPH. In contrast, application of a **nasal strip** in healthy horses constrains the normal nasal passage narrowing which occurs on inspiration, reduces the energetic cost of breathing, and significantly

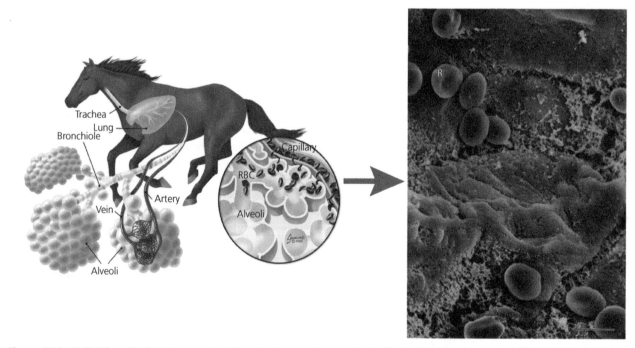

Figure 37.9 (*Left*) Schematic depicting exercise-induced pulmonary hypertension in the horse. Diagram courtesy of Flair, LLC by Brad Gilleland. (*Right*) Scanning electron micrograph of the cranial lobe of an exercised pony reveals red blood cells (R) and proteinaceous material in the alveoli. From Erickson, H.H., McAvoy, J.L. and Westfall, J.A. (1997) Exercise-induced changes in the lung of Shetland ponies: ultrastructure and morphometry. *Journal of Submicroscopic and Cytological Pathology* **29**:65–72.

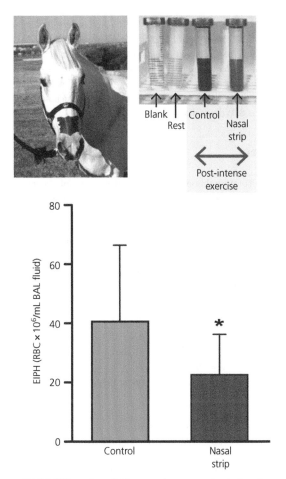

Figure 37.10 Effect of nasal dilator strip on exercise-induced pulmonary hemorrhage (EIPH) red blood cell (RBC) counts in bronchoalveolar fluid. (*Upper left*) Horse wearing the nasal strip which supports the airways and soft tissues just rostral to the nasoincisive notch. (*Upper right*) Bronchoalveolar lavage (BAL) Ringers solution under the following conditions (from left): 1, blank (no lavage); 2, from a resting horse; 3, post-exercise from a control (no nasal strip); 4, post-exercise from a horse wearing the nasal strip. Note reduction in blood from horse wearing the nasal strip). (*Bottom*) Mean EIPH reduction for horses wearing the nasal dilator strip versus control. With kind permission from Kindig, C.A., McDonough, P., Fenton, G., Poole, D.C. and Erickson, H.H. (2001) Effect of nasal strip and furosemide in mitigating EIPH in Thoroughbred horses. *Journal of Applied Physiology* **91**:1396–1400.

lessens EIPH (Figure 37.10). The complexity of EIPH etiology is emphasized by the observation that it is possible via the nasal strip, NO breathing, NO synthase inhibition and inclined running to dissociate the severity of EIPH from peak pulmonary artery pressure. Thus, while high pulmonary artery pressures are indicative of high pulmonary capillary pressures, extravascular (i.e., alveolar) pressures are also important in determining the extent of capillary rupture and EIPH. Furthermore, at a given cardiac output, high pulmonary artery pressures may arise from a pulmonary arteriolar vasoconstriction that acts to reduce transduction of pulmonary artery pressures to the fragile capillary bed and is thus protective to the integrity of

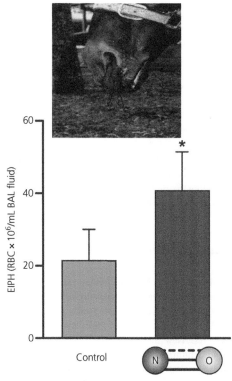

Figure 37.11 Effects of nitric oxide (NO) inhalation on exercise-induced pulmonary hemorrhage (EIPH), quantified by bronchoalveolar lavage (BAL), in maximally exercising Thoroughbred horses. Peak mean pulmonary artery pressure averaged 102 mmHg in the control trial and was significantly reduced to 99 mmHg by inhalation of 80 ppm NO. Despite this reduction in pulmonary artery pressure, the severity of EIPH was increased by NO breathing. With kind permission from Kindig, C.A., McDonough, P., Finley, M.R., Behnke, B.J., Richardson, T.E., Marlin, D.J., Erickson, H.H. and Poole, D.C. (2001) Nitric oxide inhalation reduces pulmonary hypertension but not hemorrhage in maximally exercising horses. *Journal of Applied Physiology* **91**:2674–2680.

the blood–gas barrier. In support of this notion, NO breathing at maximal exercise reduces peak pulmonary arterial pressure but concomitantly increases EIPH (Figure 37.11).

Self-evaluation

Answers can be found at the end of the chapter.

1 Viewed in cross-section, what is the most obvious structural difference between the pulmonary arteries and the systemic arteries?

2 During exercise, PVR falls as pulmonary artery pressure increases. What are the two mechanisms responsible for the fall in PVR?

3 In a Thoroughbred horse running at 15 m/s (~33 mph), the oxygen concentrations of the mixed venous (pulmonary arterial) and arterial blood are 3 and 26 ml/100 mL, respectively, and the oxygen uptake ($\dot{V}o_2$) is 70 L/min. What is the cardiac output ($\dot{Q}$)?

4 Calculate the $\dot{V}o_2$ of a greyhound running at maximal speed when $\dot{Q}$ is 20 L/min, and the oxygen concentrations of the mixed venous (pulmonary arterial) and arterial blood are 2 and 20 mL/100 mL, respectively.

5 In the arterial blood sample drawn from the horse in question 3, the pressure of oxygen (Po_2) is 55 mmHg (after temperature correction) which is substantially below alveolar Po_2. Assuming that the horse is healthy, what might account for this arterial hypoxemia?

6 Failure of the fragile blood–gas barrier is caused by high capillary transmural pressures. What two pressures summate across the capillary wall leading to capillary rupture and EIPH during exercise in the Thoroughbred racehorse?

Suggested reading

Deffebach, M.E., Charan, N., Lakshminarayan, S. *et al.* (1987) The bronchial circulation: small, but a vital attribute of the lung. *American Review of Respiratory Diseases* **135**:463–481.

Hlastala, M.P. and Berger, A.J. (1996) *Physiology of Respiration*. Oxford University Press, New York.

Leff, A.R. and Schumacker, P.T. (1993) *Respiratory Physiology: Basics and Applications*. W.B. Saunders, Philadelphia.

Marlin, D. and Nankervis, K.J. (2002) *Equine Exercise Physiology*. Blackwell Publishing, Oxford.

Murray, J.F. (1986) *The Normal Lung*. W.B. Saunders, Philadelphia.

Poole, D.C. and Erickson, H.H. (2004) Heart and vessels: function during exercise and response to training. In: *Equine Sports Medicine and Surgery* (eds K. Hinchcliff, R.J. Geor and A.J. Kaneps), pp. 697–727. Saunders Elsevier Philadelphia.

Poole, D.C. and Erickson, H.H. (2008) Cardiovascular function and oxygen transport: responses to exercise and training. In: *Equine Exercise Physiology. The Science of Exercise in the Athletic Horse* (eds K. Hinchcliff, R.J. Geor and A.J. Kaneps), pp. 212–245. Saunders Elsevier, Philadelphia.

Poole, D.C. and Erickson, H.H. (2011) Highly athletic terrestrial mammals: horses and dogs. *Comprehensive Physiology* **1**:1–37.

Robinson, N.E. (1982) Some functional consequences of species differences in lung anatomy. *Advances in Veterinary Science and Comparative Medicine* **26**:1–33.

Slonim, N.B. and Hamilton, L.H. (1987) *Respiratory Physiology*, 5th edn. C.V. Mosby, St Louis, MO.

Weibel, E.R. (1984) *The Pathway for Oxygen: Structure and Function in the Mammalian Respiratory System*. Harvard University Press, Cambridge, MA.

West, J.B. (1985) *Respiratory Physiology: The Essentials*, 3rd edn. Williams & Wilkins, Baltimore.

Answers

1 The wall of the pulmonary arteries (and also arterioles) contains relatively little smooth muscle and elastic tissue and is therefore much thinner. This means that relatively low forces within the contiguous lung parenchyma can collapse (low lung volumes, high PVR) or pull open (high lung volumes, low PVR) the vascular lumen.

2 Additional pulmonary vessels are recruited and those already recruited are distended. These processes increase the total cross-sectional area of the pulmonary vasculature for blood flow, which decreases PVR.

3 From the Fick principle,

$$\dot{Q} = \dot{V}o_2/(Cao_2 - C\bar{v}o_2)$$
$$\dot{Q} = 70{,}000/([26 - 3]/100)$$
$$\dot{Q} = 70{,}000/0.23$$
$$\dot{Q} = 304{,}000 \text{ mL/min or 304 L/min}$$

4 From the Fick principle,

$$\dot{V}o_2 = \dot{Q}(Cao_2 - C\bar{v}o_2)$$
$$\dot{V}o_2 = 20{,}000 ([20 - 2]/100)$$
$$\dot{V}o_2 = 20{,}000 \times 0.18$$
$$\dot{V}o_2 = 3600 \text{ mL/min or 3.6 L/min}$$

5 $\dot{Q}$ has increased eightfold from resting values whereas the pulmonary capillary blood volume has only increased twofold. Consequently mean red blood cell transit time has decreased to 2/8 = 25% of its resting value and there is insufficient time for oxygen loading within the pulmonary capillary.

6 High positive intraluminal pressures summate with negative alveolar pressures to cause failure of the very thin blood–gas barrier, resulting in red cells escaping into the alveoli and airways. Although frank epistaxis is rare, endoscopy and bronchoalveolar lavage demonstrate that the vast majority of Thoroughbreds suffer EIPH during racing.

38 Special Circulations

Eileen M. Hasser, Cheryl M. Heesch, David D. Kline and M. Harold Laughlin

University of Missouri, Columbia, MO, USA

Regional distribution of cardiac output

The overall function of the cardiovascular system is to provide oxygen and nutrients and remove carbon dioxide and waste products from all tissues, in accordance with the requirements of each individual tissue, and also with the demands of the body as a whole. The manner in which flow is distributed to different organs must be adaptable in order to accommodate different stressors and physiological and pathophysiological conditions. Thus, flow to specific individual organs may be adjusted to preserve overall homeostasis.

Flow to specific tissues is controlled by both global extrinsic control mechanisms and local control mechanisms (see Chapters 35 and 36). These regulatory mechanisms are separate but interrelated. In general, global control mechanisms, including the autonomic nervous system, circulating hormones and cardiovascular reflexes, are primarily responsible for maintaining overall cardiovascular function. For example, an adequate level of arterial pressure is required for both global cardiovascular homeostasis and for providing adequate blood supply to the individual organs. Local control mechanisms, on the other hand, are primarily directed toward meeting the requirements of the vascular bed in which they function. Each organ has unique features and requirements so the relative importance of global and local control mechanisms varies from tissue to tissue and even spatially within tissue. In addition, the relative importance of these different control mechanisms within a given tissue may differ depending on the tissue's immediate metabolic requirements and the overall needs of the organism.

Coronary circulation

1 What arteries supply blood to the left and right ventricular myocardium?

2 Are coronary collateral arteries uniformly present among animal species?

3 How is coronary flow to the left ventricle influenced by ventricular systole and diastole?

4 How does the myogenic response minimize changes in coronary blood flow despite changes in coronary arterial blood pressure?

5 How does myocardial metabolism alter coronary vascular resistance, flow and autoregulation?

6 What is meant by coronary flow reserve?

7 What are the effects of sympathetic nervous system stimulation on coronary blood flow?

8 What is reactive hyperemia of coronary flow?

Section VI: The Cardiovascular System

Dukes' Physiology of Domestic Animals, Thirteenth Edition. Edited by William O. Reece, Howard H. Erickson, Jesse P. Goff and Etsuro E. Uemura.
© 2015 John Wiley & Sons, Inc. Published 2015 by John Wiley & Sons, Inc.
Companion website: www.wiley.com/go/reece/physiology

> **9** Why must one evaluate both oxygen supply and oxygen demand to know whether coronary blood flow is adequate?
>
> **10** What are the determinants of myocardial oxygen demand?

Functional anatomy of the coronary circulation

The heart receives approximately 5% of cardiac output at rest (about 100 mL/min per 100 g of tissue), and coronary flow can increase fourfold to sevenfold during strenuous exercise. The blood flow to the heart is supplied by the left and right coronary arteries (Figure 38.1), which arise from the aorta at the level of the **sinus of Valsalva** (aortic sinus). Large coronary arteries course along the epicardial surface and coronary artery branches then penetrate into the myocardium to supply all layers and regions of the heart. The right coronary artery supplies the majority of flow to the right atrium and ventricle while the left coronary artery supplies primarily the left atrium and ventricle and interventricular septum, although there can be overlap. The majority of cardiac venous drainage empties into the right atrium through the **coronary sinus**. In the dog, more than 80% of coronary sinus blood arises entirely from the left ventricle, with the remaining 20% originating from other parts of the heart. Consequently, the collection and analysis of coronary sinus blood has been a valuable tool for the study of left ventricular metabolism. However, caution must be used in extending this technique to other species because of anatomic differences. In the bovine, for example, coronary sinus blood consists of a mixture of venous blood from the heart and from the azygous vein, which carries venous blood from noncardiac tissues and empties into the great cardiac vein. Venous coronary blood from the right ventricle of the dog heart predominantly drains into the right atrium through the right cardiac vein. Only a very small amount of venous blood drains from myocardial tissue directly into the cardiac chambers, primarily into the right atrium and ventricle, through the very small thebesian veins.

Collateral coronary arteries

The coronary arteries have long been characterized as lacking collateral arteries, or vessels connecting major arteries without an intervening capillary bed. However, the accuracy of this characterization depends on the species as well as on variations within a species. For example, the coronary circulation in the guinea pig has abundant collateral arteries, so that tissue perfusion is maintained following abrupt occlusion of a coronary artery, preventing myocardial infarction (an area of necrosis resulting from inadequate coronary arterial flow) or tissue damage. In most species, however, collateral coronary arteries are absent or so small in size or number that collateral blood flow is inadequate to prevent infarction following sudden coronary occlusion. For example, coronary collateral arteries in the dog heart are typically thin-walled vessels of very small diameter, and therefore conduct only a very low volume of collateral coronary blood flow. In addition, the dog also illustrates the fact that substantial variability in the extent of collateral coronary arteries may exist among individuals within a species, and in some cases specifically among breeds within a species. The purebred beagle dog, for instance, tends to have an extensive collateral coronary circulation, so that ligation of a major coronary artery may fail to produce a myocardial infarct, or produces a substantially smaller infarct than would have been anticipated.

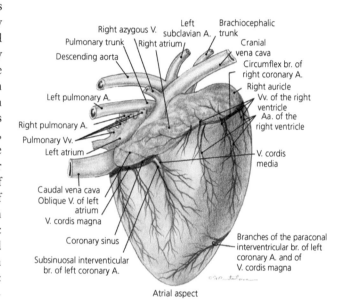

Atrial aspect

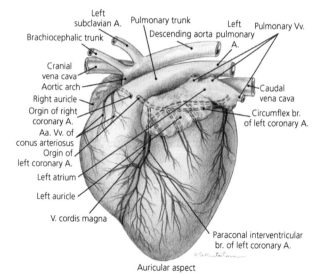

Auricular aspect

Figure 38.1 Anatomy of the coronary circulation in the dog, showing arteries (red) and veins (blue) as seen from the atrial or auricular aspects.

Despite the lack of a significant preexisting coronary collateral circulation, in most cases mammals will develop collateral coronary arteries if a major coronary artery is occluded slowly and gradually, as occurs in atherosclerosis. Initially, this newly developed collateral circulation has little reserve capacity, or ability to increase flow in response to an increase in myocardial oxygen demand. However, collateral development and expansion continue well beyond the time of occlusion, so collateral flow capacity 6 months after occlusion may approach that of the coronary artery prior to occlusion. Much of what is known about coronary collaterals has come from work in dogs. Collateral coronary arteries in the dog heart develop through a process of enlargement and expansion of preexisting epicardial arterioles (**arteriogenesis**). Arteriogenesis is stimulated by shear stress due to increased flow velocity proximal to the occlusion and involves participation of adhesion molecules and growth factors. It begins with dilation and thinning of existing collateral channels, followed by DNA synthesis and mitosis of vascular endothelial and smooth muscle cells. The final stage consists of remodeling of the collateral arterial wall, ultimately producing collateral coronary vessels primarily on the epicardial surface of the heart that are very similar to normal arteries except they are often tortuous rather than straight. The process of collateral development by arteriogenesis is not significantly influenced by the presence or absence of physical exercise.

Noncanine species vary widely in their ability to develop coronary collateral vessels and in the location and nature of these collateral vessels. In humans and the pig, collateral vessels arise as microvascular connections between capillary beds of an occluded and a nonoccluded artery, and are located within the myocardium or in the subendocardium. The development of collateral vessels in porcine and human hearts occurs through a process of **angiogenesis** or the sprouting of new capillaries from preexisting capillaries. Capillaries develop in response to factors such as vascular endothelial growth factor (VEGF), which is stimulated by hypoxia, in part via hypoxia-mediated adenosine release. It is unresolved how VEGF may contribute to arteriogenesis.

In view of the prevalence and significance of coronary artery disease in humans, it is not surprising that factors influencing arteriogenesis and angiogenesis in the coronary circulation have been of great interest. In particular, the study of vascular growth factors and their influence on the coronary circulation has led to the development of therapeutic approaches ranging from gene therapy to the administration of specific growth factors.

Control of coronary blood flow
Basal tone
The heart exhibits a high level of oxygen extraction, yet coronary blood flow in most mammals is relatively high at rest (around 100 mL/min per 100 g of tissue). In addition, substantial coronary flow reserve exists in that coronary blood flow can increase fourfold to sixfold with intense exercise. While α-adrenergic stimulation can produce coronary vasoconstriction, the importance of neural mechanisms in establishing or maintaining basal coronary tone is minimal compared to other tissues such as skin and gastrointestinal vascular beds.

The terms **myogenic tone** or **myogenic response** refer to the intrinsic tendency of vascular smooth muscle to shorten in response to stretch produced by arterial distending pressure (see Chapter 36). The myogenic response is believed to minimize changes in coronary flow despite significant changes in coronary arterial pressure. In the coronary circulation the magnitude of the myogenic response is inversely related to the size of the vessel, and is best demonstrated in arterioles of less than 200 μm in diameter. The myogenic response of arterioles also varies to some degree with their transmural location in the ventricular wall. The myogenic response of coronary arterioles in hypertensive humans has been shown to be greater than the response of these vessels in normotensive individuals, indicating that the magnitude of the myogenic response may be altered by pathophysiological conditions.

Physical factors influence coronary flow
In most systemic vascular beds, the pattern of blood flow follows that of aortic pressure, with the greatest flow occurring during systole, when pressure is highest. However, during the cardiac cycle coronary blood flow, specifically to the left ventricle, is significantly influenced by both the perfusion (aortic) pressure and by the fact that intramyocardial coronary arteries are surrounded by contracting myocardium. During systole, the high extravascular forces generated by the contracting ventricle compress the vessels and impede flow, so that left coronary artery flow may actually reverse during early systole (Figure 38.2). As aortic pressure rises during the ejection phase of systole, flow also increases. Nevertheless, peak left coronary flow occurs during early diastole, when aortic pressure is still high but the ventricle has relaxed, eliminating extravascular compressive forces. Approximately 80% of left coronary flow occurs during diastole in normal mammals.

Right ventricular pressures are normally much lower than left ventricular pressures, exerting less compressive force on the vessels. As a result aortic pressure is sufficient to overcome these forces and drive right coronary flow during systole. Therefore, the pattern of right coronary flow follows aortic pressure as in other vascular beds, and peak flow occurs during systole (Figure 38.2).

As previously noted, the left ventricular wall is supplied by penetrating intramural arteries arising from epicardial conductance vessels. Myocardial contraction creates extravascular compressive forces that are particularly high in the subendocardial layers of the ventricle, and decrease flow reserve in these layers. However, anatomic characteristics and physiological regulation of the coronary circulation in normal mammals compensate for these features, so that coronary blood flow is uniformly distributed across the ventricular wall.

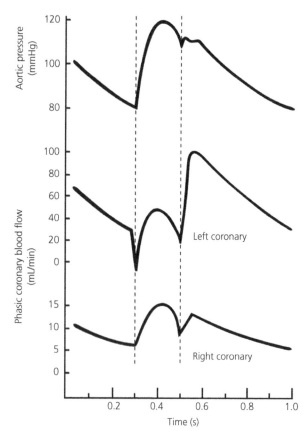

Figure 38.2 Effects of cardiac contraction on blood flow in the left and right coronary arteries. Note that the majority of flow to the left ventricle occurs during diastole, while the majority of flow to the right ventricle occurs during systole (see text for details). Ventricular systole is represented by the period between the dotted lines. From Fig. 20.3, Buss, D.D. (2004), in *Dukes' Physiology of Domestic Animals*, 12th edn (ed. W.O. Reece). Cornell University Press, Ithaca, NY. Reproduced with permission from Cornell University Press.

Myocardial metabolism is a primary controller of coronary flow

The myocardium relies on aerobic metabolism, rendering cardiac function dependent on a continuous delivery of oxygen and metabolic fuels and elimination of metabolic waste products. Oxygen extraction by the myocardium is very high (approximately 75%) in comparison to other tissues. Although oxygen extraction may increase up to 90%, an increase in oxygen demand by the myocardium must be met primarily by an increase in coronary blood flow. As a result, an important characteristic of the coronary circulation is the direct relationship between coronary blood flow and myocardial oxygen consumption ($M\dot{V}O_2$). $M\dot{V}O_2$ is determined by factors including heart rate, level of myocardial contractility, and myocardial tension or ventricular wall stress, which is related to afterload (aortic pressure or resistance) and, to a lesser degree, to preload (diastolic ventricular volume). Thus, altering any of these factors will influence $M\dot{V}O_2$ and therefore coronary blood flow (Figure 38.3).

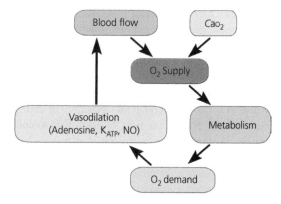

(Rate, Preload, Afterload, Contractility)

Figure 38.3 Interaction between oxygen supply and demand in determining coronary blood flow. Oxygen supply is determined by the coronary blood flow and the arterial oxygen content (Cao_2). The balance of oxygen supply and demand determines the extent to which vasodilator metabolites are present, which in turn influences blood flow, serving to match supply to demand.

The factors mediating the matching of coronary blood flow to $M\dot{V}O_2$ have not been fully delineated but appear to be related primarily to metabolic mechanisms. An increase in the ratio of oxygen demand to blood flow (due either to increased $M\dot{V}O_2$ or decreased flow or arterial oxygen content) results in release of vasodilator substances, decreasing coronary resistance. Important vasodilator mechanisms include production of **adenosine** and **nitric oxide** (NO), and activation of K_{ATP} **channels**, although their interaction is complex and other factors likely also play a role (Figure 38.3). Among these factors, substantial attention has focused on adenosine. Increased oxygen demand or reduced coronary flow leads to increased release of adenosine, which acts at purinoceptors to cause vasodilation, restoring or increasing flow. In vascular smooth muscle cells, activation or opening of K_{ATP} channels due to reduced ATP produces hyperpolarization, reducing calcium inflow through voltage-sensitive calcium channels in the cell membrane. This reduction in calcium influx decreases intracellular calcium concentration and produces smooth muscle relaxation. In endothelial cell membranes, opening or activation of K_{ATP} channels appears to be coupled to increased endothelial NO release. Consequently, coronary vasodilation due to K_{ATP} channel activation is a consequence of effects on both vascular smooth muscle and endothelial cells.

Systemic hypoxia causes an increase in coronary flow, a response that also appears to involve, in part, activation of K_{ATP} channels. In contrast, hyperoxia results in coronary vasoconstriction, produced by closure of K_{ATP} channels. Both respiratory and metabolic acidosis result in vasodilation and an increase in coronary flow. One mechanism for this vasodilator response is that of an acidosis-induced increase in adenosine production and stimulation of purinoceptors.

The adequacy of coronary blood flow at any time represents a balance between oxygen supply and demand. This balance is critical since myocardial dysfunction results when coronary flow is inadequate to meet the metabolic demands of the myocardium. The normal coronary circulation has great flexibility in meeting cardiac metabolic needs, and oxygen supply is directly related to the level of coronary blood flow. While oxygen demand is considered to be equivalent to the $\dot{M}VO_2$ under normal conditions, in humans limitations of coronary blood flow caused by obstructive coronary lesions may result in a mismatch so that myocardial oxygen demand exceeds oxygen supply. The primary sites of regulation of coronary blood flow under most circumstances are the small arteries and arterioles. The large epicardial coronary arteries, frequently termed conductance arteries, contribute little resistance to flow under normal circumstances.

Neural regulation of coronary flow

The coronary circulation is relatively independent of central neural regulation, with a predominance of local vasoregulatory mechanisms. However, both α (constrictor) and β (dilator) adrenoceptors are present in coronary vessels. Thus, adrenergically stimulated coronary vascular effects may modify or limit local mechanisms of coronary regulation. Different classes of adrenergic receptors tend to be preferentially located in various segments of the coronary circulation. For example, while α_1 **receptors** are distributed in coronary arteries and arterioles, α_2 **receptors** are found primarily in small coronary arterioles less than $100\,\mu m$ in diameter. Sympathetic nervous system stimulation generally produces a mild α-receptor-mediated vasoconstriction in the coronary circulation.

Under most circumstances activation of sympathetic nerves to the heart increases heart rate and contractility and thus cardiac metabolic activity, resulting in increased coronary blood flow. This response of coronary blood flow to generalized sympathetic stimulation is a combination of the direct constrictor effect of α-adrenergic activation on the coronary circulation and an indirect coronary vascular effect, related to β-adrenergic-mediated changes in cardiac metabolism and vasoactive tissue metabolites. Under normal circumstances the metabolic effects on cardiac muscle predominate, so that sympathetic stimulation produces an overall increase in coronary flow. However, during β-adrenergic blockade to eliminate effects of sympathetic activation on heart rate and contractility, vasoconstriction is unmasked during activation of sympathetic nerves, resulting in coronary vasoconstriction and a decrease in flow. Parasympathetic effects on the coronary vasculature are minor and vagal activation primarily has an effect to decrease heart rate.

Autoregulation and coronary reserve

The heart displays substantial **autoregulation**, or relatively constant coronary blood flow despite changes in perfusion pressure (see Chapter 36). The degree of autoregulation and the range of pressure over which autoregulation occurs are subtly

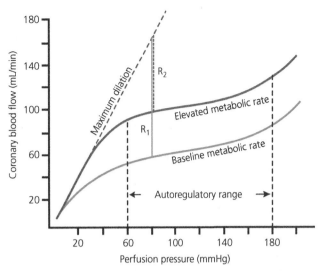

Figure 38.4 Autoregulation of coronary blood flow and coronary flow reserve. Coronary blood flow is maintained relatively constant despite a change in perfusion pressure (over a given range of pressures; autoregulatory range). Increasing myocardial oxygen consumption increases coronary flow, but autoregulation is maintained (upper curve). However, during maximal coronary vasodilation, the pressure–flow relationship becomes linear. The difference between flow during autoregulation and that observed during maximal dilation is the coronary flow reserve (R_1). Flow reserve is less (R_2) during increased metabolism. Adapted from Fig. 20.4, Buss, D.D. (2004), in *Dukes' Physiology of Domestic Animals*, 12th edn (ed. W.O. Reece). Cornell University Press, Ithaca, NY. Reproduced with permission from Cornell University Press.

less in the right than in the left coronary circulation of the dog, but the mechanisms responsible for these differences have not been identified. Many potential mechanisms have been proposed as mediators of autoregulation, including tissue P_{O_2}, P_{CO_2} and pH, adenosine, endothelium-derived NO, K_{ATP} channel activity, myogenic tone, and others. However, no single mechanism or hypothesis has fully explained the process of coronary autoregulation.

While changes in myocardial oxygen demand will shift the position of the pressure–flow relationship, autoregulation is preserved just at a different level of blood flow. For example, increases in cardiac metabolism increase coronary flow, but flow continues to exhibit autoregulation around that new higher blood flow (Figure 38.4). In contrast, maximal coronary vasodilation typically produces a fourfold to fivefold increase in coronary blood flow. In addition, the relatively flat pressure–flow relationship observed during autoregulation shifts to one that is steep and linear, with flow increasing substantially in response to increased perfusion pressure (Figure 38.4). The term **coronary flow reserve** refers to the difference between coronary flow at rest and that measured during maximal coronary vasodilation at the same perfusion pressure. Technically, coronary reserve is often expressed as the ratio of coronary resistance during the control state to coronary resistance during maximal coronary vasodilation. The concept of coronary reserve emphasizes the remarkable capacity of the normal coronary circulation to increase flow in response to increasing $M\dot{V}O_2$. The increase in coronary flow produced by increased $M\dot{V}O_2$ is often referred to as active or functional hyperemia (see Chapter 36).

Reactive hyperemia

The term **reactive hyperemia** refers to the large temporary increase in coronary flow that follows the release of a brief coronary occlusion induced experimentally (see Chapter 36). Following release, coronary flow rapidly increases to a maximum (peak reactive hyperemia flow), and then gradually declines to control level (see Figure 36.4, Chapter 36). Coronary flow during peak reactive hyperemia may exceed basal coronary flow by fivefold, and is directly proportional to the duration of occlusion, up to approximately 30 s. Reactive hyperemia can also be demonstrated after a very brief occlusion, lasting only a fraction of a single diastolic period. The coronary reactive hyperemia response is not produced by a single mechanism or mediator, but by several factors such as the myogenic response, metabolic mediators, and biophysical factors, with each factor varying in significance depending on the duration of occlusion.

Cerebral circulation

1 What is the physiological advantage of a complete vascular ring (circle of Willis)?

2 What produces the blood–brain barrier?

3 How is the blood–brain barrier influenced by histamine?

4 What is the relative importance of neural and local control mechanisms in regulating cerebral blood flow?

5 What is the response of cerebral resistance vessels to hypercapnia and hypocapnia?

6 What are some of the metabolic vasodilators associated with an increase in cerebral blood flow in response to hypoxia?

7 What is the neurovascular unit?

Anatomic considerations

The blood supply to the brain arises primarily from the circulus arteriosus cerebri (**circle of Willis**, Figure 38.5), a vascular ring located ventral to the hypothalamus. The degree to which this is a complete vascular ring varies among species. In species where the circle of Willis is complete, blood flow to the brain is maintained even in the face of an obstruction at any single point in the vascular circle. In some species, the arterial circle is supplied by the internal carotid arteries and the basilar artery, which in turn is supplied primarily by the vertebral arteries. In other species, however, the internal carotid arteries connect with other vessels in the head before entering the arterial circle. These vascular connections form a complex network of vessels, the rete mirabile. The rete mirabile may facilitate maintenance

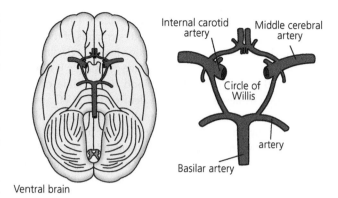

Ventral brain

Figure 38.5 Circle of Willis and primary arterial supply to the brain.

of a constant brain temperature in the face of either high or low temperature stress.

Cerebrospinal fluid

The cerebral circulation is important for the production of **cerebrospinal fluid (CSF)**, primarily formed at the choroid plexus through processes of filtration and active cellular secretion. CSF fills and bathes the cerebral ventricles, the subarachnoid space, and the central canal of the spinal cord, and is primarily reabsorbed at the dural sinuses. The primary role of CSF is to protect the brain. The brain is effectively suspended in CSF, so that its movement in response to a blow to the head is limited. CSF thus serves to cushion the brain, limiting damage in response to trauma. CSF pressure is determined by the relative rates of formation and drainage, so any obstruction to drainage, whether a consequence of trauma or tumors or other space-occupying lesions, may increase CSF pressure, with important clinical signs and consequences.

Blood–brain barrier

The capillaries of the brain exhibit very limited permeability, a feature known as the **blood–brain barrier**. A blood–brain barrier was originally postulated because intravascular injection of acidic dyes such as trypan blue stained all body tissues except brain and spinal cord. Later research showed that water, carbon dioxide, oxygen, and steroid hormones cross cerebral capillaries easily, while passage of strongly ionized substances, protein-bound substances, or those with molecular masses exceeding 40 kDa is limited or nonexistent. Importantly, certain substances, such as glucose and insulin, gain access to the brain via carrier-mediated and active transport systems present in cerebral capillaries.

Structurally, the blood–brain barrier is due to anatomic features including very tight junctions and a paucity of pores and pinocytotic vesicles in cerebral vascular endothelial cells. The limited permeability of the blood–brain barrier aids in maintaining a constant composition of brain interstitial fluid;

however, it also limits the penetration of many therapeutic agents into the brain and spinal cord.

Pathological processes may locally alter or break down the blood–brain barrier. Furthermore, its permeability may be altered physiologically by histamine via actions at H_1, H_2, and H_3 receptors. In the cerebral circulation, the response to histamine is biphasic. Relatively low concentrations increase permeability of pial venular vessels by activation of H_2 receptors on endothelial cells. In contrast, higher concentrations of histamine reduce permeability, apparently through activation of H_1 receptors. Histaminergic neurons have been demonstrated in the hypothalamus, and may, under certain pathophysiological circumstances, represent a source for local histamine release and alterations in vascular permeability.

Circumventricular organs

Specific small regions of the brain have fenestrated capillaries and are therefore permeable to large molecules. These brain regions devoid of a blood–brain barrier typically border the ventricular system and are termed **circumventricular organs (CVOs)**. The CVOs include the posterior pituitary, area postrema, organum vasculorum of the lamina terminalis, and the subfornical organ. Secretory CVOs, such as the posterior pituitary, serve as sites from which secreted peptides such as vasopressin and oxytocin can enter the circulation. Other CVOs contain receptors for various peptide hormones, such as angiotensin II, and serve as a means by which these circulating hormones can communicate with the brain.

Control of cerebral blood flow: local control mechanisms predominate

Cerebral blood flow is regulated primarily by local mechanisms, with autonomic vascular regulatory mechanisms playing only a secondary and comparatively minor role. A unique aspect of the cerebral circulation is related to the fact that the brain is extremely intolerant of ischemia. As a result, interruption of flow to the brain results in unconsciousness within seconds and irreversible tissue damage can occur within a few minutes. Importantly, therefore, cerebral blood flow is controlled primarily by local mechanisms related to brain metabolism.

Neural control factors

Cerebral blood vessels are innervated primarily by the sympathetic nervous system, which mediates vasoconstriction due to release of norepinephrine and also neuropeptide Y (NPY). However, the density of α-adrenergic receptors in the cerebral circulation is low relative to other vascular beds. As a result, sympathetic control of cerebral blood vessels is relatively weak. Innervation by the parasympathetic nervous system arises from the facial nerves but its effects on blood flow are minor.

Sensory nerves containing substance P and calcitonin gene-related peptide (CGRP) also supply the distal cerebral vessels. Both substance P and CGRP are potent vasodilators. Local perturbations result in their reflex release from perivascular nerves,

activating ATP-sensitive potassium (K_{ATP}) channels, thereby producing hyperpolarization and relaxation of cerebral arteries.

Local control mechanisms

Local control mechanisms are the primary regulators of cerebral blood flow, particularly in response to changing levels of local metabolism as well as systemic alterations in blood gases. Neural activity and increased metabolism result in reductions in ATP accompanied by adenosine release as well as decreases in tissue P_{O_2}, increased P_{CO_2}, and decreased pH. Each of these factors likely contributes to cerebral vasodilation.

Hypoxia-stimulated cerebral vasodilation Cerebral blood flow increases in response to hypoxia, likely due to increased concentrations or release of a wide variety of vasodilators, including adenosine, potassium and hydrogen ions, prostaglandins, excitatory amino acids, and NO. Adenosine, in particular, increases at the onset and remains elevated throughout hypoxic exposure. However, the significance of each of these factors depends on the severity and duration of hypoxia and the species in question. The cumulative effects of these varied mechanisms of metabolic vasodilation account for only about half of the total increase in cerebral flow noted with hypoxia.

Hypoxia also has direct effects on cerebrovascular myocytes, including modest reductions in ATP. While the magnitude of reduction of ATP appears to be too small to directly inhibit vascular smooth muscle contraction, it may alter calcium transport across the cell membrane. In addition, activation of the K_{ATP} and other potassium channels appears to play an important role in hypoxic cerebral vasodilation.

Hypoxia may result in formation of NO from nitric oxide synthase (NOS)-containing neurons and dendrites, microvascular endothelial cells, or astrocytes. However, the significance of NO in producing hypoxic cerebral vasodilation is far less than its role in hypercapnia-induced vasodilation.

The relative importance of the many mechanisms leading to cerebral vasodilation depends significantly on the size of the vessel. For example, the degree of reduction of ATP is greater in larger thicker arteries than in smaller-diameter arteries, while the importance of local vasodilator metabolites is greater in smaller vessels.

Hypercapnia-stimulated cerebral vasodilation Carbon dioxide is one of the most potent dilators of cerebral vessels in mammals, and cerebral resistance vessels are extremely sensitive to even minor elevations in arterial P_{CO_2}. For example, breathing 7% CO_2 is capable of doubling cerebral flow. NO plays a role in hypercapnia-induced cerebral vasodilation, although it may be permissive and modulatory rather than primary in nature. Further, NO is important in the hypercapnia-induced vasodilation of small cerebral arteries, while hypercapnia-induced vasodilation of large cerebral vessels occurs through other mechanisms.

In contrast, graded reductions in arterial P_{CO_2} due to hyperventilation produce parallel reductions in total cerebral blood flow. These reductions in cerebral flow may result in physiological responses such as fainting, but do not appear to provoke cell injury or death in the absence of other abnormalities. CO_2-induced changes in cerebral flow appear to be related primarily to alterations of pH in extracellular fluid within the brain.

These mechanisms can be clinically important, as mechanical hyperventilation is occasionally used deliberately to reduce intracranial pressure in acute traumatic brain injury when conventional methods fail. Reduced intracranial pressure during hyperventilation is produced by hypocapnia-induced reduction in cerebral blood flow and volume. Because of the cerebral response to changes in extracellular pH, however, such benefit is likely of very limited duration. Moreover, withdrawal of hyperventilation must be very gradual to avoid a rebound increase in cerebral blood flow, volume, and intracranial pressure.

Intracranial pressure The brain and cerebral blood vessels are encased in the rigid cranium. The contents of the skull are incompressible so that, unlike in most tissues, the total volume is relatively fixed. Therefore, any increase in arterial inflow must be balanced by an accompanying increase in venous outflow so that total cerebral blood flow remains relatively constant. As a result, brain perfusion pressure is often considered to be the difference between arterial pressure and intracranial venous pressure. Any increase in intracranial pressure, for example due to head injury or tumor, can markedly decrease cerebral blood flow. Under these conditions brain ischemia elicits the **Cushing reflex**, which involves a large increase in sympathetic nerve activity, peripheral vasoconstriction and arterial blood pressure, presumably in an attempt to increase cerebral flow.

Autoregulation Autoregulation (see Chapter 36) is a significant feature of the cerebral circulation, although the ability to autoregulate is diminished by hypercapnia. The range of perfusion pressures over which autoregulation occurs is not fixed. For example, a prolonged increase in arterial pressure, such as with hypertension, results in a "resetting" of the autoregulatory range to higher pressures, helping to maintain a continuous supply of oxygen and nutrients to the brain. The upper limit of autoregulation is also increased by increased activity of cervical sympathetic nerves.

Cerebral flow autoregulation during arterial hypotension is achieved by vasodilation. CGRP, from pial arteries and periarterial nerve fibers, contributes to vasodilation of the pial microvasculature during hypotension via activation of K_{ATP} channels. A number of other substances, including adenosine, endothelium-dependent hyperpolarizing factor, vasoactive intestinal peptide (VIP), cyclic AMP, prostacyclin, and norepinephrine-stimulated β-adrenoceptors, also vasodilate cerebral vessels, in part via activation of K_{ATP} channels. In addition, in hypertensive rats administration of an angiotensin-converting enzyme inhibitor, which reduces formation of the vasoconstrictor angiotensin II, results in vasodilation and reduces the lower limit of cerebral autoregulation.

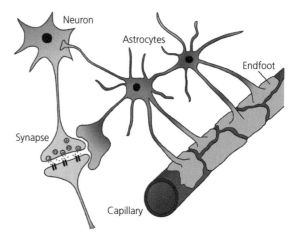

Figure 38.6 Neurovascular unit. The distribution of blood flow in the brain is determined by interactions among neurons, astrocytes and blood vessels, matching blood flow to metabolism.

Despite the importance of metabolic factors, none of these can completely account for autoregulation of cerebral blood flow. Thus, myogenic mechanisms likely contribute importantly to cerebral autoregulation. Resistance vessels in the cerebral circulation respond robustly to increases in pressure with vasoconstriction and to decreases in pressure with relaxation.

Distribution of blood flow Although total cerebral blood flow is held relatively constant by autoregulation, the regional distribution of flow within the brain varies with rate of metabolism. For example, muscle contraction or sensory stimulation in a given limb is associated with increased blood flow to the appropriate region of the motor or sensory cortex, respectively. These changes in flow are likely mediated by release of vasodilator compounds and involve an interaction with astrocytes.

Neurovascular unit Coupling of flow to metabolism in the brain involves a unique interaction among neural activity, the cerebral vasculature, and the action of astrocytes. This **neurovascular coupling** complements metabolic control mechanisms discussed previously. Astrocytes contact neurons and their endfeet form a discontinuous sheath around capillaries (Figure 38.6). Neurotransmitters such as glutamate can activate astrocytes, resulting in increased astrocyte calcium, ultimately producing vasodilation due to direct relaxation of vascular smooth muscle as well as release of vasodilators such as NO and metabolites of arachidonic acid. Overall, synaptic activity induces vasodilation via mediators related both to neurons and to astrocytes.

Cutaneous circulation

1 How does cutaneous blood flow through arteriovenous anastomoses differ from cutaneous nutritional blood flow?

2 Where are cutaneous arteriovenous anastomoses most prominent?

> 3 How does cooling and warming of the skin affect vasomotor tone in cutaneous vessels?
>
> 4 What is meant by neurogenic inflammation?

The primary function of the skin is to protect the body from external factors and preserve the internal environment. The oxygen and nutrient demands of the skin are relatively low. As a result, metabolic factors influencing blood flow are comparatively unimportant in the cutaneous circulation. Rather, neural factors, especially in response to changes in temperature, are the primary controllers of skin blood flow.

Total blood flow through the cutaneous circulation is composed of both nutritional flow perfusing the capillary beds of the skin, and flow directed through **arteriovenous anastomoses (AVAs)**, which shunt flow between arteries and veins. AVAs are plentiful in the cutaneous circulation and particularly prominent in tissues that play a role in thermoregulation, such as the rabbit ear, where flow through AVAs may markedly exceed nutritional flow. Because of the large flow capacity of AVAs, the degree of AVA vasomotor tone profoundly affects total skin blood flow and indirectly influences nutritional flow. Vasomotor tone in AVAs primarily depends on the level of sympathetic vasoconstrictor activity, mediated by both α_1 and α_2 adrenoceptors. In contrast, vasoconstriction in the precapillary arterioles that control nutritional blood flow is primarily mediated by α_1 adrenoceptors. Differential density of α_1 and α_2 adrenoceptors in AVAs and arterioles may provide some degree of selectivity in controlling the relative proportions of AVA shunt flow and nutritional blood flow.

The sympathetic neural control of anastomotic vessels is crucial in temperature regulation by providing for heat exchange. Sympathetic vasoconstriction is substantial under resting euthermic conditions. In response to cold, further increases in sympathetic nervous system activity can nearly eliminate flow through the AVAs, reducing overall skin blood flow and conserving heat. In contrast, during increases in temperature sympathetic nerve activity to skin is inhibited, markedly dilating AVAs and increasing blood flow as much as fourfold above normal levels. This increased skin blood flow allows heat loss, contributing to maintenance of body temperature.

In contrast to AVAs, resistance vessels in the skin exhibit local regulation of flow. For example, these vessels exhibit autoregulation mediated primarily by myogenic mechanisms. In addition, these vessels exhibit responses including reactive hyperemia. Despite the presence of these local control mechanisms, neural control predominates even in these cutaneous vessels.

In addition to sympathetic nerve fibers, mammalian skin contains small-diameter unmyelinated and thinly myelinated nerve fibers with nociceptive receptors that can contribute to vasodilation in response to pain or injurious stimuli. These afferent fibers contain substances such as CGRP, and release

CGRP at a basal level under normal circumstances. Activation of these receptors markedly increases CGRP release, which appears to contribute to local vasodilation. Basal sympathetic vasoconstrictor nerve activity opposing such vasodilation is of low intensity and can be overridden locally, with a net result of vasodilation. The relative significance of these opposing vasoconstrictor and vasodilator stimuli depends on the depth of the skin layers.

The balance between sympathetic vasoconstrictor activity and vasodilation produced by activation of unmyelinated and thinly myelinated nerve fibers can be altered by many factors, including temperature. As discussed above, in response to cooling, sympathetic nerve activity to the cutaneous circulation markedly increases and produces a marked reduction in blood flow. In addition, this increase in sympathetic activity may reduce or eliminate the local vasodilation ordinarily produced by stimulation of small-diameter afferent fibers. Conversely, warming produces a steep reduction in sympathetic vasoconstrictor activity, leading to a more pronounced vasodilation when small-diameter afferent fibers are activated. In addition to neurally mediated effects, the cutaneous circulation dilates or constricts in response to local heating or cooling, respectively.

Local vasodilation is also an element of the response of the skin to injury. Other elements include local increases in capillary permeability, resulting in the extravasation of plasma and the formation of a wheal. Once again, activation of small-diameter afferent fibers is important in producing these responses. In addition to CGRP, when activated these nerve fibers release substance P, VIP, and neurokinin A, which also increase microvascular permeability. These neuropeptides also stimulate adhesion of leukocytes to the capillary wall, their migration into interstitial tissue, and subsequent release of multiple substances from mast cells, basophils, and monocytes. Many of these substances are, in themselves, vasodilators or increase vascular permeability. This combination of local vasodilation, plasma leakage, and the accumulation of leukocytes in tissue has been termed **neurogenic inflammation**. Continued progress in our understanding of neurogenic inflammation is important to better define the pathophysiology of disease states and to design unique pharmacological agents to alter the inflammatory response of the skin.

Skeletal muscle circulation

> 1 What factors regulate vasomotor tone in skeletal muscle at rest?
>
> 2 What is the skeletal muscle pump, and how does it contribute to the increase in cardiac output during exercise?
>
> 3 What are the cardiovascular responses associated with the anticipation of exercise?
>
> 4 What is meant by "rapid-onset vasodilation" in reference to skeletal muscle blood flow?
>
> 5 What factors produce the increase in blood flow to skeletal muscle during moderate exercise?

6 What is the net effect of functional sympatholysis?

7 What are the primary factors that maintain an elevated level of skeletal muscle blood flow during moderate exercise?

8 Why may limits to vasodilation in the vasculature of muscle during intense exercise be advantageous?

9 What structural changes occur in the skeletal muscle vascular bed in response to exercise training?

Blood flow to skeletal muscle varies with muscle fiber type. For example, slow-twitch highly oxidative muscle exhibits greater flow and capillary density compared with fast-twitch glycolytic muscle in conscious mammals. Blood flow is low at rest in most muscles, although it is relatively high in postural muscles of animals maintaining posture (standing). An important aspect of the skeletal muscle circulation is that the volume of blood flow to skeletal muscle is intimately linked to the level of muscle metabolic activity (Figure 38.7). As a result, the range of flow is very large. Muscle blood flow can increase by 100-fold during strenuous exercise. The relative importance of vascular control mechanisms also varies with level of activity.

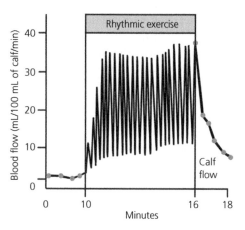

Figure 38.7 Skeletal muscle blood flow is related to level of physical activity. Skeletal muscle blood flow is low at rest but increases markedly with exercise. Note the pulsatile changes in blood flow associated with rhythmic muscle contractions, due to periodic extravascular compression with muscle contraction. Adapted from Barcroft, H. and Dornhorst, A.C. (1949) The blood flow through the human calf during rhythmic exercise. *Journal of Physiology* **109**:402–411.

Blood flow to skeletal muscle at rest

The level of vasomotor tone in blood vessels perfusing skeletal muscle at any time reflects the balance between vasoconstrictor and vasodilator effects. At rest, blood flow to skeletal muscle is low, and a substantial number of capillaries are not perfused. This low flow reflects a high level of vasomotor tone related to factors such as the vascular smooth muscle myogenic response and sympathetic vasoconstrictor activity mediated by α_1- and α_2-adrenergic receptors. While these effects are balanced by the

presence of local vasodilator substances, the concentrations of vasodilators under resting conditions is relatively low and they have little influence on flow under these conditions.

Autoregulation is a characteristic feature of the skeletal muscle circulation at rest and during exercise. The pressure range over which skeletal muscle exhibits autoregulation is small in resting muscle but during exercise, when flows are high, the range of pressures over which muscle maintains flow constant is increased. Autoregulation in the skeletal muscle circulation appears to depend on several mechanisms, with the significance of each mechanism varying from rest to exercise and with the level of exercise. For example, the myogenic response appears to play an important role in autoregulation in the skeletal muscle circulation at rest, while metabolic factors play a greater role during exercise.

Blood flow during the anticipation of exercise

Many of the cardiovascular responses associated with exercise can be produced merely by the anticipation of exercise, and the magnitude of the response is dependent on the level of exercise anticipated. For example, dogs trained to run at moderate and high intensities were conditioned with specific cues prior to each level of exercise. When these dogs are at rest, but provided with the exercise cues, blood pressure, heart rate, and muscle blood flows increase and are higher when intense exercise is anticipated than when moderate exercise is anticipated.

The increase in muscle blood flow during the anticipation of exercise is due to increased arterial blood pressure and decreased skeletal muscle vascular resistance. In some species a sympathetic cholinergic system increases muscle blood flow as part of the defense reaction, and it has been proposed that this system may play a role in hyperemia in anticipation of exercise (see Chapter 35).

Blood flow during the transition from rest to exercise

Blood flow to muscle increases immediately with onset of exercise ("on response" or **rapid-onset vasodilation**, ROV). ROV begins at the onset of exercise and its magnitude is unrelated to the level of metabolic activity in the exercising muscle. ROV appears to be significantly related to the skeletal **muscle pump** (Figure 38.8). The force of rhythmic muscle contraction is transmitted to local blood vessels and compresses them. This phasic compression of vessels during exercise, along with prevention of backflow due to venous valves, produces an increase in venous outflow from the muscle during muscle contraction, while muscle relaxation promotes an increase in arterial inflow.

The potential role of NO from vascular endothelial cells in ROV has not been conclusively determined. However, it has been hypothesized that the increase in blood flow produced by the muscle pump might produce a sufficient increase in shear stress to result in production of NO. Initiation of muscle contraction also releases K^+, resulting in dilation of proximal arterioles. The electrical signal then spreads through endothelial gap junctions into smooth muscle cells. This **conducted**

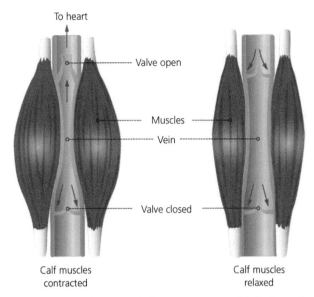

To heart

Valve open

Muscles

Vein

Valve closed

Calf muscles
contracted

Calf muscles
relaxed

Figure 38.8 Muscle pump. Rhythmic contraction of skeletal muscle increases venous return to the heart. While the muscle is relaxed, the valves are closed, preventing backflow. Muscle contraction compresses the vessel, forcing blood through the upper valve toward the heart; closure of the lower valve prevents backflow. Source: Intervention IQ. © Intervention IQ, www.iqonline.eu reproduced with permission.

vasodilation then causes upstream vessels to dilate, further increasing blood flow.

Blood flow during moderate exercise

Muscle blood flow during submaximal exercise depends on the intensity of exercise and muscle metabolic activity. Increased blood flow is produced by a combination of increased cardiac output, increased arterial blood pressure, reduced muscle vascular resistance, and constriction of other vascular beds. Cardiac output increases due to both increased heart rate and cardiac contractility. The muscle pump enhances venous return to the heart, also contributing to increased cardiac output via the Frank-Starling mechanism, and may account for up to half the energy required to pump blood. The increase in muscle blood flow is preferentially directed toward those muscles actively involved in exercise.

Reduced vascular resistance in exercising muscles is heavily dependent on local vascular control mechanisms, including metabolic factors produced by exercising muscle cells, alterations in neural activity, and the muscle pump. Vasodilator factors include reduced tissue P_{O_2} and pH and increased tissue P_{CO_2}, along with changes in osmolality, K^+, histamine, kinins, phosphates, and prostacyclin. Also, ATP and its metabolites (ADP, AMP, adenosine) are potent vasodilators found at relatively high concentrations in venous blood draining exercising muscle. The literature on adenosine as a local regulator of blood flow in muscle is complex and contradictory. However, a substantial amount of the evidence suggests that adenosine plays a major role in vascular regulation under conditions where the oxygen supply is compromised. It is generally believed that these metabolites act directly on vascular smooth muscle, or via

endothelial cells to induce vasodilation. In a physiological setting, multiple metabolic substances operate simultaneously, and the significance of individual metabolites likely varies depending on the time-course of exercise. It should be noted that no single metabolite has been shown to individually produce the degree of vasodilation seen with exercise. There appears to be substantial redundancy among these different dilator signals so that if one is blocked the others continue to produce normal blood flows.

Exercise is associated with an increase in sympathetic nerve activity proportional to the intensity of exercise. While increased sympathetic activity would be expected to produce vasoconstriction through norepinephrine release at α_1 and α_2 receptors, local metabolites inhibit this effect, a condition termed **functional sympatholysis**. With functional sympatholysis, adrenergic vasoconstriction is inhibited by metabolic substances in muscle. In addition, skeletal muscle vessels possess β_2 receptors that produce vasodilation in response to moderate levels of circulating epinephrine. The net effect of functional sympatholysis and β_2-receptor activation is to spare the circulation of exercising muscle from vasoconstriction typically produced by a generalized increase in sympathetic nervous system activity.

Outside the skeletal muscle circulation, sympathetic vasoconstriction during exercise and increased cardiac output lead to a moderate increase in systemic arterial blood pressure. Increased arterial pressure, combined with constriction of other vascular beds but vasodilation in exercising muscle and the effect of the muscle pump, helps elevate blood flow to exercising skeletal muscle during moderate exercise. As previously noted, this increase in muscle blood flow is preferentially distributed to those muscles actively engaged in exercise and especially to muscles with a high proportion of high-oxidative fibers.

Blood flow during very intense exercise

Exercise at a very high level of intensity may result in additional increases in muscle blood flow. However, the increase in flow during heavy exercise is significantly less than that which can be achieved with maximal vasodilation of isolated muscle. This apparent physiological limitation on increases in muscle blood flow during intense exercise is important in preserving arterial blood pressure. When large masses of skeletal muscle are involved in exercise, maximal vasodilation of such a large proportion of the peripheral vasculature would produce a large reduction in arterial blood pressure and thus be physiologically undesirable. Because of limitations in increasing maximal muscle blood flow, the metabolic demands of muscle during very intense exercise may exceed the level of arterial blood flow.

Effects of exercise training

Exercise training does not result in changes in resting muscle blood flow. However, the anticipation of exercise produces a greater increase in muscle blood flow and a more marked redistribution of flow within the muscle of exercise-trained animals. In addition, exercise training enhances autoregulatory mechanisms.

Section VI: The Cardiovascular System

Exercise training produces both structural and functional changes in the skeletal muscle circulation. Structurally, capillary density increases in those muscles that experience the greatest increase in activity during training and, functionally, blood flow capacity is increased in trained muscle.

During submaximal exercise, total muscle blood flow in exercise-trained animals is not different from, or is less than, flow in untrained animals. However, both endurance and sprint types of exercise training result in greater increases in blood flow to muscle during heavy exercise than occur without exercise training. Endurance and sprint types of exercise training result in different patterns of muscle recruitment, and in either type of exercise training the increase in muscle blood flow capacity is located in those muscles with high levels of metabolic activity during training bouts.

The larger increase in maximal muscle blood flow in exercise-trained animals requires greater increases in cardiac output compared with untrained animals. The redistribution of cardiac output away from nonexercising tissues toward active muscle is similar when compared at similar relative intensities of exercise (i.e., greater absolute intensity after training). Thus, after exercise training an animal has a higher maximal exercise capacity. However, if untrained and trained animals run at 100% of their own capacity, visceral blood flows decrease by the same amount but flow to exercising muscle will be higher because of the greater cardiac output. The ability to sustain a higher maximal cardiac output is dependent on enhanced cardiac function and increased ability of the skeletal muscle pump to promote venous return to the heart. The increase in total muscle blood flow during exercise is accompanied by increased redirection of flow within muscle to fibers with high metabolic activity, and may be influenced by the type of exercise training. For example, sprint-type training results in preferential redirection of flow within a muscle to low-oxidative fibers, while endurance exercise appears to result in redirection of flow toward high-oxidative fibers. Aerobic training also increases the effects of endothelium-mediated vasodilation due to NO, through increased expression of endothelial cell NOS. However, exercise does not alter the vascular responsiveness to endothelium-independent vasodilators.

Splanchnic circulation

> 1 What are the components of the splanchnic circulation?
>
> 2 How is splanchnic blood flow related to metabolic activity?
>
> 3 What are the primary vasodilators that may be released during the processes of digestion?
>
> 4 What are some stimuli that shift blood volume from the splanchnic capacitance bed to the central circulation and how does the spleen contribute to this response?
>
> 5 What happens to splanchnic blood flow during exercise?
>
> 6 What are the sources of blood supply to the liver?

> 7 What is the hepatic arterial buffer response?
>
> 8 How does a reduction in portal vein flow lead to hepatic arterial dilation?

The splanchnic circulation includes the vascular beds of the gastrointestinal tract, spleen, pancreas, and liver. Blood flow to the splanchnic bed, similar to the renal circulation, has two primary functions. It is important both in supplying oxygen and nutrients to the tissues, and in supporting the absorption of substances from the gastrointestinal tract. This circulation is unique in that it contains two capillary beds in series; venous flow from the capillary beds of the gastrointestinal tract, spleen, and pancreas combine to provide a major source of blood flow, through the portal vein, to the liver capillaries.

Intestinal circulation
Anatomic considerations
The blood supply to the gut is provided by the celiac and cranial and caudal mesenteric arteries (Figure 38.9A). There is an interconnecting network among the small arteries of the gut, likely reducing the possibility that specific regions of the gastrointestinal system may become ischemic. However, within the gut villi, the vessels form a countercurrent exchange system, in which the arteries and veins travel in opposite directions (Figure 38.9B). This arrangement, along with highly permeable capillaries, supports the absorption of solutes and water by the gut. However, when flow is low, oxygen can also diffuse from the arteries to the veins, producing hypoxia at the tips of the villi. For this reason, extensive and prolonged reductions in intestinal blood flow, as in hemorrhage, can produce necrosis in the gut.

Autoregulation
Splanchnic blood flow is relatively well maintained despite fluctuations in arterial blood pressure (autoregulation), although the degree of autoregulation in the splanchnic circulation is less than that in the heart and kidney. The primary mechanism for autoregulation is likely metabolic, related to mediators such as adenosine which potently dilates the mesenteric circulation, as well as K^+ and increases in osmolality. Myogenic responses likely also play a role.

Intestinal blood flow is related to metabolism
Splanchnic blood flow is directly linked to metabolic activity. Flow is low in the unfed animal but can increase as much as eightfold following food ingestion (**postprandial hyperemia**). Digestive activity increases metabolism, increasing concentrations of local vasodilator mediators such as adenosine and CO_2 and, consequently, augmenting blood flow. Adenosine may cause vasodilation by direct effects via purinoceptors, or indirectly via release of NO. NO appears to be an important mediator of feeding-induced increases in blood flow. Furthermore, absorption of nutrients increases osmolality, which also stimulates blood flow. In the case of ruminants, consideration of

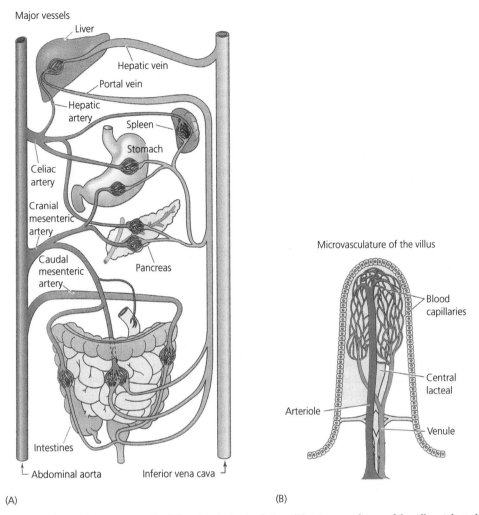

Major vessels

Liver

Hepatic vein

Portal vein

Hepatic artery

Spleen

Stomach

Celiac artery

Cranial mesenteric artery

Caudal mesenteric artery

Pancreas

Intestines

Abdominal aorta

Inferior vena cava

(A)

Microvasculature of the villus

Blood capillaries

Central lacteal

Arteriole

Venule

(B)

Figure 38.9 Splanchnic circulation: (A) major vessels of the splanchnic circulation; (B) microvasculature of the villus. Adapted from Boron, W.F. and Boulpaep, E.L. (eds) (2012) *Medical Physiology*, 2nd edn, updated. Saunders Elsevier, Philadelphia. With permission from Elsevier.

blood flow regulation is further complicated by the fact that various products of rumen fermentation, such as CO_2 and fatty acids, also act as vasodilators of the rumen circulation.

Secretion of certain gastrointestinal hormones during digestion also contributes to postprandial hyperemia. For example, cholecystokinin and neurotensin, in addition to their gastrointestinal actions, both produce vasodilation. Vasodilator kinins are also released from the intestine. In addition, prostaglandins may contribute to the increase in blood flow, although it is possible that these effects may be mediated indirectly, via an increase in metabolites due to increased transport and metabolism. Finally, the presence of fat in the gastrointestinal lumen causes the release of the vasodilator neurotensin. These factors act in concert in a complex manner to produce postprandial hyperemia.

The processes of digestion result in release of chemical mediators from nerves and local tissues of the gastrointestinal tract. Mechanical stimulation of the small intestine of the cat increases blood flow through release of serotonin from enterochromaffin

cells. Serotonin, in turn, stimulates the release of the vasodilator VIP from nerve endings.

A wide variety of other chemical mediators can alter gastrointestinal blood flow under specific circumstances. Substance P is released from the peripheral terminals of primary afferent neurons and produces vasodilation via NK_1 receptors. Similarly, CGRP is a vasodilator in intrinsic neurons and peripheral terminals of spinal afferent neurons. Although substance P- and CGRP-induced vasodilation appears to be important in producing increased blood flow with inflammation or noxious stimulation of the gut lumen, their significance under normal circumstances is unclear.

Neural control factors

Reciprocal changes in the autonomic nervous system also contribute to postprandial hyperemia. Feeding and digestion are associated with diminished sympathetic nerve activity, reducing α-adrenoceptor-mediated vasoconstriction. Concomitantly, parasympathetic nervous system activity and release of acetylcholine increase, which indirectly produce vasodilation due to increased secretory activity, motility, and metabolism in gastrointestinal tissues.

NPY is present in the gastrointestinal tract intrinsic (enteric) nervous system (see Chapter 42) and sympathetic postganglionic neurons, where it is colocalized with norepinephrine. The direct effect of NPY on blood vessels is vasoconstriction, but at higher levels, similar to norepinephrine, NPY acts at autoreceptors on presynaptic terminals to inhibit transmitter release. Consequently, NPY and norepinephrine under most physiological circumstances produce a combined vasoconstrictor effect; however, at high levels NPY (and norepinephrine) may depress further transmitter release.

Hepatic circulation
Anatomic considerations
The hepatic circulation is characterized by a dual blood supply from the hepatic artery and the **portal vein**, which supplies approximately 75% of its flow. However, because the portal flow has already passed through the intestinal capillaries, most of the oxygen supply to the liver is delivered via the hepatic artery. The total blood supply and blood volume contained in the liver constitute approximately 25% of cardiac output, and the liver accounts for 20% of total body oxygen consumption. Consequently, regulation of total hepatic blood supply and circulatory capacitance are very important for normal liver function and for stability of the cardiovascular system.

Another unique aspect of the hepatic circulation is that the capillary network in the liver is composed of **sinusoids**, which converge to form hepatic venules. Resistance upstream from these sinusoids is much greater than downstream resistance, so that sinusoidal pressure is low and only slightly greater than that of venous pressure. The sinusoids are highly fenestrated and therefore very permeable, allowing rapid exchange between the blood and hepatocytes. However, they are also very sensitive to changes in central venous pressure that alter capillary pressure and thus produce large alterations in fluid exchange through the sinusoids (see Chapter 36). For example, the increase in central venous pressure that occurs in right-sided heart failure produces substantial movement of fluid across the sinusoids into the peritoneal cavity, resulting in ascites.

Reciprocal relationship of hepatic arterial and portal vein flow
Hepatic arterial blood flow is inversely related to the level of portal vein flow (**hepatic arterial buffer response, HABR**). The HABR is sufficiently potent that doubling of portal vein flow can lead to maximal constriction of the hepatic artery, and low portal vein flow may produce maximal hepatic artery dilation. Furthermore, the HABR can account for up to a 60% reduction in portal vein flow with increases in hepatic artery flow. Adenosine plays a key role. Adenosine is released into the perivascular space of Mall where it is washed out at a rate

proportional to portal flow. Thus, reduced portal vein flow results in less adenosine being washed out into portal blood, with the resultant increase in adenosine leading to hepatic arterial dilation. Conversely, increases in portal vein flow increase adenosine washout, resulting in increased hepatic artery resistance and decreased flow. This reciprocal flow relationship is an important mechanism for maintaining the overall capacitance of the hepatic circulation at a relatively constant level.

Autoregulation
Because the portal vein is unable to control the rate at which it receives its blood flow from visceral organs, autoregulation does not occur in the portal circulation. However, hepatic artery blood flow is autoregulated in an effort to maintain total hepatic perfusion at a constant rate. Adenosine is an important component of hepatic arterial autoregulation. As already described, a decrease in arterial pressure decreases hepatic arterial flow, resulting in less adenosine washout, hepatic arterial vasodilation, and maintenance of hepatic arterial flow at a relatively constant level. Given this autoregulatory mechanism to maintain constant hepatic perfusion (~1 mL/min per gram of tissue), the liver is unique in that it responds to increased metabolic demand through increased oxygen extraction rather than increased blood flow. Maintaining total hepatic blood flow relatively constant in turn stabilizes many aspects of liver function.

Nitric oxide
NO from vascular endothelial cells is not thought to play a major role in regulation of hepatic circulatory capacitance. In addition, the portal vein does not appear to be sensitive to NO. However, NO contributes to regulation of hepatic arterial resistance under basal conditions, and may increase in significance under certain pathophysiological circumstances. Both hepatocytes and liver endothelial cells normally possess constitutive calcium-dependent NOS, and may release modest amounts of NO. In certain types of portal hypertension, the amount of NO release from constitutive NOS can increase to cytotoxic levels. In addition, calcium-independent NOS can be induced in hepatocytes by stimuli such as inflammation, exposure to endotoxin or cytokines, and by reperfusion after ischemia. The large increase in NO released by hepatocytes through this inducible pathway may produce cytotoxicity under these circumstances.

The splanchnic circulation contributes to cardiovascular homeostasis
The splanchnic circulation serves as an important blood reservoir and site of vascular resistance. The splanchnic vascular bed of the dog normally contains more than 20% of the blood volume, particularly on the venous side of the circulation. Sympathetic α-adrenoceptor stimulation significantly reduces venous capacitance, without a change in hepatic arterial blood flow, and may mobilize up to half of this volume in response to

severe hypoxia, heavy exercise, or hemorrhage. The spleen, particularly in species such as the dog, horse, sheep, cat, and guinea pig, is an important component of this response and transfers red cell-rich blood to the central circulation. Splenic contraction associated with heavy exercise in the dog, horse, and sheep increases the hemoglobin concentration of circulating blood by 20–50%, with a corresponding increase in oxygen-carrying capacity.

Constriction of the splanchnic bed also contributes importantly to circulatory adjustments to exercise and hemorrhage. Sympathetic vasoconstriction can decrease splanchnic blood flow to less than 25% of its resting value. Increased circulating angiotensin II and vasopressin may also contribute to this response. Together, these mechanisms allow redistribution of flow to other vascular beds such as brain and cardiac and skeletal muscle.

Fetal and neonatal circulation

1 What is the shunt provided by the ductus arteriosus during fetal life?

2 What is the mechanism of functional closure of the foramen ovale after birth? How does this differ from anatomic closure of the foramen ovale?

3 What is the location and function of the ductus venosus?

4 How does the pulmonary and systemic arterial resistance and blood pressure of the fetus differ from that of the adult?

5 What is the primary mechanism that causes the ductus arteriosus to close?

6 What are two major changes that occur in the fetal hemodynamic pattern at the time of parturition?

7 Where is the oxygen content of the fetal blood the highest?

8 What percentage of fetal cardiac output goes to the placenta via the umbilical arteries?

Circulation in the fetus

The physiology of the fetal cardiovascular system offers numerous contrasts with that of the postnatal infant or adult. An important aspect of this system is that the fetus derives oxygenated blood and nutrients from the placenta rather than the lungs. Consistent with this, flow to the fetal lungs is low whereas the amount of blood perfusing the placenta is high. Fetal pulmonary vascular resistance and arterial pressure are high, with pulmonary arterial pressure exceeding aortic pressure. High fetal pulmonary vascular resistance is related primarily to hypoxic pulmonary vasoconstriction (see Chapters 23 and 37) and to some extent to lack of expansion of the fetal lung. On the other hand, systemic vascular resistance and arterial blood pressure of the fetus are low, related largely to very low vascular resistance in the placental circulation. The hemodynamic effect of low placental vascular resistance is particularly prominent because a substantial percentage (approximately 45% of cardiac output) of the combined output of both ventricles flows through

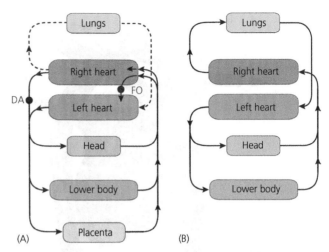

Figure 38.10 The circulatory pattern in the fetus (A) and in the adult (B). DA, ductus arteriosus; FO, foramen ovale. Note that in the fetus, the right and left ventricles pump in parallel, whereas in the adult they are arranged in series.

the umbilical cord to the placenta, the structure serving as the "fetal lung."

The fetal circulation is also characterized by the presence of several important shunts. Two of these shunts, the **foramen ovale** and the **ductus arteriosus**, cause the fetal right and left ventricles to operate as parallel pumps rather than pumps in series as in the adult (Figure 38.10). The third shunt in the fetal circulation is the **ductus venosus**, a low-resistance conduit that allows a significant fraction of relatively oxygenated blood in the umbilical vein to bypass the fetal liver and directly enter the caudal vena cava. These shunts and the pathway of blood are illustrated in Figures 38.10 and 38.11).

Relatively oxygenated blood from the ductus venosus joins blood from the lower extremities and hepatic veins in the caudal vena cava and continues to the heart (Figure 38.11). Pressure in the fetal right atrium is normally higher than pressure in the left atrium, allowing blood to flow through an open flap in the foramen ovale from the right to the left atrium. Anatomically, the foramen ovale lies in the pathway of blood from the caudal vena cava carrying the relatively well oxygenated blood from the ductus venosus. The tendency for this relatively oxygenated blood from the caudal vena cava to preferentially stream toward the foramen ovale is further accentuated by the crista dividens of the inter-atrial septum. Consequently, the majority of blood from the caudal vena cava is directed through the foramen ovale into the left atrium, and subsequently into the left ventricle. As a result, the P_{O_2} and oxygen saturation of blood in the fetal left ventricle is relatively high (Figure 38.11). In contrast, the oxygen saturation of blood in the cranial vena cava is much lower due to high oxygen consumption in the developing brain. The anatomic location of the entry of the cranial vena cava into the right atrium leads to preferential streaming of the majority of the cranial vena cava blood into the right ventricle. Consequently,

Section VI: The Cardiovascular System

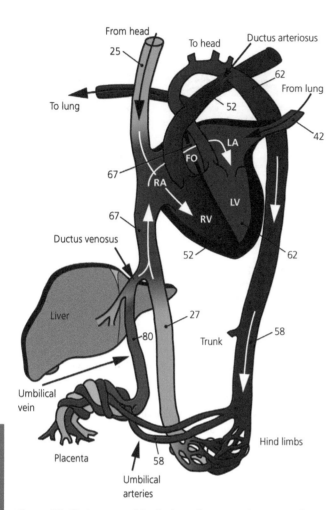

Figure 38.11 Anatomy of the fetal circulation. FO, foramen ovale; LA, left atrium; LV, left ventricle; RA, right atrium; RV, right ventricle. Numbers indicate percent oxygen saturation. Adapted from Cunningham, J.G. (1997) *Textbook of Veterinary Physiology*, 2nd edn. W.B. Saunders, Philadelphia. With permission from Elsevier. Values for oxygen saturation are from Dawes, G.S., Mott, J.C. and Widdicombe, J.G. (1954) The foetal circulation in the lamb. *Journal of Physiology* **126**:563–587.

include the coronary arteries and the brachiocephalic trunk (not shown in Figure 38.11), and they primarily receive this flow, so that the developing heart and brain benefit from receiving comparatively well oxygenated blood. This relationship would seem teleologically to be advantageous to these organs, but it is not essential for fetal survival or continued development, since fetuses lacking this preferential direction of flow due to congenital malformations continue to develop to term. The foramen ovale is also important for normal left ventricular development. By increasing the volume provided to the left ventricle, flow through the foramen ovale is important in promoting the normal growth and development of the fetal left ventricle.

Circulatory changes at parturition

Parturition is associated with marked and rapid changes from the fetal hemodynamic pattern. Expansion of the lung and the associated increase in alveolar and arterial Po_2 after birth contribute to a marked reduction in pulmonary vascular resistance and pulmonary arterial blood pressure. Pulmonary arterial pressure continues to decline over the next 1–2 weeks. In contrast, systemic arterial pressure rises after birth. The umbilical vessels are highly sensitive to trauma, catecholamines, angiotensin, bradykinin, and changes in Po_2. They constrict strongly at birth, reducing the risk of hemorrhage in newborn animals. An immediate increase in systemic arterial pressure at birth is due partly to elimination of the low-resistance placental vascular bed and partly to an increase in cardiac output. A continued rise in systemic arterial blood pressure over a period of weeks after birth is due largely to a gradual increase in peripheral vascular resistance.

After birth, the fall in pulmonary vascular resistance leads to a dramatic increase in pulmonary arterial blood flow and, consequently, to a marked increase in pulmonary venous flow returning to the left atrium. The increase in left atrial volume, combined with increased peripheral vascular resistance and blood pressure, causes left atrial pressure to increase above right atrial pressure. This change in the pressure gradient causes a passive closure of the flap of the foramen ovale, creating a physiological or functional closure. True and permanent anatomic closure of the foramen ovale is due to fibrosis, which requires a period of weeks after birth. In a minority of instances, true closure fails to occur, resulting in a patent foramen ovale. It is important to note that a patent foramen ovale may not be functionally open during life, providing that left atrial pressure continues to exceed right atrial pressure.

The ductus arteriosus and ductus venosus normally close shortly after parturition, although the precise timing of closure varies among species. The primary mechanisms of constriction of the ductus arteriosus appear to involve changes in blood oxygen and a decrease in prostaglandins from the placenta. The mechanisms by which oxygen induces closure have not been fully delineated. However, a role for the cytochrome P450 system and endothelin-1 has been postulated. Another

the oxygen saturation of blood in the right ventricle is lower than that in the left ventricle.

The ductus arteriosus forms a vascular conduit between the pulmonary artery and aorta. In the fetus, the ductus arteriosus allows blood to flow from the high-pressure pulmonary artery to the lower-pressure aorta. Physiologically, the ductus arteriosus provides a pathway for blood in the fetal pulmonary artery to bypass the high-resistance vascular bed of the fetal lung and instead to flow into the aorta distal to the origin of the coronary arteries and the brachiocephalic trunk. In fact, only 10–12% of the blood flows through the lungs in the fetus.

The roles of the foramen ovale and ductus arteriosus in the fetus are closely interrelated. During ventricular systole, the relatively well oxygenated blood in the left ventricle is ejected into the aortic root. The first vessels arising from the aorta possibility is generation of reactive oxygen species that inhibit a specific class of voltage-gated K^+ channels, producing depolarization. This would increase calcium influx across the vascular smooth muscle cell membrane via voltage-dependent calcium channels, producing smooth muscle cell constriction and physiological closure of the ductus arteriosus. The placenta normally releases prostaglandin E_2 (PGE_2), which contributes to ductus relaxation in the fetus. An abrupt decrease in PGE_2 immediately after birth, accompanied by decreased responsiveness to PGE_2, is critical for ductus closure. In fact, failure to reduce PGE_2 is often associated with a patent ductus arteriosus, and prostaglandin synthesis inhibitors such as indomethacin sometimes are used as a treatment.

Physiological closure of the ductus arteriosus is followed by anatomic closure from scarring and sclerosis over a period of weeks and results in formation of the ligamentum arteriosum. Abnormal, persistent patency of the ductus arteriosus after birth is termed **patent ductus arteriosus** and is one of the most frequently noted forms of congenital cardiovascular disease in the dog. Should the ductus arteriosus remain patent after delivery, changing pressures in the pulmonary artery and aorta change the direction of blood flow across the ductus arteriosus from a right-to-left pattern (pulmonary artery to aorta) in the fetus to a left-to-right pattern (aorta to pulmonary artery) in the neonate.

The ductus venosus closes before or at birth depending on the species, although the mechanisms of closure and the incidence of failure of closure are not well delineated.

Cardiac changes from fetus to adult

The newborn heart, especially the left ventricle, must cope with significant hemodynamic challenges including a rapid rise in systemic arterial blood pressure and a marked increase in pulmonary venous return to the left atrium. In view of the structural and biochemical immaturity of the newborn heart, the ability of the newborn left ventricle to support a twofold to threefold increase in cardiac output, increased stroke volume, and high heart rate is remarkable. This response is supported by an increase in the left ventricular contractile state. Since propranolol, used to block β-adrenergic receptors, only partially blunts this increase in contractility, thyroid hormone and other substances may contribute to the postnatal increase in contractility. The newborn left ventricle demonstrates a high level of contractility, but operates more nearly at maximal contractile capacity than does the adult heart. Hence, the contractile reserve of the newborn ventricle is much less than in the adult heart. This limits the ability of the newborn heart to respond to further increases in diastolic volume or arterial blood pressure. The clinical consequences of these findings are that the newborn heart can compensate for increases in arterial pressure only within a limited range, and is less able than the adult heart to respond to a volume load by increasing cardiac output.

Myocardial mass increases rapidly during the neonatal period. At birth, the thickness of the right ventricular wall may be equal to that of the left ventricular wall, reflecting the high right ventricular pressure in the fetus. The left ventricle gradually increases in thickness after birth, related to general body growth and to increasing arterial pressure, cardiac output, and left ventricular workload. Consequently, the normal relationship of the adult heart, where left ventricular muscle mass is approximately double right ventricular muscle mass, is gradually established over a period of weeks after delivery. Although there may be a limited amount of hyperplasia early in life, the increase in myocardial mass after birth is primarily due to hypertrophy.

Self-evaluation

Answers can be found at the end of the chapter.

1 Left ventricular coronary blood flow tends to be high:
  A When parasympathetic nerves are activated
  B During early systole
  C When myocardial oxygen consumption is high
  D When myogenic tone is high

2 Cerebral blood flow:
  A Is highly autoregulated
  B Decreases when CO_2 levels are high
  C Increases greatly during locomotion
  D Is primarily controlled by sympathetic nerves

3 Blood flow to the skin:
  A Is related primarily to metabolic activity in the skin
  B Is increased during increases in body temperature
  C Exhibits a high degree of autoregulation
  D Is decreased on exposure to light
  E Decreases during exercise

4 In the skeletal muscle vascular bed:
  A Increased α-adrenergic activation increases flow during exercise
  B Resistance to flow is less during exercise
  C Basal flow is very high compared to other organs
  D Flow to slow oxidative muscle is much less than to fast glycolytic muscle at rest
  E Is primarily under local regulation under resting conditions

5 In the splanchnic vascular bed:
  A There is very low capacitance
  B Gastrointestinal hormones contribute to vasoconstriction
  C Hepatic artery and portal vein flow are directly related
  D Feeding is associated with increased blood flow

6 In the fetal circulation:
  A Blood flow to the placenta is greater than flow to the lungs
  B The ductus arteriosus is a shunt whereby blood flows from the aorta to the pulmonary artery
  C Pressure in the left atrium is greater than pressure in the right atrium
  D Oxygen saturation is greater in the right ventricle compared to the left ventricle

Suggested reading

Barrett, K.E., Barman, S.M., Boitano, S. and Brooks, H.L. (2012) Circulation through special regions. In: *Ganong's Review of Medical Physiology*, 24th edn, ch. 33. McGraw-Hill Companies, Inc., New York.

Buss, D.D. (2004) Special circulations. In: *Dukes' Physiology of Domestic Animals* (ed. W.O. Reece), 12th edn, pp. 275–302. Cornell University Press, Ithaca, NY.

Coceani, F. and Baragatti, B. (2012) Mechanisms for ductus arteriosus closure. *Seminars in Perinatology* **36**:92–97.

Dunn, K.M. and Nelson, M.T. (2014) Neurovascular signaling in the brain and the pathological consequences of hypertension. *American Journal of Physiology* **306**:H1–H14.

Faraci, F.M. and Heistad, D.D. (1998) Regulation of the cerebral circulation: role of the endothelium and potassium channels. *Physiological Reviews* **78**:53–97.

Hall, J.E. (2010) Muscle blood flow and cardiac output during exercise: the coronary circulation and ischemic heart disease. In: *Guyton and Hall Textbook of Medical Physiology*, 12th edn, ch. 21. Saunders Elsevier, Philadelphia.

Johnson, A.K. and Gross, P.M. (1993) Sensory circumventricular organs and brain homeostatic pathways. *FASEB Journal* **7**:678–686.

Kiserud, T. and Acharya, G. (2004) The fetal circulation. *Prenatal Diagnosis* **24**:1049–1059.

Laughlin, M.H., Davis, M.J., Secher, N.H. *et al.* (2012) Peripheral circulation. *Comprehensive Physiology* **2**:321–447.

Laughlin, M.H., Bowles, D.K. and Duncker, D.J. (2012) The coronary circulation in exercise training. *American Journal of Physiology* **302**:H10–H23.

Nowicki, P.T. (2006) Physiology of the circulation in the small intestine. In: *Physiology of the Gastrointestinal Tract*, 4th edn (eds K.E. Barrett, F.K. Ghishan, J.L. Merchant, H.M. Said and J.D. Wood), Vol. **2**, ch. 63. Academic Press, Burlington, MA.

Pappano, A.J. and Wier, W.G. (2013) *Cardiovascular Physiology*, 10th edn. Elsevier Mosby, Philadelphia.

Segal, S.S. (2012) Special circulations. In: *Medical Physiology*, 2nd edn (eds W.F. Boron and E.L. Boulpaep), pp. 577–592. Saunders Elsevier, Philadelphia.

Straub, S.V. and Nelson, M.T. (2007) Astrocyte calcium signaling: the information currency coupling neuronal activity to the cerebral microcirculation. *Trends in Cardiovascular Medicine* **17**:183–190.

Toda, N., Ayajiki, K. and Okamura, T. (2009) Cerebral blood flow regulation by nitric oxide: recent advances. *Pharmacological Reviews* **61**:62–97.

Westerhof, N., Boer, C., Lamberts, R.R. and Sipkema, P. (2006) Cross-talk between cardiac muscle and coronary vasculature. *Physiological Reviews* **86**:1263–1308.

Answers

1 C. Myocardial metabolism is the major regulator of coronary blood flow, with neural factors playing a lesser role. Thus under normal circumstances coronary blood flow is matched to myocardial metabolism, primarily due to release of vasodilator metabolites. Activation of parasympathetic nerves decreases heart rate and, to a small extent, contractility; as a result myocardial metabolism is low and flow will not increase. Unlike other vascular beds, left ventricular flow actually decreases during early systole due to the compressive effect of the contracting ventricle on the vessels. Myogenic tone is related to vasoconstriction, tending to reduce flow.

2 A. Total cerebral flow is held relatively constant despite changes in arterial pressure. This is important, because the incompressible tissue of the brain is contained in the rigid cranium, so that total volume must be held constant in order to prevent damage due to increased pressure. Despite the presence of autoregulation, increases in CO_2 tend to increase, rather than decrease, cerebral blood flow. Locomotion will not increase overall cerebral blood flow, but flow will be distributed to active areas of the brain, such as the motor cortex. Cerebral vessels are innervated by sympathetic nerves but the density of α-adrenergic receptors is relatively low and metabolic factors override, so that the effects of sympathetic activation are relatively weak in the cerebral circulation.

3 B. Changes in body temperature strongly influence sympathetic nervous system control of arteriovenous anastomoses in the cutaneous vascular bed. Heating results in vasodilation in the skin due to autonomic and local effects, increasing skin blood flow and promoting heat loss. The metabolic rate of the skin is relatively low, and metabolic factors have only a weak influence on skin blood flow. Similarly, autoregulation is weak in the skin. Light alone has little effect on skin blood flow, unless it influences temperature. Skin blood flow increases during exercise as body temperature rises.

4 B. During exercise, local vascular control mechanisms predominate, overriding sympathetic nervous system-mediated constriction, causing vasodilation and substantially increasing blood flow. Sympathetic α-adrenergic activation tends to cause vasoconstriction, but is inhibited by accumulation of metabolites during exercise (functional sympatholysis). Baseline skeletal muscle blood flow (at rest) is relatively low, and is higher in oxidative compared with glycolytic muscle. The sympathetic nervous system is the primary regulator of the skeletal muscle circulation during resting conditions, while local vasodilator mechanisms predominate during exercise.

5 D. Feeding increases gut metabolism, increasing the presence of local vasodilators. In addition, several gastrointestinal hormones, in addition to their gastrointestinal effects, produce vasodilation. As a result, blood flow increases markedly in response to feeding (postprandial hyperemia). The splanchnic vascular bed has an important capacitance function, and reduced capacitance during exercise is an important factor in mobilizing volume, increasing cardiac output and oxygen-carrying capacity during exercise. As mentioned above, several gastrointestinal hormones are potent vasodilators. Hepatic artery and portal vein flow are inversely related (hepatic arterial buffer response).

6 A. In the fetus, blood becomes oxygenated in the placenta and the placenta receives a high proportion of cardiac output. The lungs provide no oxygen and flow is low due to high pulmonary vascular resistance. Only 10–12% of blood flow goes to the lungs in the fetus. Blood flows from the higher-pressure pulmonary artery in the fetus to the lower-pressure aorta through the ductus arteriosus. Pressure in the fetal right atrium is greater than pressure in the left atrium, allowing relatively oxygenated blood to flow through the foramen ovale into the left atrium and ventricle. The left ventricle has a higher oxygen saturation than the right ventricle, because it receives a greater proportion of flow from the relatively oxygenated ductus venosus while the right ventricle receives the majority of less-oxygenated blood from the cranial vena cava.

39 Heart Sounds and Murmurs

Michele Borgarelli[1] and Jens Häggström[2]

[1] Virginia-Maryland Regional College of Veterinary Medicine, Blacksburg, VA, USA
[2] Faculty of Veterinary Medicine and Animal Science, Swedish University of Agricultural Sciences, Uppsala, Sweden

Heart sounds

> 1 Define the term "auscultation."
> 2 What is the relationship of the heart sounds to the electrocardiogram?
> 3 Name the components of the stethoscope and how to use it.

Cardiac auscultation is the act of listening to the heart. Contraction of the normal heart generates vibrations by direct and indirect mechanisms. Many of these vibrations are transmitted to specific locations on the surface of thorax, but only a portion possesses sufficient frequency or amplitude to be audible. Groups of audible vibrations are perceived as **heart sounds** when the ear or a **stethoscope** is placed at appropriate locations on the thoracic surface.

The phonocardiogram (PCG) is a graphic recording of the heart sounds after they have been transduced to an electrical signal with a microphone. An electrocardiogram (ECG), and in some instances one or more pressure events, are recorded simultaneously with the PCG to identify phases of the cardiac cycle. This permits the student or clinician to visualize the temporal relationships among sound, electrical, and mechanical events of the cardiac cycle. The ability to judge the duration of the intervals separating sounds is essential to auscultation. Figure 39.1 shows the relationship between the timing of all four heart sounds, the ECG, and events of the cardiac cycle.

Stethoscope

There are many types of stethoscope. Traditionally, they have a diaphragm and a bell. The tube of the stethoscope should not be unnecessarily long (an appropriate length is 36–46 cm or 14–18 inches), and it is important that the earpieces of the stethoscope fit the ears snugly and comfortably to avoid air leakage. Auscultatory sounds range in frequency and intensity. The diaphragm accentuates higher-frequency sounds (first and second sounds and murmurs) and filters out low-frequency sounds. The bell is used to listen to low-frequency sounds, such as the third and fourth heart sounds. The same-size stethoscope is not appropriate for all animals. A pediatric size is best for cats and small animals while an adult stethoscope is better for larger animals. However, there are now electronic, often sensor-based, stethoscopes available, which allows amplification of the sound as well as their recording. These newer stethoscopes improve auscultation considerably, but are more expensive than the traditional types.

Classification of heart sounds

> 1 What is the difference between transients and murmurs?

Traditionally, cardiovascular sounds have been categorized as normal or abnormal. However, no sound is an abnormality in itself; each "extra" sound has to be judged in view of the circumstances under which it occurs. While an audible third heart sound often indicates heart disease in the dog, it is commonplace in normal horses. So-called innocent or functional murmurs are prevalent in apparently normal animals, particularly horses and puppies.

Categorizing all cardiovascular sounds as either transients or murmurs seems to be less ambiguous than the aforementioned

Dukes' Physiology of Domestic Animals, Thirteenth Edition. Edited by William O. Reece, Howard H. Erickson, Jesse P. Goff and Etsuro E. Uemura.
© 2015 John Wiley & Sons, Inc. Published 2015 by John Wiley & Sons, Inc.
Companion website: www.wiley.com/go/reece/physiology

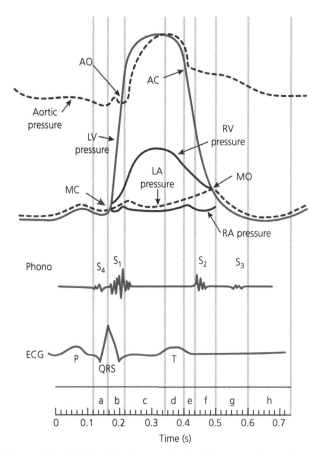

Figure 39.1 Relationships between timing of heart sounds, cardiac events, and electrocardiogram. Electrical activity depicted on the ECG precedes cardiac mechanical activity shown by the phonocardiogram (Phono). The QRS complex represents ventricular activation. The atrioventricular valves close (MC) as the ventricles eject blood through the semilunar valves and the first heart sound (S_1) occurs at the R-wave downstroke. The second heart sound (S_2) occurs at the end of ventricular contraction (i.e., ventricular systole) when the semilunar valves close (AC), approximately at the time of the T wave. The third heart sound (S_3) occurs during the first half of diastole, during passive ventricular filling (e.g., between the T wave and the ensuing P wave). The fourth heart sound (S_4) occurs late in diastole after atrial activation (P wave) and contraction. LA, left atrium; LV, left ventricle; RA, right atrium; RV, right ventricle.

classification. Transients are sounds of brief duration, such as the **first, second, third,** and **fourth heart sounds. Murmurs** are prolonged groups of vibrations that occur during normally silent intervals of the cardiac cycle.

Transient sounds

1 What are the four normal heart sounds or transients?

2 What causes the normal heart sounds?

3 What causes splitting of the heart sounds?

4 What are some factors that influence the intensity of the heart sounds?

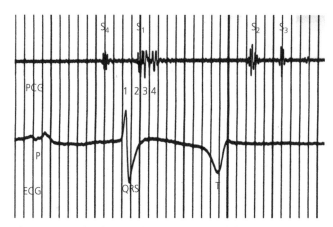

Figure 39.2 The phonocardiogram (PCG) and electrocardiogram (ECG) from a normal horse. The four components of S_1 are indicated by numbers 1–4. The somewhat accentuated fourth component could be considered an ejection sound. S_3 follows the onset of S_2 by 0.14 s. S_3 is followed by a soft low-frequency sound. Vertical lines occur at 0.04-s intervals. From Smetzer, D.L., Hamlin, R.L. and Smith, C.R. (1977), in *Dukes' Physiology of Domestic Animals*, 9th edn (ed. M.J. Swenson), p. 96. Cornell University Press, Ithaca, NY. With permission from Cornell University Press.

Each normal heartbeat generates at least two transients, the first (S_1) and second (S_2) heart sounds. These are described onomatopoeically as "lub-dub." In addition to S_1 and S_2, two other heart sounds sometimes occur during ventricular diastole. These are the third (S_3) and fourth (S_4) heart sounds.

First heart sound

The first heart sounds signals the start of ventricular ejection and begins approximately with the QRS complex of the ECG (Figure 39.1). The first sound is associated with closure and tensing of the atrioventricular (AV) valves with sudden deceleration of the blood being pushed against the valves. Sudden development of tension in the AV valves at the time of closure is generally cited as the major factor in the genesis of the first sound. Factors of less importance include vibrations generated within the contracting ventricular myocardium, opening of the semilunar valves, and vibrations generated within the wall of the aorta and pulmonary artery as blood is ejected into the arteries at the onset of systole. The first heart sound is longer and has lower frequency than the second heart sound. The first heart sound is usually best heard over the cardiac apex. Phonocardiographically, there are usually four components or groups of vibrations recognizable in S_1 (Figure 39.2).

First component

The first component is attributed to vibrations generated by the contracting ventricular myocardium, slight AV valvular regurgitation occurring at the onset of ventricular systole, and coaptation of leaflets of the AV valves prior to complete closure and distension. Vibrations of the first component are of low frequency and low amplitude.

Second and third components

It is generally believed that sudden development of tension in the closing mitral valve and then in the tricuspid valve generates the second and third components of S_1, respectively. Vibrations of the second and third components of S_1 are of higher frequency and amplitude.

Fourth component

The fourth component of S_1 occurs at the onset of ventricular ejection. It is probably caused by the sudden ejection of blood into the great arteries, which generates vibrations within the walls. Vibrations of the fourth component are of low frequency and low amplitude.

Intensity of first sound

In the dog, S_1 is usually more intense than S_2. The opposite is true for many horses under basal conditions. Furthermore, a marked beat-to-beat variation in intensity of S_1 is not unusual in horses under basal conditions.

Numerous extracardiac and cardiac factors influence the intensity of S_1 and other sounds. Since heart sounds tend to project to specific locations on the thoracic wall, proper placement of the stethoscope is important and will affect intensity of sound. The most common reasons for decreased intensity of S_1 are obesity, pericardial or pleural effusions, hypervolemia, pronounced first-degree AV block, diaphragmatic hernia, peritoneal pericardial diaphragmantic hernia, and barrel conformation of the thorax.

Intensity of S_1 is increased in animals during periods of excitement and immediately after exercise. More vigorous closing and tensing of the AV valves related to increased sympathetic activity probably accounts for increased intensity of S_1 under these circumstances. Other common reasons for increased intensity of S_1 are deep thorax, anemia, fever, hypertension, and chronic mitral valve disease.

Splitting of first heart sound

Split of heart sound is a rare event in all species. Split of S_1 is determined by a delayed closure of one of the AV valves. It can be occasionally heard in animals with severe right or left bundle branch block.

Second heart sound

The second heart sound signals the end of mechanical systole and coincides with the T wave of the ECG. The second heart sound is generated by the closure of the semilunar valves. Each semilunar valve contributes to the generation of S_2. The pulmonic component of S_2 normally follows the aortic component (Figure 39.3). However, they are usually heard as a single sound. S_2 is a shorter higher-pitched sound than S_1. Decreased intensity of S_2 has been associated with pericardial and pleural effusion, diaphragmatic and peritoneal pericardial diaphragmatic hernia, thoracic masses, myocardial failure, and severe chronic mitral valve degeneration. The most common cause of

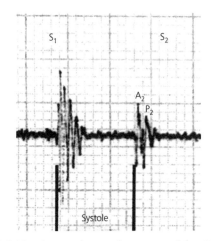

Figure 39.3 The phonocardiogram from a normal dog. S_1 is the first heart sound. A_2 is the aortic component of the second heart sound (S_2), while P_2 is the pulmonic component and normally follows A_2. However, these two components are usually heard as a single sound. Adapted from Kvart, C. and Häggström, J. (2002) *Cardiac Auscultation and Phonocardiography in Dogs, Horses and Cats*, p. 14. TK i Uppsala AB, Sweden. Reproduced with permission from C. Kvart and J. Häggström.

increased intensity of S_2 are fever, anemia, pulmonary hypertension, and conditions associated with high-ouput status such as hyperthyroidism.

Splitting of second sound

Splitting of S_2 occurs when the semilunar valves close out of phase. The split of S_2 is difficult to auscultate in dogs and cats due to the short interval between A_2 and P_2, while it is a common auscultatory finding in horses. The most common reason for splitting of S_2 is delayed closure of the pulmonic valve, and for this reason is usually best heard over the pulmonic area of auscultation. Splitting of S_2 can be physiologic or pathologic. Physiologic splitting of S_2 is a respiratory-related phenomenon appearing during inspiration and disappearing during expiration (Figure 39.4). During inspiration increased venous return to the right side of the heart occurs as a consequence of decreased intrathoracic pressure. The resultant lengthening of right ventricular ejection time causes the pulmonic valve to close later. Simultaneously, the act of inspiration hinders venous return to the left side of the heart and this in turn abbreviates left ventricular ejection time and causes the aortic valve to close earlier. During expiration, right ventricular ejection time returns to normal and left ventricular ejection time lengthens to handle the increased amount of blood delivered to the lungs during the preceding inspiration. Therefore S_2 becomes a single sound. Respiratory-related splitting of S_2 is detectable in some normal dogs, particularly if the heart rate is slow and pronounced sinus arrhythmia is present. Splitting of S_2 is detectable by auscultation in most normal horses, and it tends to be fixed rather than vary with respiration.

Pathologic splitting of S_2 is a characteristic of certain cardiac abnormalities in the dog. These abnormalities include pulmonary hypertension, pulmonic stenosis, right bundle branch block, and interatrial septal defect. Pathologic split tends to be fixed differently from physiologic one. When the split of S_2 is due to delayed closure of the aortic valve, it is defined as paradoxical splitting of S_2. Diagnosis of the paradoxical split of S_2 requires a PCG recording. Left bundle branch block or aortic/subaortic stenosis are the most common conditions associated with this finding.

Third heart sound

Third heart sound (S_3) occurs early in diastole near the end of rapid ventricular filling (see Figure 39.1). It is associated with sudden tensing of the chordae tendineae, deceleration of the filling wave of blood, and vibrations arising in the walls of the ventricles.

Although S_3 is detectable in PCGs of apparently normal dogs, it is rarely audible because it is mainly formed of low-frequency sounds. However, the third heard sound can be easily recognized in dogs afflicted with myocardial disease such as dilated cardiomyopathy. In these patients the presence of S_3 may be the only auscultatory abnormality and is generated by increased myocardial stiffness and elevated filling pressure. An audible S_3 may also be present in cats with end-stage cardiomyopathy. Occasionally, S_3 is more intense than either of the two major heart sounds, S_1 and S_2. The third sound is readily audible in many apparently normal horses (see Figure 39.2). The sound is quite intense and clicking in some horses; in others, it is soft and dull. As in dogs, S_3 in horses with congestive heart failure is frequently very intense.

Fourth heart sound

The fourth or atrial sound is generated by vibration of cardiac structures associated with atrial contraction and can be recognized on the PCG after the P wave on the ECG (see Figure 39.1). Although the fourth heart sound is seldom heard in dogs, it can be recognized in normal giant breeds. Fourth heart sound is common in apparently normal horses.

Pronounced first-degree AV block is found in many of the animals that exhibit S_4. A longer AV conduction time allows for completion of the sequence of events leading to its generation. The interval between the P wave of the ECG and S_4 in the PCG tends to remain constant at about 0.32–0.36 s in the horse (see Figure 39.2) and about 0.17 s in the dog (Figure 39.5). If the AV conduction time varies from one beat to the next, then the interval between S_4 and S_1 varies accordingly. Such a phenomenon is common in horses under resting conditions. Slight separation of S_4 and S_1 can be mistaken during auscultation for pronounced splitting of S_1. When the timing of S_4 is such that S_4 extends into S_1, the intensity of S_1 is usually reduced. This finding indirectly supports the theory that S_4 is

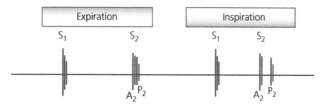

Figure 39.4 Schematic diagram showing physiologic split of S_2. During expiration, aortic (A_2) and pulmonic (P_2) components of S_2 are heard as a single sound. During inspiration the two components become separated and a split of S_2 can be heard (see text for detailed explanation).

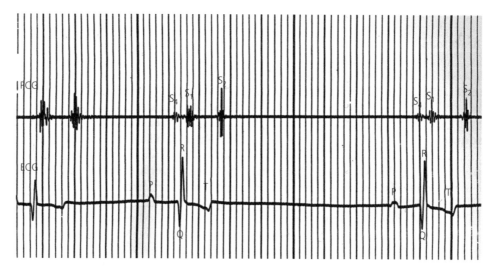

Figure 39.5 The phonocardiogram (PCG) and electrocardiogram (ECG) from a dog with first-degree AV heart block. Note that the PR interval of the second and third beats is 0.2 s. A prominent S_4 occurs on these beats. Vertical lines occur at 0.04-s intervals. From Smetzer, D.L., Hamlin, R.L. and Smith, C.R. (1977), in *Dukes' Physiology of Domestic Animals*, 9th edn (ed. M.J. Swenson), p. 99. Cornell University Press, Ithaca, NY. With permission from Cornell University Press.

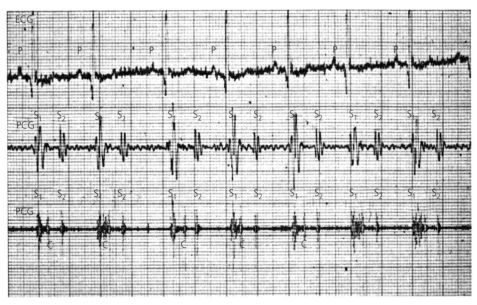

Figure 39.6 Phonocardiogram (PCG) and electrocardiogram (ECG) from a dog with mid-systolic click (C). This extrasystolic sound occurs in mid-systole between S_1 and S_2. It is a common finding in dogs with mitral valve prolapse.

generated by transient closing and tensing of the AV valves. Pathologic S_4 is present in animals with myocardial disease characterized by diastolic dysfunction such as hypertrophic cardiomyopathy. In this condition early diastolic filling is reduced because of the reduced cavity of the left ventricle. For this reason there is an increased volume of blood in the atria at the onset of their contraction. This, accordingly to the Frank–Starling law, induces a more energetic atrial contraction and S_4 might become audible. Other conditions associated with the presence of a detectable S_4 are advanced second-degree and third-degree AV block.

Gallop rhythm

Gallop rhythm occurs during tachycardia when S_3 and S_4 merge into a single heart sound. This rhythm is so-called because the sequence of S_1, S_2, and fusion of S_3 and S_4 resembles the sound of a galloping horse. As the period of diastole shortens with an increase in heart rate, atrial systole becomes superimposed upon the rapid filling phase of the ventricles. In small animals the presence of a gallop rhythm is associated with significant myocardial failure. In cats, gallop rhythms are present in animals with hypertrophic cardiomyopathy or hyperthyroidism. It should be remembered that excessive pressure of the stethoscope on the thorax of a cat can produce a gallop rhythm.

Other systolic sounds

Two "extra" sounds sometimes occur between S_1 and S_2. One of these, the ejection sound or ejection click, is an accentuation of the terminal component of S_1. It often coexists with abnormalities that cause dilation of either the aorta or pulmonary artery of the dog, but is common in normal horses and in young small animals.

The other extra systolic sound is the systolic click (Figure 39.6). This sound is often intermittent and may be best heard using the diaphragm of the stethoscope. Systolic click is a common finding in early stages of chronic mitral valve disease in dogs. The origin of the systolic click has been hypothesized to be caused by the tensing of redundant chordae tendineae and rapid deceleration of blood against the mitral valve leaflets at maximum prolapse into the left atrium. The sound is usually mid-systolic but the timing can vary and can be closer to S_1 or S_2.

Cardiac murmurs

1 What is the cause of cardiac murmurs?
2 How are murmurs classified?
3 Explain how murmurs are graded by intensity.
4 What are some systolic murmurs?
5 What are some diastolic murmurs?
6 Which murmur is often continuous?

A murmur is a prolonged series of auditory vibrations emanating from the heart or blood vessels that may occur at different times during the cardiac cycle. Turbulence in flowing blood is generally accepted as the major source of murmurs, or prolonged vibrations. Causes of turbulent blood flow include (i) alteration of the morphology of any one of the four heart valves (insufficiency or stenosis), (ii) abnormal communication between the two sides of the heart and/or great vessels (interatrial septal defect, interventricular septal defect, or patent ductus arteriosus), (iii) increased blood flow velocity through a normal valve

Table 39.1 Auscultation of heart sounds and common cardiac murmurs.

Auscultatory finding	Timing	PMI (valve area)
Normal heart sounds		
First heart sound	Onset systole	Left apex (mitral valve)
Second heart sound	End systole	Left base (aortic valve)
Pulmonic component	End systole	Left base (pulmonic valve)
Third heart sound	Early diastole	Left apex (mitral valve)
Fourth (atrial) sound	Late diastole	Ventricular inlet (left)
Valvular regurgitation		
Mitral regurgitation	Systole	Left apex (mitral valve)
Tricuspid regurgitation	Systole	Right hemithorax (tricuspid valve)
Aortic regurgitation	Diastole	Left base (aortic valve)
Pulmonary insufficiency	Diastole	Left base (pulmonic valve)
Ventricular septal defect	Systole	Right sternal border/left cardiac base (pulmonic valve)
Patent ductus arteriosus	Continuous	Dorsal left base over the pulmonary artery

PMI, point of maximum intensity.
Source: adapted from Bonagura, J.D. (1990) Clinical evaluation and management of heart disease. *Equine Veterinary Education* **2**:31–37. Reproduced with permission from Wiley.

orifice or vessel, and (iv) changes to the blood viscosity, usually occurring as a consequence of other, noncardiac, disease such as severe anemia. Murmurs are classified based on the following criteria: location, timing, quality, radiation, and intensity. The point of maximum intensity (PMI) of a cardiac murmur is generally located over the site of turbulence and gives an indication of the origin of the murmur (Table 39.1). The cause of murmurs can be further differentiated from their timing within the cardiac cycle. Murmurs occur during systole, during diastole, or during both systole and diastole. The frequency or pitch of a murmur may also aid diagnosis of the underlying cause. The direction in which a murmur radiates over the body surface also helps in localizing the site of origin. The intensity of murmurs is most commonly graded on a 1 to 6 scale, with a grade 1 murmur being the softest and a grade 6 the loudest. The heart murmur may be palpated as a precordial thrill in animals with a grade 5 or grade 6 murmur. Figure 39.7 shows the various terms used to describe cardiac murmurs and their relationship to the heart sounds. In Figure 39.8 the normal heart sounds and common abnormal murmurs and transients are depicted schematically.

Systolic murmurs

Systolic murmurs (between S_1 and S_2) result as blood regurgitates through incompetent AV (mitral and tricuspid) valves, or as blood is ejected through the semilunar (aortic and pulmonary) valves or through a ventricular septal defect.

Aortic stenosis

Subaortic stenosis is the most common form of congenital heart disease in dogs. However, aortic or subaortic stenosis is unusual in horses and in cats the aortic stenosis is usually a consequence of hypertrophic cardiomyopathy. The principal hemodynamic consequence of aortic stenosis is an increased resistance to left ventricular outflow, with a proportional

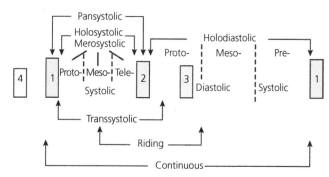

Figure 39.7 Various terms employed in describing cardiac murmurs. A pansystolic murmur begins before the end of S_1 (the first heart sound) and ends after the onset of S_2 (second heart sound). A holosystolic murmur fills the systolic period but does not encroach on S_1 and S_2. Merosystolic murmurs occupy only a part of systole: protosystolic the first third, mesosystolic the middle third, and telesystolic the final third. Holodiastolic murmurs fill the diastolic period: a protodiastolic the first third, mesodiastolic the middle third, and presystolic the last third. A transsystolic murmur is a holosystolic murmur that continues into diastole. A riding murmur begins before and ends after S_2. A continuous murmur lasts throughout the cardiac cycle from one heartbeat to the next. From Detweiler, D.K., Riedesel, D.H. and Knight, D.H. (1993), in *Dukes' Physiology of Domestic Animals*, 11th edn (eds M.J. Swenson and W.O. Reece), p. 162. Cornell University Press, Ithaca, NY. With permission from Cornell University Press.

elevation of left ventricular systolic pressure if flow remains constant. Aortic stenosis usually causes a systolic murmur with a crescendo–decrescendo character (i.e., diamond shaped); that is, the intensity of the murmur increases until mid-ventricular systole and then decreases during the remainder of ventricular systole (Figure 39.9). The PMI of the murmur is over the aortic ostium (heart base) and its intensity and quality is dependent on the severity of stenosis, ranging from a soft low-intensity

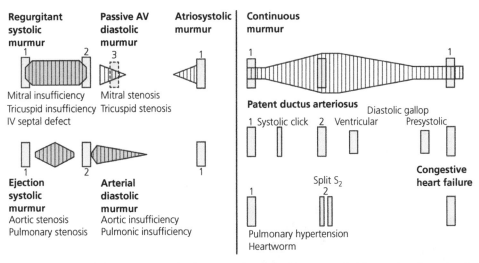

Figure 39.8 Some common abnormal murmurs. 1, 2 and 3, first, second, and third heart sounds. Murmurs are shown in relation to heart sounds by figures with vertical lines. Widening of these figures indicates crescendo and narrowing decrescendo of sound intensity. Cardiac lesions or clinical syndromes associated with each murmur are listed below each diagram. (*Left*) The regurgitant murmur of mitral or tricuspid insufficiency is of constant intensity; the others shown vary in intensity. (*Right*) The continuous murmur of patent ductus arteriosus is often called a machinery murmur. It is caused by the waxing and waning of the intensity of sound vibrations set up by the continuous but pulsatile flow of blood from the aorta through the ductus arteriosus to the pulmonary artery. Splitting of the second heart sound occurs when the contraction of the two ventricles is asynchronous (as in bundle branch block) or when closure of the pulmonic valve is delayed because of pulmonic hypertension. From Detweiler, D.K., Riedesel, D.H. and Knight, D.H. (1993), in *Dukes' Physiology of Domestic Animals*, 11th edn (eds M.J. Swenson and W.O. Reece), p. 162. Cornell University Press, Ithaca, NY. With permission from Cornell University Press.

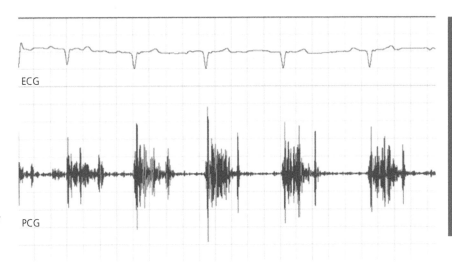

Figure 39.9 Phonocardiogram (PCG) and electrocardiogram (ECG) from a dog with a heart murmur caused by moderate subaortic stenosis. The recorded systolic heart murmur shows a crescendo–decrescendo character, and both the first (S_1) and the second (S_2) heart sounds may be identified.

murmur to very loud murmurs of harsh quality. Since left ventricular ejection time is lengthened, paradoxical splitting of S_2 may be evident in more severe forms of this congenital anomaly.

Pulmonic stenosis

The characteristics of pulmonic stenosis (Figure 39.10) are very similar to those of aortic stenosis, and it may be very difficult using auscultation to distinguish murmurs caused by pulmonic stenosis from those caused by aortic stenosis in dogs and cats. The murmur is systolic and usually of a crescendo–decrescendo character and its intensity and quality is dependent on the severity of stenosis, ranging from a soft low-intensity murmur

to very loud murmurs of harsh quality. Right ventricular ejection time may be prolonged with more severe forms of pulmonic stenosis, and splitting of S_2 may be present. Pulmonic stenosis is a common congenital lesion in dogs and humans, but is less common in cats (compared to dogs) and is extremely rare in horses.

Mitral insufficiency

Mitral insufficiency or regurgitation may be primary (i.e., caused by an abnormal mitral valve) or secondary (i.e., caused by left ventricular dilatation that leads to separation of the mitral valve leaflets). Primary mitral insufficiency is the cause

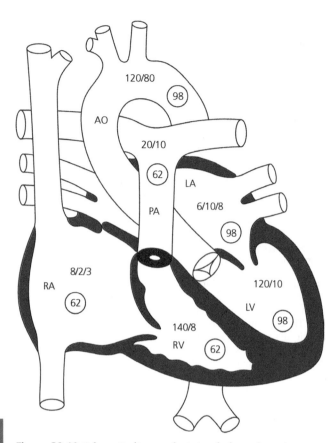

Figure 39.10 Schematic diagram depicting the hemodynamic alterations associated with severe valvular pulmonic stenosis. The resistance to flow at the pulmonary valve leads to an increase in right ventricular systolic pressure. The resultant concentric hypertrophy may lead to a mild increase in right ventricular diastolic pressure and right atrial pressure. Left-sided pressures remain normal. In the absence of an interatrial communication, both pulmonary and systemic hemoglobin remain normal. Intracardiac pressures are indicated in mmHg as systolic/diastolic for LV, RV, PA, and AO, and as a-wave/v-wave/mean for LA and RA. Circled numbers indicate percent oxygen saturation. RA, right atrium; RV, right ventricle; LA, left atrium; LV, left ventricle; PA, pulmonary artery; AO, aorta. From Kittleson, M.D. and Kienle, R.D. (1998) *Small Animal Cardiovascular Medicine*, p. 241. Mosby, St Louis, MO. With permission from Elsevier.

forms of mitral insufficiency, the murmur can often be augmented by physical maneuvers, such as a short run. With further progression, the sound becomes holosystolic, more intense, and harsher in quality, and may radiate over to the right side of the thorax. Less commonly, mitral insufficiency can cause "musical" murmurs ("whoop" sounds), composed of a fundamental frequency and overtones of the fundamental frequency of high intensity. This type of murmur does not indicate the severity of mitral insufficiency (see Figures 39.4, 39.7 and 39.11).

Tricuspid insufficiency

The characteristics of the systolic murmur of tricuspid insufficiency are very similar to those of mitral insufficiency (see Figure 39.7), but with the exception that the PMI is located over the tricuspid ostium on the right side of the thorax. The intensity of the murmur may increase during inspiration and decrease during expiration. Generally, the intensity of tricuspid regurgitation murmurs is lower than that of mitral valve insufficiency murmurs because of the lower pressure gradient between the right ventricle and the right atrium compared with the left side. Conditions associated with increased right ventricular pressure, such as pulmonary arterial hypertension, can cause louder tricuspid insufficiency murmurs.

Interventricular septal defect

Interventricular septal defect (VSD) is the most common congenital heart defect in cats and horses. The systolic murmur associated with a VSD is generated as blood flows from the left ventricle into the right ventricle. This murmur tends to be holosystolic and of uniform intensity throughout its course (see Figure 39.7); it is a plateau type of murmur like the systolic murmurs of mitral insufficiency and tricuspid insufficiency. It is usually high-pitched and blowing. The PMI of the VSD murmur is located on the right side of the thorax. Shunting of a large volume of blood through a large defect frequently causes an additional systolic murmur. This murmur is most intense on the left side of the thorax at the pulmonic area and is caused by relative pulmonic stenosis.

Interatrial septal defect

A systolic murmur is associated with an interatrial defect. In this congenital anomaly, blood flows from the left atrium to the right atrium during atrial systole (i.e., during late ventricular diastole), thereby increasing the stroke volume of the right ventricle and causing relative pulmonic stenosis. Therefore, the systolic murmur is caused by relative pulmonic stenosis rather than by blood flow through the defect itself.

Functional (physiological) systolic murmurs

Soft systolic murmurs are common in puppies, kittens, and horses having apparently normal valve orifices and great arteries (Figure 39.12). Turbulent blood flow stemming from increased blood velocity is thought to be of prime importance in the generation of these innocent murmurs. Severe anemia can also

of most systolic murmurs in middle-aged to old dogs and horses, and it occurs as a consequence of chronic progressive lesions of primarily the AV valves, referred to as myxomatous valve disease. It is also the most common cause of congestive heart failure in dogs and horses. Primary mitral insufficiency is uncommon in cats, but it may, like aortic stenosis, develop as a consequence of hypertrophic cardiomyopathy. The PMI in mitral insufficiency is over the mitral (apical) ostium on the left side of the thorax. The timing of the murmur in mild early forms of mitral insufficiency is most frequently early systolic, but may be late systolic, or may vary between the two. With progression, the murmur becomes holosystolic. The sound begins as a soft apical systolic murmur on the left side of the thorax and may be intermittent, and sometimes audible only during inspiration. In mild

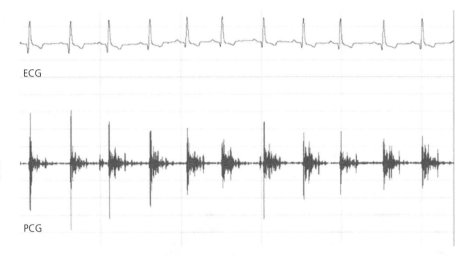

Figure 39.11 Phonocardiogram (PCG) and electrocardiogram (ECG) from a dog with a heart murmur caused by moderate to severe mitral valve insufficiency. The recording shows a first heart sound (S_1) followed by a systolic heart murmur, and the second heart sound (S_2) is reduced in amplitude.

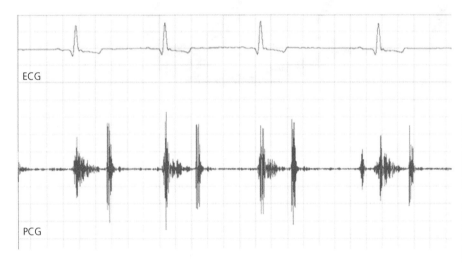

Figure 39.12 Phonocardiogram (PCG) and electrocardiogram (ECG) from a young dog with a physiologic heart murmur, i.e., a heart murmur not associated with any structural or functional heart disease. The recording shows a first heart sound (S_1) followed by a systolic heart murmur of short duration and crescendo–decrescendo character and the second heart sound (S_2).

cause a functional systolic murmur by changed blood viscosity. A functional murmur is usually of low intensity (grade 1–3) and is composed of mid- or high-frequency sounds. The murmur is usually timed to early systole and ends early or in the middle of systole. They are usually of decrescendo, but sometimes crescendo–decrescendo, character. The intensity of the murmur may vary with the heart rate and respiration.

Tetralogy of Fallot

Tetralogy of Fallot is an uncommon congenital disease in dogs, but slightly more common in cats and horses. Tetralogy of Fallot is a shunting defect in which there is usually no resistance to flow between the left and right ventricles. Consequently, blood flows to the right and left circulations proportional to systemic and pulmonary resistances (Figures 39.9 and 39.13). The pulmonic stenosis in tetralogy may be so severe that resistance to flow through the pulmonic valve is

greater than systemic vascular resistance. Consequently, a significant amount of blood flows from the right ventricle, through the ventricular septal defect, and out the aorta. The murmur associated with tetralogy of Fallot is primarily caused by the pulmonic stenosis. Thus, the intensity and character of the murmur will be dependent on pulmonic stenosis characteristics.

Diastolic murmurs

A murmur heard after S_2 is designated as diastolic. While pure diastolic murmurs are extremely rare in dogs and cats, they are not uncommon in horses (Figure 39.14).

Mitral or tricuspid stenosis

Although pathology of the AV valves, particularly the mitral valve, leading to AV stenosis is prevalent in humans, it is virtually nonexistent in domestic animals. On the other hand, lesions

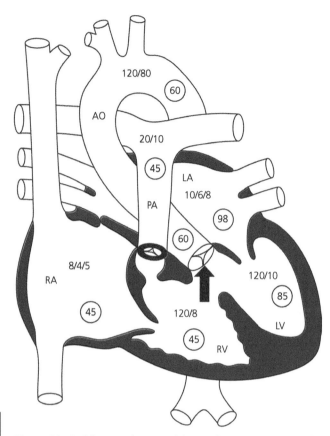

Figure 39.13 Schematic diagram of the circulation in a patient with tetralogy of Fallot with severe right ventricular (RV) outflow obstruction. The course of the circulation, oxygen saturations (circles), and pressures are shown. Systolic pressures in the right ventricle, left ventricle (LV), and aorta (AO) are identical (120 mmHg). There is a pressure gradient of 100 mmHg across the region of the pulmonic valve. Resistance to flow through the ventricular septal defect and systemic circulation is less than the resistance across the pulmonic valve region. Consequently, deoxygenated (oxygen saturation, 45%) blood from the right ventricle shunts into the left ventricle and systemic circulation. This results in systemic hypoxemia (oxygen saturation, 60%). Pulmonary blood flow is reduced to approximately 70% of systemic blood flow. Right atrial (RA) pressure is normal. PA, pulmonary artery; LA, left atrium. From Kittleson, M.D. and Kienle, R.D. (1998) *Small Animal Cardiovascular Medicine*, p. 241. Mosby, St Louis, MO. With permission from Elsevier.

such as interatrial septal defect, mitral insufficiency, or tricuspid insufficiency can result in an increased rate of blood flow through the appropriate AV valve during early diastole in domestic animals as well as humans. The resulting relative AV stenosis can cause an early diastolic murmur, often referred to as a diastolic rumble (see Figure 39.7).

Pulmonic insufficiency

Although mild to moderate pulmonic insufficiency is very common in all species, diastolic murmurs due to pulmonic insufficiency are rare in animals. Occasionally, dilatation of the pulmonary artery with attendant incompetence of the pulmonic valve resulting from pulmonary hypertension is the cause of a diastolic murmur in the dog. Likewise, a diastolic murmur of pulmonic insufficiency sometimes appears after surgical correction of pulmonic stenosis. The murmur of pulmonic insufficiency tends to be soft and blowing (see Figure 39.7).

Aortic insufficiency

Like pulmonic insufficiency, mild aortic insufficiency is common particularly in dogs. It either occurs as a consequence of myxomatous lesions or, less commonly, bacterial growth on the aortic valve leaflets (bacterial endocarditis), or as a consequence of congential aortic stenosis. In dogs and cats the aortic insufficiency must be moderate to severe before it can be auscultated, which means that it is comparably uncommon in these species. On the contrary, diastolic murmurs caused by aortic insufficiency are common in old horses. Most are "noisy," with a blend of a wide range of vibration frequencies. They tend to be high-pitched and decrescendo in configuration (see Figure 39.7). Less frequently, the diastolic murmur of aortic insufficiency in the horse is "musical." These murmurs have a groaning, whining, or buzzing quality. Some are decrescendo in configuration, others are crescendo in configuration, and some are most intense in mid-diastole. Some have both musical and noisy components.

Innocent diastolic murmurs

It is not unusual to find soft diastolic murmurs in apparently normal horses under 5 years of age. These are high-pitched and very brief in duration. They occur immediately after S_2 and their cause is unknown.

Continuous murmurs

Patent ductus arteriosus (PDA) is one of the most common congenital lesions in dogs; it occurs in cats and horses, but less commonly than in dogs. In PDA the fundamental pathophysiologic event is shunting of blood through the patent duct. The flow direction is usually from the left (aorta) to the right (pulmonic artery) side because of the pressure gradient, but with larger ducts, which are uncommon, the flow ceases or can even be from the right to the left side (so-called reversed PDA). Individuals with nonshunting or right-to-left shunting often do not present with any murmur. In the case of left-to-right shunting PDA, which is by far the most common presentation, the abnormality usually causes both a systolic and a diastolic murmur (see Figures 39.6, 39.7 and 39.15). Turbulence in blood flowing through the PDA is responsible for generating the murmur. Since the abnormal blood flow is continuous during systole and diastole, the murmur is likewise continuous during systole and diastole. The intensity of the murmur increases during systole, attains a peak at the time of S_2, and decreases during diastole. The murmur of PDA is frequently referred to as a "machinery" murmur. The murmur is audible over the left hemithorax at the aortic and pulmonary valve areas (heart base).

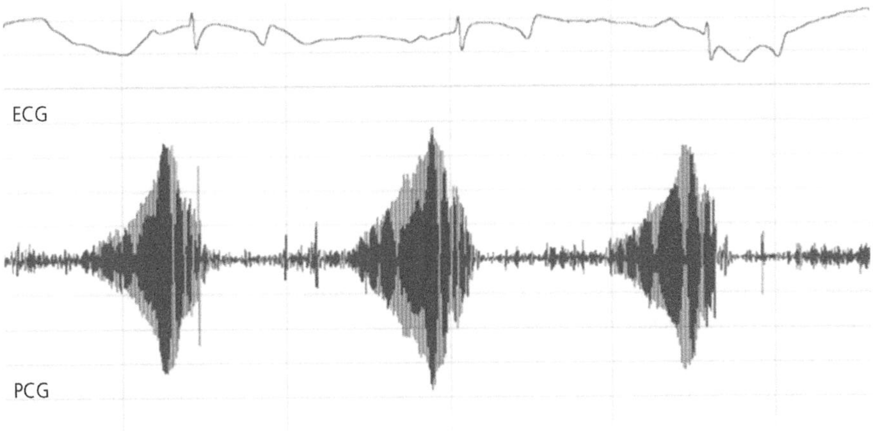

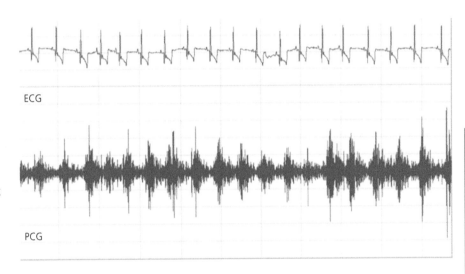

Figure 39.14 Phonocardiogram (PCG) and electrocardiogram (ECG) from an old horse with a loud diastolic heart murmur of musical character. The recording shows a very loud diastolic heart murmur of crescendo–decrescendo character with maximal intensity timed at the onset of atrial depolarization (as timed by the ECG). The first (S_1) and second (S_2) heart sounds are difficult to identify on this recording.

Figure 39.15 Phonocardiogram (PCG) and electrocardiogram (ECG) from a dog with left-to-right shunting persistent ductus arteriosus. The recording shows a continuous heart murmur with maximal intensity timed to the second (S_2) heart sound.

Section VI: The Cardiovascular System

Self-evaluation

Answers can be found at the end of the chapter.

1 An 8-year-old Poodle is presented with a grade V/VI holosystolic mitral valvular murmur and a history of nocturnal coughing. The grade V/VI murmur is most likely:
  A A very faint murmur
  B A faint murmur
  C An intermediate murmur
  D A very loud murmur

2 Which of the following murmurs is not a systolic murmur:
  A Tricuspid regurgitation
  B Mitral regurgitation
  C Pulmonic stenosis
  D Aortic stenosis
  E Mitral stenosis
  F Ventricular septal defect

3 The bell of the stethoscope is used primarily to listen to which particular frequency sounds, as exemplified by which heart sound?
  A Low frequency, first heart sound
  B High frequency, first heart sound
  C Low frequency, second heart sound
  D High frequency, second heart sound
  E Low frequency, third heart sound
  F High frequency, third heart sound

4 You examine a 7-year-old Cocker spaniel and find evidence of a systolic murmur (no diastolic murmur), pulmonary edema (rapid noisy respiration, cough), left ventricular hypertrophy, and exercise intolerance. The most likely explanation for the symptoms is:
  A Mitral stenosis
  B Mitral insufficiency
  C Aortic regurgitation
  D Pulmonic stenosis
  E Ventricular septal defect

5 In a dog with a patent ductus arteriosus, there is often a shunt in blood flow:

 A From right to left during systole only
 B From left to right during diastole, and right to left during systole
 C From right to left during systole and diastole
 D From left to right during systole and diastole
 E From right to left during diastole, and left to right during systole

Suggested reading

Blissitt, K.J. (1999) Auscultation. In: *Cardiology of the Horse* (ed. C. Marr). W.B. Saunders, Philadelphia.

Bonagura, J.D. and Reef, V.B. (1998) Cardiovascular diseases. In: *Equine Internal Medicine* (eds S.M. Reed and W.M. Bayly). W.B. Saunders, Philadelphia.

Detweiler, D.K., Riedesel, D.H. and Knight, D.H. (1993) Mechanical activity of the heart. In: *Dukes' Physiology of Domestic Animals*, 11th edn (eds M.J. Swenson and W.O. Reece). Cornell University Press, Ithaca, NY.

Geddes, L.A., McCrady, J.D. and Hoff, H.E. (1965) The contributions of the horse to knowledge of the heart and circulation. II. Cardiac catheterization and ventricular dynamics. *Connecticut Medicine* **29**:864–876.

Holmes, J.R. (1986) *Equine Cardiology*. School of Veterinary Science, University of Bristol, Langford, Bristol, UK.

Kittleson, M.D. and Kienle, R.D. (1998) *Small Animal Cardiovascular Medicine*. Mosby, St Louis, MO.

McCrady, J.D., Hoff, H.E. and Geddes, L.A. (1966) The contributions of the horse to knowledge of the heart and circulation. IV. James Hope and the heart sounds. *Connecticut Medicine* **30**:126–131.

Smetzer, D.L., Hamlin, R.L. and Smith, R.C. (1977) Cardiovascular sounds. In: *Dukes' Physiology of Domestic Animals*, 9th edn (ed. M.J. Swenson). Cornell University Press, Ithaca, NY.

Stephenson, R.B. (1997) The heart as a pump. In: *Textbook of Veterinary Physiology*, 2nd edn (ed. J.G. Cunningham), pp. 180–197. W.B. Saunders, Philadelphia.

Yoganathan, A.P., Hopmeyer, J. and Heinrich, R.S. (1995) Mechanics of heart valves. In: *Biomedical Engineering Handbook* (ed. J.D. Bronzino). CRC Press, Boca Raton, FL.

Answers

1 D. A very loud murmur. Murmurs are graded from I to VI, with I being a very faint murmur and VI a very loud murmur.

2 E. Mitral stenosis is a diastolic murmur. The murmur is rare in domestic animals, but common in the human.

3 E. The diaphragm accentuates higher-frequency sounds (first and second sounds) and filters out low-frequency sounds. The bell is used to listen to low-frequency sounds, such as the third and fourth heart sounds.

4 B. Mitral insufficiency causes an increase in left atrial pressure and an increase in pulmonary artery pressure which leads to edema. The volume workload of the left ventricle also increases leading to left ventricular hypertrophy.

5 D. From left to right during systole and diastole. Pressure is nearly always higher in the aorta than in the pulmonary artery, resulting in a left-to-right shunt during both systole and diastole.

40 Hypertension, Heart Failure, and Shock

Scott A. Brown
University of Georgia, Athens, GA, USA

Hypertension

1 What are the three determinants of **systemic arterial blood pressure** and what mechanisms contribute to the regulation of each?

2 What is the rationale for the clinical measurement of systemic arterial blood pressure in veterinary practice and how is it done?

3 What factors or conditions make an animal more likely to develop an elevated systemic arterial blood pressure?

4 What are the general mechanisms of, and target organs for, hypertensive injury?

5 What are the general physiological principles of antihypertensive therapy?

Persistently elevated systemic arterial blood pressure, often referred to as systemic hypertension, is a frequent problem in dogs and cats where it is associated with complications in the urinary system (e.g., progressive renal disease), eyes (e.g., retinal and choroidal injury), cardiovascular system (e.g., heart failure), and central nervous system (e.g., hypertensive encephalopathy). Unfortunately, systemic hypertension is usually asymptomatic initially and goes unrecognized for months or years until irreversible tissue damage becomes evident as organ failure ensues.

Definitions

Systemic hypertension is often defined as persistently elevated systemic arterial blood pressure (ABP) and is distinct in location, cause, and pathophysiology from pulmonary hypertension (see Chapter 37). **Idiopathic hypertension** exists when ABP is elevated yet a careful diagnostic evaluation fails to identify the cause of the hypertension. **Secondary hypertension** occurs when there is a known cause, generally a disease process altering renal or neurohumoral functions. Idiopathic hypertension comprises most cases of hypertension in people but secondary hypertension appears to be the most common form in dogs and cats.

Blood pressure regulation

The ABP is the product of **cardiac output** and **total peripheral vascular resistance**. Cardiac output may be further factored as the product of **heart rate** and **stroke volume**:

$$ABP = (\text{heart rate} \times \text{stroke volume}) \times \text{total peripheral vascular resistance}$$

Thus any factor or process that persistently elevates any of these three determinants of ABP can cause systemic hypertension. For a thorough discussion of the factors that affect stroke

Section VI: The Cardiovascular System

Dukes' Physiology of Domestic Animals, Thirteenth Edition. Edited by William O. Reece, Howard H. Erickson, Jesse P. Goff and Etsuro E. Uemura.
© 2015 John Wiley & Sons, Inc. Published 2015 by John Wiley & Sons, Inc.
Companion website: www.wiley.com/go/reece/physiology

volume, heart rate, and total peripheral vascular resistance, refer to Chapters 34 and 41.

There are many feedback control systems that regulate ABP, such as the arterial baroreceptor system, and these are discussed in Chapters 34 and 41. These feedback regulatory systems generally maintain ABP within a physiologic range ("set point") through adjustments in heart rate, stroke volume, or total peripheral resistance. It follows that the presence of systemic hypertension indicates an abnormality of these control systems, leading to inappropriate levels of heart rate, stroke volume, or total peripheral resistance. In particular, high ABP should produce sodium and water excretion by the kidneys ("pressure natriuresis") to lower extracellular fluid volume. A reduction in extracellular fluid volume will decrease venous return and thus stroke volume through the Frank–Starling relationship (see Chapters 34 and 41), restoring ABP toward normal. This response of the kidney, modified and enhanced by the renin–angiotensin–aldosterone system (RAAS), emphasizes the key role of renal involvement in the genesis and maintenance of systemic hypertension. This analysis demonstrates that the maintenance of high ABP requires participation by the kidney. The involvement of the kidney in systemic hypertension is generally due to a change in renal function brought about by circulating hormones, neural influences, renal vascular disease, or renal parenchymal disease.

Causes of persistently elevated systemic arterial blood pressure

Approximately 95% of hypertensive people have essential or idiopathic hypertension. In dogs and cats, idiopathic hypertension is generally believed to be uncommon. Most identified cases of hypertension in these species are associated with another disease process, being referred to as secondary hypertension. Examples of conditions associated with the development of hypertension in dogs and cats include chronic kidney disease (CKD), hyperthyroidism, diabetes mellitus, hyperadrenocorticism, pheochromocytoma, and hyperaldosteronism. A variety of medications may also elevate ABP. Examples include corticosteroids (which are normally produced and released by the adrenal cortex and used as pharmacological agents for their anti-inflammatory and immunosuppressive properties), cyclosporine (an immunosuppressive agent employed in organ transplantation), phenylpropanolamine (an α-adrenergic agonist used to treat some causes of urinary incontinence), and erythropoietin (recombinant DNA product used to stimulate increased production of red blood cells, particularly in CKD). The role of dietary factors in causation of hypertension is unclear in veterinary medicine, although normal dogs and cats are generally not susceptible to hypertension caused by increased dietary salt ingestion, unless the salt intake is massive or there is a preexisting cause of secondary hypertension. Although omega-3 polyunsaturated fatty acids (e.g., certain fish oils) appear to be antihypertensive in humans, this does not appear to be the case in dogs and cats.

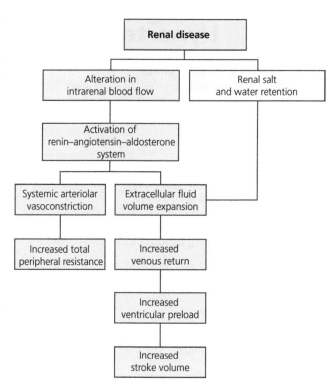

Figure 40.1 In veterinary medicine, systemic hypertension is usually secondary and related to the coexistence of chronic kidney disease. While the cause–effect nature of this relationship between high systemic arterial blood pressure and renal disease is often unclear, it is apparent that several changes commonly observed in chronic kidney disease may contribute to the genesis of systemic hypertension. In particular, activation of the renin–angiotensin–aldosterone system and renal retention of salt and water lead to increased total peripheral vascular resistance and stroke volume, raising blood pressure in affected animals.

Most cases of systemic hypertension in dogs and cats are associated with CKD. In CKD, several factors may contribute to the development of elevated ABP (Figure 40.1). First, abnormal patterns of intrarenal blood flow or renal artery stenosis may lead to reduced pressure within renal afferent arterioles, causing increased renin release. Resulting activation of the RAAS will lead to angiotensin II-induced constriction of systemic arterioles, which increases total peripheral vascular resistance. Enhanced renal reabsorption of salt and water occurs through actions of angiotensin II in the proximal tubule and aldosterone in the distal tubule. Normally an increase in ABP leads to sodium and water excretion by the kidney, a property referred to as pressure natriuresis and diuresis. Parenchymal renal disease may alter this inherent property of the kidney, increasing renal sodium and water reabsorption. The resultant increase in extracellular fluid (and blood) volume increases stroke volume and ABP rises accordingly.

Pheochromocytomas are rare tumors of the neuroendocrine cells of the adrenal medulla. Overproduction of epinephrine and norepinephrine leads to peripheral vasoconstriction, tachycardia, and an increase in cardiac contractility, which elevates stroke volume. Often, the release of these hormones from the tumor is episodic, causing periodic "attacks" of tachycardia and hypertension. Therapy is often surgical, although temporary relief may be induced by the administration of antagonists to α-adrenergic receptors (e.g., phenoxybenzamine, prazosin) and β_1-adrenergic receptors (e.g., atenolol, metoprolol).

Excess circulating glucocorticoids may result from adrenocortical overproduction or exogenous administration. The former condition is common in dogs and is referred to as Cushing syndrome or hyperadrenocorticism and usually involves overproduction of glucocorticoids, but not mineralocorticoids (i.e., aldosterone). These animals suffer from increased blood volume and overproduction of renin, both contributing to the development of systemic hypertension.

In cats, the most common adrenocortical disorder is primary hyperaldosteronism. This may be idiopathic and due to bilateral hyperplasia or caused by a unilateral tumor that is typically a benign adenoma rather than a malignant adenocarcinoma. Excess production of aldosterone leads to sodium retention and potassium depletion; it is the sodium retention which expands blood volume, increasing stroke volume and thus ABP. Unilateral disease is usually treated surgically while bilateral disease may be managed by aldosterone antagonists (e.g., spironolactone or eplerenone).

Hyperthyroidism is relatively common in geriatric cats. The condition is generally due to a benign tumor (adenoma) of the thyroid gland. Thyroid hormone enhances cardiac function and the sensitivity of the myocardium to catecholamines. The result is tachycardia and increased stroke volume, resulting in systemic hypertension. Appropriate short-term symptomatic therapy may involve β_1-adrenergic receptor antagonists (e.g., atenolol, metoprolol) to reduce cardiac hyperactivity, but definitive therapy requires surgical removal of the tumor, destruction of the tumor cells by radioiodine therapy, or administration of pharmacological agents that block the production or release of thyroid hormone (e.g., methimazole).

Animals with diabetes mellitus may develop systemic hypertension as a result of overproduction of renin and blood volume expansion associated with hyperglycemia. Careful management of the diabetic condition, generally by judicious administration of insulin, is an effective therapy in many cases.

Measurement of systemic arterial blood pressure

In contrast to clinical examination of people, the usual physical examination in veterinary clinical practice does not include measurement of ABP. Pulse pressure, the difference between systolic and diastolic ABP, is often indirectly assessed during physical examination by digital palpation of a peripheral artery. However, the character of peripheral arterial pulsations primarily reflects the pulse pressure and not the absolute level of ABP. Thus a horse with a systolic/diastolic ABP of 100/60 mmHg may have a facial artery pulsation that is very similar to that of another horse with ABP of 180/140 mmHg. Thus, assessment of the level of ABP (i.e., diagnosis of systemic hypertension) requires measurement of ABP.

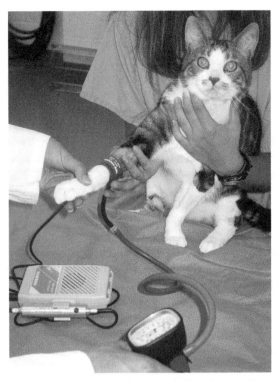

Figure 40.2 Systemic arterial blood pressure (ABP) measurement in a cat. Management of elevated ABP requires measurement of ABP in a conscious animal, accomplished here with an indirect device that utilizes a cuff and the Doppler ultrasonic principle.

The ABP may be measured in animals by direct or indirect techniques. Direct techniques rely on penetration of a peripheral artery with a catheter or a needle and connection via a fluid-filled tube to a pressure transduction system. This technique generally provides an accurate and precise measure of ABP and is useful in anesthetized animals, particularly large animals. However, because anesthetics and sedatives alter ABP, they are not used for screening of animals for the presence of systemic hypertension and indirect techniques are usually employed in veterinary practice for this purpose (Figure 40.2).

Indirect techniques rely on the placement of a cuff over an extremity (limb or tail). The cuff is inflated to occlude a peripheral artery. As pressure is automatically or manually reduced in the cuff, the restoration of arterial flow can be detected distally by a variety of methods. These devices generally utilize ultrasonic Doppler, oscillometric, or photoplethysmographic principles to detect the restoration of flow distal to the cuff. Systolic ABP may then be estimated from cuff pressure at the time of restoration of flow. Some indirect devices (e.g., ultrasonic Doppler flowmeters) are generally used only to estimate systolic ABP, while other devices often provide an estimate of systolic, mean, and diastolic ABP. Anxiety-induced elevations of ABP during the measurement process are referred to as the "white-coat effect" as this response was first identified in people and was attributed to the presence of medical personnel (in white coats). Excitement and anxiety during measurement of ABP leads to input to the cardiovascular regulatory center from higher neural centers with consequent sympathetic nervous systemic activation. Tachycardia, increased stroke volume, and peripheral vasoconstriction are responsible for an increase in ABP, which can lead to a false diagnosis of systemic hypertension. This white-coat effect occurs in dogs and cats, making it important to limit excitement and anxiety in veterinary patients during measurement of ABP. While cuff-utilizing indirect devices are less accurate and precise than direct techniques, they are less invasive and may produce less artifactual elevation of ABP from anxiety.

It is important to recognize that ABP varies considerably throughout the day. Some veterinary species have a diurnal variation. For example, in primates, ABP is 10–30 mmHg higher during daylight hours. Such a pronounced diurnal variation in ABP is not present in normal dogs and cats but ABP does vary considerably from minute to minute in all animals that have been carefully studied. These variations are due to changes in ABP associated with physical activity, higher neural center activation of the cardiovascular regulatory center, oscillations of the activity of the autonomic nervous system, and various other neurohumoral cycles. As a result of the white-coat effect and other variations in ABP, a diagnosis of systemic hypertension should not be based on a single measurement of ABP.

The importance of systemic hypertension in common metabolic diseases such as CKD and feline hyperthyroidism has led to increased awareness of the importance of ABP measurement in select populations of small animal patients. However, routine screening of all patients or even all geriatric patients of any species is rarely practiced in veterinary medicine except during general anesthesia (where systemic hypotension is the primary concern). While Stephen Hales was the first to measure ABP in 1733 when he utilized a horse for his first studies, it remains uncommon to measure ABP in large animals, except during anesthesia or in experimental studies.

Consequences of persistently elevated systemic arterial blood pressure

Persistently elevated systemic ABP causes no clinical signs directly but it can lead to substantial damage to a variety of tissues and body systems over time. In particular, the eyes, kidneys, central nervous system, and cardiovascular system may be affected by persistent high ABP and these four tissues are commonly referred as the target organs of systemic hypertension.

Eyes

Perhaps because routine screening of animals for hypertension by ABP measurement is uncommon, sudden onset of blindness from hypertensive retinopathy is one of the most common presenting complaints for animals with systemic hypertension. As with other microvascular beds, the rise in arteriolar and capillary pressure in choroidal vessels leads to plasma leakage into vessel walls, with resultant abnormalities including retinal edema, hemorrhage, and detachment. These abnormalities are often referred to as **hypertensive retinopathy/choroidopathy**.

Kidneys

Hypertension and CKD are integrally linked in humans, with hypertension serving as a leading cause of renal disease and renal disease frequently contributing to the genesis and maintenance of systemic hypertension. This represents an example of a deleterious positive feedback loop in cardiovascular pathophysiology. Recently it has been shown that systemic hypertension can contribute to renal injury in dogs with CKD and the same is likely to be the case in cats. Very little is known about other veterinary species. As in other vascular beds, high pressure in renal arterioles leads to thickening of small artery and arteriolar walls by the processes of hyaline arteriosclerosis and smooth muscle hypertrophy. This process can be unevenly distributed within the renal parenchyma, resulting in interspersed areas of ischemia and hyperperfusion. Areas of ischemia may result in overproduction of renin with resultant increases in circulating levels of angiotensin II, further raising total peripheral resistance and stroke volume, and worsening systemic hypertension. In areas of hyperperfusion, there is an alteration in Starling forces in the glomerular capillary bed, with an elevation in glomerular capillary hydrostatic pressure. The glomerular capillary bed is susceptible to hypertensive injury, which unfortunately leads to obliterative extracellular matrix production by glomerular mesangial cells, a process referred to as glomerulosclerosis. Chronically sustained hypertension can lead to nephron destruction and contribute to progression of CKD.

Central nervous system

Circulation to the brain is generally well regulated locally, resulting in the property of **blood flow autoregulation**. This autoregulatory control of blood flow is mediated primarily by small arteries and arterioles, which constrict in response to a rise in ABP. This will protect the central nervous system from many of the adverse effects of systemic hypertension across a broad range of ABPs. However, there is a limit to the ability of these arterioles to prevent the transmission of elevated arterial pressures to the local microcirculation (arterioles, capillaries, and venules). Further rises in ABP above this autoregulatory limit lead to increases in pressure and flow within the microcirculation, which alters Starling forces across the capillary wall. The subsequent rise in intracapillary hydrostatic pressure, in particular, tends to increase transcapillary fluid filtration, promoting the development of interstitial edema within the brain parenchyma. If the pressure rises far enough, especially if the rise is acute, local edema formation occurs. Because the brain is "compartmentalized" within the bony cranium, this increase in interstitial volume can lead to a rise in intracranial pressure, causing neurological dysfunction. Clinical signs caused by brain edema may include disorientation, ataxia, stupor, coma, and seizures. If severe, this edema increases intracranial pressure, which can lead to cerebral herniation under the tentorium or cerebellar herniation through the foramen magnum. Brain herniation is generally a fatal complication. This syndrome of neurological dysfunction caused by cerebral edema associated with systemic hypertension is often referred to as **hypertensive encephalopathy.**

Hypertensive encephalopathy is more likely to occur with a rapid severe rise in ABP, and is a well-recognized complication of renal transplantation in cats. The rapidity of rise of ABP affects the likelihood of development of edema, as chronic hypertension (weeks to months in duration) allows adaptation by arterioles, leading to an increase in the upper limit of tolerable ABP.

Hypertension may also lead to damage to medium and small arteries with rupture and resultant localized ischemia ("stroke" or cerebrovascular accident) and tissue death (infarct). A cerebrovascular accident can occur as a result of small artery rupture within the cerebral vasculature (hemorrhagic stroke) or from vessel thrombosis (thrombotic stroke). In both cases, affected portions of the brain suffer infarction and the animal may exhibit clinical signs such as ataxia, disorientation, seizure, stupor, or coma. These do occur in veterinary medicine but seem to be less common perhaps because atherosclerosis and arteriosclerosis, which promote the development of these lesions in people, are far less prevalent in veterinary species.

Cardiovascular system

The most commonly observed effect of hypertension in the cardiovascular system is **left ventricular hypertrophy.** Left ventricular hypertrophy may be observed by thoracic radiographic studies or cardiac ultrasound. Cardiac muscle responds to increased **afterload** by concentric hypertrophy (increased wall thickness without luminal dilation). Left ventricular hypertrophy can cause a loss of ventricular compliance. Resultant ventricular stiffness and reduced diastolic filling can elevate left ventricular diastolic pressure leading to pulmonary congestion, although this effect is minor in most hypertensive dogs and cats.

High pressures in small arteries and arterioles leads to extravasation of plasma into the vessel wall, producing a thickening of the vessel wall referred to as hyaline arteriosclerosis. Chronic hypertension also induces vascular smooth muscle hypertrophy. These two processes can be particularly significant in systemic arterioles, where they can reduce luminal diameter producing local ischemia or a generalized increase in total peripheral vascular resistance. This exacerbates the systemic hypertension, an example of a deleterious positive feedback loop. These vascular changes may contribute to vascular rupture ("stroke") in the central nervous system.

Atherosclerotic plaques are commonly observed in medium and small arteries of people with long-standing hypertension. Since increased afterload or **preload** commonly observed in systemic hypertension places an increased oxygen demand on the left ventricular muscle mass, atherosclerosis contributes to the high prevalence of significant cardiac disease (e.g., myocardial infarction, heart failure) in hypertensive people.

Atherosclerosis is uncommon in veterinary species. This may be related to differences in lifespan or, more likely, differences in lipid metabolism. Dogs and cats, for example, tend to have low plasma concentrations of cholesterol in low-density lipoprotein particles, which have been implicated in the pathogenesis of atherosclerosis in primates. As a result, heart failure and coronary artery occlusion associated with myocardial infarction are uncommonly (<5%) observed in veterinary patients with systemic hypertension.

Prevalence of persistently elevated systemic arterial blood pressure

Since idiopathic hypertension is rare in veterinary medicine but comprises 95% of cases of identified hypertension in people, systemic hypertension is anticipated to be uncommon in veterinary medicine. On the contrary, diseases associated with secondary hypertension are quite common in certain veterinary species. In particular, CKD is frequently observed in geriatric cats and dogs, with prevalence reaching nearly one in three cats in select populations. Feline hyperthyrodisim is also a common disease entity. Approximately 20–40% of these animals exhibit systemic hypertension, making it an important physiological and clinical entity, affecting approximately 0.6% of all cats for example.

Management of persistently elevated systemic arterial blood pressure

The severity of future target organ damage is directly related to the magnitude of the elevation of ABP. Consequently, in dogs and cats, instead of using threshold values for ABP to establish or reject the diagnosis of systemic hypertension, recommendations for treatment are based on the degree of elevation of ABP (Table 40.1). The therapeutic approach generally relies on the use of pharmacological agents (Table 40.2) that alter the determinants of ABP, i.e., total peripheral vascular resistance, stroke volume, or heart rate. Frequently, dietary salt restriction is part of the initial approach to therapy. The goal of dietary salt

Table 40.1 Treatment recommendations for persistently elevated systemic arterial blood pressure (systemic hypertension) based on measurement of diastolic and systolic pressure in conscious dogs and cats.

Systolic (mmHg)	Diastolic (mmHg)	Risk of future target organ damage	Should patient be treated?
<150	<95	Minimal	No
150–159	95–99	Mild	Yes, but only if there is clear evidence of ongoing target organ damage
160–179	100–119	Moderate	Yes, if suspect there is ongoing target organ damage
≥180	≥120	Severe	Yes

Section VI: The Cardiovascular System

Table 40.2 Physiological basis of treatment of systemic hypertension.

Treatment	Primary effect	Blood pressure determinants reduced
Dietary salt restriction	Decreased extracellular fluid volume	Stroke volume
Loop (e.g., furosemide) or thiazide (e.g., hydrochlorothiazide) diuretic	Decreased extracellular fluid volume	Stroke volume
Calcium channel blocker (e.g., amlodipine)	Vascular smooth muscle relaxation (± reduced cardiac contractility)	Total peripheral vascular resistance (± stroke volume)
Angiotensin-converting enzyme inhibitor (e.g., benazepril or enalapril)	Decreased plasma concentrations of angiotensin II and aldosterone	Total peripheral vascular resistance and stroke volume
Angiotensin receptor blocker (e.g., telmisartan or losartan)	Decreased binding of angiotensin II to AT_1 receptors; decreased plasma concentration of aldosterone	Total peripheral vascular resistance and stroke volume
Centrally acting α_2 agonists (e.g., moxonidine)	Decreased sympathetic output to heart and blood vessels from the cardiovascular regulatory center	Total peripheral vascular resistance, stroke volume, and heart rate
β_1 antagonists (e.g., atenolol or metoprolol)	Decreased cardiac β_1-receptor activation	Stroke volume and heart rate
α_1 antagonists (e.g., phenoxybenzamine or prazosin)	Decreased arteriolar α_1-receptor activation	Total peripheral vascular resistance
Hydralazine	Arteriolar vasodilation (direct effect)	Total peripheral vascular resistance

restriction is to reduce extracellular fluid volume and thus curtail cardiac output, though this dietary maneuver rarely produces a significant reduction in ABP in dogs and cats by itself.

In general, a decline in ABP could reduce renal functions such as glomerular filtration rate, if not for renal autoregulatory adjustments. However, in animals with renal disease, renal autoregulation may be disrupted. Lowering ABP may thus tend to reduce renal function, including glomerular filtration rate. In this setting, there is a theoretical advantage to vasodilatory agents for controlling hypertension in animals with coexistent systemic hypertension and chronic renal failure because these agents also produce intrarenal vasodilation while lowering ABP. These two effects tend to offset each other and sustain renal function. Considering the high prevalence of renal disease in hypertensive animals, antihypertensive therapy in dogs and cats is usually accompanied by the use of vasodilating agents, generally inhibitors of RAAS or calcium channel blockers.

Calcium channel blockers reduce calcium entry into myocardial cells and vascular smooth muscle cells, producing a reduction in cardiac output and vascular smooth muscle relaxation. Some classes of calcium channel antagonists preferentially affect the vascular smooth muscle cells, having little cardiac effect. Calcium channel antagonists in clinical use for the management of systemic hypertension (e.g., amlodipine) generally do have less cardiac effect and preferentially produce systemic arteriolar vasodilation and a generalized decline in total peripheral resistance.

Until recently, inhibition of the RAAS has relied on inhibitors of angiotensin-converting enzyme (ACE) such as enalapril and benazepril. Angiotensin II receptors are generally of two principal subtypes: AT_1 or AT_2. In vascular smooth muscle, most receptors are of the AT_1 subtype and there are now pharmacological agents that serve as AT_1 antagonists or **angiotensin receptor blockers** (e.g., telmisartan or losartan). The goal of RAAS inhibition with either or both classes of agents is to reduce angiotensin II-mediated increases in total peripheral vascular resistance and to reduce blood volume by decreasing renal sodium and water retention (known effects of angiotensin II and aldosterone).

The net effects of these two pharmacological approaches for inhibiting RAAS on the plasma concentrations of each component of the RAAS point out interesting differences. Both **ACE inhibitors** and AT_1 receptor blockers should lead to high circulating plasma concentrations of renin, as feedback mechanisms controlling renin release are interrupted by effective antihypertensive therapy. However, with use of ACE inhibitors the ratio of angiotensin I to angiotensin II will be high, while the opposite is the case with the use of angiotensin receptor blockers. An important question about drug efficacy concerns the net effects of the binding of accumulated angiotensin II to AT_2 receptors in patients given angiotensin receptor blockers. The answer to this question in veterinary medicine remains unknown. This is a good example of how pharmacological manipulation of physiologic systems often produces complex interactions in veterinary patients, emphasizing the importance to veterinarians of maintaining a full understanding of physiologic principles as they treat clinical disease.

Other approaches to the management of systemic hypertension include the use of centrally acting α_2-adrenergic agonists, which reduce central sympathetic outflow to the heart, blood vessels, and kidney. The result is a reduction in heart rate, stroke volume, total peripheral resistance, and renin secretion. However, side effects with these agents are common in people and these agents are rarely used in veterinary medicine for this purpose. Alternatively, systemically active adrenergic antagonists (β_1 and α_1) may be used. The former reduce cardiac output and the latter reduce total peripheral resistance. Direct-acting arteriolar vasodilators, such as hydralazine, have been used effectively in veterinary medicine to lower total peripheral resistance and thus ABP.

Heart failure

1 Know the definition and classification system for heart failure.

2 What are the major mechanisms for the development of heart failure?

3 Explain the distinction between systolic and diastolic failure, forward and backward signs of failure, and pressure and volume overload.

4 Describe the physiologic principles of, and rationale for, therapy in heart failure.

5 When does the Frank–Starling relationship between stroke volume and preload contribute to heart failure?

Definitions

Circulatory failure occurs whenever cardiac output does not meet tissue perfusion needs. Circulatory failure that is acute and severe is often termed **circulatory shock** (see corresponding section below). In veterinary medicine, circulatory failure is often caused by a marked reduction in stroke volume due to a cardiac abnormality. **Heart failure** is cardiogenic circulatory failure with sustained inability of the heart to produce a stroke volume that adequately meets tissue metabolic demands. Early heart failure is said to be present when the heart meets tissue perfusion demands only with markedly increased preload.

As heart failure is caused by inadequate stroke volume, a brief overview of factors that affect stroke volume is in order. A decrease in stroke volume can be brought about by a decline in myocardial contractility or preload or by an increase in afterload (see Chapters 34, 35, and 41). Briefly, **left ventricular contractility** is the ability of this chamber of the heart to generate force and is an inherent property of its myocardium. Contractility

may be increased by sympathetic stimulation or administration of a **positive inotropic agent** (e.g., pimobendan or digitalis glycosides) or decreased by various cardiac lesions producing **myocardial failure** (e.g., hypoxia, myocarditis, or cardiomyopathy). **Preload** is the degree of stretch of myocardial fibers prior to contraction and, in the normal animal, a reduction in ventricular preload tends to decrease stroke volume. Conditions that interfere with anterograde flow of blood into the ventricles, such as atrioventricular valvular stenosis, will reduce ventricular preload. Similarly, lesions that limit ventricular enlargement during diastole will reduce preload and thus stroke volume. Since preload is dependent on ventricular filling during diastole, it may also be reduced by arrhythmias that shorten the duration of diastole excessively. Afterload is the load against which the myocardial fibers shorten during contraction and can be thought of as the opposition to ejection faced by the ventricle. Left ventricular afterload, for example, is increased by an elevation in ABP, total peripheral vascular resistance, or hematocrit and by semilunar valvular stenosis.

Classification of heart failure

Heart failure may be classified in a variety of ways. It is often classified, on the basis of which ventricle is failing, as right-sided, left-sided, or bilateral heart failure. It is useful from a pathophysiological perspective to categorize heart failure on the basis of where the primary defect occurs in the cardiac cycle. **Systolic dysfunction** or **systolic failure** refers to heart failure in which diastolic filling of the ventricle is normal but cardiac output (usually stroke volume) is still decreased. **Diastolic dysfunction** or **diastolic failure** refers to heart failure due to abnormal cardiac filling with normal ventricular contractility (normal systolic function).

It is not accurate to presume that all patients with failing hearts have cardiac hypofunction. Cardiac failure may actually be classified according to whether stroke volume is reduced (**low-output cardiac failure**) or increased (**high-output cardiac failure**). Remember that heart failure has been defined as sustained failure of cardiac output to meet tissue perfusion needs. Some clinical patients with heart failure are affected with conditions characterized by excessive need for tissue perfusion. Heart failure may be present in these patients because a normal, or even high, cardiac output cannot meet tissue needs. Feline hyperthyroidism, chronic anemia, congenital left-to-right shunts (e.g., patent ductus arteriosus), and arteriovenous fistulas are examples of conditions observed in veterinary patients that may result in high-output heart failure.

Causes of systolic dysfunction

While severe bradycardia, as seen with third-degree atrioventricular block for example, may produce systolic dysfunction, most cases of systolic dysfunction are due to a primary reduction in stroke volume. A readily grasped cause of this type of systolic dysfunction is myocardial failure in which failing ventricular contractility reduces stroke volume (Table 40.3). A frequent cardiac disease producing systolic failure in veterinary medicine is dilated cardiomyopathy, which may be heritable (e.g., Doberman Pinscher cardiomyopathy) or acquired (e.g., dietary taurine deficiency in cats). Other acquired causes of myocardial failure, such as myocarditis or myocardial infarction, are occasionally observed in veterinary patients. In all these diseases, the primary defect is a decline in cardiac contractility that reduces stroke volume.

Consideration of the various factors that contribute to the regulation of stroke volume highlights the fact that not all animals with systolic heart failure have abnormal ventricular contractility. Valvular insufficiencies can reduce stroke volume by allowing retrograde flow of blood (e.g., systolic regurgitation due to atrioventricular valvular insufficiency), abnormal shunting of blood (e.g., arteriovenous fistula or patent ductus arteriosus), or tissue perfusion needs may rise excessively (e.g., feline hyperthyroidism producing high-output cardiac failure). All these conditions share one characteristic: the volume of blood presented to the affected ventricle is increased, producing what is termed a **volume overload**. Initially, the increase in preload is beneficial. However, as the condition progresses, there is an excessive increase in ventricular volume and pressure that produces failing contractility and **venous congestion**.

Heart failure may be caused by increasing afterload (e.g., narrowing of the outflow tract in aortic stenosis and systemic hypertension for the left ventricle and heartworm disease for the right ventricle). Conditions producing excessive afterload are often referred to as **pressure overload** and generally produce compensatory cardiac hypertrophy, which provides adequate tissue perfusion initially. This hypertrophy leads to a thickened ventricular wall, narrowing of the ventricular lumen, and reduced ventricular compliance. This cardiac response is referred to as concentric hypertrophy. Concentric hypertrophy can exacerbate heart failure by reducing ventricular preload, thereby adding diastolic dysfunction to preexisting systolic dysfunction.

Causes of diastolic dysfunction

Some conditions reduce cardiac output by interfering with ventricular filling, producing diastolic dysfunction (Table 40.3). These may be lesions that reduce inflow during diastole or conditions that limit cardiac compliance. A restrictive condition, such as excessive hypertrophy of ventricular muscle mass in hypertrophic cardiomyopathy or in response to pressure overload, can reduce chamber compliance and limit preload. Similarly, pericardial diseases (e.g., constrictive pericarditis or pericardial hemorrhage) may limit cardiac expansion and reduce cardiac filling. A space-occupying lesion (e.g., inflammatory or neoplastic mass) within the heart or pericardium or any lesion obstructing the normal cardiac inflow of blood (e.g., vena caval thrombosis or atrioventricular valvular stenosis) may limit cardiac filling. A decrement in preload will reduce stroke volume according to the Frank–Starling relationship.

Compensatory responses to heart failure

In heart failure, cardiac output falls and by itself this tends to reduce systemic ABP. A variety of compensatory mechanisms act as part of cardiovascular system regulation to sustain ABP and these are discussed in detail in Chapters 34, 35, and 41. These compensatory responses are either inherent properties of the kidney and cardiovascular system or neurohumoral responses. Initially these adaptations are beneficial but later they produce, or contribute to, many of the clinical signs commonly observed in patients with heart failure.

Frank–Starling relationship

Within physiologic limits, added preload will prestretch myocardial fibers leading to an increase in the force of contraction and an increase in stroke volume (Figure 40.3). The Frank–Starling relationship (see Chapter 34) between preload and stroke volume is present even in a failing heart, initially providing a beneficial effect in most animals with early heart

Table 40.3 Physiological mechanisms producing heart failure.

Type of failure	Primary defect	Pathogenesis	Clinical examples
Systolic dysfunction	Decreased stroke volume	Decreased myocardial contractility	Dilated cardiomyopathy Myocarditis Myocardial infarction
		Excessive afterload (pressure overload)	Systemic hypertension Polycythemia Semilunar valvular stenosis
		Excessive preload (volume overload)	Patent ductus arteriosus Atrioventricular valvular insufficiency Thyrotoxicosis
	Decreased heart rate	Uncontrolled bradycardia	Sinoatrial nodal dysfunction Third-degree atrioventricular block
Diastolic dysfunction	Decreased stroke volume	Decreased preload (constrictive): impaired diastolic relaxation	Hypertrophic cardiomyopathy Constrictive pericardial disease
		Decreased preload (obstructive): impaired venous return	Atrioventricular valvular stenosis Intracardiac neoplasia

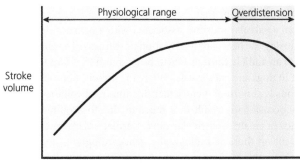

Figure 40.3 Frank–Starling relationship between ventricular preload and stroke volume. The initial portions of this curve contribute to the control of stroke volume in physiological situations. However, with extreme ventricular distension there is a failure of force generation due to disruption of actomyosin cross-bridge formation. Dramatic increases in blood volume from renal salt and water retention in the setting of a failing myocardium or volume overload can lead to overdistension. Accordingly, excess preload may lead to a declining stroke volume in advanced heart failure (right-hand portion of the curve).

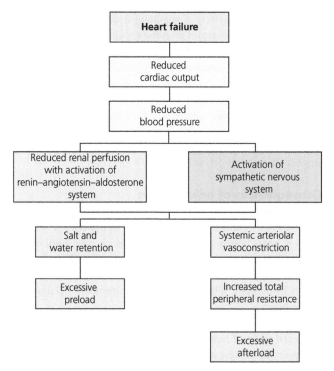

Figure 40.4 In heart failure, normal compensatory mechanisms can contribute to the development of deleterious positive feedback loops. In this setting, the sympathetic nervous system and the renin–angiotensin–aldosterone system participate in the generation of excessive ventricular preload and afterload, further reducing stroke volume and exacerbating heart failure.

failure. In fact, with the exception of primary myocardial failure, normal or increased contractility is present in most cases of early heart failure. However, this relationship between preload and stroke volume operates within limits. Excessive preload that actually lowers stroke volume may develop with the marked expansion of extracellular fluid volume that is commonly observed in the latter stages of heart failure (see following sections). The limitations of this relationship are apparent if one considers the effects of excess stretch on actomyosin cross-bridge formation, as the overstretched myocardium loses the ability to generate a forceful contraction. Simply put: if the ventricle is overdistended, there will actually be a fall in contractile force due to failure of cross-bridge formation resulting in a decline in stroke volume. This declining stroke volume may be detected during ultrasonographic studies of myocardial function in clinical patients.

Neurohumoral response to heart failure

A central adaptation to cardiac failure is detection of a decrement in ABP by **arterial baroreceptors** in the carotid sinus, aortic arch, and other large arteries. Input to the cardiovascular regulatory center results in enhanced sympathetic outflow to the heart, peripheral arterioles and veins and reduced parasympathetic outflow to the heart (Figure 40.4). This results in an increase in heart rate, cardiac contractility (increase in stroke volume), venous return, and total peripheral resistance. Initially, this results in beneficial maintenance of ABP. However, as heart failure progresses and cardiac output declines further, this response of the arterial baroreceptor system becomes counterproductive, leading to tissue ischemia in nonvital organs due to sympathetic vasoconstriction that reduces perfusion without regard for tissue needs (e.g., viscera). Eventually, skin and splanchnic viscera and to some extent the kidneys suffer from

reduced perfusion due to the consequences of this high vascular resistance and low cardiac output. Further, the rising total peripheral resistance reduces stroke volume by presenting the left ventricle with excessive afterload.

Antidiuretic hormone secretion may also be enhanced in heart failure due to direct stimulation of secretion by angiotensin II and through the arterial baroreceptor reflex. This contributes further to expansion of extracellular fluid volume, which initially increases stroke volume through the Frank–Starling relationship but later adds to volume overexpansion and reduction of stroke volume in the late stages of heart failure.

Renal response to heart failure

In heart failure, renin release is increased by reduced ABP and a decline in chloride delivery to the macula densa region of the distal tubule. This is because of enhanced tubular reabsorption of NaCl and water in heart failure due to inadequate perfusion pressure, which is exacerbated by sympathetic nervous system stimulation of β_2-adrenergic receptors within the juxtaglomerular apparatus. Activation of the RAAS leads to increased generation of angiotensin II (see Chapter 18) with resultant afferent and systemic arteriolar vasoconstriction (angiotensin II mediated). Initially beneficial by sustaining ABP, this system eventually becomes counterproductive as intense vasoconstriction increases afterload thereby reducing stroke volume. The extracellular fluid volume-enhancing effects of angiotensin are mediated through direct effects of angiotensin II in the proximal tubule and indirectly through enhanced sodium reabsorption in the distal tubule stimulated by aldosterone. As already noted, increasing extracellular fluid volume will initially increase stroke volume but in the latter stages of heart failure volume overload produces excess preload, reduces stroke volume (see section Frank–Starling relationship), and increases venous congestion and capillary hydrostatic pressure, favoring the formation of interstitial edema. This stage is often referred to as congestive heart failure.

Consequences of heart failure

A variety of organs and tissues are affected adversely in heart failure caused by either systolic or diastolic dysfunction. **Forward signs of heart failure** refers to signs that occur as a result of the failure to provide adequate tissue perfusion and **backward signs of heart failure** or venous congestion refers to effects of the elevation in diastolic filling pressure that commonly occurs in a failing heart.

Forward signs of heart failure (inadequate perfusion)

Except in the earliest stages, tissue perfusion is compromised in heart failure. Forward signs of heart failure caused by inadequate tissue perfusion are common to all causes of heart failure. In early heart failure, tissue perfusion may be inadequate only during times of high tissue perfusion needs such as intense physical activity. This is because local vasodilation within skeletal muscle diverts cardiac output from other tissues, including the vital tissues of brain, heart, and kidneys. As heart failure advances, clinical signs due to inadequate tissue perfusion (e.g., weakness) will be present even in the absence of physical activity.

Autoregulation is the ability of a tissue to sustain its own blood flow despite variations in ABP and neurohumoral activation (extrinsic factors). Blood flow autoregulation is due to the predominance of local or intrinsic factors in the regulation of vascular resistance in these tissues. Because vital tissues (e.g., brain, heart, and kidney) autoregulate more effectively, these tissues will have preservation of perfusion in early heart failure while skin and splanchnic viscera may suffer poor perfusion. Cold skin and mucous membrane pallor may be observed during clinical examination of affected animals. Other evidence of tissue underperfusion may be present as cardiac failure advances. For example, azotemia may occur as result of renal hypoperfusion. This azotemia is often termed "pre-renal" because its proximate cause is not primary renal disease (renal azotemia) or lack of integrity of the urinary conduit system (post-renal azotemia). With further progression of heart failure, even the brain may suffer from hypoperfusion. Confusion, dizziness, or syncope may be present as a result of cerebral hypoxia.

Tachycardia, a compensatory response of cardiovascular regulatory systems to a fall in stroke volume, will usually be observed on physical examination of veterinary patients with heart failure. Cardiac arrhythmias, caused by myocardial disease

or hypoperfusion, may be present. Cardiac auscultation may reveal a valvular murmur associated with a primary defect that is causing the heart failure. Dilation or stiffness of a ventricle can cause an audible third or fourth heart sound (S_3 or S_4) to be present in dogs and cats, species where the presence of such cardiac sounds is abnormal. Ventricular dilation from volume overload may occasionally result in a murmur due to acquired insufficiency of an atrioventricular valve. Cardiac enlargement may be evident on thoracic radiography, echocardiography, or electrocardiography in these patients. Myocardial failure leading to a declining stroke volume can usually be evaluated during ultrasonographic studies of myocardial function in clinical patients.

Backward signs of heart failure (venous congestion)

As a result of the failure of ejection, ventricular end-diastolic volume and pressure rise. This leads to increases in hydrostatic pressure in the corresponding venous system (i.e., passive venous congestion). In animals with either systolic or diastolic dysfunction, this venous congestion may eventually lead to an increase in intracapillary hydrostatic pressure and disrupt the balance of Starling forces in the microcirculation. Increased fluid filtration across the capillary wall will occur. Untreated, this situation will progress to the point where fluid filtration exceeds the capacity of the lymphatic system to return this accumulated interstitial fluid to the circulatory system. Depending on which ventricle is failing, the accumulation of interstitial fluid (edema) may interfere with pulmonary gaseous exchange (left ventricular failure with pulmonary edema) or produce peripheral edema, ascites, or hydrothorax (right ventricular failure).

With left ventricular failure, pulmonary edema will interfere with gaseous exchange. A careful evaluation of thoracic radiographs may reveal changes in the pulmonary vasculature and lungs consistent with pulmonary venous congestion and edema in patients with advanced left ventricular failure. Affected animals develop hypoxia and hypercapnia, which leads to chemoreceptor-mediated tachypnea and hyperpnea. Small airways that are closed from the presence of edema fluid may suddenly "pop" open during the respiratory cycle, producing a crackling sound. In affected animals, thoracic auscultation will reveal pulmonary crackles. (Wheezes, caused by narrowing of small to medium airways, are less common with pulmonary edema.)

With right-sided heart failure, hydrothorax may produce tachypnea and hyperpnea with an absence of lung sounds on thoracic auscultation ("silent lung"), ascites may lead to abdominal distension, and swelling from peripheral edema may be observed in extremities.

Management of heart failure

The clinical treatment of cardiac failure should consider the underlying defect. The principles of cardiac physiology allow an ordered approach to this clinical condition. While specific therapy may be appropriate to correct a known defect in some cases, this is rarely possible. Valve replacement and cardiac transplantation are not generally available in veterinary medicine and therapy designed to enhance cardiac performance is the most typical clinical approach. A few generalities can be applied to the therapeutic approach to most cases of cardiac failure.

It is important to recognize that nearly all advanced cases of heart failure are characterized by (i) excessive total peripheral resistance due to activation of the RAAS and increased sympathetic outflow from the cardiovascular regulatory center (excessive afterload); and (ii) overexpansion of extracellular fluid volume due to renal retention of salt and water and activation of the RAAS (excessive preload). Many, but not all, cases of heart failure are also characterized by (iii) systolic dysfunction associated with poor cardiac contractility.

While traditional therapy in veterinary medicine had been to employ loop diuretics such as furosemide to reduce extracellular fluid volume in the initial treatment of heart failure, the importance of alternative strategies has received increasing attention in recent years. Thus, inhibitors of RAAS (i.e., ACE inhibitors such as enalapril and benazepril or angiotensin receptor blockers such as telmisartan and losartan) as well as positive inotropic agents (i.e., phosphodiesterase inhibitors such as pimobendan) are now considered first-line therapy in animals with heart failure. The former agents are used to (i) reduce total peripheral resistance and thus afterload and (ii) reduce venous constriction and blood volume and thereby lower preload. The latter is administered to increase cardiac contractility, shifting the Frank–Starling curve upwards.

Clinical correlations: management of heart failure

You are presented with a 5-year-old intact male Doberman Pinscher with dyspnea. Thoracic radiographs reveal pulmonary edema and cardiac ultrasound findings a reduced stroke volume associated with poor left ventricular contractility. You diagnose low-output heart failure with pulmonary venous congestion caused by systolic dysfunction of the left ventricle, consistent with a disease you have read about in Doberman Pinschers: dilated cardiomyopathy. There are two key questions: how might you improve the dog's cardiac function and is there something else you can do that might help reduce the dog's pulmonary edema? You decide to treat the dog with a positive inotrope (pimobendan, a phosphodiesterase inhibitor) to enhance cardiac contractility, which should increase the stroke volume. You recognize that congestive heart failure is associated with extracellular fluid volume expansion, partly due to overactivity of the RAAS. This volume expansion distends the left ventricle, further reducing stroke volume, and increases venous pressure, worsening the pulmonary edema. Thus you decide to administer a diuretic (furosemide) to enhance renal excretion of salt and water and an inhibitor of the RAAS (enalapril). This latter agent should help to reduce both afterload (less angiotensin II-mediated arteriolar vasoconstriction) and preload (less aldosterone-mediated renal salt and water retention).

Shock

---

1 What are the major classifications of circulatory shock affecting animals in veterinary medicine?
2 What factors contribute to decompensation in septic or endotoxic shock?
3 What are the characteristics of each stage of shock?
4 What factors contribute to the progression of shock and what are the goals of interventional therapy?

Definitions

Circulatory shock is the severe acute failure of tissue perfusion resulting in cardiovascular collapse leading to organ and tissue dysfunction. It is generally characterized by systemic hypotension, inadequate tissue perfusion, oliguria, cellular hypoxia, and generalized dysfunction of cells, tissues, and organs. Shock and its consequences are often reversible with appropriate therapy in its early stages. Eventually, however, sustained tissue hypoperfusion leads to irreversible cell injury progressing to cell death and organ dysfunction. In the absence of effective interventional therapy, shock generally progresses through defined stages, frequently resulting in fatality.

Classification of shock

There are many causes of circulatory shock, which may be classified into three main types: cardiogenic, hypovolemic and septic shock. Cardiogenic shock is the end-stage result of progressive heart failure (see previous section), with the primary causative mechanism being a failure of cardiac output that cannot be compensated for by other factors. Low cardiac output due to a decrease in circulating blood volume (e.g., severe dehydration or hemorrhage) is the cause of most cases of hypovolemic shock. Septic shock is caused by the presence of blood-borne microorganisms or microbial toxins.

Shock may also be classified on the basis of the level of cardiac output as low- or high-output shock. Low-output shock is generally either cardiogenic or hypovolemic in origin. High-output shock is generally associated with septicemia or endotoxemia (septic shock).

Cardiogenic shock

Cardiogenic shock is caused by a severe decline in cardiac output. As discussed in the previous section and in Chapters 34, 35, and 41, there are a variety of feedback mechanisms that serve to maintain ABP within normal limits, despite a decline in cardiac function. However, if the disease process causing heart failure progresses in severity, these compensatory mechanisms may fail to sustain ABP. The consequent systemic hypotension can lead to tissue hypoperfusion and cellular hypoxia, initiating the early stages of cardiogenic shock. In the absence of effective intervention, death may result.

Hypovolemic shock

Hypovolemic shock is caused by a precipitous fall in cardiac output due to a decrease in blood volume due to hemorrhage, fluid loss, or fluid sequestration leading to a precipitous fall in preload and stroke volume. Hemorrhage and fluid loss (e.g., vomiting, diarrhea, and thermal burns) are the usual causes of hypovolemic shock in veterinary medical patients. However, circulatory collapse from decreased effective circulating blood volume may also be caused by peripheral vasodilation with venous pooling of blood. Mechanisms causing this latter form of hypovolemic shock include **neurogenic shock**, which may occur secondary to central nervous system injury, **anaphylactic shock**, which is caused by a systemic allergic response associated with IgE-triggered histamine release, and **anesthetic shock**, which is caused by anesthetic overdose. Hypovolemic shock is relatively common in veterinary medicine and is often associated with trauma-induced blood loss or excessive contraction of the extracellular fluid volume from diarrhea or vomiting. The proximate cause of the cardiovascular collapse in hypovolemic shock is the inadequacy of blood volume to sustain venous return and cardiac preload. With a marked decrement in preload, stroke volume declines precipitously and tachycardia cannot restore cardiac output. In the early stage of hypovolemic shock, peripheral vasoconstriction sustains perfusion of vital organs (i.e., brain, heart, and kidney) at the expense of nonvital tissues (e.g., skin and abdominal viscera). Later, cell and organ dysfunction ensue and, untreated, hypovolemic shock is generally terminal.

Septic shock

The presence of microorganisms or microbial toxins in the blood is the proximate cause of circulatory collapse in all of forms of **septic shock**. Circulatory shock caused by endotoxigenic Gram-negative bacilli is relatively common in all veterinary species. Endotoxins are derived from bacterial wall lipopolysaccharides, which are released when the bacterial cell wall is destroyed. Endotoxin is composed of an outer O polysaccharide component, a core polysaccharide, and a central fatty acid region (lipid A). Lipid A is the toxic component. Circulatory shock produced by endotoxemia is referred to as **endotoxic shock**. There are molecules similar to endotoxins in the walls of various Gram-positive bacteria and some fungi that can produce septic shock quite similar in clinical course to the endotoxic shock produced by Gram-negative bacilli.

Endotoxic shock is the most common form of septic shock. It is initiated by a complex interaction between endotoxin and monocytes that results in a cascade of events. The earliest stage of endotoxic shock is generally a hyperdynamic, or high-output, stage in which increased cardiac output predominates. Generally, peripheral vasodilation occurs secondary to a variety of inflammatory mediators produced by activated monocytes in what is often referred to as the **systemic inflammatory response syndrome (SIRS)**. Although cardiac output may be normal or elevated initially, extreme peripheral vasodilation and cardiac depressant factors eventually lead to hypotension

and cardiovascular collapse as the syndrome progresses, ultimately leading to death (in the absence of effective intervention). The involved mediators include arachidonic acid metabolites, tumor necrosis factor, a variety of interleukins, nitric oxide, platelet-activating factor, procoagulant factors, and a variety of other substances.

Stages of shock

Based largely on research with hypovolemic shock in dogs, circulatory shock has been divided into three stages. The staging system is based on the response to therapy. While these stages are most evident in shock due to hypovolemia from blood loss, they can be applied to all types of shock.

Stage 1: compensated circulatory shock

In this stage tissue perfusion is inadequate. With cardiogenic and hypovolemic shock, hypotension is also present. In compensated septic shock, cardiac hyperfunction is generally present and ABP is normal (or possibly elevated).

In this stage neurohumoral responses maintain adequate tissue perfusion to vital organs, preventing their hypoxia. Adapting control mechanisms include the arterial baroreceptor system, RAAS, and antidiuretic hormone. The result is tachycardia, heightened sympathetic stimulation of the ventricular myocardium, peripheral vasoconstriction with increased total peripheral resistance, reduced venous capacitance, and oliguria with renal retention of salt and water. Untreated, an animal in this stage of shock often advances to the second, progressive stage.

Stage 2: progressive circulatory shock

With failure of adequate treatment of an animal with compensated shock or with further insult to the circulatory system, progression to stage 2 often occurs. Compensatory mechanisms now fail to sustain ABP and tissue perfusion falls precipitously. Without intervention, cellular hypoxia and organ dysfunction will predominate. At this stage, appropriate therapy (e.g., intravenous fluid or transfusion therapy in hypovolemic shock; therapy for heart failure in cardiogenic shock; or intravenous fluid and antimicrobial therapy in septic shock) may restore cardiovascular function. Untreated, this stage advances to terminal cardiovascular collapse.

Clinical correlations: progressive circulatory shock

You are called to a farm to treat a 3-year-old foal. The horse owner wants you to repair a severe laceration of its left hindleg. You note a significant amount of active hemorrhage but the owner is convinced that the wound just occurred, so you repair the laceration and control the hemorrhage. As you are about to leave the farm, the owner discovers a large pool of blood in the back of the stall so you decide to reexamine the foal. It is now weak, tachycardic, has pale mucous membranes, and you suspect that its systemic ABP is very low and that the foal is in stage 2 of hypovolemic shock. You know that in this stage appropriate intervention is necessary and can reverse the foal's condition. The appropriate therapy you administer includes the intravenous administration of fluids to return the animal's blood volume to normal. As you restore the foal's blood volume, venous return to the heart increases and, via the Frank–Starling relationship, this acts to return the foal's stroke volume and systemic ABP to normal.

Stage 3: irreversible circulatory shock

There appears to be a critical threshold beyond which intervention will universally be unsuccessful. This may be very difficult to predict on the basis of clinically measured parameters and is often a retrospective acknowledgment in clinical cases.

Without therapeutic intervention, shock tends to progress inexorably toward this irreversible stage and death. In stage 3, widespread cellular injury due to hypoxia causes a failure of vascular smooth muscle, endothelial cells, and the ventricular myocardium. This leads to a loss of vascular tone, extravasation of fluid into the intestinal lumen in some species (e.g., dogs), and stasis of blood in vascular beds. Blood stasis causes intravascular activation of the clotting cascade producing a syndrome known as disseminated intravascular coagulation (DIC). Intestinal ischemia disrupts the mucosal barrier, leading to entry of bacteria or bacterial byproducts (e.g., endotoxin) into the circulation, ultimately superimposing endotoxic shock on all forms of shock in this terminal, irreversible stage. Once systolic ABP falls below 50 mmHg as a result of these processes, there is a tendency for the positive feedback effects already outlined to overcome homeostatic negative feedback loops. Despite efforts at therapeutic intervention at this stage, death of the patient results.

Self-evaluation

Answers can be found at the end of the chapter.

1 Which of the following statements about the role of cardiac preload in the progression of heart failure are correct?
  A In the earliest stages of heart failure, the Frank–Starling relationship between stroke volume and preload plays an important role to sustain stroke volume
  B In the later stages of heart failure, ventricular overdistension reduces stroke volume. This leads to systemic hypotension and further renal retention of salt and water, becoming a deleterious positive feedback loop
  C Both statements are correct

2 A dog presents for evaluation of weakness during exercise. On physical examination you note a prominent systolic heart murmur. Cardiac ultrasonography indicates normal ventricular contractility but marked retrograde blood flow across the left atrioventricular (mitral) valve during systole. What mechanism(s) do you believe are causing the heart failure?
  A Myocardial failure
  B Inadequate preload

  C Excessive afterload
  D Myocardial overdistension due to volume overload
  E Retrograde flow of blood causing a reduction in stroke volume
  F C, D, and E

3 Which of the following disease conditions can increase stroke volume to produce a persistently elevated systemic arterial blood pressure (systemic hypertension)?
  A Chronic kidney disease
  B Pheochromocytoma
  C Feline hyperthyroidism
  D Cushing syndrome (hyperadrenocorticism)
  E All of the above

4 How are the physiological determinants of arterial blood pressure affected by the use of an ACE inhibitor in a hypertensive animal?
  A Stroke volume is decreased
  B Preload is reduced
  C Total peripheral vascular resistance and afterload are reduced
  D Renal retention of salt and water is reduced
  E All of the above

5 In a dog in the initial stage of hypovolemic shock (compensated circulatory shock), what observations might you make on thorough physical examination?
  A Tachycardia
  B Weak arterial pulse
  C Pale mucous membranes
  D Increased respiratory rate
  E All of the above

Suggested reading

Brown, A.J. and Mandell, D.C. (2009) Cardiogenic shock. In: *Small Animal Critical Care Medicine* (eds D.C. Silverman & K. Hopper), pp. 146–149. Saunders Elsevier, Philadelphia.

Brown, S. (2009) Hypertensive crisis. In: *Small Animal Critical Care Medicine* (eds D.C. Silverman & K. Hopper), pp. 176–179. Saunders Elsevier, Philadelphia.

Hall, J.E. (2011) Cardiac failure. In: *Guyton and Hall Textbook of Medical Physiology*, 12th edn, pp. 255–264. Saunders Elsevier, Philadelphia.

Hall, J.E. (2011) Circulatory shock and its treatment. In: *Guyton and Hall Textbook of Medical Physiology*, 12th edn, pp. 273–284. Saunders Elsevier, Philadelphia.

Henik, R.A. and Brown, S.A. (2008) Systemic hypertension. In: *Manual of Canine and Feline Cardiology*, 4th edn (eds L.P. Tilley, F.W. Smith, M.A. Oyama and M.M. Sleeper), pp. 277–287. Saunders Elsevier, Philadelphia.

Petrie, J. (2010) Diastolic dysfunction. In: *Consultations in Feline Internal Medicine*, 6th edn (ed. J.R. August), pp. 410–419. Saunders Elsevier, Philadelphia.

Answers

1 C. Early in cardiac disease, an animal operates within the physiologic range of the Frank–Starling relationship such that increases in preload appropriately enhance the stroke volume. In the late stages of

heart failure, as extracellular fluid volume and preload expand dramatically, distending the myocardium and reducing the effectiveness of contraction, stroke volume falls. This leads to a fall in systemic ABP and additional retention of salt and water by the kidney – a deleterious positive feedback loop.

2 F. The retrograde flow of blood causing a reduction in stroke volume is the primary cause of the problem. However, myocardial overdistension contributes as this animal suffers from volume overload of the left ventricle. Additionally, excessive afterload is present in most clinically apparent cases of heart failure due to overactivity of the RAAS and sympathetic nervous system, which cause systemic arteriolar vasoconstriction and increases in total peripheral vascular resistance, raising afterload.

3 E. Changes in the determinants of ABP and associated diseases producing secondary hypertension in veterinary species include stroke volume (e.g., renal failure, pheochromocytoma, feline hyperthyroidism, hyperaldosteronism, Cushing syndrome, diabetes mellitus), heart rate (e.g., pheochromocytoma, feline hyperthyroidism), and total peripheral resistance (e.g., renal failure, pheochromocytoma).

4 E. Preload, and thus stroke volume, are reduced due to a decrease in angiotensin II- and aldosterone-mediated retention of salt and water by the kidney; total peripheral resistance, and thus afterload, are reduced due to decrease in angiotensin II-mediated contraction of vascular smooth muscle cells.

5 E. Tachycardia (compensatory response of the arterial baroreceptor reflex to systemic hypotension), weak arterial pulsations (ABP is low and peripheral vasoconstriction reduces pulse pressure), mucous membrane pallor and cool skin (peripheral vasoconstriction of nonvital organs), and tachypnea (hypoperfusion and hypoxia are present) are typical findings at this stage of shock. The ABP would be low if measured.

41 Exercise Physiology of Terrestrial Animals

David C. Poole and Howard H. Erickson

Kansas State University, Manhattan, KS, USA

Section VI: The Cardiovascular System

Dogs and horses have developed into elite athletes through domestication and genetic selection for specific tasks; first hunting, farming, and warfare and then, more recently, leisure activities. The greyhound originated in Babylon and Egypt over 5000 years ago. It is the fastest breed within the canine species and is capable of attaining speeds near 1000 m/min over 400 m with peak speeds reported over 1300 m/min. In contrast, nomadic tribes used sled dogs in Siberia some 4000 years ago. In contrast to the greyhound, the Siberian husky has tremendous endurance capacity: it is capable of speeds of 12–15 mph while racing over 1700 km in 12–14 days.

Tribes in Mesopotamia and China domesticated horses over 4500 years ago. Domestic horses were recorded in ancient Greece in 1700 BC and in Egypt in 1600 BC. The Romans standardized horses as a means of sport and recreation. In comparison to the dog, development of the horse for true speed is more recent. The British organized horse racing and developed the Thoroughbred from Arabian horses, which have been selectively bred only within the last 300 years. The American Quarter Horse was developed in America during the early 1700s, largely from the Thoroughbred, and can attain speeds up to 55 mph over 400 m.

The maximum speed of the horse and dog with respect to other species is depicted in Figure 41.1. The physiology of four species have been studied quite extensively: the human athlete, the racehorse, the greyhound, and the camel. Exercise physiology studies have been conducted on both the track and on mechanical treadmills. Whereas an article in *Scientific American* in 1891 documents the use of a mechanical treadmill in a theater to simulate a horse race, scientific studies have been primarily confined to the last 30–40 years.

The elite racing greyhound and equine athlete both possess maximal oxygen uptakes ($\dot{V}_{O_{2max}}$) in excess of 200 mL/kg per min, indicative of a high aerobic capacity. It is not known which physiological characteristics make the greyhound, Quarter Horse, and Thoroughbred faster than other breeds within their

Dukes' Physiology of Domestic Animals, Thirteenth Edition. Edited by William O. Reece, Howard H. Erickson, Jesse P. Goff and Etsuro E. Uemura.

© 2015 John Wiley & Sons, Inc. Published 2015 by John Wiley & Sons, Inc.

Companion website: www.wiley.com/go/reece/physiology

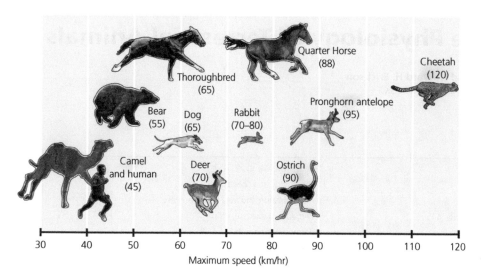

Figure 41.1 Maximum speed of the horse and dog with respect to other species. Note that the horse and camel are the only ones measured while carrying a rider. Adapted from Figure I-2, Kubo, K. (1991) The science for training of Thoroughbred horses. In: *The Race Horse*. Equine Research Institute, Japan Racing Association, Tokyo.

respective species. However, whereas there is probably no single factor that limits exercise and performance, superb equine and canine athletes are characterized by large hearts in relation to body mass. Peak performance capacity depends on maximizing the capacity of each body system to produce an overall maximal result. Physiological adaptation associated with exercise physical conditioning is a mechanism by which exercise capacity can be optimized. Progressive stress produces remarkable adaptations, enabling the individual to cope with increased physical demand and to attain maximum performance. In addition, considerable evidence suggests that genetic predetermination may be involved in setting the upper limit for performance potential.

The purpose of this chapter is to provide a basic understanding of the integrated physiological response to exercise and physical conditioning. The horse and dog will be used as examples; parallels will be made between the physiology of the horse and dog, and the human, where appropriate.

The blood

1 What is the role of the spleen in the horse during exercise?
2 How does spleen weight vary in different breeds of horses?
3 How does blood volume change with exercise?
4 What effect does training have on red cell volume?

Red blood cell mobilization

Limits are imposed on muscular performance by the capacity to deliver oxygen and metabolic substrates to the working muscles and the efficiency of removal of waste products from the muscles. Blood is the pathway by which oxygen and substrates are supplied to the musculature and by which waste products, including heat, are removed. When an animal exercises, the changes observed in circulating blood are remarkably rapid. Most notable is a sharp increase in the unit volume of erythrocytes, leucocytes, and platelets.

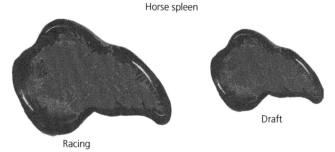

Figure 41.2 Spleen size and capacity as a percentage of body weight (spleen ratio) is far greater in racing than draft horses. Adapted from Figure 2, Kline, H. and Foreman, J.H. (1991), in *Equine Exercise Physiology 3* (eds S.G.B. Persson, A. Lindholm and L.B. Jeffcott), pp. 17–21. ICEEP Publications, Davis, CA.

Splenic contraction

The cardiovascular system has the ability to transport large quantities of oxygen to working muscle. In the horse and dog, as well as several other species, the spleen acts as a reservoir for erythrocytes. The average spleen weight is larger in the horse than in most other species and larger in racing breeds than other breeds of horses (Figure 41.2). Blood cells stored in the spleen can be mobilized into the circulation when there is an increased demand (Table 41.1). The release of stored erythrocytes from the spleen into the systemic circulation is under the influence of the sympathetic nervous system and circulating **catecholamines**. The smooth muscle capsule of the spleen is innervated by **postganglionic sympathetic neurons**. Any factor that increases sympathetic nervous activity or plasma catecholamines, such as **asphyxia**, hemorrhage, excitement, and especially exercise, will result in splenic contraction and increase the number of circulating erythrocytes. Consequently, exercise, as well as excitation, causes an increase in the circulating erythrocyte volume at an essentially unchanged or reduced plasma volume, resulting in an increase in the **packed cell volume or hematocrit**, hemoglobin concentration, and red blood cell count.

Table 41.1 Splenic response to exercise in the Thoroughbred horse and greyhound.

	Thoroughbred		Greyhound	
Variable	Rest	Exercise	Rest	Exercise
Hemoglobin (g/dL)	10–13	21–24	19–20	23–24
Hematocrit (%)	30–40	60–70	50–55	60–65

Source: data from Evans, D.L. and Rose, R.J. (1988) Cardiovascular and respiratory responses to submaximal exercise training in the thoroughbred horse. *Pflugers Archiv* **411**:316–321; Snow, D.H., Harris, R.C. and Stuttard, E. (1988) Changes in haematology and plasma biochemistry during maximal exercise in greyhounds. *Veterinary Record* **123**:487–489.

Other sites

Contraction of the spleen does not fully explain the increase in hematocrit following exercise. In the horse after exercise, the hematocrit may increase from 30–40% to about 60–70% (Figure 41.3). A concomitant rise in blood viscosity also occurs at this time. A marked alteration in the cell/plasma ratio of the peripheral venous blood takes place during exertion, with an associated shift of intravascular to extravascular fluid. Erythrocytes can also be sequestered in other organs, such as the liver, gut, and lungs. In general, Thoroughbreds have resting **erythrocyte indices (mean corpuscular volume, mean corpuscular hemoglobin, and mean corpuscular hemoglobin concentration)** that are higher than those of Standardbred trotters and pacers or endurance horses. Hematologic values for greyhounds are also higher than those of other breeds. This adaptation enables increased oxygen carriage to the tissues during exercise, which more than offsets the exercise-induced arterial hypoxemia (see section Blood gas tensions and acid–base balance).

Blood volume

The potential of the spleen to increase the circulating red cell volume is impressive in both the dog and horse. At rest, about one-third to half of the erythrocytes are stored in the spleen. The increase in hematocrit is a function of exercise intensity; a linear relationship between hematocrit and speed exists up to a hematocrit of approximately 60–70%. This **autotransfusion** of erythrocytes during exercise boosts the oxygen-carrying capacity of the blood and is thought to be a significant factor contributing to the very high, maximal, oxygen consumption of the horse and dog compared with other species. Total blood volume therefore increases dramatically during exercise, as a result of the contribution of the splenic reservoir. However, exercise also causes some reduction in plasma volume, which is attributed to fluid shift from the intravascular to extravascular compartment and also as a result of fluid loss through sweating.

Physical training and oxygen transport capacity

Physical training induces adaptations to increased metabolic demands in several respects. One limiting factor for fitness and endurance is the oxygen transport capacity of the blood. This

Horse Hematocrit

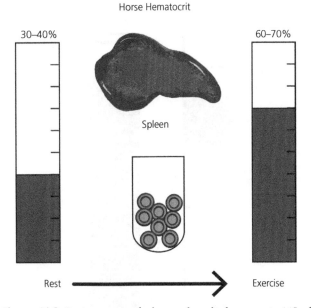

Figure 41.3 During exercise the horse spleen discharges up to 14 L of concentrated red blood cells, raising systemic hematocrit from a resting value of 30–40% to 60–70%.

capacity is enhanced during training by an increase in the total volume of red cells. A relationship between state of training, cell volume, and other erythrocyte indices is well established in both human and the horse. **Plasma viscosity** and **fibrinogen** levels are normally unaffected by training. Plasma viscosity values in the Thoroughbred are lower than in other breeds of horses and possibly all other animals.

When training is prolonged, however, the increase in **red cell mass** may become excessive. This increase in hematocrit results in reduced racing performance and has been attributed to over-training. The increased blood viscosity may be associated with a reduction in capillary perfusion and inadequate oxygen delivery to the tissues.

Cardiovascular system

> 1 How does cardiac output contribute to the increase in oxygen transport during exercise?
>
> 2 What is the range in heart rate in the horse and dog from rest to exercise?
>
> 3 What are the mechanisms involved that result in an increase in stroke volume during exercise?
>
> 4 What are the main changes in the distribution of blood flow during exercise?
>
> 5 What changes occur in blood pressure during exercise?
>
> 6 What cardiovascular adaptations occur with physical conditioning?
>
> 7 What arrhythmias are common in the racehorse at rest and during exercise?

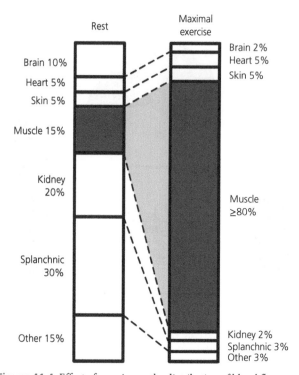

Figure 41.4 Effect of exercise on the distribution of blood flow (cardiac output) among skeletal muscle and other organs in the dog and horse. Note proportional shift toward skeletal muscle. Adapted from Figure 22.5, Erickson, H.H. and Poole, D.C. (2004), in *Dukes' Physiology of Domestic Animals*, 12th edn (ed. W.O. Reece). Cornell University Press, Ithaca, NY. With permission from Cornell University Press.

During strenuous exercise, the metabolic needs of working muscle increase dramatically. The ability of the heart to pump sufficient blood to meet the needs of the exercising horse and provide effective redistribution of the blood to working skeletal muscle is essential to maintaining performance (Figure 41.4). The extent to which oxygen delivery to active muscles can be increased is thought by many to be a limiting factor in whole body exercise.

Cardiac output

Exercise demands an increased **cardiac output** to meet the oxygen requirements to fuel working muscle energetics. The increase in cardiac output (Figure 41.5) during exercise is a primary factor in the large increase in **oxygen delivery** in the canine and equine species. Cardiac output is the product of heart rate and stroke volume as follows:

$$Cardiac\ output = Heart\ rate \times Stroke\ volume$$

Because maximal heart rate is attained during severe exercise, stroke volume may limit the increase in cardiac output during exercise. During submaximal exercise, cardiac output increases close to linearly with workload (and $\dot{V}o_2$) and this is principally due to increased heart rate. The threefold to fourfold increase in

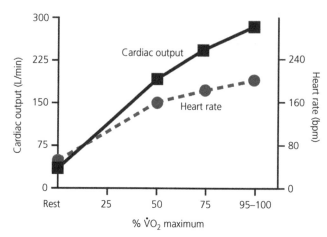

Figure 41.5 Cardiac output and heart rate responses in the horse during exercise on a high-speed treadmill. Data from Hopper, M.K., Pieschl, R.L., Pelletier, N.G. *et al.* (1991), in *Equine Exercise Physiology 3* (eds S.G.B. Persson, A. Lindholm and L.B. Jeffcott), pp. 9–16. ICEEP Publications, Davis, CA.

Table 41.2 Cardiovascular responses to exercise in 500-kg horse.

Variable	Rest	Exercise	Exercise/rest ratio
Heart rate (bpm)	30	210–250	7–8
Cardiac output (L/min)	30	150 to >500	5–16
Systolic/diastolic arterial blood pressure (mmHg)	130/80	230/110	1.6
Pulse pressure (mmHg)	50	150–200	3–4
Pulmonary artery pressure (mmHg)	20–30	80 to >90	3–4
Hemoglobin concentration (g/dL)	13	17–24	1.3–1.6
Oxygen uptake (mL/min per kg)	2.5–4	120–220	30–88

Source: data compiled from Poole, D.C. and Erickson, H.H. (2011) Highly athletic terrestrial mammals: horses and dogs. *Comprehensive Physiology* **1**:1–37.

cardiac output during maximal exercise in ponies is similar to that in dogs and humans. However, during maximal work in horses, cardiac output can increase 5–16 times that at rest and the elite greyhound may be better still.

The Thoroughbred and racing Quarter Horse can augment their $\dot{V}o_2$ 80-fold between rest and maximal exercise, representing one of the highest **aerobic scopes** in mammals. This is achieved by means of an up to 16-fold increase in cardiac output (Table 41.2), combined with an approximately fivefold increase in **oxygen extraction (arteriovenous oxygen content difference, a-vo$_2$ difference)** by the tissues. The a-vo$_2$ difference in Thoroughbred horses can exceed 23 volumes percent (vol%), whereas top human athletes can reach only 17–18 vol% when running at maximal intensity. Arterial oxygen content is a function of hemoglobin concentration of the blood and the efficiency of **alveolar ventilation** and gas exchange as these set the number of oxygen-binding sites and also hemoglobin saturation. An exercising horse can increase its oxygen-carrying capacity over 60% through splenic contraction and still not increase viscous resistance enough to impede cardiac output. A high cardiac output is also aided in the elite athlete by a high ratio of heart weight to body weight (g/kg) (Figure 41.6). Heart weight to body weight may range between 0.9 and 2%,

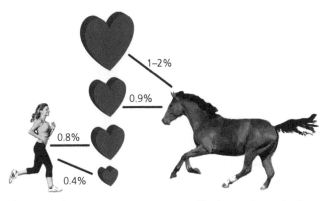

Figure 41.6 Heart mass as a percentage of body mass in a trained and untrained Thoroughbred horse compared with a human. Data in part from Kubo, K. (1974) Equine Research Institute, Japan Racing Association, Tokyo.

for the Thoroughbred and greyhound, compared with only 0.4–0.8% for humans. Within elite athletes, the best-performing or elite animals (and human endurance athletes) tend to possess values at the upper ends of these ranges.

Heart rate

The large increase in cardiac output is primarily due to the very high heart rates that can be attained in the horse and dog. In the trained Thoroughbred, resting heart rates are in the mid twenties; however, the average is around 35 bpm. During maximal exercise, heart rate can increase to 240–250 bpm (Table 41.2) in the racing Thoroughbred. In the dog, resting heart rates can be less than 100 bpm, particularly in the racing greyhound, rising to 300 bpm or more during maximal exercise (Table 41.3). Heart rate rises rapidly at the onset of exercise, reaching a maximum in 30–45 s, and then often drops before reaching a plateau during steady-state work.

The anticipatory response to exercise is evidenced by an increased resting heart rate in the canine and equine athlete, as in humans. In addition, heart rate during submaximal exercise is affected by apprehension and anxiety. The psychogenic component of the heart rate response to exercise is proportionately larger at lower, relative workloads. At a heart rate of less than 120 bpm in the horse there may be psychogenic factors such as

Table 41.3 Cardiovascular characteristics of greyhounds and mongrels.

Variable	Conditioned greyhound*	Unconditioned mongrel*
Heart weight/body weight ratio (g/100 g)		
Adult	1.3–1.7	0.94
Neonatal	1.20	0.76 (coonhounds)
6 months	1.14	
Myocardial cell diameter (μm)	18.3	12.5
Mean arterial blood pressure (mmHg)	118	98
Cardiac output (L/min) (resting/exercise)	4.4/8.1	2.7
Cardiac index (L/min per m²) (resting)	4.3	3.1
Stroke volume (mL) (resting/exercise)	55/116	27
Peripheral resistance (10 dynes·s·m⁻⁵)	2.3	3.4
Carotid sinus OP† (mmHg)	137	123
Plasma volume (mL/kg)	54	54
Blood volume (mL/kg)	114	79
Heart rate (bpm)		
Rest	29–48	61–117
Maximum exercise	290–420	220–325
Oxygen uptake (mL/kg per min)		
Rest	8	8
Maximum exercise	240	85

*Mean body weight for greyhounds 26 kg; for mongrels 20 kg.
†OP, operating point (the level at which carotid sinus perfusion pressure and systemic arterial pressure remain equal).
Source: data from Courtice, F.C. (1943) *Journal of Physiology* **102**:290–305; Donald, D.E. & Ferguson, D. (1966) *Proceedings of the Society for Experimental Biology and Medicine* **121**:626–629; Detweiler *et al.* (1974) *Federation Proceedings* **33**:360; Cox, R.H. *et al.* (1976) *American Journal of Physiology* **230**:211–218; Alonso (1972) Thesis, University of Pennsylvania; Carew, T.E. & Covell, J.W. (1978) *American Journal of Cardiology* **42**:82–88; Staaden (1980) *Current Veterinary Therapy VII. Small Animal Practice*, pp. 347–351. W.B. Saunders, Philadelphia. For elite greyhound values see Poole, D.C. and Erickson, H.H. (2011) Highly athletic terrestrial mammals: horses and dogs. *Comprehensive Physiology* **1**:1–37.

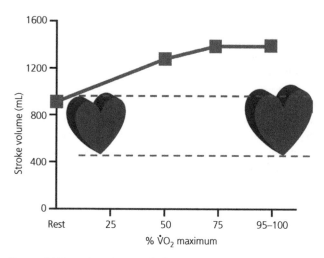

Figure 41.7 Stroke volume in the horse increases as a function of exercise intensity (expressed here as percent of maximum oxygen consumption, $V_{O_{2max}}$) during exercise on a high-speed treadmill. Data from Table 2, Hopper, M.K., Pieschl, R.L., Pelletier, N.G. *et al.* (1991), in *Equine Exercise Physiology 3* (eds S.G.B. Persson, A. Lindholm and L.B. Jeffcott), pp. 9–16. ICEEP Publications, Davis, CA.

fear; heart rates above 210 bpm begin to plateau with incremental workload as maximal heart rate is approached. Therefore, the heart rate response to graded exercise in the equine athlete is linear only between 120 and 210 bpm. Following exercise, the heart rate decreases rapidly within the first minute or two after stopping.

Stroke volume

The literature contains contradictory statements concerning the changes in stroke volume during exercise. Stroke volume has been reported to be increased or unchanged during exercise in the dog and increased during submaximal exercise in the horse (Figure 41.7). Maintenance of stroke volume during exercise occurs by several physiological mechanisms. Increased sympathetic nervous activity during exercise results in both tachycardia and reduced end-systolic ventricular volumes by increasing myocardial contractility, so that ventricular emptying is more effective. Venous return during exercise is supplemented by mobilization of the splenic reserve of blood volume, muscle movement, and increased negativity of intrathoracic pressure. Increased stretch of myocardial fibers within physiologic limits leads to an increase in developed pressure and stroke volume through the **Frank–Starling mechanism**. The observed increases in **left ventricular end-diastolic pressure** and contractility during exercise, along with the increased venous return, assist in the maintenance of stoke volume, despite the decreased filling time associated with shortened diastole at increased heart rates. During severe exercise in free-running dogs, increases in end-diastolic left ventricular diameter and pressure have been observed, with a reduction in end-systolic diameter. Therefore, stroke volume generally increases during exercise to aid in the augmentation of cardiac output and oxygen delivery to the body.

Myocardial contractility

During strenuous exercise in the dog and pony, marked augmentation of myocardial contractility is observed, along with pronounced increases in both **ventricular preload (increased end-diastolic volume)** and **afterload (mean arterial pressure)**. The net result is an increase in myocardial oxygen consumption, which is met by increases in both coronary blood flow and increased oxygen extraction. Because the right ventricle extracts less oxygen at rest than the left ventricle, at elevated heart rates the right ventricle can increase its oxygen uptake by increasing fractional oxygen extraction as well as blood flow. In contrast, the left ventricle extracts about 80% of the arterial oxygen at resting heart rates and must therefore rely predominantly on elevated blood flow to meet the increasing oxygen demands of exercising heart rates.

Blood flow

The main changes in distribution of blood flow during exercise are (i) increased pulmonary blood flow from opening of previously closed pulmonary capillaries, (ii) coronary vasodilation resulting in increased coronary flow to provide oxygen for myocardial contraction, (iii) vasodilation in working skeletal muscles that elevates capillary red blood cell flux, (iv) vasoconstriction in the nonworking muscles and the splanchnic vasculature, and (v) increased blood flow to the skin (see Figure 41.4). These cardiovascular adaptations elevate the oxygen supply to tissues with increased oxygen requirements during exercise and body thermoregulation. Blood flow to the skin is dependent on body temperature as well as environmental temperature and humidity.

Blood pressure

Ultrasound systems are often used to measure systemic arterial pressure at rest; however, during exercise, **solid-state catheter transducer systems** using an exteriorized carotid artery provide more accurate measurements. During submaximal exercise, systemic arterial blood pressure is maintained relatively constant by arterial baroreceptors in the wall of the aortic arch and in the carotid sinus. Light treadmill exercise has no significant effect on mean arterial pressure. However, during more strenuous treadmill exercise, significant increases in mean systemic arterial pressure occur (Table 41.2 and Figure 41.8). Chronic hypertension in ponies has been reported to result in an enlarged heart, particularly the left ventricle, which is a pathological increase in myocyte cross-sectional area as opposed to the increased myocyte length found after exercise training that results in augmented stroke volumes.

During strenuous exercise, cardiac output (equal to total pulmonary blood flow) increases up to 16-fold in the horse. This increase in pulmonary blood flow raises pulmonary arterial pressure from 20–24 mmHg at rest to as much as 80–90 mmHg or higher during exercise (see Table 41.2 and Figure 41.8). If left atrial pressure remains constant or increases (as it does substantially during exercise in the horse), calculated pulmonary vascular resistance decreases. Presumably in the horse, as in

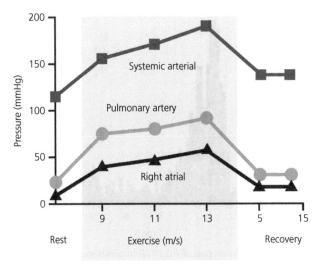

Figure 41.8 The responses of systemic arterial pressure, mean pulmonary arterial pressure, and mean right atrial pressure in the horse to progressively increasing intensities of exercise on a high-speed treadmill and during recovery. Adapted from Figures 2–4, Olsen, S.C., Coyne, C.P., Lowe, B.S. *et al.* (1992) Influence of furosemide on hemodynamic responses during exercise in horses. *American Journal of Veterinary Research* **53**:742–747.

Table 41.4 Cardiovascular effects after physical conditioning in the greyhound and Thoroughbred horse.

Variable	At rest	Maximum exercise
Heart rate	No change	Decreased
Stroke volume	Increased	Increased
Oxygen uptake	Increased?	Increased
Arteriovenous oxygen difference	No change	Increased
Heart volume	Increased	Increased
Blood volume	Increased	Increased
Blood pressure	Decreased	Decreased

Source: data from Gillespie, J.R. and Robinson, N.E. (eds) (1987) *Equine Exercise Physiology 2*. ICEEP Publications, Davis, CA; McKeever, K.H. *et al.* (1987) *Medicine and Science in Sports and Exercise* **19**:21–27; Rose, R.J. (1985) *Veterinary Clinics of North America: Equine Practice* **1**(3):437–617.

other species, the decrease in resistance results from a combination of dilation of perfused vessels and recruitment of previously unperfused vessels. Significant increases also occur in right atrial pressure (Figure 41.8).

The racing greyhound possesses multiple differences in systemic hemodynamics when compared with its mongrel counterpart. Mean arterial pressure is significantly higher in greyhounds in association with increased cardiac index and lower peripheral resistance.

Cardiovascular adaptations to physical conditioning
Heart rate
In humans, physical conditioning or training results in sinus bradycardia at rest and a decreased heart rate during submaximal work. Most studies indicate that the resting heart rate of the horse does not change significantly after training (Table 41.4), although lower resting heart rates have been observed in endurance horses after training. This effect may result, in large part, from decreased apprehension and nervousness rather than to a training-induced bradycardia as seen in humans. Like their human counterparts, horses and dogs, exhibit heart rates during submaximal exercise that are lower after training. However, maximal heart rate is not increased.

Stroke volume
Cardiac enlargement is a well-recognized adaptation of highly conditioned human athletes and may be due to increased cardiac mass or left ventricular volume leading to increases in stroke volume. Thus, cardiac output is maintained during

submaximal exercise in the face of the reduction in heart rate after exercise training. The incidence of **valvular insufficiency**, especially **mitral and tricuspid**, increases with exercise training in the Thoroughbred horse.

Blood pressure
Following training, lower left ventricular and arterial pressures, as well as higher left ventricular contractility at rest and during exercise have been reported. In contrast to the decrease in left-sided pressures during exercise following training, mean right atrial pressure, which at rest is slightly lower than at pretraining, increases steeply to significantly higher levels with increasing intensity of exercise; this effect may be consequent to the increased blood and plasma volume.

Blood volume
Chronic exercise training produces an expansion of blood and plasma volume. This adaptation to training provides an enhanced vascular volume to meet the increased cardiovascular and thermoregulatory needs during exercise. In the greyhound after 14 days of training on a treadmill, plasma volume increases 27.5%, water intake 33%, and urine output 20.8%. The primary mechanism for the exercise training-induced hypervolemia is a net positive water balance via increased water consumption without significant contribution from an increase in renal water reabsorption. The same increase in plasma volume occurs in the horse after 14 days of training; however, daily water intake does not change during training. Hematocrit and hemoglobin concentrations are lower in horses when they are in peak track condition and the values increase when the horses are removed from the track.

Electrocardiographic findings in racehorses
In the resting horse, heart rate is comparatively slow, and normal irregularities may occur in rhythm. The irregularities often disappear when heart rate increases, so that performance is not

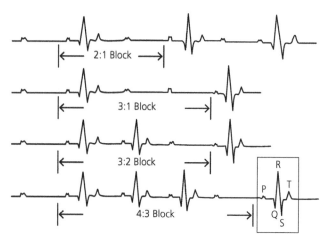

Figure 41.9 Conduction ratios in second-degree AV block in the horse at rest. A 2 : 1 block reduces the pulse or ventricular rate by half the regular rate. A 3 : 1 block results in double blocked ventricular beats which are often accompanied by single missed beats. An R–R interval plot would show normal/long/normal/long intervals with a 3 : 2 block, while a 4 : 3 block is characterized by two normal intervals then a long interval. Adapted from Figure 25, Holmes, J.R. (1988) *Equine Cardiology*, Vol. **IV**, Cardiac Rhythm. School of Veterinary Science, University of Bristol, UK.

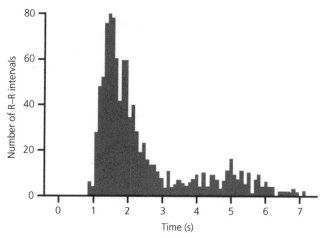

Figure 41.10 A histogram of 1024 R–R intervals measured at rest in a 20-year-old coach horse with atrial fibrillation. The histogram shows a wide distribution of R–R intervals. The resting heart rate averaged 26 bpm with some intervals of up to 7.9 s between beats. During these long periods of systolic standstill the jugular veins filled. During trotting and lunging, tachycardia occurred and the rhythm was regular. The arrhythmia was present almost immediately after work stopped. Adapted from Case Study 601, Holmes, J.R. (1988) *Equine Cardiology*, Vol. **IV**, Cardiac Rhythm. School of Veterinary Science, University of Bristol, UK.

impaired. However, the persistence of arrhythmias at high heart rates during or immediately after exercise justifies a guarded prognosis, for circulatory efficiency is of major importance at these times.

Exercise has minimal effects on the **QRS complex**. However, the **PR and QT intervals** are shortened, and P waves are superimposed on the T waves that precede them. T waves can also change form during exercise, such as increasing in amplitude; this is associated with an increased potassium. During recovery from exercise, **premature ventricular beats** or **sinus arrhythmia** may occur. Measurement of the QRS interval has been used to determine heart size in racehorses and greyhounds.

Second-degree atrioventricular block

Second-degree partial atrioventricular (AV) block is the most common rhythm irregularity observed in horses at rest. It is clinically recognizable by the appearance of missed ventricular beats (Figure 41.9). In the majority of cases, the **atrial or fourth heart sound** can be heard. It is often accompanied by **first-degree AV block** and is generally **Wenckebach type I** with variations in PR interval, which often progressively lengthen to a missed beat. On **auscultation**, a corresponding increased separation can be noticed between the atrial contraction sound and the first heart sound.

One practice in assessing the cardiac response to work is to gradually increase the exercise intensity, first at a trot, then a canter, and later a gallop. In most horses with partial AV block at rest, the missed beats disappear with exercise and do not recur until heart rate again approaches a resting value. **Radiotelemetry** or a treadmill may be used to detect missed beats, singles, and sometimes doubles for a short period

immediately after exercise in horses with partial AV block at rest. This transient period is usually followed by a regular rhythm until heart rate approaches resting rate, when partial AV block reappears. The transient nature of this arrhythmia suggests that it may be a manifestation of excessive vagal action associated with the onset of heart rate slowing, just as vagal influence may explain the frequency of partial AV block in horses at slow resting heart rates.

Whether second-degree AV block has a physiological or pathological basis is unresolved. It is the most common arrhythmia in the horse and is probably of little clinical significance. However, some regard second-degree AV block as a condition that may impair racing performance. Marked pathological changes have been noted in the myocardium of some horses with second-degree AV block. This condition can be minimized with **atropine** or exercise.

Atrial fibrillation

On auscultation, profound irregularity, absence of atrial contraction sounds, and variation in intensity of first and second heart sounds are indicative of **atrial fibrillation**. Figure 41.10 shows the variation of R–R intervals in a horse with atrial fibrillation. During exercise at high heart rates, the arrhythmia persists, but is less obvious. It quickly becomes more apparent again as heart rate begins to slow immediately after exercise. This cardiac abnormality is often associated with a history of poor performance and "fading" while racing and occurs more often in big horses. Horses showing atrial fibrillation also have a significantly higher incidence of T-wave abnormalities and second-degree AV block. Atrial fibrillation occurs more readily and probably with less serious underlying heart disease in the horse than in the dog. This arrhythmia may be complicated with murmurs, usually systolic and associated with the mitral valve. Mitral valve lesions may lead to atrial enlargement and atrial fibrillation.

Respiratory system

1 What is aerobic scope and how does it change in the horse with exercise?

2 How is gait related to $\dot{V}o_2$ and energy expenditure?

3 What are the component/links in the **oxygen transfer chain**?

4 What is the relationship between respiratory frequency and step frequency?

5 What is the cause of acidosis during exercise?

6 Why does arterial hypoxemia occur during strenuous exercise?

7 What is the incidence of exercise-induced pulmonary hemorrhage in the horse and why does it occur?

Respiratory function during exercise

The primary function of the respiratory system is the exchange of oxygen and carbon dioxide (CO_2) at a rate that is matched to metabolism. Horses have a very high aerobic scope, with the impressive ability to increase their $\dot{V}o_2$ by about 30–80-fold between rest and maximal exercise (see Table 41.2). Gas exchange involves ventilation of the lungs, perfusion of the pulmonary capillaries with blood, matching of ventilation and blood flow, diffusion of gases between air and blood, and transport of gases to and from the muscles.

Ventilation

Ventilation is the bulk flow of gas into and out of the lungs. The resting horse is unusual in that it has a biphasic exhalation and occasionally a biphasic inhalation. Maximal expiratory flow has been measured in healthy horses to determine if dynamic events in the pulmonary airways limit ventilation during maximal exercise. During maximal exercise peak expiratory flow rates for a 540-kg horse range between 80 and 100 L/s and are generated at high respiratory frequencies and relatively low tidal volumes (Figure 41.11). Catecholamine release, which accompanies exercise, dilates the bronchial tree and decreases resistance to airflow. Convective cooling associated with ventilation is also important in the regulation of body temperature in the horse. Environmental factors such as ambient temperature and humidity influence respiratory rate.

Horses change gait to minimize energy expenditure for any given running speed. At each gait, there is an optimal speed at which $\dot{V}o_2$ is minimal. Both ponies and horses select a gait that maximizes their efficiency of movement. Despite this selection of gait to minimize energy expenditure, $\dot{V}o_2$ increases almost linearly as speed increases (Figure 41.12). To accommodate this

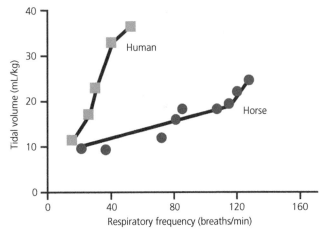

Figure 41.11 Breathing patterns at rest and up to near-maximal exercise in Thoroughbred horses and humans. Note that horses achieve their high exercising mass-specific ventilations by preferential increase in respiratory frequency in contrast to humans, in whom mass-specific tidal volume increases preferentially. Human data are from Clark, J.M., Sinclair, R.D. and Lenox, J.B. (1980) Chemical and nonchemical components of ventilation during hypercapnic exercise in man. *Journal of Applied Physiology* **48**:1065–1076. Horse data are from Hornicke, H., Meixner, R. and Pollmann, U. (1983) Respiration in exercising horses. In: *Equine Exercise Physiology 1* (eds D.H. Snow, S.G.B. Persson and R.J. Rose), pp. 7–16. Granta Editions, Cambridge, UK; and Pelletier, N. and Leith, D.E. (1995) Ventilation and carbon dioxide exchange in exercising horses: effect of inspired oxygen fraction. *Journal of Applied Physiology* **78**:654–662.

increase in $\dot{V}o_2$, minute ventilation, cardiac output, and the amount of hemoglobin in blood increase. As exercise intensity increases, there is increased oxygen extraction so that the up to 80-fold increase in $\dot{V}o_2$ occurring during maximal exercise is satisfied by a 40-fold increase in minute ventilation combined with a 16-fold increase in cardiac output.

As running speed increases, minute ventilation increases linearly. This increase can be accomplished by an increase in either tidal volume or respiratory frequency or both. At the walk and trot, respiratory frequency is usually not related to step frequency. However, at the canter and gallop, respiratory frequency and step frequency are synchronized though this is not requisite for achieving very high ventilations.

Oxygen uptake ($\dot{V}o_2$)

The response of the oxygen transport system during locomotory exercise represents one of the most striking adaptations shown by horses for aerobic performance. Thoroughbreds are able to augment their $\dot{V}o_2$ by more than 80-fold between rest and maximal exercise; with the exception of the pronghorn antelope, this may be the highest aerobic scope in mammals (Figure 41.13). Endurance-trained humans can increase $\dot{V}o_2$ 18–24 times higher than resting values in response to strenuous exercise. Maximal $\dot{V}o_2$ of Thoroughbreds may reach more than 220 mL/min per kg (or ~100 L/min for a 440-kg animal, Figure 41.13) with an a-vo_2 difference of 23 vol% and a maximal

Section VI: The Cardiovascular System

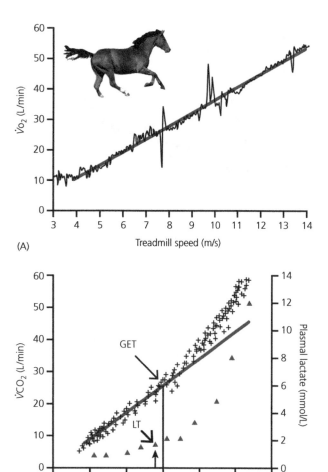

(A)

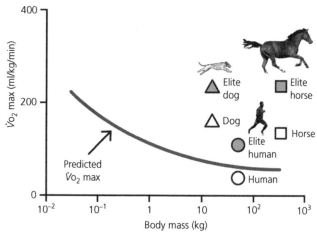

Figure 41.13 Body mass-specific maximal oxygen uptake ($\dot{V}_{O_{2max}}$) plotted as a logarithmic function of body mass for a selection of mammals with body masses differing over five orders of magnitude: solid line adapted from Linstedt, S.L., Hokanson, J.F., Wells, D.J. *et al.* (1991) Running energetics in the pronghorn antelope. *Nature* 353:748–750. Notice the extraordinary values plotted for the horse and dog (foxhound and elite dog, greyhound) compared with human. Adapted from Poole, D.C. and Erickson, H.H. (2011) Highly athletic terrestrial mammals: horses and dogs. *Comprehensive Physiology* 1:1–37.

(B)

Figure 41.12 (A) Oxygen uptake ($\dot{V}_{O_2}$) response to an incremental exercise test where treadmill speed was increased by 1 m/s each minute (from a 3 m/s baseline) until volitional fatigue ($\dot{V}_{O_{2max}}$, ~55 L/min) in a nonelite Thoroughbred horse. Note highly linear (solid line) increase of $\dot{V}_{O_2}$ as a function of speed despite trot–canter–gallop transitions. Adapted from Langsetmo, I., Weigle, G.E., Fedde, M.R. *et al.* (1997) V_{O_2} kinetics in the horse during moderate and heavy exercise. *Journal of Applied Physiology* **83**:1235–1241. (B) Determination of lactate (LT) and gas exchange (GET) thresholds in the Thoroughbred horse during same test as in (A). GET was discriminated by the nonlinearity of $\dot{V}_{CO_2}$ with respect to $\dot{V}_{O_2}$ which detects the additional CO_2 produced consequent to HCO_3^- buffering of H^+ emanating from the exercising muscles.

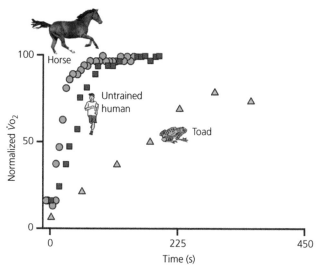

Figure 41.14 Comparison of $\dot{V}_{O_2}$ response (i.e., $\dot{V}_{O_2}$ kinetics) among the Thoroughbred horse, untrained human, and toad following a stepwise increase in metabolic demand (i.e., moderate-intensity exercise. Note the astonishingly fast kinetics in the horse (solid circles). Adapted from Poole, D.C. and Jones, A.M. (2012) Oxygen uptake kinetics. *Comprehensive Physiology* 2:933–996.

cardiac output of over 450 L/min. $\dot{V}_{O_{2max}}$ of trained humans does not exceed 100 mL/min per kg (or 5–6 L/min for a 70-kg individual). Therefore, Thoroughbred horses have an outstanding aerobic capacity with a mass-specific $\dot{V}_{O_{2max}}$ over twice as high as the best human athletes.

The kinetics of gas transport are more rapid in the dog and horse compared with humans (Figure 41.14). The rapidity of the increase in $\dot{V}_{O_2}$ with the onset of exercise in these athletes is coordinated with a rapid increase in ventilation and cardiac output, together with the release into the circulation of

erythrocytes stored in the spleen. At exercise intensities below the lactate threshold, steady-state values in $\dot{V}_{O_2}$ are reached in 50–60 s for the horse, compared with 2–3 min in humans. However, above the lactate threshold, there is a $\dot{V}_{O_2}$ slow component which elevates end-exercise $\dot{V}_{O_2}$ substantially and reduces exercise efficiency.

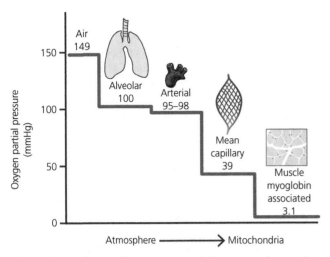

Figure 41.15 The complete oxygen cascade from atmosphere to the muscle tissue during maximal exercise in normoxia. Adapted from Figure 7, Richardson, R.S., Noyszewski, E.A., Kendrick, K.F., Leigh, J.S. and Wagner, P.D. (1995) Myoglobin O_2 desaturation during exercise. Evidence of limited O_2 transport. *Journal of Clinical Investigation* **96**:1916–1926.

The oxygen transfer chain facilitates the movement of oxygen down its pressure gradient from outside the body to metabolizing tissues (Figure 41.15). This transfer chain includes oxygen uptake and diffusion (upper and lower respiratory tract function), oxygen binding to hemoglobin in red cells, oxygen transport (cardiac pump function and circulation through the vascular system), oxygen delivery to the tissues (dissociation and diffusion), and oxygen utilization in mitochondria (oxidizable substrates and enzymes). The oxygen transfer chain is only as strong as its weakest link.

Oxygen delivery from the lungs to the tissues can be increased by three strategies during exercise: (i) increased cardiac output, (ii) increased oxygen-carrying capacity of the blood (increased hematocrit), and (iii) increased extraction of oxygen from the blood at the tissues (increased a-vO_2 difference). The prodigious 80-fold increase in $\dot{V}O_2$ during maximal exercise in the horse occurs with about a 16-fold increase in cardiac output. However, each aliquot of blood has approximately a > 50% increase in the amount of hemoglobin (oxygen capacity) over that seen at rest because of splenic discharge of erythrocytes. The remainder of the increased fractional oxygen demand is met by increasing oxygen extraction from the blood.

When a horse gallops from a standing start, the respiratory system responds almost instantaneously to stimuli arising from within the motor cortex, the exercising limbs and muscles, and also the elevated pulmonary blood flow. Ventilatory responses during exercise are under neural control by **proprioceptors** in the locomotor apparatus, **feedforward mechanisms** from the motor cortex and are also sensitive to the rate of CO_2 exchange across the lungs, which increases with cardiac output and mixed venous CO_2 concentration. **Cardiac accelerator stimuli** originate both from the autonomic nervous system and from humoral catecholamines. Withdrawal of parasympathetic inhibition

helps increase the heart rate to around 110 bpm. Increases in heart rate above this value are due to sympathetic stimulation and to circulating catecholamines. Erythrocyte mobilization is likewise under both neural and humoral control.

Respiration and locomotion

Respiratory frequency of mounted horses at rest varies between 15 and 45 breaths/min, depending on the degree of pre-exercise restlessness of the animal. No relationship between respiratory frequency and step frequency is observed at the walk or the trot but the respiratory and limb cycles are synchronized in phase (1 : 1) at the canter and gallop. Thus, horses respire up to 130–140 times per minute during a fast gallop.

Tidal volume approximately doubles during the trot. When changing from the trot to the canter, most horses exhibit a slight decrease in tidal volume, as a consequence of the higher respiratory frequency. Respiration in running horses differs from respiration in running humans. **Bipedal locomotion** has little repercussion on thoracic mechanics. Therefore, humans can choose the most efficient combination of tidal volume and respiratory frequency. When running medium distances at near maximum speed, human athletes respire with a frequency of 50–60 breaths/min at a tidal volume of about 50% of vital capacity. In contrast, the galloping horse respires at a very high rate (>120 breaths/min) with relatively shallow breaths and the tidal volume (12–15 L per breath) rarely exceeds one-third of vital capacity (see Figure 41.11).

Blood gas tensions and acid–base balance

Horses develop a **metabolic and respiratory acidosis** during strenuous exercise. The respiratory response to intense exercise results in a fall in arterial PCO_2 in many species; however, PCO_2 increases in the horse. **Arterial hypoxemia** (low PO_2) occurs during intense exercise in the horse and in highly trained human athletes. The reasons for the development of hypoxemia (and hypercapnia) include the following, in order of importance.

1 A decrease in red blood cell transit time (as pulmonary blood flow increases to a far greater extent than capillary blood volume; see Table 41.2 and Figure 41.16) results in **alveolar–capillary oxygen diffusion limitation**. This is exacerbated by the **temperature-induced rightward shift (Bohr effect)** of the **oxygen dissociation curve**. This shift results in a decreased affinity of hemoglobin for oxygen and facilitates the release of oxygen to the tissues but impairs oxygen loading in the lungs.

2 Alveolar hypoventilation elevates alveolar PCO_2 thereby reducing PAO_2.

3 Mild ventilation–perfusion mismatch (see Chapter 23).

4 Blood that is shunted around the lungs. Normally about 1% of cardiac output represents venous blood from the bronchial and **thebesian vasculature** that mixes with arterial blood downstream of the lungs.

5 There may be increases in the blood–alveolar diffusion distance associated with the development of **interstitial pulmonary edema and diffusion limited gas exchange**.

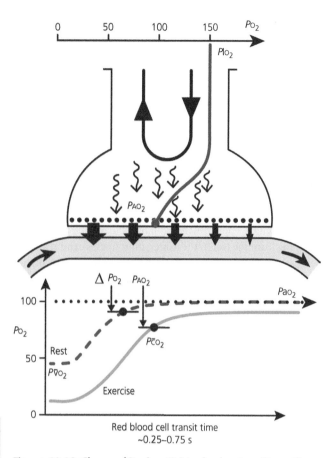

Figure 41.16 Change of Po_2 (mmHg) in alveolar air and in capillary blood along the path from the pulmonary artery (venous blood) to the pulmonary vein (arterial blood). Heavy vertical arrows in lower part of upper illustration represent a decreasing flow rate of oxygen across the alveolar–capillary barrier as incoming venous blood equilibrates with alveolar gas and becomes arterialized. Arrows in the top part of the upper illustration show the movement of air (gas) in and out of the alveoli with each respiratory cycle. The lower illustration shows that pulmonary capillary blood for a person at rest (transit time about 0.75 s) is equilibrated with alveolar air after the first third of the capillary path, whereas during exercise (transit time about 0.25 s) the entire length of capillary path may be required for equilibration. As shown, the partial pressure at various locations is represented by Po_2 (inspired oxygen 149 mmHg), Pao_2 (alveolar oxygen), $P\bar{v}o_2$ (mixed venous oxygen), $P\bar{c}o_2$ (mean capillary oxygen), and Pao_2 (arterial oxygen). In a healthy lung of the human and most animals at rest and during maximal exercise, Pao_2 is very close to Pao_2 and arterial hemoglobin is close to 100% saturated. However, for very athletic species such as the horse and greyhound during high-intensity exercise, red blood cell transit time in the pulmonary capillaries may become too short for alveolar–capillary equilibration and arterial hypoxemia results (see Chapter 37 for more details). Reprinted by permission of the publishers from Figure 12.4, Weibel, E.R. (1984) *The Pathway for Oxygen*. Harvard University Press, Cambridge, MA. Copyright by the President and Fellows of Harvard College.

Horses exercised at a lower speed (4 m/s) do not show significant changes in arterial Po_2 during exercise. In heavily exercising healthy human males, arterial Po_2 is maintained at resting or at only slightly lower levels. However, in highly trained male athletes and a significant population of healthy females, arterial

Po_2 during maximal exercise may fall significantly below resting values. The combined effect of a falling arterial Po_2 and pH and rising body and blood temperature during exercise is a gradual fall in the oxygen saturation, restoration of which (inspired hyperoxia) improves oxygen transport and exercise performance.

Hypercapnia may further negatively impact the horse's exercise performance by elevating H^+ particularly in the working muscles.

Exercise-induced pulmonary hemorrhage

Exercise-induced pulmonary hemorrhage (EIPH) is defined as bleeding from the lungs associated with exercise. **Epistaxis** or "bleeding" is a clinical sign which may be observed in performance horses during or following exercise. A direct correlation exists between a horse's age, the distance raced, and the incidence/frequency of EIPH. Thus, older horses and those enduring prolonged intense exercise bouts have a greater tendency to suffer EIPH.

EIPH is characterized by pulmonary hypertension, edema in the gas-exchange region of the lung, rupture of the pulmonary capillaries, intra-alveolar hemorrhage, and the presence of blood in the airways. Endoscopic surveys and **bronchoalveolar lavage (BAL)** studies suggest that hemorrhage occurs in essentially all Thoroughbred horses during racing or training.

Numerous causes and pathophysiologic mechanisms have been proposed for EIPH, including pulmonary hypertension, alveolar pressure swings, small airway disease, **upper airway obstruction (laryngeal hemiplegia)**, **exercise-induced blood hyperviscosity**, and the mechanical stresses of respiration and locomotion. The preponderance of evidence suggests that stress failure of the pulmonary capillaries results from pulmonary vascular hypertension in combination with very negative intrapleural pressures, which create a **high capillary transmural pressure** that ruptues the fragile blood–gas barrier. Pulmonary hypertension may be a physiologic response to excessive workloads or a response to pathology. Elevated left atrial pressure during intense exercise suggests a problem with compliance of the left ventricle or the valves of the heart.

Furosemide has traditionally been used to prevent EIPH; it reduces plasma volume and pulmonary vascular pressures. A **nasal strip** has recently been implemented to prevent EIPH; it supports the nasal passages and decreases nasal resistance, a major source of pulmonary resistance. Figure 41.17 shows the reduction in EIPH in Thoroughbred horses during exercise by furosemide and the nasal strip.

Muscular system

1 How does the percentage of live weight occupied by muscle in racehorses and greyhounds compare to that in other horses and dogs?

2 What are the different types of muscle fibers and how do they vary across different breeds of horses?

3 How are muscle fibers recruited during exercise?

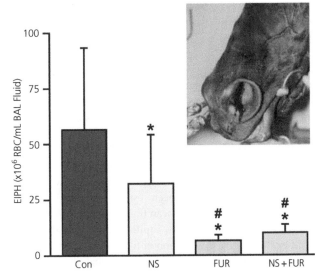

Figure 41.17 Exercise-induced pulmonary hemorrhage (EIPH), measured by bronchoalveolar lavage (BAL), was reduced significantly (*, $P < 0.05$) in the nasal strip (NS), furosemide (FUR), and NS + FUR trials compared with the control (CON). Furosemide (FUR and NS + FUR) further lessened (#, $P < 0.05$) the EIPH response compared with NS administration; however, simultaneous NS and FUR use offered no further benefit. Adapted from Figure 2, Kindig, C.A., McDonough, P., Fenton, G., Poole, D.C. and Erickson, H.H. (2001) Efficacy of nasal strip and furosemide in mitigating EIPH in Thoroughbred horses. *Journal of Applied Physiology* **91**:1396–1400.

Table 41.5 Percentage of live weight occupied by muscle, bone and fat, and the muscle/bone ratio in the horse, dog and human.

	Muscle	Bone	Fat	Muscle/bone
Thoroughbreds*	52	12	1.12	4.3
Other horses*	42	12	2.11	3.5
Greyhounds*	57	12	0.28	4.7
Other dogs*	44	12	0.94	3.6
Human (male athlete)	40	12	10	3.3

*Adapted from Gunn (1987), in *Equine Exercise Physiology 2* (eds J.R. Gillespie and N.E. Robinson), pp. 253–264. ICEEP Publications, Davis, CA.

Skeletal muscle adaptations

Adaptations in skeletal muscle occur at the gross, microscopic, and biochemical levels during exercise and following a period of exercise training. In the racing greyhound, muscle comprises 57% of body mass (Table 41.5), considerably higher than the 44% found in other dogs and 40% in most mammals studied. Similarly, skeletal muscle comprises 52% of total body weight in the Thoroughbred compared with 42% in other horses.

Muscle fiber types

Two distinct types of fibers have been identified. The **type I (or slow-twitch) fibers** have a smaller cross-sectional area and a slower contraction and relaxation time than **type II (fast-twitch)**

Table 41.6 Middle gluteal muscle fiber composition from different breeds of untrained horses (percent fiber type, mean ± SEM).

	Slow twitch (type I)	Fast twitch (type IIA)	Fast twitch (type IIB)
Quarter Horse	8.7 ± 0.8	51.0 ± 1.6	40.3 ± 1.6
Thoroughbred broodmares			
Elite	11.0 ± 0.7	57.1 ± 1.3	32.0 ± 1.3
Moderate 2 year olds	14.7 ± 0.4	65.1 ± 0.5	20.2 ± 0.5
Arabian	14.4 ± 2.5	47.8 ± 3.2	37.8 ± 2.8
Standardbred	18.1 ± 1.6	55.4 ± 2.2	26.6 ± 2.0
Shetland pony	21.0 ± 1.2	38.8 ± 1.9	40.2 ± 2.7
Heavy hunter	30.8 ± 3.1	37.1 ± 3.3	32.1 ± 3.4
Donkey	24.0 ± 3.0	38.2 ± 3.0	37.8 ± 2.8

Source: adapted from Table 2, Snow, D.H. (1983), in Snow, D.H., Persson, S.G.B. and Rose, R.J. (eds) *Equine Exercise Physiology*, pp. 160–183. Granta Editions, Cambridge, UK.

fibers. In general, type I fibers are highly oxidative and are more fatigue-resistant than type II fibers. Type II fibers can be further subdivided into subtypes IIA, IIB, and IIC fibers. Type IIA represents more oxidative fibers, whereas type IIB is more glycolytic and type IIC appears to be intermediate in both oxidative and glycolytic capacity. In contrast to many species including horses, all the type II muscle fibers in dogs are highly oxidative. Within and across species, muscle oxidative capacity (**mitochondrial volume density**) and myoglobin concentration are correlated and thus oxidative muscles appear redder than their less oxidative or more glycolytic counterparts.

Differences in the fiber composition of limb muscles can be seen among breeds of both species. These differences relate to performance characteristics for which the particular breed has been selected. In the horse, this difference is most prominent in the middle gluteal muscle, one of the largest and most important muscles for the generation of propulsive force (Table 41.6). Variations also exist between and within breeds in fiber cross-sectional area and oxidative capacity.

Although the proportions of slow-twitch and fast-twitch fibers are predominantly the result of genetic endowment, some evidence suggests that alterations in the properties of these fibers and their subtypes occur in response to training. The transition is usually toward increases in the proportions of the more oxidative type IIA fibers (i.e., increased ratio of type IIA/IIB). Dramatic increases in the volume density of mitochondria and concomitant increases in the oxidative enzymes involved in the oxidative production of ATP have been reported in horses undergoing various forms of training.

Elite endurance horses show higher percentages of type I and IIA fibers and lower percentages of type IIB fibers in their middle gluteal muscles than average competitors. In human endurance events, several reports have equated a high proportion of slow-twitch fibers in active muscles with superior performance. In contrast, sprint athletes usually display a greater percentage of type IIB muscle fibers in their locomotory muscles.

Section VI: The Cardiovascular System

Muscle fiber recruitment

For the maintenance of posture and at low exercise intensities, only type I and some type IIA fibers must be recruited; hence, it is desirable for these fibers to be fatigue-resistant. As the workload increases, development of more tension is necessary, and more type IIA fibers are recruited. The very forceful contractions required for rapid acceleration and power generation result in the recruitment of more type IIB fibers. Increased exercise intensity will lead to progressive recruitment of the faster-contracting, more powerful fibers. However, if prolonged low-intensity exercise is performed, a progressive recruitment from I through to IIB fibers takes place to maintain the required work level as the recruited muscle fibers fatigue. As the animal approaches exhaustion, all the motor units, regardless of type, may be used. This suggests that during prolonged submaximal exercise, some motor units become exhausted and drop out of the contractile process as others are added. In contrast, under conditions of exercise in which production of maximal muscle tension is required, for example Quarter Horse or Thoroughbred racing, all or nearly all muscle fiber types are recruited from the commencement of exercise.

Alterations in muscle fiber types

Skeletal muscle has the capacity to adapt to a wide variety of contractile patterns in the everyday life of an animal. One property of this tissue that allows these adaptations is the greater suitability of some motor units than others to certain types of activity. For example, the higher oxidative potential of type I and IIA motor units, relative to type IIB units, makes them more suitable to prolonged activity, when fuel reserves can be used to greatest advantage. Conversely, type IIB fibers are best suited for short intense contractile patterns in which the production and tolerance of lactate are required. Thus, it is not surprising that elite endurance horses have been found to have high proportions of type I and IIA fibers, whereas animals performing high-speed exercise (e.g., racing Quarter Horses and Thoroughbreds) tend to have higher proportions of type IIA and IIB muscle fibers.

Fiber area

In addition to the importance of the proportions of type I and type II fibers to muscle function and in assessing athletic ability, the cross-sectional area of individual fibers also plays a significant role because it influences force output. The greater the cross-sectional area of a muscle fiber, the greater the potential for force output. Therefore, where explosive acceleration is needed, recruitment of larger type IIB fibers rather than smaller type IIA fibers is desirable. However, as they are usually of low oxidative capacity and rely primarily on very limited carbohydrate reserves (glucose, glycogen), they are rapidly fatigued and of little use for powering endurance exercise, for which highly oxidative fibers are required which can better utilize energetically plentiful fat reserves. The Quarter Horse has the largest cross-sectional area of type IIB fibers, constituting about 54%

of the muscle mass, whereas the contributions of type IIB fibers in Thoroughbreds and Standardbreds are 46% and 37%, respectively.

Capillary density

Capillaries are the interface between skeletal muscle and the vascular supply that makes the exchange of metabolic substrates and waste materials possible. Increases in the size of the capillary bed in parallel with mitochondrial proliferation with endurance training have been well documented in humans. However, studies in the horse and dog are less conclusive. In equine muscle, a correlation of fiber type distribution with gross performance capacity has been established. The capillary density is determined by the mean fiber area and the **capillary-to-fiber ratio**. To some extent, **capillary density** is also influenced by the relative distribution of fiber types, which differ in oxygen diffusional capacities. Of the individual fiber types, the highest diffusional capacity (small fibers surrounded by many capillaries) is displayed by type I fibers and the lowest by type IIB fibers, which is in accordance with their respective capacities for aerobic metabolism. It is now thought that a high capillary volume density in muscle is more important for increasing red blood cell transit time and the number of red blood cells available to facilitate oxygen off-loading than for reducing oxygen diffusion distances.

Myoglobin

The overall evidence seems to be that myoglobin levels are highest in those species that engage in high levels of muscular activity. The Thoroughbred has at least twice as much myoglobin in its muscle as other species. Myoglobin possesses an oxygen dissociation curve that is shifted to the left relative to hemoglobin. This feature facilitates the movement of oxygen from the blood into the myocyte and may play a considerable role in oxygen delivery to the tissues. In addition, myoglobin concentrations in animals increase with prolonged endurance training (in concert with oxidative enzymes), thus demonstrating an enhanced potential to support aerobic metabolism by increasing oxygen uptake.

Biochemical changes

A general increase in mitochondrial volume and oxidative enzymes occurs after an aerobic training program. The enzyme activities in limb muscles in Thoroughbred horses have been examined after a 10–15 week training period involving predominantly submaximal, but some high-speed exercise. The activities of nearly all enzymes increase. Thus, substantial increases in both aerobic and anaerobic potential occur with training. The major effects of endurance training are increased use of fat with concomitant sparing of muscle glycogen, reduced blood lactate accumulation, and increased work capacity during prolonged submaximal and also maximal work.

In resting muscle samples, type I fibers have lower glycogen content than either the IIA or IIB fibers. Following endurance exercise, type I fibers show the most glycogen depletion. As the distance or the intensity increases, progressive recruitment of type IIA and IIB fibers occurs. The mechanism for the progressive fiber-type recruitment appears to be related to fiber contractile properties already discussed. Glycogen repletion occurs in the reverse pattern to depletion, with preferential repletion of type IIB relative to type I fibers.

Histochemistry, biochemistry, and morphometry

Training regimes that improve performance in humans and animals have been shown to induce changes in the cardiovascular system and also in the skeletal muscles involved in exercise. Growth itself and spontaneous activity, rather than any kind of controlled superimposed activity, seem to be the most important factors inducing the changes in muscle characteristics.

In humans, lactate has been suggested as the major contributor in promoting muscle fatigue during intense short-term exercise. In the horse, dog, and other species, exercise depletes the muscle of glycogen. The prime precursor of lactate formation in skeletal muscle during intense short exercise is intramuscular glycogen. The fuels used in exercise are dependent on the involvement of the different muscle types. The greater the speed, the greater the rate of glycogen utilization and lactate production, and as the energy demands exceed the aerobic capacity of the muscle fibers involved, there is an **obligatory anaerobiosis** (reliance on non oxygen-related energy sources).

$\dot{V}\text{O}_{2\text{max}}$ and quantifying the blood lactate response to submaximal exercise are generally recognized to be excellent descriptors of aerobic performance and capacity. Endurance exercise induces a considerable increase in the volume density of mitochondria and lipids in humans. Mitochondrial volume densities are higher in trained racehorses than in untrained ones. The volume of mitochondria closely relates to the $\dot{V}\text{O}_{2\text{max}}$ potential of skeletal muscle tissue.

Energy considerations

Maintenance of muscular contraction during exercise requires the provision of large amounts of chemical energy. Although various sources of energy are available, **adenosine triphosphate (ATP)** is the universal intracellular vehicle of chemical energy within skeletal muscle.

Energy for muscular contraction

During muscular work, ATP is hydrolyzed to adenosine diphosphate (ADP) in skeletal muscle, with the release of inorganic phosphate and energy by the myosin ATPase. During this process, a large amount of chemical potential energy is released as kinetic energy. Once this energy is liberated, it can be utilized by the muscle contractile proteins to generate force. However, under normal conditions, only a limited amount of ATP is present in skeletal muscle and this is sufficient to maintain muscular contraction for only a few seconds. There are two distinct processes that provide the intracellular replenishment of ATP: (i) **oxidative (aerobic) phosphorylation** in which the major substrates are circulating **nonesterified fatty acids (NEFA)** and glucose, together with intramuscular glycogen and triglycerides; and (ii) **anaerobic phosphorylation**, in which ATP is regenerated from creatine phosphate depletion, circulating glucose, and local glycogen stores.

Depending on the type of exercise, a balance occurs between the contributions of oxidative and anaerobic phosphorylation. Therefore, during short-term intense exercise such as sprinting, energy liberation will heavily involve anaerobic pathways. In contrast, beyond the initial transient (first minute) endurance exercise relies almost exclusively on oxidative phosphorylation.

Regulation of substrate utilization

Regulation of substrate utilization involves complex metabolic regulation within muscle cells. During periods when blood flow to muscle is adequate to provide oxygen and NEFA, fatty acids appear to be the preferred metabolic substrate. As a result, glucose and glycogen metabolism is partially inhibited. However, when fatty acid oxidation is unable to meet the energy needs of the muscle cells, whether because of high muscle energy expenditures or because of inadequate blood flow (oxygen delivery), the inhibition of glucose/glycogen metabolism is relieved and glycolysis proceeds.

Substrate utilization in the exercising horse

During exercise, the metabolic requirements of muscle vary according to the duration and/or intensity of the work. As a result of the fine metabolic control that occurs in skeletal muscle, a highly regulated system operates in which the most effective contribution of the various energy-producing pathways occurs at any given time. These contributions are directly related to the force and speed of muscular contraction, the availability of substrates, and/or the presence of metabolites. As exercise commences, the immediate energy source is locally available ATP. However, skeletal muscle ATP stores are very limited and during physiological contraction ATP concentrations are maintained close to resting levels at the expense of **creatine phosphate** stores. Creatine phosphate is able to donate its high-energy phosphate and therefore becomes an important source of energy for working muscle. Creatine phosphate levels are also limited in skeletal muscle, and if exercise continues other mechanisms for the provision of energy are required. Glycolysis, with the production of pyruvate and, to some extent, lactate, provides the ongoing energy supply. Within approximately 30 s from the onset of exercise, the glycolytic processes reach peak energy production. Because equine muscle has a large capacity for glycogen storage, this substrate is able to provide a considerable source of energy especially during short bouts of high-intensity exercise. However, during low-intensity exercise, fat represents a major source of energy. Thus, according to the intensity of exercise, a balance between anaerobic (glucose/glycogen) and aerobic (glucose/glycogen/fat) pathways occurs. The oxygen pressure in the contracting myocytes, activities of the mitochondrial/cytosolic enzymes, and the hormonal and physicochemical intramuscular environment determine the extent to which glycolytic and oxidative metabolic processes contribute to muscle energetics.

Morphology and speed

Visual observations suggest that animals noted for their high speed of running are characterized by having long legs in relation to their body length, whereas animals noted for their strength rather than fleetness have proportionately shorter legs. Comparisons of bulldogs with greyhounds, leopards with cheetahs, and draft horses with Thoroughbreds are examples of this phenomenon.

In the greyhound, Quarter Horse, and Thoroughbred, the proportion of muscle in the femoral region is greater than in other breeds of these species. Thoroughbreds and Quarter Horses have a greater mass of their hindlimb nearer the hip joint than other breeds. This feature favors a high natural frequency of hindlimb movement and facilitates a higher stride frequency and, consequently, a faster speed of running in these breeds compared with others. This greater muscle mass may be explained by both higher fiber numbers and cross-sectional areas. In contrast, in the dog, fiber areas are relatively small.

Thermoregulation and fluid balance

> 1 What are the principal means by which the body dissipates heat?
> 2 What is the composition of sweat in the horse?

Muscular activity requires the transduction of chemical energy to mechanical energy. Traditionally, the superior human athlete (and presumably the canine and equine athlete) have been assumed to have a maximal metabolic efficiency of approximately 25%. That is, only about 25% of the available chemical energy is convertible to work. This compares with 1–3% for the gasoline engine. The remaining energy is converted to heat, which must be conducted to the environment if body temperature is to remain unchanged. When exercise is performed in environments where temperature and/or humidity are high, the competing demands for evaporative cooling and energy output may limit performance and, in some instances, lead to serious heat-associated disturbances.

Energetics of exercise

As mentioned above, exercise energetics may be differentiated into aerobic and anaerobic processes. $\dot{V}o_2$ is a reliable and measurable indicator of the rate of aerobic metabolism. $\dot{V}o_2$ and heat production continue to be elevated during the recovery period and may remain elevated for an hour or more. At very high work intensities (i.e., short-term anaerobic exercise), the rate of heat production may exceed basal levels by 40–60 times. The thermoregulatory responses to the heat load generated at this work rate may limit performance, particularly when environmental temperature and humidity are high.

Thermoregulation

During exercise, the burden of dissipating the increased production of metabolic heat is placed on the thermoregulatory mechanisms. There are four principal means by which the body dissipates heat: conduction, convection, radiation, and evaporation. The evaporative route is the most efficient means of heat loss during exercise and may be the only means of heat dissipation in hot environments.

An essential function of the blood circulation is the transport of excess heat from the interior of the body to the surface. As the body's heat content increases in response to the increased metabolism associated with exercise, the cutaneous blood vessels dilate. Venous return from the extremities takes place through more superficial veins, thus increasing heat conductance of the tissues. The increased cutaneous circulation elevates skin temperature, facilitating heat loss by both convection and radiation, provided environmental temperature is lower than skin temperature. In addition, evaporative heat loss is facilitated by cutaneous vasodilation. The circulatory system must accommodate the competing demands for increased cutaneous blood flow and the increased metabolic requirements of working muscles.

If the heat load is sufficiently large, sweat glands are activated, particularly in the horse. Sweating induced by exercise occurs in response to both circulating epinephrine and the sympathetic nervous system, but only the latter is involved in thermal sweating. Epinephrine-induced sweating in the horse is mediated by β_2 receptors. Sweat promotes heat loss only when the sweat evaporates. At extremely high environmental temperatures, evaporative heat loss may not be able to keep pace with the exercise-induced heat load and the animal will gain heat from the environment. High humidity prevents complete evaporation. With incomplete evaporation, sweat production results in little or no heat transfer, but can contribute to dehydration. In controlled endurance rides of 60 km, the mean weight loss in a horse may be 5–6% of body weight. Conditions of high environmental temperature and humidity thus pose a serious risk to the equine athlete, particularly when performing protracted submaximal exercise. Although sweating is the principal means of evaporative cooling in exercising horses, the respiratory tract also contributes to heat and water loss.

In the dog sweating is insignificant in thermoregulation and panting is more important. Panting is more specifically discussed in Chapter 25 and is more generally discussed in Chapter 14. It is an important temperature-regulating mechanism in many species, particularly in dogs. The respiratory frequency increases to 200–400 breaths/min and the tidal volume decreases during panting so alveolar ventilation remains constant and arterial CO_2 levels do not fall.

The thermoregulatory responses to exercise-generated heat loads are not always sufficient to prevent elevation of body temperature. Muscle, rectal, and blood temperatures increase dramatically in the horse with increasing work intensity and duration; rectal temperatures as high as 41–43 °C have been recorded in the horse (Figure 41.18). Racing greyhounds in hot

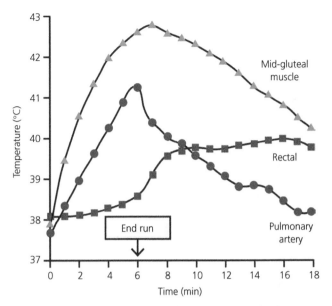

Figure 41.18 Temperatures recorded with thermocouples during and after a 6-min run in a Standardbred horse exercising at 98% maximal rate of oxygen consumption. Triangles indicate temperatures 2.5 cm deep in the middle gluteal muscle; circles indicate temperatures in the pulmonary artery; squares indicate temperatures 25 cm deep in rectum. Note that far higher rectal temperatures have been recorded in the exercising horse without untoward health consequences. From Figure 1, Jones, J.H., Taylor, C.R., Lindholm, A., Straub, R., Longworth, K.E. and Karas, R.H. (1989) Blood gas measurements during exercise: errors due to temperature correction. *Journal of Applied Physiology* **67**:879–884.

climates often exhibit symptoms of **heat stroke, azoturia, exertional rhabdomyolosis**, and/or cardiac failure during the summer racing season. During a 500-m race, ear canal or tympanic membrane temperatures can increase from 36.5 to 41.6 °C and rectal temperature from 38.0 to 41.6 °C.

Sweat composition
Sodium (Na⁺) is the principal cation in horse sweat and is present at concentrations similar to or higher than those in serum. Potassium ion (K⁺) concentrations in the sweat are typically 10–20 times greater than those of the serum. There is also a very high concentration of chloride ion (Cl⁻) in equine sweat. The relatively high ionic composition of equine sweat is in contrast to human sweat, which is almost invariably hypotonic relative to plasma. These differences in sweat composition are important in fluid and electrolyte alterations resulting from heavy sweat losses during exercise in human and equine athletes. They are also important in the provision of fluid electrolyte supplements, particularly for endurance horses.

Fluid balance
During exercise, sweating is the principal route of both fluid and electrolyte loss in the horse. Sweat rates may approach 10–12 L/hour during prolonged exercise in a hot environment. With massive fluid and electrolyte losses in sweat, excretion by other routes is probably altered. When sweat electrolyte losses are

large, renal mechanisms for electrolyte conservation are brought into play in an attempt to maintain homeostasis.

Endurance-trained horses tend to maintain a lower resting hematocrit than horses trained for shorter, faster races. The lower hematocrit is not due to a decreased erythrocyte count or an increased storage of erythrocytes in the spleen, but to an increased plasma volume. Both human and equine athletes develop an expanded plasma volume in response to endurance exercise training, which may serve to defend against excessive water losses during protracted work and heat stress.

Hormonal responses

> 1 What are the two major sites of action of thyroid hormones?
> 2 What hormones are produced by the adrenal gland during exercise?
> 3 What other hormones are involved during exercise?

The supply, uptake, and utilization of substrates for the production of energy in working skeletal muscles are integral components of an organism's ability to carry out physical exercise. The adaptation by the organism to repeated bouts of exercise is reflected in the use it makes of the different substrates available. The onset of exercise is associated with changes in the plasma concentration of energy substrates and/or their delivery to working muscles in association with the changes that occur in cardiac output and blood flow distribution. The hormones produced by the various endocrine glands are important components of the control mechanism regulating substrate supply and energy production. Excessive or inadequate levels of several hormones place constraints on exercise performance. In addition, the plasma levels of several hormones are increased with exercise, as part of the integrated response to stress.

Signals from either the working muscles or via reflexes originating from higher motor centers in the brain can modify the response of the glands of the endocrine system directly via pituitary hormones or indirectly via the **sympathoadrenal system**. The initial response to the onset of exercise is enhancement of sympathoadrenal activity and secretion of pituitary hormones, which result in a reduction in the plasma concentration of insulin and a rise in virtually all other hormones.

Thyroid gland
Thyroid hormones are essential for maximal exercise performance and act at two major sites. In the mitochondria, thyroid hormone stimulates cellular respiration, leading to an increased rate of oxygen utilization and energy production. This is most evident in skeletal and cardiac muscle. At the nucleus, thyroid hormones increase the rate of RNA synthesis, which in turn leads to an increase in protein synthesis and in the concentration of many enzymes. There is probably a coordinated pituitary–thyroid response to repeated daily exercise that

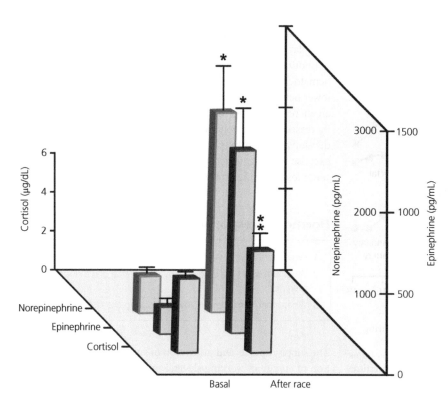

Figure 41.19 Plasma cortisol and catecholamine levels in the Thoroughbred horse before and after racing. Values are expressed as the mean of 10 determinations ± standard error of the mean. Significant differences from basal values are represented by * ($P < 0.0001$) and ** ($P < 0.05$). Adapted from Figure 2, Martinez, R., Godoy, A., Naretto, E. *et al.* (1988) Neuroendocrine changes produced by competition stress on the Thoroughbred race horse. *Comparative Biochemistry and Physiology A* **91**:599–602.

is largely influenced by the intensity of the exercise and is reflected in an increased production and turnover of thyroid hormones.

Adrenal gland

In common with other steroid hormones, **glucocorticoids** exert their effect at the nuclear level by increasing the production of RNA that supplies the code for protein synthesis. Among the enzymes produced are several that deaminate amino acids and stimulate glucose synthesis, **hepatic glycogenolysis**, and **lipolysis**. These actions facilitate metabolism to provide additional fuel for prolonged submaximal exercise, which might be compromised by inadequate levels of glucocorticoids. In the horse, the dominant glucocorticoid is **cortisol**. Cortisol levels are increased during and immediately after exercise in most species, including the horse (Figure 41.19). In addition to the role of physical stress, psychological stress may also influence the induction of cortisol secretion.

Circulating epinephrine initiates many of the metabolic events required for the maintenance of vigorous exercise. Epinephrine stimulates the conversion of muscle glycogen to glucose phosphate and ultimately pyruvate, activates tissue lipases, inhibits insulin release, stimulates the heart to increase rate and cardiac output, is involved in the redistribution of blood flow during exercise, facilitates neuromuscular transmission in skeletal muscle, stimulates contractile processes in fast-twitch fibers, relaxes bronchioles, and increases respiratory rate. Unlike thyroid and steroid hormones, catecholamines exert their effects within minutes.

The response of the sympathetic nervous system during exercise is reflected in the plasma concentrations of epinephrine and norepinephrine (Figure 41.19). This response is generally proportional to the intensity of the work performed, with norepinephrine levels being significantly increased at lower work intensities than epinephrine levels. A ninefold increase in plasma norepinephrine has been noted after brief maximal exercise in the horse and a 50% increase after an endurance ride. In contrast, there is little increase in plasma epinephrine during low-intensity work, whereas a marked increase occurs during heavy exercise, especially if it is accompanied by emotional stress. Although basal levels are unchanged, catecholamines increase less in trained subjects during submaximal exercise, unlike the adrenocortical hormones.

Other hormones

In the horse, as in humans and other species, both the intensity and the duration of exercise influences the changes in **insulin** and **glucagon**. It seems appropriate that each component contributes to an integrated response to stress. Adrenocorticotropic hormone (ACTH) stimulates cortisol release, which plays an important role in combating stress and also increases the release of epinephrine. **Lipotropic hormones** mobilize lipids, which provide the fuel for prolonged muscular activity. **Endorphins** may suppress the pain of fatigue and trauma. A rapidly growing body of evidence suggests that the **analgesia,** euphoria, and motor stimulation of **endogenous opioids** play an important role in exercise performance in humans.

Evaluation of exercise tolerance and fitness

> 1 What variables are used to evaluate exercise tolerance and fitness?
>
> 2 How do these variables change with training?

Exercise tolerance is related to the functional capacity of both the cardiopulmonary and musculoskeletal systems. Both the dimensional and functional capacities of these organ systems can be limiting factors for $\dot{V}o_{2max}$ and consequently for exercise performance. Aerobic energy production predominates during work lasting more than about 1 min. However, during heavy exercise, both aerobic and anaerobic energy production contribute to the work output. An increasing demand on energy production caused by continuous physical training induces a corresponding dimensional and functional adaptation of the cardiovascular system. It is possible to predict the degree of adaptation to physical work (i.e., exercise tolerance) from variables indicative of cardiovascular function, such as the post-exercise total hemoglobin level.

Blood volume is important to maintain or achieve high cardiac outputs which, in conjunction with elevated hemoglobin, facilitate tissue oxygen delivery. It is oxygen delivery to exercising muscles that primarily limits aerobic capacity.

In the horse, blood lactate generally does not increase significantly above the resting level until the heart rate exceeds 155–160 bpm. This indicates that a workload causing a heart rate of 150 bpm is performed almost aerobically in most horses and thus **V150, the running velocity at 150 bpm**, is an expression for the aerobic capacity of the animal. A very steep increase in blood lactate occurs above an exercise heart rate of about 200 bpm, indicating that above this level anaerobic energy release starts to play a significant role in work output.

In summary, the cardiovascular system provides the link between pulmonary ventilation and oxygen usage at the cellular level. During exercise, efficient delivery of oxygen to working skeletal and cardiac muscles is vital for maintenance of ATP production by aerobic mechanisms. The equine cardiovascular response to increased demand for oxygen delivery during exercise contributes largely to the over 80-fold increase in $\dot{V}o_2$ that occurs during maximal exercise. The large increases in cardiac output during exercise are primarily attributable to the relatively high heart rates achieved.

Higher work rates and $\dot{V}o_2$ at a given submaximal heart rate after training imply an adaptation to training that enables better oxygen delivery to and/or utilization by the working muscles. Such adaptations can be in either blood flow or a-vo_2 difference. Increases in blood hemoglobin concentrations during exercise after training are recognized but, at maximal exercise, hypoxemia may reduce arterial oxygen content. More effective redistribution of cardiac output to muscles by increased capillarization and better oxygen diffusion to cells may also be important means of increasing $\dot{V}o_2$ after training. Typically, training results in substantial elevations in maximal cardiac output (consequent to elevated stroke volume) and muscle oxygen diffusing capacity. Overall, however, the elevated maximal cardiac output rather than increased a-vo_2 difference after training accounts for the majority of increased $\dot{V}o_{2max}$.

Nutrition

> 1 How does the source of energy influence performance?
>
> 2 How does fat influence performance in sled dogs over long distances?
>
> 3 What is the value of glycogen loading in the horse?

Energy

The amount of additional energy required during exercise depends on the type of work, rate and length of work, condition of the animal, and the environmental temperature. Exercise conditioning increases the resting metabolism, most likely due to an increase in lean body mass; the anticipation of exercise also increases energy metabolism and raises dietary energy requirements.

The basic needs of the greyhound for racing are not vastly different from maintenance requirements. The average caloric intake is only 30–40% above estimated daily requirements. Food requirements for physical fitness involving short bursts of intensive exercise do not necessarily involve a high food intake.

Source of energy

The source of energy can influence performance. Energy requirements for horses are met with forage and forage–grain mixtures. A horse with high energy requirements cannot obtain all energy from bulky hay. Endurance horses need more roughage; this dilates the intestinal volume and increases the intestinal water and electrolyte reserve. There is controversy on the effect of type of grain on performance in horses. Corn contains twice as much energy as oats per volume; however, digestive upsets and metabolic problems may occur if corn is substituted for oats. Fat has been suggested for athletic horses; the NEFA are a primary source of energy for horses during prolonged exercise. Fat also improves the performance of sled dogs racing over prolonged distances. These animals may have average daily caloric expenditures over 10,000 kcal. Feeding high levels of fat during training may condition an animal to use fat more efficiently during endurance exercise because the enzymes are adapted to fat metabolism. During endurance events, fat is more likely to be a source of energy than glycogen. The addition of fat to equine diets protects against a decline in blood glucose during exercise.

Glycogen storage

Endurance capacity in the human athlete is directly related to the content of glycogen in the working muscles. Prolonged heavy exercise may result in almost total depletion of muscle glycogen

Section VI: The Cardiovascular System

and this contributes to muscle fatigue. Increased glycogen storage is accomplished in humans by eating high-fat, high-protein diets during training in order to severely deplete glycogen stores. The athlete then eats a high-carbohydrate diet 3 days prior to the event to enhance storage. In the horse, studies of glycogen loading regimens are very limited. Glycogen loading in horses appears to have limited value, particularly in short events because glycogen stores are not depleted. Increased glycogen stores may be of value in endurance horses competing over long distances. Excessive glycogen loading may predispose a horse to exertional myopathy and considerable elevation of body weight.

Protein

In the horse, there is little or no increase in dietary protein requirements during exercise. A small amount of nitrogenous compounds including protein are lost in sweat; however, the increased intake required to meet energy requirements provides sufficient protein. Plasma concentrations of urea and creatinine are consistently increased in endurance horses. The increase in urea is primarily due to a significant increase in the rate of protein catabolism. High-protein diets may actually be detrimental. Horses on a high-protein diet sweat more profusely and pulse and respiration rates are higher after long endurance events. If water is limited, a high-protein diet is not recommended because additional water is needed for the excretion of nitrogen.

Amino acid intake may affect the racing performance of greyhounds. Muscular work increases amino acid uptake and protein synthesis in muscle. Beef is the main source of protein in many kennels which is supplied as a broth. Fluid balance is critical in the racing greyhound, which does not drink very much water. Therefore, fluid needs to be supplied in the diet. Greyhounds dehydrate rapidly under hot summer conditions unless water is added to the diet.

Minerals

The exercising horse loses water, sodium, potassium, chloride, and other elements in sweat. The heavily sweating horse may develop a negative electrolyte balance. During severe sweating, muscle may be the main source to replace potassium losses by sweat. Magnesium requirements are also increased in an exercising horse because it is lost in sweat; magnesium is important in the muscle cell for ATPase activity. A growing horse that is being worked needs a higher level of calcium and phosphorus than normally required for maintenance. A growing horse that is working is more susceptible to mineral deficiency than a growing horse that is not working, because exercise increases the rate of bone turnover. Selenium is required for the integrity of muscle and is used to treat exertional myopathy.

Vitamins

Vitamin supplements for athletes are popular, but their value questionable. Good-quality hay contains an adequate level of vitamins to meet requirements in the horse, but poor-quality hay may require vitamin supplementation. Hay that is weathered or stored for over 2 years may have a low level of vitamin A activity. Grains such as oats also contain little vitamin A. Racehorses are more susceptible to thiamin deficiency than other horses; thiamin is required for energy utilization. Vitamin E is important for exercise capacity; vitamin E deficiency decreases endurance significantly.

The nutritional requirements for dogs are well documented, including recommended minimal and maximal daily intakes of both minerals and vitamins; however, the exact requirements for the racing greyhound have not been established. Nevertheless, considering the diet, physical stress of repeated racing, and parasites, greyhounds may benefit from supplementary vitamins and other additives.

Self-evaluation

Answers can be found at the end of the chapter.

1 A 3-year-old gelding named Cat Thief has just won the Kentucky Derby. A venous blood sample drawn from the jugular vein within 5 min of completion of the race would show that the hemoglobin and hematocrit have:
   A Both decreased
   B Both increased by less than 5%
   C Both increased by approximately 10–20%
   D Both increased by approximately 50%

2 A Quarter Horse named Shoot Yeah has a heart rate of 30 bpm at rest and a stroke volume of 1 L per beat. During exercise, the heart rate increases to 220 bpm and the stroke volume increases to 1.3 L per beat. What is the cardiac output at rest and during exercise?

3 What arrhythmia is common in the racehorse at rest, but disappears during exercise?

4 If you were asked to conduct an endoscopic survey of exercise-induced pulmonary hemorrhage (EIPH) in Thoroughbred racehorses at a race track near you, what would you anticipate the incidence to be?
   A 0–5%
   B 10–20%
   C 20–40%
   D 50–70%

Suggested reading

Evans, D.L. (1985) Cardiovascular adaptations to exercise and training. *Veterinary Clinics of North Americ: Equine Practice* **1**:513–531.

Gillespie, J.R. and Robinson, N.E. (eds) (1987) *Equine Exercise Physiology 2*. ICEEP Publications, Davis, CA.

Hodgson, D.R. and Rose, R.J. (1994) *The Athletic Horse*. W.B. Saunders, Philadelphia.

Holmes, J.R. (1988) *Equine Cardiology*, Vol. **IV**. School of Veterinary Science, University of Bristol, UK.

Jeffcott, L.B. (1999) Equine exercise physiology 5. Proceedings of the Fifth International Conference on Equine Exercise Physiology, Utsunomiya, Japan, 20–25 September 1998. *Equine Veterinary Journal* Suppl. 30.

Langsetmo, I., Weigle, G.E., Fedde, M.R. *et al.* (1997) $\dot{V}$o2 kinetics in the horse during moderate and heavy exercise. *Journal of Applied Physiology* **83**:1235–1241.

Lindstedt, S.L., Hokanson, J.F., Wells, D.J. *et al.* (1991) Running energetics in the pronghorn antelope. *Nature* **353**:748–750.

Marlin, D. and Nankervis, K. (2002) *Equine Exercise Physiology.* Blackwell Publishing, Oxford.

Neary, J. (2013) New thoughts on pulmonary hypertension. In: *Nebraska Veterinary Medical Association Summer Convention Proceedings, June 17–19, 2013,* pp. 120–5. Available at http://www.nvma.org/assets/site/Proceeding_Files/June%202013%20Proceedings%20.pdf

Persson, S.G.B., Lindholm, A. and Jeffcott, L.B. (eds) (1991) *Equine Exercise Physiology 3.* ICEEP Publications, Davis, CA.

Poole, D.C. and Erickson, H.H. (2008) Cardiovascular function and oxygen transport: responses to exercise and training. In: *Equine Exercise Physiology: The Science of Exercise in the Athletic Horse* (eds K. Hinchcliff, R.J. Geor and A.J. Kaneps), pp. 212–245. Saunders Elsevier, Philadelphia.

Poole, D.C. and Erickson, H.H. (2011) Highly athletic terrestrial mammals: horses and dogs. *Comprehensive Physiology* **1**:1–37.

Poole, D.C. and Erickson, H.H. (2014) Heart and vessels: function during exercise and training adaptation. In: *Equine Sports Medicine and Surgery* (eds K. Hinchcliff, A.J. Kaneps and R.J. Geor), pp. 667–694. Saunders Elsevier, Philadelphia.

Poole, D.C. and Jones, A.M. (2012) Oxygen uptake kinetics. *Comprehensive Physiology* **2**:933–996.

Richardson, R.S., Noyszewski, E.A., Kendrick, K.F., Leigh, J.S. and Wagner, P.D. (1995) Myoglobin O2 desaturation during exercise. Evidence of limited O2 transport. *Journal of Clinical Investigation* **96**:1916–1926.

Robinson, N.E. (1995) Equine exercise physiology 4. Proceedings of the Fourth International Conference on Equine Exercise Physiology, Kooralbyn, Queensland, Australia, 11–16 July 1994. *Equine Veterinary Journal* Suppl. 18.

Rose, R.J. (1985) Symposium on exercise physiology. *Veterinary Clinics of North America: Equine Practice* **1**(3):437–617.

Snow, D.H., Persson, S.G.B. and Rose, R.J. (eds) (1983) *Equine Exercise Physiology.* Granta Editions, Cambridge, UK.

Weibel, E.R. (1984) *The Pathway for Oxygen.* Harvard University Press, Cambridge, MA.

Answers

1 D. In the horse and dog, as well as several other species, the spleen acts as a reservoir for erythrocytes. Blood cells stored in the spleen can be mobilized into the circulation when there is an increased demand. The release of stored erythrocytes from the spleen into the systemic circulation is under the influence of the sympathetic nervous system and circulating catecholamines.

2 The cardiac output is the product of heart rate and stroke volume. Therefore, at rest, the cardiac output would be 30 bpm × 1 L/beat = 30 L/min. During exercise, the cardiac output would be 220 bpm × 1.3 L/beat = 286 L/min.

3 Second-degree AV block. Second-degree AV block is the most common rhythm irregularity observed in horses at rest. It is clinically recognizable by the appearance of missed ventricular beats. In the majority of cases, the atrial or fourth heart sound can be heard. In most horses with partial AV block at rest, the missed beats disappear with exercise and do not recur until heart rate again approaches a resting rate.

4 D. The diagnosis of EIPH is usually confirmed by endoscopic observation of blood in the tracheobronchial airways within 30–90 min after the completion of exercise. Endoscopic surveys have demonstrated that EIPH occurs in a high percentage (50–75%) of horses. Tracheal lavage has been used to detect EIPH by determining the presence of hemosiderophages in the aspirated fluid. BAL studies suggest that hemorrhage occurs in essentially all Thoroughbred horses.

Section VI: The Cardiovascular System

Digestion, Absorption, and Metabolism

Section Editor: Jesse P. Goff

42 Gastrointestinal Motility

Jesse P. Goff

Iowa State University, Ames, IA, USA

The digestive tracts of all animals have evolved to perform several major functions. The obvious function is to serve as a means to digest and absorb the nutrients of the diet needed to sustain the rest of the body. It is important to recognize that the lumen of the digestive tract is actually contiguous with the exterior environment. As such the lumen of the gut serves as an ecological niche for a wide variety of bacteria and, in some species, fungi and protozoa to thrive in. A major function of the gut is to identify and prevent entry of pathogens across the gut epithelium barrier. It is also critical for the immune system of the gut to have tolerance for commensal organisms, many of which aid the animal in digestion of dietary components. Another major function of the digestive tract is the elimination of wastes. This includes undigested material from the diet and removal of toxicants from the blood, carried out primarily by the liver which excretes various substances into the lumen of the gut within bile. Input from both the voluntary and autonomic nervous systems and a wide variety of hormones are required to coordinate motility and digestive processes of the gut. Nature has evolved a wide variety of methods for animals to perform the functions of the gut. Three basic types of digestive tract systems are described in detail: **simple-stomached** animals (including dogs and cats), **forestomach fermenters** (ruminants and camelids), and **hindgut fermenters** (such as the horse and rabbit).

The oral cavity

1 How are the tongue and teeth used in prehension of food in various species?

2 What are the differences between hypsodont and brachydont teeth?

The structures of the oral cavity are necessary for prehension of food, mastication of the food material, and swallowing of the material while protecting the animal from inhalation of the foodstuffs. Many strategies for moving food into the oral cavity have evolved. In horses upper and lower lips are quite flexible and sensitive and they grasp herbivorous material and draw it into the mouth far enough that the incisors can clip the stems. Pigs use their lower lips in a similar fashion. Ruminant lips are not very flexible and have limited ability to grasp food. Instead they have tongues that are long and flexible that grasp herbivorous material to be brought into the mouth to be clipped by pressing the lower incisors against the dorsal hard palate (ruminants have no incisors in their upper dental arcade). Camelids do have upper incisors but prehension of food is very similar to that in more traditional ruminants. Dogs, cats, and many other carnivores do not utilize their lips to any great extent to help them move food into their oral cavity. They generally grasp food

Section VII: Digestion, Absorption, and Metabolism

Dukes' Physiology of Domestic Animals, Thirteenth Edition. Edited by William O. Reece, Howard H. Erickson, Jesse P. Goff and Etsuro E. Uemura.
© 2015 John Wiley & Sons, Inc. Published 2015 by John Wiley & Sons, Inc.
Companion website: www.wiley.com/go/reece/physiology

with their teeth, toss food into the air and move their open mouth forward to catch the food in the more caudal aspect of their oral cavity until it can be swallowed. Most birds and reptiles also utilize a toss and catch movement of the jaws and head to move food to the back of the oral cavity. Species also differ in how they drink water. Horses and cattle, like humans, can create a negative pressure within the oral cavity that allows suction of water to the back of the oral cavity. Cats, dogs, and their wild relatives cannot develop negative pressure within their oral cavity due to elongated snouts and inability to tightly close the lips at the commissure of the mouth. These species must lap water. They turn the tip of the tongue ventrally to form a ladle which is extended into the water to lift a column of water up, followed by dropping the head down and closing the mouth to catch the water column so it can be moved to the back of the oral cavity for swallowing. This is done rapidly and repeatedly, since a dog for example may draw up just 10–15 mL of water with each lap. Birds dip their beak into the water and lift the head to allow gravity to deliver water to the back of the oral cavity.

The tongue is integral to many aspects of prehension. It has bundles of muscles that run in nearly all directions that allow great flexibility and direction of movement. There are also muscles attached to the posterior tongue that help retract or protrude and depress or elevate the tongue. The motor functions of the tongue are nearly all controlled by motor neurons of the hypoglossal or cranial nerve XII. In addition to movement, the tongue has a major sensory role. The rostral two-thirds of the tongue is innervated by the sensory lingual branch of the trigeminal (cranial nerve V), which is sensitive to temperature, touch, and pain, and the facial nerve (cranial nerve VII), which transmits a sensation of taste and carries parasympathetic fibers to the base of the taste buds. The caudal one-third of the tongue is innervated by the lingual branch of the glossopharyngeal nerve (cranial nerve IX) which carries taste sensation from taste buds, and parasympathetic efferent fibers to the taste buds. Tongues have various types of papillae, depending on species. These are mainly used to help propel food to the back of the oral cavity, though they are also useful for grooming (cat). A unique feature of the tongue is the taste bud. Figure 42.1 shows taste buds along a papilla in a rabbit tongue. Food particles proceed into the cleft between tongue papillae and can enter each taste bud through an opening pore. Inside the taste bud specialized cells react to one of five tastes (salty, sour, sweet, bitter, and umami) that might be entering the taste pore. This creates a sensory nerve impulse that is carried to the gustatory centers of the brain via the facial (VII) or glossopharyngeal (IX) cranial nerves.

Mastication of the diet can greatly aid the digestibility of the ingested material. The incisors of the dental arcade are important for cutting foodstuffs into a size that can be brought into the oral cavity. The premolars and molars are capable of reducing the ingested material into much smaller and finer particles that increase the surface area available for digestive enzymes to act upon. This is particularly important for

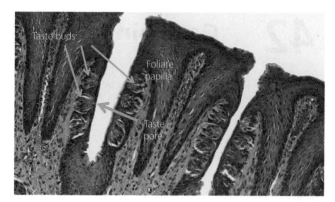

Figure 42.1 Taste buds on a foliate papilla of rabbit tongue. Note the taste pore visible as an opening of the taste bud to the lumen.

digestion of herbivorous materials. Plant cell walls need to be broken open and chewing with molars can initiate this process in the larger herbivores. Ruminants and horses have molars that are classified as **hypsodont teeth**: they emerge from the gums at a continuous rate as the animal ages (though in very old animals this process can reach an end point). Dogs, cats, and humans have **brachydont teeth**: once they emerge, they begin to wear and are not replaced. Brachydont molars are covered entirely on the occlusal surface by enamel. This hard layer must protect the softer dentin and pulp cavity throughout the life of the animal. Once the enamel is breached the tooth develops caries, which can lead to loss of the tooth. Hypsodont teeth have enamel, dentin and even pulp cementum at the occlusal surface. Because the enamel is harder than dentin, which is harder than cementum, the occlusal surface has irregular and very sharp edges to it, making hypsodont molars much more effective at grinding and shearing plant cell walls. The occlusal surface is replaced continuously as the hypsodont tooth emerges from the gum line. Rodents and rabbits have hypsodont incisors that grow continuously. In domesticated rodents and rabbits, overgrown incisors (and molars in the rabbit) constitute a leading reason for inappetance, weight loss, and the necessity for veterinary care. Individual species have great variation in tooth structure and emergence patterns, but is not discussed further in this chapter as many anatomy textbooks discuss this subject in great detail.

Salivary secretions

> **1** How is saliva secretion and composition controlled by the parasympathetic system and the hormone secretin?

As a bolus of food is being chewed, saliva is added. **Saliva** is produced by acinar glands located along the mandible and maxilla of most species. The secretions of the acinar cells are conducted by a series of ducts, beginning with intercalated ducts that lead to slightly larger striated ducts which then join with intralobular

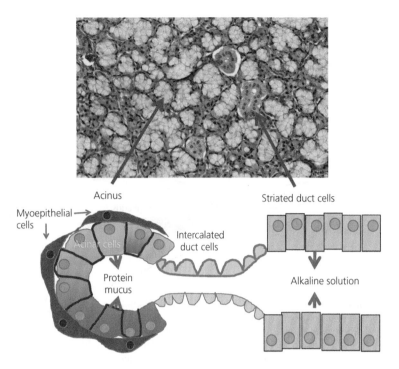

Figure 42.2 Photomicrograph of a salivary gland. Acinar cells produce proteins and antibacterial peptides. Secretion is stimulated by parasympathetic fibers that enhance metabolic activity of acinar cells and also stimulate contraction of myoepithelial cells to expel fluid into ducts. The ducts add an alkaline secretion to the saliva in response to the hormone secretin synthesized in the duodenum.

and interlobular ducts until finally the secretions reach the oral pharynx (Figure 42.2). The secretions of individual salivary glands range from a watery composition referred to as a serous secretion to a more mucoid secretion. For instance in the dog the parotid gland produces a serous secretion laden with amylase, which begins the process of starch digestion, and buffers to help control the pH of the ingesta. A lipase enzyme is also present to initiate fat digestion. Serous glands also secrete IgA and antibacterial substances such as lysozyme that also help keep bacterial numbers in check within the oral cavity. The sublingual glands of a dog produce a mucus-type saliva. The mucin helps lubricate the bolus as it passes down the esophagus. The submaxillary gland of the dog produces a mixed secretion that has both serous and mucous attributes. A 20-kg dog produces approximately 0.5–1 L of saliva daily, more when fed a dry dog food. All saliva is hypotonic to help reduce the osmotic concentration of the ingesta.

Salivary secretions are under the control of the glossopharyngeal nerve (parotid glands) and the facial nerve (submaxillary and sublingual glands). These nerves carry parasympathetic fibers and it is the parasympathetic tone that determines the rate of saliva production and secretion. Secretion occurs when myoepithelial cells (a type of epithelial cell that is able to contract) respond to parasympathetic stimulation and squeeze the acinus to propel saliva down the ducts. There is no sympathetic innervation of the salivary glands. As Pavlov demonstrated, higher centers of the brain can activate parasympathetic pathways to cause a dog to drool in anticipation of a meal. In ruminants, saliva composition can also be altered to help the animal maintain rumen pH at a more constant level. When actively chewing, the pH of ruminant saliva can increase to about 8.5. In an adult cow the amount of saliva secreted can be 100–180 L daily.

In all species, the cells lining the striated ducts of the salivary glands are capable of increasing secretion of sodium and potassium into the saliva to increase its alkalinity in order to enhance its buffering activity. These cells increase saliva pH in response to a hormone called **secretin**. Secretin is produced by enteroendocrine cells within the duodenum when the pH of the duodenum decreases.

Deglutition (swallowing)

> **1** The pathway for food and air cross each other. Describe the steps taken to insure that food does not enter the trachea or the nasopharynx.

Once the bolus of food has been chewed and is moistened by saliva and moved to the back of the oral cavity it is ready to be swallowed. **Deglutition** or swallowing is a highly complex reflex that must deliver ingesta or fluids to the esophagus while keeping such material out of the respiratory tract. Keep in mind that the pathway of airflow into the trachea and the pathway for food entering the esophagus intersect within the pharynx. The first step in swallowing is voluntary: the animal uses motor neurons to push the bolus of food to the back of the tongue. Pharyngeal receptors sense the presence of the bolus and afferent fibers of cranial nerves V, IX and X carry this information to the medulla. From this point on, the swallowing reflex is involuntary.

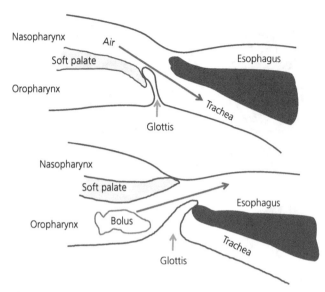

Figure 42.3 Swallowing reflex. (*Top*) Normally the glottis is open and the soft palate is down to allow air to move through the nasopharynx and oropharynx into the trachea. The upper esophageal sphincter is kept closed to reduce air entry. Once food has moved to the back of the oropharynx by voluntary muscles, an involuntary reflex causes the glottis to close over the trachea and the dorsal soft palate to be elevated to close off the nasopharynx. The hyoid apparatus lifts and the upper esophageal sphincter relaxes and the bolus enters the esophagus.

Clinical correlations

Whenever administering a pill to an animal, one must also succeed in getting the pill to the back of the tongue if it is to be actually swallowed by the patient.

The medulla coordinates the rest of the swallowing reflex. Respiration efforts are inhibited by the medulla, reducing the danger of food inhalation. Efferent motor neurons carried by cranial nerves VII, IX, X and XII carry out the following steps. The back of the tongue and floor of mouth elevate to drive the bolus to the caudal pharynx. The soft palate is elevated dorsally to close off the nasopharynx, preventing food from exiting via the nose (Figure 42.3). The hyoid apparatus elevates and the epiglottis moves downward to cover the opening to the glottis. Laryngeal muscles tighten around the glottis as well to prevent food from entering the trachea. At this point the upper esophageal sphincter relaxes allowing the bolus to enter the esophagus. Snakes have an interesting adaptation that allows them to take minutes to hours to swallow their meal. In addition to unhinging their jaw to swallow objects many times wider than they are, snakes can extend their glottis and trachea forward and out the side of the mouth. This allows them to take in air during the entire swallowing process.

Difficulties with swallowing can signal a variety of problems in animals. Failure to close the glottis during the swallowing reflex can lead to aspiration pneumonia. Anesthetized or very weak animals can inhale vomitus or saliva because reflex centers

are depressed and do not respond to pharyngeal receptor stimulation that initiates the reflex. In horses, guttural pouch infections can damage cranial nerves IX, X and XII interfering with the swallowing reflex. Animals born with cleft palates are unable to close off the nasopharynx and milk will be seen coming out of the nose during suckling. In all species, problems with swallowing can signal tumors within the medulla. As veterinarians, we must always consider rabies and other neurological diseases as a possible cause of swallowing difficulty in animals.

MOVEMENT OF INGESTA THROUGH THE GASTROINTESTINAL TRACT

Once the bolus of food has entered the esophagus the bolus takes a path through a long tube that varies in width and functions, but which essentially consists of at least two muscle layers that will act to propel the bolus down the tract. In some areas these muscles contract to prevent movement of material, forming sphincters or valves that open only occasionally. The contraction of these muscles is controlled by a novel and unique collection of neurons that form the enteric nervous system, the so-called "brain of the gut." This system can autonomously control many actions within the gut. However, its actions are often coordinated over long distances in the gastrointestinal tract by input from the autonomic nervous system and by input from endocrine or paracrine hormones produced within the intestinal tract.

The enteric nervous system

---

1 Describe the location of the myenteric and submucosal plexuses.
2 What kinds of neurotransmitters are made by neurons of the enteric nervous system?
3 Describe how stretch of a segment of intestine can result in a localized segmental contraction without any input from nerves outside the intestine.

The enteric nervous system (ENS) functions from esophagus to anus. It consists of two layers of nerve cell bodies named on the basis of their location (Figure 42.4). The cell bodies of the **submucosal plexus** (Meissner's plexus) lie within the submucosa below the tunica mucosa. The cell bodies of the **myenteric plexus** (Auerbach's plexus) lie between the inner circular smooth muscle layer that stretches around the circumference of the intestine and the outer longitudinal smooth muscle cells that runs parallel the length of the intestine. These nerve cell bodies extend sensory fibers to the secretory, absorptive, and enteroendocrine cells lining the lumen of the gut, as well as sensory fibers within the lamina propria, submucosa, and muscle layers. These sensory neurons can detect a variety of changes within the gut,

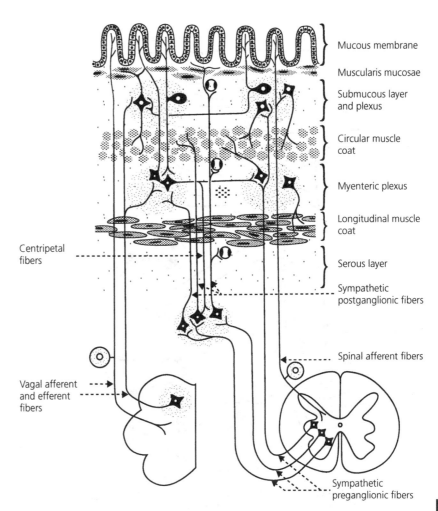

Mucous membrane

Muscularis mucosae

Submucous layer and plexus

Circular muscle coat

Myenteric plexus

Longitudinal muscle coat

Serous layer

Sympathetic postganglionic fibers

Spinal afferent fibers

Sympathetic preganglionic fibers

Centripetal fibers

Vagal afferent and efferent fibers

Figure 42.4 Scheme of the extrinsic and intrinsic innervation of the intestine. From Reece, W.O. (ed.) (2004) *Dukes' Physiology of Domestic Animals*, 12th edn. Cornell University Press, Ithaca, NY. Reproduced with permission from Cornell University Press.

including distension (stretch receptors), pH of the luminal contents, osmolarity, and even the presence of certain toxins. These sensory neurons can then relay that information to other neurons within the submucosal or myenteric plexus which may in turn activate efferent neurons within the submucosal and myenteric nerve plexuses to respond to the detected change. The efferent neurons of the ENS can secrete a wide variety of neurotransmitters to interact with receptors on their target cells. These include acetylcholine, norepinephrine (discussed in the section on neurotransmitters of the autonomic nervous system), dopamine, serotonin, and at least 30 other neurotransmitters and bioactive substances such as gastrointestinal peptide, vasoactive intestinal peptide (VIP), and calcitonin gene-related peptide which have very specific actions within the gastrointestinal tract. Some of these actions are stimulatory and some inhibitory. Responses modulated by these widely varied transmitters might include contraction of the muscle layers in response to distension, secretion of fluids to neutralize acidity, and secretion of mucus to flush toxins away from an area. Interneurons can convey information between the submucosal and myenteric plexuses, so they are always in communication with one another. The ENS can control many of the actions of the gastrointestinal tract autonomously. However, its actions tend to be rather

localized and for coordinated actions over long sections of the gut, input from the autonomic nervous system is required.

Autonomic nervous system and the gastrointestinal tract

1 Describe the location of the presynaptic parasympathetic neurons that affect the intestinal tract.

2 How does the parasympathetic nervous system interact with the enteric nervous system to effect coordinated actions within the intestinal tract?

3 What are the major actions of the sympathetic nervous system on the intestinal tract?

The efferent parasympathetic system is the predominant player when considering the effects of the autonomic nervous system on the gastrointestinal tract (Figure 42.5). The efferent sympathetic nervous system is often referred to as the "fight or flight" system for its action on heart and respiratory function. The parasympathetic system in contrast is referred to as the "rest and digest" system.

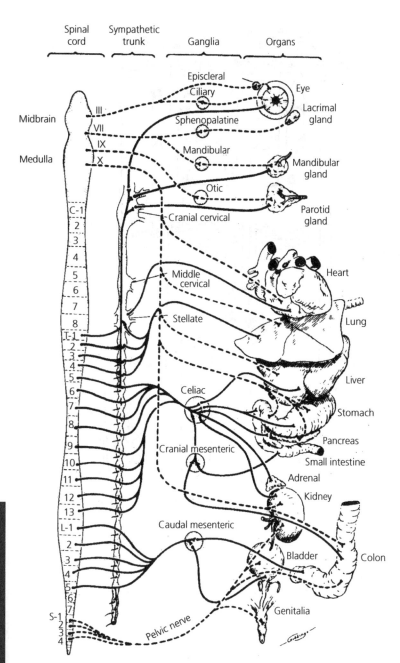

Figure 42.5 Diagrammatic representation of the efferent autonomic nervous system of a domestic animal. Lumbar and sacral cord segmentation may vary by species. Sympathetic nerves are indicated by solid lines; parasympathetic nerves by broken lines. The paravertebral ganglia and the parasympathetic ganglia of the head are paired structures, while the sympathetic prevertebral ganglia are unpaired. From Reece, W.O. (ed.) (2004) *Dukes' Physiology of Domestic Animals*, 12th edn. Cornell University Press, Ithaca, NY. Reproduced with permission from Cornell University Press.

Parasympathetic nervous innervation of the gastrointestinal tract

From the esophagus to the end of the descending colon cranial nerve X, the vagus, carries the parasympathetic efferent fibers that help control many of the functions of the gastrointestinal tract. The vagus parasympathetic nervous system is simply an efferent pathway that comprises two neurons. The cell body of the first neuron lies within the medulla, the lower half of the brainstem. This neuron is referred to as the preganglionic parasympathetic neuron. This cell body receives input from higher centers of the brain and from afferent sensory neurons that may ascend to the medulla along various sensory nerve

pathways. This input may stimulate or inhibit action potentials within the preganglionic parasympathetic neuron. The preganglionic neuron sends an axon from the medulla, down the jugular foramen and on to various viscera in the thorax (esophagus, heart, lungs) and abdomen (stomach and forestomachs in ruminants, small intestine and ascending large intestine). These axons then meet the second parasympathetic neuron and form a ganglion (or synapse) with this postganglionic neuron. This junction or ganglion is found within the wall of the organ to be acted upon. The preganglionic parasympathetic axon releases the neurotransmitter acetylcholine (ACh) to diffuse across the cleft between the two cells, where it interacts with receptors on the postganglionic nerve cell body that recognize and react to ACh. These receptors are referred to as nicotinic receptors, as they were discovered by observing the action of nicotine on these cells. Once ACh binds to the nicotinic receptor on the postganglionic cell, it stimulates that cell to secrete ACh from its axon terminus. Since these postganglionic nerve cell bodies are already within the wall of the target organ, their axons tend to be rather short. They typically end on nerve cell bodies of neurons within the submucosal and myenteric nerve plexuses, or they interact directly with the same target tissues (muscle, mucosal secretory and absorptive cells, etc.) previously described as targets for the ENS effector neurons. The postganglionic parasympathetic neurons release ACh from their nerve terminals to diffuse toward the cell membrane of target tissues. The ACh then binds to receptors on these target cell membranes referred to as muscarinic receptors. These muscarinic receptors are G protein-coupled receptors so that once ACh binds its receptor, activation of the G-protein complex initiates action within the target tissue. There are a variety of subclasses of muscarinic receptors that exist on the various tissues innervated by the postganglionic parasympathetic fibers, but all respond to ACh.

In addition to the vagus, parasympathetic efferent neurons arising from the sacral spinal cord can affect function within the transverse and descending colon. These are also sometimes referred to as the pelvic splanchnic nerves. The preganglionic nerve cell bodies reside in the sacral spinal cord between segments 1 and 4. Their axonal fibers pass out of the sacral spinal cord and run to the walls of the transverse and descending colon to form a ganglia with the postganglionic parasympathetic neuron, which releases ACh onto muscarinic receptors on the surface of target cells in the transverse and descending colon. This also includes the internal anal sphincter muscle. Recall that the urinary bladder and bladder sphincters are influenced by parasympathetic efferents arising from the sacral spinal cord.

Sympathetic nervous innervation of the gastrointestinal tract

The sympathetic efferent nervous system is also a system requiring two neurons to effect a change in function of the target cell. The major nerves carrying sympathetic preganglionic and postganglionic fibers to the gastrointestinal tract include the cranial and caudal splanchnic nerves originating from the thoracic spinal cord and the lumbar splanchnic nerves. The fibers for these neurons synapse or pass through the paravertebral sympathetic chain and then the celiac, cranial or caudal mesenteric ganglia and on to the target organ.

The first neuron is the preganglionic neuron. All preganglionic sympathetic neuron cell bodies lie within the spinal cord between vertebra T1 and L2. They send axons from the spinal cord to form a synapse or ganglion with a second, postganglionic sympathetic neuron. The site of this junction between preganglionic and postganglionic sympathetic fibers can be within the paravertebral sympathetic chain, within the abdomen in sites such as the celiac ganglion, or within the wall of the target organ.

The preganglionic sympathetic fiber releases ACh onto nicotinic receptors located on the postganglionic nerve cell body, just as in the parasympathetic nervous system. The postganglionic nerve cell body then sends out axon fibers that typically end on nerve cell bodies of neurons within the submucosal and myenteric nerve plexuses, or they interact directly with the same target tissues (muscle, mucosal secretory and absorptive cells, etc.) previously described as targets for the parasympathetic and ENS effector neurons. The postganglionic sympathetic neurons typically release norepinephrine from their nerve terminals to diffuse toward the cell membrane of target tissues. Norepinephrine is recognized by and interacts with receptors on the surface of the target cells that are referred to as adrenergic receptors. These are often further defined as α or β classes of adrenergic receptor that recognize norepinephrine, and can be further classified as α_1, α_2, β_1, and β_2 receptors. Target cells tend to have one or another of these various categories of adrenergic receptor, but in all cases these receptors respond to norepinephrine.

A few sympathetic postganglionic fibers secrete alternative neurotransmitters such as neuropeptide Y and somatostatin which are recognized by neuropeptide Y or somatostatin receptors. A few secrete ACh onto muscarinic receptors on their target cells, just like parasympathetic postganglionic fibers. These target cells include sweat glands and piloerector muscles on hair follicles.

Autonomic nervous system summary

The parasympathetic efferent system is the primary controller of functions associated with motility, secretion, and digestion within the gastrointestinal tract, by directly acting on target cells or by indirectly modulating the activity of the ENS. Most of the actions of the gastrointestinal tract are controlled by parasympathetic tone. For instance, contraction of the smooth muscles of the outer longitudinal muscle layer increases with increased parasympathetic stimulation or tone and decreases when parasympathetic stimulation is reduced. In theory the sympathetic efferent system counteracts the stimulatory actions of the parasympathetic efferent system. In practice, the sympathetic efferent action on most functions within the gastrointestinal tract is minor. An exception is the effect of the sympathetic efferents on blood flow through the gastrointestinal tract. During a "flight or fight" response, the sympathetic efferents quickly shunt blood away from the gastrointestinal tract toward the musculature. The veterinary student must also keep in mind that anatomical nerves carry both efferent and afferent neurons. The vagus nerve carries sensory afferent fibers from the viscera to the medulla in addition to parasympathetic efferent fibers. These afferent signals are received by neurons within the medulla which then may affect parasympathetic efferent activity. About 80–90% of the fibers within the vagus nerve are sensory afferent neurons. The parasympathetic sacral nerves also contain sensory afferent neurons carrying information from the transverse and descending colon to the spinal cord where the information can modulate activity of the sacral parasympathetic efferent neurons or be transmitted to the medulla and higher brain areas. Similarly, the splanchnic nerves emerging from the thoracic and lumbar spinal cord carry sensory afferent neuron information from the viscera to the spinal cord in addition to carrying the sympathetic efferent fibers. About 70% of the fibers within these nerves are sensory afferent fibers.

Nicotinic receptors recognizing ACh are found on both parasympathetic and sympathetic postganglionic fibers. Antagonists of the nicotinic receptor, such as hexamethonium, can block the action of ACh on nicotinic receptors, inhibiting both sympathetic and parasympathetic function. Recall that ACh is the neurotransmitter released by postganglionic parasympathetic neurons onto muscarinic receptors. Muscarinic receptors can be blocked by anticholinergic drugs such as atropine and glycopyrrolate. Glycopyrrolate is often administered prior to surgery to dry up secretions from the saliva in order to decrease the risk of aspiration pneumonia. Some compounds interact with the muscarinic receptor to cause activation of the receptor and are referred to as agonists or cholinomimetics.

Syndrome of special significance to veterinary medicine

The equine veterinary practitioner will often encounter horses affected by an alkaloid toxin called slaframine that is produced by a mold (*Rhizoctonia leguminicola*) found in moldy red clover. This toxin acts on salivary muscarinic receptors causing extreme salivation and drooling. The toxin is generally destroyed by exposure to stomach acids so its effects are restricted to the salivary glands. It can also affect the cow and sheep, but the horse seems particularly sensitive and can lose as much as 40 L of saliva a day from drooling.

Smooth muscles of the gastrointestinal tract

1 How do gap junctions facilitate coordinated contraction of intestinal smooth muscle?

2 Describe the location and function of the three smooth muscles in the gastrointestinal tract.

3 How does parasympathetic stimulation alter slow wave depolarization of smooth muscle Cajal cells so they are more likely to result in an action potential that results in smooth muscle contraction?

Three anatomic smooth muscles can be identified microscopically in all sections of the gastrointestinal tract (Figure 42.6). The first is the submucosal muscle (muscularis mucosae), which is within the tunica mucosa and extends into the lamina propria. In the small intestine it is responsible for movement of villi. During digestion villi are constantly shortening and lengthening as submucosal muscles contract and relax. It is a very small band of muscle. Below the submucosa run two large bands

of smooth muscle. The layer closest to the lumen or inner layer is the **circular smooth muscle**, with fibers running at right angles to the long axis of the intestine. The outer layer is the **longitudinal smooth muscle**, with fibers running parallel to the long axis of the intestine.

These two large smooth muscle layers conduct two types of muscle contraction within the gastrointestinal tract. Segmental contractions involve squeezing of the bolus of food so that it is continually being mixed as it moves down the intestinal tract. This is mediated primarily by contraction and relaxation of the circular smooth muscle. These mixing and grinding actions facilitate contact between digestive enzymes and the ingesta. It also constantly moves lumen material against the mucosal surface cells that will absorb the nutrients. The second type of contraction is known as **peristalsis**, which can propel a bolus of ingesta down the gastrointestinal tract aborally (away from the oral cavity). This requires coordinated contraction of the outer longitudinal muscle and inner circular muscle just behind the bolus and relaxation of these muscle layers just ahead of the bolus.

Smooth muscles react much more slowly than do striated skeletal muscles. However, they generally have longer actin filaments than do skeletal muscle cells so that an individual smooth muscle cell can contract three to four times the distance a striated muscle cell can. Another major difference between striated and smooth muscle is that contraction of smooth muscle requires entry of calcium into the cell from the extracellular fluid. Hypocalcemia can greatly affect smooth muscle function. Smooth muscle cells can contract as a syncytium, i.e., when one smooth muscle cell contracts many others in the same area will also contract. This is mediated by gap junctions between adjacent smooth muscle cells. These are proteinaceous tubes connecting the individual cells to form a low-resistance pathway for ion movement between adjacent cells. This allows an action potential initiated in one cell to propagate and spread through all the cells within that syncytium. Thus it does not require an individual neuron to stimulate each individual cell as does each skeletal muscle.

Certain smooth muscles within segments of the gastrointestinal tract aboral to the esophagus undergo rhythmic depolarization caused by variations in conductance of sodium and calcium across the cell membrane at regular intervals. They are known as the **interstitial cells of Cajal**. Depolarization waves may occur 16–20 times each minute in the stomach. The rate of these slow waves decreases in the small intestine and there may be just two to three slow waves of depolarization per minute in the colon. These waves of depolarization are purely electrical phenomena (Figure 42.7). Leakage of sodium and calcium into the cell will raise the membrane potential 10–15 mV during each wave. At rest, the electrical potential difference across the membrane of the Cajal cells may be −50 mV. As sodium and calcium leak into the cell, the potential difference may be reduced to just −35 mV. The leakiness of the membrane to sodium and calcium is short-lived and the sodium and calcium

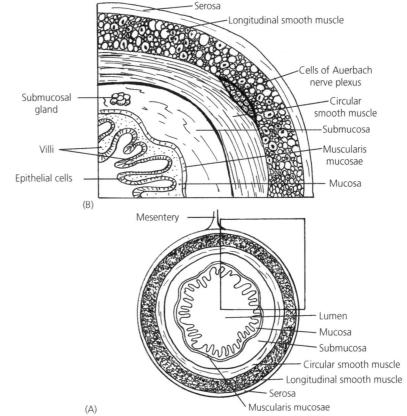

Figure 42.6 Schematic representation of the general organizational features of the mammalian gastrointestinal tract. (A) Cross-section of small intestine with its mesenteric suspension that envelops the intestine as its serosa. (B) Boxed section from (A) to show greater detail. The myenteric or Auerbach nerve plexus controls gastrointestinal movements. The submucosal or Meissner plexus (not shown) is in the submucosa and controls secretions and blood flow. The muscularis mucosae produces folds in the mucosa for amplification of surface area. From Reece, W.O. (2009) *Functional Anatomy and Physiology of Domestic Animals*, 4th edn. Wiley-Blackwell, Ames, IA. Reproduced with permission from Wiley.

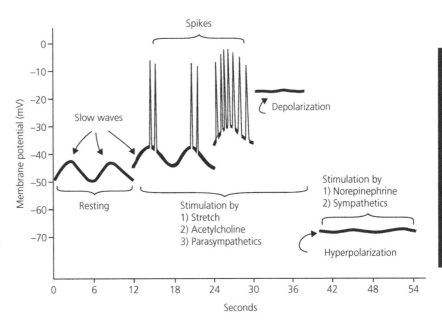

Figure 42.7 Membrane potentials in mammalian intestinal smooth muscle. Note the slow waves, spike potentials, and directions of depolarization and hyperpolarization. From Guyton, A.C. and Hall, J.E. (2000) *Textbook of Medical Physiology*, 10th edn. W.B. Saunders, Philadelphia. With permission from Elsevier.

Section VII: Digestion, Absorption, and Metabolism

are pumped out of the cell, reestablishing the resting membrane potential of –50 mV. If the threshold potential to initiate an action potential is –35 mV, this rhythmic depolarization does not result in any muscular contractions. However, the resting membrane potential of these Cajal cells can be altered by nervous, hormonal, and mechanical influences. If a segment of

intestine is stretched by the presence of a bolus of food, or if muscarinic receptors on these cells have been activated by parasympathetic stimulation, the resting membrane potential may be reduced to just –40 mV. Now as the slow wave of depolarization proceeds and sodium and calcium leak into the cell altering the potential difference by 10 mV, the membrane potential difference is now –30 mV. This is above the threshold potential and action potentials will occur. This will result in contraction of the Cajal cell, which will be carried to all the other cells within that syncytium via the gap junctions. Action potentials will continue to be elicited at maximum rate (depending on membrane ability to recover from an action potential, i.e., the **refractory period** for the Cajal cell) so long as the slow wave potential difference does not fall below the threshold potential. The greater the parasympathetic stimulation, the longer the resting membrane potential remains close to threshold and the more action potentials that will be initiated during a slow wave of depolarization. The more action potentials, the stronger the strength of the contraction of the smooth muscle cells within that syncytium. Sympathetic nervous innervation and the action of certain hormones can increase the potential difference across the cell membrane so that resting membrane potential may be –60 mV. In this case, slow wave depolarization increases potential difference across the membrane to only –45 mV, well below the threshold and little muscle contraction will occur.

Voluntary striated skeletal muscles do exist at the pharynx and proximal esophagus (entire esophagus of ruminants and some other species) as well as the external anal sphincter. Their function is discussed in later sections.

Movement of the bolus down the esophagus

> 1 What forces allow a bolus of food to move down the esophagus even if you are standing on your head?
> 2 Which factors are responsible for opening and closing the lower esophageal sphincter?

The esophagus is simply a conduit that conducts ingesta from the oropharynx to the stomach (or forestomach in the case of ruminants). The cricopharyngeus muscle forms a strong band of striated muscle encircling the orad end of the esophagus. This striated muscle is normally kept closed to prevent reflux of esophageal contents into the pharynx. This allows a slight negative pressure to be developed within the esophagus which helps ingesta enter the esophagus when the cricopharyngeus muscle is relaxed during swallowing. The presence of the bolus stimulates peristaltic contractions that move the bolus toward the stomach. The lower esophageal sphincter is normally kept tightly shut to prevent stomach contents and acid from entering the esophagus. As with most sphincters of the gastrointestinal tract, the lower esophageal sphincter consists of a greatly enlarged inner circular smooth muscle. Gastrin, a hormone synthesized by enteroendocrine cells in the pyloric stomach when the stomach is distended, and vagal parasympathetic stimulation act together to keep the sphincter muscle tightly shut. Relaxation of the lower esophageal sphincter is mediated by VIP, a neurotransmitter produced by local ENS neurons in response to the presence of a bolus of food distending the area just orad of the sphincter muscle. In most species, opening of the lower esophageal sphincter is accompanied by a peristaltic wave within the esophagus, which pushes the bolus into the stomach, and relaxation of the musculature of the stomach, reducing pressure within the stomach so that as the lower esophageal sphincter relaxes material is not ejected into the esophagus. Distensibility of the stomach can be a factor limiting the size of meals. Carnivores like wolves and lions have very distensible stomachs, allowing them to ingest very large meals, especially important if meat from prey is available only once every few days. At the other end of the spectrum is the horse which has a relatively small stomach with a very limited capacity for distension.

Movement of the bolus through the stomach

> 1 Where does contraction of the stomach begin?
> 2 Why does only a small amount of chyme enter the duodenum with each contraction of the stomach?
> 3 Describe the neuronal and hormonal factors controlling stomach emptying.

The stomach musculature has an additional smooth muscle layer inside the inner circular layer that runs transversely to the inner circular and outer longitudinal smooth muscles. This oblique muscle layer provides another dimension for stomach contraction that greatly increase mixing activities within the stomach. Distension of the fundus activates ENS and vagal afferent sensory neurons that cause ENS and vagal efferent activation of stomach muscle contraction. Contraction of the stomach begins mid-fundus as a peristaltic wave that propels ingesta toward the small intestine. As the peristaltic wave reaches the aboral or pyloric end of the stomach, the pyloric sphincter controlling movement of material from the stomach to the small intestine relaxes momentarily. A small amount of the most digested and liquid material (chyme) passes into the duodenum. The pyloric sphincter quickly contracts again before the peristaltic wave has been completed. This causes the more solid material within the chyme to hit the pylorus and be shunted back toward the fundic area of the stomach. This creates a churning action that helps break down solids in the chyme, ensuring good mixing with stomach acid and proteolytic enzymes. It also causes dietary fat to form emulsions with water in preparation for digestion in the intestine.

Stomach motility is increased by the hormone gastrin, synthesized by enteroendocrine cells in the pyloric region of the stomach in response to distension. The vagus parasympathetics also respond to distension by increasing stomach contractility. Vagal parasympathetic stimulation of stomach contractility can also be initiated by higher centers in the brain in response to the sight, smell, or taste of food. These same factors can cause the pyloric sphincter to relax.

Stomach motility is decreased when chyme enters the duodenum and causes distension of the duodenum or when there is an increase in osmolarity of the fluids within the duodenum. Vagal sensory afferents return this information to the medulla, causing a reduction in vagal parasympathetic efferent stimulation of stomach contraction. Two hormones synthesized by enteroendocrine cells in the upper duodenum can also act on the stomach muscles to slow contractility. These are cholecystokinin (CCK), secreted in response to the presence of fats and amino acids in the duodenum, and secretin, released in response to a reduction in pH in the duodenum. These hormones are secreted into the blood and the portal circulation, eventually reaching the muscles of the stomach. These hormones also act on the pyloric sphincter and cause it to constrict more tightly to reduce further entry of chyme to the duodenum.

Contraction and relaxation of the pyloric sphincter determines the rate of emptying of the stomach. The pyloric sphincter also works to prevent duodenal contents from entering the stomach. It relaxes in response to vagal stimulation and contracts in response to CCK and secretin. High-fat diets greatly increase CCK secretion, slowing emptying of the stomach. High-protein diets also stimulate some secretion of CCK. High-carbohydrate diets do not stimulate CCK secretion at all. Sugar and starch pass very quickly into the duodenum so they can be rapidly absorbed. Unfortunately, since stomach distension acts as a stimulus to the satiety centers of the brain, high-carbohydrate diets do not elicit a feeling of stomach fullness in the same way as high-fat diets do and the animal will feel "hungry" more quickly. Pyloric stenosis prevents the stomach from emptying properly. This can occur in neonates as a congenital lack of development of the myenteric plexus in the pyloric region. More commonly it can be caused by scarring of the tissues in the pyloric area secondary to ulcers. This results in projectile vomiting of ingesta following a large meal.

Eructation contractions of the stomach and esophagus in monogastric species

> **1** What is the role of the conscious brain in an eructation reflex, i.e., how much of the reflex is voluntarily controlled?

Gases can be swallowed during ingestion of a meal or they can be formed as a result of the action of acid on the ingesta. The distension of the stomach caused by the accumulation of gas can be painful. Fortunately, it can be removed by eructation or "burping." During the course of normal stomach contractions solid and liquid components are forced toward the pylorus by peristaltic contractions. By default the gases tend to accumulate at the more orad portion of the stomach. A peristaltic contraction can then raise the pressure of the gas to such a point that the lower esophageal sphincter is overcome and gas escapes into the esophagus. However, peristaltic waves within the esophagus will ordinarily force the gas back into the stomach. However, if the animal consciously contracts its abdominal muscles just as the lower esophageal sphincter is overcome, the escaped gas can develop enough pressure to overcome esophageal peristalsis and be forced out of the esophagus to the mouth to escape. Eructation in ruminants is a very different reflex, and is discussed in Chapter 45.

Vomition

> **1** What is the relationship between the chemoreceptor trigger zone and the vomiting center?
>
> **2** Why does the animal preparing to vomit exhibit tachycardia and increased salivation?
>
> **3** Why are abdominal muscles involved in the vomition reflex?

Carnivores and most omnivore mammals have the ability to vomit (also called emesis) or expel the contents of their stomach through the oral cavity. Some species may use the stomach as a means of conveyance of food to their offspring. They may vomit the contents of the stomach on stimulation by the sight and sound of their offspring. This is generally referred to as regurgitation rather than vomition or emesis. In most species vomition serves primarily as a means of removing toxic material from the stomach. Vomition is a rather complex reflex controlled by collections of neurons (nuclei) residing in the medulla (Figure 42.8). A collection of nerve cells in the reticular formation of the medulla comprise the **vomiting center**. These neurons receive sensory information directly from the gastrointestinal tract via vagal and sympathetic afferent fibers. Stomach and oropharynx irritants, such as hydrogen peroxide, syrup of Ipecac, and salt, can activate the vomiting reflex within the vomiting center. The vestibular apparatus can also release histamine to activate H_1 histamine receptors on vomiting center neurons to cause motion sickness.

A second collection of nerves within the floor of the fourth ventricle forms the **chemoreceptor trigger zone**. These neurons have receptors that recognize blood-borne chemicals or toxins that reach them. One chemical recognized by the chemoreceptor trigger zone and used by veterinarians to induce vomiting is the opiate apomorphine, which has the ability to act as a potent dopamine agonist within chemoreceptor trigger zone nuclei and initiate vomition. Xylazine, an α_2-receptor agonist, is also a reliable emetic agent, particularly in cats. The chemoreceptor trigger zone can also receive input from higher centers of the brain so that certain smells or sights can initiate vomition. The vestibular apparatus also sends signals to the chemoreceptor trigger zone, and **motion sickness** or disturbances within the middle ear, such as infection, can cause vomition. Once the chemoreceptor trigger zone is activated, it can only stimulate

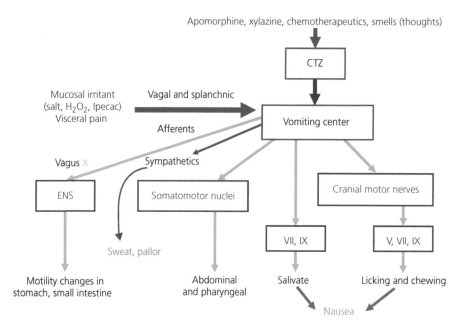

Figure 42.8 Vomition. Neurons within the chemoreceptor trigger zone (CTZ) respond to blood-borne chemicals and send input to a vomiting center in the medulla. The vomiting center also receives direct input from vagal and splanchnic afferents that indicate the presence of some irritant in the stomach. The vomiting center initiates widespread parasympathetic and sympathetic discharge resulting in sweating, nausea, and salivation. Finally the coordinated contraction of the stomach and abdominal muscles forces stomach contents up the esophagus and out of the mouth.

vomition by sending signals for vomition through the vomiting center first. It cannot carry out the vomiting reflex by itself.

The vomiting reflex begins when the vomiting center neurons have been stimulated. These neurons, which utilize dopamine and serotonin as their neurotransmitters, initiate widespread discharge by the autonomic neurons and motor neurons residing in the medulla and the spinal cord. The parasympathetic discharges lead to increased salivation, and contractions within the esophagus, stomach and even the upper duodenum. The sympathetic discharges cause the heart rate to increase and can cause sweating and a reduction in blood flow to the skin (pallor in humans). Cranial nerve motor neurons to the pharynx initiate chewing and tongue movements. The animal will have a feeling of discomfort known as **nausea**. The muscles in the pyloric end of the stomach and sometimes even the upper duodenum contract, sending ingesta toward the esophageal end of the stomach. The rest of the stomach and the lower esophageal sphincter relax allowing some stomach contents into the esophagus. However, at least initially, the esophagus responds by initiating peristaltic contractions to push the stomach contents back into the stomach. This process is called **retching** and will occur several times before true vomition occurs. During one of the next contractions that arise from the pyloric stomach the reflex will also induce strong contractions of the diaphragm and abdominal muscles that raise the pressure inside the stomach and esophagus and overcome esophageal peristalsis to propel the stomach contents out of the mouth. At the same moment, the upper esophageal sphincter relaxes, the nasopharynx closes to prevent material exiting via the nasal cavities, and the glottis closes to prevent entry of material into the trachea.

Severe vomiting can also have an earlier component whereby the pyloric sphincter relaxes to allow duodenal contents to enter the stomach for vomiting. This material will often contain bile and will have a greenish color. Antiemetic drugs work by decreasing afferent input from sensory neurons in the stomach or by inhibiting efferent components of the vomiting reflex. This generally involves use of sedatives, which may also increase the risk of aspiration of stomach contents so these are reserved for patients that have not consumed food recently. Some drugs (dopamine antagonists like acepromazine or serotonin antagonists such as metoclopramide) work by counteracting the stimulatory effects of dopamine or serotonin on vomition. Antihistamines block the effect of histamine released by the vestibular apparatus on the H_1 histamine receptors of the chemoreceptor trigger zone and vomiting center.

Some species of animals are unable to vomit. Rats are unable to vomit because they do not have nuclei within their medulla that form the vomiting center. They are therefore unable to coordinate diaphragm and abdominal muscle contraction with contraction of the stomach. They also cannot coordinate contraction of the stomach and opening of lower and upper esophageal sphincters. Rabbits cannot vomit either. They do have a vomiting center in the medulla but have a lower esophageal sphincter that they cannot relax enough to allow vomition. Horses also cannot vomit, despite having a vomiting center. Some researchers suggest that they also have a lower esophageal sphincter that will not relax. Other researchers have suggested that the angle of entry of the esophagus into the stomach becomes even more acute (kinked) when the stomach is full, preventing the horse from vomiting an excessive meal of grain for example. The horse stomach does not distend very much and the full stomach can distend to the point of initiating a vomition reflex. The stomach will try to contract (causing colic pain) and the abdominal muscles will contract but stomach contents cannot pass the lower esophageal sphincter. The horse's abdominal muscles are so strong that prolonged attempts to vomit can cause the stomach wall to rupture. Interestingly, the veterinarian can pass a nasogastric tube through the lower esophageal sphincter into the stomach and can remove stomach contents to relieve colic symptoms.

Movement of the bolus through the small intestine

> **1** What is the difference between a segmental and a peristaltic contraction of the intestine?

The primary stimulus for contraction in the small intestine is distension of the small intestine. Shortly after meals, mixing or segmental contractions predominate within the small intestine (Figure 42.9). Movement of ingesta through the small intestine involves peristaltic contractions of the circular and longitudinal muscles. This can be mediated over short distances (a few centimeters) by ENS afferent and efferent neurons alone. Peristaltic contractions that move boluses of food much longer distances require coordination by the vagal sensory afferents and parasympathetic efferent fibers (Figure 42.10). Peristaltic contractions convey material distances of 10–20 cm in the dog as it digests its meal. Between meals, once digestion is complete it is not uncommon for peristaltic waves to propel boluses of material the entire length of the small intestine. It is believed

that this action sweeps the small intestine clean of undigestible material, protecting the small intestine from becoming populated with high numbers of bacteria and reducing the risk of toxin production within the lumen.

The hormone gastrin, secreted by enteroendocrine cells of the pyloric stomach when the stomach is full, can stimulate small intestinal motility, presumably to provide more room for stomach emptying. CCK, secreted by enteroendocrine cells in the duodenum on sensing fat or amino acids in the lumen, can also stimulate contractions within the small intestine. Secretin, a hormone produced by duodenal enteroendocrine cells in response to decreased pH, slows intestinal motility. Severe distension of the intestine can sometimes occur due to blockage or necrosis of a segment of intestine. Pain from this distension elicits sympathetic discharge and release of epinephrine from the adrenal medulla, which causes the cessation of intestinal motility (ileus) and sweating.

Movement of the bolus through the large intestine

> **1** Which segments of the colon are innervated by sacral spinal parasympathetic fibers?
> **2** What is the path of a bolus of food through the horse cecum and colon? Determine the sites most likely to suffer impaction causing colic.

For material to enter the large colon it must move from the ileum to the colon (ruminants, cat and dog) through the ileocolic sphincter (valve). In some species the ileum empties into the cecum through the ileocecal sphincter (horse, pig, rabbit,

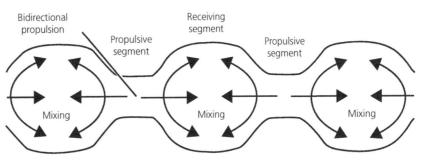

Same length of intestine later in time

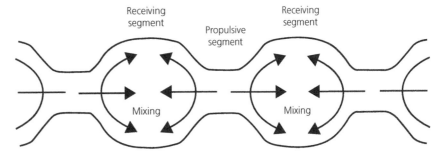

Figure 42.9 Segmental contractions of the small intestine. Movement of chyme into the receiving (relaxed) segment by the propulsive (contracting) segment results in mixing. The receiving segment then becomes the propulsive segment, and mixing continues. From Rhoades, R.A. and Tanner, G.A. (2003) *Medical Physiology*, 2nd edn. Lippincott Williams & Wilkins, Baltimore. Reproduced with permission from Lippincott Williams & Wilkins.

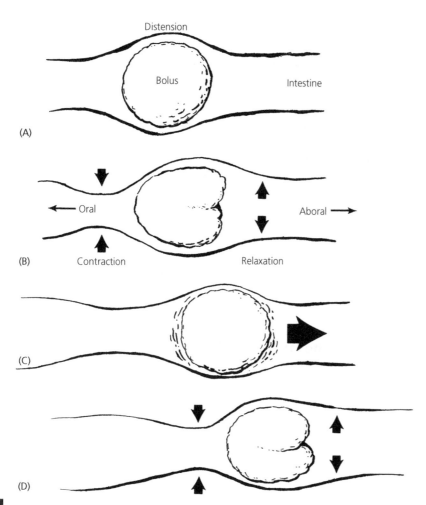

Distension

Bolus

Intestine

(A)

Oral

Aboral

Contraction

Relaxation

(B)

(C)

(D)

Figure 42.10 Intestinal peristalsis and movement of contents. (A) Original distension. (B) Contraction occurs cranial to the distension and relaxation caudal to the distension. (C) Contraction and relaxation followed by movement of contents in an aboral direction. (D) A new distension point initiates a new locus of contraction and relaxation, which continues aborally as a wave.

elephant and rat). These sphincters are normally kept closed. Distension in the ileum, and the hormone gastrin produced in response to a full stomach, cause the sphincter to relax. Distension of the colon or cecum will cause these sphincter muscles to contract more tightly to stop further entry of ingesta into the large intestine. Within the ascending colon of monogastric and ruminant species the contractions can be segmental mixing contractions or peristaltic contractions. The peristaltic contractions can be both antegrade (moving material toward the anus) and retrograde, which often moves material into the cecum or allows it to remain longer in the colon for extraction of more water and electrolytes. Cecal contractions can be both segmental and peristaltic and the peristaltic contractions generally move material out of the cecum. Segmental mixing contractions predominate in the transverse colon and both segmental and antegrade peristaltic contractions occur in the descending colon. In some species the segmented contractions of the descending colon become exaggerated, forming haustra. This allows more resident time in the descending colon to remove even more water from the ingesta before excretion. These species excrete pelleted feces. In the dog and cat (and human), between meals there can be mass aboral movement of material beginning near the ileocolic sphincter to the end of the descending colon.

As with the other segments of the gastrointestinal tract the ENS plays a role in segmental and peristaltic contractions and sensory afferent and parasympathetic input from the vagus (ascending colon) and sacral nerves (transverse and descending colon) control motility in the colon.

Megacolon may develop whenever the nerves conducting sensory afferent and parasympathetic fibers are compromised. In dogs and cats this may be due to damage to the pelvic splanchnic nerves following a traumatic experience (vehicle accident) that breaks the pelvic or sacral bones. The colon loses its parasympathetic tone and becomes greatly distended.

Horse cecum and colon

The horse is a hindgut fermenter with a cecum and ascending colon specially adapted to allow fermentation of plant cellulose and hemicellulose, providing the horse with energy in the form of volatile fatty acids. The hindgut strategy for obtaining energy from plant structural carbohydrates is also found in the rabbit, chinchilla, koala, elephant, and rhinoceros.

The cecum and ascending large colon of the horse are composed of three physiologically separate fermentation vats: the cecum, the ventral colon, and the dorsal colon (Figure 42.11). The dorsal colon empties into the transverse colon and then on

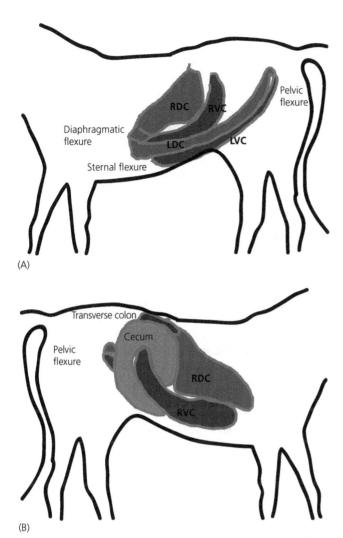

gentle curve of the ventral colon is known as the sternal flexure and the ventral colon is now called the left ventral colon. The ventral colon then follows the left ventral abdominal wall toward the pelvis. Mixing contractions can occur throughout the ventral colon and peristaltic contractions move ingesta back and forth from left to right ventral colon and back to the left, again to promote better fermentation of the ingesta. Peristaltic contractions can also propel material on to the next segment of the colon called the dorsal colon. The left ventral colon takes a sharp turn dorsally and cranially to enter the left side of the dorsal colon. This turn is particularly sharp and is known as the pelvic flexure.

Clinical correlations

The turn is so acute that the pelvic flexure is a common site of impaction in the horse and can cause distension of the ventral colon and colic. The proximity of the pelvic flexure to the pelvis allows the veterinarian to rectally palpate this structure to determine if it is impacted.

The left dorsal colon then extends cranially along the left abdominal wall until it reaches the diaphragm where it turns to the right, becoming the right dorsal colon. This gentle turn is referred to as the diaphragmatic flexure. The right dorsal colon then extends caudally and joins with the transverse colon. Segmental mixing and orad and aborad peristaltic contractions ensure thorough fermentation within this section of the large colon. The right dorsal colon narrows sharply as it converges onto the relatively small-diameter transverse colon. This narrowing is another site of possible obstruction that will cause distension of the dorsal colon and colic. The transverse colon and descending colon are similar to those in other species. Horses have haustrations within their descending colon that hold fecal material a little longer to extract more water. This forms a dry fecal ball that is passed out of the rectum during defecation.

Motility in the cecum and large colons of the horse is controlled by the ENS and the vagus. This reflects the embryologic origin of the ventral and dorsal colons as modifications of the ascending colon. The motility of the transverse and descending colon is controlled by the ENS and pelvic splanchnic nerves carrying sensory afferent and parasympathetic efferent fibers.

The rabbit is very similar to the horse, but relies on a large cecum for the bulk of its fermentation. The ascending colon is not as greatly modified for fermentation as is the horse, although it does ferment ingesta in its large colon. The rabbit has an interesting feature found in just a few animals including humans: it has an appendix at the end of its cecal blind sac. This small thin tube extends about 10–13 cm from the end of the cecum. It has a relatively small volume (a few milliliters) so it likely contributes little to fermentation efficiency. However, it is a highly lymphoid tissue and may play a role in immune responses within the cecum and large intestine. It may also serve as a reservoir for

Figure 42.11 Horse hindgut. (A) Left-sided view of ventral and dorsal colons of horse. Cecal matter enters the right ventral colon. Cecum removed for clarity. (B) Right-sided view of cecum, right ventral and right dorsal colon leading into the transverse colon. LDC, left dorsal colon; LVC, left ventral colon; RDC, right dorsal colon; RVC, right ventral colon.

to the descending colon, similar to other species. The ileum of the horse empties into the base of the cecum, which is located in the dorsal abdomen near the pelvis. The cecum is a blind sac extending cranially and ventrally from the pelvic inlet region and the apex lies near the xiphoid process. The cecum fills by gravity in the horse. Segmental contractions assure mixing of ingesta with bacteria to promote fermentation, and peristaltic contractions beginning near the apex can move material up and out of the cecum to the right side of the ventral colon. The orifice joining the cecum and colon is the cecocolic orifice and is a relatively small opening. This point of resistance to the flow of material can result in obstruction of cecal emptying and the ensuing cecal distension is a common cause of colic in horses. The right ventral colon extends cranially along the right ventral abdominal wall to the xiphoid process and turns to the left. This

Section VII: Digestion, Absorption, and Metabolism

commensal bacteria or be involved in allowing the rabbit to develop immune tolerance to commensal bacteria.

Many other animals utilize the cecum and large colon for fermentation as well, including pigs and cattle. However, the hindgut is not as well developed or relied on as the main source of energy in these species. Birds generally have two cecal out-croppings from the point where small and large intestine inter-sect. In several species of birds the fermentation of plant structural carbohydrates in the ceca supply the animal with energy in the form of volatile fatty acids.

Defecation

> **1** Describe the interplay between involuntary control of the internal anal sphincter and voluntary control of the external anal sphincter in allowing an animal to delay defecation.

Defecation is a temporary reflex that interrupts anal continence as the muscles comprising the anal sphincters are normally kept tightly shut. The rectum of most mammals is normally kept empty. At some point a peristaltic wave within the descending colon is initiated by pelvic splanchnic nerve parasympathetic efferent fibers (Figure 42.12). This sends fecal matter into the rectum and the rectum then propels this material on to the internal anal sphincter. The internal anal sphincter is an

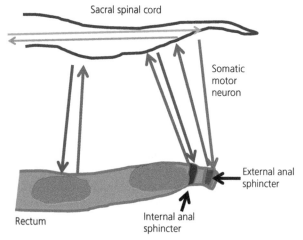

Figure 42.12 Defecation reflex. Peristalsis waves, controlled by sacral parasympathetic efferent fibers and sensory afferent fibers, move fecal material into the rectum. Sensory afferent fibers (orange arrows) sense contact of feces with internal anal sphincter smooth muscle. Sacral parasympathetic fibers (blue arrows) cause relaxation of the internal anal sphincter. The fecal matter now contacts the external anal sphincter composed of striated muscle. This information is conducted back to the spinal cord and brain by sensory afferent fibers. The animal will either consciously relax the external anal sphincter and defecate or make a conscious effort to tighten the external anal sphincter to delay defecation. This is mediated by somatic motor neurons (green arrows).

enlarged segment of the inner circular smooth muscle layer. The fecal material presses on the internal anal sphincter and afferent sensory fibers convey this information along the pelvic splanchnic nerves to the spinal cord. Pelvic splanchnic parasympathetic efferent fibers then reduce their discharge rate and the internal anal sphincter muscle relaxes. The fecal matter now reaches the external anal sphincter. Sensory afferent fibers convey this information to the spinal cord and to the brain. The animal now has a conscious urge to defecate. The external anal sphincter is composed of striated skeletal muscle and is nor-mally kept tightly shut under the control of somatic motor neu-rons exiting the sacral spinal cord. These neurons reduce their discharge, allowing the external anal sphincter muscle to relax. The animal can then consciously contract abdominal muscles to enhance the action of rectal peristalsis in discharge of rectal contents through the relaxed internal and external anal sphinc-ters. Certainly for dogs and cats, the human expectation is that defecation should not occur every time fecal matter reaches the rectum. The external anal sphincter allows some choice in halt-ing the defecation reflex. By consciously tightening the external anal sphincter the animal can resist defecation during a rectal peristaltic wave. The rectum relaxes and the internal anal sphincter regains normal tone until the next rectal peristaltic wave. Eventually, the pressure within the rectum becomes greater than the animal can bear and defecation will ensue. This is a common "complaint" faced by many of today's dog owners who work 8–10 hours a day and expect the dog to maintain anal continence all day. The fact that many do demonstrates the degree to which we have molded dog behavior. No one expects the cat or cow to maintain such control of its defecation reflex.

Self-evaluation

Answers can be found at the end of the chapter.

1 A rabbit is brought to your office. It has wet matted hair and slimy drool around its mouth and on its chest. Its hair coat is in general matted and the rabbit is in a thin condition. It has been eating a high legume/corn mix diet. What are you likely to see on examining the rabbit carefully?

2 During the swallowing reflex, the dorsal soft palate is elevated. Why?

3 The premolars of a horse are classified as (**A**) _____ teeth. Enamel ridges wear more slowly than the ridges composed of (**B**) _____ and (**C**) _____ that keep the occlusal surface sharp.

4 What kind of receptors does the neurotransmitter released by post-ganglionic fibers of the vagus nerve stimulate?

5 A horse consuming red clover hay is drooling several liters of foamy drool per hour.
  A What is in the clover?
  B And what is it doing/acting on? Be specific

6 _____ exist between muscle cells that form a syncytium. These structures allow ion fluxes to pass freely from one cell to another within the syncytium.

7 How does vasoactive intestinal peptide affect the lower esophageal sphincter?

8 How does gastrin affect the lower esophageal sphincter?

9 Arrange the following possible sites of impaction in a horse in order, with 1 being first (most orad) and 6 being last.
  A Pelvic flexure of colon
  B Pylorus of stomach
  C Sternal flexure
  D Entrance to transverse colon
  E Cecocolic orifice
  F Diaphragmatic flexure

10 Arrange the steps (A–G) involved in defecation in order from first (1) to last (7).
  A Conscious decision is made to defecate and signals are sent back down spinal column to somatic motor nerves which reach the external anal sphincter via the pudendal nerve
  B Peristalsis in descending colon sends fecal material to rectum
  C Stretch receptors in vicinity of internal anal sphincter sense presence of matter and send afferent impulses to sacral spinal cord via sacral spinal nerves
  D Sacral spinal parasympathetic efferent fibers to internal anal sphincter are activated and the sphincter relaxes
  E Pressure on external anal sphincter is sensed by receptors in vicinity of external anal sphincter sending afferent impulses to the higher centers of the brain

  F External anal sphincter relaxes and with abdominal muscle contraction raising intra-abdominal pressure the fecal matter is passed out
  G Rectum is normally devoid of feces

Suggested reading

Elwood, C., Devauchelle, P., Elliott, J. *et al.* (2010) Emesis in dogs: a review. *Journal of Small Animal Practice* **51**:4–22.

Sellers, A.F. and Lowe, J.E. (1986) Review of large intestinal motility and mechanisms of impaction in the horse. *Equine Veterinary Journal* **18**:261–263.

Answers

1 Malocclusion of the molars or incisors
2 To prevent ingesta from entering the nasopharynx and coming out the nose
3 (A) Hypsodont, (B) dentin and (C) cementum
4 Muscarinic receptors on target cells
5 (A) Slaframine. (B) Salivary muscarinic receptors
6 Gap junctions
7 Relaxes it to allow entry of bolus
8 Tightens it close
9 1, B; 2, E; 3, C; 4, A; 5, F; 6, D
10 1, G; 2, B; 3, C; 4, D; 5, E; 6, A; 7, F

43

Secretory Activities of the Gastrointestinal Tract

Jesse P. Goff

Iowa State University, Ames, IA, USA

Role of saliva in digestion

1 Which cells produce which components of saliva?

2 How is the alkalinity of salivary secretions controlled?

3 Diagram the essential parts of a salivary gland.

4 What is the role of the myoepithelial cells of salivary gland acini?

Saliva serves many functions. It moistens and lubricates the bolus of food ingested so that it is easier to swallow. It also provides water to dilute the osmolarity of the ingested material. In general the ingesta is hyperosmotic at this point and eventually it must be made isotonic within the lumen of the gut. Saliva is also slightly alkaline which provides some ability to neutralize acids that might be consumed. Salivary pH in ruminants can be considerably higher than in nonruminants, and saliva can help neutralize and buffer acids produced during bacterial fermentation in the rumen. Salivary secretions contain small amounts of an enzyme called α-amylase. This enzyme can begin to break the α1→4 linkages between glucose molecules in starch. Saliva also contains lipase, an enzyme that begins the process of fat digestion. Saliva also contains a variety of antibacterial substances such as lysozyme to control bacterial populations in the oropharynx.

The mucous and serous secretions of the salivary glands are produced in the acini. The alkalinity of the saliva is produced by the cells comprising the striated ducts of the salivary glands.

The secretion of saliva was discussed in the previous chapter. Remember that the parasympathetic efferent fibers control saliva secretion and that the alkalinity of the saliva can be increased in response to secretin, a hormone synthesized in the duodenum whenever the pH of the duodenal contents decreases.

Stomach secretions

1 What are the four categories of mucosa that might be encountered in a stomach?

2 Describe the location and secretions produced by cells of the gastric pits, chief cells, and parietal cells.

3 How is acid produced by the parietal cells?

4 Why is the reabsorption of potassium from the stomach lumen critical to developing a very low pH in the stomach lumen.

5 How do gastrin and histamine increase stomach acid secretion?

6 How do prostaglandins and cholecystokinin decrease stomach acid secretion?

7 Does secretin affect stomach acid production?

8 Why does chronic use of aspirin cause ulcers to develop?

Anatomically, the mammalian stomach (ruminant abomasum) is the organ between the esophagus (or forestomachs in ruminants) and the duodenum. Physiologically, the stomach can

Dukes' Physiology of Domestic Animals, Thirteenth Edition. Edited by William O. Reece, Howard H. Erickson, Jesse P. Goff and Etsuro E. Uemura.

© 2015 John Wiley & Sons, Inc. Published 2015 by John Wiley & Sons, Inc.

Companion website: www.wiley.com/go/reece/physiology

Section VII: Digestion, Absorption, and Metabolism

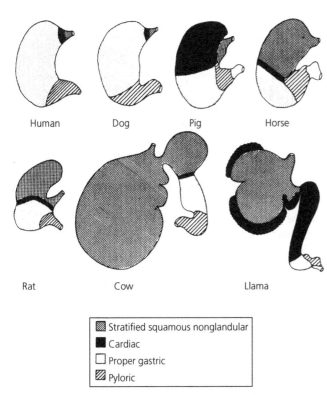

Figure 43.1 Variations in the type and distribution of gastric mucosa. Stomachs are not drawn to scale, for example the capacity of the adult bovine stomach is approximately 70 times that of the human stomach, or 14 times the capacity per kilogram of body weight. From Reece, W.O. (2004) *Dukes' Physiology of Domestic Animals*, 12th edn. Cornell University Press, Ithaca, NY. Reproduced with permission from Cornell University Press.

divided into four distinct functional compartments (Figure 43.1). Not all species have all four compartments.

1 The **esophageal stomach** is lined by stratified squamous epithelium and is often called "nonglandular" as no mucus, acid, or proteolytic enzymes are produced. The horse has a rather large esophageal stomach compartment but it is very small in the dog, pig, and cow.

2 The **cardia stomach** is considered a glandular stomach. Invaginations in the submucosa form short glands lined by simple columnar epithelial cells that produce a thick mucus and buffer that adheres to the cells to protect the epithelium from the proteolytic enzymes and acid produced in another compartment of the stomach. The pig has a very large cardia, the dog has a very small cardia, and the horse and cow have no cardia.

3 The third type of stomach compartment is also glandular and is the proper or **fundic stomach**. It has very deep invaginations in the submucosa lined by a variety of cells that produce acid, proteolytic enzymes, hormones, and mucus. All mammals have a fundic stomach and it is generally the largest compartment within the stomach.

4 The glandular **pyloric stomach** has moderately deep glands lined by epithelial cells that produce mucus and buffer, but

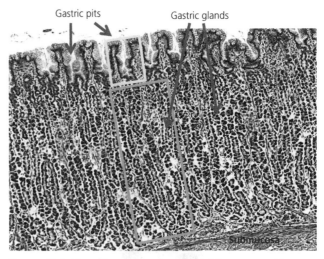

Gastric pits   Gastric glands

Submucosa

Figure 43.2 Photomicrograph of a section of the mucosa of the fundic stomach (canine).

not acid or proteolytic enzymes. It also has a notable population of enteroendocrine cells. One enteroendocrine cell type, the G-cells, produce the hormone gastrin in response to distension of the stomach or a rise in pH in the stomach. All mammals have a pyloric stomach that has at its terminus a pyloric sphincter to control the rate at which the stomach empties.

Fundic stomach secretions

The fundic stomach has **gastric pits** lined with mucus-secreting cells at the luminal surface (Figure 43.2). The mucus forms a thick gel that adheres tightly to the gastric pit to protect the stomach from acid and proteolytic enzymes. The mucus also incorporates a sodium bicarbonate buffer to provide further protection from stomach acid. Each gastric pit leads into a deep **gastric gland** that extends a long distance to reach the submucosa. Two cell types unique to the fundic stomach are found interspersed along the lining of the gastric glands (Figure 43.3).

The first is the **chief cell**, which secretes the proteolytic enzyme precursor pepsinogen into the lumen of the gastric gland, which is rapidly conveyed into the lumen of the stomach. The enzyme is secreted in an inactive form to avoid digestion of the chief cell, which might occur if it was in an active state within the cell. Pepsinogen is cleaved to the active enzyme pepsin by the hydrochloric acid it encounters in the gastric glands and lumen. Chief cells also produce a proteolytic enzyme known as rennin, which is particularly important in neonates as it helps digest milk proteins and forms milk curds within the stomach.

Parietal cells (or oxyntic cells) also line the gastric glands. These cells form the stomach acid, which aids in hydrolytic breakdown of diet components and also kills many of the bacteria that might be residing in the ingesta. In most species the parietal cells also produce a protein known as intrinsic

Gastric gland

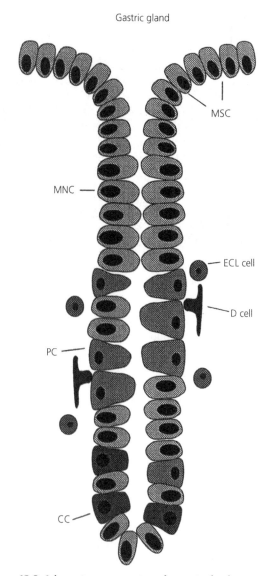

MSC

MNC

ECL cell

D cell

PC

CC

Figure 43.3 Schematic representation of a gastric gland indicating mucous surface cells (MSC), mucous neck cells (MNC), enterochromaffin-like (ECL) cells, somatostatin-containing D cells (D cell), parietal cells (PC), and chief cells (CC). From Reece, W.O. (2004) *Dukes' Physiology of Domestic Animals*, 12th edn. Cornell University Press, Ithaca, NY. Reproduced with permission from Cornell University Press.

factor. This protein binds vitamin B_{12} in the diet and carries the vitamin B_{12} to the ileum, where a specific transport system exists for endocytic absorption of the intrinsic factor–vitamin B_{12} complex.

Toward the base of the fundic gastric glands it is common to find enteroendocrine (also called enterochromaffin) cells among the chief and parietal cells and in the lamina propria under them. These enteroendocrine cells produce hormones that act in both an endocrine and paracrine fashion to control acid and proteolytic enzyme production in gastric glands throughout the fundic stomach.

Parietal cells and acid secretion

Parietal cells absorb chloride from the blood and actively pump it into the lumen of the stomach (Figure 43.4). Chloride crosses the basolateral membrane to enter the cell down its concentration gradient. Chloride may enter the cell in exchange for a bicarbonate ion or blood chloride may be cotransported into the parietal cell along with a sodium or potassium ion. Chloride concentration in the lumen of the gastric glands and stomach is ordinarily kept well above that inside the parietal cell. To move more chloride ions into the lumen requires expenditure of energy and active transport processes to pump the chloride across the apical membrane. Some pumps move chloride alone into the lumen of the gastric glands. Other pumps cotransport potassium (or a small amount of sodium) with the chloride into the lumen of the gastric glands. Chloride pumping is more or less a continuous process at the apical membrane of the parietal cell. This baseline secretion of chloride keeps the pH in the lumen of the gastric glands around 1.6. However, when greater acid secretion is needed hormonal and parasympathetic efferent innervation can greatly increase activity of the various chloride pumps. Potassium pumps are also activated to increase the removal of potassium from the gastric gland fluid. (In some textbooks the potassium reabsorbing pump is presumed to exchange the potassium ion for a hydrogen ion and is therefore called a **proton pump**.) The small amount of sodium in the lumen is also resorbed. Together the actions of these pumps can reduce the pH to about 0.9. Interestingly, despite their low pH, the osmolarity of the secretions in the gastric gland lumen is nearly isotonic (Table 43.1).

Control of parietal cell acid secretion

Three factors are known to activate mechanisms to enhance chloride secretion into and sodium and potassium removal from the gastric gland fluids in order to increase the acidity of the secretions produced by the parietal cells (Figure 43.5). The first is histamine produced by enteroendocrine cells at the base of the gastric glands when the pH of the gastric gland fluid rises too high. The histamine diffuses through the lamina propria to reach nearby parietal cells and binds to histamine H_2 receptors on the parietal cell basolateral membrane. The histamine H_2 receptors are classical G protein-coupled receptors and increase cyclic AMP production inside the cell to trigger increased acid production. (The histamine H_2 receptor is not to be confused with the histamine H_1 receptor associated with allergic responses.) The hormone gastrin, produced by enteroendocrine cells in the pyloric region of the stomach is secreted into the blood in response to distension of the pylorus or a rise in pH in the pyloric stomach.

Gastrin reaches the parietal cell via the circulation and binds to gastrin receptors on the basolateral membrane of parietal cells and this stimulates increased acid secretion. Gastrin can also bind to gastrin receptors on the histamine- producing enteroendocrine cells of the fundic gastric glands and cause them to secrete more histamine.

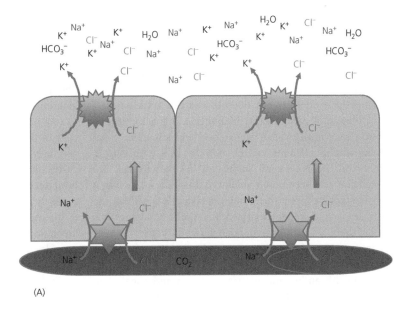

(A)

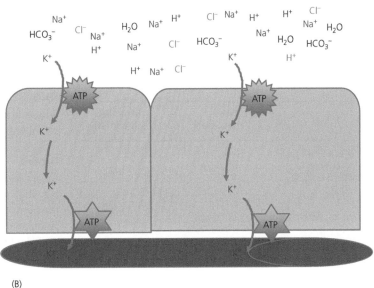

(B)

Figure 43.4 Parietal cells transfer chloride into the lumen of the gastric glands of the stomach and remove sodium and potassium from the gastric gland lumen fluid to generate a low pH in the gastric gland juices. (A) Cl⁻ pumped into lumen from blood. Cl⁻ moves with a K⁺ to maintain electroneutrality and to utilize force generated by K⁺ moving down its concentration gradient to the lumen. This does not create a change in the strong ion difference in the lumen if K⁺ accompanies Cl⁻, so there is no change in lumen pH at this point. (B) Potassium is pumped from the lumen into blood. Sometimes referred to as the "proton pump" because movement of a positive charge (K⁺) from lumen means an H⁺ will dissociate from lumen water to maintain electroneutrality and this makes lumen fluid much more acid. (C) Cl⁻ can also be pumped into lumen from blood in exchange for a Na⁺ to maintain electroneutrality. The overall result is that most of the potassium and sodium have been resorbed from the lumen fluids and a high amount of chloride is present. The strong ion difference becomes much more negative and the pH decreases.

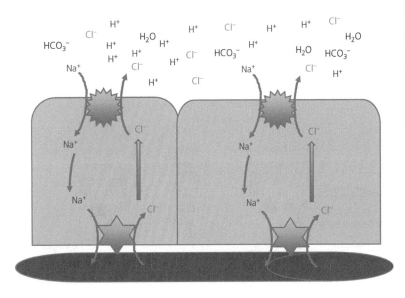

(C)

The third activator of parietal cell acid secretion is the vagus nerve. Vagal afferents can detect stretch of the stomach or alterations in osmolarity of stomach contents and transmit this information to the medulla. This may then activate parasympathetic efferent vagal fibers that extend to the basolateral membrane of parietal cells. In addition, higher centers of the brain may anticipate or smell food and stimulate vagal parasympathetic efferents to the parietal cells. Muscarinic receptors on the basolateral surface of the parietal cell are activated and acid secretion is enhanced. In addition, the vagal parasympathetic efferent fibers can stimulate the G-cells in the pyloric stomach to secrete more gastrin. It quickly becomes evident that there are multiple redundancies in the control of acid secretion to insure that acid production by the parietal cell can be increased on demand.

Reducing histamine and gastrin secretion and vagal tone serve as means to reduce acid production. However, when excessive acid has been produced and resulted in damage to any epithelial cells lining the stomach wall, the damaged cells respond by producing prostaglandin (PG)E$_1$, PGE$_2$ and PGI$_2$.

Table 43.1 Gastric juice composition (includes secretions of mucous, parietal, and chief cells).

	Basal secretion	Histamine stimulated
Chloride (mEq/L)	125	160
Sodium (mEq/L)	85	20
Potassium (mEq/L)	10	18
H$^+$ (mEq/L)	25	125
pH	1.6	0.9
Strong ion difference	−30 mEq/L	−122 mEq/L
(Na + K) − Cl	(−0.03 Eq/L)	(−0.122 Eq/L)
pH (mathematic)	1.52	0.91

Damage to the cell, caused by excessively low pH or any other trauma, stimulates the activity of the cyclooxygenase (COX)-1 enzyme. COX-1 converts arachidonic acid, liberated from phospholipids in cell membranes, to prostacyclin and then to prostaglandins. The prostaglandin diffuses through the basal lamina to reduce histamine and gastrin secretion by enteroendocrine cells in the vicinity of the damaged area. The stomach wall is normally protected from the acid and pepsin produced in the gastric glands by a heavy coating of mucus. In addition to its inhibitory actions on stomach acid secretion, prostaglandins cause increased mucus secretion by nearby epithelial cells. One of the most important functions of prostaglandin released following cell damage is to increase blood flow to the area. This provides nutrients needed for rapid repair or replacement of the damaged cells.

Cholecystokinin (CCK) and several other hormones produced in the duodenum in response to the entry of fats and amino acids or changes in osmolarity have a minor role in inhibiting acid production by binding to their respective receptors on parietal cells. Surprisingly, secretin, a hormone synthesized in the duodenum in response to low pH, does not inhibit parietal cell acid production. Secretin always works to correct low pH in the duodenum by increasing the production of alkaline secretions by the salivary glands, pancreas, and duodenal submucosal glands (Brunner's glands) that neutralize or buffer the acid.

Ulcers

Ulcers are erosions of the mucosal lining of the stomach. In the pig, they are most commonly found in the cardia region of the stomach. In the horse, ulcers are most common in the nonglandular esophageal compartment of the stomach. Excessive acid production can overcome the protective mucus layer on the stomach wall, particularly in animals that have not been

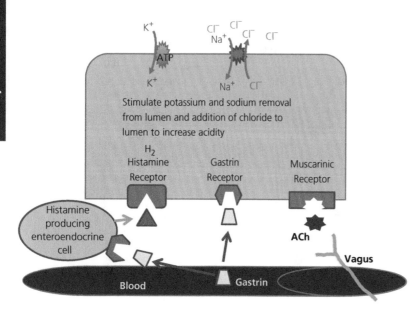

Figure 43.5 Factors stimulating acid secretion by fundic parietal cells. Histamine produced by local enteroendocrine cells interacts with H$_2$ histamine receptors. Gastrin produced in the pyloric stomach circulates through the blood to interact with gastrin receptors on parietal cells to directly stimulate acid production. Gastrin also interacts with gastrin receptors on the histamine-producing enteroendocrine cells to stimulate histamine production and indirectly increase parietal acid secretion. Acetylcholine (ACh) released by vagal parasympathetic postganglionic neurons activates muscarinic receptors to stimulate acid secretion.

consuming feed which helps neutralize acid produced. Many factors are involved in ulcer development, but one worth discussing is the effect of nonsteroidal anti-inflammatory drugs (NSAIDs). NSAIDs are generally administered to relieve pain caused by inflammation, particularly in joints. In arthritic joints, the enzyme COX-2 is expressed. Normally no COX-2 is active in joints, but in response to wear and tear or trauma this enzyme can be expressed. COX-2 catalyzes the production of prostaglandins from arachidonic acid, just as COX-1 does in the cells lining the digestive tract. However, the prostaglandins produced in these locations are proinflammatory and activate nociceptors (pain) in the affected joint. NSAIDs such as aspirin, ibuprofen, and flunixin meglumine are potent COX-2 inhibitors. By blocking production of prostaglandins in the affected joint, inflammation and pain are reduced. Unfortunately, these NSAIDs also are potent inhibitors of COX-1. This prevents prostaglandin production by cells that are damaged within the digestive tract. NSAID use removes the inhibitory effect of prostaglandins on stomach acid production. More importantly, without the local prostaglandin production by damaged cells, mucus secretion is reduced and blood flow to the damaged area will not increase to allow repair or replacement of the cells. Prolonged use of NSAIDs greatly increases the risk of ulcer development in the stomach and throughout the digestive tract. Horses are very likely to also develop ulcers in the colon where acids of fermentation can damage cells and prostaglandins produced by COX-1 are needed to permit repair of colon cells. Newer NSAIDs such as carprofen are primarily COX-2 inhibitors with only minor inhibition of COX-1 activity. This greatly reduces, but does not eliminate, their effect on COX-1-mediated production of prostaglandins in the digestive tract.

In humans many ulcers of the stomach and duodenum are caused by the presence of *Helicobacter pylori* in the stomach. This bacteria weakens the barrier layer of mucus, and it also appears that this bacterium secretes a toxin that acts as an agonist of gastrin receptors, increasing stomach acid secretion. Many *Helicobacter* species have been found in animals but a causative link between the presence of these bacteria and ulcers in animals is still weak. An exception is the cheetah, where the presence of *Helicobacter acinomyx* has been linked to gastritis.

Treatment of ulcers focuses on reducing the action of those factors known to affect stomach acid secretion. Cimetidine is a drug that blocks the histamine H_2 receptors on parietal cells. Omeprazole is a drug that slows the pump that reabsorbs potassium from the lumen of the gastric glands, which is vital to production of a very low pH gastric gland secretion (these drugs are often referred to as proton pump inhibitors). Surgically cutting the branches of the vagus nerve to the fundic stomach (vagotomy) has been used as well. Since prostaglandins are helpful in reducing acid secretion and allowing more mucus production and blood flow to the damaged area, synthetic analogs of PGE and PGI (misoprostol) can be administered.

Liver

> 1 Describe the major proteins produced by the liver.
> 2 What is the flow of blood through the liver?
> 3 Which structures are found in the portal triad?
> 4 Where are the central vein and sinusoids of a hepatic lobule?
> 5 Describe the space of Disse.
> 6 What are the functions of Kupffer cells and stellate cells and where is each located?
> 7 What is the general structure of a bile salt?
> 8 How does the body remove bilirubin from the bloodstream?

The liver is considered an accessory organ to the digestive tract. It sits outside the digestive tube, but its secretions in the form of bile are vital to fat digestion. The liver also receives all the blood leaving the viscera via the portal vein. The portal vein conducts blood from the capillary beds within the lamina propria and submucosa of the intestinal tract to the capillary beds known as sinusoids of the hepatic lobules. This portal vein blood is carrying the end products of the digestion of carbohydrates and proteins directly to the liver for processing. Some of the sugars absorbed by the intestine are removed and used to supply energy for the metabolic processes of the liver. Some are converted to glycogen for later use by hepatocytes between meals. A high percentage of the amino acids in the portal vein blood are extracted by the liver and used to make a variety of proteins, such as albumin, α_1-globulins, α_2-globulins and β-globulins, clotting factors, and acute-phase proteins. Lipids absorbed during digestion are packaged into chylomicrons that are taken up by the lymphatic circulation and reach the liver via the hepatic artery. The lipids can be oxidized within the liver to provide energy needed for the various metabolic pathways or they can be packaged into very low density lipoprotein (VLDL) particles for transport of lipid to other organs for energy use. Another major action of the liver is to detoxify potential poisons and waste products via biotransformation and excretion into the bile for elimination with the feces. The liver also acts as a site of storage for lipids and the fat-soluble vitamins A, D, and E. The liver is also home to unique macrophages known as Kupffer cells that guard the liver against bacterial and viral antigens that may enter the portal circulation.

Microscopic anatomy of the liver

A pig's liver serves as our guide to the functional anatomy of the liver (Figure 43.6). The basic structure in the liver is the **hepatic lobule**. Other species have similar functional anatomy but the hepatic lobules are not as clearly defined. In the pig, the hepatic lobules are often hexagonally shaped structures with a large **central vein**. At each corner of the hexagon there will be an arteriole derived from the hepatic artery, a venule from the portal vein, and a small bile ductule that will eventually join with other ductules to form the bile duct (Figure 43.7). These

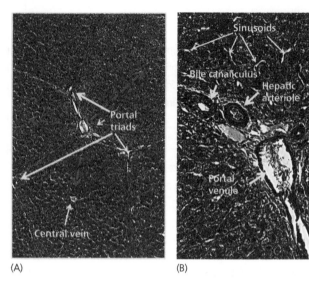

(A)   (B)

Figure 43.6 Pig liver histology. (A) A 5× view of hepatic lobule. These hexagonal lobules are not easily delineated in other species. A mixture of portal vein blood, carrying absorbed nutrients, and oxygenated hepatic arteriole blood flows from the portal triad area through sinusoids to reach the central veins. Each portal area can send blood to portions of several hepatic lobules (red dashed lines). (B) A 20× view. Portal triad with hepatic arteriole and portal vein and bile canaliculus. Portal triads can be found at each corner of the hexagonal lobules in the pig liver.

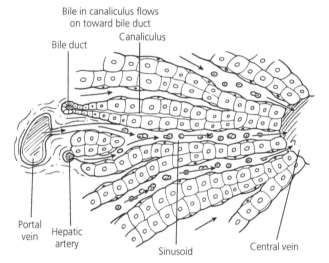

Figure 43.7 Portion of a liver lobule (highly magnified). Blood from the portal vein and hepatic artery flows into sinusoids (lined with Kupffer cells) and empties into the central vein. Bile travels in the opposite direction in canaliculi to empty into bile ducts in the triad areas. From Ham, A.W. (1974) *Histology*, 7th edn. J.B. Lippincott, Philadelphia. Reproduced with permission from Lippincott Williams & Wilkins.

three structures are commonly referred to as the **portal triad**. The hepatic arteriole is bringing highly oxygenated blood to the liver. It is also carrying chylomicrons containing the lipids absorbed during digestion of dietary fats. The portal venule is bringing poorly oxygenated blood to the hepatic lobule along with the sugars, volatile fatty acids, and amino acids derived from the digestion and absorption of dietary carbohydrates and proteins. The hepatic arteriole and the portal venule each contribute blood to capillary beds that run between the portal triad and the central vein. Each hepatic lobule receives blood from each of the portal triads at its boundaries. And each portal triad may provide blood to several adjacent hepatic lobules. Pathological infections and toxins are often brought to the liver with the blood flow, so it is common to see pathological changes in areas serviced by a portal triad.

The capillary beds carrying the portal venule and hepatic arteriole blood are lined by a highly fenestrated and leaky endothelium known as a **liver sinusoid**. Specialized macrophages known as **Kuppfer cells** roll along the sinusoids, patrolling the area in the event a bacterium may have also been brought to the liver with the portal blood. The sinusoids are lined on either side by hepatocytes. Between the sinusoid endothelial layer and the hepatocytes is a small space known as the **space of Disse**. Ions and nutrients leaving the sinusoids must cross the space of Disse before they can reach the hepatocytes. Within the space of Disse lies another unique cell type known as a **stellate cell**. These cells are normally inactive, but should any damage occur to the hepatocytes as a result of toxins or infection the stellate cells will produce fibrous scar tissue to wall off the area to prevent spread of the disease. When this fibrous scarring occurs over a wide area it is referred to as sclerosis of the liver.

The hepatocytes remove some portion of the nutrients from the mixed portal and hepatic arteriole blood in the sinusoids, depending on their need. They can return these nutrients to the sinusoid in the form of new proteins or glucose. Triglycerides produced in the liver can be packaged with apolipoproteins to form VLDL for export. The sinusoidal endothelium has large fenestrae (windows) to allow the large proteins and lipoprotein particles made in the hepatocytes to move into the blood. The hepatocytes also remove many toxins or waste materials from the blood for processing and eventual excretion into the bile. The sinusoid blood eventually reaches the central vein where it will converge on other veins to form the hepatic vein, which eventually joins the caudal vena cava leading to the heart.

Bile secretion

The cell membranes of adjacent hepatocytes develop a small space between them known as a canaliculus. Each hepatocyte excretes bile into this space which eventually carries that bile to a bile canal behind each row of hepatocytes. The bile canal joins the bile ductule at the portal triad area.

Hepatocytes perform many detoxifying actions to help rid the body of wastes, such as steroid hormones and bilirubin and toxins that may have been ingested. Many drugs are also removed from the blood by hepatocytes and excreted in the bile. Toxins or wastes generally undergo a two-phase process before they are excreted into the bile. In phase 1, the compound undergoes an oxidation reaction. Phase 1 generally adds one or more hydroxyl groups to various points in the molecule in order

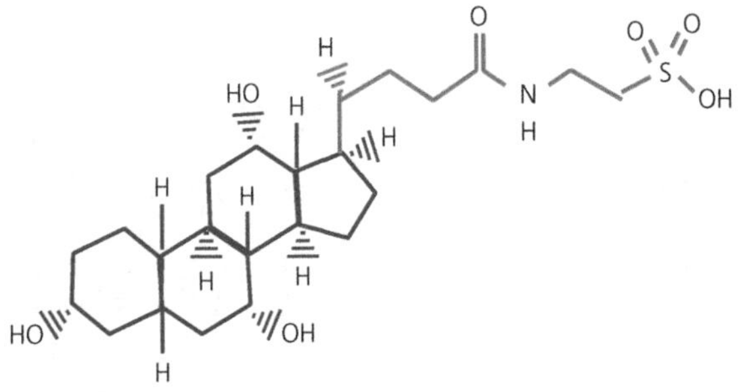

Figure 43.8 Taurocholic acid, a bile salt composed of cholesterol and the amino acid taurine. The blue section is lipophilic and will be on the inside of the micelle. The green portion is hydrophilic and will be on the outer surface of the micelle.

to change its structure sufficiently so that it is no longer a danger. The enzymes performing these reactions are often members of the family of cytochrome P450 monooxygenases. They insert one atom of oxygen into the aliphatic position of an organic substrate, R–H, to form R–OH. In the second phase of detoxification, the compound is often conjugated to a glucuronide or sulfate molecule by enzymes in the hepatocyte. This makes the molecule much more water-soluble and permits it to remain soluble in the bile as it moves through the bile ductules.

An example of a waste material excreted in the bile is bilirubin. Bilirubin is a very water-insoluble product of the metabolism (breakdown) of hemoglobin. The bilirubin is carried in blood bound to albumin and is removed from sinusoidal blood by the hepatocytes. Bilirubin is yellowish in color, and is responsible for the yellow color of bruises and the yellow discoloration seen in the jaundice of liver failure. Hepatocytes then conjugate the bilirubin with glucuronic acid to form a more water-soluble bilirubin diglucuronide which is excreted into the canaliculi. This gives bile its greenish color. Conjugated bilirubin can be converted by colonic bacteria to urobilinogen and to stercobilin, which is responsible for the brown color of normal feces. Some of the urobilinogen produced by bacteria in the intestine is reabsorbed into the blood and removed by the kidney. The urobilinogen gives urine a distinct yellow color.

The final important components of bile are bile salts. Bile salts are formed within hepatocytes by conjugating an amino acid with cholesterol. Taurine is one of the amino acids most commonly used and when bound to cholesterol it forms the bile salt taurocholic acid (Figure 43.8). Bile salts are highly polar molecules and very water-soluble. They have a hyrophobic end, provided by cholesterol, and a hydrophilic end, provided by the amino acid. This gives them the ability to form specialized structures called micelles within the intestine that aid in fat digestion and absorption.

Secretion of bile (choleresis) is a continuous process. In many species the bile is collected in a gallbladder so that it can be released following meals. The horse and the rat do not have a gallbladder and bile flows into the duodenum of these species continuously. In most species the bile duct joins with the

pancreatic duct and this common bile/pancreatic duct delivers bile and pancreatic secretions to the upper duodenum. Bile production by hepatocytes and contraction of the gallbladder can be stimulated by the hormone CCK produced by enteroendocrine cells of the duodenum in response to the presence of fats and amino acids in the duodenum (calcium and low pH in the duodenum also have minor stimulating effects on CCK secretion).

Bacterial infection of the bile ducts or gallbladder can result in gallstones or choleliths. Bacteria break the glucuronide bond between the glucuronic acid and compounds like bilirubin. Loss of the glucuronide molecule renders the bilirubin less soluble in water and it can form crystals and precipitate, especially if free cholesterol is also present in the bile. Choleliths can be found in all species.

Pancreas

1 Identify the exocrine and endocrine portions of the pancreas.

2 What factors affect the secretion of digestive enzymes?

3 Describe the factors involved in altering the pH of pancreatic secretions.

4 Why is it necessary to secrete digestive enzymes in an inactive form?

The pancreas is both an exocrine and an endocrine gland. The endocrine function of the pancreas will be discussed in other chapters, but the endocrine cells comprise less than 10% of the mass of the pancreas. The endocrine cells tend to be found in small collections of cells known as the **islets of Langerhans** that are scattered throughout the parenchyma of the pancreas.

The exocrine pancreas consists of many tubuloalveolar glands (Figure 43.9). These glands have an acinus and a duct system. The acinus is surrounded by a myoepithelial cell that can contract to send the contents of the acinar alveoli into the duct system. The exocrine functions of the pancreas provide enzymes needed for digestion of starches, proteins, and triglycerides. These enzymes are produced within acinar cells of the glands. Many of these enzymes are secreted in an inactive form. They become active only when in the duodenum. This avoids self-digestion of the pancreatic cells and ducts. Occasionally some of these enzymes are prematurely activated, resulting in a condition known as pancreatitis. Production and secretion of the pancreatic enzymes is stimulated by the hormone CCK produced in response to the presence of fats and amino acids in the duodenum.

The cells that comprise the ductule of each acinus function to increase the alkalinity of the pancreatic secretion. They secrete sodium and some potassium into the fluid secreted by the acinar cells and remove chloride from those secretions. The net effect is a rise in the pH of the fluids. Pancreatic juices will normally be slightly alkaline, with a pH of 7.8. However, under the influence of the duodenal hormone secretin, produced in response to a

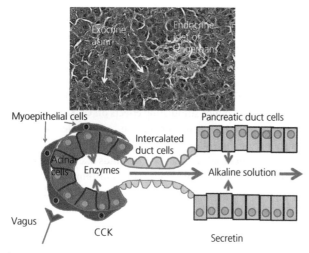

Myoepithelial cells

Pancreatic duct cells

Figure 43.9 Pancreatic acini and ducts: histomicrograph and schematic diagram. Cholecystokinin (CCK), produced in the duodenum in response to fat and amino acids, and vagal parasympathetic neurons stimulate acini to produce and secrete pancreatic enzymes, many in an inactive form. Secretin, produced in the duodenum in response to low pH, is the major factor controlling duct cell alkali secretion.

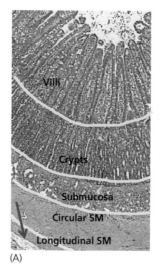

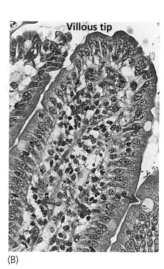

(A)   (B)

Figure 43.10 (A) Duodenum of a cat. Lines demarcate the villi from the crypts. The submucosa contains numerous Brunner's glands. The smooth muscle (SM) layers are labeled and the serosa is at the end of the red arrow. (B) Close-up of the villous tip lined by absorptive enterocytes. Several goblet cells are intermingled with the enterocytes (blue arrow). The lamina propria consists of fibroblasts and collagen fibrils. It also contains numerous lymphocytes (red arrows) and the muscularis mucosae (yellow arrow). Though not visible, blood vessels and a lymphatic lacteal also reside in the lamina propria.

low pH in the duodenum, the amount of chloride removed from the acinar fluid by the ductule cells is greatly increased and the pH of the pancreatic juices can rise to 8.2. This fluid plays a major role in neutralizing the low-pH chyme leaving the stomach. This must be done to protect the intestinal mucosa and also to optimize enzyme activity as most of the pancreatic enzymes operate most effectively at a pH between 7 and 8.

Small intestine

1 Describe the difference in function between the crypt and villous cells of the small intestine.

2 What are the major anatomic differences between duodenum, jejunum, and ileum?

3 What is the source of the cells that will become villous cells?

4 List the cell types of the crypt and their major functions.

5 Which cell types migrate up the crypt lining to become villous cells?

6 Which cells produce mucus in the small intestine?

7 Which cells contain enzymes needed for the final phases of digestion?

8 How do M-cells function?

9 Can water cross the tight junctions?

10 What happens to crypt cells as they mature?

11 What happens to older villous cells?

12 How do the crypt and villus respond to destruction of mucosal cells by a viral pathogen?

13 Why are cells at the tip of the villus most likely to experience hypoxia?

14 How is crypt secretion of chloride normally controlled to aid absorption of nutrients by the villous cells?

15 How is crypt secretion of chloride utilized in the inflammatory process to flush pathogens or toxins from a section of the intestine?

16 Describe how crypt secretion of chloride can be activated pathologically by certain bacteria to cause a severe watery diarrhea.

17 Describe how intestinal cells aid the humoral immune response in the intestinal tract.

The **tunica mucosa** of the small intestine is composed of projections from the mucosa into the lumen called **villi** and invaginations into the mucosa referred to as **crypts** (crypts of Lieberkuhn) (Figure 43.10). This greatly increases the surface area available for digestion and absorption of nutrients (Figure 43.11). The cells lining the crypts and villi are a single layer of simple columnar epithelium. The apical surface of each cell is thrown into folds known as microvilli that further increase the surface area for digestion and absorption (Figure 43.12). The apical surface is in contact with the lumen of the intestine and the basolateral membrane is attached to the basal lamina. The length of the villi is greatest in the jejunum and shortest in the ileum. A loose connective tissue called the lamina propria can be found below the basal lamina. Arterioles, venules, and lymphatic lacteals run throughout the lamina propria. Lymphocytes are commonly interspersed among the fibroblasts

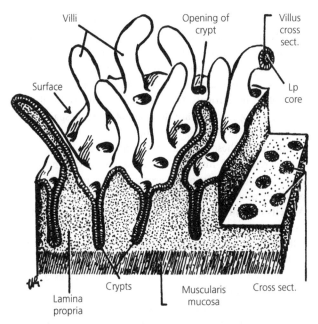

Figure 43.11 Three-dimensional representation of the small intestine lining. The villi are finger-like processes with cores of lamina propria that extend into the lumen. The crypts of Lieberkühn are depressions in the lamina propria (Lp). From Ham, A.W. (1974) *Histology*, 7th edn. J.B. Lippincott, Philadelphia. Reproduced with permission from Lippincott Williams & Wilkins.

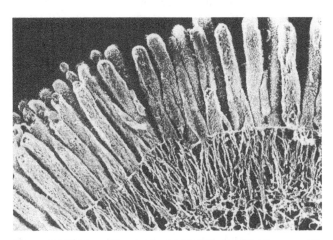

Figure 43.12 Photomicrograph of microvilli extending from a small intestine epithelial cell. The cord-like structures extending downward from the microvilli are contractile actin filaments. From Fawcett, D.W. (1986) *Bloom and Fawcett: A Textbook of Histology*, 11th edn. W.B. Saunders, Philadelphia. Courtesy of N. Hirokawa and J. Heuser. With permission from Elsevier.

in the lamina propria. A thin smooth muscle, the muscularis mucosae, also extends up into the villi and can be used to shorten and lengthen each villus during the digestive process.

Below the mucosa lies the **submucosa**. Neurons comprising the **submucosal nerve plexus** of the enteric nervous system can be found in the submucosa of all regions of the gastrointestinal tract. In the upper duodenum, the submucosa contains many

glands known as **Brunner's glands**. These are typical compound tubular glands with acinar structures with a duct system that conveys their secretions ot the base of the crypts. The acinar cells secrete mucus and the duct cells add sodium and potassium to, and remove chloride from, the secretions to form an alkaline secretion. This alkaline fluid is used to flush the crypts and then the villi with this acid-neutralizing fluid. Secretion by the Brunner's glands is controlled by the hormone secretin, released by enteroendocrine cells within the crypts of the duodenum when the pH of the fluid in the crypts falls too low. The submucosa of the lower duodenum and jejunum are not remarkable. However, the submucosa of the ileum contains unique aggregates of B and T lymphocytes, macrophages and dendritic cells known as **Peyer's patches**. They occupy large sections of the submucosa and can also extend into the mucosa of the ileum. Peyer's patches are an important component of the mucosa-associated lymphoid tissue (MALT) and provide immune surveillance of the intestinal lumen, facilitating the generation of immune responses within the mucosa.

The **tunica muscularis** is below the submucosa and comprises the inner circular and outer longitudinal smooth muscle layers. The nerve cell bodies of the neurons comprising the **myenteric nerve plexus** of the enteric nervous system reside between the two muscle layers. Outside this layer is the **tunica serosa**, a single cell layer of squamous epithelium on a loose connective tissue or adventitia.

Cells within the small intestine crypts
Six cell types exist within the crypts.

Crypt stem cells
The base of the crypts contain a pluripotent stem cell population that persists throughout the life of the animal. These cells undergo regular division and give rise to the majority of the cells in the crypt. Crypt secretory cells, mucus-secreting goblet cells, enteroendocrine cells, and Paneth cells all arise from these stem cells. The stem cells do not migrate from the base of the crypts.

Crypt enterocytes
The majority of cells lining the crypts are crypt enterocytes. These cells have microvilli at their apical surface that increase their surface area tremendously. Their primary function is to secrete chloride, sodium and water into the lumen of the crypt to facilitate absorption by absorptive enterocytes in the villus. The crypt enterocytes migrate up the basal lamina toward the villus and eventually up onto the villus itself. Once on the villus, the crypt cells stop being secretory cells and their phenotype switches to that of an absorptive enterocyte. The crypt cells migrate up the lamina propria propelled by means of lamellipodia, small actin monomers extending from the basaolateral membrane that interact with integrin proteins on the basal lamina. This allows them to "walk" up the crypts and onto the villus. The crypt cell requires 1–2 days to migrate up the crypt

and another 3–4 days to reach the tip of the villus. At that point they die and are sloughed off.

Goblet cells

These cells are derived from the crypt stem cells. They also migrate out of the crypts to populate the villi. They become more and more numerous from duodenum to ileum. They secrete mucus. They move onto the tip of the villi at the same rate as crypt enterocytes, and they too are shed shortly after arrival at the villus tip.

Enteroendocrine cells

These cells are derived from crypt stem cells but remain near the base of the crypts. These cells have contact with the lumen of the crypt at their apical surface, allowing them to monitor pH, osmolarity, and composition of the ingesta in the lumen. They contain secretory granules containing the hormone they will secrete which, when properly stimulated ,will be secreted into the lamina propria to enter the postcapillary venules and be distributed throughout the circulation. In some cases, these hormones have paracrine effects on neighboring cells rather than endocrine effects. A multitude of hormones are produced by the enteroendocrine cells, many of them unique to the gastrointestinal tract. The veterinary student should be aware of the most important hormones and their function, such as CCK and secretin. Realize that somatomedins, vasoactive intestinal peptide, serotonin, enteroglucagon, and other hormones also play important roles in gastrointestinal physiology.

Paneth cells

These cells are derived from crypt stem cells but do not migrate from the base of the crypts. They are relatively long-lived cells that are believed to provide protection for the crypt stem cells. They produce antibacterial substances such as lysozyme, phospholipases, and defensins which they release into the lumen of the crypt. These substances provide protection against a wide spectrum of bacteria, fungi, and even some enveloped viruses. Interestingly, the dog, cat and pig do not have Paneth cells.

M-cells or dome cells

These are not derived from the crypt stem cells and their origin remains unknown. They can be found interspersed among the enterocytes in the crypt and even villous areas. They are particularly common in the mucosal lining over the tops of the Peyer's patches. They should be considered cells of the immune system. They capture particles (bacterial and viral antigens) and pass them on unchanged to the dendritic cells and lymphocytes within the lamina propria and within the lymphoid follicles in the mucosa and submucosa.

Cells within the villus of the small intestine

Three cell types line the small intestinal villi.

1 **Villous absorptive enterocytes**: these cells are derived from the crypt secretory enterocytes. At some point in their migration up the villus, the crypt cells quit their secretory activity and begin to elaborate enzymes within their apical membrane microvilli, often referred to as the brush border. These enzymes are needed for the final phases of digestion. The cells also begin to express the transport proteins necessary for absorption of nutrients. On reaching the villous tip, the cells undergo apoptosis and are sloughed off. The lifespan of a villous absorptive cell is less than 4 days.

2 **Goblet cells**: these migrate up the crypt and are responsible for secretion of mucus. Mucus secretion can be greatly increased on stimulation by prostaglandins released by damaged mucosal cells in the area.

3 **M-cells or dome cells**: same as in the crypts, though not as numerous in the villi.

All the cells lining mucosal surfaces of the intestinal tract (esophagus to anus) have an apical and a basolateral membrane. Adjacent cells are linked to one another on all sides by "tight junctions" that form a seal between cells that is relatively impermeable to bacteria, viruses, and large molecules that have been ingested. The tight junctions also provide resistance to the passage of small ions and water. However, this resistance can be overcome if the electrochemical forces are great enough to drive the ions to the opposite side of a tight junction. Water channels (likely consisting of claudin proteins) can allow passage of water through the tight junction. They provide paths of lower resistance for water molecule passage that are utilized only when there is a great difference in osmolarity on one side of the tight junction.

Populating and repopulating the crypts and villi

A typical crypt of the small intestine contains about 250–300 enterocytes and goblet cells covering its surface (Figure 43.13). A typical villus may require 3000 cells to completely cover its basal lamina. There are approximately 30 pluripotent crypt stem cells at the base of the crypt and 40–50 Paneth cells guarding them. Even fewer enteroendocrine and dome cells are found among the crypt and villous cells. It is estimated that about 1400 cells slough off the normal villous tip each day. The crypt stem cells must produce an equal number of replacement cells each day. Keep in mind that there may be multiple crypts surrounding each villus and supplying cells to that villus. It also means each crypt is supplying cells to more than one villus.

Some viruses, such as the coronavirus causing porcine epidemic diarrhea, can destroy nearly all the cells on a villus. This leaves the basal lamina completely exposed and invites bacterial invasion of the lamina propria. The villus must be covered with new cells rapidly. The crypt stem cells divide even more rapidly and the crypt enterocytes and goblet cells migrate onto the villus more rapidly than normal. The muscularis mucosae proves its value by contracting and shrinking the length of the villus. If the villus normally required 3000 cells to completely cover its normal full length, it may take just 2000 to cover the shortened villus. The object is to ensure the villous basal lamina is covered

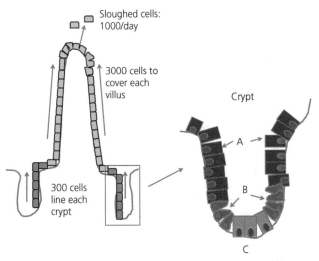

Figure 43.13 Several crypts will contribute the cells needed to cover the villus. Shortly after leaving the crypt zone the migrating crypt enterocytes, which were primarily secretory cells, change their phenotype to become villous absorptive cells. It takes 4–5 days for a crypt cell to reach the villous tip. Once there, they last only a period of hours before they are sloughed off into the lumen of the intestine. The crypts contain rapidly dividing stem cells (B), which multiply and differentiate to give rise to secretory crypt enterocytes and goblet cells (A). At the base of the crypts reside enteroendocrine and Paneth cells that were derived from crypt stem cells (C). They do not migrate up to the villi.

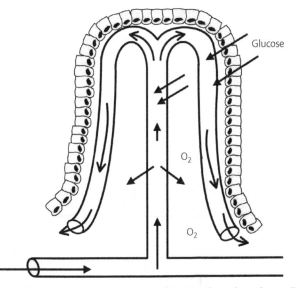

Figure 43.14 A functional schematic of the blood supply to the small intestinal villus. A central arteriole emerging from the submucosal artery carries oxygenated blood upward toward the villous tip, where a capillary network ramifies outward and is collected into venules and veins, which progress downward at the periphery just beneath the mucosal epithelium. An exchange of oxygen and nutrients can occur in such a hairpin countercurrent arrangement. From Reece, W.O. (2004) *Dukes' Physiology of Domestic Animals*, 12th edn. Cornell University Press, Ithaca, NY. Reproduced with permission from Cornell University Press.

quickly. The new cells are unlikely to be fully functional as it takes several days for brush border enzymes to be elaborated. It may take weeks for the villus to recover its full length.

Blood flow within the lamina propria of the villus

An arteriole carries blood to the tip of the villus and this arteriole is in close proximity to a venule carrying blood away from the capillary beds at the tip of the villus (Figure 43.14). The arteriole is carrying oxygenated blood that has a Po_2 of about 90 mmHg. The venule will have a Po_2 of about 40 mmHg. The arteriole and the venule are in such close proximity that a countercurrent process develops. Oxygen diffuses from the arteriole as it ascends the villous tip and the venule picks up this oxygen as it moves blood away from the villous tip. The net result is that the Po_2 in the arteriole decreases to about 75 mmHg by the time it reaches the villous tip. The villous tip cells have a huge role in absorption of nutrients and electrolytes and conduct this work in a relatively oxygen-poor environment. An interesting outcome of this situation is that whenever there is a problem with oxygenation of the blood due to pneumonia or heart disease, the villous tip cells receive even less oxygen and can die and slough off faster. Ischemia or disruption of blood flow to a section of intestine will also result in death of the villous tip cells first. The denuded villus can then allow bacterial invasion through the exposed basal lamina.

Crypt enterocyte secretion of chloride, sodium, and water

While the enterocytes are in the crypts their main function is to secrete chloride, sodium, and water into the lumen of the crypts. This serves two critical functions. The sodium excreted into the lumen of the crypts provides the electrochemical force needed to allow absorption of amino acids, sugars, phosphate, and other nutrients by the villous absorptive cells (described in detail in Chapter 44). There is generally not enough sodium in the diet to perform this critical function, so the crypt cells provide the sodium that allows the villous cells to perform many of their absorptive functions. The water secreted into the lumen by the crypt cells acts to reduce the osmolarity of the digesta, as well as ensuring the digesta remains sufficiently moist to solubilize ions, sugars, and amino acids. Understanding how the crypt enterocytes secrete these ions and water and how this process is controlled will allow the veterinary practitioner to understand the etiology of the "secretory" components of diarrhea.

During digestion within the small intestine, particularly in the duodenum and jejunum, vagal and enteric nervous system sensory afferent neurons sense changes within the lumen such as increased osmolarity, stretch, presence of amino acids in the lumen, or reduced pH and the medulla initiates vagal parasympathetic efferent stimulation of the crypt cells (Figure 43.15). Vagal postganglionic parasympathetic neurons release acetylcholine (ACh) that interacts with muscarinic

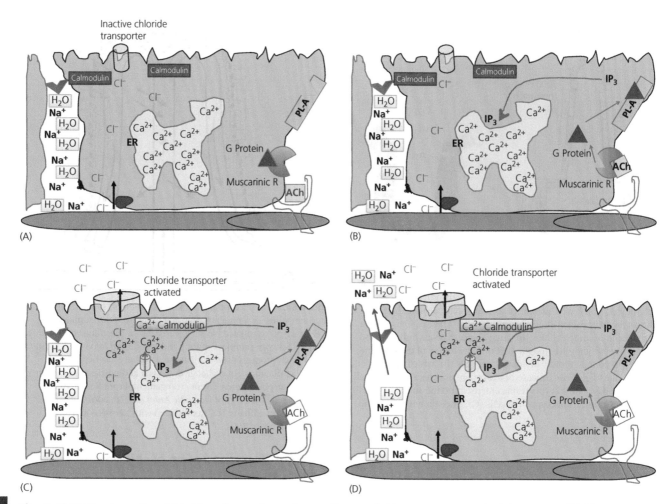

Figure 43.15 Crypt secretion of chloride, sodium, and water is normally controlled by vagus parasympathetic innervation. (A) The vagus responds to stretch or osmotic changes in the intestine and releases acetylcholine (ACh). The G protein-coupled muscarinic receptor resides in the basolateral cell membrane. (B) Activation of muscarinic receptor stimulates G-protein activation of phospholipase A (PL-A), which catalyzes production of inositol trisphosphate (IP_3). (C) The IP_3 moves to the endoplasmic reticulum (ER) and binds to an IP_3 receptor causing a Ca^{2+} channel to open in the ER membrane. (D) Ca^{2+} binds to calmodulin and the Ca^{2+}–calmodulin complex activates the chloride channel to become active. Cl^- is actively pumped out of the cell into the lumen at the expense of ATP. Sodium follows through the tight junction between cells to maintain electroneutrality. Water will also cross the tight junction, pulled by the osmotic gradient created by Cl^- and Na^+ in the lumen.

receptors on the basolateral membrane of the crypt cells. These receptors are G protein-coupled receptors linked to phospholipase A, so on activation the intracellular concentration of inositol trisphosphate (IP_3) rises. IP_3 acts on the membrane of internal cell organelles that store calcium, such as the endoplasmic reticulum, and causes calcium channels to open in the the membrane. This releases Ca^{2+} to the cytosol of the cell where it becomes bound to calmodulin, an important cell regulatory protein, and causes it to become activated. The Ca^{2+}–calmodulin complex then interacts with a Cl^- channel pump protein at the apical membrane and causes it to open. It also causes an ATP to donate the energy of a phosphate bond to supply the energy needed to transport the chloride from the inside of the cell, which has a relatively low Cl^- concentration (<30 mmol/L), to the lumen of the crypt where Cl^- concentration

is substantially higher. This Cl^- channel pump is also known as the cystic fibrosis transmembrane conductance regulator protein. The Cl^- pumped into the lumen is rapidly replaced by entry of a chloride into the cell from the extracellular fluid ([Cl^-] ~105 mmol/L) across the basolateral membrane, alone or cotransported with Na^+ or K^+. Once chloride has been secreted into the lumen, the negative charges of the Cl^- ions in the lumen of the crypt, together with the high Na^+ concentration in the extracellular fluid, cause Na^+ ions to move from the extracellular fluid to the lumen across the tight cell junctions separating adjacent crypt enterocytes. Water then follows the solute into the lumen using water channels in the tight cell junctions. In this way, the secretory activity of the crypt cells is coordinated to occur only at the time the villous cells need sodium ions to accomplish absorptive activities.

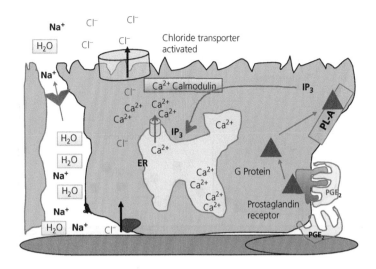

Figure 43.16 (A) Prostaglandin E (PGE₂), produced in response to damage or reactive oxygen species in the area around the crypt cell, binds to a G protein-coupled PGE₂ receptor. This results in activation of phospholipase A (PL-A) and production of inositol trisphosphate (IP₃). The IP₃ causes opening of Ca⁺² channels in the endoplasmic reticulum (ER) resulting in formation of the Ca²⁺–calmodulin complex and activation of the apical membrane chloride transporter. This same mechanism can be used by tumor necrosis factors, interleukins, and other cytokines to initiate secretory activity that might help flush away harmful compounds or bacteria. This same mechanism works in goblet cells to stimulate mucus secretion.

Crypt cell secretion as a response to inflammation or pathogens

Certain toxins, pathogens, and poisons can cause damage to cells in an area of the intestine. The damaged tissues respond by producing and secreting prostaglandins, primarily PGE₂ and PGI₂. The prostaglandins diffuse through the lamina propria to reach crypt cells. Crypt enterocytes possess receptors for prostaglandin on their basolateral membrane. These are G protein-coupled receptors link to phospholipase A (Figure 43.16). When prostaglandin binds to its receptor, it causes intracellular concentrations of IP₃ to increase in the cytosol of the crypt enterocyte. This causes Ca²⁺ channels on the endoplasmic reticulum to open and Ca²⁺ floods the cytosol. Ca²⁺–calmodulin complexes form and interact with the apical membrane chloride pump and Cl⁻ is actively pumped out of the cell into the lumen. Extracellular fluid Na⁺ and water move across the tight junction to follow the Cl⁻ out into the lumen. This action brings large volumes of fluid into the crypt and to surrounding villi to flush the offending toxin away from the area.

Inflammation in a segment of the intestine can also activate crypt secretion activity, presumably to help flush a pathogenic substance away from an area of inflammation. For example, lymphocytes that have become activated by the presence of some "pathogen-associated molecular pattern" can respond by producing a variety of cytokines. Cytokines such as tumor necrosis factor (TNF)-α, interleukins, and interferons bind to their respective receptors at the base of the crypt cells and activate adenylyl cyclase or guanylate cyclase. The resulting cyclic AMP or cyclic GMP causes Ca²⁺ ions to leave intracellular stores and bind to calmodulin. This complex then causes the chloride channel pump to be activated, driving Cl⁻ into the lumen with Na⁺ and water following through the tight junctions. A slightly different way of stimulating crypt chloride secretion is provided by the action of serotonin (Figure 43.17). Serotonin can be released from enteroendocrine cells in the crypt by the presence of toxins or bacterial cell walls in the lumen of the crypt. The released serotonin diffuses through the lamina propria to

activate nearby crypt cells in a paracrine fashion. Serotonin binds to its receptor, which is linked to a Ca²⁺ channel in the basolateral cell membrane. The Ca²⁺ channel opens and extracellular Ca²⁺ floods the cytosol. Again, the Ca²⁺–calmodulin complex forms and binds to the chloride channel pump, activating secretion of Cl⁻ into the lumen and extracellular Na⁺ and water cross the tight junction to follow the Cl⁻ into the lumen.

Receptors for all the factors discussed (prostaglandins, cytokines, and serotonin associated with cell damage and inflammation) can also be found on goblet cells in the crypts and villi. They respond to these substances by markedly increasing mucus secretion, thought to be a response for flushing away the offending material and coating it with mucus so it will not be as likely to reach the mucosal cells.

Secretory diarrhea caused by bacterial enterotoxins

The crypt cell secretion activities described so far have been localized to small areas of the intestine that might require Na⁺ for absorption of sugars and amino acids (described in Chapter 44) or which might use the secretions to flush away pathogens. However, certain bacteria produce toxins that can hijack the normal crypt cell secretion process and cause widespread uncontrolled activation of crypt cell secretion. The classic example of this is cholera toxin produced by *Vibrio cholerae* ingested with contaminated water. The bacteria produce a toxin that is released into the lumen of the small intestine. The cholera toxin binds to proteins (receptors?) at the apical membrane of the crypt enterocyte (Figure 43.18). It is not known why these receptors for cholera toxin exist – it seems logical that there is some natural compound found in the lumen they recognize but none have been identified. Once cholera toxin binds this apical membrane protein, it stimulates activation of guanylate cyclase. Cyclic GMP levels rise inside the cell, causing the Ca²⁺ channels on the endoplasmic reticulum to open and Ca²⁺ ions flood the cytosol. This permits Ca²⁺–calmodulin complexes to form and activate the chloride channel pump. Cl⁻ is secreted into the

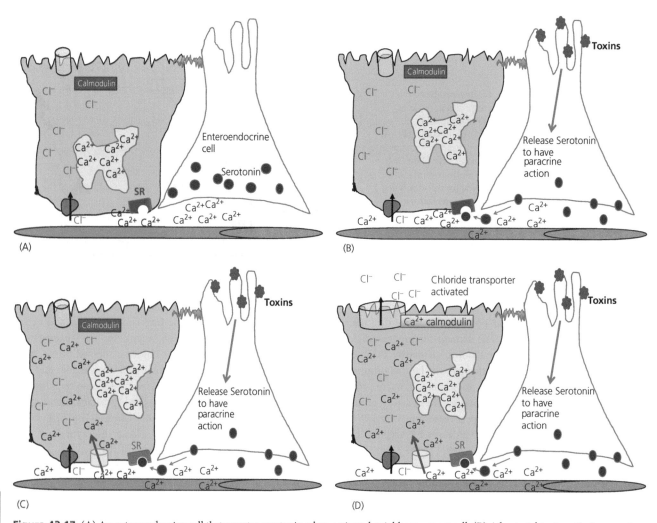

Figure 43.17 (A) An enteroendocrine cell that secretes serotonin when activated neighbors a crypt cell. (B) A bacterial toxin activates receptors at the apical membrane of the enteroendocrine cell causing serotonin vesicles to fuse with the basolateral membrane and secrete serotonin into the lamia propria, where it diffuses toward a serotonin receptor (SR) in the basolateral membrane of the crypt cell. (C) Binding of serotonin causes a conformational change in the receptor allowing it to open Ca^{2+} channels in the basolateral membrane. Extracellular Ca^{2+} enters the cell. (D) The rise in cytosolic Ca^{2+} results in formation of the Ca^{2+}–calmodulin complex and activation of the apical membrane chloride transporter. Sodium and water follow the chloride into the lumen across the tight junctions.

lumen and Na^+ and water follow. These toxins spread throughout the intestinal tract and activate huge numbers of crypt cells for a prolonged period. To make matters worse, the toxin can also bind to cholera toxin "receptors" on the villous absorptive enterocytes. Again this causes cyclic GMP production and a rise in intracellular Ca^{2+} and formation of Ca^{2+}–calmodulin complexes. However, in this instance the Ca^{2+}–calmodulin complex binds to the Na^+/Cl^- cotransporter used to absorb lumen Na^+ and Cl^- across the apical membrane of the villous cells. Shutting down this mechanism for absorption of Na^+ and Cl^- also reduces the amount of water that can be absorbed. The end result is that crypts are in a state of tremendous hypersecretion and the villous cells have a reduced capacity to absorb, causing a massive loss of fluids and electrolytes with the feces.

In veterinary medicine, the offending bacteria producing entertoxins are likely to be certain strains of *Escherichia coli*. At least two enterotoxins have been described. One is heat stable (ST toxin) and when it binds to receptors on the apical membrane of crypt cells (and villous cells) it activates cyclic GMP production just like cholera toxin, causing a similar severe watery diarrhea. The other enterotoxin produced by a different strain of *E. coli* is a heat-labile toxin (LT). This toxin binds to its receptor on the apical surface of enterocytes (crypt and villus) and activates adenylyl cyclase, causing intracellular cyclic AMP levels to rise, triggering increased secretion of Cl^- by crypt enterocytes and decreased absorption of Na^+ and Cl^- by villous enterocytes (Figure 43.19). A notable difference is that when the LT toxin binds to the receptor protein that recognizes

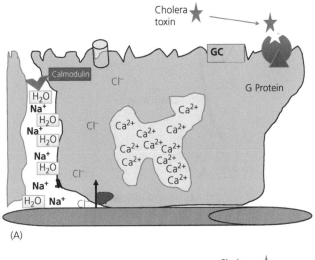

(A)

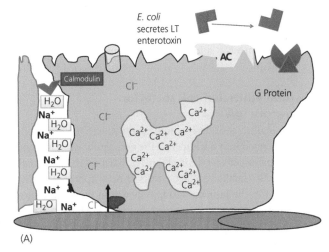

(A)

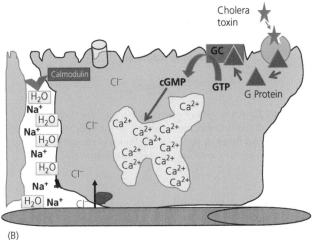

(B)

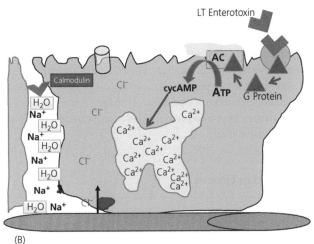

(B)

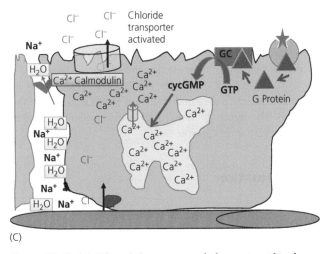

(C)

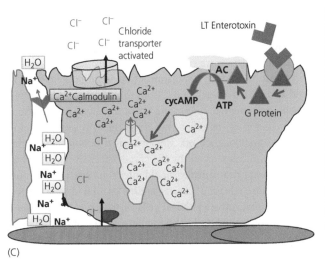

(C)

Figure 43.18 (A) *Vibrio cholerae* secretes cholera toxin within the lumen of the intestine. A G protein-coupled receptor that responds to this toxin resides in the apical membrane of the cell. (B) On binding to the receptor, the G protein activates guanylyl cyclase (GC). The GC converts guanosine triphosphate (GTP) to cyclic guanosine monophosphate (cyclic GMP). (C) The cyclic GMP activates kinases and pathways that cause Ca²⁺ channels in the endoplasmic reticulum to open. This results in formation of the Ca²⁺–calmodulin complex and activation of the apical membrane chloride transporter. Sodium and water follow the chloride into the lumen across the tight junctions.

Figure 43.19 (A) Certain strains of *Escherichia coli* secrete enterotoxin (LT toxin) within the lumen of the intestine. A G protein-coupled receptor responds to this toxin in the apical membrane of the crypt (and villus) cells. (B) On binding to the receptor, the G protein activates adenylyl cyclase (AC). The AC converts adenosine triphosphate (ATP) to cyclic adenosine monophosphate (cAMP). (C) The cAMP activates kinases and pathways that cause Ca²⁺ channels in the endoplasmic reticulum to open. This results in formation of the Ca²⁺–calmodulin complex and activation of the apical membrane chloride transporter. Sodium and water follow the chloride into the lumen across the tight junctions. In villous cells, the toxin's action is similar but results in blockade of the Na⁺/Cl⁻ absorption cotransporter in the apical membrane.

it, it binds irreversibly: the affected cell will hypersecrete Cl⁻ and fail to absorb Na⁺ and Cl⁻ until it is finally sloughed from the villous tip.

Intestinal epithelial cell secretion of secretory IgA

The intestinal mucosa derives some protection from immunoglobulin secreted into the lumen of the gut. Antibodies can bind toxins and pathogens rendering them less harmful to the animal. Antibodies also facilitate phagocytosis by neutrophils and other cells present in the lumen. Plasma cells within the lamina propria synthesize dimers of immunoglobulin A (IgA). Special proteins called secretory piece extend from the basolateral surface of the enterocytes and act as IgA receptors. Once the IgA dimer binds to the secretory piece it stimulates endocytosis of the IgA dimer bound to the secretory piece. The endosome traverses the enterocyte and fuses with the apical membrane. The attachment of the secretory protein to the membrane vesicle is severed and the IgA dimer enters the lumen of the intetine with a piece of the secretory protein attached. The presence of secretory protein on the IgA dimer provides it with resistance to proteolysis by digestive enzymes in the lumen of the intestinal tract.

Large intestine

> **1** Identify the major layers found in the colon.

The cecum and colon are very similar in their microscopic appearance. The mucosa contains crypts (but not villi) lined primarily by goblet cells that secrete a slighlty alkaline mucus. There are also some absorptive epithelial cells (Figure 43.20). As in the small intestine, a small population of colon crypt stem cells is found at the base of each crypt. Both the goblet and absorptive epithelial cells migrate toward the top of the crypt. After a short time at the top of the crypt (1–2 days) the cells undergo apoptosis and are sloughed off. Under normal circumstances the amount of mucus secreted by the crypts is relatively small but that can change dramatically should infection damage the colon cells and cause release of prostaglandins or inflammatory cytokines. The absorptive epithelial cells of the crypts can absorb some electrolytes and the last remnants of water from the ingesta.

Acid–base secretion summary

> **1** How is it possible to neutralize stomach acid in the upper small intestine?

A 20-kg dog would be expected to produce about 600 mL of gastric juice with a pH of about 1.2. That same dog will secrete

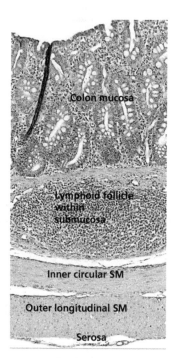

Figure 43.20 A 10× view of colon tissue from a dog. Lymphoid follicles serve an important role in protecting the body from bacteria and viruses that might be present in the lumen of the colon. Lymphocytes are also common in the lamina propria of the colon mucosa.

about 300 mL of saliva, 600 mL of pancreatic juice, 300 mL of bile, and 300 mL from the Brunner's glands and crypt cell secretory efforts. These secretions are slightly alkaline and have a pH of about 8.0. All these secretions are essentially isotonic. It would seem unlikley that 1500 mL of secretions with a pH of 8.0 could neutralize 600 mL of gastric fluid with a pH of 1.5. The gastric juices will also be partially neutralized by components in the diet as well. The chyme leaving the stomach will generally have a pH of 2.0–2.25. A major aid to the increase in pH of duodenal contents is the rapid reabsorption of Cl⁻ ions from the chyme by the upper duodenal villous absorptive enterocytes (described further in Chapter 44).

Self-evaluation

Answers can be found at the end of the chapter.

1 What kind of cells produce histamine within the gastrointestinal tract?

2 Giving nonsteroidal anti-inflammatory drugs for long periods can cause ulcers to develop because many NSAIDs block (**A**) _____, resulting in failure of damaged cells to produce (**B**) _____. This leads to failure to increase (**C**) _____ needed for cell repair.

3 The alkalinity of pancreatic fluid is achieved by pancreatic duct cells that resorb (**A**) _____ ions from the pancreatic acinar secretions and add (**B**) _____ ions to those secretions.

4 Many enzymes produced by pancreatic acinar cells are secreted in an inactive form. What happens if they accidentally become activated within the acinar cells or the interlobular pancreatic ducts?

5 Within a single functional unit of the liver the hepatocytes that are closest to the portal vein are receiving (**A**) the least or (**B**) the most oxygenated blood. Choose one option.

6 Bilirubin and many drugs are excreted via the biliary system. Generally, the process involves hepatocytes removing water-insoluble compounds bound to plasma albumin and increasing their water solubility by _____ and then releasing them into the bile canaliculus.

7 What is the function of M or dome cells in the intestine?

8 Chloride is actively secreted into the lumen of the small intestine by _____ cells.

9 A clostridial bacterial toxin is ingested by a dog who got loose and obtained dinner from the neighbor's garbage can. The toxin activates receptors on (**A**) _____ cells located at the base of the crypts, which secrete serotonin in response to the toxin. The serotonin acts on neighboring cells and causes (**B**) _____ channels in the basolateral membrane of (**C**) _____ cells to open.

10 Between meals, crypt cells are largely inactive. Crypt secretion of chloride increases shortly after a meal causes distension of the stomach. The crypt secretory process in this case is controlled by the (**A**) _____ which releases (**B**) _____ onto (**C**) _____ receptors of the crypt cells.

11 Many horses harbor adult strongyle nematode parasites within their gut. In their larval stage these parasites can migrate outside the digestive tract (not a long-term survival strategy for the parasite but

they occasionally do this). A young horse raised in relative isolation was put into a pasture with 50 other foals, all on a nonexistent to poor deworming program. Within weeks this foal has a strongyle larva migrate into a tributary of the cranial mesenteric artery where the foal's immune response kills the larva and the dead larva and immune cells block that small section of artery. Blood flow to a section of intestine is greatly reduced. This causes which cells to die first?

Suggested reading

Dubreuil, J.D. (2012) The whole shebang: the gastrointestinal tract, *Escherichia coli* enterotoxins and secretion. *Current Issues in Molecular Biology* **14**:71–82.

Malarkey, D.E., Johnson, K., Ryan, L., Boorman, G. and Maronpot, R.R. (2005) New insights into functional aspects of liver morphology. *Toxicologic Pathology* **33**:27–34.

Answers

1 Enteroendocrine cells of the fundic stomach
2 (A) Cyclooxygenase 1, (B) PGE and PGI, (C) blood flow
3 (A) Chloride, (B) sodium and potassium
4 Digestion of body tissues leading to pancreatitis
5 B
6 Hydroxylating them at various sites and conjugating them to a water-soluble compound like glucuronic acid
7 Present antigens from the lumen to lymphocytes and dendritic cells residing in the lamina propria
8 Crypt enterocyte
9 (A) Enteroendocrine, (B) calcium, (C) crypt
10 (A) Vagal parasympathetic, (B) acetylcholine, (C) muscarinic
11 Cells at the villous tip

Section VII: Digestion, Absorption, and Metabolism

Digestion and Absorption of Nutrients

Jesse P. Goff
Iowa State University, Ames, IA, USA

Most of the components of a diet are too large to be absorbed directly across the intestinal epithelium and into the blood. Digestion is the process of breaking these dietary compounds into small fragments that can be absorbed. The process of moving these digested fragments across the gastrointestinal tract requires the secretion of various digestive enzymes and absorption aids such as bile. This chapter describes those processes. As an introduction to this process the chapter starts with a review of the basic chemical and biological processes used to move materials across lipid bilayer membranes.

Movement of particles across cell membranes

1 How is diffusion affected by the charge of particles in a compartment?

2 What is the driving force that allows facilitated diffusion to operate?

3 Does a pH of 3.4 promote nonionic diffusion of propionic acid better than a pH of 7.0 at the absorptive surface to be crossed?

Dukes' Physiology of Domestic Animals, Thirteenth Edition. Edited by William O. Reece, Howard H. Erickson, Jesse P. Goff and Etsuro E. Uemura.
© 2015 John Wiley & Sons, Inc. Published 2015 by John Wiley & Sons, Inc.
Companion website: www.wiley.com/go/reece/physiology

Section VII: Digestion, Absorption, and Metabolism

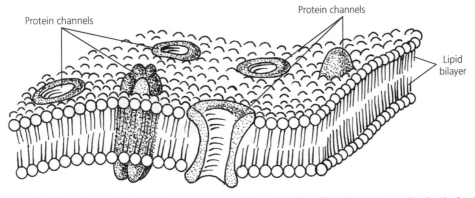

Figure 44.1 Structure of a cell membrane. The lipid bilayer is represented by a thin film of lipid that is two molecules thick. The protein channels (pores) may be composed of a single protein or a cluster of proteins. The channels may have specificity for certain substances, or they may be restrictive because of size. Virtually all water diffuses through the protein channels. From Reece, W.O. (2009) *Functional Anatomy and Physiology of Domestic Animals*, 4th edn. Wiley-Blackwell, Ames, IA. Reproduced with permission from Wiley.

When considering absorption of nutrients across the intestinal tract it must be kept in mind that there are two membranes that need to be crossed to move material from the lumen of the intestine to the blood. Absorptive epithelial cells lining the intestine have an apical membrane in contact with the luminal contents and a basolateral membrane in contact with extracellular fluids. The apical membrane of enterocytes has microvilli that project into the lumen to increase the surface area for absorption. These cell membranes are composed of a bilayer of phospholipids (Figure 44.1). Phospholipids have a hydrophilic head extending into the water on the outside and inside of the cell and a hydrophobic region between the two hydrophilic surfaces. Interspersed among the phospholipids are cholesterol molecules and various types of proteins. These proteins are often glycoproteins and they can extend varying distance in or out of the cell membrane. Some are important as receptors for hormones or neurotransmitters. Many are enzymes in the intestinal tract and some also serve as membrane channels to allow or facilitate entry of material across the lipid bilayer. Lipid-soluble hydrophobic compounds can easily cross the lipid bilayer of the cell membranes. As a rule, water and hydrophilic materials cannot easily cross the lipid bilayer without some accommodation in the form of a protein-based transporter. Like all cell membranes, a thin layer of glycoproteins, oligosaccharides, and glycolipids covers the lipid bilayer to form the glycocalyx. A thin layer of water, the unstirred water layer, adheres to the glycocalyx by surface tension forces. The unstirred water layer and glycocalyx do not impede absorption of water-soluble solute, but do form a barrier to the entry of larger lipophilic substances that might ordinarily cross the apical membrane unimpeded.

Very often the mechanisms utilized to move solute from the lumen of the gut across the apical membrane and into the enterocyte are not the same as the mechanisms used to move the solute from the interior of the cell across the basolateral cell membrane into the extracellular fluid. The bulk of absorption is performed by the villous absorptive enterocytes in the small intestine. Absorptive enterocytes also exist in the large intestine, but they lack many of the enzymes and transport molecules of the small intestinal villous enterocyte, which limits what they can absorb. The basic principles involved in developing the forces required for movement of material across a lipid bilayer are described next.

Diffusion

Diffusion is a process in which particles in solution move from an area of high concentration to an area of low concentration. When a gram of salt is placed into a glass of water the salt dissolves into its components, sodium and chloride ions, and both particles move throughout the solution from areas of high concentration to areas of lower concentration until they are evenly distributed within the glass of water and the concentration of sodium and chloride ions is exactly the same anywhere one samples within the glass of water. Particles will also move from one compartment where they are in high concentration to another compartment of low concentration if the barrier between the two compartments is permeable to the substance (Figure 44.2). Concentration can signify chemical concentration (as in moles) or electrical concentration. Compounds that are positively charged will move toward areas that are more negatively charged and vice versa. The combined concentration and electrical forces involved in movement of a material by diffusion constitute the electrochemical gradient. The presence of charged ions on one side of a membrane that is not permeable to that ion will limit or prevent the amount of a similarly charged ion that can cross into that compartment even if the membrane separating the compartments is completely permeable to the second ion.

Charged water-soluble particles such as ions will not cross the lipid bilayer freely. Small uncharged particles can freely cross the lipid bilayer membrane down their concentration gradient. Their only limit to diffusion across the lipid bilayer is their size and lipid solubility. In general, uncharged compounds that have a molecular weight (MW) below 100, such as urea (MW 60),

Section VII: Digestion, Absorption, and Metabolism

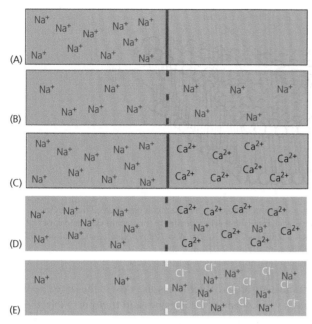

Figure 44.2 Diffusion. (A) 10 Na⁺ atoms in one compartment are separated from a second compartment by a Na⁺-impermeable membrane. (B) Simple diffusion. The membrane becomes permeable to Na⁺ and the Na⁺ diffuses into the second compartment until the concentrations on both sides of the membrane are equal. (C) Eight Ca^{2+} atoms and 10 Na⁺ atoms are separated by an impermeable membrane. There are 16 positive charges on the Ca^{2+} side and 10 positive charges on the Na⁺ side. (D) The membrane becomes permeable to Na⁺ but not Ca^{2+} and Na⁺ tries to move down its concentration gradient into the compartment without Na⁺ atoms. However, the great number of positive charges provided by Ca^{2+} already in that compartment limits the movement of any more positively charged particles into that compartment. (E) If instead, there are 10 Cl⁻ ions in the compartment without Na⁺ and the membrane separating them is permeable to Na⁺ but not Cl⁻, the negative charges in the Cl⁻ compartment will cause more Na⁺ ions to move into that compartment than simple diffusion down its concentration gradient would predict.

can freely cross the lipid bilayer. Monosaccharides such as glucose (MW 180) are uncharged but too large to pass through pores within the lipid bilayer. Fatty acids and triglycerides are very large and can be charged; however, because they are very lipid-soluble they can freely cross the lipid bilayer down their concentration gradient once they cross the unstirred water layer.

Facilitated or carrier-mediated diffusion

Solutes that are too large or which carry a charge can utilize carrier proteins to facilitate their diffusion across the cell membrane. These carrier proteins recognize very specific molecules and form a channel of low resistance that allows the molecules to move down their electrochemical gradient to the other side of the membrane (Figure 44.3). Often these carrier proteins are regulatable – they may be under hormonal or neural control. In some cases ions will be transported together using a transporter. This involves a transporter that facilitates movement of one ion

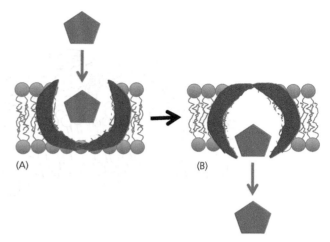

Figure 44.3 Facilitated diffusion. (A) A large molecule that is too large or too highly charged to diffuse across the cell membrane moves into a specific site in a carrier protein. (B) This triggers a conformational change that allows the molecule to exit the carrier protein on the other side of the membrane. No energy is expended in this process; it is powered by the concentration gradient.

against its electrochemical gradient by pairing it with another ion that is moving down its electrochemical gradient. An example of this is the chloride–bicarbonate exchanger (see Figure 44.7). In this example chloride anion will be moving down its concentration gradient inside the cell, despite some electrical resistance to this movement. The strength of this force provided by chloride can be used to also move a bicarbonate anion out of the cell against its concentration gradient but perhaps with the aid of its electrical gradient.

This strategy is repeatedly used to absorb materials across the intestinal cell membranes. For instance, sodium is normally in much higher concentration within the lumen of the intestine than inside the intestinal epithelial cell. The amino acid aspartate has a negative charge and is much too large to cross the cell membrane even though it will also be in much higher concentration in the lumen of the intestine than inside the epithelial cell. Since the inside of the cell is negatively charged compared to the outside of the cell, sodium will have both an electrical and a concentration gradient pushing it to move into the cell. Aspartate will be moving into the cell down its concentration gradient but against its electrical gradient. Carrier proteins in the apical membrane of the intestinal epithelial cell recognize aspartate and sodium and can open up when both are bound to the carrier protein. The combined electrochemical force supplied by sodium moving down its electrical and concentration gradient and aspartate moving down its concentration gradient will help drive the aspartate molecule across the membrane against its electrical gradient and through the membrane despite its large size. The sodium atom also enters the cell. Keep in mind that it was the extra push provided by sodium moving down its electrochemical gradient that allowed the transporter to also bring aspartate across the cell membrane.

Active transport across the cell membrane

Active transport across membranes implies that energy will have to be provided, usually in the form of ATP, to move ions or molecules. Active transport is usually required when moving a substance against its electrochemical gradient. The cell membrane proteins that carry out this function are often referred to as pumps since they are generally moving ions from an area of low concentration to an area of higher concentration. The active transport pumps are generally highly specific in the substance they will pump, but can develop very high concentration gradients across membranes.

An example of such a pump is the electrogenic Na^+/K^+-ATPase pump. This pumping protein utilizes the energy in one ATP molecule to move three sodium atoms from inside the cell to the outside of the cell against sodium's electrical and concentration gradient in exchange for two potassium atoms moving into the cell down their electrical gradient but against the concentration gradient. This pump keeps extracellular sodium concentration high and intracellular potassium concentration high. It also generates an electrical potential difference across the cell membrane, keeping the inside negative relative to the outside of the cell.

Nonionic diffusion

Weak acids and weak bases are compounds that exist in both a dissociated and a nondissociated state. In the nondissociated state they are both water- and lipid-soluble. In this state they have no charge and being lipid-soluble they can freely cross the lipid bilayer of cell membranes. In the dissociated state their charge makes them unable to cross the lipid bilayer and that charge also makes them soluble in water only. The nondissociated and dissociated forms of weak acids and weak bases are in equilibrium and the concentration of nondissociated and dissociated forms is dependent on the pH of the solution they occupy. The pH at which 50% of the weak acid or base is in the dissociated form and 50% is in the nondissociated form is called the pK_a for the compound. How this affects the equilibrium and concentrations of nondissociated and dissociated forms is best illustrated using acetic acid as an example. Acetic acid in water exists in the nondissociated state, HAc, and in the dissociated state, Ac^-, as described by the following equation:

$$HAc \leftrightarrow H^+ + Ac^-$$

The pK_a for acetic acid is 4.76. In a pH 4.76 solution, 50% of the acetic acid will exist in the nondissociated state, designated HAc, and 50% will exist in the dissociated state as Ac^-. If the pH of the solution is 5.76 (and remembering that pH is a logarithmic scale), the reduction in H^+ ions shifts the equilibrium further to the right and now just 10% of the acetic acid is in the HAc form while 90% is in the Ac^- dissociated form. If the solution has a pH of 6.76, not unlike the pH in the colon of the horse, just 1% of the acetic acid is in the nondissociated form, while 99% is in the dissociated form. Using the horse colon cell membrane as an example, the small amount of HAc in the nondissociated form will freely cross the apical membrane down its concentration

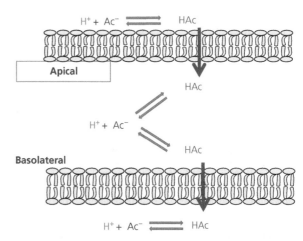

Figure 44.4 Nonionic diffusion. Assume a high concentration of acetic acid in the lumen of the colon. It establishes an equilibrium, with a portion existing in the uncharged nondissociated state (HAc) and a portion in the charged dissociated state (Ac^-). The lipid bilayer cell membrane is freely permeable to weak acids such as acetate when they are in the nondissociated uncharged state (HAc). Once HAc has crossed the apical membrane it again establishes an equilibrium, with a portion of the acetic acid in the HAc and Ac^- states. This equilibrium is also established at the basolateral membrane. The HAc can then cross the basolateral membrane. Once in the extracellular fluid the HAc reestablishes an equilibrium, with some in the HAc and some in the Ac^- form. The acetic acid in the charged Ac^- form is trapped in the extracellular fluid as it cannot recross the lipid bilayer.

gradient to the interior of the cell (Figure 44.4). By removing HAc from the lumen the equilibrium of acetic acid dissociation will be shifted toward the left to replace the lost HAc, allowing another HAc to cross the cell membrane. Once on the other side of the membrane the HAc quickly dissociates to form H^+ and Ac^-. The Ac^- is now trapped inside the cell. However, as long as HAc is being produced in the lumen and is crossing the apical membrane, there will be a second equilibrium set up for acetic acid at the opposite side of the cell near the basolateral membrane. Here Ac^- and H^+ will again be in equilibrium with HAc. As HAc is formed it will move out to the extracellular fluids down its concentration gradient as it is lipid-soluble and able to freely cross the basolateral cell membrane.

Weak bases also set up similar equilibria when placed in solution:

$$BaseOH \leftrightarrow Base^+ + OH^-$$

Their pK_a will generally be in excess of 8.0 and their dissociation is promoted by placing them in more acid solutions. This system is surprisingly efficient and can operate even when the nondissociated form would be expected to comprise less than 0.01% of the total amount of weak acid or weak base present. Nonionic diffusion is the main method used by ruminants and hindgut fermenters to absorb the volatile fatty acids (VFAs) produced by bacterial fermentation of cellulosic plant materials. Most of the drugs utilized in veterinary medicine are weak acids or weak bases and this is the method they utilize to cross cell membranes.

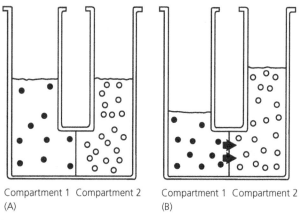

Compartment 1   Compartment 2
(A)

Compartment 1   Compartment 2
(B)

Figure 44.5 Osmosis. (A) Before osmosis. Equal volumes of aqueous solutions (solutes represented by black circles and open circles) are placed in compartments that are separated by a membrane permeable to water but not to the solutes (semipermeable membrane). The aqueous solution in compartment 1 has the highest concentration of water (lowest concentration of solute). (B) During osmosis. Osmosis (diffusion of water) occurs from compartment 1 to compartment 2 (highest water concentration to lowest water concentration) and the water level rises in compartment 2. From Reece, W.O. (2009) *Functional Anatomy and Physiology of Domestic Animals*, 4th edn. Wiley-Blackwell, Ames, IA. Reproduced with permission from Wiley.

Osmosis

A critical concept in biology is the concept of osmosis. Water will always try to move from an area or compartment of low solute concentration to an area of high solute concentration (Figure 44.5). Each ion or particle within a solution acts as an osmotic particle, regardless of its charge. The osmolarity of a compartment or solution is determined by the concentration or number of moles of particles in that solution: 1 mol of sodium in a solution will provide just as much osmotic pull for water as 1 mol of albumin. Thinking another way, 10 g of sodium (atomic weight 23) will provide 0.43 osmol of particles to a solution. Adding 10 g albumin (MW 60,000) to the solution provides just 0.00016 osmol of particles to a solution. The key to absorption of water across the intestinal tract is to absorb solute. Water will follow the solute across the cell membranes.

Solvent drag or convection of solute

Small solutes such as electrolytes can be swept from one compartment to another by the bulk flow of water. The water is moving from one compartment to another due to hydrostatic pressure or osmotic pull. The smaller the particle and the less charge it carries, the greater the chance it can be dragged along with the water into the next compartment.

Pinocytosis

In some circumstances, very large or highly charged particles can be moved across cell membranes via a process called **endocytosis**. The substance to be transported comes in contact with the cell membrane and an endocytic membrane forms around the substance. It is taken into the cell as a membrane-surrounded

vesicle and very often the membrane will cross the membrane on the opposite side of the cell by exocytosis. This process is used to absorb immunoglobulins, very large proteins in colostrum that provide passive immunity from mother to neonate.

Paracellular versus transcellular transport

> **1** How do paracellular and transcellular transport processes differ?
>
> **2** Which process works well when there is a large concentration gradient favoring transport? Which system is required to be used if pumping of a substance against its electrochemical gradient is required?

Paracellular absorption

All the mucosal cells lining the intestinal tract have an apical and a basolateral membrane. Adjacent cells are linked to one another on all sides by "tight junctions," also known as occluding junctions and zonula occludens. The tight junctions are composed of several proteins that form a seal between cells that is relatively impermeable to bacteria, viruses, and large molecules that have been ingested. The tight junctions also provide resistance to the passage of small ions and water. However, this resistance can be overcome if the electrochemical forces driving the ions to the opposite side of a tight junction are great enough. Water channels and ion channels do exist in the tight junction. They provide paths of lower resistance for water and ions that are utilized only when there is a great difference in osmolarity or concentration on one side of the tight junction. Movement across the tight junctions is only significant for the smaller ions such as Na^+, Cl^-, K^+, Ca^{2+}, PO_4^- and Mg^{2+}. Absorption of solute across the tight junctions between enterocytes, from the lumen directly into the extracellular fluid, is referred to as paracellular transport (Figure 44.6). It is also possible for solute to move from extracellular fluid to the lumen across the tight junctions. Very high concentrations of some solutes in the lumen of the intestine, such as Ca^{2+}, can put so much electrochemical force on the tight junction that it is damaged and develops holes and becomes leaky.

Transcellular absorption

Most of the nutrients of the body are too large to cross the tight junctions and must be moved across the absorptive enterocytes of the villus by a variety of transport mechanisms (Figure 44.6). Transport proteins can facilitate passive diffusion or allow active transport (pumping) of solute against its electrochemical gradient at the expense of ATP. The process involves moving solute from lumen to cytosol of the enterocyte across the apical membrane and movement of solute from the cytosol to extracellular fluid across the basolateral membrane. The mechanism used to transport a solute across the apical membrane is often quite different from that used to transport the solute across the basolateral cell membrane.

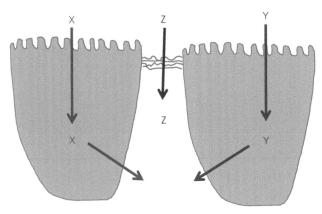

Figure 44.6 X and Y ions are transported across the intestine by transcellular mechanisms: they have to cross both the apical and basolateral cell membranes. These mechanisms are efficient even if relatively low amounts of solute are present in the lumen compared with extracellular fluid. Ion Z is traversing the tight junction and is absorbed by a paracellular process. Paracellular transport is concentration driven and only functions when solute concentration in the lumen is far higher than ion concentration in the extracellular fluid.

ABSORPTION OF DIETARY MINERALS AND REABSORPTION OF SECRETED ELECTROLYTES

Dietary electrolytes (Na^+, K^+ and Cl^-) and minerals must be in solution within the fluids of the digestive tract if they are to be absorbed. Fortunately, many minerals that might be in an insoluble form within the diet components become soluble after exposure to the acid in the stomach. The stomach can absorb some sodium and potassium, but these electrolytes are likely to have been placed in the gastric glands from the blood and not the diet. For monogastric species the bulk of mineral and electrolyte absorption occurs in the small and large intestine. The colon can also absorb electrolytes quite well if they are still present in the lumen. The major site of absorption and the mechanisms used to absorb the electrolytes are listed in Table 44.1.

Sodium

> 1 How do sodium atoms cross from the lumen of the gut to the interior of the villous cell?
>
> 2 How do sodium atoms cross from the interior of the cell to the extracellular fluid?

Sodium concentration in the lumen of the gastrointestinal tract and in the extracellular fluid is generally higher than inside the enterocyte. The inside of cells is negative in relation to the outside of cells.

Apical membrane transport

Intracellular Na^+ concentration is about 12–15 mmol/L. Lumen Na^+ concentration will vary but except for the final sections of the colon will generally exceed 15 mmol/L. Na^+ will be moved across the apical membrane down its concentration and electrical gradient in most of the tract and down its electrical gradient even when Na^+ concentration is very low in the distal colon.

1 Cotransported with chloride to maintain electrical balance. All sections of the small and large intestine have these Na^+/Cl^- cotransporters (Figure 44.7).

2 Cotransport of Na^+ with sugars and amino acids liberated during digestion. The electrochemical force provided by Na^+ moving down its electrical and concentration gradient will help push these larger molecules across the apical membrane. These transporter proteins are found in the villous cells of the duodenum and upper jejunum.

Basolateral membrane transport

Extracellular Na^+ concentration is about 140 mmol/L. Na^+ will be moving out of the cell against its electrical and concentration gradient into the extracellular fluid.

1 Electrogenic pump: $3Na^+$ ions will be pumped out of the cell in exchange for $2K^+$ ions moving into the cell. This pump will require the energy from an ATP molecule to power it. All cells of the body have electrogenic pumps (Figure 44.7).

2 Na^+/Cl^- pump: sodium and chloride can be actively pumped across the basolateral membrane at the expense of an ATP. This mechanism is used primarily in the lower intestine (Figure 44.7).

Chloride

> 1 How do chloride atoms cross from the lumen of the gut to the interior of the villous cell?
>
> 2 How do chloride atoms cross from the interior of the cell to the extracellular fluid?
>
> 3 Where is paracellular absorption of chloride most likely to occur and why?

Apical membrane transport

The concentration of Cl^- in the lumen is variable. Chyme leaving the stomach contains close to 120 mmol/L Cl^-. The concentration of Cl^- in the distal large intestine will be closer to zero. Intracellular Cl^- concentration is variable and can be as low as 4 mmol/L in the colon and as high as 30 mmol/L in the upper small intestine.

1 Cotransported with Na^+ to maintain electrical balance. All sections of the small and large intestine have these Na^+/Cl^- cotransporters (Figure 44.7).

2 One Cl^- ion is brought into the cell in exchange for one HCO_3^- ion moved into the lumen to maintain electrical neutrality. This process requires the energy of an ATP. This mechanism is especially important in the colon where lumen Cl^- concentration is expected to be low (Figure 44.7).

3 Na^+/K^+/$2Cl^-$ cotransporter: the electromotive force of Na^+ moving down both its electrical and concentration gradient helps move the more reluctant K^+ and Cl^- ions across the apical membrane (Figure 44.7).

Table 44.1 Major mechanisms utilized for absorption of electrolytes, hexoses, amino acids, and water in various segments of the intestinal tract.

Mechanism	Duodenum	Upper jejunum	Middle jejunum	Lower jejunum	Ileum	Colon
Na$^+$/Cl$^-$ cotransporter	+	+	+	+	++	+++
Na$^+$/hexose cotransporter	++++++	++++	+	+	–	–
Na$^+$/amino acid cotransporter	++++++	++++	+	+	–	–
Cl$^-$/HCO$_3^-$ exchange	–	–	–	–	++	+++
Paracellular Cl$^-$ absorption	++++	–	–	–	–	–
Paracellular K$^+$ absorption	–	–	–	–	+	+++
Water	+++	+++	+	+	++	+

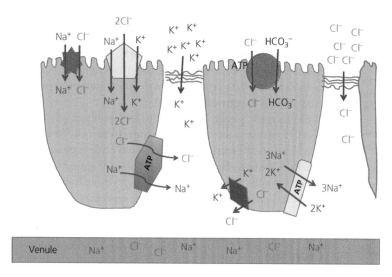

Figure 44.7 Major electrolyte absorption mechanisms. The apical membrane has a Na$^+$/Cl$^-$ cotransporter, a Na$^+$/K$^+$/2Cl$^-$ cotransporter, and a Cl$^-$/HCO$_3^-$ ATPase pump to bring electrolytes from the lumen into the cytosol. The basolateral membrane uses a Na$^+$/Cl$^-$ ATPase pump, a K$^+$/Cl$^-$ cotransporter, and the 3Na$^+$/2K$^+$ exchange ATPase pump (the electrogenic pump) to move electrolytes from the cytosol into the extracellular fluid. In the lower small intestine and colon most of the K$^+$ is absorbed paracellularly. In the uppermost duodenum Cl$^-$ can also be absorbed paracellularly.

Basolateral membrane transport

Chloride concentration in the extracellular fluid is about 102–108 mmol/L. Inside the enterocyte the Cl$^-$ concentration might get as high as 30 mmol/L. Cl$^-$ will move to the extracellular fluid against its concentration gradient but with its electrical gradient.

1 Cl$^-$/K$^+$ cotransporter: K$^+$ will be moving into the extracellular fluid down its concentration gradient but against its electrical gradient. The combined force of K$^+$ moving down its concentration gradient and Cl$^-$ moving down its electrical gradient permits both molecules to overcome the forces resisting this movement (Figure 44.7).

2 Cl$^-$ pump: chloride can be actively pumped across the basolateral membrane at the expense of an ATP. This mechanism is used primarily in the lower intestine (Figure 44.7).

3 Na$^+$/Cl$^-$ pump: sodium and chloride can be actively pumped across the basolateral membrane at the expense of an ATP. This mechanism is used primarily in the lower intestine (Figure 44.7).

Paracellular absorption into the extracellular fluid

When Cl$^-$ concentration is very high, as in the uppermost duodenum (110–120 mmol/L), the concentration gradient between the lumen and the extracellular fluid (102–108 mmol/L) will allow Cl$^-$ to pass through the tight junctions between adjoining enterocytes directly into the extracellular fluid. This mechanism is important in the first few centimeters of the duodenum and quickly removes a large amount of chloride from the chyme; this action also increases the pH of the digesta in the duodenum (Figure 44.7).

Potassium

1 How do potassium atoms cross from the lumen of the gut to the interior of the villous cell?

2 How do potassium atoms cross from the interior of the cell to the extracellular fluid?

3 Where is paracellular absorption of potassium most likely to occur and why?

Paracellular K$^+$ transport

The bulk of K$^+$ absorption occurs across the tight junctions and K$^+$ moves between cells directly into the extracellular fluid, particularly in the lower small intestine. K$^+$ concentration in extracellular fluid is low (4–6 mmol/L) while the concentration of K$^+$ in the lumen can be many fold higher. The concentration of K$^+$ in the lumen actually increases as the digesta moves down the tract from the upper to lower small intestine as water is removed from the ingesta and concentrates the remaining potassium (Figure 44.7).

Transcellular K⁺ transport

Transcellular K^+ transport is a relatively minor contributor to overall K^+ absorption.

Apical membrane

K^+ concentration inside the cell is about 139 mmol/L. Lumen K^+ must cross the apical membrane against its concentration gradient but with its electrical gradient.

1 $Na^+/K^+/2Cl^-$ cotransporter: the electromotive force of Na^+ moving down both its electrical and concentration gradient helps move the more reluctant K^+ and Cl^- ions across the apical membrane (Figure 44.7).

Basolateral membrane

K^+ will be moving down its concentration gradient but against its electrical gradient.

1 Cl^-/K^+ cotransporter: K^+ will be moving into the extracellular fluid down its concentration gradient but against its electrical gradient. The combined force of K^+ moving down its concentration gradient and Cl^- moving down its electrical gradient permits both molecules to overcome the forces resisting this movement (Figure 44.7).

Calcium

> 1 How do calcium atoms cross from the lumen of the gut to the interior of the villous cell?
>
> 2 How do calcium atoms cross from the interior of the cell to the extracellular fluid?
>
> 3 Where is paracellular absorption of calcium most likely to occur and why?

Depending on the amount of Ca^{2+} in the diet and its solubility (highly variable), Ca^{2+} can be absorbed by a paracellular passive transport system or it can be actively transported across the enterocyte transcellularly.

Transcellular Ca²⁺ transport
Apical membrane

Ca^{2+} concentration in the lumen of the intestinal tract is always higher than the concentration inside the cell (0.0002 mmol/L) so Ca^{2+} will move across the apical membrane down its concentration and electrical gradients. However the membrane is impermeable to Ca^{2+}.

1 Entry through Ca^{2+} channels: production of these channels within the apical membrane depends on stimulation of the epithelial cells by the hormonal form of vitamin D, 1,25-dihydroxyvitamin D_3, abbreviated as $1,25(OH)_2D$ (Figure 44.8).

2 Free Ca^{2+} ions within the cytosol can have many effects on the cell since free Ca^{2+} ions are utilized as the second messenger by many G protein-coupled receptors. Therefore the Ca^{2+} must be chelated to another $1,25(OH)_2D$-dependent protein called calbindin-9K for transport across the enterocyte to the basolateral membrane.

Basolateral membrane

Ionized Ca^{2+} concentration in the extracellular fluid (~1.25 mmol/L) is nearly 5000-fold higher than the Ca^{2+} concentration inside the enterocyte. Ca^{2+} will have to exit the enterocyte against its concentration and electrical gradient.

1 $Ca^{2+}/3Na^+$ exchange ATPase pump: this is another $1,25(OH)_2D$-dependent protein. The pump uses the energy in ATP and the electrochemical force provided by allowing $3Na^+$ ions into the cell to drive a Ca^{2+} atom into the extracellular fluid against a huge concentration gradient.

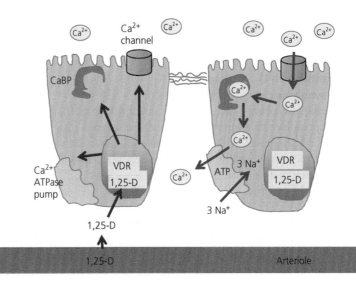

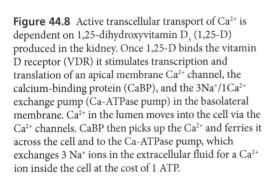

Figure 44.8 Active transcellular transport of Ca^{2+} is dependent on 1,25-dihydroxyvitamin D_3 (1,25-D) produced in the kidney. Once 1,25-D binds the vitamin D receptor (VDR) it stimulates transcription and translation of an apical membrane Ca^{2+} channel, the calcium-binding protein (CaBP), and the $3Na^+/1Ca^{2+}$ exchange pump (Ca-ATPase pump) in the basolateral membrane. Ca^{2+} in the lumen moves into the cell via the Ca^{2+} channels. CaBP then picks up the Ca^{2+} and ferries it across the cell and to the Ca-ATPase pump, which exchanges 3 Na⁺ ions in the extracellular fluid for a Ca^{2+} ion inside the cell at the cost of 1 ATP.

Paracellular Ca^{2+} transport

A second, vitamin D-independent mechanism for the absorption of Ca^{2+} also exists. This mechanism involves movement of Ca^{2+} from the lumen of the intestine to the extracellular fluid between intestinal epithelial cells. This is known as **paracellular Ca^{2+} transport** and the mechanism is driven purely by the concentration of soluble Ca^{2+} reaching the epithelial cells. When ionized Ca^{2+} concentration in proximity to the tight junctions between epithelial cells substantially exceeds the ionized Ca^{2+} concentration in the extracellular fluid (~1.25 mmol/L), Ca^{2+} flows across the tight junctions directly into the extracellular fluid and blood. It likely becomes significant only when the ionized Ca^{2+} concentration over the intestinal epithelium exceeds 4 mmol/L. This mechanism is a factor when dietary Ca^{2+} is high and only in the upper duodenum. Since milk is very high in available Ca^{2+}, passive paracellular absorption of Ca^{2+} occurs for a short period following suckling.

In ruminants both passive and active Ca^{2+} transport mechanisms have been described in the rumen. Passive transport of Ca^{2+} across the rumen wall may be an important means of Ca^{2+} transport in these species. In both monogastrics and ruminants, paracellular Ca^{2+} transport is thought to be the mechanism used to absorb between 30 and 60% of dietary calcium on normal diets. When dietary calcium is low or of poor availability, the animal will rely more on the active transport mechanisms. In at least two hindgut fermenters, the horse and rabbit, the active transport of Ca^{2+} across the intestine is not regulated by the hormone $1,25(OH)_2D$. In these species the active transport mechanisms for dietary calcium absorption are always turned on.

Phosphate (HPO_4^-)

> 1 How do phosphate molecules cross from the lumen of the gut to the interior of the villous cell?
>
> 2 How do phosphate molecules cross from the interior of the cell to the extracellular fluid?
>
> 3 Where is paracellular absorption of phosphate molecules most likely to occur and why?

Transcellular HPO_4^- transport
Apical membrane

Intracellular phosphate concentration is about 100 mmol/L. Luminal phosphate concentration is generally lower than this, even with a high-phosphate diet so phosphate will move across the apical membrane against its concentration gradient and against its electrical gradient.

1 $HPO_4^-/2Na^+$ coupled transport: several different types of cotransporter protein can perform this function. The most efficient of these is only produced in the enterocytes on stimulation by $1,25(OH)_2D$. Without $1,25(OH)_2D$, the animal cannot absorb phosphate well from a low-phosphate diet and can develop rickets. The driving force for phosphate

absorption is provided by the entry of the $2Na^+$ atoms cotransported with the phosphate anion.

Basolateral membrane

Extracellular phosphate concentration is about 0.8 mmol/L so phosphate anion can cross the basolateral membrane into the extracellular fluid down its concentration and electrical gradient, i.e., passive diffusion through phosphate channels in the basolateral membrane.

Paracellular HPO_4^- transport

Because dietary phosphate can cause intraluminal phosphate concentrations to be considerably higher than extracellular phosphate concentration (0.8 mmol/L), a large amount of phosphate does manage to cross the tight junctions and enter the extracellular fluid. Perhaps 60–80% of dietary phosphate is absorbed paracellularly when animals are fed a typical diet.

Digestion and absorption of dietary proteins

> 1 Which enzymes are involved in protein digestion in the stomach?
>
> 2 Which enzymes are involved in protein digestion in the upper intestine?
>
> 3 What is the maximum length of a peptide that can be absorbed across the villous apical membrane?
>
> 4 How are single amino acids brought across the apical membrane? What purpose does sodium cotransport play in this process?
>
> 5 What is the fate of dipeptides absorbed across the apical membrane?
>
> 6 How do amino acids cross the basolateral membrane?

Proteins in the diet tend to be very large molecules and often consist of hundreds of amino acids linked by peptide bonds. For example, casein, the major protein in milk, has a molecular weight of 23,000 and is about 200 amino acids in length. These molecules need to be broken down to at least the dipeptide and tripeptide level before they can cross the enterocytes. Protein digestion begins in the stomach. Here the very acidic environment alone can hydrolyze some of the peptide bonds. The chief cells of the gastric glands secrete **pepsinogen**, an inactive proteolytic enzyme. It is secreted in an inactive form to prevent autodigestion of the chief cells and gastric gland cells. Gastric gland acid mixes with the pepsinogen and cleaves off a fragment of the pepsinogen to form pepsin, the active enzyme. Pepsin cleaves peptide bonds next to hydrophobic amino acids with aromatic side chains (phenylalanine, tryptophan, tyrosine). **Rennin** is another enzyme produced by chief cells. It cleaves between phenylalanine and methionine residues on proteins, and is especially important for digestion of casein by neonatal

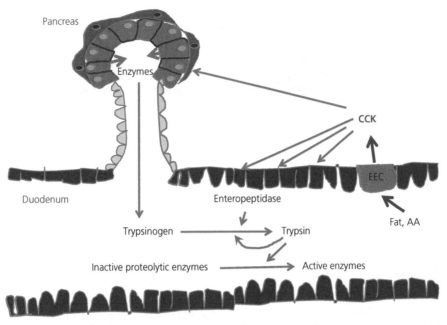

Figure 44.9 Many of the enzymes secreted by the pancreas are in an inactive form. Activation begins when an enteroendocrine cell (EEC) secretes cholecystokinin (CCK) in response to the presence of fats or amino acids (AA) in the duodenum. The CCK stimulates the pancreas to secrete enzymes, many of which are in an inactive form. The CCK also acts on nearby villous enterocytes and causes them to secrete enteropeptidase. Enteropeptidase converts pancreatic trypsinogen to the active enzyme trypsin. Trypsin then cleaves off portions of all the other inactive pancreatic enzymes allowing them to become active in the intestinal lumen. Trypsin can also cleave trypsinogen to form more trypsin enzyme.

mammals. Both pepsin and rennin function optimally when the pH is between 2 and 3. The net result is that proteins that were hundreds of amino acids long when they entered the stomach enter the duodenum as fragments that may be 25–100 amino acids long.

As peptides reach the small intestine they activate receptors of enteroendocrine cells lining the duodenum crypts, stimulating them to secrete cholecystokinin (CCK). The CCK enters the circulation and reaches the pancreatic acinar cells and myoepithelial cells surrounding each acinus. This triggers secretion of pancreatic enzymes into the upper duodenum via the pancreatic ducts (Figure 44.9). The proteolytic enzymes of the pancreas are produced and secreted into the pancreatic ducts in an inactive form. This prevents autodigestion of the pancreas and pancreatic ducts. The proteolytic proenzymes secreted by the pancreas incude trypsinogen, chymotrypsinogen, pro-elastase, and pro-carboxypeptidases A and B.

The CCK secreted by crypt enteroendocrine cells in response to peptides (and fats) entering the duodenum also reaches the villous enterocytes. This causes the enterocytes to secrete an enzyme called enteropeptidase (also called enterokinase) into the lumen of the duodenum. Enteropeptidase seeks out trypsinogen that has entered the duodenum and cleaves off a fragment to form the active proteolytic enzyme trypsin. Trypsin then cleaves off portions of each of the other proteolytic enzymes secreted by the pancreas causing them to become active as well. Trypsin can actually convert trypsinogen to active trypsin in an example of positive feedback regulation. The action of

enteropeptidase quickly causes all the inactive proteolytic enzymes in the pancreatic secretions to become active in the lumen of the gut. Each of these different proteolytic enzymes (trypsin, chymotrypsin, elastase, and the carboxypeptidases) cleave peptide bonds between specific amino acids so that when the luminal phase of digestion is finished the protein has been converted to peptides that are generally just 1–12 amino acids long.

These single amino acids and longer peptides then move to the brush border. They are very soluble in water and have no problem crossing the unstirred water layer and entering the glycocalyx, adhering to the microvilli forming the brush border of the villous enterocytes. Several intestinal peptidases project from the brush border into the glycocalyx, but these enzymes are not released into the lumen of the intestine. These intestinal peptidases hydrolyze the peptide bonds, reducing the length of the peptides to no more than three amino acids in length. The next obstacle to their absorption is moving across the apical membrane of the villous enterocyte.

Crossing the apical membrane of villous enterocytes

The single amino acids develop a large concentration gradient above the apical membrane of duodenal and jejunal villous cells following ingestion of a meal. Thanks to the secretory efforts of the crypt enterocytes, high amounts of sodium are also found above the apical membrane. At least four facilitated carriers are known to exist in the apical membrane of the villous cells. These transporters seem to be specific for the basic, acidic, or neutral amino acids.

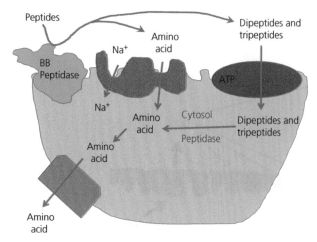

Figure 44.10 Brush border digestion and absorption of proteins and amino acids. A brush border peptidase (BB peptidase) of villous cells can break down any peptides greater than three amino acids that reach the glycocalyx. Single amino acids then use one four known types of Na$^+$/amino acid cotransporters to cross the apical membrane. These facilitated diffusion carriers utilize the driving forces provided by the high concentration of amino acid in the lumen following a meal and high lumen Na$^+$ provided by crypt cell secretions to move the large charged amino acids across the brush border. Dipeptides and tripeptides can be transported by special active transport proteins that do not require Na$^+$, but do expend an ATP to move such large molecules across the membrane. Once inside the cell the dipeptides and tripeptides are converted to single amino acids by intracellular peptidases. Transporters unique to the basolateral membrane then facilitate diffusion of the amino acids into the extracellular fluid.

Proline seems to have its own unique carrier. All these single amino acid carriers are facilitated carriers that bind the amino acid and a Na$^+$ atom (Figure 44.10). The combined force of the amino acid moving down its concentration gradient and Na$^+$ moving down its electrical and concentration gradient helps drive the large amino acid molecule across the apical membrane.

The dipeptides and tripeptides at the brush border can be absorbed by active transport mechanisms. They are so large that it takes the force supplied by an ATP molecule along with a transporter protein to pump them across the apical membrane. Research suggests that the bulk of amino acids is transported across the apical membrane in the form of dipeptides and tripeptides. Once these arrive in the cytosol of the villous enterocyte they are hydrolyzed to single amino acids by intracellular peptidases.

Crossing the basolateral membrane of the villous enterocyte

As the single amino acids accumulate at the basolateral side of the enterocytes, their concentration becomes much higher than that of free amino acids in the extracellular fluid. Transporters unique to the basolateral membrane facilitate the diffusion of amino acids across the basolateral membrane, independent of Na$^+$. The amino acids enter the extracellular fluid and are transported in the portal circulation to the liver. The Na$^+$ ions that accompanied the single amino acids across the apical membrane are pumped into the extracellular fluid by the 3Na$^+$/2K$^+$

electrogenic pump residing in the basolateral membrane at the expense of an ATP. The sodium may be removed from the blood by crypt secretory cells and returned to the lumen to assist facilitated transport of other amino acids by villous cells.

Absorption of intact proteins

In rare instances some very specific proteins can be absorbed intact across the intestinal villous cells. The most important of these are the colostral antibodies that provide passive immunity for the neonatal mammal. In the case of colostral immunoglobulins, the antibodies found in colostrum have unique properties that allow them to resist degradation by stomach acid and the proteolytic enzymes. Neonatal proteolytic enzyme secretion and activation processes do not seem to be fully developed, which also helps the protein avoid digestion. Villous cells of the neonate have specific receptors that recognize the immunoglobulins. Once the immunoglobulin binds its receptor, it activates endocytosis of the immunoglobulin: it is enclosed in a section of the apical membrane, transported to the basolateral membrane, and released into the extracellular fluid by exocytosis. The presence of these receptors on the neonatal villous enterocytes is short-lived: most mammals lose these immunoglobulin receptors and stop absorbing immunoglobulin within 24 hours of birth.

Digestion and absorption of nonstructural carbohydrates

Plant starches and glycogen from ingestion of muscle and liver comprise large numbers of glucose molecules linked together by

---

1 What is the difference between starch, glucose, fructose, and lactose?

2 Where does amylase come from and what does it do?

3 Can disaccharides cross the apical membrane?

4 Which enzymes are found within the glycocalyx attached to the brush border membrane? What is their primary function?

5 How do single molecules of galactose and glucose cross the apical cell membrane? How does fructose cross the apical membrane of villous cells?

6 Does sugar absorption from the intestinal tract require insulin?

---

bonds at the $\alpha(1{\rightarrow}4)$ or $\alpha(1{\rightarrow}6)$ position. The most common plant sugar in the diet is sucrose, a disaccharide composed of a glucose molecule linked to a fructose molecule. Milk sugar or lactose is a disaccharide of glucose and galactose linked in the $\beta(1{\rightarrow}4)$ position. Digestion of plant structural carbohydrates (cellulose and hemicellulose) is critical to the survival of ruminants and hindgut fermenters and is discussed in Chapter 45.

On ingestion, starches in the diet will begin to be broken down by salivary α-**amylase**. This process breaks some of the $\alpha(1{\rightarrow}4)$ linkages, but the enzyme does not have time to break down very much of the starch molecule before the bolus enters

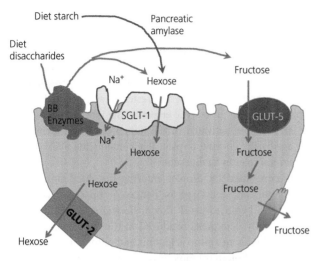

Figure 44.11 Starch is converted to glucose, maltose, and limit dextrins by amylase in the lumen of the intestine. Brush border enzymes (BB enzymes) such as maltase, lactase, sucrase, and dextrinase convert dietary disaccharides (e.g., maltose, lactose, sucrose) and limit dextrins to single hexose (glucose and galactose) or pentose (fructose) molecules. Hexoses in the brush border are brought into the cell using a Na^+-linked glucose transporter (SGLT-1). Pentose sugars use a Na^+-independent facilitated transporter (GLUT-5). At the basolateral membrane, both hexose (GLUT-2 transporter) and pentose sugars use facilitated transport diffusion to enter the extracellular fluid down their concentration gradient.

the stomach where the amylase will be destroyed by the low pH. Stomach acids and proteolytic enzymes have no effect on starches and they continue into the duodenum. The osmolarity change caused by entry of starch and acids into the duodenum causes vagal parasympathetic stimulation of pancreatic secretion. The pancreas secretes α-amylase in an active form that attacks the $\alpha(1\rightarrow4)$ links between glucose molecules and is highly efficient. The bulk of starch is broken down to maltose (two glucoses) and maltotriose (three glucoses) and limit dextrins ($\alpha1\rightarrow6$ linked glucoses) within minutes of entry to the duodenum. These starch breakdown products then move to the brush border: they are very water-soluble and have no problem crossing the unstirred water layer to reach the glycocalyx. A wide variety of enzymes extend into the glycocalyx from the brush border and these complete the digestive process (Figure 44.11). Some of these enzymes include **sucrase**, which converts sucrose to glucose and fructose; **maltase** and **maltotriase**, which convert maltose and maltotriose to their constitutive glucose molecules; and **lactase**, which converts milk lactose to glucose and galactose. Lactase is found on the villous enterocyte brush border of all mammalian neonates, but often disappears after the animal is weaned. Sucrase, on the other hand, is often lacking in neonates and is expressed only after the animal is several weeks old. Trehalase is an enzyme that breaks down trehalose, a sugar found in insect bodies. The brush border also has its own form of α-amylase to degrade any starch that fails to be broken down by pancreatic α-amylase . An

α-**dextrinase** is also found in the brush border to break down the $\alpha(1\rightarrow6)$ links between glucose molecules in the limit dextrins liberated during starch digestion by pancreatic α-amylase in the lumen of the intestine. In the typical monogastric diet about 80% of ingested nonstructural carbohydrate is glucose, and the rest is fructose (or galactose in young milk-fed animals).

Crossing the apical membrane of villous enterocytes

The hexose (e.g., glucose and galactose) and pentose (e.g., fructose) sugars liberated by the brush border enzymes are too large to cross the apical membrane easily. Their concentration over the apical membrane rises following a meal so there is a concentration gradient that can help them cross into the cytosol. Glucose and galactose can be transported using a hexose transporter molecule (SGLT-1) in the apical membrane (Figure 43.11). This protein binds hexose sugars and also binds a Na^+ ion (provided by secretions of the crypt enterocytes). The combined force provided by the hexose concentration gradient and the electrochemical force of Na^+ moving into the cytosol can push the glucose to the interior of the cell. Fructose is also a six-carbon sugar but its ketone group gives it slightly different properties. Fructose can be absorbed with the help of a pentose transporter protein (GLUT-5) in the apical and basolateral membranes, allowing it to cross into the cytosol by facilitated diffusion independent of Na^+.

Crossing the basolateral membrane of villous enterocytes

The concentration of hexoses and pentoses will increase within the cytosol of the enterocytes and at the basolateral membrane to concentrations that exceed the concentration in the extracellular fluid. Both hexoses and fructose diffuse across the basolateral membrane into the extracellular fluid facilitated by a transporter molecule (GLUT-2 for hexoses, GLUT-5 for fructose). The Na^+ ions that accompanied the hexose sugars across the apical membrane are pumped into the extracellular fluid by the $3Na^+/2K^+$ electrogenic pump residing in the basolateral membrane at the expense of an ATP. The Na^+ may be removed from the blood by crypt secretory cells and returned to the lumen to assist facilitated transport of other hexoses and amino acids by villous cells.

It is important to consider why the intestine does not digest all dietary starch and disaccharides to their constituent hexoses and pentoses in the lumen. The reason digestion is completed at the brush border is to prevent the osmolarity of the lumen contents from rising too high and drawing excessive amounts of water into the lumen. By liberating the hexoses and pentoses in the brush border they can be absorbed almost as soon as they are liberated, preventing a rise in osmolarity of the lumen contents. It is also important to note that SGLT-1, GLUT-2, and GLUT-5 are insulin-independent transporters: the intestinal cells absorb sugars during insulin deficiency as well as they do during insulin sufficiency.

Digestion and absorption of fat

> **1** What happens to fat in the stomach?
>
> **2** Colipase is secreted from the pancreas as pro-colipase. What is its function and why is it not secreted in an active form?
>
> **3** What are the end products of lipase digestion of fat?
>
> **4** What is the function of bile salts in the process of fat digestion? How do they function in fat absorption?
>
> **5** What happens after the micelle contacts the apical surface of the villous cell?
>
> **6** Why are monoglycerides and fatty acids converted back to triglycerides inside enterocytes?
>
> **7** What is an apolipoprotein and what does it do?
>
> **8** What is HDL?

Dietary fats are generally in the form of triglycerides. Their digestion may begin in the mouth as lingual glands produce pharyngeal lipase that converts triglycerides to fatty acids, monoglycerides, and diglycerides. This enzyme is relatively stable in acid and is thought to play a role in digestion of milk fat by neonates that may not be producing the full complement of pancreatic enzymes and liver bile. In general, the amount of fat that is digested by pharyngeal lipase has a negligible effect in normal fat digestion. The first step in fat digestion takes place in the stomach where the dietary fats are subjected to the churning action of stomach contractions. This causes dietary fats to form an emulsion with water – a suspension of fine droplets of fat in water. This is often aided by incorporation of dietary phospholipids into the emulsion. The emulsified fat droplets then enter the duodenum (Figure 44.12). The presence of fats in the duodenum elicits secretion of CCK by crypt enteroendocrine cells. CCK causes the pancreas to secrete enzymes and also causes contraction of the gallbladder (not present in the horse or rat). Several critical enzymes can be found in pancreatic secretions: pancreatic lipase, secreted in an active form; colipase, secreted in an inactive pro-colipase form; phospholipases, secreted in an inactive form (cleave phospholipids of cell membranes); and cholesterol esterase, secreted in the active form. Just as with proteolytic enzymes, the inactive lipid-digesting enzymes are activated in the lumen of the duodenum on cleavage by the enzyme trypsin. Bile contains the bile salts that play several roles in fat digestion.

The emulsified fat droplet entering the duodenum is too hydrophobic and too large for pancreatic lipase to access the droplet and begin to break down the triglycerides. Bile salts are essentially detergents produced in the liver by combining cholesterol with an amino acid. One end of the molecule, composed of the cholesterol moiety, is hydrophobic which allows it to form ionic bonds with hydrophobic fatty acids. The other end is very hydrophilic due to the amino acid component. Bile salts surround the emulsified fat droplet and break it into smaller fat droplets suspended in the water in the lumen. This increases the surface area available for enzymatic degradation of the triglycerides to occur. Colipase must bind to pancreatic lipase to allow it to be fully active and this complex then begins to digest triglycerides to monoglycerides and two fatty acids at the surface of the small fat droplet created by the bile salts. Cholesterol esterase may free cholesterol from the droplet and phospholipase liberates fatty acids and monoglyceride from phospholipids. As the lipolytic action of these enzymes progresses, more bile salts surround the liberated fatty acids, monoglycerides, cholesterol, and fat-soluble vitamins (e.g., vitamins A, D, and E) that were in the diet to form small bile salt-covered structures known as micelles.

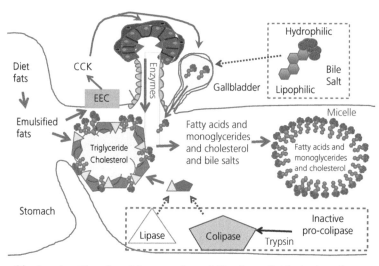

Figure 44.12 Luminal phase of fat digestion. Churning of the stomach emulsifies dietary lipids. As these fats enter the duodenum they stimulate enteroendocrine cells (EEC) to secrete cholecystokinin (CCK). CCK stimulates the pancreas to release digestive enzymes including lipase and pro-colipase needed for fat digestion. CCK also stimulates the gallbladder to contract causing secretion of bile salts into the lumen. Pro-colipase is cleaved by trypsin to form active colipase, which is a cofactor needed for full activity of lipase. Lipase, colipase, and the bile salts work together on the emulsified fat to convert the triglycerides to monoglycerides and free fatty acids. The liberated fatty acids and monoglycerides, as well as cholesterol and fat-soluble vitamins, are surrounded by bile salts to form micelles. Micelles are several hundred fold smaller than the emulsified fat droplet.

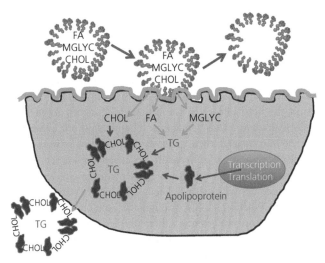

Figure 44.13 Brush border phase of lipid digestion and absorption. Lipids packaged into the micelle are able to cross the unstirred water layer above the enterocytes. On making contact the fatty acids (FA), monoglycerides (MGLYC), cholesterol (CHOL), and fat-soluble vitamins diffuse across the apical membrane to the cytosol. The FA and MGLYC are combined to reform triglycerides (TG), encouraging further diffusion of FA and MGLYC from the micelle. The empty micelle bile salts return to the lumen to collect another load of FA and MGLYC. The enterocyte produces apolipoproteins that are combined with cholesterol to form a chylomicron structure which surrounds cytosol TG and fat-soluble vitamins. The chylomicron is then exocytosed across the basolateral membrane. It is too large to enter venules so it enters the lacteal and lymphatics to reach the thoracic duct.

Moving lipids across the apical membrane of villous enterocytes

Fatty acids and monoglycerides alone are not able to access the apical membrane of the villous enterocytes for absorption as they cannot cross the unstirred water layer and glycocalyx due to their hydrophobic nature. However, the micelle, carrying its load of lipids, is surrounded by bile salts with their hydrophilic end protruding. This allows them to traverse the unstirred water layer and glycocalyx to reach the apical surface of the enterocyte. The micelle comes in direct contact with the apical membrane and the lipophilic contents of the micelle diffuse through the apical cell membrane into the cytosol down their concentration gradient (Figure 44.13). The bile salts themselves are too water-soluble to enter the the cell. The bile salts reenter the lumen and collect another load of lipids to be carried to another villous enterocyte. They can do this numerous times before they are finally swept to the ileum. In the ileum, specific bile salt transporters absorb the bile salts via receptor-mediated endocytosis and carry them in the portal circulation back to the liver where they can be absorbed by hepatocytes and be again excreted into the bile. In humans, it is estimated that each bile salt is recycled twice to absorb the fat in one meal.

At the brush border of the apical membrane any diglycerides or triglycerides that managed to be incorporated into the micelle are broken down by a brush border lipase to monoglyceride and fatty acids, which quickly diffuse into the cell. Once the monoglycerides and fatty acids enter the cell, they are quickly taken to the smooth endoplasmic reticulum and converted back into triglycerides. This serves two purposes: it reduces the osmolarity of the cytosol and it removes fatty acids and monoglycerides from the cytosol. This maintains the fatty acid and monoglyceride gradient forcing the fatty acids and monoglycerides across the apical membrane so that the entire lipid load of the micelle can diffuse into the cytosol compartment.

Moving lipids across the basolateral membrane of villous enterocytes

The newly formed triglycerides and cholesterol (and fat-soluble vitamins) in the cytosol are too water-insoluble to move out of the cell across the basolateral membrane and too insoluble to circulate in the blood (Figure 44.13). The solution that has evolved is to package these lipid materials with lipoproteins (apolipoproteins). An apolipoprotein has hydrophilic and hydrophobic ends and forms a special structure that has many of the properties of cell membranes, i.e., contains phospholipids and cholesterol. The apolipoproteins surrounding a collection of triglyceride molecules form a structure called a chylomicron. The chylomicron comprises about 80% triglyceride, which forms the interior of the chylomicron. The outer surface is composed of phosphoglycerides (9%), cholesterol (3%), and apolipoprotein B (2%). It is believed that chylomicrons cross the basolateral membrane of the villous enterocytes by exocytosis into the extracellular fluid. They are too large (400–1200 nm) to enter the portal circulation so instead they enter the lacteal vessels within the lamina propria and then the lymphatic circulation to join the blood circulation via the thoracic duct.

Fate of chylomicrons in the circulation

When the chylomicron is released from the enterocyte the main lipoprotein on its surface is apolipoprotein B48. As the chylomicron circulates in the blood it will encounter high-density lipoproteins (HDLs) released by the liver. The HDLs are covered with apolipoproteins C and E on their surface. When the chylomicron encounters HDL, it unloads some of its triglyceride to the HDL and in turn receives some apolipoprotein C and E, which is incorporated on the surface of the chylomicron. Apolipoprotein C receptors exist on adipose, mammary, and skeletal and cardiac muscle. As the chylomicrons pass through these tissues, the apolipoprotein C on the surface can bind the chylomicron to its receptor on these tissues. The triglycerides are transported into the tissue and the now empty chylomicron remnant is released back into the circulation. As it passes through the liver sinusoids, the apolipoprotein E on the surface of the chylomicron remnant becomes bound to apolipoprotein E receptors on the hepatocytes and the chylomicron remnant is taken into the hepatocyte by endocytosis. The liver can use the remaining triglycerides for energy and can store vitamins A, D, and E that were in the chylomicrons or the liver can repackage the triglyceride with the cholesterol and phospholipids into other lipoprotein particles such as very low density lipoproteins (VLDL) and HDL. VLDL can deliver triglyceride to peripheral tissues such as adipose, muscle, and mammary gland. The remnant of a VLDL is called a low-density lipoprotein (LDL). It still contains a large amount of cholesterol and has the unhealthy habit in humans of delivering cholesterol to endothelial cells lining arteries. This is why LDL is often referred to as "bad cholesterol." The HDL particles released from the liver can actually remove triglyceride and cholesterol from arteries and other peripheral tissues and take these materials to the liver for processing. This property has earned them the moniker of "good cholesterol."

Absorption of water

1 What are aquaporins? Do they allow water to move down or against its osmotic gradient?

2 Why is movement of solute critical for absorption of water?

3 Can water cross the tight junctions? Under what circumstances?

4 How does the flow of blood at the villous tip affect water absorption?

5 Where is the bulk of water absorbed in the digestive tract?

6 Can the colon compensate for malabsorption in the upper intestine? What can it absorb that might help with water absorption?

Two forces are at work to move water (Figure 44.14): **osmotic pressure** is generated by the movement of solute from one compartment to another creating an osmotic gradient; **hydrostatic pressure** is a physical force created when water is moved into a confined area. Aquaporin channels exist in the apical and basolateral membranes of enterocytes that allow water to move across the lipid bilayer of the cell membranes to follow the osmotic gradient. These aquaporin channels do not allow any charged ions through them. The key to absorption of water is to absorb solute. Solute is typically absorbed across the apical membrane and crosses the basolateral membrane to enter the lateral space between epithelial cells. This draws water into the lateral space between cells through the aquaporins. As more solute and more water enters this confined space it increases hydrostatic pressure. Distension of the elastic cell membranes of the lateral space also allows the hydrostatic pressure to increase. Under normal circumstances the path of least resistance for this water will be to cross the basement membrane of the fenestrated capillary endothelium to enter the circulation. A critical fact is that the tight junction offers more resistance to flow of water than the fenestrated endothelial basement membrane of the capillary bed. The tight junctions are not impermeable to water, just less permeable than the capillary endothelium. Water channels formed by claudin proteins (not the same as aquaporins) in the tight junction generally resist the flow of water, but this

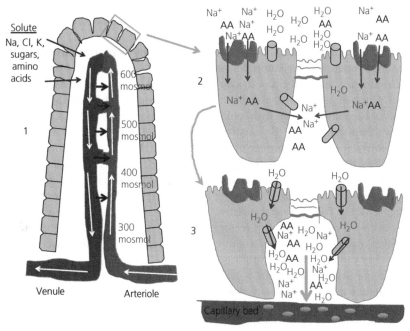

Figure 44.14 Water absorption. Water is pulled into areas high in solute. (1) In the villous tip the countercurrent flow of arteriole and venule blood causes solute in the descending venule to diffuse into the ascending arteriole to be carried back to the villous tip. The osmolarity at the villous tip can approach 600 mosmol. (2) At the level of individual enterocytes, water utilizes aquaporin to follow its osmotic gradient, created by absorption of solutes such as Na^+ and amino acids (AA) into the extracellular fluid through the enterocytes. Aquaporins are specialized water channels that allow water but not charged ions through their channels. (3) As water moves into the lateral spaces, hydrostatic pressure builds up between the cells causing distension and bulging of the cell walls below the tight junction. The hydrostatic pressure then drives the water and solute into the fenestrated capillaries, which have lower resistance to the flow of water than do the tight junctions.

resistance can be overcome if osmotic forces are great enough on one or another side of the membrane.

A phenomena that aids absorption of water at the villous tip is the countercurrent movement of solute from vein to arteriole in the lamina propria of a villus. Recall that an arteriole carries blood to the tip of the villus and this arteriole is in close proximity to a venule carrying blood away from the tip of the villus. During digestion and absorption of a meal, the postcapillary venules bring large amounts of absorbed solute into the venules. As the venule passes down the villus, solute can diffuse from the venule into the arteriole down its concentration gradient (see Figure 44.14). The arteriole brings this solute to the villous tip and eventually the osmolarity of the lamina propria at the villous tip can reach 500–600 mosmol, about twice the osmolarity of plasma. This draws water from the lumen of the intestine into the villous tip and on to the extracellular fluid.

Water balance in the gastrointestinal tract

Nearly all the water that enters the gastrointestinal tract is removed, so that feces generally contain only small amounts of water. A 20-kg dog might drink (or ingest with its diet) 600 mL water each day. Salivary glands add 300 mL, gastric juices 600 mL, bile 300 mL, pancreatic secretions 600 mL, small intestine (Brunner's glands and crypt cell secretions) add another 600 mL, and the colonic mucus adds 50 mL water to the lumen of the gastrointestinal tract for a total of 3050 mL water entering the lumen (Table 44.2). Only about 35 mL, about 1%, of this water exits the tract with the feces. The bulk of the water, about 2650 mL, is absorbed by the small intestine. The duodenum and jejunum absorb about 1600 mL or 52%. The ileum absorbs about 1060 mL or about 35%, and the colon absorbs 365 mL or 12% of the water entering the gastrointestinal tract. Water is absorbed with close to 99% efficiency. The water balance for the dog is therefore ingested 600 mL, retained 565 mL (which was likely used for respiration humidity and urine production).

Water balance in the horse (and other hindgut fermenters) is somewhat different. A 500-kg horse would be expected to ingest about 40 L of water each day (Table 44.3). Salivary and gastric juices add 41 L of water, and pancreatic, bile, and small and large intestine secretions add another 63 L for a total of 144 L of water entering the gastrointestinal tract. The small intestine absorbs 79 L of water daily. The cecum absorbs 18 L, the ventral colon absorbs 13 L, the dorsal colon absorbs 18.5 L, and the transverse and descending colon absorb another 8 L of water, for a total of 57.5 L for the large intestine. The horse colon absorbs a much greater amount of water than the monogastric colon. It uses the osmotic force of VFA absorption to absorb much of this water. The net loss of water to the feces is about 7.5 L/day. On balance the horse retains 32.5 L of the 40 L ingested.

Malabsorptive diarrhea

Bacteria and viruses can damage the tight junctions and/or villous absorptive cells and can interfere with absorption of solute, both the solute that was in the diet and the solute secreted

Table 44.2 Water secretion and absorption in a 20-kg dog.

	Into lumen (ingested and secreted)	Out of lumen (absorbed)
Food and drink	600 mL	—
Salivary glands	300 mL	—
Gastric juice	600 mL	—
Bile	300 mL	—
Pancreatic secretions	600 mL	—
Small intestine	600 mL	2650 mL
Colon	50 mL	365 mL
Totals	3050 mL	3015 mL = 35 mL in feces

Table 44.3 Water secretion and absorption in a 500-kg horse.

	Into lumen (ingested and secreted)	Out of lumen (absorbed)
Food and drink	40 L	—
Salivary glands	30 L	—
Gastric juice	11 L	—
Bile	5 L	—
Pancreatic secretions	10 L	—
Small intestine	47 L	79 L
Colon	1 L	57.5 L
Totals	144 L	136.5 L = 7.5 L in feces

from crypt cells and in pancreatic, and salivary secretions. The inability to absorb solute will also cause some loss in efficiency of water absorption. If water absorption efficiency in the 20-kg dog drops from nearly 99% to 90% due to enteritis in a section of the intestine, fecal water content will increase from 35 to 275 mL, which will create a very watery feces. If damage to the gastrointestinal tract is restricted to the colon and no water is absorbed by the colon, fecal water content will only increase by the 365 mL the colon is expected to absorb. However, damage to large segments of the small intestine can cause loss of up to 2650 mL water.

Bacterial and viral infections can not only destroy villous absorptive cells, they can initiate inflammation reactions that generally cause hypersecretion by the crypt and goblet cells in an attempt to flush away the offending pathogens. This can greatly increase the amount of fluid lost with the feces. Bacterial infections tend to be fairly localized and cause local damage to either the small or large intestine. Rotaviruses attack the cells at the tips of villi causing some malabsorption. Coronaviruses, such as the causative agents of transmissible gastroenteritis and porcine epidemic diarrhea, kill villous entrocytes the full length of the villus and are therefore much more severe infections. Parvoviruses causing canine parvo and feline panleukopenia attack rapidly dividing cells – in the intestine these are the crypt cells. Since these cells are destined to replace senescent villous cells, both the crypt and villous cells can be lost over a few days. Almost no absorption can occur in the small intestine. This also exposes great lengths of denuded basal lamina and allows bacterial entry. The bacteria will erode the lamina propria to cause widespread hemmorhage, and often septicemia ensues.

Osmotic diarrhea

Ingestion of solute that cannot be absorbed causes water to remain in the intestine. Prune juice contains sorbitol, an alcohol sugar that mammalian cells cannot absorb. Milk of magnesia contains $Mg(OH)_2$, supplying an amount of Mg that exceeds intestinal absorption capacity for this element, and this also causes more water to be retained in the lumen. This concept can be useful in treating constipation.

Osmotic diarrhea can also follow overfeeding, particularly in young animals. Milk contains lactose and neonates possess the enzyme lactase within the brush border of villous enterocytes. However, when fed a very large milk meal, the ability of lactase to successfully break down all the lactose for absorption is exceeded and the unabsorbed lactose will osmotically drag water with it as it exits in the feces.

Principles of oral rehydration therapy to treat diarrheal diseases

In nearly all forms of diarrhea more Na^+ and K^+ are lost in the feces than Cl^-. The colon does a better job of absorbing Cl^- than Na^+ and K^+, though large amounts of all three ions are lost during diarrhea. This causes metabolic acidosis in the animal. This is exacerbated by dehydration, which reduces cardiac output and the delivery of oxygen to tissues of the body. Poor tissue perfusion causes anaerobic end products like lactic acid to build up in the blood, which can also exacerbate metabolic acidosis. Rehydration formulas often contain alkalogenic ingredients such as sodium acetate or sodium bicarbonate to help combat acidosis.

Surprisingly, many of the viruses and bacteria that affect villous cells do not infect the colon, though the colon has plenty of its own pathogens to deal with. Because the colon is generally intact, it can often compensate for lost villous absorption by increasing the amount of fluid that it absorbs. The colon does not possess the enzymes needed for breaking down sugars or peptides and has no transporters for sugars and amino acids. However, the colon can still absorb Na^+, Cl^-, K^+, and HCO_3^-. The colon can also absorb VFAs very well. If the animal is old enough, colonic bacteria can break down sugars in the lumen of the colon and convert them to VFAs. If solute can be absorbed by the colon, water will follow. While the colon of a 20-kg dog normally only absorbs 365 mL of water each day (Table 44.2), it can absorb two to three times this amount if water and electrolytes are presemt in colonic lumen fluids. In less severe cases of small intestine enteritis, the colon can almost totally compensate for disruption of absorption in the small intestine.

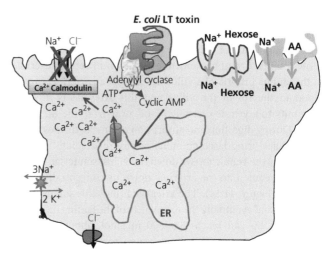

Figure 44.15 Enterotoxigenic *Escherichia coli* can elaborate a toxin that recognizes a receptor on the apical membrane of villous cells. This activates adenylyl cyclase and cyclic AMP is produced. The cyclic AMP causes Ca^{2+} channels in the endoplasmic reticulum (ER) to open releasing Ca^{2+} to the cytosol where it forms a complex with calmodulin. The Ca^{2+}–calmodulin complex blocks the activity of the Na^+/Cl^- cotransporter in the apical membrane. It has no effect on the Na^+/hexose or Na^+/amino acid cotransporters.

Most viruses and bacteria that cause enteritis do not destroy all villous cells. Some can be used to absorb solute. During an outbreak of enterotoxigenic secretory diarrhea the enterotoxin may affect a great majority of the cells. These toxins bind receptor proteins on the apical surface and activate adenylyl cyclase. The resulting cyclic AMP causes intracellular Ca^{2+} stores to release Ca^{2+} into the cytosol. The resulting Ca^{2+}–calmodulin complex blocks Na^+/Cl^- cotransporters in villous cells. They do not affect the Na^+/glucose or Na^+/amino acid transporters (Figure 44.15). Since these transporters remain intact, they can be utilized to advantage to rehydrate the animal.

A fluid that can be used to rehydrate animals with diarrhea will include Na^+, K^+, and Cl^-. If absorbed in the small intestine or colon, these electrolytes bring water with them to restore the circulation. Sodium bicarbonate is typically added to alkalinize the solution to help combat the metabolic acidosis of diarrhea. Glucose and amino acids are also generally added to take advantage of Na^+/sugar and Na^+/amino acid transport mechanisms that may remain intact. They also provide energy and amino acids to help the animal avoid starvation. Very often salts of VFAs or lactic acid are also added since the VFAs and lactose supply alkalinizing Na^+, energy and osmotic pull for water once they are absorbed. Research demonstrates that these solutions should be isotonic (~290 mosmol) or slightly hypotonic for best rehydration results. However, in many cases hypertonic solutions (up to 600 mosmol) can be used, especially if frequent handling of the animal to administer the fluid is difficult. In animals such as piglets that will drink ad libitum, the more isotonic fluids are used. In suckling calves that may only be fed three to four times daily, it is more common to use rehydrating solutions that are hypertonic (Table 44.4).

Summary

Digestive physiology involves a complex series of events that provide nourishment to the animal while preventing invasion by bacteria and viruses in the lumen of the gastrointestinal tract. Table 44.5 outlines the actions of the major hormones of the gastrointestinal tract. Another function that only becomes clear once the complex mechanisms have been revealed is the role of crypt cell secretion. Amino acids and hexose sugars are liberated from dietary proteins and carbohydrates during the luminal and brush border phases of digestion. These molecules, critical for sustaining the life of the animal, are too large or too highly charged to pass through the cell membrane lipid bilayer. Transporter proteins facilitate diffusion of these molecules across the apical membrane of duodenal and upper jejunal villous enterocytes. However, it is the driving force provided by Na^+ moving from the lumen, where its concentration is high, into the cytosol, where its concentration is very low, that allows these large molecules to traverse the apical membrane of villous enterocytes. Many of the diets fed to animals are relatively low in Na^+, so the animal cannot rely on the diet to provide Na^+ in the lumen for absorption of amino acids and sugars. Thus crypt cells are essential for maintaining a high concentration of Na^+ over the villous enterocyte brush border (Figure 44.16). Saliva and pancreatic and bile secretions also contribute substantial amounts of Na^+ to the lumen. The crypt enterocytes pump Cl^- out into the lumen to be followed by Na^+ and water. The Na^+ diffuses to the villous area and is used to absorb amino acids and sugars. The Na^+ not used to absorb amino acids and sugars is returned to the venous blood at the villous tip by Na^+/Cl^- cotransporters. The Cl^- and water also diffuse up to the villous area and can be absorbed by villous cells into the venous circulation. It is important to remember that there are additional Cl^- absorbing mechanisms in the ileum and colon that will absorb the Cl^- that is not cotransported with Na^+ in the upper intestine. As the venous blood passes through the crypt area, the Na^+, Cl^-, and water diffuse out to the crypt cells which pump them into the lumen again. This provides Na^+ needed for absorption of more sugars and amino acids. The same Na^+ atom may be recycled from the crypt to the villus and back to the crypt several times during a meal. This normal function of the crypt cells is under tight control: normally the vagus parasympathetic innervation determines when crypt secretory

Table 44.4 Common formulas for oral rehydration fluids for piglet (allowed ad libitum access to rehydrating fluid) and suckling calf (offered rehydrating fluids three to four times daily).

Compound	Piglet	Suckling calf
Glucose (mmol/L)	100	160
Sodium (mmol/L)	90	120
Potassium (mmol/L)	20	25
Chloride (mmol/L)	65	55
Citrate (mmol/L)	10	50
Amino acid (glycine) (mmol/L)	15	120
Acetate (mmol/L)	10	45
Osmolarity (mosmol/L)	310	575

Table 44.5 Location of major gastrointestinal hormones, their stimulus for release, and their primary actions.

	Site of secretion	Stimulus for release	Action on stomach	Action on liver and pancreas	Action on small intestine
Gastrin	Pyloric stomach	Stomach distension Rising pH in stomach Peptides in stomach	Stimulates acid secretion Stimulates motility Relaxes pyloric sphincter	—	—
Histamine	Fundic stomach	Rising pH in stomach Gastrin	Stimulates acid secretion	—	—
Cholecystokinin	Duodenum	Fats, peptides in duodenum	Inhibits motility Closes pyloric sphincter	Stimulates bile secretion and gallbladder contraction Stimulates pancreatic enzyme secretion	—
Secretin	Duodenum	Low pH in duodenum	—	Stimulates alkaline secretion by pancreas (and saliva)	Stimulates alkaline secretions of Brunner's glands
Prostaglandins	Gastrointestinal tract	Mucosal damage Inflammation	Inhibits histamine secretion Inhibits acid secretion Stimulates mucus production Stimulates blood flow for repair	—	Stimulates mucus production Stimulates blood flow for repair

Section VII: Digestion, Absorption, and Metabolism

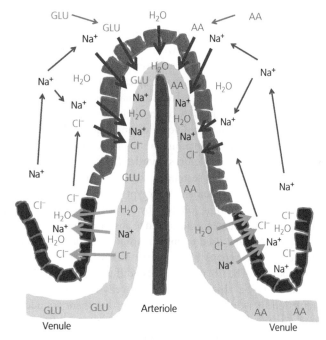

Figure 44.16 Electrolyte circulation from crypt to villus and back to crypt. Crypt cells pump extracellular fluid Cl⁻ into the lumen. The Cl⁻ is followed by Na⁺ and water. The Na⁺ diffuses to the villous cell area where it is utilized to help drive facilitated diffusion of hexose sugars (GLU) and amino acids (AA) across the apical membrane of villous cells. Some of the Na⁺ and Cl⁻ are cotransported across the villous cells and enter the venous blood of the villus. As the venous blood flows past the crypt area, the crypt cells can pump the Cl⁻ out into the lumen and cause the Na⁺ and water to again enter the lumen to be reused to absorb more GLU and AA.

efforts should be activated. As veterinarians we often deal with diarrheal conditions caused by excessive crypt secretion. The *Escherichia coli* enterotoxigenic diarrheas are an example of this. Even when dealing with malabsorptive types of diarrheal disease, the inflammatory response induced by the virus or bacterium will cause cytokines to be released that will generally instigate a strong crypt secretory response to flush away the pathogens and toxins.

Self-evaluation

Answers can be found at the end of the chapter.

1 With regard to digestion and absorption of dietary proteins:
   A Trypsinogen first becomes converted to trypsin by what?
   B Which cells produce this substance?
   C What stimulates these cells to produce the trypsin activating factor?

2 With regard to the gallbladder:
   A Contraction of the gallbladder is stimulated by which hormone?
   B Made by which cells?
   C Located where?
   D Made in response to what stimulus?

3 A micelle consists of fatty acids, monoglycerides, and cholesterol surrounded by what?

4 Two proteolytic enzymes are produced by (**A**) _____ cells of the fundic gastric glands. One is secreted as an inactive enzyme called (**B**) _____. It is activated to its proteolytic form by (**C**) _____. The other proteolytic enzyme is especially important to the neonatal mammal trying to digest its milk meals and is called (**D**) _____.

5 Facilitated diffusion of tryptophan across the apical membrane of a villous cell in the jejunum requires which of the following. List all correct answers.
   A Amino acid carrier protein
   B Sodium
   C Calcium
   D GLUT-2 transporter
   E ATP (directly)
   F Tryptophan cannot be transported across jejunum

6 Name three brush border membrane-bound enzymes involved in the final stages of carbohydrate digestion in the villi of the jejunum.

7 Number, in the order in which they occur (1, first to 9, last), the steps in fat digestion in a dog.
   A CCK stimulates gallbladder contraction and secretion of pancreatic enzymes including pro-colipase
   B Micelles are formed, allowing the lipophilic contents to cross the unstirred water layer and glycocalyx of the villous enterocyte
   C Chylomicrons exocytose through basolateral membrane and enter the lacteals
   D Stomach contractions emulsify ingested fat
   E Fat entering duodenum stimulates CCK release by enteroendocrine cells
   F Pro-colipase is activated to colipase by trypsin in the lumen of the intestine
   G Colipase, lipase and bile salts act together on emulsified fat to begin triglyceride breakdown
   H Triglycerides are reformed and packaged in cholesterol–apolipoprotein B48 structures known as chylomicrons
   I Micelles contact brush border membrane and fatty acids, monoglycerides, cholesterol and fat-soluble vitamins cross cell membrane lipid bilayer into cytosol

8 Magnesium citrate ingestion relieves constipation since Mg is not readily absorbed across the intestinal epithelium. This causes an increase in _____ of the chyme, causing water to remain in the intestinal lumen and exit with the feces.

9 Chloride is actively secreted into the lumen of the jejunum by which cells?

10 Secreted by the cells of question 9, chloride enters the cell from the blood/extracellular fluid:
   A With its concentration gradient and with its electrical gradient
   B With its concentration gradient and against its electrical gradient
   C Against its concentration gradient and with its electrical gradient
   D Against its concentration gradient and against its electrical gradient

11 Glucose molecules are unable to cross the apical membrane by simple diffusion because they are (**A**) _____. Fortunately, glucose can be cotransported across the apical membrane because of several forces that aid its movement. These include the force generated by high glucose concentrations above the apical membrane during the final phases of brush border digestion. The rest of the force needed to permit facilitated diffusion of glucose into the cell is provided by (**B**) _____ moving (**C**) with or against (choose one) its concentration gradient and (**D**) with or against (choose one) its electrical gradient.

12 Volatile fatty acids are the end product of anaerobic bacterial fermentation within the rumen and colon of herbivores and are absorbed across the epithelium to serve as major energy sources for these species. Many of the drugs you will utilize are also weak acids or weak bases. These compounds are absorbed by a process known as (**A**) _____. The weak acid or weak base only crosses the lipid bilayer membrane of absorptive cells when it is in the (**B**) _____ state. For a weak base with a pK_a of 10.8, absorption across the epithelium would be expected to occur most readily in the (**C**) stomach or jejunum (choose one).

13 A 5-kg cat is brought into your clinic first thing in the morning and has diarrhea. You are busy and put it into a clean stainless steel cage with a collection pan underneath; 4 hours later you return to look at the cat and notice there is loose fecal matter in the collection pan. You skillfully measure the volume and discover there is about 40 mL of fluid fecal matter in the pan. You feel confident that the problem in this cat is located in which section of the gastrointestinal tract?

Suggested reading

Goodell, G.M., Campbell, J., Hoejvang-Nielsen, L., Stansen, W. and Constable, P.D. (2012) An alkalinizing oral rehydration solution containing lecithin-coated citrus fiber is superior to a nonalkalinizing solution in treating 360 calves with naturally acquired diarrhea. *Journal of Dairy Science* **95**:6677–6686.

Karasov, W.H. and Douglas, A.E. (2013) Comparative digestive physiology. *Comprehensive Physiology* **3**:741–783.

Saif, L.J. (1999) Comparative pathogenesis of enteric viral infections of swine. *Advances in Experimental Medicine and Biology* **473**:47–59.

Answers

1 (A) Enteropeptidase, (B) villous enterocytes, (C) cholecystokinin
2 (A) Cholecystokinin, (B) enteroendocrine cells, (C) duodenum, (D) fats and peptides entering the duodenum
3 Bile salts
4 (A) Chief, (B) pepsinogen, (C) acid of stomach, (D) rennin
5 A and B
6 Lactase, sucrase, maltase, trehalase, dextrinase, enterocyte amylase
7 1, D; 2, E; 3, A; 4, F; 5, G; 6, B; 7, I; 8, H; 9, C
8 Osmolarity
9 Crypt cells
10 B
11 (A) Too large, (B) Na$^+$, (C) with its concentration gradient and (D) with its electrical gradient
12 (A) Nonionic diffusion, (B) nondissociated (uncharged) state, (C) jejunum
13 Small intestine. This volume of fluid (240 mL/day) could not come from the colon, even if it was unable to perform any absorption duties

45 Ruminant Digestive Physiology and Intestinal Microbiology

Jesse P. Goff

Iowa State University, Ames, IA, USA

Ruminants are a widespread and diverse group of mammals. Domesticated species such as the cow, sheep, goat, water buffalo, and camel utilize plant structural carbohydrates that humans cannot digest to provide the energy to produce milk and meat for human consumption and fiber for our clothes. In many areas of the world ruminants still supply much of the "horsepower" for farm work and transportation. Ruminants all have a common feature: they have specially adapted outcroppings of the esophagus called forestomachs that allow storage of ingesta and permit bacterial fermentation to digest materials that mammalian enzymes cannot break down. There are variations in the shape and size of the various esophageal structures utilized as fermentation vats by ruminants. The cow's anatomy will be used to illustrate basic principles shared by most of the ruminants.

Forestomachs of the cow

> **1** What is the function of the rumen and reticulum and to a lesser extent the omasum?
>
> **2** What is the function of the abomasum?

The esophagus proper of the cow carries material into a large fermentation vat that is composed of the rumen and the reticulum (Figures 45.1 and 45.2). The **rumen** is the largest compartment and is lined with papillae resembling "shag carpeting" that extend from the rumen wall to increase the surface area for absorption (Figure 45.3). Rumen papillae are practically absent from the neonatal rumen. The length and width of rumen papillae increases as the rumen becomes populated with bacteria and as the neonate is placed on a diet that promotes production of butyrate in the rumen. Butyrate is a volatile fatty acid (VFA) that is vital to the integrity of the epithelium of the rumen. The type of diet that best promotes butyrate production and development of rumen papillae in the young ruminant is high in grains as opposed to forage.

The most cranial section of the large fermentation vat is called the **reticulum**. It is distinguishable from the rumen by the unique honeycomb-shaped projections from its wall. Functionally, the rumen and reticulum are the same: both serve as sites of storage of ingesta and provide a safe haven for the bacteria unique to the rumen that will ferment the plant cellulose and hemicellulose of their diet. They are both lined by stratified squamous epithelium that is capable of absorbing VFAs and some electrolytes and minerals. After fermentation in the rumen–reticulum, the more liquid portion of the fermentation mixture moves to the third forestomach, the **omasum**, through the reticulo-omasal orifice. The omasum is built very much like an automobile oil filter (Figure 45.3). It has long leaves covered by a stratified squamous epithelium that the juices leaving the rumen and reticulum must pass over on their way to the true stomach, known as the **abomasum** in ruminants The leaves of the omasum can also absorb VFAs and water. The abomasum of ruminants may have more folds in its inner surface than the stomach of monogastrics, but functionally is the same as a monogastric stomach as are the ruminant small and large intestines.

Dukes' Physiology of Domestic Animals, Thirteenth Edition. Edited by William O. Reece, Howard H. Erickson, Jesse P. Goff and Etsuro E. Uemura.

© 2015 John Wiley & Sons, Inc. Published 2015 by John Wiley & Sons, Inc.

Companion website: www.wiley.com/go/reece/physiology

Section VII: Digestion, Absorption, and Metabolism

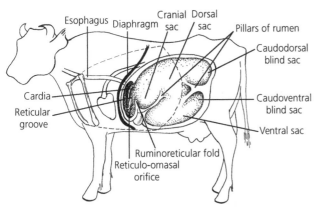

Figure 45.1 The stomach of cattle (left side view). The rumen and reticulum (shown) are two of the three compartments of the forestomach that precede the true stomach (abomasum). The reticulo-omasal orifice is the passageway to the third compartment known as the omasum. The rumen is divided into a number of sacs by muscular pillars. Pillar contraction is essential for movement of rumen content. The dashed line illustrates the extent of the ribcage. From Reece, W.O. (2009) *Functional Anatomy and Physiology of Domestic Animals*, 4th edn. Wiley-Blackwell, Ames, IA. Reproduced with permission from Wiley.

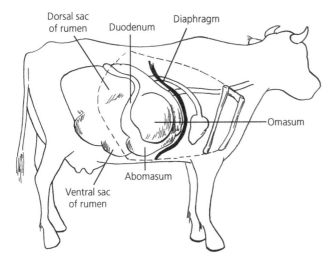

Figure 45.2 The stomach of cattle (right side view). The omasum is the third compartment of the forestomach, which has a short omasal canal that connects the reticulo-omasal orifice with the omaso-abomasal orifice. The dashed line illustrates the extent of the ribcage. From Reece, W.O. (2009) *Functional Anatomy and Physiology of Domestic Animals*, 4th edn. Wiley-Blackwell, Ames, IA. Reproduced with permission from Wiley.

Rumen fermentation

> 1 How does a ruminant derive energy from plant structural carbohydrates consisting of β-linked sugar units?
>
> 2 How many kilocalories of energy can a dog derive from 1 g of glucose? How will dietary glucose be metabolized in the ruminant? How is glucose metabolized in the horse?

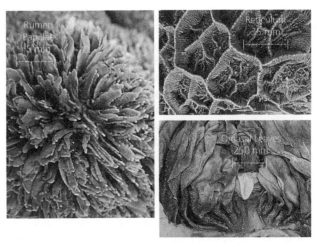

Figure 45.3 Mucosal surfaces of the forestomachs of a cow showing rumen papillae, reticulum honeycomb, and omasal leaves. Photos obtained post-mortem. Note the difference in scale for each photo.

> 3 How many kilocalories of energy can a dog derive from 1 g of cellulose? How will dietary cellulose be metabolized in the ruminant and how much energy can be derived from cellulose? How is cellulose metabolized in the horse and how much energy can be drived from dietary cellulose?
>
> 4 Is it worthwhile to feed a cow a very high quality protein like egg white (albumen)? What if that protein is able to bypass the rumen? Is this true in the horse? Can we feed a nitrogen source like urea to a dairy cow and expect to see it converted to milk proteins?
>
> 5 What is the normal pH of the rumen fluids?
>
> 6 What are rumen protozoa? What is the significance of their absence from rumen fluid?

From the cow's perspective, a major advantage of having a rumen is to provide a home to the bacteria that possess the enzymes needed to break the β1→4) linkages between the various sugars that make up cellulose (mostly hexoses such as glucose) and hemicellulose (mostly pentoses such as xylose and arabinose). Mammalian enzymes cannot perform this task. The **cellulolytic** bacteria that can break these bonds are very **strict anaerobes** and most are members of the *Bacteroides*, *Ruminococcus* and *Butyrovibrio* genera. They break the β(1→4) linkages of plant cell wall structural carbohydrates and utilize the liberated hexoses and pentoses to provide them with energy. However, because they are anaerobes living in an anaerobic environment, the end products of their fermentation are primarily the VFAs acetate, propionate, and butyrate. The VFAs are rapidly absorbed by nonionic diffusion across the forestomach epithelium and used by the ruminant for energy (discussed in more detail in the section on VFA absorption). The normal pH of rumen fluid varies with diet. High-forage diets promote higher rumen pH, typically around 6.5–7.0. High-grain diets decrease pH as VFA production is generally greater. The rumen stays "healthy" so long as average pH stays above 5.7.

Section VII: Digestion, Absorption, and Metabolism

A disadvantage to being a ruminant is that the starches and simpler monosaccharides and disaccharides in the ruminant diet are utilized by rumen bacteria as an energy source. Very little starch or sugar escapes the rumen for absorption in the small intestine. While many bacteria can break the $\alpha 1 \rightarrow 4$) linkages in starch, the **amylolytic genera** such as *Streptococcus* and *Ruminobacter* are particularly adept at digesting starch and sugar. Under the strict anaerobic conditions within the rumen these bacteria ferment the starches and sugars to lactic acid, with some VFAs also produced. The action of the amylolytic bacteria can be a particular concern to ruminants fed high-grain diets. Beef cattle are sometimes switched from high-forage (grass) diets to high-grain (corn, wheat, barley) diets on entering feedyards. The amylolytic bacterial populations can multiply very quickly in response to the starch in the diet and they produce large amounts of lactic acid. Lactic acid has a pK_a of 3.86, making it nearly 10 times stronger acid than acetate (pK_a 4.75), propionate (pK_a 4.87) and butyrate (pK_a 4.83). High amounts of lactic acid and other VFAs in the rumen fluid can cause rumen pH to fall below 5.7. At this pH the cellulolytic bacteria begin to die and the rumen epithelium can be damaged by the accumulation of acid. The dying bacteria release endotoxins that enter the blood and can cause shock. This condition is known as rumen acidosis. This is particularly likely to occur in cattle that have not been allowed time to acclimate to the high-grain diet. When the amount of grain in the diet is increased slowly over a period of weeks, it allows populations of bacteria known as lactate utilizers to populate the rumen. These bacteria metabolize the rumen fluid lactate as an energy source. The lactate utilizers belong to the *Selenomonas* and *Megasphaera* genera. Animals with very high populations of these bacteria in the rumen can be fed very high starch diets with little risk of rumen acidosis. Horses and other hindgut fermenters have essentially the same types of cellulolytic bacteria living in their cecum and colon as cows have in their rumen. However, in these species starches and sugars are absorbed by the small intestine before they reach the colon so the risk for very low pH is reduced.

Energetic considerations

Energetically, a monogastric animal should be able to obtain about 4 kcal of metabolizable energy per gram of starch or glucose digested. The ruminant will only obtain about 2.2 kcal of metabolizable energy per gram of starch or glucose and this will be in the form of the VFAs remaining from anaerobic fermentation. However, the monogastric animal derives no energy from cellulose and hemicellulose, whereas the ruminant can still obtain close to 2.2 kcal of metabolizable energy per gram of cellulose and hemicellulose in the diet. These $\beta(1 \rightarrow 4)$ linked plant structural carbohydrates do not supply the same amount of energy as the $\alpha 1 \rightarrow 4$) linked starches but they are so much more plentiful that the ruminant survives well. Perhaps the animals with the best of both worlds are the hindgut fermenters. They obtain 4 kcal of metabolizable energy per gram of $\alpha(1 \rightarrow 4)$

linked starches in their small intestine, and can also obtain about 2 kcal metabolizable energy per gram of $\beta(1 \rightarrow 4)$ linked plant structural carbohydrates after microbial fermentation in the cecum and colon.

Protein considerations

Another possible advantage to being a ruminant is that it is possible for the rumen bacteria to provide very high quality protein to the animal. Rumen bacteria have the ability to combine nitrogen from ammonia or urea with carbon skeletons liberated from dietary carbohydrates to form all the amino acids that make up their protoplasm. When the bacteria die or move into the small intestine with other digesta, the proteins within the bacteria can be digested by mammalian proteolytic enzymes and the amino acids used by the cow. Microbial protein is considered very high quality: its amino acid profile is almost identical to that of muscle and milk, permitting great conversion into meat and milk by the cow. A disadvantage of being a ruminant is that much of the protein that is fed to the cow can be utilized by rumen bacteria. They find it energetically more efficient to use preformed amino acids when available rather than making them *de novo*. Dietary protein that the rumen bacteria can break down is referred to as **rumen-degradable protein**. In monogastric animals it is critical to feed high-quality proteins to supply the animal with essential amino acids. In ruminants, if the protein is rumen degradable the essential amino acids are lost to the animal unless they can be recovered in the form of microbial protein that enters the small intestine. Not all the dietary protein fed to a cow is degraded by the rumen bacteria for their use. Dietary ingredients vary in the rumen degradability of the protein they contain. Most of the proteins found in typical feedstuffs contain between 25 and 80% rumen-degradable protein. The protein that bypasses the rumen bacteria, known as **rumen-undegradable protein**, can be digested in the small intestine and, if it is of high quality, can be an excellent source of essential amino acids. Horses and other hindgut fermenters digest and absorb protein and amino acids in the small intestine. However, the microbes in their hindguts do contain amino acids. Amino acid transporters have been identified in the horse's colonic mucosal epithelium but the contribution of microbial protein to the essential amino acid needs of the horse is unclear. Certainly in hindgut fermenters that practice coprophagy, such as rabbits, the ingested microbial protein will be digested and amino acids absorbed by the small intestine.

Rumen fungi and protozoa

The rumen is an ecosystem. In addition to a wide variety of anaerobic and facultative anaerobic bacteria, the rumen also contains small populations of fungi. Some of these fungal species may help degrade lignin, a woody and indigestible constituent of plant cell walls. Other quite noticeable inhabitants of the rumen are the protozoa. These eukaryotes can be quite large and generally live by ingesting bacteria and each other in the rumen (Figure 45.4). There is little evidence this is

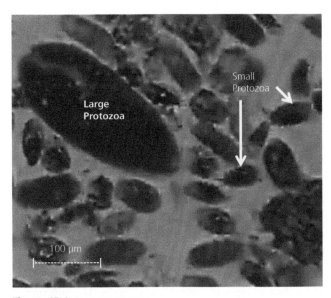

Figure 45.4 Rumen protozoa.

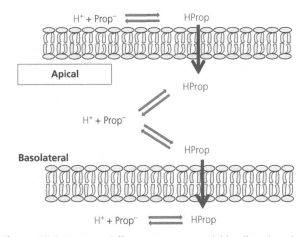

Figure 45.5 Nonionic diffusion. Propionic acid, like all weak acids, exists in a charged dissociated state (Prop⁻) and an uncharged nondissociated state (HProp). The amount of each species depends on the pK_a of the acid and the pH of the solution. In the HProp state the acid freely crosses membranes. Once across the membrane it dissociates to reestablish the dissociation equilibrium.

helpful to the cow. The practicing veterinarian can make an easy diagnosis of excessive rumen acidosis by passing a tube into the rumen of the cow and extracting a small amount of rumen fluid for microscopic examination. The larger protozoa die rapidly when the rumen pH falls too low. Protozoa and fungi also live in the cecum and colon of hindgut fermenters.

Absorption of volatile fatty acids across the rumen wall

1 What is meant by the pK_a of a weak acid or base?
2 The equilibrium of dissociation of a weak acid can be shifted toward or away from dissociation by the pH of the solution containing the weak acid. Would acetate absorption be more complete in the abomasum or the small intestine?
3 How does the rumen epithelium manage to make the process of VFA absorption more efficient?

The VFAs produced in the rumen are weak acids that exist in both a dissociated and a nondissociated state. In the nondissociated state they are both water- and lipid-soluble. In this state they have no charge and being lipid-soluble they can freely cross the lipid bilayer of cell membranes. In the dissociated state their charge makes them unable to cross the lipid bilayer and that charge also makes them soluble in water only. The nondissociated and dissociated forms of weak acids and weak bases are in equilibrium and the concentration of nondissociated and dissociated forms is dependent on the pH of the solution. How this affects the equilibrium and concentrations of nondissociated and dissociated forms is best illustrated using propionic acid as an example. Propionic acid in water exists in the nondissociated

state, designated HProp, and in the dissociated state, Prop⁻, as described by the following equation:

$$HProp \leftrightarrow H^+ + Prop^-$$

The pK_a for propionic acid is 4.87. In a pH 4.87 solution, 50% of the propionic acid will exist in the nondissociated state, HProp, and 50% will exist in the dissociated state, Prop⁻. If the pH of the solution is 5.87 (and remembering that pH is a logarithmic scale), the reduction in H⁺ ions shifts the equilibrium further to the right and now just 10% of the propionic acid is in the HProp form while 90% is in the Prop⁻ dissociated form. If the solution has a pH of 6.87, not unlike the pH in the rumen, just 1% of the propionic acid is in the nondissociated form, while 99% is in the dissociated form. The small amount of HProp in the nondissociated form will freely cross the apical membrane down its concentration gradient to the interior of the cell (Figure 45.5). By removing HProp from the lumen, the equilibrium of propionic acid dissociation will be shifted to the left to replace the lost HProp, allowing another HProp to cross the cell membrane. Once on the other side of the membrane the HProp quickly dissociates to form H⁺ and Prop⁻. The Prop⁻ is now trapped inside the cell. However, as long as HProp is being produced in the lumen and is crossing the apical membrane, there will be a second equilibrium set up for propionic acid at the opposite side of the cell near the basolateral membrane. Here Prop⁻ and H⁺ will again be in equilibrium with HProp. As HProp is formed it will move across the basolateral membrane to the extracellular fluid. To cross from rumen fluid into the extracellular fluid, the VFA must cross through all layers of cells that form the stratified squamous epithelium covering the rumen papillae. It would seem a gargantuan and inefficient process to establish these equilibria at both the apical and basolateral membrane of each layer of squamous cells. The rumen

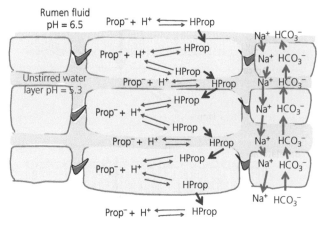

Figure 45.6 Rumen absorption of volatile fatty acids. The rumen wall is composed of stratified squamous epithelium. Absorption of volatile fatty acids is enhanced by the absorption of Na^+ and secretion of HCO_3^- across the rumen epithelium. This creates a small zone of lower pH within the unstirred water layer above and between epithelial cells. The lower pH greatly increases the amount of volatile fatty acids in the nondissociated uncharged state, promoting absorption across the apical membranes.

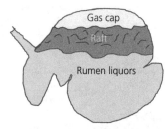

Figure 45.7 The ingested forages and grains comprise two distinct layers of ingesta within the rumen of the cow and some other ruminants. The longer forage particles float in a raft of material in the top layer. A pocket of gas, composed of CO_2 and some methane produced during bacterial fermentation, is dorsal to the rumen raft. The finer particles released from forage breakdown are in suspension within the rumen liquor below the rumen raft. In the majority of smaller ruminants (browsers), the ingested material does not form layers during fermentation.

epithelium has a clever way of improving the efficiency of this process. Above each layer of squamous epithelium there is an unstirred water layer held in place by surface tension (Figure 45.6). The rumen epithelial cell will remove (absorb) a Na^+ atom from this unstirred water layer in exchange for secretion of an HCO_3^- anion into this space. This reduces the pH in the unstirred water layer so that it is generally 1–1.5 pH units lower than the rumen fluid pH. The lower pH in this fluid promotes the equilibrium of propionate and the other VFAs away from dissociation, so much more of it is in the nondissociated state and ready to cross the apical membranes into the cells. This greatly improves the efficiency of absorption of VFAs from the rumen. A similar mechanism for enhanced VFA absorption is thought to occur in horse colon as well.

Ruminant forestomach motility

1 What is the purpose of mixing contractions of the rumen? How often should you be able to auscultate the rumen contractions in a normal cow?

2 Why is eructation important?

3 Why is it important for the ventral sac of the rumen to relax in order to allow eructation?

4 What is frothy bloat?

5 What are the steps needed for a cow to "chew her cud"?

6 What is hardware disease and why does it occur?

7 What is a displaced abomasum and why does it occur?

8 How do young ruminants avoid having the high-quality proteins found in milk destroyed by rumen fermentation?

Three distinct types of contractions occur in the cow's rumen and reticulum and serve three different purposes: **mixing of digesta** with rumen bacteria, **removal of gases** produced during fermentation, and **regurgitation of rumen contents** so that they can be more thoroughly chewed to aid their degradation by rumen bacteria. Each type of contraction is controlled as a distinct programmed reflex within the medulla in response to vagal sensory afferent information and is initiated by the vagus efferent nerves. A regurgitation reflex contraction will not allow passage of gas from the rumen and an eructation reflex will not permit fibrous material to enter the esophagus. The ruminant esophagus cranial to the forestomachs has inner circular and outer longitudinal muscle composed of striated skeletal muscle. It is unique in that it is capable of both antegrade and retrograde peristalsis. In cows and sheep, the rumen ingesta form distinct layers in the rumen. A thick mat of the longer fibrous particles in the diet floats on top of the rumen fluids (Figure 45.7). Below the rumen raft the size of the particles suspended in the rumen fluid decreases, until near the ventral part of the rumen the material is almost entirely liquid with only small particles suspended in the fluids. In the great majority of ruminants there is no layering of rumen ingesta: all sizes of fibers and particles are continuously mixed and evenly distributed throughout the fermentation fluids.

Mixing contractions

These contractions serve to keep the rumen contents well mixed to promote effective fermentation. They begin with contraction of the rumen near the cardia (site of entrance of the esophagus) and move across the dorsal surface to the caudal aspect of the rumen. The contractive wave then proceeds down to the ventral rumen and to the reticulum and then back toward the cardia region (Figure 45.8). Material is moved from the dorsal sac of the rumen to the ventral sac and then on to the caudal dorsal blind sac and back to the dorsal sac again. Each mixing contraction requires 30–50 s to complete and they occur one after the other. Auscultation of rumen is accomplished by placing a

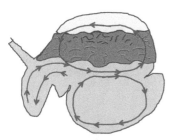

Figure 45.8 Mixing contractions within the rumen. These contractions move material from rumen to reticulum and back as well as from front to back of rumen. The raft and the liquor move in opposite directions. The coordination of motility of the rumen depends on vagal parasympathetic efferent input. In a normal cow there will be three complete rumen motility cycles every 2 min.

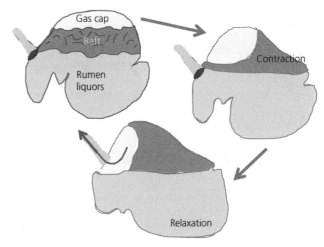

Figure 45.9 Eructation reflex. Gases formed during bacterial fermentation in the rumen must be removed. The reflex begins with contraction of the caudodorsal rumen. This pushes the gas cap forward toward the cardia (purple) or opening to the esophagus. At this point the ventral sac of the rumen relaxes, allowing the fluid level of the rumen to fall below the cardia. Receptors within the cardia sense the absence of fluid and presence of gas and vagal afferents trigger the medulla to cause vagal efferent neurons to open the lower esophageal sphincter and gas is propelled up the esophagus by reverse peristalsis.

stethoscope in the left paralumbar fossa region. The veterinarian should hear about three rumen rumblings every 2 min in a normal cow. Mixing contractions are interrupted only by eructation or regurgitation contractions in normal healthy cows. The presence of fibrous material (the rumen raft) seems to be the major factor stimulating rumen contractions. The raft material is sometimes referred to as "scratch factor" as the presence of a thick rumen raft promotes both mixing and regurgitation contractions of the rumen and reticulum.

A notable feature of the reticulum is that during contraction of the rumen and reticulum heavy materials and foreign objects will generally end up lodged in the reticulum. Because cows consume their diet very quickly before they find a quiet place to ruminate, they may not be very discriminating about what they swallow. It is not uncommon for cows to swallow nails and pieces of wire that then take up residence in the reticulum. Further contractions of the reticulum can cause such objects to pierce the cranial wall of the reticulum and enter the peritoneum, causing peritonitis. This is known as **hardware disease**. Occasionally, the object pierces the diaphragm to cause pleuritis as well. Most dairy cows are administered a magnet orally, which is swallowed and ends up in the reticulum. The magnet holds any iron-containing material like wire to prevent it from moving through the wall of the reticulum.

Eructation contractions

During fermentation about 2 L of gas, primarily carbon dioxide with small amounts of methane , is produced each minute. These gases must be removed to prevent distension of the rumen that could interfere with the ability of the diaphragm to expand the thoracic cavity. The eructation reflex is initiated by vagal afferents that sense distension of the dorsal rumen by gas (Figure 45.9). Contractions start in the caudal rumen and move forward from the caudodorsal blind sac to the dorsal sac. At the same time the caudoventral sac of the rumen is relaxed. This has the important effect of dropping the fluid level around the cardia region so that the entrance to the lower esophagus is free of fluid. Only if the cardia is free of fluid will the lower esophageal sphincter relax and allow gas into the esophagus. The gas is

then propelled up the esophagus by an inspiratory effort against a partially closed nasopharynx. This causes a portion of the eructated gas to enter the trachea and into the lungs. The rumen gas is then expelled through the nostrils during the next exhalation. Each eructation contraction takes about 30 s to complete and one typically occurs after every three to five mixing contractions. It is suggested that the inspiration of eructated gases into the lungs by the ruminant may help to muffle the noise that might be generated by gases escaping directly out of the mouth. Emitting loud burps might lead to easy detection by predators.

Bloat

Bloat occurs when the gases cannot leave the rumen. This could be caused by blockage of the esophagus (choke) due to ingestion of some food item. It can also occur in animals with diseases affecting vagal nerve function or medullary function. As veterinarians, rabies should always be considered a possibility in a cow exhibiting bloat. However, bloat is more typically caused by ingestion of certain types of plant material. The classic example is bloat caused by ingestion of legumes such as alfalfa. These plants have waxy saponins in their leaves. When mixed with rumen fluid these saponins can form very stable bubbles that float on the surface of the rumen fluid (Figure 45.10). This froth interferes with the eructation reflex. The vagal afferent sensory fibers in the region of the cardia interpret the froth as fluid and will not stimulate relaxation of the lower esophageal sphincter. This might ordinarily be a mechanism to protect the ruminant from inhalation of rumen fluids during the eructation reflex. However, the cardia can never be cleared of this froth, the gases

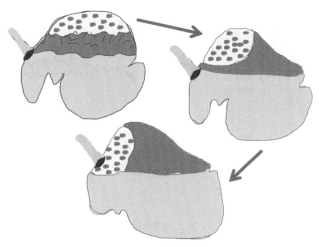

Figure 45.10 Frothy bloat. Legumes such as alfalfa can contain high amounts of waxy substances known as saponins. These compounds, when churned within the rumen, form a frothy bloat. These froth bubbles are very stable and are interpreted by receptors within the cardia as fluid. These receptors signal the medulla that the cardia is still covered with fluid. As a result the lower esophageal sphincter (purple) will not relax. The eructation reflux cannot be completed and gas cannot escape. The rumen becomes greatly inflated and this interferes with respiration.

of fermentation cannot be removed, and the pressure of the gas build-up causes distension of the rumen and prevents diaphragm expansion and the ruminat eventually suffocates. Bloat can also occur in cattle fed high-grain diets, particularly those containing wheat and barley grains. In this case amylolytic bacteria produce a dextrin slime that causes froth to develop in the rumen. This froth is also perceived by the sensory receptors in the cardia as failure to clear the cardia of fluid and the lower esophageal sphincter will not open.

Regurgitation contractions

This reflex allows the cow to bring large-particle material from the rumen to the mouth so that it can be chewed to reduce particle size and increase the surface area available for bacterial attachment. It is often referred to as **chewing the cud**. The presence of a rumen raft (the fibrous material that floats on the rumen fluid) promotes initiation of this reflex. Regurgitation begins with contraction in the middle of the dorsal sac (Figure 45.11). This forces raft material toward the cardia and the gas pocket moves to the caudal part of the rumen. Coinciding with this is an inspiratory effort against a closed nasopharynx and open upper esophageal sphincter that creates great negative pressure in the esophagus to bring the bolus of fibrous material (cud) into the esophagus past a relaxed lower esophageal sphincter. The presence of the cud initiates retrograde antiperistaltic contractions of the esophagus that propel the cud up into the mouth. That cud is chewed for a couple of minutes, swallowed, and another bolus is brought up. Regurgitation has some voluntary component to it. Cows chew their cud when they are relaxed. The amount of fiber (neutral detergent fiber) in the diet

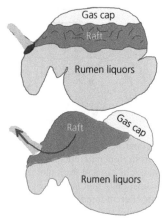

Figure 45.11 Regurgitation reflex. This reflex begins with contraction at the mid-dorsal rumen with some elevation of the ventral rumen. This pushes the gas cap caudally and pushes the rumen raft toward the cardia. The lower esophageal sphincter relaxes and a bolus of raft material (the cud) enters the esophagus. It is propelled up the esophagus by reverse peristaltic contractions. It is chewed for 1–2 min to reduce particle size and swallowed.

affects the rate of regurgitation. Fibrous material can spend 3 days being digested in the rumen. Chewing the cud also stimulates saliva secretion and saliva serves as an important source of rumen buffer that helps prevent the development of rumen acidity. Normally, a regurgitation contraction occurs every 2–3 min between mixing contractions and eructation contractions. When the veterinarian observes a herd of cattle at rest, at least 60% of cows should be actively chewing the cud. Fewer than 60% could be indicative of a lack of fiber in the diet, which could lead to rumen acidosis.

Abomasal contraction

In ruminants, material is sent to the abomasum at a fairly steady rate. As with the true stomach of monogastric species, the contractions of the abomasum allow material entering the abomasum to be thoroughly mixed with the acids and enzymes of the abomasum. Contractions also allow some material to exit to the small intestine.

A great amount of carbon dioxide is produced during bacterial fermentation and some remains dissolved in the rumen fluid. However, carbon dioxide is almost insoluble in low pH solutions and so a large amount of gas is liberated when the rumen fluid meets the acid of the abomasum. A unique action of abomasal contraction in ruminants is to drive gases back into the omasum and rumen for regurgitation. The abomasum normally contracts about 2.25 times each minute. It is coordinated with rumen contractions so that there are about two contractions of the abomasum for every rumen mixing contraction. If rumen contractions are slowed by the absence of rumen raft material, the abomasum contractions also slow. Unfortunately, if abomasal contractility is greatly reduced, the abomasum can fill with gas and "float" to the top of the abdominal cavity, a condition known as **displacement of the abomasum**. It is particularly common in dairy cows shortly after calving. It is often associated with a diet poor in fiber or a diet that promotes hypocalcemia (milk fever). Abomasal muscle, like all smooth and skeletal muscle, loses contractile strength when blood calcium is low.

Reticular groove reflex of neonatal ruminants

While suckling milk many young ruminants initiate a reflex that shunts the milk from the esophagus directly into the omasum. It is sometimes erroneously referred to as the esophageal reflex. This avoids having milk enter the rumen where it might sour and possibly destroy colostral antibodies. As the calf ages and develops a population of rumen bacteria, this reflex shunts the high-quality proteins of milk to the abomasum to supply essential amino acids to the calf rather than to the rumen bacteria. Suckling action and the presence of milk proteins and electrolytes causes pharyngeal afferent neuronal pathways to initiate this reflex. A fold of the reticulum moves dorsally to form a groove between the esophagus and the reticulo-omasal orifice that guides liquids directly from the esophagus to the omasum.

Camelids

1 What is the function of the three chambers of a camelid stomach?

2 What is the function of the saccules found in the ventral portions of chambers 1 and 2 in camelid stomachs?

3 Does the ingesta form distinct layers in the camelid stomach?

Llamas, guanacos, and camels are also ruminants with a slightly different forestomach design. They possess three chambers (named chambers 1, 2 and 3) including the abomasum, rather than the four-chamber forestomach and stomach of more traditional ruminants. The first two chambers are large fermentation vats and material passes from Chamber 1 to 2 and on to 3 (Figure 45.12). Camelids have unique saccules in the ventral portion of Chamber 1 and Chamber 2 that are invaginations into the chamber wall. These saccules greatly increase the surface area available for absorption and they can absorb VFAs from the fermentation fluid about three to four times faster than traditional ruminants. These saccules fill with fermented fluid and then contractions of the chamber wall completely evert the saccule, dumping the contents back into the fermentation chamber. The ingesta are not found neatly layered by fibrous material content; instead they are kept homogeneously mixed with chamber fluid. Camelids eructate more often than ruminants, which may explain why they are less prone to bloat. They also have the ability to regurgitate material from Chamber 1 to chew the cud. And as anyone who has worked with camelids soon learns, they can eject this malodorous material beyond the mouth with force and some accuracy. Chamber 3 is somewhat

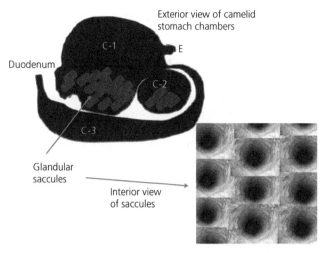

Figure 45.12 The camelid fermentation chambers. Camelids generally have three chambers to their forestomach and true stomach area. Chambers 1 and 2 are fermentation vats. The ingesta do not form layers as they do in large ruminants. These chambers have specialized saccules on their ventral surface that can take in and expel fermentation fluid. This greatly increases their surface area for absorption and is thought to enhance the rate of digestion of cellulosic materials. Chamber 3 is divided into two physiologically distinct zones. The cranial portion of Chamber 3 is a continuation of the fermentation vat. The final third or less of Chamber 3 is the true stomach of the camelid, analogous to the abomasum of ruminants.

analogous to the abomasum, although only the last one-third of this compartment is truly glandular stomach. Fermentation continues in the cranial portion of Chamber 3.

Microbial ecology of the digestive tract

1 Is the gastrointestinal tract colonized by bacteria *in utero*?

2 What are the primary sources of intestinal bacteria in the neonate?

3 Which types of bacteria predominate in the lower intestines of the dog and cat? What about the rabbit and rat?

4 Why are lactobacilli commonly found in probiotic products?

All neonatal animals are born or hatch with a sterile intestinal tract; there are no bacteria, fungi or protozoa present. Within weeks the young animal will ingest bacteria from the mother's oral cavity (licking and grooming the neonate) or through contact with feces in the environment and the process of colonization will begin. Ruminant and hindgut fermenters develop a functional microbial population in their respective fermentation vats in about 2–3 months. Even in monogastric species, colonic bacteria can greatly affect health of the gut through butyrate production and many monogastric animals can obtain some energy from production of VFAs in the cecum and colon.

Section VII: Digestion, Absorption, and Metabolism

Many types of bacteria can be found in the mouth and oropharynx. Their numbers are kept relatively low by enzymes, antibacterial substances, and antibodies found in saliva. Periodontal disease (dogs and cats) or an infection below the gumline may be sequelae of poor control of these bacteria. Duodenum and upper jejunum have relatively low numbers of bacteria. The stomach acids and proteolytic enzymes kill most ingested bacteria (90%, which still leaves 10% that grow exponentially) and the flushing action of digesta keeps numbers relatively low in the upper gastrointestinal tract. Typically, the duodenum contains about 10^5 bacteria per gram contents. Many of the bacteria in the jejunum are descended from bacteria found in the ileum. As populations in the ileum grow they migrate up the tract. The ileum contains about 10^8 bacteria per gram. In the lower intestine and colon the oxygen levels in the lumen of the gut fall much lower and this allows some anaerobes to grow. The cecum and colon contain about 10^{10} bacteria per gram contents. There are some notable species differences in the types of bacteria colonizing the intestine. In humans, dogs, and cats, Gram-negative bacteria such as *Escherichia coli* tend to predominate in the small intestine and colon. There are also many lactobacilli (Gram positive). Lactobacilli seem to be associated with improved health of the gut, hence the popularity of using yogurt with live cultures as a probiotic.

Lactobacilli (Gram positive) and segmented filamentous bacteria predominate in rodent and rabbit small intestine. There are also more cellulolytic anaerobes in their colon than in monogastric species.

> Administering antibiotics of the penicillin family to rabbits and rats can kill Gram-positive bacteria and allow *E. coli* to overgrow the intestine. This is generally deadly for these animals.

Most of the inhabitants of the intestinal tract are not harmful and likely beneficial. However, certain bacteria are pathogens: some all the time, as exemplified by most *Salmonella* species that produce toxins and cause tissue destruction or systemic inflammation; some only when conditions are right. For example, *Clostridium perfringens* is likely present in the intestine of most young lambs and causes no difficulty. However, when the lamb is placed on a high-grain diet, some starch escapes rumen fermentation and makes its way to the lower small intestine. The availability of starch as an energy source enables *C. perfringens* to proliferate. It then produces enterotoxins that damage the enterocytes and cause hemorrhage into the bowel. Colonization by normal bacteria can help prevent colonization by pathogenic bacterial species. **Probiotics** are mixtures of "normal" intestinal bacteria such as lactobacilli that fill an ecological niche and thus competitively exclude a pathogen from occupying that area of the intestine. **Prebiotics** are diet ingredients fed to provide nutrients preferred by the beneficial bacteria in hopes of promoting their growth.

Self-evaluation

Answers can be found at the end of the chapter.

1 What is the fate of glucose in the dog?

2 What is the fate of glucose in the ruminant?

3 What is the fate of glucose in the horse?

4 What is the fate of urea if fed to the dog?

5 What is the fate of urea if fed to the cow?

6 What is the fate of urea if fed to the horse?

7 Why does bloat develop in some animals grazing alfalfa pastures?

8 What happens if a cow eats a piece of wire?

9 How many chambers are found in the camelid "stomach."

10 What will happen if you treat a rabbit with pneumonia with penicillin?

Answers

1 The glucose will reach the small intestine and be absorbed by Na^+/glucose cotransporters. Glucose provides about 4 kcal metabolizable energy per gram.

2 The rumen bacteria will anaerobically utilize the energy in glucose by glycolysis. The end products of anaerobic glycolysis will be a mixture of VFAs and lactic acid, depending on the type of bacteria that takes up each glucose molecule. The ruminant will derive about 2.2 kcal metabolizable energy per gram glucose.

3 The glucose will reach the small intestine and be absorbed by Na^+/glucose cotransporters. Glucose will provide about 4 kcal metabolizable energy per gram.

4 The urea will likely be absorbed from the small intestine and some will be immediately excreted in the urine. The rest may be converted to ammonia in the liver. If a large amount is fed, the dog will eventually exhibit ammonia toxicity.

5 The bacteria in the rumen will break down the urea to ammonia and then utilize the ammonia to synthesize amino acids, provided there is also a carbohydrate source fed with the urea. The bacteria use the amino acids to form the various proteins needed for survival. As the bacteria die or are flushed into the small intestine, the cow's small intestinal enzymes digest these bacterial proteins to provide essential amino acids.

6 The urea will likely be absorbed from the small intestine and some will be immediately excreted in the urine. A smaller amount will leave the blood and diffuse into the lumen of the large intestine, where it can be used by bacteria to produce microbial protein. It is uncertain how much benefit, if any, the horse can obtain from microbial protein produced in the cecum and colon.

7 Saponins in alfalfa cause frothy bubbles to develop in the rumen. These very stable bubbles are present throughout the gas pocket. During the eructation reflex the cardia must be cleared of fluids completely before the lower esophageal sphincter will relax and allow gas

to enter the esophagus. Unfortunately, the froth is interpreted by cardia receptors as a liquid and the eructation reflex will not continue to completion. Gases cannot escape the rumen and distension of the rumen prevents adequate expansion of the pleural cavity and the animal slowly suffocates.

8 Since cows eat their meals quickly without chewing (they chew later; regurgitation reflex), they are likely to swallow wire if it is accidentally present in the diet. The wire will enter the reticulum or quickly reach the reticulum as rumen contractions push material into the reticulum. The wire can be pushed through the reticulum wall and cause peritonitis or be pushed through the diaphragm and cause pleuritis.

9 Three, the final chamber also contains glandular true stomach.

10 The pneumonia may respond but the penicillin kills the Gram-positive bacteria that predominate in the rabbit large intestine. This will likely kill the rabbit as pathogenic Gram-negative bacteria fill the void left by the death of the Gram-positive bacteria.

46 Avian Digestion

William O. Reece and Darrell W. Trampel
Iowa State University, Ames, IA, USA

There are approximately 9700 species of birds and each is adapted for survival in their own unique environment and habitat. Veterinary interests related to the diversity that exists among the species are those associated with the food production industry, pet bird industry, and aspects of wildlife care and management. While all birds have some characteristics in common, there are unique features applicable to each of the above interests wherein veterinary specialties exist. Accordingly, this chapter will relate to the domestic species associated primarily with the food industry

The digestive tract

1 What are the choanal clefts and what does each communicate with?

2 Where is the crop relative to the esophagus?

3 Which one of the two avian stomach chambers is the glandular stomach and which one is the muscular stomach?

4 Are there lacteals in the lamina propria of the avian small intestine?

5 What structure marks the end of the small intestine ileum?

6 What are the two parts of the large intestine?

7 What appears to be the function of the well-developed villi near the ileocecal junction?

8 What are the three compartments of the cloaca? Which one is most cranial and which one is most caudal?

9 Are gallbladders present in domestic birds?

The digestive organs of domestic birds are obviously different in several respects from mammals. In general, the intestines of birds are relatively shorter than those of mammals. Presumably, such adaptations are important in reducing overall body weight in birds that fly. In adult chickens the length of the entire digestive tract may be 200 cm or more (Table 46.1). Teeth are absent, a well-developed two-chambered stomach is present, the **cecum** is double, and the **rectum (colon)** is short, linking the **ileum** with the **cloaca**, which is a common pathway for excretory and digestive wastes and the reproductive tract. These anatomical differences signify differences in the digestive processes.

Oropharynx

The **oropharynx (mouth and pharynx)** is the combined cavity that extends from the beak to the esophagus. The roof of this cavity is formed by the **palate**, which has a long median cleft (**choana**) that connects with the nasal cavity. A shorter cleft (**infundibular cleft**) more caudally located is the common opening of the **auditory tubes**. The floor of the oropharynx is

Section VII: Digestion, Absorption, and Metabolism

Table 46.1 Length of the digestive tract of chickens (five birds).

	At 20 days (cm)	At 1.5 years (cm)
Entire digestive tract	85	210
Duodenum (complete loop)	12	20
Ileum and jejunum	49	120
Cecum	5	17.5
Colon and cloaca	4	11.25

Source: Reece, W.O. (ed.) (2004) *Dukes' Physiology of Domestic Animals*, 12th edn. Cornell University Press, Ithaca, NY. Reproduced with permission from Cornell University Press.

formed by the mandible, tongue, and **laryngeal mound**, which is caudal to the base of the tongue. The laryngeal mound has a median slit (**the glottis**). There is no epiglottis guarding the glottis. The triangular tongue moves a bolus within the oropharynx, propelling it into the esophagus when the bird swallows. Very little muscle tissue exists in the tongue; its movements are produced by the well-developed hyoid muscles. **Taste buds** are variably located in the oropharynx. Chickens may have as many as 300 taste buds. **Salivary glands** are present and are well developed in chickens and turkeys but the secretion contains little amylase. Abundant saliva moistens ingested food and provides lubrication for boli when swallowed.

Esophagus and crop

A schematic of the digestive tract beyond the oropharynx that begins with the esophagus is shown in Figure 46.1. The avian esophagus consists of a cervical and a thoracic region. It is wide and dilatable, thus serving to accommodate bulky unmasticated food. Near the thoracic inlet of the cervical esophagus there is a dilatation that forms a pouch known as the **crop (ingluvies)**, which has a food storage function. In the thoracic region the postcrop esophagus terminates in the **proventriculus** (see Figure 46.1). Mucous glands are abundant in the esophagus to provide lubrication for food being swallowed.

Stomach

The proventriculus is the first of two chambers that comprise the avian stomach. The second chamber is the **ventriculus**, also known as the **gizzard** (see Figure 46.1). The proventriculus is the glandular stomach and the ventriculus is the muscular stomach. The ventriculus is composed of opposing thin and thick muscle pairs (smooth muscle). The deep red color is due to a high concentration of myoglobin. The mucosal surface of the ventriculus is lined with a thick **cuticle**, called **koilin**, a carbohydrate–protein complex. Koilin is formed when the mucosal secretion solidifies on the surface following exposure to the low pH in the ventriculus. The cuticle protects the ventriculus from acid and proteolytic enzymes secreted by the proventriculus. The cuticle is continuously secreted at its base and is continuously eroded away on its surface. Clusters of hard rodlets on the surface create an abrasive surface similar to sandpaper.

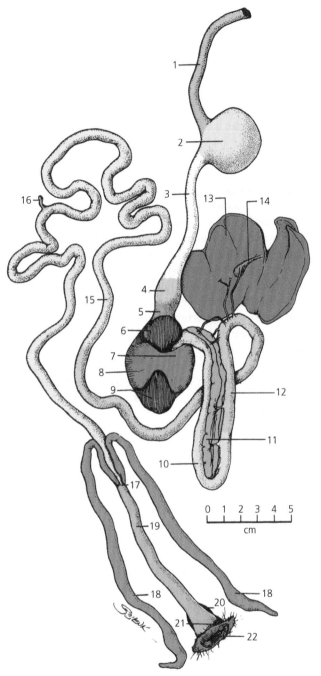

Figure 46.1 Digestive tract of a turkey. 1, Precrop esophagus; 2, crop; 3, postcrop esophagus; 4, glandular stomach (proventriculus); 5, isthmus; 6–9, muscular stomach (gizzard); 10, proximal duodenum; 11, pancreas; 12, distal duodenum; 13, liver; 14, gallbladder; 15, jejunum; 16, Meckel's diverticulum (remnant of yolk sac); 17, ileocecocolic junction; 18, ceca; 19, colon; 20, bursa of Fabricius; 21, cloaca; 22, vent. See text for description of the various parts. From Trampel, D.W. and Duke, G.E. (2004) Avian digestion. In: *Dukes' Physiology of Domestic Animals*, 12th edn (ed. W.O. Reece). Cornell University Press, Ithaca, NY. Reproduced with permission from Cornell University Press.

The greenish or brownish color of the cuticle is due to the reflux of bile pigments from the duodenum.

Grit (i.e., small stones) is present in the ventriculus (gizzard) of most graniverous and herbivorous birds. It is used for grinding hard foods between the thick muscles of the ventriculus. Grit apparently is not essential for normal digestion, but digestion of hard foods is slower and the digestibility of a diet may be decreased without it. Normally, grit is ingested regularly, but if it is not available food is retained for a longer period in the gizzard.

Small intestine

The small intestine is continued caudally from the ventriculus by the duodenum (see Figure 46.1). Divisions of the small intestine into **duodenum**, **jejunum**, and **ileum** are indistinct. There is a duodenal loop as found in mammals. The vestige of the yolk sac (**Meckel's diverticulum**) is about midway in the small intestine and is used to indicate the division between jejunum and ileum (see Figure 46.1). A well-defined network of blood capillaries, connective tissue, smooth muscle, and nerve fibers are present in the lamina propria, but no there are lacteals (blind beginnings of lymph capillaries). The ileum ends with a circular ring of muscle tissue projecting into the rectal lumen that appears to serve as a valve at the **ileocecocolic junction** (see Figure 46.1). Entrances to the ceca are located immediately caudal to this ring.

Large intestine

The large intestine comprises the ceca and the rectum (colon) (see Figure 46.1). In most birds, a right and left ceca arise at the junction of the small and large intestines and pursue retrograde courses beside the ileum to which they are attached by ileocecal folds. There appears to be no correlation between diet and cecal development nor between the size of the ceca and the length and width of the rectum. In chickens, a cecum can be divided into three regions depending on development of their villi and the presence or absence of longitudinal and/or transverse folds. Near the ileocecal junction, villi are well developed and interdigitate to form a filter that excludes coarse intestinal contents and allows fluids to enter. While early opinions considered their function to be mainly for absorption, a greater understanding and importance of the ceca is presently recognized. In this regard, cecectomy results in reduced metabolism of food, lower digestibility of crude fiber, and greater loss of amino acids. Also, bacterial breakdown of cellulose occurs in the ceca.

Rectum and cloaca

The **rectum (colon)** is relatively short and links the ileum with the coprodeal compartment of the cloaca (Figure 46.2). The **coprodeum** is the most cranial of the three cloacal compartments followed in order by the **urodeum** and **proctodeum**. The three compartments are continuous with each other and are separated only by two annular folds, the coprourodeal and the uroproctodeal folds. Urinary and reproductive tracts empty

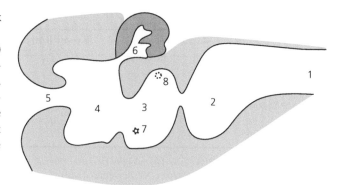

Figure 46.2 Median section of the cloaca of a 6-month-old female domestic fowl. 1, Colon; 2, coprodeum; 3, urodeum; 4, proctodeum; 5, vent; 6, cloacal bursa; 7, position of oviduct bursa, on left side only; 8, ureteric orifice.

into the urodeum and the proctodeum opens externally through the **anus (vent)**. The **bursa of Fabricius (cloacal bursa)**, which is involved in immune function, projects dorsally from the proctodeum.

Liver and pancreas

The **liver** (right and left lobes) and **pancreas** are **accessory organs** to avian digestion. The pancreas is located within the duodenal loop. There are three pancreatic ducts in domestic fowl that drain into the distal part of the distal duodenum. Gallbladders are present in chickens, turkeys, ducks, and geese and bile is transported to the duodenum by two ducts (one from each liver lobe). The duct from the right lobe is the only one connected to the gallbladder. Bile ducts drain into the distal duodenum near the location of the pancreatic ducts.

Prehension and deglutition

1 How is prehension accomplished by chickens and turkeys?

2 How do the tongue and caudally projected papillae assist swallowing in the oral phase?

3 What actions accomplish the pharyngeal phase of swallowing?

4 How does the fullness of the ventriculus influence the destination of a swallowed bolus during the esophageal phase?

Food is grasped by the beak and brought into the mouth by repeated upward and downward movements of the head. Following **prehension**, swallowing is accomplished in three phases, oral, pharyngeal, and esophageal. In the oral phase, the food bolus moves caudally into the pharynx by rapid rostrocaudal movements of the tongue. Bolus movement is assisted by caudally directed papillae. During the pharyngeal phase, the glottis and choanal and infundibular clefts are closed when the pharyngeal roof or tongue are stimulated. The distance between the oropharynx and esophagus is decreased by a forward movement of the esophagus coupled with the hyoid apparatus becoming concave, and the tongue moving backward. Food particles are propelled from the tongue to the esophagus by further head raisings and tongue movements that are assisted by rostrocaudal movements of the laryngeal mound that contains rows of caudally directed cornified papillae. During the esophageal phase, peristalsis within the esophagus moves the bolus toward the stomach. Swallowed boli enter the ventriculus when it is not filled. When the ventriculus is filled with food, esophageal muscles in the region of the crop relax and food enters the crop. Domestic fowl depend on gravity to assist in getting water into the pharynx for swallowing.

Motility

> 1 Within a gastroduodenal contraction sequence, is the movement of ingesta oral or aboral when the thick ventriculus muscles contract? What does that fill?
>
> 2 What is filled when the thin ventricular muscles contract during the contraction sequence?
>
> 3 What is remixed with a less frequent contraction in turkeys?
>
> 4 What are the functions of the antiperistaltic contractions of the colon? Are they frequent?
>
> 5 What is the difference between the major and minor contractions of the ceca?

Gastroduodenal motility

In chickens and turkeys there is a rhythmic gastroduodenal contraction sequence that occurs at the rate of about three contractions per minute. A sequence includes the following, in order of occurrence:

1 contraction of thin ventricular muscles;
2 two or three peristaltic waves through the duodenum;
3 contraction of thick ventricular muscles;
4 a peristaltic wave through the proventriculus.

During each sequence, ingesta flows aborally into the duodenum by contraction of the thin ventricular muscles and continues aborally by peristaltic waves of the duodenum. Ingesta flows orally into the proventriculus by contraction of the thick ventricular muscles, which allows further mixing with proventricular secretions. This latter flow produces pressure changes in the proventriculus that precede its contraction, whereby ingesta are returned to the ventriculus. The next sequence begins with contraction of the thin ventricular muscles and flow of ingesta into the duodenum.

Contractions of the proventriculus and duodenum are dependent on intrinsic neural connections with the ventriculus. Extrinsic innervation does not appear to be involved in the initiation of contractions or to be significant in the regulation of the sequence.

In addition to the above sequence of contractions that move contents orally and aborally, there is another oral movement of luminal content that occurs about four times per hour in turkeys. It involves a reflux of duodenal and upper jejunal contents into the ventriculus. This activity permits the remixing of intestinal content with gastric secretions.

Ileal, colonic, and cecal motility

Peristalsis and segmenting contractions have been observed radiographically in the ileum. In the turkey, these normally occur at a mean frequency of about four per minute and about six per minute in periods of more intense activity.

The colon links the ileum with the coprodeal compartment of the cloaca. Antiperistalsis occurs almost continuously in the colon. Functions of the antiperistaltic contractions are (i) to move urine from the cloaca into the colon and ceca for water reabsorption and (ii) filling of the ceca. Antiperistaltic contractions arise from the cloaca and occur at a rate of 10–14 per minute in chickens and turkeys. Antiperistalsis ceases immediately before defecation, and the entire colon contracts to evacuate the feces.

There are major and minor contractions that occur in the ceca. The major contractions are associated with peristaltic contractions in the colon, whereby a series of major contractions is associated with cecal evacuation, and a single major contraction is associated with defecation. The minor contractions perform a mixing function.

Cecal droppings have a chocolate brown color, homogeneous texture, and are distinguished from **intestinal droppings**, which that have a greenish, granular-textured appearance. One or two cecal droppings occur per day, while 25–50 intestinal droppings are formed.

Secretions and digestion

> 1 What appears to be the major function of the salivary and esophageal secretions?
>
> 2 What accounts for the digestion that occurs in the crop?
>
> 3 What are the secretions of the proventricular glands? What is the function of pepsin?
>
> 4 What is the function of the gizzard?
>
> 5 What are the secretions of the exocrine pancreas?
>
> 6 What ensures proteolytic inactivation within the pancreas? Why is this important?
>
> 7 What is the function of enterokinase?
>
> 8 What is the role of bile salts in the hydrolysis of fats?
>
> 9 What is accomplished by microflora in the ceca?

Salivary, crop, and esophageal secretions

The salivary glands in chickens and turkeys are mucus-secreting cells that primarily assist lubrication. Chickens secrete 7–30 mL of mucinous saliva per day. The mucosal surface of the esophagus contains glands that secrete mucus for lubrication of its surface.

Mucus is also secreted by the crop in gallinaceous birds but amylase is not. A significant amount of starch digestion occurs in the crop as a result of bacterial action. Nonbacterial digestion of carbohydrates also occurs in the crop and results from amylase activity at this site that comes from intestinal reflux. A more thorough mechanical and chemical digestion occurs in the stomach and intestines.

Gastric secretions

Two types of glands are predominant in the proventriculus: (i) **simple mucosal glands** that secrete mucus and (ii) **compound submucosal glands**, which are functionally homologous to the chief and parietal cells of the mammalian stomach, that secrete mucus, HCl, and pepsinogen. **Pepsinogen** is converted to **pepsin** in the acid environment, and the pepsin produced begins the hydrolysis of protein molecules to polypeptides. The pH of the gastric juice (0.5–2.5) is appropriate for good peptic activity. The pH of gastric content is higher (4.8) due to the presence of ingesta.

The grinding action of the ventriculus (gizzard) not only reduces food particle size but also mixes digestive fluids with the food. Grinding is facilitated by the presence of grit (i.e., sand or small stones) in diets containing large particles (i.e., cracked or whole kernel corn). The presence of grit is not a necessity when commercially prepared feeds are fed because the feed-grinding process adequately reduces the size of ingredients, thereby facilitating gizzard activity.

Intestinal, pancreatic, and biliary secretions

The small intestine is the primary site of chemical digestion, accomplished by pancreatic enzymes and microbial activity, as well as by intestinal secretions. The **exocrine pancreas** secretes lipase, amylase, and precursors of the proteolytic enzymes **trypsinogen, chymotrypsinogen A, B, and C,** and **procarboxypeptidase A and B.** The proteolytic enzymes are not activated until secreted into the intestinal lumen because trypsin inhibitor is secreted by the pancreas to ensure proteolytic inactivation within the pancreas, thereby preventing autodigestion. Trypsinogen is activated within the intestinal lumen to trypsin by **enterokinase**, an intestinal enzyme secretion. Following activation, trypsin activates other proteolytic enzyme precursors. Trypsin and the chymotrypsins hydrolyze specific bonds within large protein molecules and polypeptides to produce **oligopeptides** (peptides with more than two but not more than 10 amino acids). In the intestinal lumen, carboxypeptidases release free amino acids from the oligopeptides. **Aminopeptidases** and **dipeptidases** are synthesized in the cytoplasm of enterocytes and perform brush border hydrolysis of oligopeptides.

The primary carbohydrate in poultry feed is starch, of which there are two forms, **amylose** and **amylopectin.** Both forms are rapidly hydrolyzed by α-amylase secreted by the pancreas to form **maltose**, a disaccharide composed of two glucose units. The principal carbohydrate enzymes are **maltase** and **isomaltase** (substrates maltose and dextrins, respectively), which generate glucose, and **sucrase** (substrate sucrose), which generates glucose and fructose.

Fats are hydrolyzed to fatty acids and glycerol before absorption. This hydrolysis is accomplished by pancreatic lipase and by the action of bile salts that emulsify fats and activate pancreatic lipase.

In addition to digestive enzymes secreted by the exocrine pancreas, an aqueous solution of bicarbonate is also secreted which acts to neutralize the acidic gastric **chyme.** The pH of the avian intestinal tract increases from oral to aboral, from about 5.6 to 7.2. A pH of 6–8 is considered optimal. Secretion of bile into the duodenum also aids in neutralization of chyme. Bile salts are readily absorbed through the intestinal wall, allowing their recirculation and reuse.

Factors affecting secretion

Pancreatic secretion is controlled by nervous and hormonal components. The nervous component has a cephalic phase whereby the sight of food increases secretion. This response is mediated by cholinergic fibers of the vagus nerve. Pancreatic juice refers to both aqueous and enzyme components. Pancreatic aqueous secretion is stimulated by **vasoactive intestinal peptide (VIP)** in response to entry of acidic chyme into the duodenum. Avian VIP is involved in secretory regulation analogous to secretion in mammals. Release of **cholecystokinin (CCK)** initiates the secretion of pancreatic enzymes. VIP does not stimulate pancreatic enzyme secretion. In addition, distension of the proventriculus with **peptones** (products of partial protein digestion) not only stimulates pancreatic enzyme secretion but also secretion of the aqueous component. This effect is mediated by **gastrin-releasing peptides (GRP).**

Diet can influence the secretion rate of pancreatic enzymes. If the content of carbohydrate and fat in the diet are increased, pancreatic amylase and lipase secretions are increased. Also, increasing protein content of the diet increases chymotrypsin activity in the duodenum and jejunum.

Cecal function

Little or no digestion takes place in the large intestine and only about 10% of most diets receive cecal digestion. The most noticeable digestive functions of the ceca are reabsorption of water from refluxed urine and microbial digestion of cellulose. The ceca are filled by the antiperistaltic activity of the colon. A circular muscular ring of the ileum projects into the colon and its contraction (sphincter-like action) effectively prevents reflux of colonic material into the ileum.

Urine is refluxed from the cloaca into the colon and it enters the ceca via colonic antiperistalsis. The nitrogenous component of avian urine is **uric acid**, which is degraded for utilization of the nitrogen by the microflora. Water reabsorption from the refluxed urine is an important function of the ceca.

Regulation of motility and secretion

> 1 How is movement of food into or out of the crop regulated?
> 2 How do the cephalic and gastric phases regulate gastric motility and secretion?
> 3 What is the mediator of the cephalic phase of gastric secretion and motility?
> 4 What is the mediator of the gastric phase of gastric secretion and motility?
> 5 What stimulates secretin release and what does it cause after its release?
> 6 What is the stimulus for the release of cholecystokinin and what does it cause after its release?

The presence of food in the mouth and esophagus increases the respective salivary and mucus secretions and also motility in these areas. Regulation of food movement into or out of the crop is controlled reflexively by the fullness of the digestive tract distal to the crop.

Both a cephalic and a gastric phase regulate gastric motility and secretion. The sight of food (cephalic phase) results in significant increases in the frequency of gastroduodenal contractions, while the ingestion of food (gastric phase) that follows results in further increases in not only frequency but also amplitude of gastric contractions. There is also a direct relation between the protein content of a diet and the proteolytic activity and rate of production of gastric secretions, a further indication of the presence of a gastric phase.

The cephalic phase of gastric secretion and motility is likely mediated by hypoglycemia. The gastric phase is mediated by the vagus nerve, inasmuch as it has been shown to initiate or enhance proventricular secretion and gastric motility. There is also a duodenal phase of gastric regulation whereby distension of the duodenum causes a decrease in gastric secretion and motility. **Gastrin**, a peptide, stimulates acid secretion from the proventriculus.

The cephalic phase is associated with pancreatic secretion, whereby secretion begins immediately following eating. Two hormones that are secreted when stomach contents enter the duodenum are **secretin** and CCK. Secretin release is stimulated by acid perfusion of the duodenum and causes the pancreas to secrete bicarbonate. The hormone CCK is secreted in response to the presence of protein and fat in the duodenum and causes the pancreas to secrete enzymes and proenzymes. Avian VIP is more potent than avian secretin in stimulating bicarbonate secretion. Intestinal motility and secretions are increased by vagal stimulation (parasympathetic).

Absorption

> 1 Where does most of the absorption of carbohydrates and amino acids occur?
> 2 What is the location for absorption of fatty acids?
> 3 What are portomicrons?
> 4 Why are portomicrons absorbed directly into the hepatic portal blood supply rather than lacteals?
> 5 What is the origin of the volatile fatty acids?

Most absorption of carbohydrates, amino acids, and fatty acids occurs in the duodenum and proximal jejunum. Glucose absorption occurs predominantly in the duodenum and jejunum via passive transport (high concentration to low concentration). Active transport of glucose (carrier-mediated, Na^+/K^+-ATPase dependent) occurs primarily in the ileum, where luminal glucose concentrations are lower than in the duodenum and jejunum.

Significant active absorption of glucose also occurs in the proximal cecum. Amino acids and peptides are also absorbed from the duodenum and jejunum via Na^+/K^+-ATPase energy-dependent cotransport processes. Carbohydrates and proteins are rapidly digested and glucose and amino acids can be analyzed in portal blood within 15 min after eating.

Fatty acid absorption occurs in the distal half of the jejunum, and to a lesser extent in the ileum, rather than duodenum and proximal jejunum as noted for carbohydrates and amino acids. This is due to the location of the bile duct entrance near the distal duodenum. Accordingly, emulsification of fats is delayed. Fatty acids enter the enterocytes and are re-esterified to triglycerides, given a protein covering that makes them water-soluble, and packaged into **portomicrons**. Portomicrons facilitate transport of water-insoluble triglycerides. In mammals, re-esterified triglycerides are packaged into **chylomicrons**, which enter the central lacteal (lymphatic capillary) of the villus for delivery to the blood. Birds do not have lacteals in their villi, so portomicrons are absorbed directly into the hepatic portal blood supply.

Volatile fatty acids (VFAs) arise from microbial decomposition of uric acid in the ceca. Acetate is predominant but some propionate and butyrate are present. VFAs are absorbed from the ileum and ceca by passive transport.

Yolk utilization

> 1 What provides the energy requirements for avian embryos during incubation?
> 2 When does the utilization of yolk content begin as a process of absorption into the blood, and how long does that endure?
> 3 What is the process whereby yolk material is utilized after hatching?
> 4 How long after hatching is yolk material utilized as an energy source by the combined processes of endodermal absorption and secretion into the small intestine?

Energy requirements of avian embryos during incubation are fulfilled by lipids stored in the **yolk**. Approximately 50% of yolk material consists of lipid. Yolk contents of chicks and poults are utilized by two different concurrent processes. First, lipids are transferred from the yolk to blood following endocytosis by endodermal cells of the yolk membrane and packaging into lipoproteins for release into the bloodstream. This process begins during early embryonation, accelerates during the last week of incubation, and continues after hatching. Second, yolk material is secreted through the **yolk stalk** into the small intestine as irregular pulses during the first 72 hours after hatching in chicks and for 120 hours after hatching in turkey poults. Peristalsis and antiperistalsis of the small intestine disseminate yolk materials throughout the small intestine and gizzard. **Yolk lipids** reaching the proximal small intestine are hydrolyzed and utilized, whereas hydrolysis and therefore utilization do not occur in the ileum and cecum.

By 72 hours after hatching, lymphocytes accumulate in the subepithelial connective tissue of the yolk stalk. The lumen of the yolk stalk becomes partially occluded and passage of yolk into the intestinal lumen from the yolk sac ceases. The vitelline stalk of chicks is occluded by lymphocyte aggregations by 4 days after hatching. The yolk stalk converts to lymphopoietic tissue after 14 days and may become a site for extramedullary hematopoiesis. The embryonic remnant of the yolk stalk is often referred to as the **Meckel's diverticulum**.

Gastrointestinal ontogeny

> **1** What is the cause for the greatly increased growth rate of the gastrointestinal tract after hatching as compared to overall body weight?

A major transition occurs soon after hatching when the digestive physiology and metabolism in chicks and turkey poults must change from a yolk-based lipid food source to an exogenous carbohydrate-based diet. The developing gut becomes responsible for acquiring nutrients from the yolk sac and ingested food during the immediate posthatch period when the relative growth rate of birds is at a maximum. The avian gastrointestinal tract is physically and functionally immature at hatching. Adaptation to oral ingestion of food is associated with a rapid increase in the weight of the gastrointestinal tract and increase in the activity of digestive enzymes during the first 7–10 days after hatching. Studies in broiler chickens indicate that the small intestine is growing four times faster than the body as a whole at the age of 8 days. During the first 6 days after hatching, weights of the proventriculus, pancreas, and small intestine increase more rapidly than body weight in turkey poults.

The surface area available for absorption greatly expands during the first week following hatching due to (i) rapidly increasing length of the villi caused by an increased number of enterocytes per villus and (ii) elongation of microvilli on the apical surface of enterocytes.

Food and water factors

> **1** Where does the net absorption of water and electrolytes occur?
>
> **2** How does urine in the urodeum proceed to the ceca?
>
> **3** Is the sense of taste in domestic fowl similar to taste in humans?
>
> **4** What is the response of domestic fowl to water temperature differences?

Water balance is maintained when water intake equals water output. The greatest intake is via drinking and the greatest output is via feces and urine. The kidneys regulate the volume and composition of the body's internal environment, the **extracellular fluid (ECF)**. Regulation is provided by many osmotic exchanges between ECF and the intestinal tract. Water is absorbed throughout the small and large intestine as needed by osmosis. The principal electrolytes associated with osmotic equilibrium are Na^+, K^+, and Cl^- ions. Movement of water and electrolytes needed for water equilibrium between the ECF and intestinal tract (net absorption) occurs in the distal 25% of the small intestine, and in the ceca, colon, and coprodeum. Urine formed by the kidneys is excreted into the urodeum portion of the cloaca. Urine is refluxed from the urodeum into the coprodeum and then into the colon and ceca via antiperistalsis. Urine mixed with feces and water may be absorbed from the colon and ceca to maintain osmotic equilibrium of the ECF.

Domestic fowl do have a sense of taste, but it is characterized by a general indifference to categories humans recognize as sweet and bitter. It was mentioned earlier that taste buds are variably located in the oropharynx and that chickens may have as many as 300 taste buds. On an otherwise inadequate diet, birds are indifferent to sucrose solutions. However, if caloric intake in feed is restricted, a chick will select a sucrose solution and increase fluid intake to make up the deficiency. This nutritional choice was not made when an isocaloric solution of fat or protein was offered.

Domestic fowl depleted of protein avoid a solution of casein (protein source) and select only water, apparently because of the taste. In other tests, feed that was rendered so distasteful that it was totally avoided in a choice situation did not influence intake when there was no alternative. However, response to taste quality was modified by hunger, whereby offensiveness had to be increased almost 10-fold in a no-choice situation to effect a reduced intake over an extended period.

Domestic fowl are acutely sensitive to the temperature of water. Acceptability decreases as temperature of water increases above ambient levels. Discrimination occurs between choices where the temperature differences are only a few degrees Celsius, rejecting the higher-temperature water. Also, fowl will suffer from acute thirst rather than drink water 5°C above their body temperature (average body temperature 41°C, 107°F). At the other extreme, water is readily accepted down to the level of freezing. These findings are important for water placement in outdoor environments (avoiding direct sun) and when trying to induce intake of medicated water. Birds do have a wide range of tolerance for acidity and alkalinity in their drinking water.

Self-evaluation

Answers can be found at the end of the chapter.

1 In mammals, peristaltic waves create a unidirectional movement of ingesta from the oral cavity to the anus. In birds, movement of ingesta is bidirectional at several locations along the digestive tract. Give examples of orad movement of digestive tract contents and explain how they are beneficial to the bird.

2 Yolk material serves as a source of nutrition during the immediate posthatch period when hatchlings are adapting to an external food source. How do hatchlings access the yolk material stored within their body cavity?

3 The avian digestive tract is physically and functionally immature at hatching. Describe maturation processes that occur during the first week after hatching.

4 Fatty acids in mammals and birds are re-esterified to triglycerides, given a protein covering that makes them water-soluble, and packaged into portomicrons in birds and chylomicrons in mammals. How does delivery into the blood differ?

5 Which one of the avian digestive tract structures secretes HCl and pepsinogen?
   A Crop
   B Proventriculus
   C Gizzard
   D Ceca

6 Which one of the avian digestive tract structures is very muscular and serves to grind or break down food?
   A Crop
   B Proventriculus
   C Gizzard
   D Ceca

7 Which avian digestive tract structure provides for the microbial digestion of cellulose?
   A Gizzard
   B Ileum
   C Ceca
   D Cloaca

8 It is possible for uric acid to go from the cloaca to the ceca.
   A True
   B False

9 The avian vent:
   A Ventilates the cloaca
   B Serves as an opening for the passage of feces, feces mixed with urine, and eggs

10 The bursa of Fabricius:
   A Is part of the small intestine
   B Is associated with humoral immunity
   C Produces erythrocytes
   D Is a site for water reabsorption from the cloaca

Suggested reading

Denbow, D.M. (2000) Gastrointestinal anatomy and physiology. In: *Sturkie's Avian Physiology*, 5th edn (ed. G.C. Wittow), pp. 299–325. Academic Press, New York.

Dyce, K.M., Sack, W.O. and Wensing, C.J.G. (2010) *Textbook of Veterinary Anatomy*, 4th edn, pp. 794–802. Saunders Elsevier, St Louis, MO.

Moran, E.T. Jr (1985) Digestion and absorption of carbohydrates in fowl and events through perinatal development. *Journal of Nutrition* 115:665–674.

Pinchasov, Y. (1995) Early transition of the digestive system to exogenous nutrition in domestic post-hatch birds. *British Journal of Nutrition* 73:471–478.

Tarvid, I. (1995) The development of protein digestion in poultry. *Poultry and Avian Biology Reviews* 6:35–54.

Answers

1 During each gastroduodenal contraction sequence, ingesta flows orally into the proventriculus during contraction of the thick muscles of the gizzard. Gastroduodenal contractions also generate reflux of duodenal and upper jejunal contents into the ventriculus and occur about four times each hour in turkeys. Both of these movemetns facilitate the mixing of ingesta with digestive enzymes and hydrochloric acid. Antiperistaltic waves in the colon move ingesta and urine from the cloaca into the colon and ceca. This action facilitates water absorption and provides nitrogen for cecal bacteria.

2 First, lipids are transferred from the yolk to the blood following endocytosis by endodermal cells of the yolk membrane and packaging into lipoproteins for release into the bloodstream. Second, yolk material is secreted through the yolk stalk into the small intestine as irregular pulses during the first 3 or 4 days after hatching. Yolk nutrients reaching the proximal small intestine via antiperistaltic movements are hydrolyzed and utilized.

3 Adaptation to oral ingestion of food is associated with a rapid gain in gastrointestinal tract weight and in the activity of digestive enzymes. The surface area available for absorption greatly expands owing to further development of villi and microvilli. The capacity to transport amino acids across enterocyte membranes increases rapidly along with γ-glutamyltransferase, an enzyme required for amino acid absorption. Glucose uptake capacity rises because of increased maltase and sucrase in the apical membranes of enterocytes. The pancreas grows rapidly and pancreatic enzyme production rises accordingly.

Section VII: Digestion, Absorption, and Metabolism

4 In mammals, chylomicrons enter the central lacteal (lymphatic capillary) of the villus for delivery to the blood. Birds do not have lacteals in their villi and the portomicrons are absorbed directly into the hepatic portal blood supply.

5 B

6 C

7 C

8 A

9 B

10 B

47 Disorders of Carbohydrate and Fat Metabolism

Jesse P. Goff

Iowa State University, Ames, IA, USA

The genetic capacity to produce food for human consumption can challenge the metabolic capabilities of many of our farm animals. Bovine ketosis and ovine pregnancy toxemia are hypoglycemic conditions of ruminants in which the ability of the animal to produce glucose is outpaced by the drain of glucose from the blood by the mammary gland or developing fetus. Newborn animals can also develop hypoglycemia, especially when chilled or when they fail to nurse. The newborn pig is particularly susceptible to this syndrome as it has little body fat that it can use as an alternative source of fuel. Diabetes mellitus is increasingly diagnosed in our companion animals, just as it is in their owners. The basic etiology of diabetes mellitus in dogs and cats will be examined. Excessive mobilization of body fat can cause a build-up of triglycerides within the parenchyma of the liver. Fatty liver is a common disorder of dairy cattle, cats, and laying hens. The etiology of the fatty liver syndrome of these species is somewhat different and will be contrasted.

Energy metabolism

> **1** What does the presence of glucose in urine tell you about blood glucose concentration?

The cells of the body require a constant supply of nutrients to utilize for fuel and for synthesis of new proteins. However, nutrients are not generally constantly supplied from the diet. Energy must be obtained from the diet and stored for later use.

This is known as the absorptive phase of energy metabolism. Following a meal there is a rapid influx of sugars, fats, and amino acids into the blood. The animal must quickly remove these substances from the blood for several reasons. The presence of such a large amount of solute in the blood would greatly increase the osmolarity of the blood. Thus sugars absorbed across the intestine as monosaccharides must quickly be condensed into larger molecules, such as glycogen, to reduce their osmotic effect. For many solutes capable of being filtered across the renal glomerus there is only a finite capacity of the renal tubules to reabsorb the solute to prevent it from being lost to the urine. The maximal concentration of a solute in the blood that can be filtered by the glomerulus and fully recovered by reabsorptive processes within the renal tubules is known as the renal threshold. When blood concentration rises above the renal threshold, the solute will appear in the urine. The renal threshold for glucose is about 180 mg/dL plasma. Following a high sugar meal, plasma glucose could rise above the renal threshold were it not for the body's ability to rapidly transfer glucose from the plasma to the intracellular space of cells.

Absorptive phase

> **1** What is the role of insulin in the way the body handles absorbed carbohydrates, amino acids, and fats following ingestion of a meal?
>
> **2** What is the fate of glucose, amino acids, and fats absorbed following ingestion of a meal?

Section VII: Digestion, Absorption, and Metabolism

Dukes' Physiology of Domestic Animals, Thirteenth Edition. Edited by William O. Reece, Howard H. Erickson, Jesse P. Goff and Etsuro E. Uemura.

© 2015 John Wiley & Sons, Inc. Published 2015 by John Wiley & Sons, Inc.

Companion website: www.wiley.com/go/reece/physiology

A typical meal will supply an animal with carbohydrate, protein, and fat (as well as minerals and vitamins, discussed in Chapters 48 and 49). These nutrients cross the gastrointestinal tract and enter the blood as monosaccharides and amino acids, or enter the lymph as triglycerides. Those compounds entering the blood will first pass into the liver, which may modify them before they are passed on to the rest of the body. Triglycerides entering the lymphatics packaged in chylomicrons are able to directly enter the adipose tissue for storage. Following the ingestion of a meal there will be a rapid rise in blood and lymph concentrations of monosaccharides, amino acids, and triglycerides, especially in monogastric species. This is known as the absorptive phase of metabolism, a time when nutrients can be stored for later use. In ruminants, the passage of digesta from the rumen to the lower gut for absorption is relatively constant so that the absorptive phase is less readily apparent.

The primary hormone involved in the coordination of the events of the absorptive phase is insulin. Insulin is produced by the β cells within the islets of Langerhans of the pancreas. Insulin promotes the expression of the glucose transporter (GLUT)-4 proteins that facilitate glucose uptake by muscle, adipose, and pancreatic α cells. When insulin levels are low these tissues cannot remove glucose from the blood. Insulin does not affect, and is not required for, the uptake of glucose by cells of the brain, liver, renal tubules, erythrocytes, leukocytes, and gastrointestinal epithelium. The primary stimulus for release of insulin is a rise in blood glucose concentration, which typically occurs following the ingestion of a meal. Conversely, insulin secretion ceases once blood glucose concentration has decreased to normal limits. The normal concentration of glucose in the blood of monogastric species is 80–120 mg/dL. In ruminants the blood glucose concentration is normally 55–75 mg/dL. Other factors can also initiate insulin secretion. A rise in both amino acid and potassium concentrations in the blood, which commonly occur following a meal, will cause the secretion of insulin. And insulin, in turn, will stimulate the uptake of amino acids and potassium by tissues. Interestingly, fructose, a monosaccharide found in plant sucrose, uses a constitutively expressed GLUT-5 protein to enter cells. It also does not stimulate secretion of insulin when it is given intravenously. However, its low glycemic index is somewhat deceiving. It spares glucose so blood levels of glucose generally rise following oral administration of fructose.

Carbohydrate

While monosaccharides, such as galactose and fructose, are major portions of the carbohydrate absorbed from the diet, we shall simplify the discussion by referring only to glucose as the monosaccharide derived from digestion. The liver rapidly converts nearly all the galactose to glucose, and fructose and glucose enter essentially the same metabolic pathways for energetic purposes. Much of the glucose absorbed across the gastrointestinal tract enters the hepatocytes, but little is oxidized for energy. Some of the glucose is converted to the polysaccharide glycogen.

Insulin controls the activity of glycogen synthase, the enzyme responsible for formation of glycogen in both liver and muscle. Much of the absorbed glucose reaching the liver is converted to fat immediately after a meal (monogastric species). Glucose provides carbons needed for both the fatty acids and the glycerol backbone used for the formation of triglycerides. Some of the fat produced in the liver is stored in the liver, but the majority of triglycerides produced are packaged with very low density lipoproteins (VLDL) for export to adipose tissue. The main effect of insulin stimulation of fat synthesis is to raise intracellular glucose in the adipose tissue. The formation of fatty acids and glycerophosphate is essentially substrate driven and mass action subsequently drives the reaction toward conversion to triglyceride. The direct action of insulin on fat metabolism is to inhibit lipase, the enzyme that catalyzes triglyceride breakdown. This action allows triglyceride to accumulate in the tissues. A function of insulin in the liver is to activate pyruvate dehydrogenase, which causes pyruvate to be oxidized or converted to fat, thus making it unavailable for glucose synthesis. This makes sense as after a meal blood glucose should be relatively high and there is no need for gluconeogenesis.

Some of the absorbed glucose that bypassed the liver will enter the adipose tissue where it is stored as fat, some will be stored as glycogen in muscle and other select peripheral tissues, and some of the glucose absorbed will be oxidized to CO_2 and water within the tissues of the body as a means of supplying the cells with energy. Glucose is the body's main energy source during the absorptive phase for all tissues except the liver. It is also the exclusive (with minor exceptions) source of energy for nervous tissue during the postabsorptive phase as well.

Triglycerides

Triglycerides within the chylomicrons are taken up by adipose tissue where they are stored. A small portion of the absorbed triglyceride is oxidized during the absorptive phase by muscle (smooth, cardiac and skeletal) to provide energy, especially if the animal's diet is low in carbohydrate or the animal has been in a state of negative energy balance. Adipose tissue fat can be derived from ingested triglyceride, triglyceride synthesized in liver and transported to adipose tissue, or triglyceride synthesized from glucose within adipose tissue. The main effect of insulin on these processes is to drive triglyceride synthesis through uptake of glucose by adipose tissue and the direct inhibition of lipolysis by inhibiting the activity of hormone- sensitive lipase.

Amino acids used for energy

Amino acids, dipeptides, and tripeptides absorbed will enter the liver and be deaminated to convert them into carbohydrate (ketoacids). The ammonia liberated during deamination is converted to urea which diffuses into the blood for eventual excretion by the kidneys. The ketoacids thus produced can enter the tricarboxylic acid (TCA) cycle and be oxidized to produce energy for the hepatocytes. Amino acids provide most of the energy required by hepatocytes during the absorptive phase of metabolism. The ketoacids can also be converted to fatty acids, serving as further components of fat synthesis in the liver. Intestinally absorbed amino acids not taken up by the liver enter other cells of the body, especially muscle. After entering muscle cells, most of the amino acids will be used to synthesize new protein (especially important in the growing animal) and to replace protein catabolized during the postabsorptive phase of metabolism. Excess amino acids entering the cells are not stored as protein, but are instead converted to carbohydrate or fat. Insulin enhances the uptake of amino acids by muscle tissue and enhances their incorporation into new proteins. At the same time, it inhibits the degradation of existing protein.

Postabsorptive phase

---

1 What is the role of liver and muscle glycogen during fasting?

2 How do amino acids contribute to glucose homeostasis?

3 How does lipid stored in adipose tissue contribute to glucose homeostasis?

4 Which hormones regulate the processing outlined in questions 1–3?

During this period of fasting, no glucose is being absorbed across the gastrointestinal tract. However, normal blood glucose must be maintained because nervous tissue is unable to oxidize other nutrients for energy. (During periods of extreme energy stress, such as starvation, the nervous tissue can utilize ketone bodies derived from fatty acids by day 4 or 5 of the fasting period.) Two major actions occur during the postabsorptive phase: mobilization of sources of glucose, and utilization of other fuels to spare glucose for nervous tissue. The major hormones coordinating these efforts are glucagon, epinephrine, glucocorticoids, and growth hormone.

Glucagon is produced within the α cells of the pancreatic islets and secretion is stimulated when blood glucose concentration falls below normal levels. The mechanism for sensing the concentration of blood glucose resides in the interior of the α cell. Unfortunately, glucose entry into the α cell is dependent on insulin. Thus, in diabetic animals the secretion of glucagon continues despite the fact that blood glucose concentration is greatly elevated. High levels of fatty acids in blood inhibit secretion of glucagon, while high concentrations of amino acids in blood can stimulate glucagon secretion.

Epinephrine release from the adrenal medulla is primarily under the control of the hypothalamus and the sympathetic nervous system. Low blood glucose is sensed by hypothalamic glucose receptors which in turn impact sympathetic nervous system control of epinephrine secretion. Some sympathetic nerves contact adipose tissue and release epinephrine directly onto the tissue.

The secretion of growth hormone from the anterior pituitary is complex. Low blood glucose concentration is sensed by

hypothalamic glucose receptors that stimulate the release of growth hormone-releasing factor and subsequently growth hormone. In addition, a rise in blood amino acid concentration also stimulates growth hormone secretion.

Glucocorticoids are released by the adrenal cortex in response to adrenocorticotropic hormone (ACTH) released by the anterior pituitary. ACTH release is primarily under the control of the nervous system. Basal ACTH release occurs on a diurnal rhythm. Stress (cold, pain, etc.) can greatly increase ACTH and thus glucocorticoid secretion. Thus, glucocorticoid secretion is not directly tied to the level of any one nutrient. However, glucocorticoid effects on metabolism are widespread.

Mobilizing glucose from body stores during fasting

Glycogen stored in liver is rapidly broken down to release glucose into the blood. The amount of glucose that can be liberated is relatively small and in humans the amount of glycogen contained in the liver would supply the energy needs of the body at rest for only about 4 hours. The glycogen content of muscle and all other tissues is nearly equivalent to that contained in the liver. However, there is an important difference: muscle does not have the enzymes necessary to form free glucose from glycogen. Instead the glycogen is broken down to glucose 6-phosphate, which is then catabolized via glycolysis to pyruvate and lactate. The pyruvate and lactate can be released to the blood and are recovered by the liver where they can be converted to glucose and returned to the circulation.

The catabolism of triglycerides within adipose tissue yields both fatty acids and glycerol. The fatty acids cannot be converted to glucose. However, glycerol released into the blood circulates to the liver where it can be converted to glucose. A major source of blood glucose during the fasting period is muscle protein. Large portions of the protein in muscle serve no essential function in locomotion but are instead placed in muscle as a repository of amino acids to be utilized as energy sources during the postabsorptive phase. Release of these amino acids is stimulated by glucocorticoids. The amino acids released from the muscle are converted in the liver to glucose. Insulin is not required by the liver to take up these amino acids from the blood. While the liver is the main organ involved in these gluconeogenic processes, the renal cortex also has gluconeogenic capabilities. Glucagon and the glucocorticoids are the primary stimulants of the gluconeogenic pathways in the liver. In humans, it is estimated that the liver and kidneys produce about 180 g of glucose daily. In the dairy cow, the amount of glucose that must be made to support production of the lactose contained in 40 kg of milk would be 1.9 kg.

Glucose sparing activities

In humans, the daily production of 180 g of glucose by the liver would only provide 180 g × 4 kcal/g = 720 kcal metabolizable energy per day. If we assume the average man requires 2200 kcal energy every day to maintain body tissue function, we can see that the liver cannot supply enough glucose to meet the energy needs of the body during fasting. The brain and nervous tissue continue to oxidize glucose at similar rates during the absorptive and postabsorptive phases.

During the postabsorptive phase many tissues such as muscle turn to oxidizing fat for energy, thereby sparing glucose for use by nervous tissue. During the postabsorptive phase the adipose tissue catabolizes stored triglycerides. The glycerol released from the triglyceride enters the blood and is converted to glucose in the liver. The nonesterified fatty acids released from adipose tissue are absorbed by virtually all tissues of the body, except nervous tissue, and they enter the TCA cycle where they are oxidized to CO_2 and water to yield energy. The liver also uses fatty acids as energy source during the postabsorptive phase, switching from the amino acids it uses as its primary energy source during the absorptive phase. This action spares amino acids for use in gluconeogenesis. While most of the fatty acids entering the liver enter the TCA cycle for complete oxidation, some of the fatty acids are instead converted to ketone bodies such as acetone, acetoacetic acid, and β-hydroxybutyrate. The ketones are released into the blood and serve as an important fuel source for most tissues of the body. Nervous tissue can, when deprived of glucose for several days, begin to oxidize ketones for energy also, but it always prefers glucose.

Within adipose tissue, lipolysis is stimulated by growth hormone, glucocorticoids, epinephrine, and glucagon secreted during the postabsorptive phase. Also, insulin levels will be low during the postabsorptive phase so the inhibitory effect of insulin on adipose tissue lipolysis is removed. The uptake of glucose by adipose tissue is inhibited by glucagon, glucocorticoids, and growth hormone. This action inhibits fatty acid synthetic pathways as well. Glucagon acts directly on adipose cells to inhibit glucose uptake. Glucocorticoids and growth hormone reduce adipose uptake of glucose by making adipose tissue resistant to the effects of insulin, possibly by reducing the number of insulin receptors on adipose tissue.

Within muscle tissue, growth hormone reduces the sensitivity to insulin, thus reducing glucose uptake by muscle. Within muscle, glucocorticoids reduce muscle uptake of amino acids, reduce protein synthesis, and stimulate degradation of existing proteins. Growth hormone is actually anabolic to muscle: it stimulates amino acid uptake and protein formation, while inhibiting protein degradation. It also stimulates glycogen synthesis and inhibits glycogen breakdown in muscle. However, these effects only occur in the presence of insulin. Thus, when an animal is in positive energy balance the effect of growth hormone is anabolic. If the animal is in the postabsorptive phase, or negative energy balance, growth hormone tends to be ineffective on muscle. Epinephrine is the primary stimulant of glycogenolysis in the muscle. Glucagon has little or no direct effect on muscle metabolism.

Glycogenolysis within the liver is stimulated by epinephrine and glucagon. At the same time these hormones inhibit formation of new glycogen. Formation of new glucose within

the liver and renal cortex is primarily stimulated by glucagon and the glucocorticoids, but epinephrine and growth hormone can also stimulate gluconeogenesis. Both growth hormone and the glucocorticoids inhibit the formation of triglyceride in the liver.

In humans, it is estimated that about 160 g fat can be removed from adipose tissue each day during fasting. This can provide 160 g × 9 kcal/g = 1440 kcal metabolizable energy per day. The combined effects of gluconeogenesis and glucose sparing are so efficient that even after 1 month of complete fasting (water and electrolytes only), the blood glucose concentration will only be 25% lower than normal.

Ruminant energy metabolism

1 How do ruminants make blood glucose? What are the major substrates derived from the diet?

2 Which action requires the most blood glucose in a cow: maintenance, fetal development, or lactation?

In monogastric species, dietary starch and sugars can contribute directly to maintenance of normal blood glucose concentrations. However, the rumen bacteria that enable the cow to utilize the structural carbohydrates of plant material, such as cellulose, also degrade most of the diet starch and sugars to volatile fatty acids before they can enter the blood of the ruminant. The ability to utilize cellulose as an energy source requires ruminants to synthesize most of the glucose their body requires from gluconeogenic precursors. There are normally only a limited number of substances that can be used to produce glucose. Of the three volatile fatty acids (acetate, propionate, and butyrate) that comprise the bulk of the products resulting from fermentation of carbohydrates within the rumen, only propionate can be used to synthesize glucose. Lactic acid from fermented feedstuffs (silages) can also serve as a gluconeogenic precursor. Other compounds which can be used for gluconeogenesis include amino acids (especially aspartate, alanine, and glutamine) and glycerol, arising from hydrolysis of fats. In high-producing dairy cows fed a high-grain diet, as much as 70% of their total glucose production is from propionate. Of course, during starvation propionate does not contribute at all to maintenance of blood glucose. In monogastric species, blood glucose concentration is normally maintained between 90 and 120 mg/dL. Ruminant blood glucose concentration is normally maintained at just 55–75 mg/dL, and they can tolerate levels as low as 40 mg/dL for days at a time, a level that would place most monogastric animals into a coma.

Blood glucose is also essential if the animal is to make body fat, as it is the precursor for the glycerol backbone needed to produce triglycerides. Elevated blood glucose concentration is also required if muscle glycogen is to be produced. Fetal growth utilizes substantial amounts of glucose, especially in late gestation, when the glycogen content of fetal liver and muscle rises rapidly. Gluconeogensis is also important in the fetus. It has been estimated that the fetal calf obtains more than half of its glucose via gluconeogenesis using maternal amino acids as the gluconeogenic precursor.

Lactation imposes a great stress on glucose metabolism. Milk sugar (lactose) is a disaccharide, composed of one glucose and one galactose molecule. In most monogastric species, glucose is also called upon as a substrate for production of milk fat. Most ruminants utilize acetate from fermentation of structural carbohydrates of forages as the source of acetyl-CoA required for milk fat synthesis.

Ketosis

> **1** Is production of ketones from fatty acids bad for the cow? Explain.
>
> **2** What is the basic problem causing classical ketosis, as seen in grazing dairy cattle?
>
> **3** What is the basic problem causing ketosis in the periparturient cow fed a high-grain diet?
>
> **4** Is there a difference in how you would treat the cow with classical versus periparturient ketosis?

The typical dairy cow has been selected to produce large volumes of milk very quickly after parturition. Unfortunately, the amount of feed and the quality of the feed offered that the cow is able to eat in the first weeks after calving is limited. Virtually all high-producing dairy cows are in negative energy balance in the first month of lactation. That is to say that a calculation of the amount of energy (calories) contained in the milk and the number of calories required for the maintenance of the cow is greater than the amount of calories contained in the ration she is capable of consuming. As a result, she must utilize body tissue to support milk production. Body fat is mobilized, raising nonesterified fatty acid concentration in the blood. The fatty acids have several fates. Initially, they can be utilized as a fuel source by peripheral tissues, primarily muscle and liver. This will spare glucose for some of the more vital functions that only glucose can perform, such as a fuel for nervous tissue and production of milk lactose. Fatty acids are broken down to acetyl-CoA for entry into the TCA cycle and can be oxidized to CO_2 and water with generation of ATP and NADPH (Figure 47.1A). Unfortunately, the liver has a limited capacity to oxidize fatty acids and once this capacity is exceeded the fatty acids are instead converted to ketone bodies (acetoacetic acid, β-hydroxybutyrate, and acetone). These ketones are released into the peripheral circulation. Many tissues of the body can utilize these ketones as a source of energy (Figure 47.1B). In most species that develop severe hypoglycemia, the brain of the animal can begin to utilize alternative fuels for energy, such as ketones and free fatty acids. The ruminant brain is a little slower to adapt, but will begin to oxidize ketones as an energy source after several days of hypoglycemia.

Unfortunately, there is also a limit to the ability of the peripheral tissues to utilize ketones and when that is exceeded the ketone bodies build up to high levels in the blood of the animal. They also spill over into the urine and into the milk, a fact that veterinarians make use of by testing urine and milk for the presence of ketones as an aid in diagnosis of ketosis. This test is traditionally performed by mixing a small amount of urine or milk with nitroprusside to observe for the purple color characteristic of the presence of acetoacetic acid or acetone. Recently, blood tests for β-hydroxybutyrate have been developed that are more accurate and can detect subclinical ketosis. The presence of high levels of ketones in the blood reduces the pH of the blood, impairs the appetite of the cow, and may impair immune cell function.

The liver has only a limited capacity to produce ketones from the fatty acids that escape oxidation within the TCA cycle. Once that is exceeded, the fatty acids are re-esterified into triglycerides and the triglycerides accumulate within the hepatocytes, leading to a condition known as **fatty liver** (Figure 47.1C). Remember also that the glycerol backbone of the new triglyceride molecule is derived from a glucose molecule. So formation of triglycerides in the liver will reduce the ability to make glucose molecules, a commodity already in short supply.

In many species, triglycerides within the hepatocytes are packaged along with lipoproteins to form VLDL. The triglycerides can then be cleared from the liver by exporting them to other tissues such as muscle and adipose. Unfortunately in the ruminant (and cats, discussed in the next section) the ability to produce VLDL is very limited and it is difficult for ruminant hepatocytes to clear triglyceride (Figure 47.1D). One hypothesis is that the cow may also be deficient in protein in early lactation and may not have the essential amino acids, such as methionine, needed to produce sufficient lipoprotein for packaging into the VLDL. As the triglycerides accumulate in the hepatocytes, there is a reduction in liver cell function. Research demonstrates a reduction in the ability to detoxify ammonia and it is suspected that the ability to perform gluconeogenic steps is impaired when fat builds up in the liver.

Classical ketosis

The form of ketosis commonly observed in cows kept on pasture or fed high-forage diets develops 2–3 weeks into lactation. In this form of ketosis, the cow suffers a sudden decline in blood glucose and rise in blood ketones, followed by a dramatic reduction in milk production. The cow may exhibit neurological impairment: stumbling, circling, or head-pressing. The main problem causing the classical form of bovine ketosis is a diet devoid of sufficient gluconeogenic precursors. High-forage diets are fermented primarily to acetate, with small amounts of propionate also being produced. Acetate cannot be converted to glucose, though it does support production of milk fat. Fermentation of starches results in greater amounts of propionate being produced. The treatment for the classical form of ketosis is to supply the animal immediately with glucose, usually

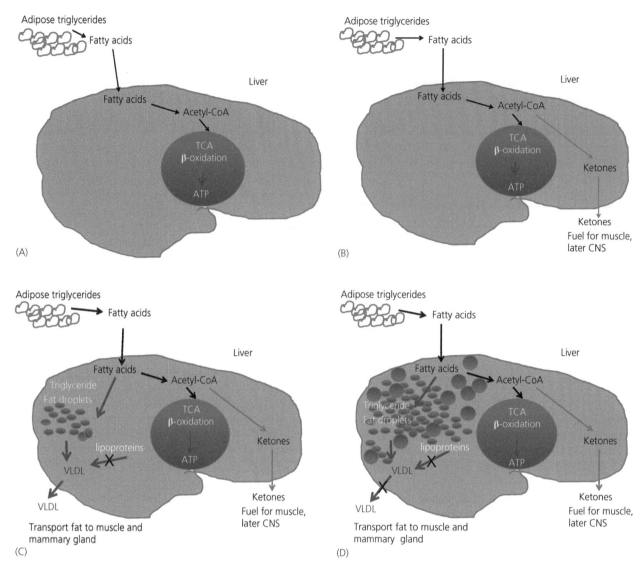

Figure 47.1 (A) During the postabsorptive phase of metabolism, the adipose tissue releases nonesterified fatty acids into the blood where they circulate bound to albumin. The liver hepatocytes take up these fatty acids where they are broken down into two-carbon units and combined with coenzyme A to form acetyl-CoA, which is oxidized via the TCA cycle and mitochondrial electron transport chain to CO_2, generating ATP. (B) The ability of fatty acids to undergo complete β-oxidation is limited and some of the acetyl-CoA is instead converted to β-hydroxybutyrate and acetoacetate for export to other tissues that can use these as an energy source. (C) As the limit for production of ketones is approached, the hepatocytes begin converting the free fatty acids into triglycerides. The triglycerides are then encased in lipoproteins to form particles known as very low density lipoproteins (VLDL) for transport out of the hepatocyte for export to other cells. (D) In some species, such as the cow and cat, the ability to produce VLDL is limited and triglycerides accumulate within the cells to pathological levels disrupting hepatocyte function, a condition known as fatty liver.

by intravenous injection of 250 g glucose, which will usually restore neurologic function and appetite. The cow's diet must then be supplemented with grains to provide propionate for gluconeogenesis.

Periparturient ketosis

In modern confinement of cows, there is a more injurious form of ketosis that appears. Ketosis often develops in these animals during the first week after calving and seems to be associated with a rapid build-up of fat in the liver. These cows are often

offered diets that are relatively high in starches, which should supply reasonable amounts of propionate to the cow. The syndrome seems to arise as a result of inappetence in the cow during the immediate postpartum period. The inappetence may be the result of the cow having dystocia, retained placenta, milk fever, or any other disorder. The dramatic reduction in feed intake at calving initiates a rapid increase in mobilization of body fat, especially in cows carrying excess body condition. It appears that the rapid mobilization of body fat leads to a rapid build-up of triglyceride in the liver. Liver fat becomes a precipitating factor for ketosis. These cows prove much more difficult to treat successfully. They often do not respond to a single injection of glucose intravenously. They are usually offered a diet that would provide a good amount of propionate for gluconeogenesis, but they remain inappetent and so cannot take advantage of the diet. They also do not seem fully capable of utilizing the propionate to produce glucose. Ancillary treatments utilized by veterinarians include injection of synthetic glucocorticoids, presumably to stimulate gluconeogenesis by the liver. Glucocorticoids also reduce milk production by the mammary gland, reducing the cause of the negative energy balance in the cow. Both of these actions can be beneficial. However, it must be kept in mind that glucocorticoids are immunosuppressive, which can increase the susceptibility of the cow to infection. Supplying gluconeogenic precursors in the form of drenches can often be helpful as well. Propylene glycol, glycerol, and sodium or calcium salts of propionate can be used for this purpose. Propylene glycol is converted in the liver to phosphoenolpyruvate and then to glucose. Glycerol is converted to diacylglycerol and then to glucose. Propionate is converted to succinate and enters the TCA cycle where it is eventually converted to glucose as well.

Limits on ability of the liver to oxidize fatty acids

Oxidation of fatty acids requires that they enter the TCA cycle. In order for acetyl-CoA to enter the TCA cycle, the acetyl-CoA must be combined with a molecule of oxaloacetate (OAA) to form citrate. One theory suggests that the demand for OAA during gluconeogenesis is so great that the liver cells are depleted of OAA. Without OAA the oxidation of acetyl-CoA cannot proceed and the acetyl-CoA is instead converted to ketone bodies. Fatty acids build up within the hepatocytes and formation of triglycerides is stimulated, resulting in fatty liver. Recent studies have been unable to demonstrate a reduced level of OAA in the hepatocytes of cows with ketosis, suggesting that the cause of the defective catabolism of fatty acids lies elsewhere.

The hepatic oxidation theory, which is gaining evidence and traction, suggests that excessive release of propionate by highly fermentable starch sources, such as high-moisture corn, may limit the duration of meals by the cow. Cows eat a limited number of meals each day. The rapid uptake of propionate by the liver sends a satiety signal to the brain. This makes each meal of shorter duration and the overall intake of dry matter by the cow is therefore reduced at a time when intake should be maximized. Propionate needed for gluconeogenesis should instead be derived from slowly fermenting sources so that each meal can be of longer duration.

HEPATIC LIPIDOSIS IN CATS

This disorder primarily affects cats that are slightly to morbidly obese. It has become the primary cause of liver disease in cats in the USA. Cats can become ill from a variety of diseases and often they become inappetant. When these cats are suddenly deprived of food calories and dietary proteins, they begin to mobilize large amounts of triglyceride from adipose stores. The nonesterified fatty acids entering the blood are taken up by the liver and are initially used as fuel. However, as with the cow the ability to oxidize the fats is rapidly overwhelmed and triglycerides build up within the hepatocytes. And again as with the cow, it appears cats have a limited ability to produce VLDL and have trouble removing triglyceride from the liver. In cats the hepatocytes rapidly lose function, causing jaundice within a couple of days. The key to treatment is to provide nutrients, intravenously if necessary. More commonly an esophageal feeding tube is placed in the cat and force feeding of highly digestible liquid diets is practiced.

Pregnancy toxemia

> **1** Why are ewes carrying twins more susceptible to pregnancy toxemia than ewes carrying a single lamb?

This is a hypoglycemic condition commonly observed in ewes and beef cows. In both cases, the disorder usually occurs in late gestation and is associated with the presence of multiple fetuses. In most cases, the plane of nutrition the animals are on in late gestation is not adequate to support the development of more than one fetus. In sheep, the amount of glucose that must be synthesized each day to maintain the body of the ewe is about 100 g. In late gestation, the amount of glucose required of the ewe to support each fetus increases by 60–80 g/day. This is complicated by reduced rumen volume, reducing feed intake in late gestation as the fetuses demand more space within the abdomen. Fat ewes and cows suddenly experiencing a period of poor nutrition seem to be at increased risk because they will mobilize large amounts of triglycerides of adipose origin that overwhelm the liver's capacity to metabolize or export the fatty acids. The disease is also often complicated by concurrent hypocalcemia, hypomagnesemia, and hypophosphatemia.

Fatty liver syndrome in poultry

> **1** Is fatty liver in birds a sequela of excess dietary energy or lack of dietary energy?

This disease is most common in laying hens. The liver and abdomen become infiltrated with fat and become friable, and a common cause of death is rupture and hemorrhage of the liver of affected birds. The disease is associated with excessive calorie intake. The typical laying hen has a very high calorie requirement while she is laying eggs. However, at the time of molting she quits laying eggs (or if she quits laying eggs before the rest of the hens in the house are induced to molt) and no longer requires the high-energy diet. The liver and adipose tissue accumulate the extra energy and deposit it as triglyceride. Caged layers seem to be at higher risk, perhaps because they do not exercise as much as floor-housed birds and thus have an even lower calorie requirement. In some cases, mycotoxins (aflatoxins) interfere with lipid metabolism and cause excessive body fat accumulation. A common practice in some countries is to force-feed high-calorie diets to poultry to induce fatty liver. Pâté de fois gras was traditionally obtained by "noodling" ducks and geese with more carbohydrate than the goose would voluntarily consume.

Diabetes mellitus

> 1 Define insulin deficiency in relation to type I and type II diabetes mellitus.
>
> 2 What is meant by exhaustion of the β cells of the pancreatic islets?

Diabetes mellitus has been reported to occur in a wide variety of species; however, it is a common ailment of humans, dogs, and cats. Animals with diabetes all exhibit the following characteristics: high blood glucose concentration and consequently large amounts of glucose in the urine. The blood glucose is increased because of reduced entry of glucose into muscle and adipose tissue and because of increased production of glucose by the liver from excessive glucagon stimulation. During diabetes, the muscles of the body are essentially starving for energy despite the fact that they are surrounded by glucose.

Insulin is required to drive glucose across the cell membrane of muscle, adipose tissue, and α cells of the pancreas. Nervous tissue, erythrocytes, hepatocytes, intestinal epithelium, mammary gland, and cells of the renal cortex are insulin-independent and do not require insulin for uptake of glucose from the blood. If insulin is not produced in adequate amounts or if it is unable to act on its target tissues, glucose does not enter the insulin-dependent tissues and they must utilize fatty acids, ketones, and amino acids as alternative sources of energy. Glucose builds up in the blood of the animal since it is not being utilized by the tissues of the body. The concentration of glucose in the blood of the diabetic animal will usually exceed the renal threshold for tubular glucose reabsorption and therefore it is common to find large amounts of glucose in the urine of the diabetic animal. The osmotic pressure exerted by the presence of so much glucose in the urine also increases water loss via the urine. This reduces blood volume and causes thirst in the diabetic patient, often one of the first clinical symptoms observed by the owner of a diabetic animal.

Exacerbating the situation is the fact that the α cells of the pancreatic islets require insulin, and when insulin is not available the α cells do not recognize that blood glucose levels are above normal. The α cells interpret the inability to take up glucose from the plasma to mean that blood glucose concentrations must be low and therefore glucagon secretion is increased. Glucagon stimulates gluconeogenesis, which acts to raise blood glucose concentrations even further.

Forms of diabetes mellitus
Type I or juvenile diabetes
In this form of diabetes, the β cells of the pancreatic islets fail to produce adequate insulin. In humans, it is well known that there is a genetic component to development of type I diabetes mellitus as the disorder tends to follow familial lines. However, it is also recognized that the disease appears to be a disorder with an autoimmune component. The β cells within the pancreatic islets of many type I juvenile diabetes victims become mistaken by the immune system as a foreign tissue and are destroyed. Why this occurs is unknown, though it is speculated that exposure to certain viruses may cause the body to mistake islet cell components as viral antigens. With destruction of the β cells, the ability to produce insulin is lost.

Type II or adult-onset diabetes
In this form of diabetes, the β cells do produce insulin (at least initially). However, the tissues fail to respond to insulin as they usually do. In humans, the failure to respond to insulin is associated with a decline in the number of receptors for insulin on the surface of target cells. In most cases, this is associated with obesity. The tissues of the body can still respond to insulin but the concentration in the blood must be raised considerably over normal levels to allow adequate uptake of glucose by the tissues. Initially, the β cells of the pancreas respond by producing the higher levels of insulin needed to maintain normal blood glucose concentrations. However, prolonged production of high amounts of insulin eventually leads to exhaustion and atrophy of the β cells. It is at this point that the patient develops hyperglycemia. Initial treatment may consist of drugs such as tolbutamide, which stimulate the remaining β cells to increase their production of insulin. However, in most cases, therapy will involve the exogenous administration of insulin. This is generally the situation in veterinary medicine as the condition is rarely diagnosed before the β cells of the pancreas are reduced to numbers that will not sustain adequate insulin production. In people diagnosed very early in the course of this disease, simply losing weight will improve the insulin responsiveness of the tissues.

In human medicine, the success of therapy with insulin is often determined by monitoring blood glucose concentration. Also, it is the general practice in human medicine to administer insulin after each meal to help drive absorbed glucose into the cells. In veterinary medicine, it is common to give the diabetic patient just one meal per day and to administer insulin just once each day at the time of the meal. Most protocols involve feeding and administering insulin in the morning. Monitoring blood glucose is generally impractical and is only used in the veterinary hospital to establish a dose of insulin to be administered to the animal. After being released from the hospital, the status of the animal is generally assessed by the owner who monitors urine glucose appearance each morning. It is assumed that if there is no glucose in the urine that blood glucose remained below the renal threshold (180 mg/dL) during the night hours. When glucose appears in the urine, it is assumed that the animal is getting an inappropriate insulin dose.

The initial assumption would be that the animal was not being given enough insulin. This is not always a safe assumption. It is also possible that the animal has been given too much insulin. When too much insulin has been given the animal develops hypoglycemia 6–12 hours after the insulin injection. The body reacts by increasing secretion of cortisol and glucagon to increase blood glucose. Since this effect begins about the time the effects of the insulin injection are wearing off, the animal can develop hyperglycemia during the night that results in the appearance of glucose in the morning urine. This phenomena is known as the **Somogyi overswing**. Misinterpreting the appearance of glucose in the urine as an automatic indication of insulin underdosing could lead the veterinarian or owner to increase the dose of insulin administered to the animal, possibly resulting in fatal hypoglycemia as a result of insulin shock.

Neonatal hypoglycemia

> 1 Why is it critical for newborn mammals to nurse shortly after birth?

Neonates of most species have very few glycogen reserves in their muscle and liver tissues. As a result, they can only sustain normal blood glucose concentrations for a short period of time before they must have a meal to raise blood glucose and tissue glycogen concentrations. Clinically, the development of severe hypoglycemia is most important in piglets, but puppies and kittens can also be affected. The condition is especially evident whenever neonates are chilled, which unfortunately can occur commonly on concrete floors of older farrowing facilities. When exposed to colder temperatures the piglet must use more energy to produce body heat. Unlike some other species, the piglet does not have large amounts of body white or brown fat that it can utilize for energy. Neonates of many species have substantial amounts of a special fat known as brown fat, which is specifically metabolized within the mitochondria to produce heat. When chilled, the piglet must resort to glucose for nearly all its heat production. This rapidly reduces blood glucose levels. In addition, the chilled piglet is lethargic and may fail to have the energy required to nurse the sow properly. As a result, the piglet is unable to replenish blood glucose, and eventually hypoglycemia progresses to the point of inducing coma in affected piglets. Chilled puppies can suffer a similar fate.

Agalactia, or failure to produce adequate milk, in any mammalian mother can also initiate the condition. Most animals will respond to the oral administration of glucose solutions, especially when provided with a warmer environment.

Self-evaluation

Answers can be found at the end of the chapter.

1 For each of the following tissues describe its major role in the absorptive and in the postabsorptive phase of metabolism: (A) liver; (B) muscle, and (C) adipose tissue.

2 Which hormones stimulate lipolysis?

3 Which hormones control muscle protein turnover?

4 How does muscle protein contribute to glucose production?

5 How does muscle glycogen contribute to blood glucose concentration?

6 Why might glucagon administration be a good idea for treating the cow with ketosis? Why might it be a bad idea?

7 Current treatment of cows with ketosis generally includes intravenous administration of a large amount of glucose solution in a short time. (A) Why might it be a good idea to give the dairy cow with ketosis an injection of insulin at the same time? (B) Why might this be a bad idea? (C) Is propylene glycol a good idea? (D) Is injecting dexamethasone (a synthetic glucocorticoid) a good idea?

8 Pregnancy toxemia in ewes is sometimes treated by inducing parturition in the ewe. Why might this be a good idea?

9 (A) What is the "Somogyi overswing"? (B) Why is it important for you to know this?

10 Why do Holstein cows maintained on pasture in early lactation often develop ketosis?

11 The typical dairy cow loses 45–68 kg body weight in early lactation as she utilizes body reserves to help supply the energy needed for milk production. (A) How will she make the needed glucose? (B) What role is body fat playing in this process?

12 In human medicine, many people with adult-onset diabetes are successfully treated with the oral hypoglycemic drug tolbutamide. Why does this not seem to be a common option in veterinary medicine?

13 It is Christmas Day, with snow on the ground, and you are on call again! The mother of a newborn litter of retriever pups is brought to you because she will not eat and is running a fever. You diagnose mastitis. You are worried about the pups housed out in the garage. Why?

Suggested reading

Herdt, T.H. (2000) Ruminant adaptation to negative energy balance. Influences on the etiology of ketosis and fatty liver. *Veterinary Clinics of North America. Food Animal Practice* **16**:215–230.

Rook, J.S. (1999) Pregnancy toxemia of ewes. In: *Current Veterinary Therapy. Food Animal Practice* (eds J.L. Howard and R.A. Smith), pp. 228–230. W.B. Saunders, Philadelphia.

Vander, A.J., Sherman, J.H. and Luciano, D.S. (1975) *Human Physiology: The Mechanisms of Body Function*, 2nd edn, pp. 393–401. McGraw-Hill Book Company, New York.

Answers

1A *Absorptive phase*: Produces glycogen, and produces triglycerides (combining glycerol from the absorbed glucose with fatty acids from the diet or produced de novo) and packages them into lipoproteins, made from absorbed amino acids, for use by peripheral tissues. Excess amino acids can be converted to fatty acids.

Postabsorptive phase: Breaks down glycogen to release glucose to blood, gluconeogenesis from amino acids, glycerol, or other three-carbon compounds like propionate, pyruvate, or lactate from muscle. Oxidation of fatty acids to fuel liver functions. Conversion of some fatty acids to ketones for export to peripheral tissues.

1B *Absorptive phase*: Stores glucose as muscle glycogen, builds muscle proteins from amino acids, stores some extra glucose (or glucose from excess amino acids) as fat.

Postabsorptive phase: Breaks down glycogen to release lactate to blood. Catabolism of muscle protein to provide liver with gluconeogenic precursors.

1C *Absorptive phase*: Takes up glucose to form fatty acids and triglycerides for storage as fat, uses fatty acids and triglycerides incorporated into chylomicrons (diet) or lipoproteins (packaged in liver) for storage as fat.

Postabsorptive phase: Releases fatty acids (alternative to glucose as energy source for some tissues) and glycerol (gluconeogenic) into circulation.

2 Epinephrine, growth hormone, glucagon, glucocorticoids.

3 Glucocorticoids increase catabolism; growth hormone and insulin promote anabolism. (Note that growth hormone is only anabolic when insulin is present. Otherwise no effect.)

4 During the postabsorptive phase, muscle proteins are degraded under the influence of glucocorticoids and release amino acids to the blood, which are taken up by the liver and used for gluconeogenesis.

5 Under influence of epinephrine, muscle glycogen is broken down to glucose 6-phosphate. Muscle lacks the enzymes necessary to metabolize glycogen all the way to glucose so the glucose 6-phosphate is used to produce pyruvate and lactate, which are released to the blood. The liver then converts these to glucose.

6 At low doses it appears able to stimulate gluconeogenesis pathways in the liver. This could help improve the glucose status of the cow. However, at higher doses or for prolonged periods the glucagon will stimulate lipolysis, which may tax the liver's ability to oxidize fatty acids, contributing to ketone production.

7 (A) The cow's tissues take up more of the injected glucose so it is not lost to the urine. (B) You could overdose the cow with insulin and drive blood glucose too low. Also she is able to make her own insulin, so is it really necessary? (C) Probably a good idea to supply the cow with glucose precursors orally as she usually is not eating on her own when she has ketosis. (D) It could stimulate gluconeogenesis, which would be helpful. It will also reduce milk production, which helps improve energy balance. Its major downside is possible suppression of the immune system.

8 It removes the fetal drain of glucose, which can improve the energy balance of the ewe allowing her to regain control of her blood glucose.

9 (A) A phenomenon that can occur when an animal is given a large dose of insulin. Instead of driving blood glucose just to normal limits, the large dose can actually drive blood glucose below normal levels in several hours. This then stimulates the body to produce epinephrine, glucagon, and growth hormone to increase blood glucose. The gluconeogenic mechanisms are activated about the time that the initial insulin dose has worn off. As a result blood glucose rises above the renal threshold for glucose and there will be glucose in the urine. (B) Most animal clinicians utilize the appearance of glucose in urine as an index of the success of their treatment of the diabetic patient. Ordinarily, the appearance of glucose in the urine might suggest the animal has not been given enough insulin. However, it is also possible that the animal has been overdosed with insulin. Thus the presence of urine glucose must be interpreted cautiously.

10 Fermentation of grass diets often fails to provide enough three-carbon propionate units to allow high-producing cows (most Holsteins today) to make the glucose needed to produce milk lactose. One might assume they would just make less milk. However, the dairy breeds will often make milk, requiring energy beyond what the diet will supply, until they become clinically ill from ketone body formation.

11 (A) From amino acids liberated from muscle protein and lactate liberated from muscle tissue. (B) It liberates fatty acids and glycerol. The glycerol can be used to make glucose directly in the liver. Peripheral tissues could use the fatty acids as an energy source to spare the blood glucose for other uses.

12 Tolbutamide can stimulate the remaining pancreatic islet β cells to increase production of insulin to overcome tissue resistance. By the time the diabetes is recognized in most canine or feline patients the condition has progressed to the point that the β cells have undergone exhaustion and will not respond to insulin secretagogues.

13 The lack of milk production by the mother means the pups may not be getting any nourishment. Unfortunately, the pup has little body fat and little stored glycogen reserves to draw on during the postabsorptive phase. The cold weather increases the energy requirement of the pup. Without a steady supply of glucose from the diet the pups are in danger of developing hypoglycemia and hypothermia.

48 Vitamins

Jesse P. Goff

Iowa State University, Ames, IA, USA

Vitamins are organic compounds that are essential to life. They function as metabolic catalysts or regulators and can generally be classified on the basis of their solubility as fat-soluble vitamins (A, D, E, and K) or water-soluble vitamins (B vitamins and C). All the vitamins are required for normal function in all animals, and often the diet must supply these compounds if the animal is to function normally. However, some of the vitamins are synthesized within the body of some animals so that there is no dietary requirement of that vitamin for that particular animal. In ruminants, the microbes are capable of producing many of the water-soluble B vitamins needed to support ruminant tissue needs.

The goals of this chapter are to familiarize the veterinary student with (i) the role each vitamin has in body functions; (ii) deficiency symptoms; (iii) toxicity symptoms; and (iv) syndromes of special concern in veterinary medicine.

Dukes' Physiology of Domestic Animals, Thirteenth Edition. Edited by William O. Reece, Howard H. Erickson, Jesse P. Goff and Etsuro E. Uemura.
© 2015 John Wiley & Sons, Inc. Published 2015 by John Wiley & Sons, Inc.
Companion website: www.wiley.com/go/reece/physiology

Section VII: Digestion, Absorption, and Metabolism

Vitamin A

> **2** What compound is the biologically active form of vitamin A?
>
> **3** What does retinaldehyde do?
>
> **4** What is the main function of vitamin A?
>
> **5** What are the classical signs of vitamin A deficiency?
>
> **6** How can you assess the vitamin A status of an animal?

The term "vitamin A" is often used to describe compounds that possess, or which can be metabolized into compounds that possess, the biological activity of **all-*trans* retinol**. One international unit (IU) of vitamin A activity is obtained with 0.3 μg of retinol. The major commercial forms of vitamin A, retinal palmitate (1 IU = 0.549 μg) and retinal acetate (1 IU = 0.344 μg), are more stable to oxidation than retinol. These retinal esters are enzymatically converted to retinol in the lumen of the gut before absorption by the intestinal cells. Retinol is not present in plant materials. However, **carotenoids** (over 50 with biological activity) exist in high concentrations in plants, especially fresh green forages. β-Carotene is the most active and most abundant of these compounds. Carotenes are absorbed by the enterocytes and partially converted to retinol within the enterocytes by 15,15′-dioxygenase (Figure 48.1). The efficiency of conversion of carotenes to retinol is much lower in herbivores than in humans and rats. For cattle, 1 mg of β-carotene is assumed to be equivalent to 400 IU of retinol, which is about one-fourth the rat value. At high dietary carotene levels, the conversion of carotene to retinol is even less efficient, perhaps representing an adaptation of herbivores to prevent toxicity from high-forage diets. Carotenes are also absorbed intact into the bloodstream of most herbivores, accounting for the yellow color of the serum and fat. The Channel Island breeds of cattle are particularly recognized for this trait. Carotenes may act as antioxidants of the blood. Retinol itself has little antioxidant activity.

Once inside the enterocyte, retinol reacts with long-chain fatty acids to re-form retinyl esters, which are incorporated into chylomicrons for transport to the liver, fat, and other tissues. The chylomicrons are taken up by the parenchymal hepatocytes and the retinyl esters are converted to retinol. The retinol is then secreted into the blood bound to **retinol-binding protein (RBP)**. A large amount of the RBP-bound retinol is also transferred directly from the parenchymal hepatocytes to the perisinusoidal stellate cells for storage as the retinyl ester.

Target cells for retinol have a receptor for RBP on their surface. It is unclear whether the retinol–RBP complex is then endocytosed into the target cell or if RBP simply acts as a transporter for retinol. Once inside the cell, a portion of the retinol is converted to one of several **retinoic acids**, the most active of which are all-*trans* retinoic acid and 9-*cis* retinoic acid. Target tissues of vitamin A contain specific intracellular retinol and retinoic acid-binding proteins that permit accumulation of retinol and retinoic acids. Target tissues differ greatly in the relative distribution of these two types of cytosolic proteins, suggesting

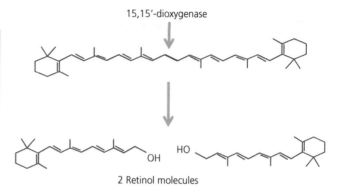

Figure 48.1 β-Carotene, commonly found in plant material, can be split into two retinol molecules by intestinal 15,15′-dioxygenase in most species.

they play a regulatory role in the metabolism of vitamin A within the cells.

Four nuclear **retinoic acid receptor** proteins have now been identified in vitamin A target tissues. Retinoic acid receptor α is expressed in high levels in cerebellum, adrenals, and testes. Retinoic acid receptor β is abundant in kidneys, prostate, and cerebral cortex. Retinoic acid receptor γ is present exclusively in the skin. These retinoic acid receptors share a great deal of homology with the steroid–thyroid hormone receptor family of proteins. The fourth nuclear retinoic acid receptor is designated retinoid X receptor α and is most abundant in visceral tissues. Little is known of its structure. Once retinoic acid binds to a retinoic acid receptor it initiates transcription and translation of certain genes. It seems reasonable to assume that each retinoic acid receptor protein binds to a distinct promoter region of different vitamin A-responsive genes. Little is known of the precise genes affected, although they are most likely involved in cell differentiation. In some cells, the retinoic acid–retinoic acid receptor complex binds to the same domain as thyroid hormone and vitamin D receptor proteins, suggesting that one effect of vitamin A is to modulate the activity of these other hormones.

In many respects vitamin A is simply a precursor to a group of hormones, the retinoic acids. Retinol in and of itself has little biological activity. It must be converted to one of the retinoic acids in order to affect gene expression.

Functions

Vitamin A, also known as retinol, is required for normal growth and development and plays a key role in differentiation of cells. Vitamin A deficiency can cause cessation of endochondral bone elongation, although periosteal bone growth is unaffected. This results in leg bones that are short and thick and skull bones that fail to grow, raising cerebrospinal fluid (CSF) pressures.

Epithelial cells line most of the mucosal surfaces and provide a physical, and sometimes mechanical (ciliated epithelium of the respiratory tract), barrier to invasion by bacterial pathogens. In vitamin A deficiency, epithelial cells that might normally be of a columnar, cuboidal, or transitional type undergo atrophy and develop a squamous type phenotype. This is termed **metaplasia** of the cells, and secretion of mucus decreases. The remaining basal epithelial cells proliferate, and the original epithelial cells are replaced by stratified keratinized epithelium. The loss of functional epithelial cells on mucosal surfaces facilitates bacterial entry and proliferation.

Vitamin A is required for vision. Vitamin A serves as the precursor for **retinaldehyde**, a component of the visual pigments needed for vision, especially when the light is dim. Retinaldehyde combines with proteins in the retinal rods and cones to form the visual pigments **rhodopsin** (rods) and **iodopsin** (cones). Light dissociates these pigments from the proteins resulting in generation of a nerve impulse to the brain. **Night blindness** (**nyctalopia** or loss of visual acuity in dim light) is common in vitamin A deficiency, and results in affected animals stumbling in the dark and failing to avoid objects placed in their path in dim light.

In addition to maintenance of host mechanical barriers to infection, vitamin A also modulates the immune system response to infection. During vitamin A deficiency primary and secondary lymphoid organs are reduced in size and antibody titers to a variety of antigens are decreased. Cell-mediated immunity is also compromised during vitamin A deficiency. Studies in mice indicate that the major effects of vitamin A in the immune system are mediated by enhancement of T-helper and natural killer cell activities.

β-Carotene may have a role in reproduction independent of other forms of vitamin A. The bovine corpus luteum has an unusually high concentration of β-carotene, which suggests that there may be specific binding of β-carotene to this tissue, although a receptor has yet to be identified. Corpora lutea from cows fed diets low in β-carotene have been found to produce less progesterone despite having more than adequate vitamin A supplementation. β-Carotene supplementation of vitamin A-replete mares has reportedly resulted in stronger heats, improved conception, and reduced embryonic mortality.

Vitamin A status

In most species, plasma retinol concentration (determined by high performance liquid chromatography) is generally maintained above 200 ng/mL (20 μg/dL) and is relatively independent of diet. As long as small reserves of vitamin A exist in the liver, the blood level remains unchanged. An exception might occur if the animal is malnourished for protein or calories. In this case, plasma levels of RBP (which carries retinol in the blood) and therefore plasma levels of retinol might be low despite adequate liver stores of vitamin A. Clinical signs of vitamin A deficiency may be apparent even though plasma retinol is still around 20 μg/dL. However, if plasma retinol falls below 10 μg/dL, a diagnosis of vitamin A deficiency can be safely made. Analysis of liver biopsy vitamin A content in conjunction with plasma retinol determinations are most fruitful in assessing vitamin A status. CSF pressure rises during vitamin A deficiency; however, determination of CSF pressure in veterinary medicine is not generally practical. Toxicity of vitamin A is dependent on the amount of vitamin A accumulated (which may be evident in liver biopsy), so the daily amount fed and the length of time fed is important. β-Carotene concentration in the plasma is well correlated with dietary β-carotene intake.

Deficiency

In vitamin A deficiency, epithelial cells that might normally be of a columnar, cuboidal, or transitional type undergo atrophy and metaplasia. Metaplasia occurs because the basal epithelial cells proliferate in an uncontrolled fashion, and the new cells fail to differentiate properly and adopt the simplest form, i.e., stratified keratinized epithelium. Goblet cells are also lost so secretion of mucus decreases. The loss of functional epithelial cells on mucosal surfaces facilitates bacterial entry and infections.

Classical lesions of the eye include **nyctalopia** (night blindness), **keratomalacia** (corneal metaplasia), and **xerophthalmia** (dryness and thickening of the conjunctiva). The skin develops excessive keratinization and drying of the epidermis with papular eruptions of the skin. The bronchorespiratory tract exhibits squamous metaplasia of the epithelium that leads to loss of mucus secretions and increased keratinization of the tract, with decreased elasticity to the lung. Increased respiratory tract infections are common. Males have impaired spermatogenesis. Females often abort or resorb their fetuses. Malformed offspring are possible. There will be reduced numbers of goblet cells and loss of mucus secretion in the gastrointestinal tract. Metaplasia of pancreatic ducts affects digestion. Bones fail to remodel properly and grow poorly. This poor bone growth constricts CSF flow and can cause greatly elevated CSF flow pressures.

Toxicity

Anorexia is common. The skin is often thickened. Congenital malformations are particularly pathognomonic of vitamin A toxicity in pregnant animals. There is often accelerated resorption of bone and cartilage and accelerated formation of new bone in tendon sheaths (**exostoses**). Bones continue to grow in length but not in thickness. There is premature closure of physes in bones of growing animals.

Syndromes of concern to veterinary medicine
Caged avian vitamin A deficiency
This is often an unrecognized malady of pet birds as a result of inferior bird feed. White plaques (hyperkeratosis) in and around the mouth, eyes, and sinuses are suggestive of vitamin A deficiency. These birds often have chronic conditions such as conjunctivitis, sinusitis, and bumblefoot (thick and irregular skin on the foot).

Vitamin A deficiency in turtles
Turtles with vitamin A deficiency will present with eyes closed shut due to swelling of the eyelids and the orbital glands, which have undergone squamous metaplasia.

Vitamin A toxicity in cats

This disease is a common sequela in cats fed high amounts of liver. Lesions are most prominent in the cervical region and involve excessive resorption of bone, subperiosteal bone formation and exostoses – bone forming in tendon sheaths, on periosteal surfaces and other places bone is not normally found – which can eventually lead to complete fusion of the spine. **Arthrodesis** or fusion of joints can also be seen radiographically.

Hyena disease of cattle

Administration of large amounts of vitamin A to young calves (often given as an adjunct treatment for scours) can induce premature closure of the physes, especially those in the hindlimbs. The result is a calf with depressed skeletal growth characterized by hindlegs that are considerably shorter than the front legs.

Vitamin D

1 What is the biologically active form of vitamin D?

2 Where does conversion of vitamin D to 1,25-dihydroxyvitamin D take place? Would this occur in an animal with renal failure?

3 How does 1,25-dihydroxyvitamin D affect intestinal calcium absorption?

4 How does 1,25-dihydroxyvitamin D affect bone formation and bone resorption?

5 Why does rickets develop during vitamin D deficiency?

6 Why is vitamin D_3 the most commonly used form of vitamin D supplementation?

7 What happens to a horse that gets no vitamin D supplementation?

Function

Vitamin D is a prohormone that becomes a required nutrient only in the absence of adequate exposure to sunlight, as occurs in northern latitudes or confinement housing. Exposure of skin to ultraviolet (UV) irradiation of sunlight converts **7-dehydrocholesterol** to vitamin D_3 (Figure 48.2). Dietary vitamin D_2 (**ergocalciferol**) and D_3 (**cholecalciferol**) are absorbed in the small intestine, where they enter the lymphatic circulation after incorporation into chylomicrons. Vitamin D circulates in the blood at 1–3 ng/mL. These low concentrations reflect the rapid uptake of vitamin D by the liver, where it is hydroxylated to form **25-hydroxyvitamin D**, and released into the blood. This metabolite is the major circulating form of vitamin D and is the best indicator of the vitamin D status of an animal. The normal range of 25-hydroxyvitamin D in the blood of most species is 15–70 ng/mL. Feeding vitamin D at 30 IU/kg live weight will generally ensure normal plasma 25-hydroxyvitamin D concentrations. Plasma 25-hydroxyvitamin D concentrations below 5 ng/mL can be considered deficiency, while plasma concentrations in excess of 130 ng/mL are indicative of toxicity.

The 25-hydroxyvitamin D circulates in plasma bound to vitamin D-binding protein and is taken up by the kidney. 1α-Hydroxylation of 25-hydroxyvitamin D in the kidney results in the formation of the steroid hormone **1,25-dihydroxyvitamin D** [1,25-$(OH)_2$D]. Production of this hormone is increased with increasing demand for calcium or phosphorus. **Parathyroid hormone** (PTH) acts as the primary stimulus for 1,25-$(OH)_2$D production. The parathyroid gland secretes PTH whenever it senses a decline in plasma calcium. During periods of calcium excess, both 25-hydroxyvitamin D and 1,25-$(OH)_2$D are hydroxylated at positions C-23 and/or C-24 to form inactive metabolites, which are ultimately excreted.

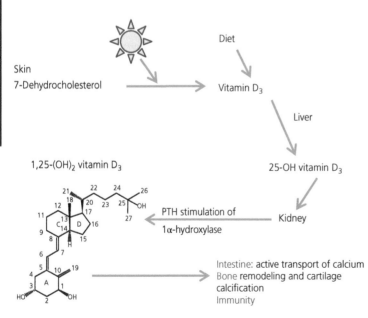

Figure 48.2 Vitamin D metabolism. Vitamin D, produced in the skin following UVB irradiation or consumed in the diet, travels via the blood to the liver where it is hydroxylated at the C-25 position. The resulting 25-hydroxyvitamin D_3 (25-OH vitamin D_3) enters the circulation and is taken up by the kidney tubule epithelium. If these cells have been stimulated by parathyroid hormone (PTH), a 1α-hydroxylase enzyme will act on 25-OH vitamin D_3 and convert it to 1,25-dihydroxyvitamin D_3 (1,25-$(OH)_2$vitamin D_3). This hormone stimulates intestinal calcium absorption and bone development. It also has widespread actions on immunity and differentiation of cells.

The kidney releases 1,25-(OH)$_2$D into the blood where it circulates bound to vitamin D-binding protein. Less than 5% of the hormone circulates in the free state, yet it is this form that readily enters cells due to its lipophilic nature. 1,25-(OH)$_2$D accumulates only in tissues that possess intracellular receptors for 1,25-(OH)$_2$D. Target tissue 1,25-(OH)$_2$D receptor number determines the biologic response to 1,25-(OH)$_2$D during calcium crisis periods. The higher a tissue's receptor concentration, the greater the response to the hormone. The formation of receptor–hormone complexes results in specific DNA or acceptor site binding, followed by induction or suppression of specific mRNA transcription. This regulates specific protein synthesis for maintenance of calcium homeostasis by the classical target tissues (bone, intestine, and kidney). Receptors for 1,25-(OH)$_2$D have been found in a wide variety of tissues in the body (notably the intestine, bone, kidney, thymus, mammary gland, and lymphoid tissues), suggesting that vitamin D modulates the function of these tissues as well.

Functions of 1,25-(OH)$_2$D

Calcium is an important component, and is required for the normal functioning, of a wide variety of tissues and physiological processes. Vertebrates have evolved a highly complex endocrine system to maintain plasma and extracellular calcium concentrations within a very narrow range. Calcium homeostasis results from an intricate balance of input, output, and calcium recycling. Mechanisms for absorption of dietary calcium, recycling of bone calcium stores, and renal conservation of calcium are primarily controlled by PTH and 1,25-(OH)$_2$D.

A limited amount of calcium can be absorbed from the lumen of the intestine, by passive diffusion between the intestinal epithelial cells, if the ionized calcium concentration in the luminal fluid over the enterocytes exceeds about 6 mmol/L. Experimental studies suggest that if animals are fed a high-calcium diet, more than 50% of the calcium absorbed will be by passive diffusion. Efficient absorption of dietary calcium, when dietary calcium is low or when demand is very high, occurs by active transport of calcium across the epithelial cells. This process requires 1,25-(OH)$_2$D. Calcium concentrations within enterocytes are about 1000-fold lower than in the lumen of the gut (even in animals fed a low-calcium diet); thus, calcium entry into the intestinal epithelial cell occurs readily down a concentration gradient through channels that are under the control of 1,25-(OH)$_2$D. 1,25-(OH)$_2$D also stimulates the synthesis of **calcium-binding protein**, which transports calcium from the luminal side of enterocytes to the basolateral membrane. Calcium is then extruded out of the enterocyte into the extracellular fluid by Ca^{2+}/Mg^{2+}-ATPase-dependent pumps, which are also under the control of 1,25-(OH)$_2$D.

Bone is highly dependent on 1,25-(OH)$_2$D for normal growth and remodeling. Vitamin D deficiency results in **osteomalacia** in adult animals (failure of mineralization of osteoid) and **rickets** in young animals (failure of mineralization of osteoid plus failure of mineralization of cartilaginous matrix at growth plates). Defective mineralization of bone and cartilage are classical histological findings of vitamin D deficiency. This results primarily from decreased plasma calcium and phosphorus levels (and secondary hyperparathyroidism) as a result of decreased intestinal calcium and phosphorus absorption. If normal plasma calcium and phosphorus concentrations are maintained in vitamin D-deficient rats by continuous intravenous infusion of these minerals, bone will mineralize normally. This suggests no direct effect on mineral deposition. The primary function of 1,25-(OH)$_2$D in bone formation may simply be to maintain adequate blood calcium and phosphorus levels for mineralization to occur. Yet, there is evidence that 1,25-(OH)$_2$D influences production of bone matrix proteins and that 1,25-(OH)$_2$D or 24,25-(OH)$_2$D plays a direct role in repair of bone fractures, indicating a role for vitamin D metabolites in bone formation. 1,25-(OH)$_2$D plays an important role in osteoclastic bone calcium resorption. 1,25-(OH)$_2$D greatly augments bone resorption once it is initiated by PTH. However, 1,25-(OH)$_2$D has little effect on bone resorption activity unless PTH is present. A minor function of 1,25-(OH)$_2$D is to act with PTH to enhance renal reabsorption of calcium from the glomerular filtrate.

Requirement

The amount of dietary vitamin D required to provide adequate substrate for production of 1,25-(OH)$_2$D is difficult to define. Animals exposed to sunlight at the lower latitudes may not require any dietary vitamin D. Sun-cured hay may also provide enough vitamin D$_2$ to prevent symptoms of vitamin D deficiency. The movement away from pasture feeding systems and toward confinement and feeding of stored feeds and byproducts has increased the need for dietary vitamin D supplementation of cows.

Deficiency

Vitamin D deficiency reduces the ability to maintain calcium and phosphorus homeostasis, resulting in a decline in plasma phosphorus and less often a decrease in plasma calcium. This eventually causes rickets in young animals and osteomalacia in adults; both are bone diseases where the primary lesion is failure to mineralize the organic matrix of bone. In young animals, rickets causes enlarged and painful joints; the costochondral joints of the ribs are often readily palpated. In adults, lameness and pelvic fracture are common sequelae of vitamin D deficiency.

Toxicity

Toxicity of vitamin D is most common following injection of vitamin D or when high amounts of vitamin D are fed for an extended time. Vitamin D intoxication is associated with reduced feed intake, polyuria initially followed by anuria, dry feces, and reduced production, all of which are secondary to the pronounced hypercalcemia and hyperphosphatemia induced by excessive vitamin D. Generally, the production of 1,25-(OH)$_2$D is inhibited during vitamin D intoxication. The actual toxic compound in many cases of toxicity is the 25-hydroxyvitamin D metabolite, which builds up to very high levels in toxic animals. At these levels, it will interact with the receptor for 1,25-$(OH)_2$D and mimic the actions of 1,25-$(OH)_2$D. On necropsy, calcification of kidneys, aorta, abomasum, and bronchioles is evident. This is known as metastatic calcification of soft tissues.

Syndromes of special concern in veterinary medicine

Vitamin D_2 versus vitamin D_3

Vitamin D_2, the form associated with plants, and vitamin D_3, the form associated with vertebrates, are both used for supplementation of diets. The biological activity of the two forms is generally considered equal; however, it is important to point out that avian species, many fish, reptiles, and the New World monkeys can only utilize vitamin D_3. Presumably, this discrimination is the result of reduced binding of vitamin D_2 metabolites to vitamin D-binding proteins in blood leading to more rapid clearance of D_2 metabolites from plasma.

Vitamin D in the horse and rabbit

The horse and the rabbit (and perhaps other hindgut fermenters) seem to have no vitamin D requirement. In these species, intestinal calcium absorption is not dependent on the actions of 1,25-$(OH)_2$D. There has never been a documented case of vitamin D deficiency in these species. They absorb a large proportion of the available dietary calcium at all times, then excrete the excess calcium in their urine, which gives the ground a characteristic chalky look where they have micturated. The horse and rabbit do remain very susceptible to vitamin D intoxication because they do have receptors for 1,25-$(OH)_2$D in their intestine.

Milk fever in dairy cattle

Certain dietary factors (potassium and sodium) alkalinize the blood, which prevents renal tissue (bone also) from recognizing PTH. Therefore, production of 1,25-$(OH)_2$D may be reduced, which prevents calcium homeostasis in the periparturient cow and leads to severe hypocalcemia known as milk fever.

Enteque secio (chronic wasting disease) of cattle, sheep, and horses

In some areas of the world, certain plants such as *Solanum malacoxylon*, *Cestrum diurnum*, and *Trisetum flavescens* cause a life-threatening hypercalcemia when ingested by grazing animals. These plants contain high amounts of a glycoside form of 1,25-$(OH)_2$D that becomes biologically active within the small intestine.

Vitamin D intoxication from rodenticide in cats and dogs

Rodents are more sensitive to vitamin D toxicity than are most of the domesticated species. Certain rodenticides utilize vitamin D as their active component. Unfortunately, dogs and cats

consuming these rodenticides directly or rats and mice killed by these rodenticides have developed vitamin D intoxication.

Vitamin E

> **1** If tocopheryl acetate is not biologically active, why is it the most commonly utilized supplemental form of vitamin E used by the feed industry?
>
> **2** What is the fate of absorbed tocopherol?
>
> **3** What is the primary function of vitamin E in the cell?
>
> **4** Do immune cells have a higher requirement for vitamin E than other tissues?
>
> **5** Why might dairy cows be fed supplemental vitamin E?
>
> **6** Unsaturated fat increases vitamin E requirement. What species does this affect most?
>
> **7** What are some of the classical signs of vitamin E deficiency in calves and in chicks?

Function

Vitamin E activity can be found in the naturally occurring **tocopherols** (α, β and γ), all of which act as chemical antioxidants. The major tocopherol in animal tissues is α-**tocopherol**, which also happens to have the greatest vitamin E activity as assessed by biological assays such as prevention of infertility in rats or nutritional muscular dystrophy in rabbits. Natural α-tocopherol of plant and animal tissue is all D-α-tocopherol. Chemical synthesis of tocopherol yields both D and L racemers, with the L-α-tocopherol possessing less than half the activity of D-α-tocopherol. Since α-tocopherol is a readily oxidized compound, most supplements are prepared as the acetate or succinate esters of DL-α-tocopherol to enhance stability. Since the acetate and succinate esters of α-tocopherol do not function as antioxidants until the ester linkage has been split off by esterases in the intestine, they are able to bypass the rumen without being oxidized.

Tocopherols must then become incorporated into micelles with bile salts in order to enter the intestinal cells. Once within the intestinal epithelial cells, tocopherol is incorporated into chylomicrons and released to the mesenteric lymphatics. Lipoprotein lipase bound to the endothelial cells of the lymphatics and blood vessels hydrolyzes the triacylglycerols in chylomicrons, reducing them to chylomicron remnants. The chylomicron remnants are taken up by the liver and the tocopherol stored, primarily in the parenchymal cells. Tocopherol is secreted from parenchymal liver cells in association with very low density lipoproteins (VLDL). These VLDL particles can also be degraded by endothelial lipoprotein lipase, converting them to high-density lipoprotein (HDL) or low-density lipoprotein (LDL). Tocopherol leaves the circulation by receptor-mediated uptake of LDL by liver and peripheral tissues.

Liver, skeletal muscle, and adipose tissue have the ability to store tocopherol and account for over 90% of the tocopherol within the body. Adrenal glands contain the highest concentration per gram of tissue, which may be due to the specific binding of HDL by adrenal glands. The testes and the cerebrum have the lowest levels of tocopherol, suggesting that they will be the first tissues depleted of vitamin E, which may account for two common signs of vitamin E deficiency, reproductive failure and neurological dysfunction.

Cells exposed to molecular oxygen risk being damaged by oxygen-derived free radicals (superoxide anion radical and hydroxyl radical) and lipid peroxidation products. Antioxidants such as vitamin E, superoxide dismutase, glutathione peroxidase (containing selenium), catalase, vitamin C, and β-carotene quench free radicals before they can damage tissues. Vitamin E is the most important fat-soluble antioxidant, making it the primary antioxidant of cell membranes. Exposure of polyunsaturated fats to oxygen can result in removal of a hydrogen atom, resulting in formation of a lipid radical. If unquenched by vitamin E, this radical can react with oxygen to form a hydroperoxide radical. If vitamin E is not able to quench this radical, hydroperoxide radicals can extract hydrogen atoms from other lipids (possibly initiating a cascade of polyunsaturated fatty acid oxidation) to form hydroperoxides, with subsequent damage to cell membranes. Vitamin E quenches free radicals by donating a hydrogen atom from position C-6. The unpaired electron left on the oxygen atom in the C-6 position can be delocalized into the aromatic ring structure, increasing the stability. The vitamin E radical may be reduced back to tocopherol by glutathione peroxidase and vitamin C, or it may go on to form tocopherol quinone and other compounds that are eventually excreted in the bile and urine. In simpler terms, the body prefers to sacrifice vitamin E to the free radicals rather than cell membranes.

Vitamin E supplementation above the amounts needed to prevent the classical deficiency symptoms can act as a stimulant of the immune system. Vitamin E supplementation leads to enhanced humoral immune responses and increased resistance to bacterial infections in mice and chickens. Vitamin E supplementation can also enhance T-helper cell activity in mice and alveolar macrophage function in rats. Addition of vitamin E to cultures of peripheral blood mononuclear cells obtained from vitamin E-deficient cows enhanced *in vitro* antibody production and secretion of interleukin-1.

Deficiency

The beneficial effects of vitamin E are classically attributed to its role as an antioxidant and the stabilizing effect this has on cell membranes. Signs of vitamin E deficiency are many and varied. In herbivores, the system that seems most at risk is skeletal muscle function. Calves and lambs are born with low reserves of vitamin E, making them particularly prone to development of degeneration and necrosis of the muscles, which is commonly described as **white muscle disease**. Anemia (red blood cell hemolysis), stunted growth, and reproductive failure are common signs of vitamin E deficiency in many species. Classical

signs in chicks include **encephalomalcia**, causing sudden prostration, outstretched legs and arched neck; **exudative diathesis**, in which the capillaries become leaky, leading to edema under the skin; and **muscular dystrophy** similar to white muscle disease in calves and lambs.

Toxicity

Vitamin E is essentially nontoxic.

Syndromes of special concern in veterinary medicine

Vitamin E and mastitis in dairy cows

Supplementation of vitamin E at 1 g/day reduced the incidence of new clinical cases of mastitis in a research dairy herd by 37%. These observations were extended into commercial herds with similar results. Maximal protection from mastitis was seen when both vitamin E and selenium were added to the diet. Udder edema and retained placenta in dairy cattle also appear to be reduced by dietary supplementation of vitamin E. Another benefit is that milk from cows fed supplemental vitamin E is less susceptible to oxidation, which improves the marketability of the product.

Steatitis (white fat disease, yellow fat disease) in cats, marine mammals, and mink

These animals are often fed fish that have been dead for some time or rancid meat. High unsaturated fat content of fish will cause hydroperoxides to build up in the stored fish. These free radicals can induce steatitis in the fat of the mammal, which is characterized by marked inflammation of adipose tissue and deposition of ceroid pigment within the fat cells. Vitamin E should routinely be added to these diets to provide antioxidant activity to these mammals. Domesticated cats are also candidates for this disease when fed high-fish diets.

Vitamin K

> **1** What proteins are not made during vitamin K deficiency? What is the main clinical syndrome caused by vitamin K deficiency?
>
> **2** What is sweet clover poisoning?

Vitamin K takes its name from *koagulation*, the Danish term for blood coagulation, which is an important function of vitamin K. The term "vitamin K" covers two related compounds: vitamin K_1, or **phylloquinone**, synthesized by plants; and vitamin K_2, or **menaquinone**, produced by bacteria. Both compounds contain a menadione ring structure with an isoprene side chain that can be variable in length. Vitamin K_3, **menadione**, is the ring structure by itself. Though not as active as vitamin K_1 and K_2, vitamin K_3 can be easily manufactured and is the form utilized in most commercial supplements.

Function

Vitamin K is required in order to synthesize many of the **calcium-binding proteins** of the body. The first ones discovered were the calcium-binding proteins involved in blood coagulation, i.e., **prothrombin** and **clotting factors VII, IX, and X**. Other calcium-binding proteins found in bone, such as **osteocalcin**, are essential for mineralization of bone tissues. Prothrombin and the other vitamin K-dependent clotting factors are produced in the liver in an inactive form, unable to bind calcium. They become active following post-translational processing. The reduced form of vitamin K works with a carboxylating enzyme to incorporate CO_2 into glutamic acid residues on the proteins to form γ-**carboxyglutamic acid**. The γ-carboxyglutamic acid gives them the ability to bind calcium. In the process of producing γ-carboxyglutamic acid, the vitamin K is oxidized to the epoxide form of vitamin K. The epoxide form can then be reduced by epoxide reductase to regenerate the reduced or active form of vitamin K so it can be reused.

Intestinal microbes produce vitamin K. Rumen microbes produce all the vitamin K required by ruminants so none needs to be added to their diet. In nonruminants, the cecum and colon microbes produce vitamin K but absorption of the vitamin K is poor. In most monogastric species, vitamin K must be added to the diet, unless the animal practices coprophagy routinely. High amounts of vitamin K are found in green leafy forages.

Deficiency

Vitamin K deficiency reduces the prothrombin content of the blood. Coagulation time will be increased and hemorrhages often occur in any part of the body, spontaneously or following a bruise. Often the only real evidence is subcutaneous hemorrhaging. On necropsy, blood can often be found in the thoracic and abdominal cavities. Vitamin K antagonists can interfere with the activity of vitamin K and induce vitamin K deficiency symptoms.

The most common cause of vitamin K deficiency is ingestion of coumarins. Dicoumarol and related compounds, found in plants such as sweet clover, bind to the enzyme epoxide reductase and interfere with regeneration of the active (reduced) form of vitamin K, quickly depleting the body of vitamin K activity. Many rodenticides are based on dicoumarol and its derivatives and dogs or cats are often poisoned by ingestion of the rodenticide or animals that have died from ingestion of the rodenticide.

Toxicity

Very high doses can cause a reduction in feed intake and depressed growth, but toxicity is uncommon.

Syndromes of special concern in veterinary medicine

Anticoagulant rodenticide poisoning

Dicoumarol and related compounds, such as **warfarin**, are utilized as rodenticides. Unfortunately, accidental poisonings occur when domesticated and wild nontarget species consume the baits or rats that have been poisoned. Dicoumarol and the first generation of anticoagulants required repeated ingestion to kill the rodents and therefore were less toxic to pets. However, the new rodenticides containing second-generation anticoagulants, such as **brodifacoum** and **bromadiolone**, will kill rodents ingesting a single dose of rodenticide, making accidental ingestion more dangerous. Treatment involves subcutaneous injections of vitamin K_1. Menadione, the feed supplement, must not be used parenterally as it is associated with a high incidence of anaphylactic reactions.

Sweet clover poisoning

A hemorrhagic disease can occur in animals that consume poorly preserved hays and silages containing significant amounts of sweet clover (*Melilotus officinalis*). Fresh sweet clover can contain large amounts of harmless natural coumarins. However, if **sweet clover in hay or silage** becomes moldy and spoils, the coumarins can be converted to dicoumarol, an antagonist of vitamin K. Cows, sheep, and horses are most susceptible.

Sulfa drugs and antibiotics

Sulfa drugs used to control microbial and coccidial infections are antagonistic to vitamin K and have induced hemorrhagic syndromes following long-term use. Long-term treatment with any antibiotic can reduce intestinal microbial production of vitamin K, which can induce vitamin K deficiency in those species that rely on intestinal microbes to supply them with vitamin K.

Anti-inflammatory use in horses

Horses consume small amounts of the coumarin type of anticoagulants in their forage, and this presents no problems. These compounds are bound to proteins within the circulation, effectively neutralizing them. Eventually they are excreted. However, many of the nonsteroidal anti-inflammatory drugs, such as phenylbutazone, can displace the anticoagulant from the proteins in blood. In horses with laminitis treated for long periods with high doses of phenylbutazone, the anticoagulants displaced by the treatment have actually induced cases of vitamin K deficiency (coumarin toxicity).

Biotin

> **1** What biochemical reactions require biotin?
>
> **2** What are typical symptoms of biotin deficiency in chickens and in cattle?

Function

Biotin is a water-soluble compound consisting of two five-membered rings with three asymmetrical carbons. It is required for **decarboxylation reactions**. Only the all-D isomers of biotin are biologically active. Microbes of the lower intestinal tract produce biotin and enough is absorbed to meet the biotin requirements of most animals. In poultry, the rate of passage of ingesta through the intestinal tract may be too rapid to allow microbial synthesis of adequate biotin and supplementation is usually required. Long-term oral antibiotic administration can reduce microbial biotin production and induce biotin deficiency.

Deficiency

Biotin deficiency is rare in animals fed corn/soybean meal-based diets. Biotin-deficient animals have poor hair coats and exhibit alopecia, scaly dermatitis, and achromotrichia (lack of hair color). Cats, mink, and foxes are species at some risk of developing biotin deficiency. In cats, anorexia, scaly dermatitis around the mouth and eyes, hypersalivation, and alopecia are observed. In cattle, poor hoof growth and lack of hoof hardness are ascribed to biotin deficiency.

In poultry, broken flight feathers and bending of the metatarsus are common. Dermatitis of the bottoms of the feet, corners of the mouth and eyes are observed. Diets containing high amounts of fat, especially if the fat is rancid, can oxidize the biotin in the diet resulting in biotin deficiency.

Syndromes of special concern to veterinary medicine
Egg whites and biotin deficiency

Raw egg whites contain a protein called avidin. **Avidin** tightly binds biotin, making it unavailable for absorption and inducing biotin deficiency. Cooking the egg white to 91°C for 5 min destroys the avidin. Biotin for use by the embryonic chick is found only in the yolk of eggs.

Choline

> **1** What role does choline play in cell physiology?
>
> **2** Is choline deficiency common in animals fed high-quality protein diets?

Function

Choline is required in relatively large amounts by the body, up to 0.1% of the diet. Most of the other vitamins are required at one-hundredth this level. Choline is required in such large amounts because it is a component of lecithin, a phospholipid found in cell membranes, and is a component of the neurotransmitter acetylcholine. Choline also serves as a donor of methyl groups in certain methylation reactions, such as the conversion of homocysteine to methionine. Some of the methyl donor functions of choline can be carried out by **methionine** in the diet.

Deficiency

Choline deficiency causes lipids to accumulate in the liver due to lack of the phospholipids required to transport fat from the liver to the tissues. Some choline can be synthesized within the body from phosphatidylserine provided there is adequate methionine to serve as a methyl donor. Most corn/soybean meal diets provide adequate amounts of choline and high-protein feed ingredients are generally good sources of choline. Choline-deficient swine exhibit incoordination and have fatty liver and kidney degeneration. The only sign that may be exhibited in choline-deficient sows is a smaller litter size.

Syndromes of special concern in veterinary medicine

Rumen-protected choline has been used as a supplement in the diet of cows around the time of calving. It may reduce the incidence of ketosis and fatty liver by permitting formation of **VLDL** necessary for the removal of fat from the liver.

Cyanocobalamin (vitamin B$_{12}$)

> **1** What is intrinsic factor?
>
> **2** Do ruminants require vitamin B$_{12}$?

Function

Cyanocobalamin incorporates cobalt as a cofactor. Cyanocobalamin is involved in the *de novo* synthesis of labile methyl groups necessary for the conversion of homocystine to re-form methionine. Ingredients of plant origin are devoid of cyanocobalamin. Only animal byproducts provide the vitamin. In ruminants, the rumen microorganisms will produce adequate cyanocobalamin if the animal is fed adequate amounts of cobalt in its diet. Cyanocobalamin is absorbed from the ileum by a very specific process. A protein produced in the stomach known as **intrinsic factor** must bind the cyanocobalamin within the upper gastrointestinal tract. The intrinsic factor–cobalamin complex then interacts with specific receptors in the ileum to allow absorption of the cyanocobalamin. In human gastrectomy patients, a lack of intrinsic factor production leads to deficiency of cyanocobalamin, causing a disease called pernicious anemia.

Deficiency

Poor growth and productivity and anemia are common. Reduced fertility is also reported. Monogastric species fed diets containing only plant materials must be fed supplemental cyanocobalamin to avoid deficiency. Deficiency is seen in ruminants fed cobalt-deficient diets. In ruminants, the **gluconeogenic** pathways seem most affected.

Folic acid

> **1** Without folic acid, which biochemicals cannot be synthesized?
>
> **2** What are the main clinical signs of folic acid deficiency?

Folic acid consists of a pteridine ring structure joined to a *p*-aminobenzoic acid ring, with a glutamic acid attached to the *p*-aminobenzoic acid ring. Folic acid exists in an oxidized and reduced form. The reduced form is **tetrahydrofolic acid**. It is a heat-labile compound.

Function

The folic acid found in many dietary ingredients has multiple glutamic acid residues attached. All but the last of these are removed during the course of digestion. The folic acid is absorbed across the intestinal tract by passive diffusion and active transport processes. It becomes bound to special folate-binding proteins for transport in the blood. These carrier proteins are upregulated during folate deficiency and also during pregnancy. Folate is taken up by the liver for storage or the folate is reduced to tetrahydrofolic acid and a methyl group is added to form N^5-methyltetrahydrofolic acid for release from the liver to the tissues.

Within tissues, tetrahydrofolic acid is required for transfer of one-carbon methyl units from one molecule to another and in hydroxylation of various compounds. Methyl-group transfer provided by tetrahydrofolic acid is necessary for the synthesis of methionine, serine, thymidine, and the purine bases needed to make nucleic acids. Tetrahydrofolic acid is necessary for hydroxylation of tyrosine to form norepinephrine and for conversion of tryptophan to serotonin.

Deficiency

Rumen microbes provide ruminants with all the folic acid they require. In swine, horses, and many other species, microbial activity in the hindgut and absorption of folate is great enough to meet most of their folic acid requirements. The high rate of passage of ingesta in poultry places them at the greatest risk of developing folate deficiency.

Folic acid deficiency causes reduced growth, poor hair coat, and poor feather development. **Macrocytic hypochromic anemia** is common. Turkey poults develop a characteristic cervical paralysis in which the neck is extended and the birds gaze at the ground.

In humans, folic acid deficiency is a major risk factor for **spina bifida** in the fetus. Folic acid deficiency may also play a role in susceptibility to myocardial infarction from atherosclerosis due to build-up of homocysteine in tissues.

Syndromes of special concern in veterinary medicine
Folic acid antagonists to treat coccidiosis
Sulfonamides and **ethopabate** are structural antagonists of *p*-aminobenzoic acid that are used to control coccidiosis in poultry and other species. Coccidia are eukaryotic parasites that produce their own folic acid for their own use, combining *p*-aminobenzoic acid with a pteridine structure. Sulfonamides and ethopabate substitute for *p*-aminobenzoic acid, resulting in biologically inactive folic acid. The coccidia become folic acid

deficient, unable to produce DNA and RNA and fail to reproduce, keeping the infection in check until immunity can develop.

Sulfa drugs can also prevent intestinal microbes from producing folate, which increases the need for dietary supplementation of folic acid.

Niacin

> **1** Why is NAD essential?
> **2** What tissues are most affected by niacin deficiency?
> **3** What role does tryptophan play in niacin deficiency?

Function

Niacin is also known as nicotinic acid and is required for the enzymes nicotinamide adenine dinucleotide (NAD) and nicotinamide adenine dinucleotide phosphate (NADP). These coenzymes are essential for the metabolism of carbohydrates, proteins, and lipids. Some animals are capable of converting some of the dietary tryptophan they ingest to niacin, but in general this is insufficient to supply the needs of the animal for niacin. Niacin present in some plant products (corn, oats, wheat) exists in a bound form that renders it unavailable to the animal unless processed to free the niacin. Niacin in soybean meal is highly available for absorption.

Deficiency

Since niacin is involved in so many metabolic pathways, deficiency of niacin most affects those tissues undergoing rapid turnover and growth. Poor weight gain and dry rough skin are common. Diarrhea occurs secondary to necrosis and ulceration within the gastrointestinal tract. Feeding a high-quality protein with surplus tryptophan can reduce reliance on dietary niacin. Rumen microbes generally supply adequate amounts of niacin to meet the needs of ruminants.

Syndromes of special concern in veterinary medicine
Pellagra (black tongue)
Pellagra is an Italian term describing the rough skin and darkened pigmentation that develops in people and animals that rely on corn as a major component of the diet. Dogs fed diets that are corn based develop a black tongue, along with rough dry skin. Corn is also a poor source of tryptophan, so the animal cannot produce niacin either. Central and South American Indians learned that treating corn with lye and lime water increases the availability of niacin and prevents development of pellagra. Modern refinement of corn and wheat to produce flour does not preserve the niacin.

Ketosis and fatty liver
Addition of niacin to diets of cows around the time of calving is sometimes of aid in the prevention of ketosis and fatty liver in dairy cows. Niacin is **antilipolytic** and it is thought that this

property may prevent build-up of liver fat leading to ketosis. It is thought that the high metabolic demands of milk production, coupled with poor feed intake around the time of calving, may lead to insufficient niacin production in the rumen.

Pantothenic acid

> 1 What enzymes require pantothenic acid?
> 2 What species must have pantothenic acid added to their ration?

Function

Pantothenic acid is a required component of **coenzyme A**. Coenzyme A is involved in enzyme-catalyzed reactions involving the transfer of acetyl (two-carbon) groups. These reactions are important in the oxidative metabolism of carbohydrates, especially gluconeogenesis. It is involved in the synthesis and degradation of fatty acids and in the synthesis of steroid hormones. This vitamin is widely distributed in feedstuffs and deficiency is uncommon.

Deficiency

Neuromuscular degeneration and adrenocortical insufficiency are common in pantothenic acid deficiency. Only in poultry is deficiency described as a practical possibility. The main effect is reduced hatchability and early embryonic death in eggs laid by brooder hens.

Pyridoxine (vitamin B$_6$)

> 1 Which enzyme catalyzing neurotransmitter production is affected by pyridoxine deficiency?

Function

Pyridoxal phosphate is an enzyme of metabolic transformations of amino acids, including decarboxylation and transamination reactions. Pyridoxine is needed for conversion of tryptophan to 5-hydroxytryptamine.

Deficiency

Certain drugs, such as **isoniazid** and **penicillamine**, speed excretion of pyridoxine and have been associated with pyridoxine deficiency. Dermatitis and convulsive seizures can occur during pyridoxine deficiency. Animals become abnormally excitable. Deficiency is rare, but has been described in newly hatched chicks.

Riboflavin (vitamin B$_2$)

> 1 What is the function of flavin adenine dinucleotide?

Function

Riboflavin is a water-soluble compound that is relatively heat-stable but which is rapidly inactivated by exposure to light. Riboflavin is absorbed by an active transport process in the intestinal tract. At high concentrations, riboflavin can be absorbed by passive diffusion.

Grain concentrates and plant proteins tend to be poor sources of riboflavin and riboflavin needs to be added to the diet of most monogastric animals. Ruminants derive adequate riboflavin from microbial synthesis in the rumen.

Riboflavin consists of a ribose sugar moiety and an isoalloxine ring structure. It is converted to flavin mononucleotide or flavin adenine dinucleotide by phosphorylation of the ribose by ATP and addition of adenine to the ribose chain.

Flavin adenine dinucleotide and flavin mononucleotide are enzymes that function in the electron transport system to oxidize substrate to generate ATP within the mitochondria. During these reactions the nitrogens of the isoalloxine ring function to transfer H$^+$ to, or accept H$^+$ from, the substrates.

Deficiency

It is difficult to reconcile the biochemical function of riboflavin with the clinical disease associated with riboflavin deficiency. In monogastric mammals, riboflavin deficiency usually presents as **dermatitis** with **alopecia** (hair loss), impotence, and **ophthalmic** problems that include catarrhal discharge, photophobia, cataracts or lens opacity. In poultry, riboflavin deficiency creates lesions in the sciatic and brachial nerves and the birds walk with the hocks in contact with the ground and their toes curled in, which is referred to as **curled toe paralysis**.

Syndromes of special concern in veterinary medicine
Equine uveitis

This disease of horses is also known as **periodic ophthalmia** or **moonblindness**. In the equine, riboflavin deficiency due to insufficient absorption of microbial riboflavin synthesized in the hindgut is an occasional cause of uveitis. It should be stressed that riboflavin deficiency is not the major cause of equine uveitis.

Thiamine (vitamin B$_1$)

> 1 In the absence of thiamine, can carbohydrates enter the TCA cycle?
> 2 Describe the three types of thiamines of concern to veterinary medicine.

Function

Thiamine is a water-soluble compound composed of a pyrimidine and thiazole ring. Within tissues the thiamine is phosphorylated by adenosine triphosphate (ATP) to form thiamine pyrophosphate. Thiamine pyrophosphate is a required cofactor of the enzyme that converts pyruvate to acetyl-CoA. This enzyme moves carbons from the glycolysis pathway into the tricarboxylic acid (TCA) cycle. Thiamine pyrophosphate is also essential within the TCA cycle, as it is a cofactor for the enzyme that converts α-ketoglutarate to succinyl-CoA. Thiamine pyrophosphate is a required cofactor for enzymes involved in metabolism of the ketoacids formed from the catabolism of the amino acids leucine, isoleucine, and valine. The transketolase enzymes of the pentose shunt also require thiamine pyrophosphate.

Thiamine is common in feedstuffs and is usually present in adequate amounts to satisfy the requirements of monogastric species. However, heat treatment of feeds will rapidly destroy thiamine activity. Pelleting of feed can generate enough heat to also destroy thiamine. Rumen microbes normally produce enough thiamine to meet the requirements of the ruminant.

Deficiency

Thiamine deficiency can occur due to inadequate amounts of thiamine in the diet or, more commonly, due to the presence of **thiaminases** in the feed which destroy the thiamine or, worse yet, convert it to an anti-vitamin. Certain plants, microbes, and fishmeal contain thiaminase enzymes. One type of thiaminase cleaves the thiazole ring destroying the biological activity of thiamine. A second type of thiaminase substitutes nicotinic acid or picolinic acid for the thiazole ring of thiamine. The resulting compound cannot be phosphorylated to make it biologically active and may tie up the enzymes required for phosphorylation of thiamine. A third type of thiaminase substitutes a hydroxyl group (OH^-) for the amino group on the pyrimidine ring. This compound, called **oxythiamine**, is a potent anti-vitamin and effectively outcompetes normal thiamine for the binding sites of thiamine-dependent enzymes. The result is rapid development of thiamine deficiency symptoms.

Thiamine deficiency prevents tissues from producing energy. Thiamine deficiency results in elevated blood pyruvate levels, since it interferes with conversion of pyruvate to acetyl-CoA. Since neurological tissue has a very high-energy requirement, neurological symptoms predominate during thiamine deficiency.

Syndromes of special concern to veterinary medicine
Chastek paralysis of fox, marine mammals, mink, and cat

This disease is associated with diets that contain certain **raw fish**. Bullhead, herring, whitefish, and carp are among the species of fish that contain high thiaminase activity. Raw-fish diets cause the animals to walk stiff-legged initially, followed by spastic convulsions and, finally, paralysis and death. The thiaminase activity is destroyed by cooking the fish.

Cats have about five times the requirements for thiamine that dogs have. The process (high heat and pressure) used to sterilize the contents of canned cat food destroys about 90%

of thiamine. Cat food manufacturers must therefore replenish canned cat food products with large amounts of thiamine to ensure that the 10% that survives canning will still be adequate to meet the needs of the cat.

Bracken-fern poisoning in horse and others

These ferns contain several toxic substances of importance to veterinary medicine. One of these toxins is a thiaminase that induces thiamine deficiency. Horses are more susceptible to thiamine deficiency than ruminants grazing the same pasture where bracken fern grows, probably because the rumen usually produces more thiamine than the cow needs. Horses with thiamine deficiency are anorexic, incoordinated, and have a typical crouching stance with an arched neck. Colonic spasms and convulsions are followed by death.

Polioencephalomalacia (cerebrocortical necrosis) in cattle (sheep)

Rumen microbial production of thiamine generally supplies the ruminant with all the thiamine it needs. However, abrupt changes in the diet, particularly the introduction of concentrates and corn silage, can interfere with microbial thiamine production or result in proliferation of microbes that produce thiaminases. High sulfite and sulfate diets may also interfere with thiamine activity in the rumen.

Low tissue thiamine levels result in energy-starved tissues, and in the brain leads to necrosis of glial cells and cortical neurons. The brain softens (**malacia**, **softening**) and the tissues **autofluoresce** under UV light, a simple diagnostic test post mortem. Affected animals are depressed and exhibit medial **strabismus** (cross-eyed) and are often blind (**cortical blindness**). In most cases, hyperesthesia, recumbency, and death follow. Intravenous thiamine treatment can save some animals.

Amprolium (coccidiostat)

Coccidia are single-celled parasites that affect the intestinal epithelium of many young animals and cause diarrhea with hemorrhage. These parasites are eukaryotes and require thiamine just like their host species. Amprolium mimics the structure of thiamine and acts as a competitive inhibitor of the mechanisms for uptake of thiamine by the coccidia. Amprolium will therefore cause a thiamine deficiency in the parasite preventing it from replicating. In small short-term doses the host animal can survive without thiamine. However, prolonged use of amprolium will induce a thiamine deficiency in the patient. Conversely, excess thiamine in the diet will reduce the anticoccidial actions of amprolium.

Vitamin C (ascorbic acid)

> **1** Describe the role of vitamin C in collagen synthesis.

Function

Ascorbic acid is involved in many of the oxidative reactions in the body. It is required for conversion of proline to hydroxyproline, a major constituent of bone and tissue collagen. It is an important antioxidant of the cytosol of cells throughout the body and this role may be especially important in immune cell function. It is also necessary for steroid synthesis in the adrenal cortex and for absorption of iron across the intestinal tract. In most species, ascorbic acid can be produced from glucose and the tissues synthesize all the ascorbic acid the animal requires. However, humans, most primates (an exception may be some prosimians), and guinea pigs lack the enzyme gulonolactone oxidase that converts L-gulonolactone to ascorbic acid.

Deficiency

Vitamin C-deficient primates and guinea pigs exhibit lethargy and muscle and joint pain. **Gingival hemorrhage**, loose teeth, and leukopenia will become evident as the deficiency progresses. In humans, these lesions were termed **scurvy** and were common in sailors who were out at sea for months at a time and who were fed no fruits. Commercial diets for primates and guinea pigs are generally well supplemented with vitamin C. However, problems are sometimes seen in diets of table scraps fed by well-meaning owners.

Self-evaluation

Answers can be found at the end of the chapter.

1 Why are animals suffering from vitamin A deficiency susceptible to respiratory infections?

2 A cat is brought in for you to examine that is exhibiting pain when walking. On radiographic examination, you notice new periosteal bone formation extending up the tendon sheaths. The cat's diet includes a large proportion of liver. What could be the problem?

3 How does vitamin D affect bone metabolism?

4 How does vitamin D affect intestinal calcium absorption?

5 What form of vitamin D is required by poultry? By New World monkeys?

6 What is the main antioxidant of cell membranes?

7 Accidental rodenticide ingestion in dogs and cats can involve two different vitamins. What are they and what is the mechanism of the toxicity?

8 Do ruminants require any of the B vitamins? Why?

9 Feeding raw eggs to your dog every day could lead to a deficiency of what vitamin? What symptoms would you expect to see?

10 Sheep that graze pasture low in cobalt may suffer from a vitamin deficiency? Why? What are the symptoms?

11 You place a group of turkey poults on a coccidiostat (drug to fight off Coccidia parasites). Two weeks later you are called because the turkey poults are acting strangely. They stand with their neck extended and gaze at the ground. What happened?

12 A group of beef steers on full feed are exhibiting neurologic signs that include circling and apparent blindness. As you stand watching them, one keels over dead. You do a necropsy and on examination of the brain you see areas of the cerebral cortex that appear soft and mushy. You pull out your black light (UV light) and the brain autofluoresces. What is your diagnosis? Explain to the owner how this occurs.

13 A child brings his guinea pig in for an examination. You examine the mouth and note that the teeth are loose and the animal has a scruffy looking hair coat. What do you suspect? How will you cure it?

Suggested reading

National Research Council (1985) *Nutrient Requirements of Dogs.* National Academy Press, Washington, DC.

National Research Council (1987) *Vitamin Tolerance of Animals.* National Academy Press, Washington, DC.

National Research Council (1998) *Nutrient Requirements of Swine,* 10th revised edn. National Academy Press, Washington, DC.

Weiss, W.P. (1998) Requirements of fat-soluble vitamins for dairy cows: a review. *Journal of Dairy Science* **81**:2493–2501.

Answers

1 Vitamin A is necessary for the maintenance of normal epithelial structure. During vitamin A deficiency the ciliated columnar epithelium of the bronchioles becomes a more squamous type, losing the ability to move mucus and the bacteria filtered and trapped within the mucus up and out of the respiratory tract.

2 Vitamin A toxicity. Sometimes liver can be a massive source of vitamin A. The calcification of tendons and spinal column is a common finding in vitamin A intoxication.

3 Vitamin D helps increase calcium and phosphorus absorption from the diet. This allows the animal to maintain normal blood calcium and phosphorus concentrations. This is necessary to allow mineralization of the organic matrix laid down by osteoblasts during bone formation.

4 The hormonal form of vitamin D, 1,25-dihydroxyvitamin D, interacts with its receptor located in the intestinal epithelial cells. This stimulates transcription and translation of genes coding for proteins involved in calcium absorption. Two examples are calcium-binding protein, which attaches to calcium at the luminal surface and carries it across the cell cytosol, and a Ca^{2+}-ATPase pump protein, which helps move calcium from the cell cytosol to the blood across the cell membrane.

5 Both have a requirement for vitamin D3. Neither can use vitamin D_2.

6 Vitamin E.

7 The first rodenticides contained coumarin types of compounds, which interfere with the action of vitamin K. This leads to blood coagulation problems causing the rodents (and dogs or cats) to die of internal hemorrhaging. The second type contains analogs of the hormonal form of vitamin D. These kill by causing excessive hypercalcemia and hyperphosphatemia, leading first to renal failure.

8 Not usually once they are fully ruminating. Rumen microbes can usually make all the B vitamins in quantities above the level required by the ruminant tissues.

9 Biotin, due to avidin in egg whites, which binds biotin making it unavailable. Biotin-deficient animals have poor hair coats and exhibit alopecia, scaly dermatitis, and achromotrichia (lack of hair color).

10 Rumen bacteria need to utilize the cobalt to produce cyanocobalamin for themselves and for the cow. Poor rumen function leads to reduced feed efficiency and growth primarily due to energy deficiency. The bacteria and the cow are unable to utilize energy-producing pathways requiring cyanocobalamin.

11 Some coccidiostats work by preventing folate production by Coccidia so that the Coccidia have no source of it thus stopping their growth. Unfortunately, occasionally it also causes folate deficiency in the animal because it can also reduce bacterial production of folate, important if no folate is added to the diet! Another important coccidiostat is amprolium. Amprolium interferes with thiamine uptake and the parasite develops thiamine deficiency preventing it from replicating. However, prolonged high doses cause thiamine deficiency. Thiamine-deficient birds exhibit opisthotonus: the head and neck are extended backwards to an extreme degree.

12 Thiamine deficiency. Occasionally, steers on full feed undergo rumen flora changes that do not favor the production of thiamine or favor the production of thiaminases within the rumen. The net effect is a lack of thiamine reaching the small intestine. Ruminant diets are generally not supplemented with B vitamins since they normally procure their B vitamins from the rumen flora. If the rumen does not deliver the thiamine to the intestine, the steers become thiamine deficient.

13 Scurvy. Start supplying the guinea pig with vitamin C every day.

SECTION VIII

Minerals, Bones, and Joints

Section Editor: Jesse P. Goff

49 Minerals

Jesse P. Goff

Iowa State University, Ames, IA, USA

Section VIII: Minerals, Bones, and Joints

Dukes' Physiology of Domestic Animals, Thirteenth Edition. Edited by William O. Reece, Howard H. Erickson, Jesse P. Goff and Etsuro E. Uemura.
© 2015 John Wiley & Sons, Inc. Published 2015 by John Wiley & Sons, Inc.
Companion website: www.wiley.com/go/reece/physiology

A number of inorganic elements have been shown to be essential for normal growth and reproduction of animals. Those required in greater quantities are referred to as **macrominerals** and this group includes calcium, phosphorus, sodium, chlorine, potassium, magnesium, and sulfur. The macrominerals are important structural components of bone and other tissues and serve as important constituents of body fluids. They play vital roles in the maintenance of acid–base balance, osmotic pressure, membrane electrical potential, and nervous transmission. Those elements required in much smaller amounts are referred to as the **trace minerals**. This group includes cobalt, copper, iodine, iron, manganese, molybdenum, selenium, zinc, and perhaps chromium and fluorine. Other elements have been suggested to be essential but these are generally not considered to be of practical importance. The trace minerals are present in body tissues in very low concentrations and often serve as components of metalloenzymes and enzyme cofactors, or as components of hormones of the endocrine system. A thorough discussion of the dietary requirements of each species for each mineral is beyond the scope of this chapter, and the reader is referred to the publications on nutrient requirements of domestic animals produced by the National Research Council of the National Academy of Science.

For all minerals considered essential, detrimental effects on animal performance can be demonstrated from feeding excessively high levels. Generally, the dietary level required for optimal performance is well below levels found to be detrimental to performance. However, toxicity from several of the essential minerals, including fluorine, selenium, molybdenum, and copper, are unfortunately problems that can occur under practical feeding conditions. The National Research Council's *Mineral Tolerance of Domestic Animals* (1980) describes signs of toxicosis and the dietary concentrations of minerals that are considered excessive. Certain elements such as lead, cadmium, and mercury are discussed because they should always be considered toxic and are of practical concern because toxicosis from these elements unfortunately occasionally occurs.

The goals of this chapter are to familiarize the veterinary student with (i) the role each mineral has in body functions; (ii) homeostatic mechanisms for each mineral; (iii) deficiency symptoms; (iv) toxicity symptoms; and (v) syndromes of special concern in veterinary medicine.

MACROMINERALS

Macrominerals are those minerals required by the body in large amounts each day. In general their concentration in a diet is expressed on the basis of percentage of the diet or in grams per kilogram diet.

Calcium

1 Where is the majority of the body's calcium stored?

2 What function does extracellular calcium have?

3 What function does intracellular calcium have?

4 What is the role of parathyroid hormone in calcium homeostasis?

5 What is the role of vitamin D in calcium homeostasis?

6 How does the horse regulate blood calcium concentration?

7 Why does the laying hen have a blood calcium concentration nearly twice that of a broiler chick?

8 What tissue is most affected when an animal is fed a low-calcium diet?

9 How does metabolic alkalosis affect calcium homeostasis in a cow at parturition?

10 What is lactation tetany?

Function

Extracellular calcium is essential for formation of skeletal tissues, transmission of nervous tissue impulses, excitation of skeletal and cardiac muscle contraction, blood clotting, and as a component of milk. Intracellular calcium, while only $1/_{10,000}$th the concentration of extracellular calcium, is involved in the activity of a wide array of enzymes and serves as an important second messenger conveying information from the surface of the cell to the interior of the cell.

About 98% of the calcium in the body is located within the skeleton where calcium, along with phosphate anion, serves to provide structural strength and hardness to bone. The other 2% of the calcium in the body is found primarily in the extracellular fluid. Normally, blood plasma calcium concentration is 2.2–2.5 mmol/L (9–10 mg/dL, or 4.4–5 mEq) in adult mammals, with slighty higher values in the young. Between 40 and 45% of total plasma calcium is bound to plasma proteins, primarily albumin, and another 5% is bound to organic components of the blood such as citrate or inorganic elements. Between 45 and 50% of total plasma calcium exists in the ionized soluble form; this value is closer to 50% at low blood pH and closer to 45% when blood pH is elevated. The ionized calcium concentration of the plasma must be maintained at a relatively constant value of 1–1.25 mmol/L to ensure normal function.

Extracellular calcium

1 Skeletal strength and hardness. Bone mineralization only occurs when plasma calcium and phosphorus concentrations are normal. Bone mineral has a chemical structure similar to the mineral hydroxyapatite, $Ca_{10}(PO_4)_6(OH)_2$. This means that 10 calcium atoms are deposited in bone for every 6 phosphate anions incorporated into bone. In addition to its structural role, the skeleton acts as a reservoir of calcium, which can be used to replenish extracellular calcium in times of need.

2 Extracellular calcium helps maintain resting nerve membrane potential. Extracellular calcium, being positively charged, increases the potential difference across the cell membrane. When extracellular calcium concentration falls, the potential difference between the positively charged extracellular fluid and the negatively charged intracellular fluid is reduced to a value that is much closer to the threshold for initiating an action potential. In many species hypocalcemia (low blood calcium) causes hyperexcitability of the nervous system resulting in tetany.

3 At the myoneural junction, when an action potential passes to the terminal end of the motor neuron the permeability of the nerve membrane to calcium is increased. The influx of calcium stimulates acetylcholine-containing vesicles to fuse with the nerve membrane, releasing the acetylcholine into the space separating the nerve and muscle cell membranes. The amount of acetylcholine released is directly related to the amount of calcium that enters the terminal end of the motor neuron, which is in turn dependent on extracellular calcium concentration. Hypocalcemia reduces the strength of muscle contraction. Magnesium competitively inhibits calcium entry into the motor neuron. The animal that is hypocalcemic and hypermagnesemic will be able to initiate only very weak muscle contractions. This condition is known as paresis.

Dairy cows often develop parturient paresis (see section Milk fever in dairy cows) as a result of hypocalcemia coupled with hypermagnesemia. Extracellular calcium concentration also influences the secretion of other substances by nerves and endocrine glands. For instance, the hypocalcemic cow is unable to secrete insulin from the pancreas and therefore becomes hyperglycemic.

4 Calcium is essential for blood clotting.

5 Action potentials in cardiac muscle involve a change in membrane conductance of sodium, potassium, and calcium. Contractions of the heart are weak during hypocalcemia due to incomplete depolarization of cardiac muscle fibrils. Clinically, the cardiac output will be reduced and the heart rate will often increase to try to compensate. On the other hand, severe hypercalcemia as occurs during intravenous administration of calcium can stop the heart in systole by preventing repolarization of cardiac muscle.

Intracellular calcium

1 Initiation of muscle cell contraction. Once an action potential is transmitted down a muscle fibril, the depolarized muscle cell releases calcium from the lateral sacs of the sarcoplasmic reticulum. The calcium binds to troponin, which permits cross-linking of actin and myosin resulting in muscle contraction.

2 Intracellular calcium serves as a second messenger to relay information from outside the cell to inside of the cell. For example, most peptide hormones cannot enter the target cell yet they initiate biological activity. However, interaction of hormones with their receptors can cause calcium channels in the cell membrane to open. Extracellular calcium rushes into the cell, raising the intracellular calcium concentration. Calcium-binding proteins such as calmodulin bind the calcium, which causes the shape of these proteins to change. Now the calcium–calmodulin complex can stimulate ion channels, enzyme activity, or DNA transcription to initiate a biological response by the cell.

Calcium homeostasis

Since calcium is so essential for life, vertebrates have evolved an elaborate system to maintain calcium homeostasis. This system attempts to maintain extracellular calcium concentration constant by increasing calcium entry into the extracellular fluid whenever there is loss of calcium from the extracellular compartment. When calcium loss exceeds entry hypocalcemia can occur. If calcium enters the extracellular compartment faster than it leaves, hypercalcemia can occur and can lead to soft-tissue deposition of calcium.

Calcium leaves the extracellular fluid during bone formation, as digestive secretions, sweat, and urine. An especially large loss of calcium to milk occurs during lactation in mammals and eggshell formation in birds. Calcium lost via these routes can be replaced from dietary calcium, from resorption of calcium stored in bone, or by resorbing a larger portion of the calcium

Section VIII: Minerals, Bones, and Joints

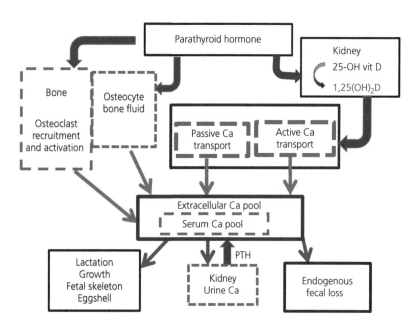

Figure 49.1 Calcium homeostasis. Parathyroid hormone is secreted in response to a decrease in serum calcium, which might be caused by the loss of calcium from the serum pool to lactation, growth, or fetal development. Calcium can also be lost in pancreatic secretions and bile, which is called endogenous fecal calcium loss. Parathyroid hormone increases renal tubular reabsorption of calcium to reduce urine calcium loss, increases osteocytic and osteoclastic bone calcium release, and stimulates the kidney to produce 1,25-dihydroxyvitamin D (1,25(OH)$_2$D). The 1,25(OH)$_2$D enhances the active transport of calcium across the intestinal tract. Calcium can also be absorbed paracellularly if diet calcium is high enough.

filtered across the renal glomerulus, i.e., reducing urinary calcium loss. Whenever calcium loss from the extracellular fluid exceeds the amount of calcium entering the extracellular fluid, there is a decrease in plasma calcium concentration. The parathyroid glands monitor carotid artery blood calcium concentration and secrete **parathyroid hormone** (PTH) when they sense a decrease in blood calcium (Figure 49.1). PTH immediately increases renal calcium reabsorption mechanisms to reduce urinary calcium loss. This will succeed in returning blood calcium concentration to normal if the loss from the extracellular compartment is small, since normally only a small amount of calcium is excreted in the urine each day. When calcium losses are larger, PTH will stimulate processes to enhance intestinal calcium absorption and resorption of bone calcium stores (Figure 49.1).

Bone osteocytes are embedded within the bone matrix. They are surrounded by lacunae and these are all interconnected by a series of canals called **canaliculi**. The fluid within the canaliculi and lacunae is relatively rich in calcium. PTH can stimulate the osteocytes to pump this calcium back into the extracellular fluid, known as **osteocytic osteolysis**. This returns a modest amount of calcium to the blood very quickly. When larger amounts of calcium are needed because a diet is not supplying adequate calcium, the animal can use **osteoclasts** to resorb solid bone. Bone is a living tissue that is constantly undergoing formation and resorption. In young animals the rate of formation by osteoblasts normally exceeds the rate of bone resorption by osteoclasts, resulting in net bone accretion. In mature animals, portions of the skeleton, presumably those traumatized with microfractures during normal wear and tear on the skeleton, are resorbed and re-formed constantly. In humans it is estimated that the entire adult skeleton is

rebuilt every 7 years. PTH can uncouple bone resorption from bone formation, stimulating resorptive mechanisms of bone osteoclasts while inhibiting formation mediated by bone osteoblasts. The net result is an efflux of calcium from bone to extracellular fluid.

Ultimately, dietary calcium must enter the extracellular fluid to permit optimal performance of the animal. Calcium absorption can occur by passive transport between epithelial cells across any portion of the digestive tract whenever ionized calcium in the digestive fluids directly over the mucosa exceeds about 1.5 mmol/L, though for practical reasons it likely must exceed 3–4 mmol/L to contribute greatly. Such concentrations are commonly reached when young animals are fed milk. In nonruminant species, studies suggest that as much as 50% of dietary calcium absorption can be passive. It is unknown how much passive absorption of calcium occurs from the diets typically fed ruminants but the diluting effect of the rumen would likely reduce the degree to which passive calcium absorption would occur.

Active transport of calcium is the second route for calcium absorption, and is especially important when diets are not high in calcium. Active transport of calcium is controlled by **1,25-dihydroxyvitamin D** [1,25-(OH)$_2$D], the hormone derived from vitamin D. Vitamin D, produced within the skin or provided in the diet, is converted to **25-hydroxyvitamin D** in the liver and can be further metabolized to 1,25-(OH)$_2$D in the kidneys. PTH indirectly stimulates intestinal calcium absorption because it is the primary regulator of renal production of 1,25-(OH)$_2$D. The 1,25-(OH)$_2$D is released to the circulation and interacts with nuclear receptors within the intestinal epithelium, primarily in the small intestine, causing transcription and translation of at least three calcium transport proteins. A **calcium channel protein** opens under the influence of 1,25-$(OH)_2D$, allowing charged Ca^{2+} ions to cross into the cytosol. They are too hydrophilic to cross the lipid membrane without the calcium channel proteins. **Vitamin D-dependent calcium-binding protein** captures calcium at the apical surface of epithelial cells and ferries the calcium to the basolateral side of the cell where it is pumped into the extracellular space against a concentration gradient by a 1,25-$(OH)_2D$-dependent **plasma membrane Ca^{2+}-ATPase pump** protein. By carefully regulating the amount of 1,25-$(OH)_2D$ produced, the amount of dietary calcium absorbed can be adjusted up or down to maintain constant extracellular calcium concentration. This is the strategy used by most mammals and birds, but not by hindgut fermenters (see next section).

If plasma calcium increases above normal concentrations, it could begin to be deposited into the soft tissues of the body (**metastatic calcification**). **Calcitonin** is a hormone produced by the thyroid gland in response to hypercalcemia. Calcitonin inhibits renal reabsorption of calcium from the glomerular filtrate, resulting in increased calcium excretion. It also inhibits bone calcium resorption, slowing entry of calcium into the extracellular fluid. Calcitonin is not often called on to restore calcium homeostasis unless a very high calcium diet such as milk is fed in a short period of time.

Special calcium homeostasis considerations

The horse and rabbit and perhaps wild hindgut fermenters use a different approach to maintain calcium homeostasis. In these species all the calcium available for absorption is absorbed from the diet independently of vitamin D. They then excrete the excess calcium via the urine to regulate plasma calcium concentration. Horse and rabbit urine tends to be high in calcium and can take on a chalky appearance. Renal excretion is regulated by PTH just as in other species and bone resorption can be stimulated if dietary calcium is too low to meet the needs of the animal. An interesting consequence of this adaptation is that vitamin D is not required by these two species, though they are still susceptible to vitamin D intoxication. Also, a common hallmark of renal failure in these species is hypercalcemia.

Birds have another special adaptation that allows them to maintain calcium homeostasis during the calcium stress associated with formation of the eggshell. Estrogen produced by the ovary stimulates the liver to produce a calcium-binding protein that circulates in the blood. As a result the blood total calcium concentration can be 20–25 mg/dL in the laying hen. Ionized calcium remains at about 5 mg/dL as in mammals and nonlaying hens. This large amount of calcium in the plasma can act as another reservoir of calcium the animal can draw on during eggshell formation.

Dietary sources

Calcium within mineral supplements such as calcium carbonate or calcium chloride is generally more available than calcium in forages and common feedstuffs. The more soluble, the better the absorbability. Grains are poor sources of calcium and animals fed high-grain diets are at risk of becoming calcium deficient. Forages are better sources of calcium, with legumes being especially high in calcium. Unfortunately, forage calcium availability can be low due to the presence of oxalates that render the calcium insoluble.

The amount of available calcium that will actually be absorbed varies with the physiological state of the animal. The efficiency of absorption of calcium decreases as animals age. Young animals absorb calcium very efficiently while very old animals absorb calcium poorly. As animals age there is a decline in vitamin D receptors in the intestinal tract, which is thought to reduce the ability to respond to 1,25-$(OH)_2D$.

Deficiency

When dietary calcium is insufficient to meet the requirements of the animal, calcium will be withdrawn from bone to maintain normal extracellular calcium concentration. If dietary calcium is severely deficient for a prolonged period, the animal will develop severe bone lesions; yet, because the desire to maintain extracellular calcium concentration is so strong, plasma calcium will only be slightly lower than normal values. Dietary calcium deficiency in young animals leads to failure to mineralize new bone and contributes to retarded growth. **Rickets** is more commonly caused by vitamin D or phosphorus deficiency but calcium deficiency can contribute to rickets as well. In older animals dietary calcium deficiency forces the animal to withdraw calcium from bone for homeostasis of the extracellular fluid. This causes **osteoporosis** and **osteomalacia** in the bones, which makes the bone prone to spontaneous fractures. Milk calcium concentration is not altered even during severe dietary calcium deficiency.

In early lactation nearly all mammals, but especially cows, are in negative calcium balance. To maintain normal blood calcium concentrations the animal will remove calcium from the bones. This is referred to as **lactational osteoporosis**. In dairy cows, between 800 and 1300 g of calcium (up to 13% of skeletal calcium) is lost in early lactation. It is replaced in later lactation provided the cow is fed adequate dietary calcium.

Low-calcium diets fed to laying hens will result in very thin shelled eggs. The hen will utilize calcium from her bone also and prolonged feeding of a diet inadequate in calcium will lead to a syndrome of osteoporosis and leg fracture known as **caged layer fatigue**.

Toxicity

Feeding excessive dietary calcium is generally not associated with any specific toxicity. Feeding excessive calcium could interfere with trace mineral absorption (especially zinc, see section Parakeratosis of swine) and replace energy or protein the animal might better utilize for increased production. In ruminants, feeding calcium in excess of requirements has been suggested to improve performance, especially on corn silage diets. Since calcium is a strong cation, addition of calcium carbonate to diets above that required to meet absorbed calcium needs may be providing a rumen alkalinizing effect to enhance performance.

Syndromes of special concern in veterinary medicine

Milk fever in dairy cows

Milk fever affects about 5% of the dairy cows in the USA each year. In these cows the calcium homeostatic mechanisms, which normally maintain blood calcium concentration at 9–10 mg/dL, fail and the lactational drain of calcium causes blood calcium concentration to fall below 5 mg/dL. This hypocalcemia impairs muscle and nerve function to such a degree that the cow is unable to rise. Intravenous calcium treatments are used to keep the milk fever cow alive long enough for intestinal and bone calcium homeostatic mechanisms to adapt.

An important determinant of milk fever risk is the acid–base status of the cow at the time of parturition. Metabolic alkalosis impairs the physiological activity of PTH so that bone resorption and production of 1,25-$(OH)_2D$ is impaired, reducing the ability to successfully adjust to the calcium demands of lactation. Evidence suggests that metabolic alkalosis induces conformational changes in the PTH receptor that prevent tight binding of PTH to its receptor. Cows fed diets that are relatively high in potassium or sodium are in a relative state of metabolic alkalosis, which increases the likelihood that they will not successfully adapt to the calcium demands of lactation and will develop milk fever. These cows exhibit a temporary pseudohypoparathyroidism at parturition. The parathyroid glands recognize the onset of hypocalcemia and secrete adequate PTH. However, the tissues respond only poorly to the PTH, leading to inadequate osteoclastic bone resorption and renal 1,25-$(OH)_2D$ production.

Since metabolic alkalosis is an important factor in the etiology of milk fever, it is important to prevent metabolic alkalosis. Dry cow diets that are high in potassium and/or sodium alkalinize the cow's blood and increase susceptibility to milk fever. Adding calcium to practical prepartum diets does not increase the incidence of milk fever. It is now recognized that addition of anions to the prepartum diet can prevent milk fever. Ammonium, calcium and magnesium salts of chloride and sulfate have been successfully used as acidifying anion sources. Chloride salts are more acidogenic than sulfate salts. Hydrochloric acid has also been successfully utilized as a source of anions for prevention of milk fever and is the most potent and palatable of the anion sources available.

A second common cause of hypocalcemia and milk fever in the periparturient cow is hypomagnesemia. Low blood magnesium can reduce PTH secretion from the parathyroid glands causing temporary hypoparathyroidism and can also alter the responsiveness of tissues to PTH by inducing conformational changes in the PTH receptor, again causing temporary pseudohypoparathyroidism.

Lactation tetany of bitches, mares, and sows

Animals that have been lactating heavily for several weeks such as Chihuahua bitches nursing several pups or white breed sows nursing many piglets may not be able to maintain calcium homeostasis. In general this is because the diet being fed is inadequate in calcium and the rate at which bone calcium stores are resorbed is inadequate to maintain normal calcium in blood. Most will exhibit varying degrees of tetany and muscle paresis. Sows often exhibit broken bones. They will respond to parenteral calcium administration and increased dietary calcium provided the bones have not already fractured.

Phosphorus

> **1** How does parathyroid hormone affect blood phosphorus concentration?
>
> **2** How does vitamin D affect blood phosphorus concentration?
>
> **3** What is the role of phosphorus in a cow's salivary secretions?
>
> **4** How does phosphorus deficiency affect bone in the young animal and in the adult?

Function

Most of the phosphorus found in the body is combined with oxygen to form the **phosphate anion**. It is second only to calcium as the major component of bone mineral. Phosphate is a component of phospholipids, phosphoproteins, nucleic acids, and energy-transferring molecules such as ATP and is therefore involved in every major metabolic pathway in the body. Phosphate anion is an essential component of the acid–base buffer system. Most references refer to blood and tissue phosphorus concentration. This would be better expressed as the phosphate concentration because that is the biologically relevant form of phosphorus.

Phosphorus homeostasis

Plasma phosphorus concentration is normally 1.3–2.6 mmol/L or 4–8 mg/dL. Intracellular phosphorus concentration is about 25 mmol/L or 78 mg/dL. About 30% of blood phosphorus is present as inorganic phosphate anion; the rest is incorporated into organic molecules such as proteins and cell membrane phospholipids. It is the inorganic phosphate anion that is measured by standard assays that determine blood phosphorus concentration. Maintaining the extracellular phosphorus pool involves replacing phosphorus removed for bone and muscle growth, endogenous fecal loss, urinary phosphorus loss, and milk production with phosphorus absorbed from the diet or resorbed from bone.

Phosphorus is primarily absorbed in the small intestine via an active transport process that is responsive to 1,25-$(OH)_2D$.

Intestinal phosphorus absorption efficiency can be upregulated during periods of phosphorus deficiency as renal production of 1,25-$(OH)_2D$ is directly stimulated by very low plasma phosphorus. Plasma phosphorus concentrations are well correlated with dietary phosphorus absorption. Phosphorus absorbed in excess of needs is excreted in urine and saliva.

PTH, secreted during periods of calcium stress, increases renal and salivary excretion of phosphorus, which can be detrimental to maintenance of normal blood phosphorus concentrations. This is one reason that hypocalcemic animals tend to become hypophosphatemic. PTH could conceivably increase blood phosphorus concentration since it stimulates bone mineral resorption. However, PTH is secreted in response to hypocalcemia not hypophosphatemia. This means that phosphorus homeostasis and calcium homeostasis are sometimes at odds.

Dietary sources

Phosphorus is found in high amounts in grain and lower amounts in forage. Unfortunately, 35–70% of the phosphorus found in plant materials is bound to **phytic acid**, an organic acid of plants. Phytate-bound phosphorus is practically unavailable to monogastric animals. Inorganic mineral sources of phosphorus such as sodium phosphate or dicalcium phosphate are highly available and often incorporated into the diet of animals.

Phosphorus utilization in ruminants

Salivary secretions remove 30–90 g phosphorus from the extracellular phosphorus pool each day, with higher amounts secreted when dietary phosphorus is high. Salivary phosphorus secretions supply rumen microbes with a readily available source of phosphorus, and this appears necessary for cellulose digestion. Most, but not all, the salivary phosphorus secreted is recovered by intestinal absorption. Rumen microbes are able to digest phytic acid so that nearly all the phytate-bound phosphorus, the major form of phosphorus in plants, is available for absorption in ruminants.

Deficiency

Moderate chronic hypophosphatemia, with plasma phosphorus concentrations of 0.64–1.3 mmol/L or 2–4 mg/dL, is generally recognized only as animals that perform poorly. Growth and fertility are impaired. With more severe hypophosphatemia, the performance of the animals becomes very poor and feed intake of the animals is depressed. The reduction in feed intake is often accompanied by **pica**, or abnormal appetite, with a particular desire for soil, flesh, and bones. Pica can cause problems for phosphorus-deficient animals. Outbreaks of **botulism** in cattle in South Africa and other parts of the world where phosphorus deficiency is endemic and the cattle are desperate for phosphate have been traced to consumption of carcasses of wild animals that had died on the veldt and contained toxin as a result of the growth of *Clostridium botulinum* during putrefaction. Recumbency and paresis can be observed once plasma phosphorus concentrations fall below 0.3 mmol/L or 1 mg/dL. This syndrome is referred to as the **downer phosphorus cow** and is occasionally seen as a sequela to milk fever.

Rickets and osteomalacia

Rickets is a disease of young growing animals in which the cartilaginous matrix at the growth plate and the osteoid matrix formed during bone remodeling fail to mineralize. In adults (no active growth plates) the term **osteomalacia** is used to describe the failure of osteoid matrix to mineralize. Calcium and phosphate ions combine in a ratio of 10 calcium ions to 6 phosphate ions at the point of mineralization of the bone cartilage or osteoid matrix. Failure to supply phosphorus in the diet will result in low plasma phosphorus concentrations, which will not support the mineralization process, and the bone matrices fail to mineralize. Bone phosphorus released during the process of bone remodeling, which is normally incorporated into the new bone being formed, is instead used to maintain plasma phosphorus concentration.

Young growing animals will exhibit joint pain and reluctance to move. Growth rate will be greatly depressed. The animals have narrow chests and the costochondral joints are enlarged and readily palpable. Adult animals with osteomalacia exhibit joint pain, joint enlargement, and lameness. Impaired pelvic bone growth in heifers raised on phosphorus-deficient diets may result in **dystocia**, or difficulty in calving, later in life.

Toxicity

Excessive dietary phosphorus can interfere with calcium absorption but the ratio of dietary calcium to phosphorus generally has to be less than 1 : 5 for this to occur. Dietary ratios are not as important as the total amounts of mineral being fed to the animal. The exception may be the horse and rabbit, where dietary phosphate seems to interfere with calcium absorption more than in other species.

Syndromes of special concern in veterinary medicine

Acute hypophosphatemia in ruminants

Beef cows fed a diet marginal in phosphorus will have a chronic hypophosphatemia of 0.6–1.1 mmol/L or 2–3.5 mg/dL. In late gestation, plasma phosphorus can decline precipitously as the growth of the fetus accelerates and removes substantial amounts of phosphorus from the maternal circulation. These animals often become recumbent and are unable to rise, though they appear fairly alert and will eat feed placed in front of them. Cows carrying twins are most often affected. Plasma phosphorus concentration in these recumbent animals is often less than 0.3 mmol/L or 1 mg/dL. The disease is usually complicated by concurrent hypocalcemia, hypomagnesemia, and in some cases hypoglycemia (see section Pregnancy toxemia in Chapter 47).

At the onset of lactation the production of colostrum and milk draws large amounts of phosphorus out of the extracellular phosphorus pools. This alone will often cause an acute decline in plasma phosphorus levels. In addition, if the animal is also developing hypocalcemia, PTH will be secreted in large amounts, which increases urinary and salivary loss of phosphorus. Cortisol, secreted around parturition, may further depress plasma phosphorus concentrations. In dairy cows, plasma phosphorus concentrations routinely fall below the normal range at parturition and in cows with milk fever plasma phosphorus concentrations are often 0.3–0.6 mmol/L or 1–2 mg/dL. Plasma phosphorus concentrations usually increase rapidly following treatment of the hypocalcemic cow with intravenous calcium solutions. This rapid recovery is due to reduction in PTH secretion, reducing urinary and salivary loss of phosphorus, and resumption of gastrointestinal motility accompanied by increased plasma concentrations of 1,25-$(OH)_2D$, which allows absorption of dietary phosphorus and reabsorption of salivary phosphorus secretions.

Some animals developing acute hypophosphatemia do not recover normal plasma phosphorus concentration. This is sometimes the case in cows that are classified as "downer cows." This syndrome often begins as milk fever but, unlike the typical milk fever cow, plasma phosphorus remains low in some of these cows despite successful treatment of the hypocalcemia. Protracted hypophosphatemia in these cows appears to be an important factor in the inability of these animals to rise to their feet, but why plasma phosphorus remains low is unclear.

Magnesium

> 1 What role does magnesium have in nerve conduction and muscle contraction?
>
> 2 Explain how renal reabsorption of magnesium regulates blood magnesium concentration.
>
> 3 Describe at least three factors that influence magnesium absorption across the rumen wall.

Function
Intracellular magnesium

Magnesium is a major intracellular cation that is a necessary cofactor for enzymatic reactions vital to every major metabolic pathway. Magnesium cation interacts with the negatively charged adenosine triphosphate (ATP) to form **Mg-ATP**, a substrate for most kinase-catalyzed reactions. **Adenylate cyclase**, responsible for producing the second messenger cyclic AMP; acyl-CoA synthetase, which plays a role in β-oxidation of fatty acids; and succinyl-CoA synthetase, a key enzyme in the citrate cycle are all magnesium-dependent enzymes. Glycolysis involves seven key enzymes that require magnesium alone or in asssociation with ATP or AMP. The intracellular magnesium concentration is about 13 mmol/L, making it the second most abundant cation found inside of cells.

Extracellular magnesium

Magnesium is vital to normal nerve conduction. Plasma magnesium concentration is normally 0.75–1.0 mmol/L or 1.8–2.4 mg/dL. Just as with calcium, a reduction in extracellular magnesium reduces the nerve membrane potential closer to the threshold for an action potential to occur. Also, an increase in the ratio of calcium to magnesium at the myoneural junction increases the release of acetylcholine into the myoneural junction. Hypomagnesemia causes tetany. Normal bone formation also requires magnesium. About one magnesium atom is substituted for every 40th calcium atom in the hydroxyapatite mineral of bone.

Magnesium homeostasis

Despite the importance of magnesium, there is no hormonal mechanism concerned principally and directly with magnesium homeostasis. The kidneys play a key role in maintaining magnesium homeostasis, but only under conditions of hypermagnesemia. If dietary magnesium is absorbed in excess of needs, plasma magnesium concentration rises above the renal threshold for reabsorption of magnesium and the excess is excreted into the urine. The **renal threshold for magnesium** (i.e., the plasma magnesium concentration at which all magnesium filtered across the glomerulus is reabsorbed) is 0.75–0.90 mmol/L or 1.8–2.2 mg/dL. Plasma magnesium concentrations below these levels indicate that dietary magnesium absorption is not sufficient and little or no magnesium will be detected in urine. PTH, released in response to hypocalcemia, raises the renal threshold for both calcium and magnesium. The result is that during hypocalcemia plasma magnesium concentrations will increase if dietary magnesium absorption is adequate. This is often the case in cows suffering from milk fever. If plasma magnesium is below 0.75 mmol/L or 1.8 mg/dL (suggesting inadequate dietary magnesium absorption), raising the renal threshold further will not increase plasma magnesium.

Bone is not a significant source of magnesium that can be utilized in times of magnesium deficit, as bone resorption occurs in response to calcium homeostasis, not magnesium status. Maintenance of normal plasma magnesium concentration is nearly totally dependent on a constant supply of dietary magnesium.

Magnesium is absorbed primarily from the ileum and colon of monogastric animals and young ruminants. Magnesium absorption is by passive absorption and is therefore dependent on the concentration of magnesium ions in the digesta. As the rumen and reticulum develop, these organs become the main, and perhaps only, site for magnesium absorption in adult ruminants. In adult ruminants the small intestine is a site of net secretion of magnesium.

Deficiency

Magnesium deficiency causes hyperexcitability and muscle twitching. Cerebrospinal fluid magnesium is in equilibrium with plasma so that when plasma magnesium concentration falls, cerebrospinal fluid magnesium concentration falls, which can lead to clonic convulsions. In many species hypomagnesemia is associated with calcification of soft tissues of the body. There is also an association between hypomagnesemia and atherosclerotic lesions.

Magnesium forms a complex with the G-proteins that interact with the PTH receptor. During hypomagnesemia the PTH receptor function is compromised so that hypocalcemia often accompanies hypomagnesemia.

Toxicity

Animals can excrete large amounts of magnesium in the urine so magnesium toxicity is not a practical problem in most species. The negative effects of high-magnesium diets are generally restricted to causing a reduction in feed intake (most magnesium salts are not very palatable, especially magnesium sulfate and magnesium chloride) and/or inducing an osmotic diarrhea.

Syndromes of special concern in veterinary medicine

Hypomagnesemic syndromes of cattle and ewes

Hypomagnesemic tetany is most often associated with beef cows and ewes in early lactation grazing lush pastures high in potassium and nitrogen and low in magnesium and sodium. This is the most common situation and is often referred to as **grass tetany**, **spring tetany**, **grass staggers** or **lactation tetany**. Magnesium deficiency occurs most often in spring or fall when pastures are growing at maximal rates, and is most common in grazing lactating ruminants as milk production removes 0.15 g magnesium from the blood for each liter of milk produced. Ewes suckling more than one lamb and higher-producing cows are at greatest risk. Magnesium must be constantly ingested as it cannot be mobilized from body tissues to maintain normal plasma magnesium concentrations. Conditions associated with hypomagnesemia as a result of feed restriction include transport over long distance (**transport tetany**) or sudden exposure to inclement weather. Cows can also develop hypomagnesemia in late gestation, which is often associated with, and complicated by, inadequate energy intake. This syndrome is sometimes referred to as **winter tetany** and is seen in animals turned out in winter to feed on crop residues such as corn stalks or straw. Animals grazing wheat pasture (**wheat pasture tetany**) or other early-growth cereal forages can develop hypomagnesemia with concurrent severe hypocalcemia, resulting in a clinical picture that more closely resembles milk fever. Hypomagnesemia can also occur in calves, especially if fed only milk or milk replacer beyond the first 2 months of age (**milk tetany**).

Magnesium deficiency is a common problem in ruminants, so some detail on magnesium metabolism in ruminants is presented. Magnesium absorption from the rumen is dependent on the concentration of magnesium in solution in the rumen fluid and the integrity of the magnesium transport mechanism, which is a sodium-linked active transport process.

The soluble concentration of magnesium in rumen fluid is dependent on the following.

1 Dietary magnesium content: low-magnesium forages and inadequate supplementation will keep soluble magnesium content low. Cool weather, common in spring and fall when pastures are growing rapidly, reduces plant tissue uptake of magnesium as does potassium fertilization of pastures.

2 The pH of the rumen fluid greatly affects magnesium solubility. Magnesium solubility declines sharply as rumen pH rises above 6.5. Grazing animals tend to have higher rumen pH because of the high potassium content of pasture and the stimulation of salivary buffer secretion associated with grazing. Heavily fertilized, lush pastures are often high in nonprotein nitrogen and relatively low in readily fermentable carbohydrates. The ability of the rumen microbes to incorporate the nonprotein nitrogen into microbial protein is exceeded and ammonia and ammonium ion build up in the rumen, increasing rumen pH. When high-grain rations are fed, rumen fluid pH is often below 6.5 and magnesium solubility is generally adequate.

3 Forage can often contain 100–200 mmol/kg of unsaturated palmitic, linoleic, and linolenic acids, which can form insoluble magnesium salts. Plants also can contain *trans*-aconitic acid or citric acid. A metabolite of *trans*-aconitic acid, **tricarballylate**, can complex magnesium and is resistant to rumen degradation, but its role in hypomagnesemic tetany is unclear.

The major factor affecting magnesium transport across the rumen epithelium is high dietary potassium, which can reduce the absorption of magnesium. Lambs switched from a low-potassium diet (0.6% K) to a high-potassium diet (4.9% K) had about a 50% reduction in apparent magnesium absorption. High potassium concentrations in the rumen fluid cause the apical membrane of the rumen epithelium to depolarize, reducing the transepithelial membrane potential responsible for propelling rumen fluid magnesium into the blood.

Feline urolithiasis syndrome

About 10% of the male cat population seen in veterinary practice will be suffering from **uroliths**. These "plugged" tom cats usually have **struvite crystals** composed of magnesium ammonium phosphate hexahydrate blocking the urethra. High-magnesium diets, especially if dietary calcium is marginal, may increase the incidence of feline urolithiasis syndrome. A high-magnesium diet alone is unlikely to cause uroliths to form. Viral infection by Manx calicivirus, feline herpesvirus, or feline paramyxovirus may also precede formation of struvite stones in cats. Unfortunately, these viruses are common among cats. The restriction of dietary magnesium has been commonly practiced as a means of preventing feline urolithiasis syndrome, though it is more important that the animal produce dilute acidic urine to prevent stone formation.

Sodium

> **1** What is the role of renin in maintenance of normal blood sodium concentration?
>
> **2** What is the role of aldosterone in maintenance of blood sodium concentration?
>
> **3** What is the role of atrial natriuretic peptide in maintenance of blood sodium concentration?

Function

Sodium is the chief cation of the extracellular fluid and plays a pivotal role in maintaining osmotic pressure and water content (extracellular volume) of the circulation. As one of the strong ions of the blood, it plays a key role in acid–base balance of the body. Sodium is the key extracellular mineral determining the electrical potential of nervous tissue and plays an important role in transmission of nerve impulses. Efficient absorption of monosaccharides and some amino acids is dependent on sodium-coupled transport processes.

Feeding sodium without chloride (e.g., sodium bicarbonate or sodium propionate) to an animal will alkalinize the blood.

Extracellular sodium concentration is tightly regulated and is generally maintained at 135–155 mmol/L, depending on the species of animal. Intracellular sodium concentration is about one-tenth that of the extracellular fluid. Maintaining this gradient is vital to maintenance of the electrical potential across cell membranes and is essential for the transport of nearly every other substance in or out of the cell. Perhaps 40% (some estimates are even higher) of the energy utilized by the body is dedicated to pumping sodium out of the cells of the body via Na^+/K^+-ATPase electrogenic pumps.

Sodium homeostasis

Detailed descriptions of the mechanisms the body uses to maintain total body sodium and plasma sodium concentration are described in Sections III and VI. Briefly, a decrease in extracellular volume or blood volume results in a decrease in renal perfusion, which causes the kidney to release **renin** from the **juxtaglomerular apparatus**. Renin is an enzyme capable of converting **angiotensinogen**, which circulates in the blood, to **angiotensin** I. Angiotensin I then undergoes conversion to **angiotensin** II within the lungs. Angiotensin II stimulates sodium reabsorption within the renal proximal tubule. More importantly, angiotensin II stimulates the secretion of **aldosterone** from the cortex of the adrenal glands. Aldosterone enhances renal reabsorption of sodium within the cortical collecting tubules and medullary collecting ducts while enhancing renal secretion of potassium.

Excessive extracellular volume stimulates the release of **atrial natriuretic peptide** from myocardial cells within the atria. Atrial natriuretic peptide inhibits renal reabsorption of sodium, resulting in a reduction in plasma sodium. It also reduces production of angiotensin II and release of aldosterone.

Dietary sodium is absorbed with about 90% efficiency at all times. About 50–60% of dietary sodium is absorbed by passive diffusion; another 20–45% is cotransported with other ions and substrates, some by passive and some by active transport processes.

Deficiency

Plants contain only small amounts of sodium, leaving herbivores at risk of becoming sodium deficient if salt is not added to the diet. Sodium-deficient animals develop an intense craving for salt leading to pica, with licking and chewing of various objects. Prolonged sodium deficiency leads to an unthrifty animal with rough hair coat, haggard appearance, and poor growth and productivity. Severe deficiency leads to shivering, incoordination, weakness, and cardiac arrhythmia. Cows will produce less milk. Horses deprived of sodium tire easily and have trouble sweating, reducing their tolerance for work.

Toxicity

Animals can tolerate very high levels of dietary salt if water is provided and the kidneys are functioning. They simply excrete the excess via the kidneys. High dietary salt (sodium chloride) will reduce feed intake in animals. Grain intake in cattle fed ad lib can be limited by including 4–5% salt into the ration.

Syndromes of special concern in veterinary medicine

Diarrhea

Sodium is lost from the body when animals suffer from diarrhea. The loss from secretory diarrheas is greater than from malabsorptive diarrheas but in either case total body sodium can fall to the point that it causes a severe decline in extracellular fluid volume, leading to circulatory collapse, and metabolic acidosis.

Wet poultry droppings

Birds fed too much sodium will excrete the sodium in their urine. A certain amount of water must accompany each sodium ion excreted making the droppings wet, a major problem when it occurs in modern poultry facilities.

Salt toxicity

The term **salt toxicity** is a misnomer as this syndrome is more properly due to lack of water. It affects many species, although swine and poultry seem particularly susceptible. It happens in summer (dry watering sources) and in winter (frozen water pipes to barns). With water deprivation, sodium concentrations within the cerebrospinal fluid increase. When the animal is then allowed unlimited access to water, the water quickly enters the cerebrospinal fluid due to its high osmolarity, causing **brain edema** and neurological impairment. Incoordination and staggering are commonly observed followed by convulsions and death. Water will cure the animal but access to water must be limited and given in small increments until the animal is rehydrated.

Chloride

> 1 Explain how chloride and bicarbonate anions work together to allow carbon dioxide to be transported by red blood cells.
>
> 2 Why do cows with a displaced abomasum often suffer from a metabolic alkalosis?

Function

Chloride is the chief anion of the extracellular fluid and plays a role in maintaining osmotic pressure and water content (extracellular volume) of the circulation. As one of the strong ions of the blood, it plays a key role in acid–base balance of the body. Chloride also plays a small role in determining the electrical potential of nervous tissue.

Chloride is pumped into the lumen of the stomach to form hydrochloric acid, which aids in digestion. Chloride also plays a vital role in oxygen and carbon dioxide transport by red blood cells, the so-called "chloride shift." As red blood cells pass through capillary beds, they pick up carbon dioxide, which is converted to the bicarbonate (HCO_3^-) anion. As bicarbonate diffuses from the red blood cell into the plasma, a chloride anion enters the cell to maintain electrochemical neutrality. On reaching the lungs the carbon dioxide leaves the plasma and red blood cells and chloride reenters the plasma.

Extracellular chloride concentration is 100–113 mmol/L, depending on the species of animal and their blood acid–base status. Intracellular chloride concentration is about one-tenth that of the extracellular fluid. This gradient is maintained largely by the electrical potential of the cells (outside positive with respect to the inside), which draws chloride out of the cells. This gradient is maintained by the Na^+/K^+-ATPase pumps.

Chloride homeostasis

Dietary chloride is absorbed with at least 80% and closer to 100% efficiency. The kidneys excrete chloride that is in excess of that needed to produce stomach acid, intestinal secretions, and sweat and to maintain acid–base balance in the animal. Often chloride anions accompany the movement of sodium cations.

Deficiency

Chloride deficiency can result in metabolic alkalosis and hypovolemia. Less severe deficiency can cause lethargy and poor performance. It rarely occurs if salt is fed. If salt is not fed, sodium deficiency will generally occur long before chloride deficiency.

Toxicity

Feeding high amounts of chloride unaccompanied by sodium or potassium (e.g., feeding ammonium chloride or calcium chloride) will induce metabolic acidosis which can be life-threatening. Fed in high amounts it can have the same toxic effects as sodium in terms of increasing the osmolarity of the blood and cerebrospinal fluid.

Syndromes of special concern in veterinary medicine
Displaced abomasum of ruminants

During **displacement of the abomasum** chloride secreted as hydrochloric acid becomes sequestered within the lumen of the abomasum. Depending on the severity of the displacement and whether or not there is also abomasal torsion, the chloride may not be available for reabsorption in the small intestine. This results in metabolic alkalosis, which adds to the depression observed in cows with this disease.

Diarrhea

Chloride along with sodium is lost from the body when animals suffer from diarrhea. The loss from secretory diarrheas is greater (toxins actually stimulate chloride secretion) than that from malabsorptive diarrheas, but in either case total body chloride can fall to the point that it causes a severe decline in extracellular fluid volume, leading to circulatory collapse. It should be noted that potassium and sodium losses tend to be greater than chloride losses during diarrhea as the colon absorbs chloride fairly well, even during many types of diarrhea.

Potassium

> 1 What is the role of potassium in extracellular fluid?
>
> 2 What is the relationship between insulin secretion and blood potassium concentration?
>
> 3 How does aldosterone secretion affect blood potassium concentration?
>
> 4 Explain why some Quarter Horse bloodlines result in hyperkalemia and spastic muscle contraction.

Potassium is the major intracellular cation of the body. It serves the same functions that sodium does in the extracellular fluid: it maintains intracellular fluid volume and acid–base balance. Inside most cells the concentration of potassium is around 150 mmol/L; outside the cells, potassium concentration in plasma and other extracellular fluids is 3–6 mmol/L.

Functions

Potassium is a major determinant of cell resting membrane potential. The inside of a cell is negative compared to the outside because the Na^+/K^+-ATPase pump moves 2 K^+ into the cell for every 3 Na^+ it moves into the extracellular fluid. The positive electrical charge of potassium tends to keep potassium within the cell. However, potassium concentration outside the cell is lower than inside the cell, which will cause potassium to flow out of the cell down its concentration gradient until the electromotive force keeping potassium within the cell is equal to the chemical gradient force moving potassium out of the cell. When this occurs the electrical potential across the cell is about –90 mV, with the inside of the cell negative. The actual electrical potential across cells is slightly less negative because sodium ions are continually leaking into the cell. The majority of ion channels that are open in the resting cell are potassium channels. Therefore variations in the potassium concentration gradient will have large effects on resting membrane potential, which can be calculated according to the Nernst equation:

$$\text{Membrane potential} = 61.5 \times \log([K]_i / [K]_o)$$

where $[K]_i$ is potassium concentration inside the cell and $[K]_o$ is potassium concentration outside the cell. A small decline in extracellular potassium concentration will have a dramatic effect on the cell resting membrane potential. For example, under normal conditions when $[K]_i$ is 150 mmol/L and $[K]_o$ is 4 mmol/L, the concentration ratio is 38 : 1 and the predicted membrane potential is –97 mV. If plasma potassium falls to 2 mmol/L, the ratio becomes 75 : 1 (150/2) and the predicted membrane potential increases to –115 mV, making the cell much less likely to reach the threshold potential for an action potential. An increase in plasma potassium to 6 mmol/L decreases the $[K]_i/[K]_o$ ratio to 25 : 1 and the resting membrane potential becomes –86 mV, closer to the threshold for opening the sodium channels in the cell to initiate an action potential.

Potassium is necessary for growth. Incorporation of amino acids into proteins is dependent on normal intracellular potassium concentration. Also potassium is required for normal secretion of insulin, so impaired growth during potassium deficiency may also be due to relative insulin deficiency.

Potassium is also important in blood acid–base balance. When blood becomes acidic, hydrogen ions enter the intracellular fluid compartment in exchange for potassium ions. This makes the blood less acidic but also causes hyperkalemia. Conversely, when the blood becomes alkaline, hydrogen ions leave the cells and enter the blood in exchange for extracellular potassium ions, which can then result in hypokalemia.

Metabolism and regulation

Nearly all the dietary potassium is absorbed across the intestinal tract as a consequence of bulk fluid absorption. Most diets contain more than adequate amounts of potassium to supply the potassium needed by the body for maintenance, growth, pregnancy, and lactation. The kidneys excrete the excess absorbed potassium. High blood potassium concentration (hyperkalemia) can directly stimulate secretion of aldosterone by the adrenal glands. The mineralocorticoid activity of aldosterone enhances renal secretion of potassium in exchange for sodium ions. Aldosterone, being a steroid hormone, must bind to a nuclear receptor and initiate transcription and translation of proteins involved in sodium and potassium transport. It is important to point out that dietary potassium can enter the extracellular fluids very rapidly following a meal, while the kidney will take several hours to excrete the excess potassium in response to the aldosterone. Gastrointestinal secretion of potassium can work with the kidneys to help prevent hyperkalemia but it is the intracellular uptake of potassium following a meal that helps buffer blood potassium concentration. This intracellular uptake of potassium is mediated by insulin, which is secreted in response to hyperglycemia induced by a meal or in response to elevated plasma potassium concentration. Insulin increases the activity of the Na⁺/K⁺-ATPase pump, particularly in the liver and skeletal muscle, increasing uptake of potassium by these cells. Under most conditions hypokalemia is corrected by reducing aldosterone secretion. However, if dietary potassium is inadequate, hypokalemia may not be corrected.

Deficiency

When total body potassium content is below normal, the animal is suffering from potassium depletion. When plasma potassium concentration is below normal the animal is hypokalemic. Hypokalemic animals are not always potassium depleted, and animals with low total body potassium stores can have normal plasma potassium concentrations.

Total body depletion of potassium leads to generalized muscle weakness. Hypokalemia, whether produced by redistribution or total body depletion, is more life-threatening. Hypokalemia adversely affects the heart: the heart rate is reduced and the size of the T wave will be diminished as a result of slow repolarization of the ventricles. Hypokalemia also interferes with insulin secretion, upsetting carbohydrate metabolism. Potassium depletion decreases renal blood flow and reduces the ability of the kidneys to concentrate the urine.

Toxicity

Excessive potassium intake or a sudden increase in potassium intake can increase potassium in the blood very rapidly. In most instances the kidneys will remove the excess potassium before severe hyperkalemia can develop. Hyperkalemia is life-threatening. A doubling of normal blood potassium concentration (4 to 8 mmol/L) can be fatal. Hyperkalemia can induce fatal arrhythmias of the heart. The electrocardiogram shows a pronounced increase in QRS duration as a result of slow depolarization of the ventricles of the heart. Peaked T waves are also diagnostic of hyperkalemia. Cardiac arrest is more common with hyperkalemia than with hypokalemia.

Syndromes of special concern in veterinary medicine
Secretory diarrhea
Many bacterial toxins stimulate secretion of both potassium and chloride from the intestinal epithelium. This can rapidly lead to depletion of total body potassium. Unfortunately, this disease is also complicated by acidosis, which causes blood potassium concentration to be elevated. Treatment must first focus on restoration of normal blood pH and then on supplying the body with potassium. Oral potassium bicarbonate can help with both problems.

Plugged tom cats

The inability to excrete potassium can lead to fatal hyperkalemia in these male cats with stones in the urethra.

Abomasal displacement in cattle

Because chloride anions become sequestered within the abomasum, the animal becomes alkalotic. This can cause hypokalemia.

Hemolytic crisis

Ruptured red blood cells can release potassium into the blood to cause acute and severe hyperkalemia. Along these same lines, blood that has been cooled and stored for transfusion will lose potassium from inside the red blood cells to the plasma and can cause hyperkalemia on transfusion. Warming the blood to normal body temperature will prevent this by activating the Na^+/K^+-ATPase pump to bring potassium back into the cells. Blood samples that are hemolyzed will have falsely elevated plasma potassium values on analysis.

Hypoadrenocorticism

Lack of aldosterone production will result in hyperkalemia.

Milk fever of dairy cattle

Excessive dietary potassium is a major factor increasing the susceptibility of dairy cattle to severe hypocalcemia at calving. The potassium absorbed from the diet induces a mild metabolic alkalosis, which interferes with the ability of the tissues to recognize PTH, interfering with calcium homeostasis.

Grass tetany and other hypomagnesemic disorders of cattle

High potassium content of forages and pastures coupled with low dietary magnesium content prevents absorption of magnesium from the rumen. High rumen potassium concentrations depolarize the apical membrane of the rumen epithelium, reducing the electromotive force that normally allows magnesium to be absorbed across the rumen wall. Ruminants do not absorb magnesium very well from the intestines, as do monogastric animals.

Hyperkalemic periodic paralysis of Quarter Horses

Hyperkalemic periodic paralysis is an autosomal codominant genetic disease of horses. It produces a muscular phenotype that has unfortunately been considered desirable by Quarter Horse show judges, which has resulted in the rapid dissemination of this disease. Clinical attacks are characterized by muscle fasciculation and spasm, and they respond to treatments for the concurrent hyperkalemia. Sweating and prolapse of the third eyelid are early signs of this disease. Skeletal muscles begin alternately to contract and relax uncontrollably. Eventually, in severe cases the animal's skeletal muscles become flaccid and the animal becomes recumbent and is essentially paralyzed. The horse becomes hyperkalemic, which can have fatal consequences on the heart. It appears that the main defect may actually be an upset in sodium conductance across the skeletal muscle cells. The increased entry of sodium forces potassium into the extracellular fluid and also alters membrane potential closer to the threshold potential. At first the cells are more likely to depolarize, causing the spasms; eventually the cells are no longer able to repolarize and the muscle becomes flaccid.

Sulfur

1 Which amino acids contain sulfur?

2 Which three diet ingredients containing sulfur cannot be made by mammalian tissues?

3 Ruminants fed excessive amounts of sulfur can develop neurological symptoms. Why?

Function

About 0.15% of body weight is sulfur. Sulfur is found in the amino acids methionine, cysteine (cystine), homocysteine, and taurine. Sulfur is also found in chondroitin sulfate of cartilage, and in the B vitamins thiamine and biotin. The disulfide bonds of the sulfur-containing amino acids are largely responsible for determining the tertiary structure of proteins. Oxidation of methionine and cysteine causes sulfur to also exist in tissues as the sulfate anion, which influences the acid–base status of the animal.

Methionine, thiamine, and biotin cannot be synthesized by mammalian tissues and these nutrients must be supplied in the diet. When provided with adequate substrates (nitrogen, energy and sulfur), rumen microbial synthesis of methionine, thiamine, and biotin can supply enough of these compounds to the ruminant to meet daily requirements, with the possible exception of very high producing cows. Therefore only ruminants can be said to have a dietary requirement for sulfur.

Metabolism

Sulfur incorporated into microbial protein is absorbed within the small intestine as cysteine and methionine. Some dietary sulfur is absorbed as the sulfate or sulfide anion. Sulfide is absorbed more rapidly and efficiently from the rumen of sheep than is sulfate. Sulfate sulfur is absorbed more efficiently in the small intestine.

Deficiency

The body has no real requirement for sulfur (or sulfate). A "sulfur deficiency" is a deficiency in the sulfur-containing amino acids, thiamine, or biotin (discussed in Chapter 48). Ruminants need a certain amount of dietary sulfur to provide the rumen microbes with the materials needed to synthesize the cysteine, methionine, thiamine, and biotin that the animal will use.

Toxicity

Excessive dietary sulfur can interfere with the absorption of other elements, particularly copper and selenium (see sections on copper and selenium). Acute sulfur toxicity causes neurological changes, including blindness, coma, muscle twitches, and recumbency. Postmortem examination reveals severe enteritis, peritoneal effusion, and petechial hemorrhages in many organs, especially kidneys. Often the breath will smell of hydrogen sulfide, which is likely the toxic form of sulfur. Sulfates are less toxic, though they can cause an osmotic diarrhea as the sulfate is only poorly absorbed. Excess sulfate added to rations can reduce feed intake and performance. Water with a sulfur concentration of more than 5000 mg/kg reduces feed and water intake. Recent observations in beef cattle have determined that a **polioencephalomalacia-like syndrome** can be induced with diets containing 0.5% sulfur using sulfate salts as supplemental sulfur sources or from drinking water high in sulfates. The strong reducing environment within the rumen can reduce dietary sulfate, sulfite, and thiosulfate to sulfide.

TRACE MINERALS

Trace minerals are required by animals in very small amounts each day. Their concentration in the diet is often expressed as parts per million (ppm), equivalent to mg/kg, or in some cases as parts per billion (ppb), equivalent to µg/kg.

Chromium

> 1 What is the role of chromium in glucose homeostasis?
> 2 What form of chromium in the diet is biologically available?

Function

Chromium is primarily found in tissues as an organometallic molecule composed of Cr^{3+}, nicotinic acid, glutamic acid, glycine, and cysteine known as **glucose tolerance factor**. Without Cr^{3+} the glucose tolerance factor is inactive. Glucose tolerance factor can potentiate the effect of insulin on tissues, either by stabilizing the insulin molecule or by facilitating the interaction of insulin with its receptor in tissues.

The essentiality of chromium as a required element necessary for normal glucose metabolism in the diet of humans is well accepted and it is recommended that the diet of adult humans supplies 50–200 µg of chromium daily. Unfortunately, the amount of chromium required in the diet for optimal performance of animals is unclear and the literature does not support a general recommendation for chromium supplementation of typical diets. It is generally thought that most animal diets supply adequate chromium.

Regulation

Studies in rats have determined that chromium is absorbed primarily from the small intestine. Inorganic forms of Cr^{3+} ($CrCl_3$, Cr_2O_3) are very poorly absorbed (hence the utility of Cr_2O_3 as a marker for digestion studies). Complexing Cr^{3+} with organic compounds greatly increases the bioavailability of chromium. Chromium nicotinate and chromium picolinate are usually considered the most available sources of supplemental chromium. Chromium from naturally occurring sources such as brewer's yeast is also high in bioavailability, with as much as 10–25% absorbed by rats.

Deficiency

Chromium deficiency causes hyperglycemia as the glucose tolerance factor is inactive. Several reports in the literature suggest that chromium is an important immune modulator. Supplementation of sow diets with chromium picolinate may improve the number of piglets born from each sow. Chromium may also improve leanness of growing pigs.

Toxicity

It is generally accepted that the levels of trivalent chromium added to diets are safe and nontoxic. Chromium toxicity is primarily associated with hexavalent Cr^{6+} exposure (chromium trioxide, chromates, bichromates). Hexavalent chromium passes into the interior of cells much more readily than trivalent chromium and is able to depress mitochondrial oxygen consumption by inhibiting α-ketoglutarate dehydrogenase. If significant amounts reach the cell nucleus, there can be a variety of pathological changes in the DNA. For livestock the maximum tolerable concentration of chromium in the diet is set at 3000 ppm for the oxide form and 1000 ppm for the chloride form of the trivalent forms of chromium. Hexavalent forms of chromium are at least five times more toxic.

Cobalt

> 1 Is dietary cobalt required by monogastric species?
> 2 Is cobalt deficiency in ruminants due to deficiency of vitamin B_{12} in the cow or lack of cobalt for rumen bacterial growth?

Function

Cobalt is a component of vitamin B_{12} (**cobalamin**), which is a cofactor for two major enzymes: **methylmalonyl-CoA mutase**, necessary for conversion of propionate to succinate, and **tetrahydrofolate methyltransferase**, which catalyzes transfer of methyl groups from 5-methyltetrahydrofolate to homocysteine to form methionine and tetrahydrofolate. Vitamin B_{12} is not found in the tissues of plants. Microbes are the only natural source of vitamin B_{12}. Rumen microbes can produce all the vitamin B_{12} required by ruminants provided adequate available cobalt is in the diet.

Regulation

A proportion of dietary cobalt can be absorbed in the cation form; however, it has no known function and once absorbed does not appear capable of reentering the rumen so microbes could utilize it. Most is excreted in the urine and a smaller amount exits with the bile.

Cobalt chloride and nitrate, and cobaltous carbonate and sulfate all appear to be suitable sources for cobalt in ruminants. Cobaltous oxide, being much less soluble, is somewhat less available. Cobaltous oxide pellets and controlled-release glass pellets containing cobalt that remain in the rumen–reticulum have been used successfully to supply cobalt over extended periods to ruminants on pasture, although regurgitation can cause loss of some types of pellets.

Deficiency

Nonruminants do not suffer from cobalt deficiency but from vitamin B_{12} deficiency (see Chapter 48). Ruminants, who depend on rumen microbes producing vitamin B_{12}, can suffer vitamin B_{12} deficiency if dietary cobalt is inadequate to allow microbial synthesis of vitamin B_{12}. Ruminants appear to be more sensitive to vitamin B_{12} deficiency than nonruminants, largely because they are so dependent on **gluconeogenesis** for meeting tissue glucose needs. A breakdown in propionate metabolism at the point where methylmalonyl-CoA is converted to succinyl-CoA may be a primary defect arising from vitamin B_{12} deficiency. The appearance of methylmalonic acid in urine may be used as an indicator of vitamin B_{12} deficiency. Vitamin B_{12} deficiency may also limit methionine production and limit nitrogen retention. The advantages and disadvantages of methylmalonic acid and vitamin B_{12} determinations for assessing vitamin B_{12} and/or cobalt status have recently been reviewed.

Without cobalt in the diet, rumen production of vitamin B_{12} rapidly (within days) declines. Vitamin B_{12} stores in the liver of adult ruminants are usually sufficient to last several months when they are placed on a cobalt-deficient diet. Young animals are more sensitive to dietary cobalt insufficiency because they have lower liver vitamin B_{12} reserves. Early signs of cobalt deficiency include failure to grow, unthriftiness, and weight loss. More severe signs include fatty degeneration of the liver, anemia with pale mucous membranes, and reduced resistance to infection as a result of impaired neutrophil function.

While the cow may have adequate stores of vitamin B_{12} to last several months, the rumen microbes apparently do not. Within a few days of a switch to a cobalt-deficient diet rumen concentrations of succinate rise, either as a result of inability of rumen microbes to convert succinate to propionate or a shift in rumen bacterial populations toward succinate rather than propionate production.

Toxicity

Cobalt toxicity causes reduced feed intake, loss of body weight, hyperchromemia, and eventually anemia, signs similar to those seen in cobalt deficiency.

Syndromes of special concern in veterinary medicine

Phalaris staggers of ruminants

Phalaris staggers, a neurological syndrome induced by alkaloids in the grass *Phalaris tuberosa*, can be prevented by supplemental cobalt. Cobalt inactivates or interferes with the absorption of this neurotoxin. The disease is reported in Australia primarily.

Copper

> 1 List three essential functions of copper.
>
> 2 What is the role of metallothionein in regulation of intestinal copper absorption?
>
> 3 What problems might occur in a lamb that accidentally ingests pig starter ration?

Function

Copper is a component of enzymes such as **cytochrome oxidas**, necessary for electron transport during aerobic respiration; **lysyl oxidase**, which catalyzes formation of desmosine cross-links in collagen and elastin necessary for strong bone and connective tissues; **ceruloplasmin**, essential for absorption and transport of iron necessary for hemoglobin synthesis; **tyrosinase**, necessary for production of melanin pigment from tyrosine; and **superoxide dismutase**, which protects cells from the toxic effects of oxygen metabolites and is particularly important in phagocytic cell function.

Absorption and metabolism

The amount of dietary copper required to supply the copper needed for maintenance, growth, and lactation will vary with the age of the animal, the chemical form of the dietary copper, and the presence of substances in the diet that interfere with dietary copper absorption. It also varies with the copper status of the animal.

Copper is absorbed primarily by mucosal cells of the small intestine. Dietary copper is generally in the Cu^{2+} state. To be absorbed it must be reduced to the Cu^+ state. This is accomplished by a **copper reductase** enzyme in the brush border. When the body is in need of copper, the enterocytes express a special copper transport protein to move the Cu^+ across the apical membrane (Figure 49.2A). The copper is transferred to a second protein to shuttle it across the cell to the basolateral membrane. Here a special copper pump will use the energy of ATP to move the copper across the basolateral membrane to the extracellular fluid, where it is captured by proteins in the portal blood such as albumin and transcuprein for transport to the liver. This is essential as free copper is a very strong oxidizing agent and free copper will cause hemolysis of red blood cells. The liver can use the copper to synthesize copper-dependent enzymes. It can also store the copper for later use or it can excrete the copper into the bile.

When copper stores are adequate, the amount of copper transporter protein in the apical membrane is reduced. Nevertheless, some dietary copper (Cu^{2+}) diffuses into the cell. The enterocyte produces a protein called metallothionein that can bind the copper diffusing into the cell, sequestering the

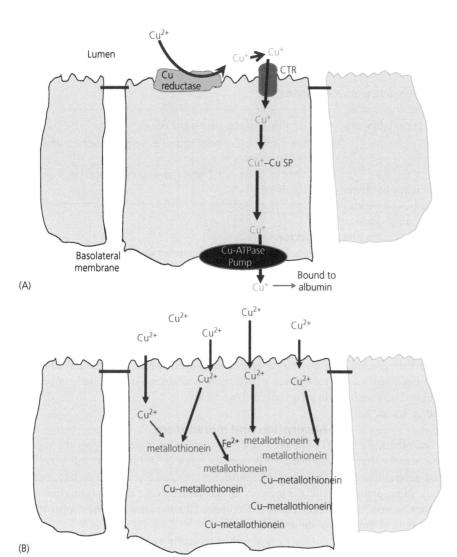

Figure 49.2 Copper absorption. (A) When copper is needed by the body, copper transporters bring reduced Cu^+ across the apical membrane and into the cytosol. A Cu-ATPase pump in the basolateral membrane then moves the Cu^+ into the blood where it is bound to albumin for transport to the liver. (B) When the body has a sufficient store of copper, the copper transporter in the apical membrane is not expressed. Any copper that diffuses into the cell becomes bound to metallothionein and remains in the cell until that cell dies of senescence and is sloughed off. This prevents copper toxicity from developing.

copper inside the cell until the cell is sloughed off the villous tip. High concentrations of metallothionein help prevent copper toxicity by reducing the amount of dietary copper absorbed (Figure 49.2B). High intracellular copper can induce intestinal metallothionein, which in theory permits regulation of copper metabolism. Unfortunately, the primary regulator of enterocyte metallothionein concentration is the zinc status of the animal. A key point to be made is that a diet high in zinc can induce high intestinal metallothionein concentrations, which effectively blocks copper absorption leading to copper deficiency.

The availability of dietary copper is reduced by the presence of sulfur and molybdenum in the diet. Sulfur and molybdenum form **tetrathiomolybdate** in the rumen digesta. Tetrathiomolybdate binds copper to form a highly insoluble complex that renders the copper unavailable for absorption. Molybdenum can reduce monogastric copper absorption as well but the effect is not as pronounced. High dietary iron and water containing high amounts of iron have also been implicated as a cause of copper deficiency but no specific recommendation on how iron affects the coefficient of absorption of copper can be made. Copper absorbed in excess of needs is stored in the liver and can be excreted from the liver within bile secretions.

Deficiency

Copper deficiency can interfere with melanin production leading to loss of hair color. An early classical sign of copper deficiency in cattle is **loss of hair pigmentation**, particularly around the eyes. The copper-containing protein hephaestin works in concert with ferroportin to allow transport of iron across the basolateral membrane of cells, so copper deficiency can cause secondary iron deficiency. Another copper-containing protein, ceruloplasmin, is needed in order for copper to be transferred from macrophages to erythroid progenitor cells. Anemia (hypochromic macrocytic), fragile bones and osteoporosis, cardiac failure, poor growth, and reproductive inefficiency characterized by depressed estrus are also observed in copper deficiency. Scours is a clinical sign of copper deficiency that seems to be unique to ruminants, though the pathogenesis of this lesion is not understood. An effect of copper deficiency that is not easily observed is loss of immune function. Neutrophils have a reduced ability to kill invading microbes, leading to increased susceptibility to infections. The dietary copper required for optimal immune function may exceed the requirement to prevent the more classical signs of copper deficiency.

Toxicity

Although copper toxicity can occur in any species, ruminants are much more susceptible than monogastric animals. While horses can tolerate diets with copper levels of 800 mg/kg, sheep can be killed by diets containing as little as 20 mg/kg. Cattle can generally tolerate diets with copper levels as high as 100 mg/kg. In general, monogastric species have a great capacity to excrete copper in the bile, but ruminants are not able to excrete copper in this way to the same degree. Cattle seem to have a greater capacity to eliminate copper from the body by way of bile than do sheep. Goats tolerate more copper than sheep but not as much as cattle. Copper toxicosis can occur in ruminants that consume excessive amounts of supplemental copper or feeds meant for monogastric animals or which have been contaminated with copper compounds used for other agricultural or industrial purposes.

Breed differences exist in sheep and cattle that increase the susceptibility to copper toxicity. Jersey cattle fed the same diet as Holstein cattle accumulate more liver copper than do Holstein cattle. It is not clear whether this reflects differences in feed intake, efficiency of copper absorption, or biliary excretion of copper. When ruminants consume excessive copper, they may accumulate extremely large amounts of the mineral in the liver before toxicosis becomes evident. Stress or inflammation may result in the sudden liberation of large amounts of copper from the liver to the blood, as part of an acute-phase response. This can overwhelm the copper transport proteins. The presence of free unbound copper in the blood acts as a strong oxidizing agent and causes hemolysis of red blood cells. The hemolytic crisis is characterized by considerable jaundice, methemoglobinemia, hemoglobinuria, generalized icterus, widespread necrosis, and often death.

Syndromes of special concern in veterinary medicine

Copper as a growth promoter in swine and poultry

Adding copper at 10–50 times the concentrations needed to meet requirements can substantially improve the rate of growth of swine and poultry and is a common practice. At these levels copper can have antibacterial properties, which appears to account for the increased growth rate. Manure from poultry fed elevated copper levels should be fed to ruminants with great care.

Neonatal enzootic ataxia (swayback) of lambs

Ewes with chronic copper deficiency can give birth to lambs that are weak and ataxic. The disease is characterized by symmetrical demyelination of the cerebrum, and degeneration of the motor tracts within the spinal cord. Unfortunately, the lesions are permanent and copper supplementation will not be of aid to these lambs. The disease has also been observed rarely in goats and cattle.

Copper-associated hepatitis in Bedlington terriers

Bedlington terriers (perhaps the majority of the dogs of this breed) can be genetically predisposed to a liver disease that is caused by a marked accumulation of copper in hepatocytes. Often following some stressful event such as whelping or being shown, the animals become acutely ill as a result of the toxic effects of the copper that accumulates in their liver. They become jaundiced and can suffer hemolytic crises as the damaged hepatocytes release copper into the circulation.

Iodine

> 1 What hormone is affected by iodine deficiency?
> 2 Describe the two major types of goitrogens present in some feedstuffs.

Function

Iodine is necessary for the synthesis of the thyroid hormones thyroxine and triiodothyronine that regulate energy metabolism. Thyroid hormone production is also increased during colder weather to stimulate an increase in basal metabolic rate as the animal attempts to remain warm.

Iodine homeostasis

About 80–90% of dietary iodine is absorbed and most of the iodine not taken up by the thyroid gland is excreted in urine and milk. Milk normally contains iodine concentrations of 30–300 µg/L and milk iodine content generally increases as dietary iodine increases, making milk iodine content a reasonable indicator of iodine status. The availability of thyroid hormone assays is allowing more accurate assessment of actual thyroid function and the causes of thyroid dysfunction.

When iodine content of the diet is more than adequate, less than 20% of dietary iodine will be incorporated into the thyroid gland. Under conditions where dietary iodine intake is marginal, the thyroid gland will incorporate about 30% of dietary iodine into thyroid hormones. When severely iodine deficient, the hyperplastic thyroid can bind up to 65% of the iodine consumed.

Most iodine sources are readily available and the iodides of sodium, potassium, and calcium are commonly used. Potassium iodide tends to be easily oxidized and volatilizes before the animal can ingest it. Pentacalcium orthoperiodate and ethylenediamine dihydroiodine (EDDI) are more stable and less soluble and commonly used in mineral blocks and salt licks exposed to the weather.

Section VIII: Minerals, Bones, and Joints

Forage iodine concentrations are extremely variable and depend on soil iodine content. Soil near the oceans tends to provide adequate iodine to plants. However, in the Great Lakes regions and northwest USA iodine concentrations in forages are generally low enough to result in iodine deficiency unless supplemented. Iodine deficiency remains a common problem in many parts of the world.

Deficiency

Iodine deficiency reduces thyroid hormone production, slowing the rate of oxidation of all cells. Often the first indication of iodine deficiency is enlargement of the thyroid, known as **goiter**, of newborn animals. Animals may be born hairless, weak, or dead. Fetal death can occur at any stage of gestation. Often the mothers will appear normal. Under conditions of marginal or deficient dietary iodine the maternal thyroid gland becomes extremely efficient in uptake of iodine from the circulation and in recycling thyroid hormone iodine. Unfortunately, this leaves little iodine for the fetal thyroid gland and the fetus becomes hypothyroid. The goiter condition is the hyperplastic response of the thyroid gland to increased pituitary thyroid-stimulating hormone production. Under mild iodine deficiency the hyperplastic thyroid gland can compensate for the reduced availability of iodine. Adult animals with iodine deficiency are unthrifty and often infertile.

Toxicity

Iodine toxicity has been reported with dietary iodine intakes of 50 mg/day or more (about 5 mg/kg dietary dry matter). Symptoms included excessive nasal and ocular discharge, salivation, decreased milk production, coughing, and dry scaly coats. High dietary iodine concentrations also increase milk iodine concentrations, and since humans are much more sensitive to iodine thyrotoxicosis than cows, the limitation of dietary iodine to cattle also is a public health issue.

Syndromes of special concern in veterinary medicine
Factors affecting iodine requirement

Goitrogens are compounds that interfere with the synthesis or secretion of thyroid hormones and cause hypothyroidism. Goitrogens fall into two main categories. **Cyanogenic goitrogens** impair ioidide uptake by the thyroid gland. Cyanogenic glucosides can be found in many feeds, including raw soybeans, beet pulp, corn, sweet potato, white clover, and millet and once ingested are metabolized to thiocyanate and isothiocyanate. These compounds alter iodide transport across the thyroid follicular cell membrane, reducing iodide retention. This effect is easily overcome by increasing supplemental iodine.

Progoitrins and goitrins found in cruciferous plants (rape, kale, cabbage, turnips, mustard) and **aliphatic disulfides** found in onions inhibit thyroperoxidase, preventing formation of monoiodotyrosine and diiodotyrosine. With goitrins, especially those of the thiouracil type, hormone synthesis may not be

readily restored to normal by dietary iodine supplementation and the offending feedstuff needs to be reduced or removed from the diet. Dietary iodine required to overcome the goitrin effects could result in milk with excessive iodine content.

Iron

> 1 What is the major clinical symptom of iron deficiency in growing animals?
>
> 2 How does ferritin protect an animal from excessive dietary iron?
>
> 3 Why is free iron in tissues so harmful?

Function

Iron primarily functions as a component of heme, found in hemoglobin and myoglobin. The presence of iron in the Fe^{2+} ferrous state allows these compounds to bind oxygen molecules. Enzymes of the electron transport chain, cytochrome oxidase, ferredoxin, myeloperoxidase, catalase, and the cytochrome P450 enzymes also require iron as cofactors.

Iron homeostasis

Iron required by the body must be obtained from the diet. Carnivores obtain the iron they need from their prey, usually in the form of the prey animal's red blood cells. Herbivores must get their iron in the form of ferrous or ferric ions.

In carnivorous species, the iron-containing heme proteins liberated by digestion of blood are extremely well utilized as a source of iron. Specific heme transport proteins exist on the apical surface of the enterocytes and once these proteins bind heme they cause endocytosis of the heme protein across the apical membrane (Figure 49.3A). Once in the cytosol the heme iron (Fe^{2+}) is liberated. As the ferrous (Fe^{2+}) iron crosses the basolateral membrane, it is oxidized to ferric (Fe^{3+}) iron and becomes bound to transferrin for transport to the liver and other tissues. Iron bound to transferrin circulates to all cells of the body, which can then take up iron from the transferrin.

In herbivores the bulk of dietary iron is in the Fe^{2+} or Fe^{3+} form. Iron in the ferric (Fe^{3+}) form is poorly absorbed from the intestinal tract. Much of the dietary iron exists within feedstuffs in the ferric form. Some of the ferric iron can be reduced to the ferrous (Fe^{2+}) form on reaction with the acid of the stomach or abomasum. During digestion, dietary nonheme iron in the Fe^{2+} state usually becomes bound to some chelator such as amino acids, mucin, or fructose. These chelators enhance iron absorption by solubilizing iron and protecting it in the ferrous state. Other chelators (oxalate, phytate, and phosphate) can inhibit iron absorption. During absorption the iron binds to a specific nonheme iron transporter within the brush border of the enterocyte and is transported into the cell (Figure 49.349.3B). Once inside the cell, the Fe^{2+} is oxidized to Fe^{3+} at the basolateral membrane by the **ferroportin complex**, a group of proteins that

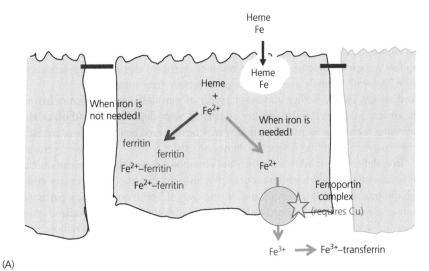

(A)

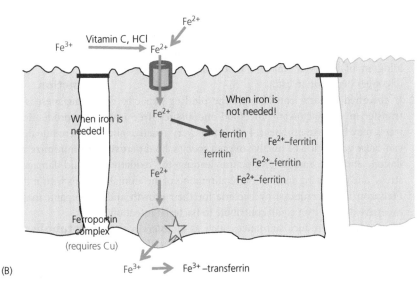

(B)

Figure 49.3 Iron absorption. (A) Heme iron in the diet (carnivores) is endocytosed into the cytosol and the Fe^{2+} iron is liberated from the heme molecule. When the body needs iron, the Fe^{2+} is moved across the basolateral membrane using the ferroportin protein complex (which includes a copper-containing protein). This complex also oxidizes the Fe^{2+} to Fe^{3+} as it is traversing the membrane so it can be transported in the blood as Fe^{3+} bound to transferrin. When iron is not needed by the body, the Fe^{2+} becomes bound to ferritin that is expressed by the cell when iron is plentiful. Ferritin binds the Fe^{2+} for the life of the cell. (B) Nonheme iron is reduced to the Fe^{2+} state and uses a specific transport molecule to traverse the apical membrane. When iron is needed, the ferroportin complex is expressed and the Fe^{2+} is transported into the blood as described above. When iron is not needed, the cell expresses ferritin to sequester the iron within the cell until it dies and is sloughed off.

includes the copper-containing protein **hephaestin**. It is then transported across the basolateral membrane by the ferroportin complex. Once the Fe^{3+} crosses the basolateral membrane, it becomes bound to transferrin for transport within the blood. Free iron cannot be permitted in the body as it is a very strong oxidizing agent, so the body takes great pains to keep iron bound to proteins.

If the iron status of the body is adequate, the Fe^{2+} entering the enterocyte is not transported to the basolateral membrane but is instead bound by **ferritin**, a protein produced by the enterocytes when iron is in surplus. Once bound to ferritin, the iron is sequestered within the enterocyte and stays in the cell until the enterocyte dies and is sloughed off the villous tip. The amount of dietary iron absorbed can be controlled by upregulation or downregulation of enterocyte ferritin content. Unfortunately, ferritin can also bind zinc and copper, so when ferritin levels are very high due to excessive dietary iron, it can reduce absorption of copper and zinc, which may cause secondary deficiencies of

these minerals. How enterocyte ferritin concentrations are regulated by iron status is unknown, though it is believed the liver produces a "hormone" that controls enterocyte ferritin production, based on liver iron stores. It is known that the liver produces a hormone called **hepcidin**, which downregulates the ferroportin complex, comprising a second way to block iron absorption.

The primary need for iron is to form hemoglobin and myoglobin for oxygen transport. The bulk of iron used for production of red blood cells in adult animals comes from recycling of iron obtained from breakdown of senescent red blood cells. Old red blood cells are phagocytosed by macrophages and the iron is released from them to transferrin for circulation through the body. The macrophages use a copper-containing enzyme called ceruloplasmin to oxidize heme iron so it can be transported out of the macrophage as Fe^{3+}. In the bone marrow and spleen the erythroprogenitor cells take up iron from transferrin and use it to form hemoglobin.

Deficiency

Iron deficiency results in **hypochromic microcytic anemia** due to failure to produce hemoglobin. The light color of veal is due to low muscle myoglobin levels as a result of restricted dietary iron. Anemic animals are listless and have poor feed intake and weight gain. Another important aspect of iron deficiency is greater morbidity and mortality associated with depressed immune responses. Increased morbidity may be observed before there is an effect of iron deficiency on hematocrit.

Iron deficiency in adult animals is not common. In part this is because their requirement is reduced, but also because iron is ubiquitous in the environment and, in the case of herbivores, soil contamination of forages (and soil ingested by animals on pasture) generally ensures that iron needs of the adult will be met or exceeded.

Toxicity

Excessive dietary iron is of concern for two reasons.

1 Iron interferes with the absorption of other minerals, primarily copper and zinc. As little as 250–500 mg of iron per kilogram of dietary dry matter has been implicated as a cause of copper depletion in cattle.

2 If absorbed dietary iron exceeds the binding capacity of transferrin and lactoferrin in blood and tissues, free iron levels may increase in tissues. Free iron is very reactive and can cause generation of reactive oxygen species, lipid peroxidation, and free radical production leading to "oxidative stress" and increasing antioxidant requirements of the animal. Free iron is also required by bacteria for their growth and excessive dietary iron could contribute to bacterial infection. The body can produce substances such as **lactoferrin** that binds free iron, making it unavailable for bacterial growth and preventing bacterial infection. Iron toxicity is associated with diarrhea, reduced feed intake, and weight gain.

Syndromes of special concern in veterinary medicine

Anemia in piglets

Piglets are born with almost no iron stores in their liver and because the piglet grows very quickly (four to five times their birthweight in the first 3 weeks of life) the piglet must retain between 7 and 16 mg of iron each day. Sow milk is a poor source of iron, supplying just 1 mg/L, placing the piglet at high risk of developing iron deficiency. This is especially true for piglets raised in confinement. Pigs raised on pasture root around in the soil and often can ingest enough iron to meet their needs. Iron-deficient piglets will have blood hemoglobin below 10 g/dL. Anemic pigs grow slowly, have rough hair coats, and pale mucous membranes. When exercised the piglets may exhibit labored breathing, often referred to as the "thumps," a spasmodic contraction of the diaphragm as the piglet battles anoxia. A common practice is to inject piglets in the first 3 days of life with 100–200 mg iron, usually in the form of iron dextran, dextrin, or gleptoferrin, which serve to slowly release iron from the

injection site. Interestingly, the same dose of iron given orally as ferrous sulfate can sometimes cause increased mortality, often from enteric infection with *Escherichia coli*, which experience a population explosion in the presence of free iron in the gut.

Hemochromatosis of pet mynahs, toucans, and black rhinoceros

These animals seem especially prone to build-up of iron within their livers, as a result of either excessive dietary iron or poor control over iron absorption. The main effects are lethargy and anorexia and **hemosiderosis**, the accumulation of iron in tissues, particularly the liver and heart. The iron build-up causes localized oxidative stress and tissue destruction. Blood-letting to remove iron from the body is the recommended treatment.

Manganese

> 1 Which tissues are most affected by manganese deficiency?

Function

Manganese is a required cofactor for several enzymes necessary for production of bone collagen, and cartilage. Manganese superoxide dismutase works in concert with other antioxidants to minimize accumulation of reactive forms of oxygen, which could damage cells. Manganese is found in highest concentrations within the mitochondria of cells. It also accumulates in the inorganic matrix of bone.

Metabolism

The great majority of the dietary manganese that is absorbed is removed from the portal circulation by the liver and ends up being excreted into the bile. A small portion is bound to transferrin within the liver and released into the circulation for transport to the tissues. Some of the absorbed manganese becomes bound to α_2-macroglobulin and albumin and bypasses the liver to remain in the circulation. The proportion of manganese absorbed from the diet is less than 4% and generally closer to 1%. A mechanism to enhance the efficiency of manganese absorption during manganese deficiency does not appear to exist. The major homeostatic control for manganese appears to be regulation of biliary excretion of manganese absorbed in excess of tissue needs. Almost no manganese is excreted in urine. Manganese accumulates in the liver in direct proportion to dietary manganese, providing a more precise index of manganese status. The liver and perhaps other tissues have a limited ability to store mobilizable manganese, which may satisfy needs for several weeks during times of manganese deficiency.

Deficiency

Manganese deficiency can cause impaired growth, skeletal abnormalities (shortened and deformed), disturbed or depressed reproduction, and abnormalities of the newborn (including ataxia due to failure of the inner ear to develop). The skeletal changes are related to loss of galactotransferase and glycosyltransferase enzymes, which are vital to production of cartilage and bone ground substance mucopolysaccharides and glycoproteins.

In one experiment, all calves born from cows fed 16–17 ppm of dietary manganese for 12 months had neonatal deformities. The deformities included weak legs and pasterns, enlarged joints, stiffness, twisted legs, general weakness, and reduced bone strength. Heifers and cows that are fed low-manganese diets are slower to exhibit estrus, are more likely to have "silent heats," and have a lower conception rate than cows with sufficient manganese in their diet.

Toxicity

Manganese toxicity is unlikely to occur and there are few documented incidences, with adverse effects limited to reduced feed intake and growth. These negative effects began to appear when dietary manganese exceeded 1000 mg/kg.

Molybdenum

> 1 Molybdenum should probably be classified as a toxic element rather than a required nutrient. Why?

Function

Molybdenum is a component of xanthine oxidase, sulfide oxidase, and aldehyde oxidase, enzymes found in milk and many tissues. Milk and plasma molybdenum concentrations increase as dietary molybdenum increases.

Absorption

Dietary molybdenum is absorbed very efficiently and occurs by unregulated passive diffusion of molybdenum across the small intestine. Absorbed molybdenum is stored in the liver, kidney, and bone. Molybdenum is eliminated from the body via the urine.

Deficiency

From a practical standpoint this is not a concern in veterinary medicine as it would seem very unlikely that animals would develop a deficiency of molybdenum on practical diets. A molybdenum deficiency state in animals has been difficult to reproduce even in laboratory animals, unless great amounts of tungsten have been added to the diet to suppress molybdenum absorption.

Toxicity

Dietary molybdenum becomes a practical concern because it antagonizes the absorption of copper (and to a lesser extent phosphorus). Signs of molybdenum toxicosis are essentially those associated with copper deficiency. Molybdenum and sulfate interact within the digestive tract to form a thiomolybdate complex, which has a high affinity for copper. Copper bound to this molybdate is unavailable for absorption (see section on copper). The toxicity of molybdenum can be overcome by increased copper supplementation and copper toxicity can be reduced by molybdenum supplementation. The critical ratio of dietary copper to dietary molybdenum needed to avoid copper deficiency ranges from 2 : 1 in reports from Canada to 4 : 1 on pastures in England with a high molybdenum content (20–100 mg/kg forage dry matter). In the USA, molybdenum is a significant problem in the western states and an area around the Everglades in Florida.

Syndromes of special concern in veterinary medicine
Teart or peat scours of ruminants

Plants grown on peat or muck soils can contain high amounts of molybdenum. Cattle and sheep ingesting these plants can become copper deficient and develop unpigmented circles around the eyes and a chronic diarrhea.

Selenium

> 1 What is the main function of selenium-containing enzymes?
> 2 What is white muscle disease?

Function

Selenium is a necessary component of **glutathione peroxidase**, an enzyme that plays a major role in protecting tissues against oxidative damage. During the course of catabolism small, but extremely dangerous, quantities of free radicals are produced, including **superoxide anion (O_2^-)**, **hydrogen peroxide (H_2O_2)**, and **hydroxyl radical (OH·)**. These substances are extremely reactive and can disrupt the function of normal proteins and lipids in the cell. Left unchecked they would quickly destroy the cell. Glutathione peroxidase catalyzes the reduction of hydrogen peroxide and hydroperoxides formed from fatty acids and other substances according to the general reaction:

$$ROOH + 2GSH \rightarrow R - OH + HOH + GS - SG$$

where R represents H if the free radical is hydrogen peroxide or a fatty acyl group if a fatty acid hydroperoxide has been formed, and GSH represents glutathione in the reduced state. Glutathione peroxidase levels in serum are somewhat correlated with dietary selenium concentrations. Vitamin E also can neutralize peroxides, but its action is limited to cell membranes. Vitamin E can replace some of the antiperoxidant function of selenium, and selenium can spare vitamin E by scavenging free radicals before they get to cell membranes.

Selenium is also critical to thyroid hormone metabolism because the enzyme **iodothyronine 5′-deiodinase** is a selenium-containing protein. A selenoprotein also seems to be important in muscle, though it is not yet identified. In selenium-replete animals a selenoprotein can be isolated from the muscle, although this protein is not present in animals that are selenium deficient. This protein seems to play a critical role in the cardiac and skeletal muscle degeneration common in the selenium deficiency referred to as **white muscle disease**.

Metabolism

The duodenum is the major site for selenium absorption. Around 90% of dietary selenite and selenate salts of selenium are absorbed from the diet. Selenium absorption is not regulated and homeostasis of selenium is regulated by controlling urinary excretion of selenium. When dietary selenium is in great excess of requirements, selenium is also expired in the breath as dimethylselenide.

Deficiency

The soil in large areas of the USA is too low in selenium and will not provide adequate selenium to meet the needs of animals fed crops grown on those soils. The states bordering the Great Lakes, the Pacific Northwest, and the Eastern Shore are all considered areas where selenium deficiency is likely to occur. Selenium deficiency causes infertility and poor growth in most species. Selenium deficiency has some species-specific effects as well. Some of these effects can be reduced by vitamin E supplementation. The dietary selenium requirement for most animals is about 0.1–0.3 mg/kg.

Toxicity

In his travels across Asia Minor, Marco Polo related that horses ingesting certain plants would lose their mane and tail hair and slough their hooves. Toxicity from selenium occurs in two forms, acute and chronic. **Acute selenium poisoning** is associated with hepatic and renal damage and can include hemorrhagic exudate in the lungs, and ascites is common. Blindness and stumbling are also common. Gastroenteritis may be present. **Chronic selenium poisoning** in horses and cattle is associated with lameness and loss of hair and hoof malformations. Animals at pasture eventually die from starvation due to impaired mobility. Selenium can be toxic at 8–10 mg/kg diet.

Syndromes of special concern in veterinary medicine

Exudative diathesis of poultry

Exudative diathesis of broilers is a generalized edema that begins in the breast, wing, and neck areas due to abnormal permeability of the capillaries. The accumulation of fluids under the ventral skin gives it a greenish-blue discoloration. Growth is slow and mortality is high. Vitamin E can prevent exudative diathesis in selenium-deficient chicks. Selenium deficiency causes atrophy of the pancreas in very young chicks, resulting in **pancreatic fibrosis**. The pancreas produces subnormal amounts of lipase and trypsin, interfering with digestion of lipids primarily. Vitamin E will not prevent pancreatic fibrosis.

Hepatosis dietetica of swine

This selenium/vitamin E deficiency syndrome is observed in growing pigs 3–25 weeks of age and is associated with **severe necrotic liver lesions**.

Mulberry heart disease of swine

Selenium deficiency causes hemorrhagic and necrotic lesions in the heart muscle leading to a red mottled "mulberry" appearance of the heart. This is accompanied by reduced heart function and transudation of fluids into serous cavities and generalized circulatory failure.

Some selenium-deficient swine show both hepatosis dietetica and mulberry heart disease at the same time but more often one syndrome predominates over the other in a particular herd, suggesting that other factors may also be involved, especially for mulberry heart disease.

White muscle disease of lambs and calves

White muscle disease is a **nutritional muscular dystrophy** that causes necrotic changes in the striated muscles of the body. It is most common in lambs and calves but also occurs in pigs, foals, and poultry. The name is derived from the white striations observed in many of the muscles of the body, particularly those in the thigh and shoulder. Lesions are bilaterally symmetrical and serum aspartic aminotransferase activity will be greatly elevated.

Retained placenta of dairy cows

Selenium deficiency is associated with an increased risk of retained placenta and perhaps mastitis. It is thought that selenium deficiency reduces the immune response in the cow. The mechanisms are largely unknown.

Blind staggers and alkali disease in cattle and horses

Certain plant species, such as princesplume, woody aster and milkvetch (*Stanleya*, *Xylorhiza*, and *Astragalus* species), found in pockets of the upper Great Plains and deserts of North America are **selenium accumulators** and can contain several hundred to a thousand milligrams of selenium per kilogram. They are generally unpalatable but animals consuming these plants can develop selenium toxicity. If consumed in high amounts the animal can exhibit acute poisoning, called **blind staggers**. More commonly in periods of drought the animals on pasture may be hungry enough to occasionally eat a few of these selenium accumulator plants or the soil (usually alkaline) may have sufficient selenium that forage plants grown in these areas provide more than 10 mg of selenium per kilogram of pasture. Over time the animals develop lameness and emaciation, called **alkali disease**. Profitable ranching is nearly impossible in these particular areas of the country.

Zinc

1 What are the main functions of zinc-containing enzymes?
2 How is zinc absorption across the intestinal epithelium controlled?
3 Why do high-calcium diets cause problems in pigs?

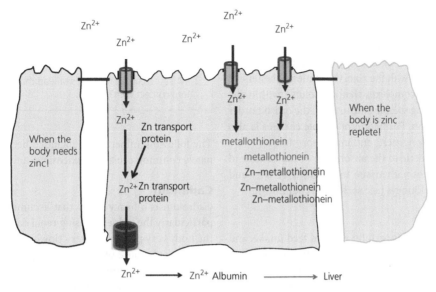

Figure 49.4 Zinc absorption. When zinc is needed by the body, zinc transporters bring zinc across the apical membrane and into the cytosol. A zinc transport protein binds the zinc as it enters the cytosol and ferries it to the basolateral membrane where it is passed on to a basolateral zinc transport protein and then into the serum where it becomes bound to albumin for transport to the liver in the portal blood. When the body has sufficient stores of zinc, the zinc transporter in the basolateral membrane is not expressed. Any zinc that diffuses into the cell becomes bound to metallothionein, expressed when zinc is plentiful, and remains in the cell until that cell dies of senescence and is sloughed off. This prevents zinc toxicity from developing.

Function

Zinc is a component of metalloenzymes such as **copper-zinc superoxide dismutase**, **carbonic anhydrase**, alcohol dehydrogenase, carboxypeptidase, alkaline phosphatase and **RNA polymerase** that affect metabolism of carbohydrates, proteins, lipids, and nucleic acids. Zinc regulates calmodulin, protein kinase C, thyroid hormone binding, and inositol phosphate synthesis. Zinc deficiency alters prostaglandin synthesis, which may affect luteal function. Zinc is a component of thymosin, a hormone produced by thymic cells that regulates cell-mediated immunity.

Absorption

Intestinal zinc absorption occurs primarily in the small intestine (Figure 49.4). In animals in need of zinc, zinc readily enters the enterocytes using facilitated diffusion and is transported across the cell by a cysteine-rich zinc transporter protein. At the basolateral membrane a second facilitated diffusion transporter permits zinc to cross into the extracellular fluid. The zinc is released into the portal circulation to be carried primarily by albumin and transferrin to the liver. Free zinc is a very strong oxidizing agent so it must be bound to a protein for transport in the blood. In animals that are zinc replete, **metallothionein**, a second cysteine-rich protein, is induced in the enterocytes. The metallothionein competes with the cysteine-rich transporter protein for zinc entering across the brush border membrane. Zinc bound to metallothionein will remain in the enterocyte and be excreted with the feces when the enterocyte dies and is sloughed. By upregulating or downregulating mucosal enterocyte metallothionein

content, the amount of dietary zinc that is absorbed can be regulated. How zinc status regulates intestinal metallothionein concentration is unknown, but it takes weeks to change metallothionein concentration in the intestine when an animal has to adjust to a low-zinc diet.

Zinc and copper are antagonistic to one another. In most cases zinc interferes with copper absorption to cause copper deficiency, but when dietary copper/zinc ratios are very high (50 : 1) copper can interfere with zinc absorption. Excessive dietary iron can also interfere with zinc absorption in humans and other species. Under practical conditions dietary iron content is often well in excess of iron requirements of herbivores and can be a factor causing zinc and copper deficiency. High dietary calcium also interferes with zinc absorption. This effect is especially pronounced in nonruminants (see section Parakeratosis of swine). The mechanism is not well understood.

Organic chelators of zinc can increase or decrease bioavailability of zinc. Those that interfere with absorption tend to form insoluble complexes with zinc. One such chelator is phytate (phytic acid), which is also an important chelator of phosphate, copper, and iron. Phytate commonly binds zinc in plant sources of zinc and greatly diminishes the availability of zinc for absorption in monogastric and pre-ruminant animals. However, rumen microbes metabolize most of the dietary phytate so it is not a factor affecting zinc absorption in ruminants.

Some naturally occurring zinc chelators improve zinc bioavailability. In most cases these complexes improve the solubility of zinc. Peptides and amino acids can form soluble complexes with zinc. Both cysteine and histidine bind zinc strongly and improve bioavailability of zinc in chicks. At the alkaline pH found in the intestine it is likely that little free zinc cation exists in solution. It will precipitate as zinc hydroxide if no other substance can form a complex with the zinc. One action of beneficial chelates is to form zinc complexes that are soluble within the small intestine, permitting soluble zinc to reach the brush border membrane for absorption. Formation of soluble chelates is also important for copper, manganese, and iron absorption.

Cadmium is antagonistic to the absorption of both zinc and copper. It also interferes with tissue metabolism of zinc and copper in the liver and kidneys (see section on cadmium).

Deficiency

Zinc-deficient animals quickly exhibit reduced feed intake, and reduced growth rate. With more prolonged deficiency the animals exhibit reduced growth of testes, weak hoof horn, and parakeratosis of the skin on the legs, head (especially nostrils), and neck. On necropsy, thymic atrophy and lymphoid depletion of the spleen and lymph nodes are evident. Zinc-deficient animals are highly immunosuppressed, making them more susceptible to many opportunistic infections.

Toxicity

High dietary zinc is fairly well tolerated by cattle, although zinc toxicity was observed in cattle fed a diet containing zinc levels of 900 mg/kg. High levels of zinc have a very negative effect on copper absorption and metabolism and it is for this reason primarily that dietary zinc content should be limited. The maximal tolerable level of dietary zinc is suggested to be 300–1000 mg/kg.

Syndromes of special concern in veterinary medicine

Parakeratosis of swine

Pigs fed diets that are deficient in zinc or that are high in calcium can develop lesions of the superficial layers of the epidermis known as parakeratosis. Early signs are limited to the skin and consist of symmetrically distributed areas of excessive keratinization of the skin. There is usually little pruritis (itching). The skin becomes scaly and can "crack" due to fissures that form in these areas. In more severe cases growth is impaired and the animals are anorexic and lethargic. The animals respond quickly to the addition of zinc to the ration or the removal of calcium from the ration.

Genetic zinc deficiency of cattle and Malamutes

A genetic defect that greatly reduces zinc absorption has been identified in Black Pied and Dutch-Friesian cattle. It has also been identified in Malamute dogs. These animals become severely zinc deficient unless fed extremely high levels of dietary zinc. Calves appear normal at birth but develop scaly thickened skin over the neck and shoulders within a few months. In dogs the skin around the eyes is most susceptible. They also grow slowly and are very susceptible to infection due to their inability to mount an immune response.

Toxic minerals

> 1 What is the danger of using sewage sludge as fertilizer for crops fed to food animals?
>
> 2 What are common sources of lead that animals might come into contact with?

The following minerals are included because they are unfortunately common causes of toxicosis in animals.

Cadmium

Cadmium is a heavy metal that accumulates within the body, particularly the kidney, causing renal damage. It is cleared from the body very poorly and very slowly. It is of particular concern to humans because of our long lifespan and because cadmium has become so commonly distributed in the environment. The maximal tolerable level of cadmium in the diet of food animals is set at 0.5 ppm in an effort to avoid adding cadmium to the diet of humans consuming food animal products.

Cadmium is antagonistic to zinc and copper, and to a lesser degree iron. Diets containing 5–30 ppm of cadmium generally decrease animal performance by interfering with copper and zinc absorption, resulting in symptoms usually associated with copper and zinc deficiency. Cadmium binds to intestinal metallothionein very tightly. Liver and kidney contain metallothionein proteins, which accumulate cadmium throughout the life of the animal.

Cadmium is a contaminant of the zinc sulfides used to galvanize iron to prevent corrosion. It is a component of nickel–cadmium batteries and is used as a stabilizer in polyvinylchloride plastics. Urban sewage sludge contains significant amounts of cadmium and should not be used as fertilizer on farmland growing crops intended for human or food animal consumption.

Less than 1% of dietary cadmium is absorbed by ruminants. Intestinal metallothionein binds cadmium tightly and limits the absorption of cadmium. Cadmium can be detected in milk in small amounts but the mammary gland limits its transport and milk cadmium concentration is not increased by high dietary cadmium concentrations.

Fluorine

While fluorine in very small amounts can increase the strength of bones and teeth, it is generally not regarded as an essential dietary component. Fluorine substitutes for OH^- in bone hydroxyapatite crystals, giving them strength when present in small quantities. Fluorine is generally regarded as a toxic element with regard to domestic livestock because in high amounts fluorine accumulates in bone and replaces so much of the OH^- in bone crystals that it actually weakens bone, increasing lameness and increasing wear of teeth. The teeth of fluorine-intoxicated cattle become mottled and stained, and are often eroded or pitted.

Soluble forms of fluoride, such as sodium fluoride, are rapidly and nearly completely absorbed by cattle. About 50% of fluorine in un-defluorinated rock phosphates is absorbed. Dietary calcium, aluminum, sodium chloride, and fat can reduce fluorine absorption. Fluorine does not pass readily into milk and milk fluorine does not increase markedly with increased dietary fluorine.

Rock phosphates from Florida [fluorapatite, $Ca_{10}F_2(PO_4)_6$] can contaminate cattle when used in feed or when applied as a fertilizer without first being defluorinated. Other potential sources of fluorine include bonemeal, deep well water, and soil near volcanoes and fumaroles. Fluorine in the form of hydrofluoric acid, silicon tetrafluoride, or fluoride-containing particulates can be released from industrial sites associated with aluminum or phosphate processing. These emissions can contaminate water, soil and plants downwind of these sites, resulting in fluorine toxicosis in animals grazing in the areas.

Lead

Lead is the most common cause of toxicoses in domestic livestock. Lead halides and lead bromochloride that were once added to gasoline engines as valve lubricants were emitted from auto exhaust during combustion and contaminated much of the American landscape. Lead-based pigments were common until legal restrictions were imposed and paint chips from older structures remain a significant source of lead contamination in cattle. Lead intoxication has also occurred in cattle consuming lead from batteries, putty from window glazing, linoleum, asphalt roofing, and used engine or crankcase oil. Between 3 and 10% of ingested lead is absorbed. Elevated dietary levels of calcium, phosphorus, iron, zinc, fat, and protein decrease the absorption and retention of lead. Lead accumulates in bone. Lead readily passes into milk so that increasing dietary lead concentrations results in increased lead concentration in milk.

Clinical intoxication interferes with normal metal-dependent enzyme functions. Lead causes derangements in porphyrin and heme synthesis, interferes with protein synthesis, causes basophilic stippling of erythrocytes, and causes microcytic hypochromic anemia.

Chronic exposure to low levels of lead is not associated with clinical symptoms in cattle because bones sequester lead and release it gradually into the blood for excretion. In humans, low levels of lead exposure are associated with a loss of cognitive powers. Acute intoxication with lead causes impaired neurological function resulting in blindness and irritability. Lead toxicity also causes intestinal pain and colic, and abortion. Lead accumulates in the kidney cortex and renal tubular inclusion bodies suggest impaired renal function. In cattle that have died from lead poisoning, concentrations in the kidney cortex are often above 50 ppm and in the liver are often above 20 ppm (fresh tissue).

In recent years lead ingestion has become a leading cause of death in eagles and other raptors. They may eat fish that contain lead jigheads released by fishermen, they may eat ducks shot by hunters and not retrieved, and they may eat waterfowl that have ingested lead shot that has fallen into the water.

Mercury

Mercury toxicity is uncommon. Most cases have been associated with ingestion of seed grain coated with an organic mercury fungicide. Fishmeal protein concentrates have also accidently caused mercury poisoning. Fish concentrate methylmercury that might be in the water. The organic mercury compounds, especially methylmercury, are more toxic than the inorganic forms of mercury. Organic mercury compounds are absorbed with greater efficiency and retained longer. Little organic or inorganic mercury is secreted into the milk.

Inorganic mercury compounds are very caustic and cause acute gastroenteritis when ingested. Low doses of inorganic mercury ingested over time cause depression, anorexia, and a stiff-legged gait followed by paresis. Alopecia, pruritus, scabby lesions around the anus and vulva, shedding of teeth, and diarrhea are typical of later stages of inorganic mercury poisoning. The primary cause of death is acute renal failure.

The organic mercury compounds (alkyl mercuries) primarily affect the nervous system and clinical signs include listlessness, incoordination, progressive blindness, and convulsions.

Self-evaluation

Answers can be found at the end of the chapter.

1 You are called to examine a Jersey cow that is unable to stand. Her newborn calf is beside her. What condition might this cow have? What role did the high potassium alfalfa hay fed to her the last days before calving play in the development of this disorder?

2 What role does high-potassium forage play in the lactating beef cow exhibiting signs of tetany?

3 Explain how a high-grain diet with no supplemental calcium added might affect the bones of a growing horse?

4 On a very hot day a farmer notices that the pigs waterer is no longer working. He fixes it and the pigs all run to the trough to drink. Three hours later you receive a call to examine the pigs. They are staggering around in circles and several have died. What is going on?

5 Why do cows with displaced abomasum have high blood pH?

6 Explain why a dog suffering from bilateral hypoadrenocorticism might develop hyperkalemia.

7 Your practice is located in an area where the soil is very rich in molybdenum. When you visit the herbivores in the area, what symptoms should you be alert for and why do these lesions develop?

8 A Bedlington terrier has just whelped. Her owner reports the dog is jaundiced and is urinating small amounts of dark urine. What is a likely diagnosis and why does this occur at whelping?

9 The throat of a stillborn hairless lamb has a large mass. The ewe has spent the winter on a kale pasture. What happened?

10 What is mulberry heart disease?

11 Pigs with scaly-looking skin and lots of itching with lesions and redness at the top of the foot are brought to your attention. Examination of the ration reveals that four times as much calcium as is required is being put into the ration. What has happened to the pigs?

12 Why is metallothionein production in enterocytes important?

Suggested reading

Ammerman, C.B., Baker, D.H. and Lewis, A.J. (1995) *Bioavailability of Nutrients for Animals*. Academic Press, San Diego, CA.

Goff, J.P. (2000) Pathophysiology of calcium and phosphorus disorders. *Veterinary Clinics of North America. Food Animal Practice* **16**:319–337.

Martens, H. and Schweigel, M. (2000) Pathophysiology of grass tetany and other hypomagnesemias. Implications for clinical management. *Veterinary Clinics of North America. Food Animal Practice* **16**:339–368.

National Research Council (2005) *Mineral Tolerance of Animals*. National Academy of Science Press, Washington, DC.

Underwood, E.J. and Suttle, N.F. (1999) *The Mineral Nutrition of Livestock*, 3rd edn. CABI Publishing, Wallingford, UK.

Answers

1 Milk fever. The high-potassium diet alkalinizes her blood, interfering with parathyroid hormone receptors on bone and kidney tissue. As a result she has difficulty maintaining calcium homeostasis at the onset of lactation.

2 It could reduce magnesium absorption across the rumen resulting in hypomagnesemia. Hypomagnesemia directly increases nervous system excitability and can contribute to hypocalcemia as well.

3 High-grain diets tend to be high in phosphorus. When coupled with low dietary calcium there is an upset in the amount of calcium that can be absorbed and then utilized for bone formation. This stimulates excessive secretion of parathyroid hormone, causing bone resorption. The normal bone osteoid is often replaced by a fibrous collagen. The result is osteodystrophy. If the matrix that has been resorbed by the activated osteoclasts is not replaced, the result is often referred to as osteoporosis.

4 Suddenly giving water to pigs that are severely dehydrated causes water to move rapidly into the brain where salt concentrations have become elevated due to the dehydration. This rapid rehydration of the animal results in brain edema and neurological dysfunction.

5 The chloride excreted into the abomasum is not reaching the small intestine due to sequestration within the displaced abomasum. This lack of chloride anions in the blood is the cause of a metabolic alkalosis.

6 Lack of aldosterone production can reduce renal potassium excretion.

7 Copper deficiency is suspected, which is causing a lack of pigmentation of the hair coat, poor growth and performance, and anemia. Molybdenum and diet sulfur form a tetrathiomolybdate–copper complex that renders diet copper unavailable for absorption leading to copper deficiency.

8 Copper toxicity. The stress of whelping causes sudden release of large amounts of copper from the liver. Free copper is such a strong oxidizing agent that it causes a hemolytic crisis.

9 The lamb developed goiter (hypothroidism). Kale contains a goitrogenic substance interfering with iodine utilization by the mother's thyroid gland. She in turn strives to save herself by increasing uptake and storage of iodine, leaving none for the developing fetus.

10 Selenium deficiency of pigs causing changes in the muscle of the heart.

11 Excessive calcium in the diet has interfered with zinc absorption causing zinc deficiency. Zinc is critical to normal keratinization processes.

12 Metallothionein is produced by enterocytes in response to high zinc and to a lesser extent copper stores in the body. The metallothionien will bind any zinc or copper that enters the enterocyte and sequester it within the cell until the cell sloughs off into the lumen. The trapped mineral then passes out with the feces. Metallothionein is a critical factor preventing toxicity from copper and zinc in many species.

50 Cartilage, Bones, and Joints

Jesse P. Goff

Iowa State University, Ames, IA, USA

Cartilage is a special type of connective tissue that is of extreme importance in embryonic development, serving as the model on which true bone is later formed. Cartilage also persists in adult animals, primarily as articular cartilage that cushions the interface between adjacent bones or joints of the body (Figure 50.1).

Bone is a hard rigid organ of the body that serves several important functions. Bones forming the skull and ribcage serve to protect vital soft tissues from external harm. The long bones of the legs, arms, and vertebral column form the appendicular skeleton, which works in concert with muscles and tendons to allow locomotion. A more subtle function of bone is to serve as a store of minerals, primarily calcium, vital to maintenance of a normal ionic environment. The purpose of this chapter is to provide the veterinary student with a basic knowledge of normal cartilage and bone physiology so that syndromes of special importance to veterinary medicine involving these tissues can be recognized and understood.

Anatomy of cartilage

> **1** Why must cartilage cells be tolerant of a low oxygen environment?

Cartilage consists of specialized cells known as **chondrocytes** entrapped within an **amorphous gel-like matrix** that the chondrocytes have secreted. The cells are isolated from other cells by this matrix and each cell resides in a small cavity within the matrix (Figure 50.2). Unlike most other tissues the number of chondrocytes within cartilage tissue is relatively small. Also, cartilage has no nerves or blood vessels within it. Chondrocytes therefore survive in a relatively hypoxic and malnourishing medium. All the oxygen and nutrients needed by the cartilage cells must diffuse through the cartilage matrix from capillary beds located outside the cartilage. Cartilage is usually enclosed within a dense fibrous connective tissue covering known as the

Section VIII: Minerals, Bones, and Joints

Dukes' Physiology of Domestic Animals, Thirteenth Edition. Edited by William O. Reece, Howard H. Erickson, Jesse P. Goff and Etsuro E. Uemura.

© 2015 John Wiley & Sons, Inc. Published 2015 by John Wiley & Sons, Inc.

Companion website: www.wiley.com/go/reece/physiology

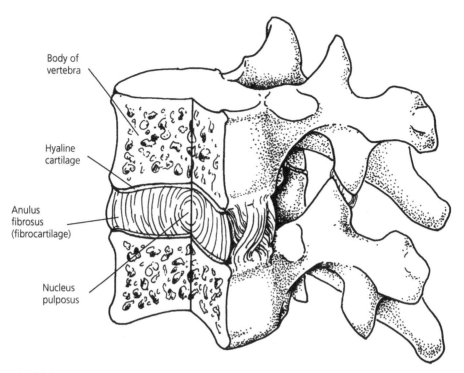

Figure 50.1 Intervertebral disk, composed of hyaline cartilage and fibrocartilage, serves to interconnect the bodies of contiguous vertebrae. From Cormack, D.H. (2001) *Essential Histology*, 2nd edn. Lippincott Williams & Wilkins, Baltimore. Reproduced with permission from Lippincott Williams & Wilkins.

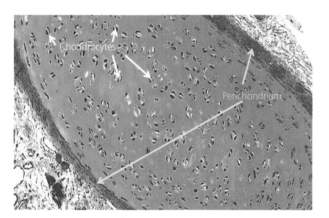

Figure 50.2 Section through the cartilage comprising a bronchiole of a cat illustrating the separation of chondrocytes from one another by the cartilage matrix. Perichondrium surrounds the cartilage and is the source of the chondrocytes that reside within the cartilage matrix. Note the absence of blood vessels within the cartilage.

perichondrium. Three types of cartilage exist, distinguished by the nature of the matrix surrounding the cells and the amount of collagen or elastin embedded in that matrix. **Hyaline cartilage** forms the bulk of cartilage in the animal and is the type most involved in veterinary pathologies. Hyaline cartilage is found on the ventral ends of ribs, within tracheal rings and the larynx, and on articulating surfaces of bones. In growing animals the cartilage comprising the physeal plates of long bones is also hyaline cartilage. The bones of the body arise from a hyaline

cartilage "model" of that bone formed in the embryonic stage of development. **Elastic cartilage** is relatively scarce but can be found in the external ear and epiglottis. **Fibrocartilage** is found at the site of insertion of many of the larger ligaments onto bone. It is also found within the intervertebral disks and the symphysis of the pubis.

Growth of cartilage

> **1** Which type of collagen is unique to cartilage?

Cartilage growth is especially important in the embryo where cartilage models exist for all the tissues that will eventually become bone in the animal. Growth also continues in the adult animal though at a much slower pace. Cartilage chondrocytes originally arise from the mesenchymal cells of the embryo. As they undergo mitosis they spread out, expanding the cartilage from within, a process known as **interstitial growth**. As cartilage cells develop and mature they surround themselves with a specialized mixture of proteins to form an interstitial matrix. The composition of the interstitial matrix distinguishes the three types of cartilage from each other. In hyaline cartilage, the interstitial matrix is composed of a mixture of mucopolysaccharides, and mucoproteins such as chondroitin 4-sulfate and chondroitin 6-sulfate. Fine fibrils of collagen also exist within the matrix. These fibrils are originally secreted into the matrix as tropocollagen by the chondrocytes. They then aggregate and assemble themselves into collagen fibrils within the matrix. Though these fibrils make up nearly 40% of the weight of hyaline cartilage matrix, they are not as visible as the bundles of collagen that exist in bone and other connective tissues. Elastic cartilage is more flexible than hyaline cartilage due to the presence of elastin fibers embedded in the ground substance forming the cartilage matrix. In fibrocartilage, the collagen content of the matrix is greatly increased and the collagen fibrils form thick tough bundles aligned in one direction to provide great tensile strength.

The **proteoglycans** and **glycosaminoglycans** that comprise the amorphous matrix function to maintain hydration of cartilage by electrostatically attracting water and provide cartilage with resilience and compressive strength. A wide variety of proteoglycans exist, but all are composed of a core protein to which an extensive variety of different carbohydrate side chains, including chondroitin sulfate, dermatan sulfate, heparan sulfate, and keratan sulfate, are attached.

The fibrous structural proteins of the cartilage matrix form a framework that provides cartilage with strength, elasticity, and shear force resistance. The main fibrillar collagen in cartilage is **type II collagen**. This protein accounts for more than 50% of the dry weight in most cartilaginous tissues. While type I collagen is the primary fibrillar collagen in bone and most other connective tissues, type II collagen is only found in cartilage. Cartilage also contains several types of collagen that do not form fibrils in the matrix. Type IX collagen has been identified on the surface of type II collagen fibers, where it may function to regulate the spatial arrangement of type II fibers. Type X collagen can be found in chondrocytes within the growth plates of long bones and may be critical to endochondral ossification (described in the section on bone formation), in which cartilage is replaced by bone.

Anatomy of bone

> 1 What structure separates the diaphysis from the epiphysis in growing long bones?
>
> 2 What are the three major bone cell types and what are their functions?

A typical long bone of the body is depicted in Figure 50.3. The ends of the bone are termed the **epiphyses**. The long compact shaft of the bone is the **diaphysis** and in growing animals a cartilaginous matrix termed the **epiphyseal plate** separates the two. The diaphysis is joined to the epiphyseal plate (or growth plate) by a transitional spongy bone termed the **metaphysis**. The diaphysis consists of a thick-walled cylinder of very dense or compact bone, with spongy bone in the middle or **medullary space**.

The medullary space is not entirely hollow. A delicate framework of bony spicules forms a lattice structure and provides

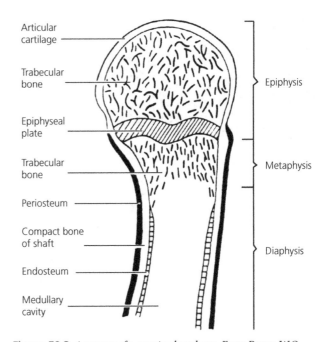

Figure 50.3 Anatomy of a growing long bone. From Reece, W.O. (2004) *Dukes' Physiology of Domestic Animals*, 12th edn. Cornell University Press, Ithaca, NY. Reproduced with permission from Cornell University Press.

space for the bone marrow, home to the hematopoietic cells of the body. This spongy or trabecular bone (also known as cancellous bone) provides great strength to the bone and allows some flexibility that would not be possible if the entire bone was compact bone. The scaffolding effect of the trabeculae also greatly reduces the weight of the bone without greatly compromising strength.

The outside of bone surfaces is covered by a layer of cells, forming the **periosteum**. This layer of cells is endowed with special properties as it can give rise to **osteoprogenitor cells** or bone-forming cells vital to growth and repair of the bone. The internal surfaces of bone trabeculae within the marrow cavity are also lined with osteoprogenitor cells and this layer is termed the **endosteum**. In the flat bones forming the skull, the outside layer analogous to the periosteum is termed the **pericranium**. **Dura mater** is the name applied to the cells lining the inner surface of the flat bones of the skull. Both layers serve as sources of osteoprogenitor cells in flat bones, though the flat bones do not seem as efficient at repair and remodeling efforts as long bones.

Three major cell types are found in bone tissue, the **osteoblasts**, the **osteocytes**, and the **osteoclasts** (Figure 50.4).

Osteoblasts

Osteoblasts are the main cells involved in the ossification process and are readily observed during new bone formation. They are usually 20–30 μm in size and are often observed forming a one-cell thick layer covering the surfaces undergoing remodeling or primary ossification. The nuclei of osteoblasts

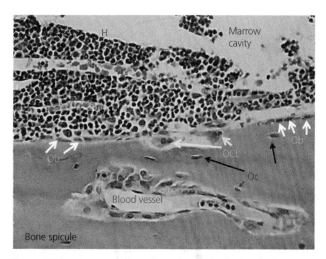

Figure 50.4 Microscopic view of a single spicule of trabecular bone. In this preparation the organic matrix of the bone is stained pink. Osteoblasts (Ob) line the bone surface forming the endosteum. Osteocytes (Oc) reside within lacunae within the bone matrix. Multinucleated osteoclasts (OCL) can be found in a resorption cavity where bone is being resorbed. Hemopoietic cells (H) outside the bone form the bone marrow and an obliquely cut blood vessel is seen passing through the bone.

are generally located at the end of the cell furthest from the bone surface and the cytoplasm is rich in rough endoplasmic reticulum, befitting a cell responsible for synthesis and secretion of the proteins that will form the organic matrix of bone. When actively involved in bone formation, the osteoblasts are intensely basophilic histologically, due to the presence of increased amounts of RNA. The intensity of basophilic staining is decreased when osteoblasts are in a resting stage.

Osteocytes

Both osteoblasts and osteocytes originate from mesenchymal cells. Osteoblasts entrapped within bone matrix become osteocytes. It is thought that osteocytes can revert to active osteoblasts when the organic matrix surrounding them is dissolved during bone resorption. Osteocytes are relatively solitary cells. The small areas or holes in the bone in which the osteocytes reside are called **lacunae**. It is believed that osteocytes are essentially osteoblasts that have been entrapped and embedded within the bone matrix during bone formation. **Canaliculi** or tunnels form a labyrinth of connections between neighboring osteocytes as they reside in their lacuna. Cytoplasmic projections from each osteocyte extend through the canaliculi allowing neighboring osteocytes to contact each other. The canaliculi extend to the surface of the bone, allowing osteocytes to also network with osteoblasts and the extracellular fluid.

The fluid within the lacunae and canicular system is relatively high in calcium. When activated by parathyroid hormone, the osteocytes can pump this bone fluid calcium into the extracellular fluid to help raise blood calcium concentrations, a process known as **osteocytic osteolysis**. It does not involve matrix dissolution as typical osteoclastic bone resorption does

and it mobilizes a relatively small amount of calcium compared with osteoclastic bone resorption. However, it is a very quick response to hypocalcemia (within hours) as compared to osteoclastic bone resorption, which takes several days to become active.

Osteoclasts

Osteoclasts are very large multinucleated cells observed at bone surfaces actively undergoing resorption. Evidence now suggests that osteoclasts are derived from the same progenitors as monocytes of the immune system. It may therefore be appropriate to consider them as macrophages of bone tissues. Their nuclei are usually located at the end of the cell furthest from the bone surface. The cytoplasm is dense with nonmembrane-bound ribosomes, and numerous lysosomes are present, befitting a cell whose origin is similar to that of a macrophage. They also have a distinct ruffled edge on the end in contact with the bone surface, composed of cytoplasmic folds. Osteoclasts are quite mobile and can migrate along surfaces of bone to sites of bone resorption.

Bone composition

1 What are the two types of bone?

2 What steps occur during formation of collagen matrix?

3 What purpose is served by the space between collagen microfibril fibers?

4 Why does vitamin C deficiency affect bone?

Long bones contain two distinct types of bone (Figure 50.5). **Compact or cortical bone** is very dense. This type of bone is found at the outer edges of long bones and at each end of the bones, under the articular cartilage. **Trabecular or spongy bone** (also known as **cancellous bone**) is found within the marrow cavity and forms a lightweight but strong scaffolding to allow the bone to bend slightly and also provides a place for hematopoietic cells to reside. Blood vessels run parallel the length of the bone and are contained in channels known as **Haversian canals** (Figure 50.6). Smaller blood vessels run perpendicular to the vessels within the Haversian canals and these channels are called **Volkmann canals**. The Volkmann canals connect the Haversian canal blood vessels to the periosteum on the outside of the bone and the medullary cavity that forms the bone marrow on the interior of the bone. In compact bone the osteoblasts form bone in concentric layers surrounding each Haversian canal. As osteoblasts become encased in the bone matrix they have produced, they become osteocytes. A system of channels known as canaliculi connects osteocytes with each other and to the periosteum and bone marrow. These canaliculi are filled with bone interstitial fluid that is relatively rich in calcium (Figure 50.7).

The spongy or trabecular bone forms a lattice within the middle of long bones. The hematopoietic bone marrow cells

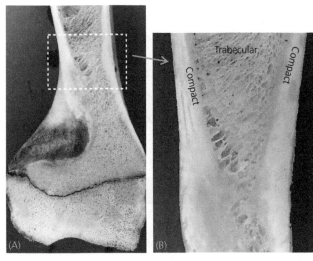

Figure 50.5 (A) Sagittal section of the distal humerus of a horse. (B) Close-up view of a section of the diaphysis highlighting the compact and trabecular bone structures.

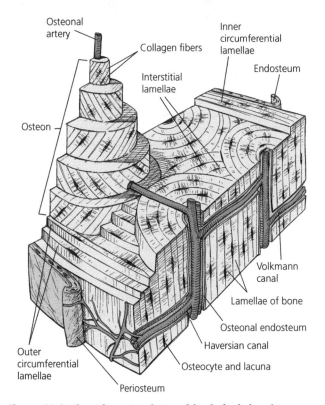

Figure 50.6 Three-dimensional view of the shaft of a long bone. From Ross, M.H. (2003) *Histology, A Text and Atlas*, 4th edn. Lippincott Williams & Wilkins, Baltimore. Reproduced with permission from Lippincott Williams & Wilkins.

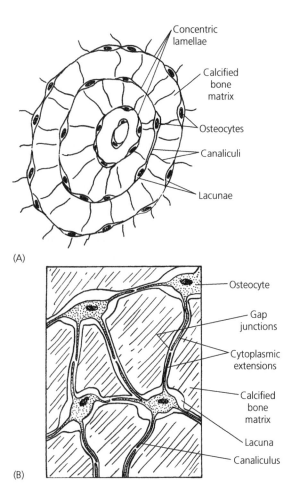

Figure 50.7 An osteon (Haversian system). (A) Concentric lamellae, showing osteocytes within their lacunae and their communicating canaliculi. (B) Cytoplasmic extensions of osteocytes into canaliculi for communication with other osteocytes. From Reece, W.O. (2009) *Functional Anatomy and Physiology of Domestic Animals*, 4th edn. Wiley-Blackwell, Ames, IA. Reproduced with permission from Wiley.

can be found within the lattice spaces between the spicules of bone that comprise the trabecular bone. In trabecular bone the spicules are lined by osteoblasts and again become osteocytes when they have surrounded themselves with the bone matrix they have produced (see Figure 50.4). The osteocytes are connected with each other by canaliculi, filled with bone interstitial fluid, that are in communication with the marrow cavity extracellular fluid.

Bone consists of inorganic salts deposited within an organic matrix composed of collagen fibrils and glycoproteins. Bone minerals include calcium, phosphorus (as the phosphate anion), magnesium, sodium, potassium, chloride, and fluoride. Trace amounts of many other inorganic elements can also be found in bone. Bone salt also contains significant amounts of citrate, hydroxyl, and carbonate anions.

A general structure for bone mineral is approximated by the formula for hydroxyapatite crystals, $Ca_{10}(PO_4)_6(OH)_2$. There are about 10 calcium cations for every 6 phosphate anions in bone. Citrate and carbonate anions are also often found on the surface of bone crystals. If fluoride ions substitute for a few of the OH^- ions in the bone crystals, the bone is given extra strength. Thus, a minute amount of fluoride added to drinking water can increase resistance of teeth to cavities. Larger amounts of fluoride actually weaken the bone structure, and in some areas grazing animals will consume enough fluoride to cause pathological changes in bone.

Other trace minerals can also intercalate themselves into bone mineral. Lead and strontium readily substitute for calcium in the crystals. In the event of a nuclear disaster, strontium-90 may present a special threat to grazing livestock. Bone will serve as a reservoir for strontium-90 that may be excreted in milk for a long period.

The organic component of bone provides toughness and resilience. If all the bone organic matrix is removed, the inorganic minerals retain the gross shape of the bone but the bone has lost its tensile strength and is as brittle as a china plate. On the other hand, if the bone mineral is removed by exposing the bone to a weak acid, the organic matrix is very flexible and has no hardness.

The major organic component of bone is the fibrous protein collagen. The main collagen of bone is referred to as type I. Type I collagen makes up 90% of the matrix of bone. In contrast, type II collagen, found only in cartilage, makes up just 40% of the matrix of cartilage. Intercalated between collagen fibrils are smaller proteins called proteoglycans. They are smaller and denser than the proteoglycans of cartilage. In cartilage there is enough space between proteoglycan and type II collagen fibrils to allow diffusion of nutrients and oxygen through the matrix. Therefore cartilage is relatively free of blood vessels. Bone proteoglycans form a much denser matrix with type I collagen of bone. Nutrients will not diffuse through bone to any great extent. Therefore all bone cells are relatively close to a blood vessel or connected to a blood vessel by the canaliculi that permeate bone tissue. Numerous smaller proteins also exist within the bone matrix. Some have important roles in controlling the mineralization process.

Type I collagen is synthesized within osteoblasts and, to a smaller extent, osteocytes. Within osteoblasts the newly translated procollagen molecule undergoes some unique post-transcriptional modification, such as hydroxylation of some of the proline and lysine residues. Vitamin C (ascorbic acid) is required for hydroxylation reactions within osteoblasts. In those species, such as guinea pigs, incapable of producing ascorbic acid, dietary deficiency of vitamin C causes weakening of the collagen matrices of bone, teeth, and skin leading to the condition known as scurvy. It is believed that three individual collagen fibrils are braided together to form a tropocollagen fibril during their extrusion from the osteoblasts and osteocytes (Figure 50.8). The three collagen molecules are braided around each other like rope and provide added strength and rigidity. Five tropocollagen fibrils come together to form a microfibril. Numerous microfibrils are in turn laid end to end in a staggered formation, all in the same direction within a single bone metabolic unit, to form the collagen matrix. The microfibril fibers are each about 64 nm in length and there is a small space between the ends of fibrils. This space seems to serve an important

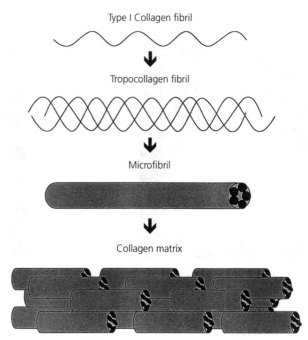

Figure 50.8 Bone collagen formation. Three type I collagen fibrils synthesized within osteoblasts are braided together to form a tropocollagen fibril during their extrusion from the osteoblasts and osteocytes. Five tropocollagen fibrils then come together to form a microfibril. Numerous microfibrils in turn are laid end to end in a staggered formation to form the collagen matrix. Each of the microfibril fibers is about 64 nm long, and there is a small space between the ends of adjacent fibrils. This space seems to serve an important function as the site of initial nucleation of mineral crystals onto collagen matrix.

function as the site of initial nucleation of mineral crystals onto collagen matrix.

Collagen contains the unique amino acid hydroxyproline. During bone resorption, the digestion of bone collagen fibrils causes hydroxyproline concentration to rise in the blood. Excretion of hydroxyproline in urine has been used as a crude estimate of bone resorption activity in certain disease states such as hyperparathyroidism. Hydroxylysine is another amino acid common in collagen but found only rarely in other proteins. Hydroxylysine forms a covalent cross-link with norleucine across adjacent collagen fibrils, stabilizing the fibrils. The staggered assembly and cross-linking of the type I collagen fibrils causes a characteristic banding pattern to the organic matrix.

Osteocalcin is protein specific to bone that contains three unique glutamate residues in which the gamma carbon has been carboxylated. This carboxylation reaction is dependent on vitamin K. The synthesis of osteocalcin is regulated by 1,25-dihydroxyvitamin D, the hormonal form of vitamin D. Osteocalcin appears to inhibit formation of hydroxyapatite precipitates and thus it may inhibit mineralization. It is a chemoattractant of blood leukocytes, suggesting it may also play a role in attracting osteoclasts to a bone site in need of resorption and remodeling.

Other small proteins within bone have been isolated and identified, although little is clear about their function.

Bone formation

> 1 How does intramembranous ossification differ from endochondral ossification?
>
> 2 Does the epiphyseal ossification center replace all the cartilage in the epiphysis?

Bone only develops on a preexisting connective tissue. Two different paths for bone formation occur in embryos and growing animals. If the bone formation occurs within primitive connective tissue, the process is known as **intramembranous ossification**. When preexisting cartilage is converted to bone, the process is referred to as **endochondral ossification**. Under pathological conditions, connective tissues that are not normally converted to bone become ossified, a process called **ectopic bone formation**.

Intramembranous ossification

Many of the flat bones of the skull, including the frontal, parietal, occipital, and temporal bones, and part of the mandible develop by intramembranous ossification. The developing embryo has areas of mesenchyme within it. Mesenchyme is tissue characterized by primordial cell types surrounded by a large amount of extracellular matrix. This matrix is a loose connective tissue. During embryonic development the mesenchyme in those areas destined to become flat bones condenses and becomes well vascularized. The mesenchymal cells begin to secrete collagen fibrils, which are randomly oriented within a gel-like ground substance. The rigid organization of collagen fibrils observed in mature bone is not yet present. As these collagen fibrils accumulate, the matrix between cells is thickened, forming strands of solid matrix. Simultaneously, the mesenchymal cells enlarge and gather on the surface of the collagen fibril strands. The cells become basophilic and differentiate into osteoblasts. They secrete additional bone matrix. The small strands of collagen become longer and thicker and form a network of strands or trabeculae. The collagen fibrils remain randomly interwoven and this early bone is referred to as **woven bone**. The random organization of the collagen fibrils means that woven bone is relatively weak. The advantage of woven bone is that it can be laid down quickly, a point that will be revisited when the student learns about fracture repair.

Shortly after the osteoblasts begin producing collagen fibrils and glycoproteins, calcium phosphate deposits build up on the matrix. As the trabeculae thicken and become calcified, some of the osteoblasts become trapped within the matrix to become osteocytes. The osteocytes reside within their lacunae and remain connected to osteoblasts at the surface by slender processes. Eventually, the canaliculi of bone are formed when matrix is deposited around these cell processes. As osteoblasts are incorporated into the matrix to become osteocytes, they are replaced by mitotic division of osteoprogenitor cells at the surface of the trabecula. Interestingly, osteoblasts themselves have only rarely been observed to divide.

Prior to birth, the randomly organized collagen of the woven bone is replaced with a more organized collagen. A distinction is that the new matrix replacing the woven bone matrix consists of collagen fibrils secreted in regularly arranged tight layers around the blood vessels so the bone in these areas comes to resemble mature lamellar bone. Lamellar bone has a regular parallel alignment of the collagen fibrils into sheets (Latin *lamellae*), giving the bone its great strength. The outside and inside surfaces of the woven bone are destined to become compact bone with a thin layer of trabecular bone between them.

The connective tissue on the outer surfaces of the bone condenses to form the pericranium. Osteoblasts on these surfaces revert to fibroblast-like cells as growth ceases. When called on to form bone again, they can be reactivated.

Endochondral ossification

Bones that first exist in the embryo as hyaline cartilage develop by a process known as endochondral ossification. These include the bones of the extremities, the base of the skull, the vertebral column, and the pelvis. This is in contrast with the intramembranous bones that develop directly from the mesenchyme with no cartilage involvement.

Endochondral ossification begins with mesenchymal cells differentiating into chondrocytes, which then lay out hyaline cartilage in the shape of the bone to be formed (Figure 50.9). The chondrocytes secrete hyaline matrix consisting of type II collagen, giving hyaline cartilage a soft and flexible consistency. While these changes are occurring in the interior of the cartilage model of the future bone, the osteogenic potential of cells within the perichondrium lining the cartilage model is activated. These cells deposit a thin collar of woven bone on the outside of the cartilage model, in a process that is very similar to intramembranous ossification.

Centers of ossification arise within the hyaline cartilage. These are distinguished by a tremendous enlargement of the chondrocytes in certain areas of the cartilaginous bone. The lacunae surrounding these chondrocytes expand and only thin strands of cartilage matrix separate adjacent lacunae. Next, these small strands of remaining cartilaginous matrix begin to accumulate calcium phosphate deposits. This appears to be initiated by factors, such as type X collagen, produced by the hypertrophied cartilage cells.

As the cartilage surrounding them calcifies, the hypertrophied chondrocytes undergo apoptosis or programmed cell death. Blood vessels arising from the newly formed periosteum invade the area containing the dying hypertrophied chondrocytes and new osteoprogenitor cells follow the blood vessels into the region. Other cells follow the blood vessels and will eventually become hemopoietic elements of the bone marrow.

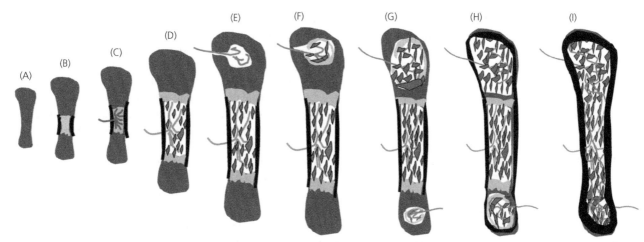

Figure 50.9 Endochondral ossification. (A) Chondrocytes form a cartilaginous model in the shape of the bone to be formed. (B) Chondrocytes hypertrophy and the cartilage matrix becomes calcified in the area of an ossification center. Osteoprogenitor cells develop within the perichondrium. (C) Blood vessels invade the calcified cartilage matrix from the newly formed periosteum. (D) Osteoprogenitor cells follow blood vessels into the area, and these give rise to osteoblasts that congregate on the surface of the calcified cartilage spicules and begin depositing bone matrix. (E) A second center of ossification begins to develop within the epiphysis as blood vessels invade the area of hypertrophied chondrocytes (shade area) and calcified cartilage. (F–I) Primary ossification of the calcified cartilage proceeds at the epiphyseal and diaphyseal ossification centers.

Osteoprogenitor cells give rise to osteoblasts that congregate on the surface of the calcified cartilage spicules and begin to deposit bone matrix, consisting of loosely organized type I collagen, on them. Therefore the earliest bone trabeculae formed within the interior of the cartilage model have calcified cartilage at their core and an outer layer of woven bone.

The actual process by which bone or cartilage matrix becomes mineralized is poorly understood. Some liken it to a solution that is supersaturated with calcium and phosphorus to which addition of a foreign substance initiates crystallization. In the case of bone, the collagen fibers (or collagen in combination with glycoproteins or chondroitin sulfate) act as a nucleation catalyst, which transforms calcium and phosphate in solution in the tissue fluids into a solid mineral deposited on the collagen fibers.

In horses and cows, centers of ossification first appear in the diaphysis of the hyaline cartilage model of each of the long bones of the skeleton by the third month of fetal development. Secondary centers of ossification appear in the epiphyses of the long bones much later. They differ from the diaphyseal ossification centers in two important ways.

1 The expansion of the epiphyseal ossification center does not replace all the epiphyseal cartilage. It does not replace that cartilage which will come in contact with another bone. This cartilage will persist as the articular cartilage throughout life.

2 A transverse disk of epiphyseal cartilage will remain between the epiphysis and diaphysis, which will give rise to the epiphyseal plate (more commonly referred to as the growth plate). Chondrocytes within the growth plate become arranged into columns that will allow growth in length of the bone as discussed later.

Growth in length of bones

> 1 What is happening in the zone of proliferation of a growth plate?
>
> 2 What is happening in the zone of maturation?
>
> 3 What is happening in the zone of provisional calcification?
>
> 4 How does the metaphysis differ from the diaphysis?

In the cartilage model of bone formation some of the chondrocytes at the epiphyseal ends of the primordial bone become arranged in columns running parallel to the length of the bone and will eventually serve as a growth plate. The long bones of the body will have a growth plate that separates the epiphyses from the diaphysis at each end of the bone (Figure 50.10). In some bones, additional growth plates form to allow growth of special features, such as the greater trochanter of the femur. The columns of chondrocytes are separated by longitudinal bars of hyaline cartilage matrix. Chondrocytes within each column are directly related to each other as they are the result of mitotic division within that column.

The cells that form the growth plate take on a distinct layered shape, with each layer representing a different stage of bone formation. Those chondrocytes within the growth plate that are the furthest from the diaphysis comprise the **zone of proliferation**. The next visible stage within the growth plate is the **zone of maturation**. Here the chondrocytes have stopped dividing and have become enlarged. This leads to great hypertrophy and vacuolation of the chondrocytes to form the **zone of hypertrophy**. The cartilaginous matrix surrounding these cells begins to calcify, causing some anatomists to refer to this area as the **zone of provisional calcification**, instead of the zone of hypertrophy.

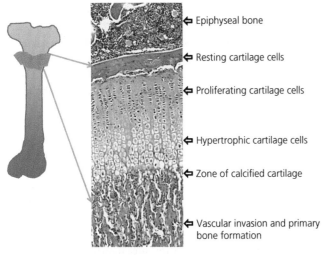

← Epiphyseal bone

← Resting cartilage cells

← Proliferating cartilage cells

← Hypertrophic cartilage cells

← Zone of calcified cartilage

← Vascular invasion and primary bone formation

Figure 50.10 Microscopic view of the growth plate from the femur of a growing cat. The bone lengthens as chondrocytes in the zone of proliferation divide and expand the plate away from the diaphysis. After the chondrocytes have proliferated they hypertrophy and begin to undergo apoptosis or programmed cell death. Shortly after this, the matrix surrounding the apoptotic chondrocytes becomes calcified. Blood vessels invade the calcified cartilage matrix and carry in the osteoblasts that will replace the calcified cartilage matrix and dead chondrocytes with primary bone or woven bone. This bone is rather weak and is eventually remodeled and replaced with more mature stronger bone.

Finally at the diaphyseal side of the growth plate the chondrocytes undergo apoptosis and degenerate. The diaphyseal ends of their large lacunae are invaded by blood vessels and osteoprogenitor cells from the marrow spaces of the primary ossification center within the diaphysis.

As the lacunae are invaded, osteoblasts differentiate and form along the irregularly shaped bars of calcified cartilage that had once separated the columns of chondrocytes. A thin layer of loosely organized collagen matrix (see Figure 50.8) is deposited on the surface of the calcified cartilage. If conditions are favorable (adequate dietary calcium, phosphorus, and vitamin D), the new bone matrix quickly calcifies. This primary spongy bone area is often referred to as the metaphysis of the bone. As the growth process finishes, osteoclasts move into the metaphysis to resorb the woven bone and calcified cartilage and new osteoblasts move in to form the organized sheets of type I collagen that comprise true lamellar bone. Thus the rapidly dividing cells of the zone of proliferation continually advance the growth plate away from the diaphysis, while osteoclasts and osteoblasts continually convert primary woven bone (also called spongiosa bone) to true lamellar bone at the diaphyseal side of the growth plate. The net result is that the growth plate and metaphysis continue to move away from the diaphyseal ossification center. This growth of long bones is largely controlled by pituitary secretion of growth hormone (somatotropin). Growth hormone causes local production of insulin-like growth factor 1 (somatomedin), which causes the chondrocytes at the zone of proliferation to continue to divide.

Once the bone has reached its mature length, proliferation of cartilage cells slows to a halt. Replacement of cartilage with bone at the diaphyseal side of the growth plate continues until the entire growth plate cartilage is replaced by bone. The bony trabeculae of the diaphysis then become contiguous with the trabeculae of the epiphyses. This process is referred to as **closure of the growth plate**. The bone has reached its mature length.

Closure of the growth plate occurs at different times in different bones and the two growth plates within each long bone can close at different times. Such information becomes valuable in assessment of radiographs and in orthopedic surgery. Injury to a growth plate can alter the stature of the animal. Excessive ingestion of vitamin A can cause premature closure of the growth plate. A condition in dairy heifers in which the growth plates of the hindlimbs close prematurely causes the front legs to be slightly longer than the hindlegs, leading to the description of this condition as **hyena disease**. It is attributed to administration of large doses of vitamin A to calves as part of the therapy for scours.

Growth in diameter of bones

> 1 How does a bone thicken?
> 2 Are chondrocytes involved?

The growth in diameter of the shaft of long bones is due to deposition of new bone on the outside surface by cells within the periosteum. In many respects this is simply a continuation of a process very similar to intramembranous ossification. The distinction is that bone resorption plays a major role in this process. The deposition of new bone under the periosteum is accompanied by the resorption of older bone at the interior edge of the shaft of the diaphysis. This allows the diameter of the bone to increase as the activities at the growth plate increase the length of the bone, and allows the marrow cavity within the bone to expand. A solid compact bone would be much heavier and less flexible than a bone with trabeculae forming a lattice of support.

During growth, the bones retain the same shape that they had in the fetal hyaline cartilage model. This implies that the rate of bone formation and resorption is somehow regulated to maintain this general shape. However, subtle changes in shape do occur during the growth process. For instance, skull bones must accommodate a growing brain. As the radius of curvature of the skull vault increases, the bones become more flattened. How this is controlled is unknown.

Stress on a bone can increase the amount of mineral and thickness of the bone matrix deposited during bone remodeling. Right-handed tennis players can have as much as 35% more bone in their right humerus than in their left humerus. In contrast, astronauts working in zero gravity and bed-ridden patients can lose close to 1% of vertebral bone mass for each week spent in these conditions. How this is controlled is not well understood.

In the areas of bone that will persist as spongy or trabecular bone, the thickening of the trabeculae ceases at some point during development and the space between trabeculae is transformed into hemopoietic tissue known as bone marrow. As animals age, and if they are well fed, adipose tissue can replace some of the hematopoietic tissue, giving the marrow a yellow appearance.

Bone remodeling

1 What is the purpose of bone remodeling?
2 What are the major steps involved in remodeling a portion of a bone?

Once fully formed and the animal reaches its adult frame size, bone does not become a totally quiescent structure. Throughout life the bone will undergo remodeling, a process in which old lamellar bone is replaced by new lamellar bone, with little or no change in bone mass (Figure 50.11).

Why does bone undergo remodeling? Stress from physical trauma over time creates microscopic fractures within the mature bone. Remodeling allows the body to continually replace small pockets of worn-out bone with new bone through a gradual process that does not interfere with bone function. How this is recognized is unknown. One possibility involves the piezoelectric property of bone mineral affixed to collagen. Forces applied to crystals within the bone matrix give rise to a very small electric potential or current in the bone crystal, which may influence bone cell metabolism locally. Interruption of this current may initiate remodeling of that section of bone. Only very small units of bone are undergoing remodeling at any one time. These units are often referred to as **bone remodeling units** (BRU). The shape of the BRU in compact or cortical bone differs from that in trabecular or cancellous bone, but the same four distinct steps – activation, resorption, reversal, formation – occur during remodeling at both sites.

Activation

This is the process that converts a resting or inactive bone surface into a surface to be remodeled (Figure 50.11A,B). How a particular bit of bone is chosen for remodeling is not clear. It appears to be a random event; however, the presence of microfractures in an area does seem to mark an area for remodeling. This "selective" remodeling appears to be directed by a signal arising from the bone. Microfractures may simply disrupt the ordered collagen fibril orientation. When collagen fibrils are oriented correctly there is a very minute electrical charge oriented along the fibrils. Microfractures upset the piezoelectric charge of that portion of bone, which may act to initiate remodeling of that area. Deterioration of bone could also

elicit secretion of autocrine or paracrine factors that locally initiate activation of the BRU.

During activation the bone lining cells, which are essentially quiescent osteoblasts, retract and shrink in the area of bone to be remodeled. This exposes the bone matrix (Figure 50.11C). Multinucleated osteoclasts move onto this site and a tight bond is formed between bone and ruffled border.

Resorption

The osteoclasts release acids and proteolytic enzymes from their ruffled border onto the bone surface, dissolving the organic matrix of the bone (Figure 50.11D). The acids include carbonic, hydrochloric, citric, and lactic acids. The proteolytic enzymes (protein degrading) include acid hydrolases, which function well at low pH. The mineral crystals are dissolved by the acids and the minerals along with the breakdown products of the organic matrix enter the osteoclast by diffusion or specific transport processes. They are then extruded into the extracellular fluid on the opposite side of the osteoclast.

In trabecular bone the osteoclasts resorb bone until they have formed a saucer-shaped depression that is around 50 μm in depth at its center and 200–300 μm in diameter (Figure 50.11E). In cortical or compact bone, the osteoclasts drill out bone to create a tunnel only about 2.5 mm deep/long and 200 μm in diameter. At this point the osteoclasts quit their bone-resorbing activity and leave the BRU.

Reversal

This phase signals the start of the rebuilding of the resorbed bone (Figure 50.11F). Osteoblasts move from the bone surface down into the depths of the resorption hollow, known as **Howship's lacuna** after the scientist who first reported it in 1816. What signals the osteoblasts to migrate into Howship's lacuna remains largely unknown. Several growth factors, such as insulin-like growth factor 2 and transforming growth factor (TGF)-β, are thought to be incorporated into bone matrix during bone formation. During resorption these peptides are released during digestion of the collagen matrix and activate the bone-lining cells to revert to osteoblasts. Both of these factors can be found in bone and both have been shown to stimulate replication of osteoblasts *in vitro*. Many other substances, including interleukin (IL)-1, platelet-derived growth factor, and insulin-like growth factor 1 (somatomedin), are also considered candidates capable of initiating the reversal phase of remodeling. Perhaps no chemoattractant factors are elaborated and it is simply the presence of exposed bone matrix when the osteoclasts leave that attracts osteoblasts into the area. Somehow osteoblasts are stimulated to assemble in the area of resorbed bone in appropriate numbers to refill the resorption cavity.

Formation

Bone matrix formation begins with deposition of osteoid by the osteoblasts. This organic matrix consists primarily of type I collagen, proteoglycans, and smaller proteins typical of

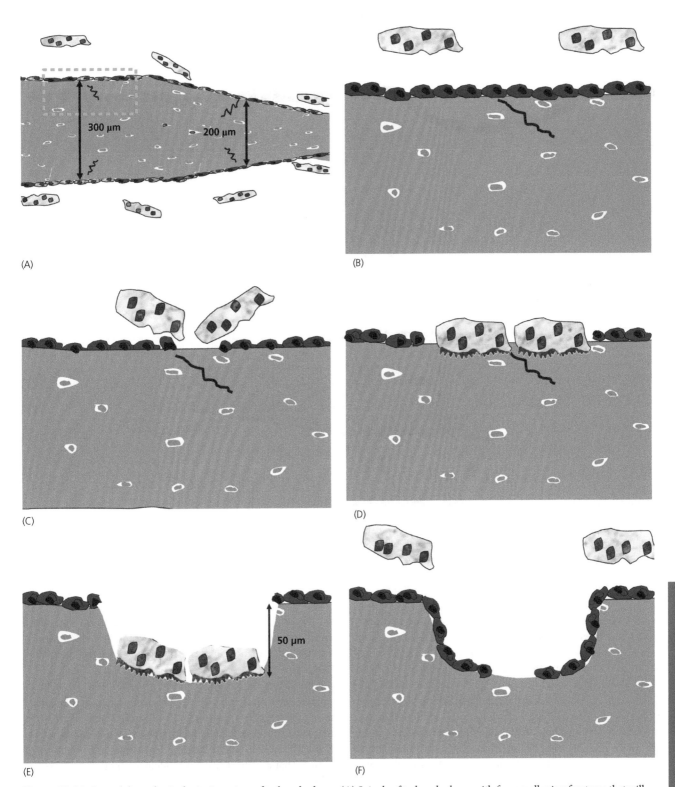

Figure 50.11 Remodeling of a single site in a piece of trabecular bone. (A) Spicule of trabecular bone with four small microfractures that will be resorbed and replaced. (B) Close-up view of endosteal surface of the spicule of trabecular bone outlined by dashed green line in (A). The osteoclasts and osteoblasts are in the resting state above a small microfracture within the bone matrix. (C) Activation: osteoblasts retract from the surface of the area of bone to be remodeled. Osteoclasts move toward the site of exposed bone. (D) Resorption: osteoclasts develop a ruffled border and form a tight seal with the exposed bone. Secretion of acids and enzymes causes dissolution of the organic matrix, freeing the minerals which enter extracellular fluid. (E) Resorption: osteoclasts scoop out bone matrix and mineral to a depth of approximately 50 μm. (F) Reversal: osteoclasts leave the area and become inactive. Osteoblasts from among the endosteal bone lining cells at the edge of the resorption site now enter the depths of the resorption cavity.

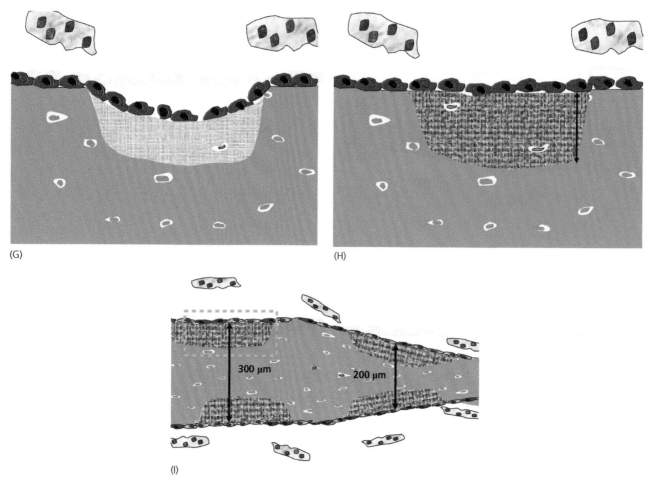

Figure 50.11 (*Continued*) (G) Osteoblasts begin producing new bone matrix to fill the resorption cavity. Some become trapped within the matrix to give rise to new osteocytes. (H) The area of new matrix becomes mineralized and that section of bone reenters a resting state. However, there is now approximately 50 μm of new bone formed to replace the microfracture with new bone. (I) The four original microfracture sites in the bone spicule have been replaced with new strong bone.

mature adult bone (Figure 50.11G). The osteoid is laid down in discrete layers or lamellae about 3 μm thick, with all the collagen fibrils within each lamella oriented parallel to each other. In cortical bone the tunnel hollowed out by the osteoclasts is filled in from the outer circumference toward the center until only a small central canal containing blood vessels is left open. The collagen fibrils within different lamellae are oriented at an angle to the layer above or below, giving the bone added strength, an idea shared by lumberyards producing plywood. In trabecular bone the osteoid layers are deposited in gently curved sheets following the curve of the resorption cavity.

Mineralization of the organic matrix is the final step in bone formation (Figure 50.11H). It occurs after a time delay, which is about 20 days in humans. Once triggered, the mineralization process is rather rapid. During the first few days of the process nearly 75% of the total bone calcium will

be deposited, with the final 25% of mineralization being completed months later. The total time for osteoblasts to complete the formation phase in a single BRU approximates 150 days.

Remodeling is necessary in large long-lived animals to replace bone that is fatigued and accumulating microfractures (Figure 50.11I). If bone remodeling came to a halt, the microfractures that accumulate would cause mechanical failure of the skeleton in about 2 years. In rodents and other small animals that are short-lived, remodeling is not as necessary as in longer-lived species but still occurs.

Bone remodeling also serves another important function. It allows the skeleton to act as a repository of minerals by allowing transfer of calcium and other ions in and out of bone as needed to maintain electrolyte balance. The hormones involved in calcium homeostasis can greatly influence the rate and extent of bone remodeling.

Repair of a broken bone

> 1 Why is angiogenesis (formation of new blood vessels) so critical to the process of bone repair?
>
> 2 Why is woven bone important to this process?

When a bone fractures, the broken ends of the bone must be brought together in close apposition if the bone is to heal properly and quickly. In less serious fractures the bone is simply cracked and the bone ends are not misaligned. In more serious breaks the ends of the bone should be realigned and stabilized by casting the limb, or pinning or wiring the ends together.

At the site of the break the periosteum (osteoprogenitor cells and osteoblasts lining the outside of the bone) and endosteum (osteoprogenitor cells and osteoblasts lining compact and trabecular surfaces inside the bone) will be torn and blood vessels in the area will be severed causing bleeding. A blood clot forms, and the interruption of blood flow causes osteocytes in the area to die (Figure 50.12A). These dying and dead tissues release proinflammatory cytokines that attract phagocytes into the area to remove the blood clot and some of the dead tissues (Figure 50.12B).

Unfortunately, in most cases apposition of bone ends is not close enough to allow good vascularization of the area containing the dead bone. In this case, osteoprogenitor cells arising from intact periosteum and endosteum in the area bordering the low oxygen zones give rise to chondrocytes. These chondrocytes then proliferate and form cartilage within this hypoxic environment to begin to bridge the gap between the bone ends (Figure 50.12C). This cartilage is eventually replaced by bone in the same way that endochondral ossification of the hyaline cartilage model occurs during bone development. That is to say, the chondrocytes hypertrophy and die, and the cartilage matrix calcifies. Blood vessels proliferate and move into the area of the calcified cartilage matrix. As blood vessels move into the calcified cartilage it is replaced with loosely organized woven bone. This is performed by osteoblasts arising from healthy osteoprogenitor cells from the undamaged periosteum and endosteum that follow the oxygen-providing vasculature into the area of the break. The osteoprogenitor cells lay this new bone on top of the calcified cartilage (Figure 50.12D). This new woven bone may also be firmly cemented to the old dead bone that has yet to be resorbed. It has very little strength at this point. As chondrocytes and osteoprogenitor cells move into the break from both sides, a callus or collar of repair tissue forms a complete bridge across the break. The portion of the callus derived from the periosteum is called the **external callus** while that derived from the endosteum is called the **internal callus**, with the external callus forming the stronger bond across the break. Eventually, the calcified cartilage is completely replaced by new woven bone. This takes several weeks and the new woven bone remains relatively weak (Figure 50.12E). The woven bone and any old dead bone is then resorbed and replaced by true lamellar bone

fragments, beginning from the existing healthy bone at the edges of the break. These dense cortical bone fragments grow across the break from each side until they eventually fuse (Figure 50.12F). Over time the cortical bone callus is resorbed and remodeled to the original shape of the bone to complete the repair.

In some cases the ends of the broken bones can be brought back into very tight apposition and stabilized. Under these, or if there is simply a hairline fracture, it is possible to get healing without formation of a callus. Blood vessels and osteogenic precursor cells from the Haversian canals simply extend across the gap through the dead bone. BRUs are formed which extend across the break. Since a BRU can be only about 2.5 mm long in cortical bone, the bone ends must be brought into very tight apposition for this to occur. The new bone formed joins the ends of the bones together in a manner similar to the way in which cabinet makers use wooden pegs to join the ends of two pieces of wood.

Bone metabolism and mineral homeostasis

> 1 How does parathyroid hormone affect osteocytic osteolysis?
>
> 2 How is this different from the effects it has on osteoclastic bone resorption?

Bone mineral is rich in calcium, phosphorus, and other minerals. During bone remodeling these minerals are released into the extracellular fluid through the action of the osteoclasts. They are also removed from blood during bone formation by the osteoblasts. Under stable conditions the rate of bone resorption is equal to the rate of bone formation, so that the mineral content of the skeleton is unchanged. During growth, the rate of bone formation exceeds the rate of bone resorption. Likewise, during conditions causing **osteoporosis** of bone, the rate of bone resorption exceeds the rate of bone formation, resulting in loss of mineral from the skeleton to the extracellular fluid.

Bone also acts as a buffer of the blood pH. Bone can release cations (calcium) to the blood in response to acidosis or release anions (phosphate) in response to excessive blood alkalosis.

Bone mineral metabolism is an essential component of calcium homeostasis. Blood calcium concentration must be maintained within narrow limits if life is to be sustained. When dietary intake of calcium is inadequate to replace calcium leaving the extracellular fluid (via urine, pancreatic secretions, milk, or fetal skeletal development), bone mineral must provide the needed calcium if hypocalcemia is to be avoided. Calcium homeostasis is discussed more thoroughly in Chapter 49, but a brief discussion of the effects of calcium-regulating hormones on bone is warranted. The primary hormone regulating calcium resorption from bone is parathyroid hormone (PTH). When released from the parathyroid glands in response to low blood calcium, PTH first acts on the osteoblasts lining the bony trabeculae.

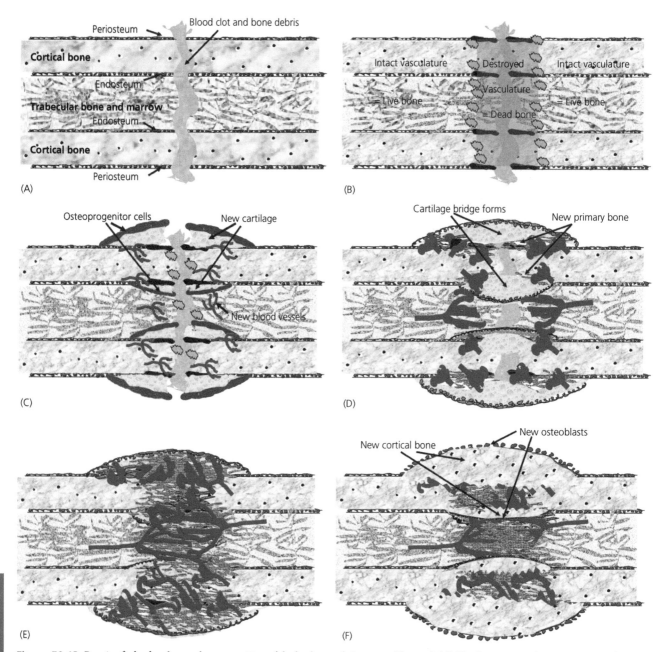

Figure 50.12 Repair of a broken bone where apposition of the broken ends is reasonably good. (A) The fracture rips the periosteum and endosteum. Torn blood vessels bleed into the fracture site and a blood clot forms. The interruption of blood flow causes osteocytes in the area to die. (B) The dying and dead tissues release proinflammatory cytokines that attract phagocytes (orange) into the area to remove the blood clot and some of the dead tissues. (C) Intact periosteum and endosteum cells in the area bordering the low oxygen zones give rise to chondrocytes (green). These chondrocytes then proliferate and form cartilage (light blue matrix) within this hypoxic environment to begin to bridge the gap between the bone ends. The phagocytes continue to remove the dead tissue. (D) The chondrocytes hypertrophy and die, and the cartilage matrix calcifies (light blue matrix). Blood vessels proliferate and move into the area of the calcified cartilage matrix. As blood vessels move into the calcified cartilage, it is replaced with trabecular bone (dark blue matrix) by osteoblasts that follow the oxygen-providing vasculature into the area of the break. (E) As chondrocytes and osteoprogenitor cells move into the break from both sides, a callus or collar of repair tissue forms a complete bridge across the break. Eventually all the calcified cartilage is completely replaced by new trabecular bone. (F) The trabecular bone is then resorbed and replaced by true cortical bone.

Release of calcium from bone stores occurs by two different mechanisms. The first is termed osteocytic osteolysis. Each osteocyte resides within a hollow lacuna in the bone. Surrounding the osteocyte within the lacuna is bone fluid. This fluid is higher in calcium content than nonbone extracellular fluid. When stimulated by PTH, osteocytes utilize the canalicular system to pump a portion of this bone fluid calcium into the extracellular fluid compartment. This bone calcium is readily and rapidly exchangeable. In an adult cow, the size of this pool of calcium is approximately 6–15 g. This is adequate for minor perturbations in calcium balance but for larger or prolonged extracellular fluid calcium deficits the skeleton must resort to osteoclastic osteolysis to supply the needed calcium. Continued secretion of PTH causes an increase in the number and activity of osteoclasts in bone. PTH does not act on the osteoclasts directly: they do not possess a receptor for PTH. However, PTH receptors do exist on osteoblasts. When stimulated by PTH the osteoblasts lining trabecular bone surfaces shrink back to expose the bone matrix to osteoclasts. The osteoblasts also elaborate local paracrine factors such as prostaglandin E_2 and IL-1 and IL-6, which stimulate osteoclast activity in the area.

It should be readily apparent that this sequence of events is similar to those occurring during the activation and resorption phases of bone remodeling. PTH increases the number of sites that are undergoing activation and bone resorption at any one time. But it also, at high doses, will uncouple bone resorption from bone formation (see section Lactational osteoporosis). PTH prevents the osteoclasts from entering the reversal phase of bone remodeling. Instead they continue to slowly erode the bone.

PTH also prevents the osteoblasts from laying down new matrix within the cavity created during bone resorption. Once the animal is in positive calcium balance (calcium entry into the extracellular fluids from diet exceeds loss of calcium from the extracellular fluid), PTH secretion subsides and the osteoblasts can finish the reversal and formation phases of remodeling in each BRU.

With continued PTH stimulation, more BRUs enter the activation and resorption phase. The loss of bone without replenishment cannot be tolerated forever. Eventually, the loss of bone can lead to weakening and a condition known as osteoporosis.

Vitamin D is a precursor to the hormone 1,25-dihydroxyvitamin D (see Chapter 48). The role of 1,25-dihydroxyvitamin D in bone formation is primarily indirect. It acts on the intestine to increase the efficiency of dietary calcium and phosphorus absorption. By maintaining normal blood calcium and phosphorus concentrations, it permits mineralization of bone matrix. Osteoblasts contain a receptor for 1,25-dihydroxyvitamin D. However, treatment of osteoblasts with 1,25-dihydroxyvitamin D does not stimulate bone matrix secretion. Instead it has some of the same effects as PTH, enhancing production of factors that augment osteoclast activity. It has been suggested that certain other metabolites of vitamin D, notably 24,25-dihydroxyvitamin D, play a direct role in the mineralization process.

Calcitonin is the third major calcium-regulating hormone. It is secreted by C-cells within the thyroid gland in response to elevated blood calcium levels. It acts directly on the osteoclasts to inhibit bone resorption. This action has aroused interest in use of calcitonin to inhibit bone resorption in osteoporotic diseases. Unfortunately, osteoclasts develop tolerance to calcitonin and bone resorption resumes so any effectiveness is short-lived.

Joints

> 1 What is the purpose of synovial fluid?
>
> 2 Where are ligaments derived from in a synovial joint?

The junction between any two bones is known as an articulation or a joint. There are several types of joints. Some are practically immovable, such as those found between the skull bones. These are sometimes referred to as fibrous joints. Others are freely movable and have articular cartilage and joint capsules and are called synovial joints. Their function is to provide a means of attaching one bone to another in such a way that the bones can withstand high impact forces yet still allow the bones to "swing" freely with little resistance. The movement of a joint is controlled and limited by the action of muscles and passive structures such as ligaments and tendons.

Synovial joints contain a capsule that has an outer fibrous layer consisting of collagen fibers that run from the periosteum of one bone to the periosteum of the other bone, lending side-to-side stability to the joint (Figure 50.13). Ligaments are special extensions of the fibrous capsule that can be located on the inside or outside of the joint capsule. The inner surface of the joint capsule is composed of the synovial membranes. The synovial membranes are involved in the production of synovial fluid, a very viscous liquid with a consistency similar to egg white. It is essentially an ultrafiltrate of blood plasma to which the synovial cells have added substances such as hyaluronic acid and proteins such as lubricin. Synovial fluid provides lubrication to the joint, reducing wear on opposing articular cartilage surfaces. **Menisci** are special areas of dense fibrocartilage that exist between the articulating cartilage surfaces of some bones, especially those that are bearing great weight. The menisci function to cushion compressive forces acting on the ends of bones. Articular cartilage covering the ends of the bones involved in the joint provides further cushioning over that which might be achieved by two ossified surfaces coming in contact with each other.

Syndromes affecting cartilage of special significance to veterinary medicine

Osteochondrosis of mammals and tibial dyschondroplasia of poultry

These disorders have the common feature of lameness caused by a lesion consisting of a small focal area of **necrotic cartilage**. In most cases of osteochondrosis in mammals, the lesion is located in or near the interface between the articular cartilage and the epiphyseal growth cartilage. In dogs, horses, and pigs, the caudal aspect of the humeral head is a common site and leads to shoulder pain. The lateral and medial femoral condyles are also commonly affected. In pigs the distal growth plate of the ulna is also commonly affected. In fast-growing broilers and turkeys, the lesion is often in the physeal growth plate of the tibiotarsus

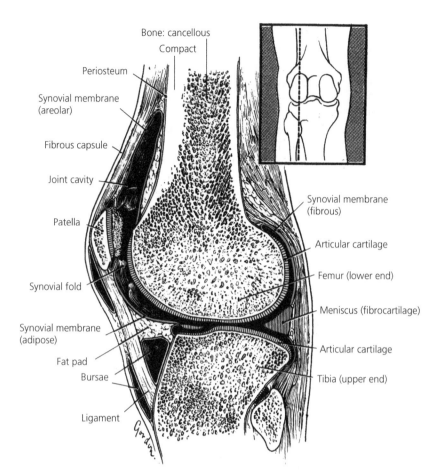

Figure 50.13 Human knee joint (sagittal section indicated by inset). This is an example of a synovial joint. From Cormack, D.H. (2001) *Essential Histology*, 2nd edn. Lippincott Williams & Wilkins, Baltimore. Reproduced with permission from Lippincott Williams & Wilkins.

bone and is termed **tibial dyschondroplasia**. The term "dyschondroplasia" may be the best term in both mammals and birds as it denotes a dysfunction of cartilage growth rather than a bone problem as conveyed by the word "osteochondrosis."

These lesions are associated with rapid growth rate, and genetic selection for growth has actually resulted in increased incidence of this skeletal disease. It has been suggested that the defect develops when cartilage grows too rapidly and the ability of nutrients and oxygen to diffuse through the cartilage matrix to all cells in the matrix is compromised. Chondrocytes in these areas die before they can undergo hypertrophy and stimulate provisional calcification of cartilage matrix. Blood vessels can only invade an area of calcified cartilage, so endochondral ossification cannot proceed where there is necrotic cartilage and a cartilage plug will remain in the bone as ossification bypasses that particular area (Figure 50.14). This necrotic cartilage is a weak point in the bone and articular cartilage and can easily fragment. Small fragments of cartilage can become separated and flake off into the joint space, where they become calcified and give rise to "joint mice" that may interfere with the smooth operation of the joint and cause lameness. Trauma or heavy compressive forces on growth plates can interrupt blood supply

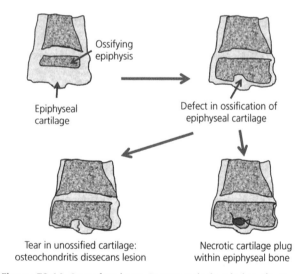

Figure 50.14 Osteochondrosis. During endochondral ossification the cartilage should be replaced with bone. In some cases the cartilage fails to ossify and is retained. This can lead to osteochondritis dissecans, where the cartilage is too soft to bear the weight of the animal and tears, causing pain and lameness. Alternatively, the retained cartilage plug undergoes necrosis within the epiphysis, again causing pain and lameness.

in an area of developing cartilage and can also cause dyschondroplasia.

Dyschondroplasia is a very common defect associated with the growth plates of meat-type chickens, ducks, and turkeys and swine. In many broiler chicken and turkey flocks, up to 30% of birds may have lesions of dyschondroplasia characterized by abnormal masses of cartilage below the growth plate (poultry) or just below the articular cartilage in the epiphyses (mammals). Though lesions can be identified in a large number of market swine slaughtered at 6 months of age, it does not always cause lameness. The major problem is manifest in breeding sows and boars, where osteochondrosis does cause lameness and is a leading cause of culling.

Syndromes affecting bone of special significance to veterinary medicine

Primary hyperparathyroidism

Occasionally, one of the parathyroid glands will give rise to a parathyroid adenoma (nonmalignant tumor). Of the species most veterinarians deal with, the dog is the most commonly affected. The adenoma produces and secretes PTH in an uncontrolled fashion. The increased PTH levels in blood will stimulate excessive bone resorption. The resorbed bone is replaced by fibrous tissue, giving rise to the pathological description of fibrous osteodystrophy for the bone. It occurs throughout the skeleton but especially affects those bones with a high proportion of trabecular bone such as the mandible and the vertebrae.

Affected animals have an abnormally high blood calcium concentration, and teeth of the lower arcade are often loose. Radiographs of the jaw and skull reveal radiolucent areas within these bones.

Pseudohyperparathyroidism

This disorder is actually more common than primary hyperparathyroidism and has been described in dogs and cats rather frequently as well as sporadically in other species. It should be considered the primary suspected disorder that can cause hypercalcemia in dogs and cats.

This disorder is caused by a PTH-like peptide secreted by malignant tumors in a variety of tissues, though most commonly in dogs these are tumors of the apocrine glands of the anal sac or lymphosarcoma. Squamous cell carcinomas have also been reported to produce this substance. One peptide recently isolated and identified is PTH-related peptide. It binds PTH receptors with high affinity and because it is secreted in large amounts by the tumor, the clinical bone disease is the same as in primary hyperparathyroidism. These animals also develop hypercalcemia, the so-called **hypercalcemia of malignancy**.

Other tumors can produce substances such as IL-1 or IL-6 which stimulate bone resorption but usually not to the same extent as PTH-related peptide.

Secondary hyperparathyroidism

This disease occurs secondary to a chronic decrease in blood calcium concentration. The parathyroid glands recognize the lower blood calcium concentration and secrete large amounts of PTH to attempt to maintain normocalcemia. This disorder has two basic forms.

Nutritional secondary hyperparathyroidism

A deficiency of dietary calcium or vitamin D can reduce the amount of calcium that can be absorbed across the intestine into the extracellular fluid. Diets severely deficient in calcium will not supply adequate calcium to replenish calcium lost from extracellular pools. As a result blood calcium concentration decreases and PTH secretion increases. PTH can act on the kidney to reduce urinary calcium loss and increase synthesis of 1,25-dihydroxyvitamin D to enhance the efficiency of intestinal calcium absorption. However, if diet calcium is very low, increasing the efficiency of intestinal calcium absorption cannot substantially increase the amount of calcium entering the extracellular pool of calcium. The only action of PTH that can improve blood calcium concentration under this situation is to enhance bone calcium resorption. The continued removal of bone without replacement results in fibrous osteodystrophy, as previously described for primary hyperparathyroidism. These animals are generally vitamin D and phosphorus replete, so the osteoblasts do produce a matrix. However, the lack of calcium and the continued effects of PTH cause this matrix to be abnormal and it will not calcify. The clinical signs of nutritional secondary hyperparathyroidism include hypertrophy of the parathyroid glands (though they can be rarely palpated) and cessation of growth in young animals as the physes are also affected. The lack of calcium available for mineralization of bone matrix causes the growth plates to be soft, weak, and swollen. The cortices of the long bones are thin, and minor or major fractures are common.

Nutritional secondary hyperparathyroidism is unfortunately common in veterinary medicine. Dog and cat owners may feel that an "all-meat" diet is best for their "carnivore." Unfortunately, meat alone is a poor source of calcium and is high in phosphorus, which can reduce passive absorption of calcium across the intestinal epithelium. Horses fed high-grain diets (especially common in the days when draft horses needed a high-energy diet to sustain them at work) were low in calcium and high in phosphorus. The characteristic fibrous dystrophy of the skull and jaw bones gave rise to the term "big-head disease" in horses with nutritional secondary hyperparathyroidism. Turtles fed hamburger diets develop a soft shell (loss of bone from the modified vertebrae that form the shell). Monkeys love fruit, but fruit diets provide little calcium (or protein, which raises other problems). Surprisingly, once recognized, dietary correction can rapidly reverse the bone changes induced by nutritional secondary hyperparathyroidism if still in the early stages.

Renal secondary hyperparathyroidism

This syndrome is due to renal failure and is common in older animals, especially dogs and cats. A major function of the kidneys in most species is to remove excess phosphate from the circulation. As renal function is lost, phosphate is retained and hyperphosphatemia develops. This only occurs when the amount of functional renal tissue is 25% or less than normal.

The hyperphosphatemia has two effects. The first effect is to reduce the ionized calcium content of the blood. This is because calcium and phosphate ions normally exist in blood at concentrations that are slightly below the levels that would cause saturation of the fluids and result in precipitation of calcium phosphate salt from the solution. However, the greatly elevated phosphate in blood of patients with renal failure can exceed the equilibrium of calcium and phosphate in solution, reducing the amount of calcium that can coexist in plasma with the extreme phosphate concentrations. This contributes to hypocalcemia. More importantly, as phosphate builds up in the blood it has a second effect on the remaining renal tissue. It blocks the activation of 1α-hydroxylase, the enzyme that catalyzes conversion of 25-hydroxyvitamin D to 1,25-dihydroxyvitamin D within the kidney. Therefore even though PTH should stimulate the remaining functional renal tissue to produce 1,25-dihydroxyvitamin D, this action of PTH is blocked by hyperphosphatemia.

As renal function is lost, the amount of renal tissue available for production of 1,25-dihydroxyvitamin D decreases, and blood concentrations of 1,25-dihydroxyvitamin D decline. This reduces dietary calcium absorption and further depresses blood calcium concentration. This in turn stimulates increased PTH secretion and, again, resorbing bone calcium reserves becomes a major means of maintaining normocalcemia. Fibrous osteodystrophy follows the prolonged secretion of PTH.

As bone calcium is resorbed, more phosphorus is also resorbed. However, the loss of renal function prevents PTH from having its usual phosphaturic effect, exacerbating the hyperphosphatemia. A vicious cycle of increasing blood phosphate, increasing PTH, and increased bone resorption ensues. The loss of renal function can rarely be reversed. However, reducing dietary phosphate (or its absorption using phosphate binders) and/or supplementing the diet with 1,25-dihydroxyvitamin D can reduce the severity of bone lesions associated with renal secondary hyperparathyroidism.

Hypoparathyroidism

Occasionally, parathyroid gland function is disrupted so as to prevent PTH secretion. Autoimmune disease in which the parathyroid gland is attacked, or tumors that encroach on the parathyroids and cause pressure necrosis can reduce PTH secretion. An unfortunately more common cause is inadvertent removal of the parathyroid glands during surgical ablation of the hyperplastic thyroid gland of cats. The immediate problem for the patient is the hypocalcemia that ensues. However, long-term lack of stimulus for bone resorption can increase cortical bone thickness and mineral content. This condition is termed

osteopetrosis. It is generally not life-threatening. The hypocalcemia that develops is life-threatening.

Nutritional hypercalcitoninism

When animals are fed diets that are much higher in calcium than is required, there can be abnormally large amounts of calcium entering the extracellular fluid as a result of passive absorption of calcium across the intestinal epithelium.

Adjusting 1,25-dihydroxyvitamin D concentration in blood only controls active transport of calcium across the intestinal epithelium. As a result blood calcium concentration can be increased above normal, which stimulates secretion of calcitonin. In the long term, the excess calcitonin secretion can cause exostoses or mineral deposits extending off the edges of bones (bone spurs). Vertebral exostoses were evident in bulls fed high-calcium diets intended for lactating dairy cows.

In large-breed dogs excessive dietary calcium has been linked to several skeletal abnormalities such as hip dysplasia and osteochondrosis dissecans. Calcitonin apparently has some significant negative effects on development and maturation of articular and epiphyseal cartilage in growing animals. The inhibitory effect of calcitonin on osteoclast function is suspected to cause abnormalities in bone formation and bone remodeling, leading to stunted growth and cartilage maturation disturbances. As with primary hypoparathyroidism, excessive diet calcium reduces PTH secretion and increases the bone density causing mild osteopetrosis.

Hereditary osteopetrosis of calves

This disease has been reported as a recessive dominant genetic defect in Angus calves. The defect appears to result in a lack of osteoclast activity in these animals. The defect is manifest *in utero* and the calves are usually stillborn. They have dense, thick, shortened bones composed of solid cortical bone and no marrow cavity.

Osteopetrosis of manatees

The bones of the manatee are normally osteopetrotic, made of solid cortical bone. Luckily, the added weight of the bone is easily buoyed by the water environment manatees live in. The absence of marrow cavities in their bones forces the manatee to rely on extramedullary hematopoiesis for blood cell formation.

Rickets and osteomalacia

Rickets is a disorder of growing animals in which the newly formed osteoid and the cartilage septa within the growth plate fail to mineralize. This is most often associated with vitamin D or dietary phosphorus deficiency. Both conditions lead to a reduction in blood phosphate concentration. When blood phosphate concentration falls below the level required to support mineralization, the cartilage and primary spongiosa within the growth plate do not mineralize. Chondrocytes within the zone of proliferation continue to elongate the cartilage model in the growth plate. However, since the cartilage does not calcify no blood vessels can invade the area to begin ossification and the growth plate elongates. It is more flexible and rubbery and gives the ends of bones an enlarged look, especially evident at the growth plates within the ribs. Blood phosphorus concentration in young animals is generally higher than in adult animals, a reflection of their greater requirement for phosphorus to support mineralization of new growing bone.

In adult animals with vitamin D or phosphorus deficiency, the blood phosphorus concentration can fall below the level needed to mineralize newly formed bone matrix during the remodeling process. Pathological changes occur much more slowly than in rickets but over a prolonged period the bones can also become more flexible, leading to extensive joint pain in these animals. In this case the sites of remodeled bone fail to mineralize. This is termed osteomalacia.

In principle, calcium deficiency differs from phosphorus deficiency in that normal osteoid is formed but fails to mineralize in phosphorus deficiency, while in calcium deficiency the normal osteoid is either not formed at all (osteoporosis) or replaced by fibrous tissue. In vitamin D or calcium deficiency it is common to see mixed lesions – osteomalacia, osteoporosis and fibrous osteodystrophy – all in the same bone.

Vitamin D deficiency also seems to reduce secretion of type X collagen by the chondrocytes within the growth plate and somehow prevents the programmed cell death of chondrocytes within the zone of provisional calcification.

Osteoporosis

Three forms of osteoporosis commonly occur: lactational, postmenopausal, and senile osteoporosis. Of these, only lactational osteoporosis is a syndrome of concern in animals. However, since at least half of the readers of this text will develop postmenopausal osteoporosis and all readers can hope to live long enough (about 80 years) to develop senile osteoporosis, all three forms will be described.

The process resulting in osteoporosis for each syndrome is described as it occurs within a spicule of trabecular bone (Figure 50.15). The same basic process also occurs in the cortical Haversian canal system. During normal bone remodeling, the osteoclasts within a BRU resorb bone to a depth of 50 μm and then the osteoblasts move into the saucer-shaped cavity to replace the 50 μm of bone removed (Figure 50.15A–C).

Postmenopausal osteoporosis

After menopause in women the ovaries fail to produce estrogens. Estrogens seem to regulate the depth to which the osteoclasts resorb bone, perhaps by regulating osteoblast production of IL-6, an osteoclast activity factor. Now during the bone remodeling process osteoclasts resorb bone down to a depth of 70 μm instead of 50 μm (Figure 50.15D–F). The osteoblasts continue to move into the resorption cavity and produce their usual 50 μm of bone. However, the net result is a loss of 20 μm of bone at each BRU. After menopause bone resorption is greatly accelerated. This unchecked osteoclast activity goes on for a period

of 5–10 years. Then, for reasons unknown, the osteoclasts resume their typical bone resorption activity and only resorb bone to a depth of 50 μm within each BRU.

Women typically lose 20–30% of their skeletal minerals during this time. For women with a high bone mass at the onset of menopause, this bone loss may not compromise bone strength too greatly. But if bone mass is low at the time of menopause, the loss of bone mineral can leave the woman at dangerous risk of fracture. The key is to build the bone mineral up while women are young.

From puberty until about age 35 years, the skeleton is actively accruing bone mass, if nutrition permits. At each BRU the osteoclasts resorb 50 μm of bone to form each resorption cavity and the osteoblasts build 51–52 μm of bone, slightly more than the osteoclasts resorbed. However, after age 35 the situation is reversed. The osteoclasts may resorb 50 μm of bone but the osteoclasts may only replace 49 μm of bone so that bone is slowly being lost from the skeleton from that time on in both men and women.

Ovariectomized dogs and cats (the laboratory rat is a favored model of osteoporosis) also undergo a period of enhanced osteoclastic bone resorption due to loss of estrogen. However, the duration of bone loss and the high starting mass of the bones of these species prevent this effect from being a significant clinical disease.

Senile osteoporosis

At very advanced age (after 80 years), in both men and women, the osteoclasts within a BRU resorb bone to the typical depth of 50 μm. However, the osteoblasts moving into the area become much less able to build back the resorbed bone. They may replace less than 30 μm, leaving a deficit of 20 μm or more at each BRU, resulting in a condition referred to as senile osteoporosis (Figure 50.15G–I). This bone loss can also lead to fracture, especially in older women who have already experienced bone loss from postmenopausal osteoporosis. Again, those people with the greatest bone mass at age 35 will be most likely to have enough total bone mass to withstand these accelerated rates of bone loss without developing clinical disease. However, few people, especially women, ingest enough calcium in their diet prior to age 35 to ensure that maximal bone mass is attained. And as we spend more and more time indoors, vitamin D insufficiency is also common. As bone is lost from the trabeculae of the vertebrae, small fractures occur and the weight of the body compresses the vertebra, leading to shortened stature of the person with painful bending of the vertebral column, creating the "dowager's hump" common in elderly women and men.

Lactational osteoporosis

During lactation in virtually all species, there is an obligatory loss of bone mass from the skeleton. In this case the osteoclasts within a BRU resorb bone to the normal 50-μm depth if diet calcium is adequate, or to even greater depths if the animal is in severe negative calcium balance. However,

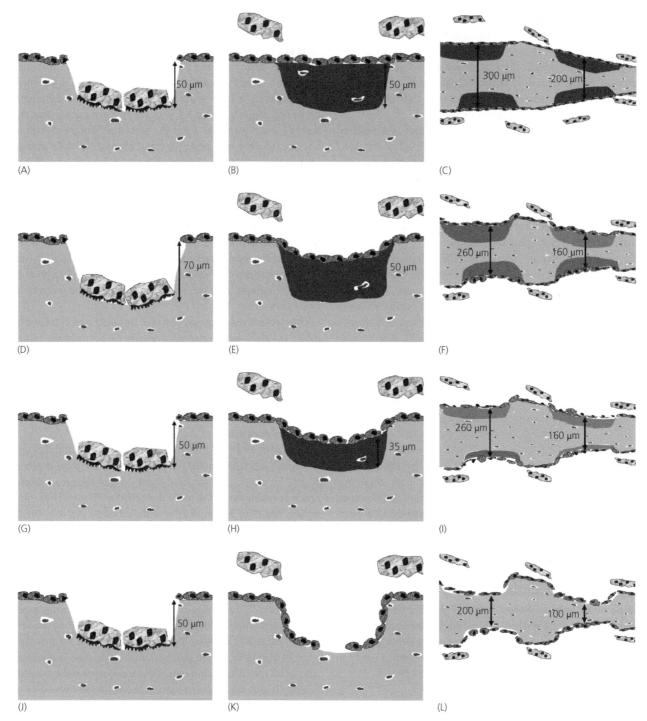

Figure 50.15 Osteoporosis. (A–C) During normal bone remodeling, the bone lost during the resorptive phase (approximately 50 μm) is completely replaced (shadowed area) during the reversal phase of remodeling, with no net loss of bone. (D–F) In postmenopausal osteoporosis, the lack of estrogen production causes excessive osteoclastic activity, resulting in approximately 70 μm of bone being resorbed. However, the reversal phase continues at its usual pace, replacing approximately 50 μm of bone. This leaves a deficit of 20 μm of bone at each remodeled site. (G–I) During senile osteoporosis, the resorptive phase of remodeling occurs at the normal pace, removing 50 μm of bone. However, fatigued osteoblasts may only replace 30 μm of the original bone, again leaving a deficit of 20 μm of bone at each remodeled site. (J–L) During lactational osteoporosis, the need for calcium to support lactation causes a disconnect between the resorptive and reversal phases of the remodeling process. Bone resorption occurs normally but osteoblasts remain inactive, leaving 50-μm divots in the bone. This resorbed bone is not replaced until some later point when dietary calcium absorption is sufficient to sustain the calcium requirements of milk production. At that time all the resorbed bone can be successfully replaced. From Reece, W.O. (2004) *Dukes' Physiology of Domestic Animals*, 12th edn. Cornell University Press, Ithaca, NY. Reproduced with permission from Cornell University Press.

osteoblast movement into the resorption cavity is temporarily put on hold (Figure 50.15J–L). This occurs to some extent in all females shortly after parturition, even when they are in positive calcium balance. However, the degree and duration can be magnified greatly by negative calcium balance. Once the animal has undergone the obligatory lactational osteoporotic bone loss, and if the animal is in positive calcium balance, the osteoblasts now return to the resorption cavity and replace the lost bone. This is the only one of the three forms of osteoporosis where the lost bone will eventually be replaced. Lactational osteoporosis can help the female meet the calcium demands of lactation by uncoupling bone formation from bone resorption. In high-producing dairy cows, dietary calcium intake is inadequate to meet lactational calcium demands the first 4–6 weeks of lactation. These animals can lose as much as 13% of their skeletal mass during this period, which is replaced in later lactation when diet calcium intake allows the cow to enter a period of positive calcium balance.

Pseudohypoparathyroidism and milk fever in dairy cows

Dairy cows begin lactating at the time they calve. The onset of lactation in dairy cows can draw enormous amounts of calcium from the extracellular fluid for use in milk production. Ordinarily, this would cause a slight drop in blood calcium concentration, which would trigger PTH secretion. The PTH would stimulate bone resorption and renal production of 1,25-dihydroxyvitamin D to enhance intestinal calcium absorption. These two actions can allow the cow to meet the calcium demands of lactation. However, in some cows these mechanisms are defective. Current evidence suggests that high-potassium diets fed to cows before calving induce a metabolic alkalosis. This interferes with the interaction between PTH and its receptor located on bone osteoblasts and renal cortical cells. Now, despite enhanced PTH secretion as hypocalcemia develops, the bone and renal tissues fail to be stimulated to enhance calcium homeostatic mechanisms. The result is a severe decline in blood calcium concentration, which often results in death of the cow if left untreated.

Growth hormone and bone metabolism

Growth hormone received its name in part because of the effect it has on the growth plate. Growth hormone stimulates chondrocytes to proliferate at the zone of proliferation within the growth plate. Animals that fail to produce growth hormone will be dwarfs, though not all dwarfism is caused by growth hormone deficiency. Excessive growth hormone results in large and often misshapen bones and is termed acromegaly.

Much of the effect of growth hormone on the growth plate seems to be mediated by insulin-like growth factor (somatomedin), which is produced by the liver in response to growth hormone. There is also some evidence that growth hormone can elicit production of insulin-like growth factor within chondrocytes, which then elicits a paracrine response by other chondrocytes located in the zone of proliferation.

Self-evaluation

Answers can be found at the end of the chapter.

1 Osteochondrosis or retained cartilage within the epiphyses that should have become bone is a common pathologic finding in several species, including dogs. Why might placing pups on a high-protein, high-energy diet result in a high incidence of osteochondrosis?

2 Why would failure of the kidneys cause the teeth of an old cat to fall out?

3 Explain how bone remodeling goes wrong in the postmenopausal woman? What about very old men? What about a cow in early lactation?

4 When a hairline fracture occurs to the bone, it heals much more quickly than a compound fracture of the bone, even if you are a great orthopedic surgeon who returned the bones to close apposition. Why?

Suggested reading

Coe, F.I. and Favus, M.J. (1992) *Disorders of Bone and Mineral Metabolism*. Raven Press, New York.

Answers

1 The high-protein, high-energy diet could cause excessively fast growth in the pups. It has been suggested that the defect develops when cartilage grows too rapidly and the ability of nutrients and oxygen to diffuse through the cartilage matrix to all cells in the matrix is compromised. Chondrocytes in these areas die before they can undergo hypertrophy, which is believed necessary to stimulate provisional calcification of cartilage matrix. Blood vessels can only invade an area of calcified cartilage, so endochondral ossification cannot proceed in this area of necrotic cartilage and a cartilage plug will remain in the bone as ossification bypasses that particular area. This necrotic cartilage is a weak point in the bone and articular cartilage and can easily fragment. Small fragments of cartilage can become separated and flake off into the joint space, where they become calcified and give rise to "joint mice" that may interfere with the smooth operation of the joint and cause lameness.

2 As kidneys fail they have a reduced ability to excrete phosphate and reduced ability to produce the hormone 1,25-dihydroxyvitamin D, vital to efficient absorption of calcium. High blood phosphate depresses the amount of calcium that can be maintained in solution within blood, so blood calcium concentration decreases. In addition, the lack of intestinal calcium absorption due to lack of 1,25-dihydroxyvitamin D also causes a decline in blood calcium. Falling

blood calcium stimulates PTH secretion, which stimulates activation of osteoclasts and bone resorption. However, the inability to utilize dietary calcium causes excesive reliance on bone for calcium homeostasis and bone resorption becomes uncoupled from bone formation. Bone tissue is replaced by fibrous tissue. This includes the bone of the jaw which hold the teeth in place. When weakened by excessive bone resorption, the jaw bones can no longer hold the teeth.

3 During normal bone remodeling the bone lost during the resorptive phase (approximately 50 μm) is completely replaced during the reversal phase of remodeling, with no net loss of bone. In postmenopausal osteoporosis the lack of estrogen production causes excessive osteoclastic activity, resulting in approximately 70 μm of bone being resorbed. However, the reversal phase continues at its usual pace, replacing approximately 50 μm of bone. This leaves a deficit of 20 μm of bone at each remodeled site. During senile osteoporosis the resorptive phase of remodeling occurs at the normal pace, removing 50 μm of bone. However fatigued osteoblasts may only replace 30 μm of the original bone, again leaving a deficit of 20 μm of bone at each

remodeled site. During lactational osteoporosis the need for calcium to support lactation causes a "disconnect" between the resorptive and reversal phases of the remodeling process. Bone resorption occurs normally but osteoblasts remain inactive, leaving 50-μm divots in the bone. This resorbed bone is not replaced until some later point when dietary calcium absorption is sufficient to sustain calcium requirements of milk production. At that time all the resorbed bone can be successfully replaced. This is not true of postmenopausal or senile osteoporosis where the bone lost is essentially permanent.

4 In a hairline fracture the ends of the bone may be close enough to allow osteoblasts to lay bone directly onto the old bone. This is strictly a function of distance from a good blood supply, as osteoblasts require oxygen to survive. In a compound fracture, blood supply within the fracture site is too compromised to supply the concentration of oxygen required by osteoblasts. In this case chondrocytes must first lay down a cartilage bridge across the gap that will eventually be replaced by bone once the blood vessels invade the calcified cartilage matrix.

SECTION IX

Endocrinology, Reproduction, and Lactation

Section Editor: Jesse P. Goff

51 The Endocrine System

Jesse P. Goff

Iowa State University, Ames, IA, USA

Hormones: basic concepts

> **1** How do peptide hormones differ from steroid hormones?

Endocrine tissues secrete **hormones** which are carried in the bloodstream to other cells of the body, where they help regulate metabolism and other functions within the cell. Processes such as digestion, reproduction, electrolyte and fluid balance, growth, and development are regulated and coordinated by hormones. Endocrine glands are ductless glands: the hormones are released into the extracellular fluid and diffuse into the bloodstream. This distinguishes them from exocrine glands that secrete substances such as saliva or milk into an alveolar structure which carries those substances through ducts to a specific site in the body.

Dukes' Physiology of Domestic Animals, Thirteenth Edition. Edited by William O. Reece, Howard H. Erickson, Jesse P. Goff and Etsuro E. Uemura.

© 2015 John Wiley & Sons, Inc. Published 2015 by John Wiley & Sons, Inc.

Companion website: www.wiley.com/go/reece/physiology

Section IX: Endocrinology, Reproduction, and Lactation

The endocrine system works in concert with the nervous system, particularly the autonomic nervous system, to regulate the body's activities. The nervous system can act on a cell within one-tenth of a second. Hormones reach their target cells via the bloodstream, necessitating at least 30 s. Hormonal action on cells is slower than nervous action on cells but tends to be more persistent, providing long-term stimulation of target tissues.

While this chapter focuses on the endocrine effects of hormones, it must be mentioned that hormones can also act locally. Hormones can be released from endocrine cells and diffuse through the extracellular fluid to act on neighboring cells. This is known as a **paracrine action** of the hormone. In extreme cases a hormone may be generated by a cell and act on that same cell, referred to as an **autocrine action** of the hormone. Paracrine actions of hormones are particularly important in the digestive system. "Hormones" of the immune system are called **cytokines** and they have a major role in regulating immune responses, having both local paracrine (e.g., site of an infection) and systemic endocrine effects. A special category of hormones are the **pheromones**, which are secreted on to body and mucosal surfaces to stimulate actions in other animals.

Hormones can be classified into two categories, based on the location of the **receptors** for the hormone in the target cell the hormone is supposed to act on. Receptors are proteins that specifically recognize and form an ionic bond with the hormone. When a receptor is thus activated by binding to the hormone, it often results in a change in shape of the receptor molecule, which then initiates some action in the cell.

Hormones acting on cell-surface receptors: peptide hormones

> **1** What are the basic types of peptide hormone?
> **2** Where do they act on a cell?
> **3** How do G protein-coupled receptors activate cells?
> **4** What is phospholipase C?
> **5** What is the function of the Gα protein?
> **6** How does a tyrosine kinase receptor activate cells?

These hormones are primarily composed of one to hundreds of amino acids and are sometimes referred to simply as **peptide hormones**. They are too large or too water-soluble to enter cells. Hormones acting on receptors located within the target cell's membrane can be grouped into the following categories based on their composition.

1 *Catecholamines*: Tyrosine is an amino acid that is used as a substrate by cells of the adrenal medulla to synthesize catecholamines, such as norepinephrine (noradrenaline), epinephrine (adrenaline), and dopamine. These are also common neurotransmitters. Technically, the adrenal medulla can be thought of as a collection of postganglionic sympathetic nerves that release neurotransmitter into the blood.

2 *Protein and peptide hormones*: these hormones consist of a string of amino acids. They are referred to as peptide hormones if the length of the amino acid chain is less than 10 amino acids, and protein hormones when more than 10 amino acids in length. In many cases the hormone is constantly being produced and stored within the endocrine cell but is secreted only when the cell is properly stimulated to secrete the hormone. Protein-based hormones are transcribed from DNA and stored within the endocrine cell as a much longer protein inside a Golgi produced **vesicle**. This version of the hormone is referred to as a **prohormone** and is essentially biologically inactive. When the endocrine cell is stimulated to secrete the hormone, the prohormone is cleaved by enzymes within the storage vesicle to form the active true hormone. The storage vesicle fuses with the cell membrane and the hormone is released into the extracellular fluid.

3 *Eicosanoids*: these hormones are derived from unsaturated fatty acids and include the prostaglandins, thromboxanes, and leukotrienes. Arachidonic acid is the most common fatty acid precursor for these types of hormones. Thromboxanes and leukotrienes are critical to the inflammatory process and aggregation of platelets, and are considered in detail in other chapters (see Chapters 12 and 35 for example). Prostaglandins are important to a wide variety of functions, especially reproduction, intestine integrity and repair, and circulation of blood through organs. The eicosanoids tend to have greater paracrine action than endocrine action. For example, prostaglandin (PG)E_2 can be made by intestinal mucosal cells in response to any factor that causes damage to them. The prostaglandins diffuse away from the damaged cell and can increase mucus secretion by neighboring cells to flush away offending factors. They can also diffuse to nearby arterioles to increase blood flow to the damaged area to facilitate repair.

As a rule, because these hormones are water-soluble, they diffuse through tissue readily and circulate freely in the bloodstream. A few, such as growth hormone, circulate through the blood bound to special carrier proteins. However, because they are not lipid-soluble they do not enter their target cells. Target cells for these hormones possess receptors located within the cell membrane that extend out into the extracellular fluid. These receptors recognize and bind their respective hormone (**ligand**) and undergo a change in shape that initiates altered function of the cell. How this is accomplished is discussed further in the next section. As a rule, the catecholamines, proteinaceous hormones, and eicosanoids have a short half-life in the bloodstream (minutes to hours) and they initiate relatively rapid but short-term actions in the cells they affect.

The number of receptor molecules on the surface of a cell is not static, and ranges from a few thousand to over 100,000 receptors depending on the hormone. The receptor number also changes with stage of development and receptor molecules can be induced or lost due to the action of other hormones. Old receptor molecules are recycled and typically receptors that have bound hormone are recycled rather quickly so that cell stimulation does not last too long.

Cell membrane-bound receptors

The peptide hormones cannot enter their target cells because of their size and charge, so require a mechanism that allows the hormonal message to enter the target cells and cause them to alter their metabolism or function. This is achieved by a process termed **signal transduction**. When a hormone binds to its receptor, it initiates a cascade of events that eventually cause the cell to alter its physiology.

Peptide hormone receptor molecules possess a segment that protrudes into the extracellular fluid and binds hormone and an intracellular portion that activates signaling pathways inside the cell. When a hormone binds its receptor it causes a change in the conformation of the receptor molecule, particularly the portion inside the cell. This causes production of a **second messenger** that alters the cell's physiology. There are several basic types of actions that occur on the inside surface of the target cell to generate each type of second messenger.

G protein-coupled receptors

These receptors have guanine nucleotide-binding **G proteins** in close apposition to their internal segment. The G protein has three subunits, α, β, and γ. The Gα subunit ordinarily has a guanosine diphosphate (GDP) bound to it. It is considered inactive in this state. When hormone binds the receptor the conformational change of the internal segment of the hormone

receptor causes a mechanical change in the G-protein complex. The Gα subunit now exchanges the GDP for a higher-energy guanosine triphosphate (GTP) molecule and is now considered to be in the **active state**. Subsequent events follow either scenario A or scenario B.

Scenario A

The Gα subunit migrates away from the receptor along the internal surface of the cell membrane until it encounters an enzyme in the membrane, such as adenylyl cyclase (Figure 51.1). It binds to a regulatory site on the enzyme and causes the enzyme catalytic site to become active. In the case of adenylyl cyclase, the enzyme converts adenosine triphosphate (ATP) to cyclic adenosine monophosphate (cyclic AMP). Thus **cyclic AMP** is the second messenger. Cyclic AMP can bind to regulatory sites on another enzyme known as protein kinase A, activating the catalytic portion of this enzyme. It also causes the protein kinase catalytic subunit to dissociate from the rest of the molecule and leave the cell membrane. The protein kinase A catalytic subunit adds phosphate molecules to other enzymes (including other protein kinases) and proteins in the cytosol, either stimulating or inhibiting their function.

After some time, the GTP bound to the Gα protein loses a high-energy phosphate to become GDP. This causes the Gα subunit to detach from adenylyl cyclase and return to the hormone receptor where it recombines with the Gβ and Gγ subunits to await the next time hormone binds the receptor. The adenylyl cyclase catalytic unit is no longer stimulated and cyclic AMP

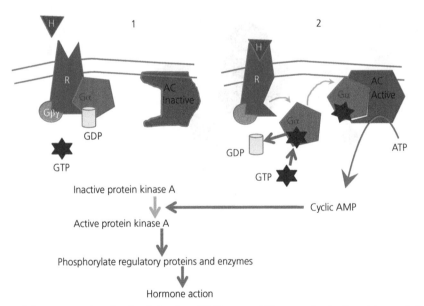

Figure 51.1 G protein-coupled receptor acting via adenylyl cyclase. (1) Hormone (H) approaches its G protein-coupled receptor (R) on the target cell membrane. The Gα, Gβ, and Gγ regulatory subunits tightly adhere to the intracellular component of the receptor. The Gα regulatory subunit is binding a GDP molecule. The nearby adenylyl cyclase (AC) is in an inactive state. (2) The ligand–receptor complex undergoes a conformational change, causing Gα regulatory unit to exchange the GDP molecule for a GTP molecule. It now separates from the receptor and moves into the regulatory site of the adenylyl cyclase, causing it to become active. The adenylyl cyclase can then convert cytosolic ATP to cyclic AMP. The cyclic AMP then fits into a regulatory site on protein kinase A, activating the enzyme which goes on to phosphorylate various proteins and enzymes that alter the physiology of the cell.

stops being produced. Cyclic AMP levels also decrease as a result of degradation by another enzyme known as cyclic AMP phosphodiesterase. When cyclic AMP levels fall sufficiently, the action of the hormone on the cell ceases.

In the example given, the Gα subunit stimulates adenylyl cyclase action. In some cases the Gα subunit can be considered inhibitory: this form of Gα subunit blocks adenylyl cyclase activity when it binds the adenylyl cyclase regulatory site. The enzyme activated or inhibited by the Gα subunit is usually adenylyl cyclase, resulting in production of cyclic AMP as the second messenger. However, the enzyme involved can also be guanylyl cyclase, resulting in production of cyclic GMP as second messenger.

Scenario B

The activated Gα subunit moves from the hormone receptor to bind to an activation site on the membrane-bound enzyme phospholipase C (Figure 51.2). This activates the phospholipase C enzyme and it splits phosphatidylinositol 4,5-bisphosphate (PIP_2), a component of the lipid bilayer of the cell membrane, into inositol 1,4,5-trisphosphate (IP_3) and diacylglycerol (DAG). The IP_3 molecule diffuses through the cytosol and binds to a receptor located on the membrane of the endoplasmic reticulum. The endoplasmic reticulum contains large amounts of Ca^{2+} ions. When IP_3 binds its receptor it causes a Ca^{2+} channel to open in the endoplasmic reticulum membrane and Ca^{2+} ions

enter the cytosol and serve as the second messenger. Ca^{2+} can bind calmodulin and the Ca^{2+}–calmodulin complex can have a variety of actions within the cell. DAG migrates along the cell membrane until it encounters an enzyme called protein kinase C. It binds to a regulatory site on the protein kinase C enzyme, partially activating the enzyme. However, the enzyme is called protein kinase C because for full catalytic activity the enzyme must also bind Ca^{2+} ions. The Ca^{2+} ions liberated from the endoplasmic reticulum by IP_3 serve as the final stimulator of protein kinase C activation. Protein kinase C then phosphorylates various proteins in the cell to alter their function. The activation of protein kinase C ends when the Gα subunit hydrolyzes the GTP to GDP and rejoins the Gβ and Gγ subunits. Phospholipase C ceases production of DAG and IP_3. The Ca^{2+} is pumped back into the endoplasmic reticulum to lower intracellular Ca^{2+} ions and the response of the cell to the hormone ceases.

The various proteins activated in these signaling pathways can themselves be protein kinases (which add a phosphate to a substrate molecule to activate or deactivate it) or phosphatases (which remove a phosphate molecule from a substrate to activate or deactivate it).

Receptor tyrosine kinases

For some hormones and growth factors, such as insulin, epidermal growth factor, and insulin-like growth factor, the binding of hormone to receptor causes the receptor molecule to

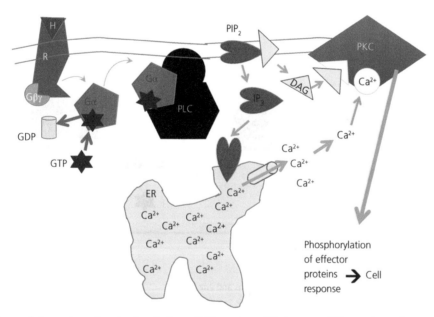

Figure 51.2 G protein-coupled receptor acting via phospholipase C. The receptor (R)–hormone (H) complex undergoes a conformational change causing Gα regulatory unit to exchange the GDP molecule for a GTP molecule. It now separates from the receptor and moves into the regulatory site of phospholipase C (PLC), causing it to become active. The active phospholipase C can then split phosphatidylinositol 4,5-bisphosphate (PIP_2) in the cell membrane to inositol 1,4,5-trisphosphate (IP_3) and diacylglycerol (DAG). The IP_3 moves into the cytosol to bind to an IP_3 receptor on the endoplasmic reticulum (ER). This opens a calcium channel in the endoplasmic reticulum membrane and calcium ions move into the cytosol. The diacylglycerol binds to a regulatory unit of protein kinase C (PKC) and partially activates it. However, it becomes fully active only after it has bound a Ca^{2+} ion released from the ER. Once fully active it can phosphorylate proteins and enzymes in the cell to alter the physiology of the cell.

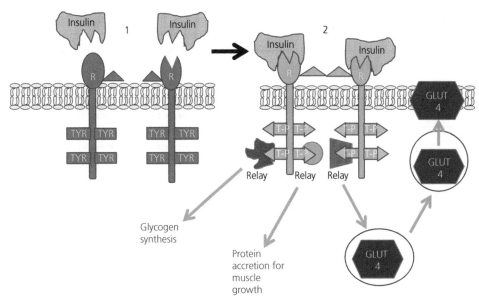

Figure 51.3 Insulin receptor tyrosine kinase. (1) Two insulin receptors are located close to one another in a target muscle cell membrane. The receptor proteins have many tyrosine residues (TYR). The receptor molecule is an inactive tyrosine kinase, unable to phosphorylate those tyrosine residues at this point. (2) The insulin binds the receptor causing a conformational change. The receptors form a dimer, cross-linking with each other. The dimer now becomes an active tyrosine kinase and it proceeds to phosphorylate all the tyrosine residues on the receptor molecules. The phosphorylated tyrosines (T-P) bind to various relay proteins, activating them. This then stimulates functions such as glycogen synthesis and protein accretion, or it might cause the GLUT-4 molecule stored in a vesicle to move into the cell membrane for glucose transport.

develop the ability to phosphorylate tyrosine residues (gain tyrosine kinase activity). The best-known example of a hormone using this second messenger system is insulin and it is used here to illustrate how these receptors function. Insulin receptors are usually in close apposition to one another in the cell membrane (Figure 51.3). They also have many tyrosine amino acids in their intracellular portion or domain. In this case binding of a molecule of insulin to receptors that are in close apposition to one another in the cell membrane allows those receptors to come together to form a dimer. The formation of this dimer, with two insulin receptors bound to two insulin molecules, causes a conformational change and the dimer becomes an active **tyrosine kinase**. The receptor turned kinase catalyzes conversion of ATP to ADP and the phosphate liberated is used to phosphorylate the tyrosine residues on the receptor molecules. When all the tyrosine residues are phosphorylated, the receptor dimer's phosphorylated tyrosines can interact with and bind various proteins diffusing throughout the cytosol known as relay proteins. The phosphorylated tyrosine can fit into regulatory units on these relay proteins to increase their signaling activity. Phospholipase C, the enzyme that converts PIP_2 to DAG and IP_3, can be activated in this manner (as well as by G protein-coupled receptor). Mitogen-activated protein (MAP) kinase-activated signaling cascades are another signaling pathway activated by the phosphorylated tyrosines on the receptor molecules and are particularly important in control of cell proliferation.

In a variation on this theme some hormones have tyrosine kinase-linked receptors. The receptor itself does not have the ability to phosphorylate tyrosine amino acids. Instead these receptors, when bound to their hormone ligand, form a dimer with an inactive tyrosine kinase in the cell membrane. The dimerization process induces conformational changes in the tyrosine kinase that activate it, and this kinase then phosphorylates the tyrosines on the receptor molecule.

Once fully phosphorylated, a receptor tyrosine kinase dimer can activate many (10 or more are known) various signaling pathways through activation of relay proteins. This allows these hormone receptors to coordinate many functions in a cell at the same time. In contrast, G protein-coupled receptors activate only one pathway in the cell.

Unfortunately, it appears that some cells develop a mutated receptor tyrosine kinase (such as MAP kinase) that may be active even in the absence of the hormone ligand. This can lead to uncontrolled growth of the cells and neoplasia.

Receptors coupled to ion channels

This mechanism is widely used within the nervous system to allow neurotransmitters to stimulate cells. The receptor for the neurotransmitter or hormone is linked to a cation channel in the cell membrane. When the receptor binds its ligand it causes a conformational change that alters membrane depolarization in that small portion of the cell membrane and causes the channel protein to open, allowing cations, often Ca^{2+} but sometimes Na^+ or even K^+, to flow into the interior of the cell and effect a change in the physiology of the cell. It is not a major method of signal transduction utilized by the major endocrine gland hormones. The reader is referred to the neurophysiology chapters in Section I for more details on ion channels.

Hormones acting on receptors located in the cell nucleus

1 Can a steroid or thyroid hormone enter a cell's nucleus?
2 Where are receptors for steroid and thyroid hormones located and what happens after formation of the hormone–receptor complex?

Steroid hormones

These compounds are all derived from cholesterol. Steroid hormones are produced by the adrenal cortex, sex glands, placenta, kidney, and other tissues. Steroid hormones are not stored within the endocrine cells making them. This means they must be made *de novo* when needed. This is controlled by regulating the enzymes involved in their production. They are lipid-soluble and diffuse from the cell as soon as they are produced. Because they are lipid-soluble they are not very water-soluble and require transport proteins to carry them throughout the body via the bloodstream. Only a small fraction, perhaps 1–10%, of the secreted hormone actually exists in the extracellular fluid not bound to the carrier proteins. This tiny fraction is extremely important as it is this free or unbound hormone that is able to diffuse into target tissues and cause an action in a target cell. Some hormones form weak ionic bonds with albumin, while other steroid hormones have unique carrier proteins to carry them in the blood. In all cases an equilibrium is established between steroid hormone bound to carrier proteins and steroid hormone that is in the free or unbound state. This equilibrium insures that as the free steroid hormone molecules enter target cells from the extracellular fluid, the carrier proteins release molecules of steroid hormone to the extracellular fluid. The overall concentration of free hormone is therefore directly linked to the concentration of hormone bound to carrier proteins in the blood.

Thyroid hormones

Thyroid hormones are derived from the amino acid tyrosine by iodination of the hydroxyl group on the phenyl ring of tyrosine. Thyroid hormones are not water-soluble and must travel in the circulation bound to a special carrier protein. Like the steroid hormones, these small thyroid hormones are lipid-soluble and diffuse into cells of the body. Their target cells will have thyroid hormone receptors in the nucleus that function in a similar manner to steroid hormone receptors.

Steroid and thyroid hormone receptors and transcription

The receptors for the steroid and thyroid hormones (iodinated tyrosine molecules) are located in the nucleus of the cell. When the steroid or thyroid hormone binds its receptor it causes a change in the shape of the receptor (Figure 51.4). In most cases the receptor then forms a bond (dimer) with a transcription-regulating protein. The dimer complex formed by the receptor-bound hormone and the transcription factor allows the complex to bind to certain segments of DNA and initiate transcription and translation of certain genes. Conversely, the formation of the dimer complex may have an inhibitory effect that prevents transcription and translation of certain genes. The newly synthesized proteins (often comprising enzymes or growth factors) constitute the response of the cell to the steroid hormone. Because it takes time to transcribe and translate genes, steroid

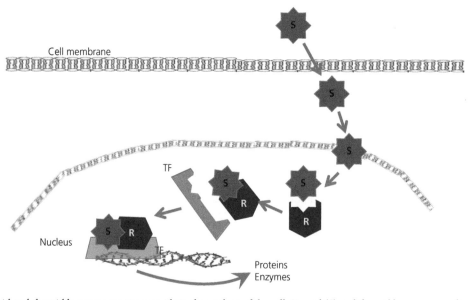

Figure 51.4 Steroid and thyroid hormone receptors reside in the nucleus of the cell. Steroid (S) and thyroid hormones are lipophilic and diffuse into the cell and cross the cytosol to bind their receptors (R). The steroid hormone–receptor complex is then able to bind to and activate a transcription factor (TF) and the entire complex binds to DNA, causing transcription of a particular set of genes coding for the proteins that will alter cell functions.

and thyroid hormones are involved in slower but much longer-term responses of cells than the peptide hormones.

Feedback control of hormone secretion

> **1** What is negative feedback?

Hormones have the ability to alter metabolism and functions of target tissues located a distance away from where the hormone is produced. How is the production of the hormone regulated? Most hormones serve to maintain homeostasis of the body or return the body to some physiologic set point. An important concept in endocrinology is the concept of **feedback control**. When a hormone is secreted it is expected to induce some physiologic change in the target tissues. The target tissue response then affects further secretion of the hormone. The most common type of feedback control is **negative feedback**. In this case, some perturbation of the physiology of the animal is sensed by regulatory centers in the endocrine or nervous system. This causes a hormone to be secreted. That hormone acts on target tissues to alter the physiology of the animal to correct the abnormal situation. The regulatory centers sense that the target cells have accomplished their mission and the regulatory centers cause hormone production to cease. A simple illustration of negative feedback can be seen with calcium metabolism (Figure 51.5). Blood calcium concentration is normally 10 mg/dL in many mammals. The cells within the parathyroid gland are very sensitive to blood calcium concentration. Any decline in blood calcium concentration causes the cells to secrete parathyroid hormone (PTH). The PTH stimulates renal tubular reabsorption of calcium, reducing urinary calcium excretion which can help increase blood calcium. If this action raises blood calcium concentration back to 10 mg/dL, the parathyroid cells will sense normocalcemia and PTH secretion will cease.

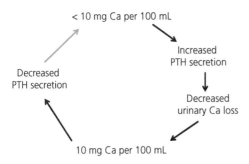

Figure 51.5 Negative feedback. The homeostatic set point for blood calcium is 10 mg/dL. If blood calcium falls below this concentration, it stimulates secretion of parathyroid hormone, which acts on renal tubular epithelium to increase renal reabsorption of calcium. This reduces calcium lost to urine and may bring enough calcium back into the blood to return blood calcium to 10 mg/dL, which is sufficient to stop parathyroid hormone secretion until the next time the calcium concentration falls below 10 mg/dL.

This is perhaps overly simplified. Often there are multiple factors which can act on the regulatory sensing centers that control secretion of a particular hormone. In general in negative feedback, when the hormone has successfully increased activity of the target organ, the response of the target organ will cause a reduction in hormone secretion.

Much less common is **positive feedback** control. In this situation a hormone is secreted to achieve a certain end point. Once the hormone is first secreted, it promotes further secretion of hormone until some physiologic end point is achieved. An example of this is the act of ovulation of an oocyte from the ovary. This process begins with the hypothalamus secreting **gonadotropin-releasing hormone (GnRH)** into the hypothalamo-hypophyseal portal system, perhaps in response to the pineal gland sensing a change in daylength. This causes luteinizing hormone (LH) to be secreted by the adenohypophysis. This hormone causes estradiol to be released from a developing ovarian follicle. The estradiol reaches the hypothalamus and causes increased secretion of GnRH, resulting in more LH secretion, and more estradiol secretion. This increased estradiol again feeds back on the hypothalamus to stimulate GnRH and LH secretion, causing more estradiol production to stimulate even more GnRH secretion. Finally, the surge in LH secretion is great enough to induce ovulation, the end point of this physiologic sequence.

Hypothalamo-hypophyseal (pituitary) axis

> **1** What is the difference between the adenohypophysis and the neurohypophysis?
>
> **2** Which hormones are secreted by the adenohypophysis and the neurohypophysis?
>
> **3** Outline the path of the hypothalamo-hypophyseal portal system and explain why it is an important conduit between the hypothalamus and adenohypophsis.

The **hypothalamus** is an area of the central nervous system that contains neurons with some of the attributes of endocrine cells. The hypothalamus receives input from nearly all regions in the brain and uses this information to control body temperature, appetite, sexual behavior, defensive reactions (fear, rage), biological rhythms, and output of the autonomic nervous system. It is the site where the nervous system meets the endocrine system. Many nuclei (groups of neurons with the same function) exist in the hypothalamus and they produce compounds (neuroendocrines) that affect the release of hormones from the pituitary gland.

The **pituitary gland** is sometimes called the "master gland" because it produces several key hormones and modulates the secretions produced by several other endocrine glands. The pituitary gland is a singular gland, also known as the **hypophysis**. It sits in a depression of the sphenoid bone called the sella turcica, which places it directly beneath the hypothalamus.

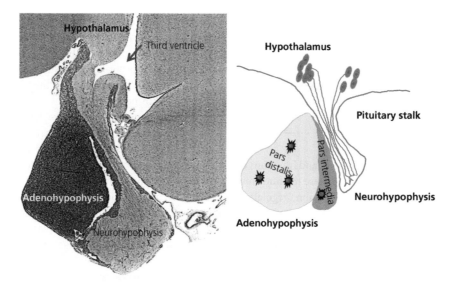

Figure 51.6 Photomicrograph (5×) of hypothalamus and hypophysis with sketch of structures.

The hypophysis is divided into two functionally different parts, the adenohypophysis and the neurohypophysis (Figure 51.6).

The **adenohypophysis** is a collection of endocrine cells that secrete a variety of hormones into the blood. It is often further subdivided into the pars distalis (anterior lobe of pituitary) and the pars intermedia (intermediate or middle lobe of the pituitary). The major hormones secreted by the pars distalis include thyroid-stimulating homone, prolactin, growth hormone, luteinizing hormone, follicle-stimulating hormone, and adrenocorticotropic hormone. The pars intermedia endocrine cells produce melanocyte-stimulating hormone, β-endorphins, enkephalins, and corticotropin-like intermediate lobe peptide, the latter being particularly prominent and important in horses.

The **neurohypophysis** is essentially where the axons of nerve cells located in the supraoptic and paraventricular nuclei of the hypothalamus terminate and secrete their neurotransmitters into the blood. The axons from these nuclei extend down the infundibular stalk (pituitary stalk) that suspends the pituitary within the sella turcica. The two principal neurotransmitters released by these axon terminals are oxytocin and antidiuretic hormone. Because they are released into the blood they are often referred to as hormones, but to be clear – they are simply special neurotransmitters that are released directly into the hypophyseal veins which empty into the general circulation.

Hypothalamo-hypophyseal portal system

A portal blood system connects the hypothalamus and the adenohypophysis. A **portal system** is a system of veins that drains one capillary bed and carries the blood to a second capillary bed. In this case, the first capillary bed exists in the ventral portion of the hypothalamus. The second capillary bed exists in the adenohypophysis. The hypophyseal portal venules link the two. Neuroendocrine substances, which we shall refer to as neurohormones, are produced by neurons within the various nuclei of the

hypothalamus and are released into the area drained by the first capillary bed. They then enter the portal venules to be carried to the sinusoids (highly fenestrated endothelium) of the second capillary bed. The neurohormones diffuse into the extracellular fluid of the adenohypophysis and can stimulate or inhibit release of the hormones of the adenohypophysis (Figure 51.7).

The advantage of the hypothalamo-hypophyseal portal system is that it allows stimulation of all the cells of the adenohypophysis without sending a nerve axon to each individual endocrine cell of the hypophysis. It also circumvents problems with dilution of the releasing hormones of the hypothalamus that would occur if they were secreted into the general circulation rather than the portal system. The neurohypophysis receives no blood from this portal system.

In summary, the hypothalamus processes afferent information from most areas of the body and brain and then secretes releasing or release-inhibiting neurohormones into the hypothalamo-hypophyseal portal system to control secretion of hormones from the adenohypophysis. The adenohypophyseal hormones are secreted into the hypophyseal veins, which convey the hormones to the general systemic circulation. They then affect the secretion of hormones by secondary endocrine glands.

Growth hormone

1 What are the main effects of growth hormone?
2 What is the role of insulin-like growth factors?
3 How is growth hormone secretion controlled?

Growth hormone (GH), a 191-amino-acid protein also known as **somatotropin**, is produced by somatotropes in the pars distalis of the adenohypophysis. It promotes growth in length of

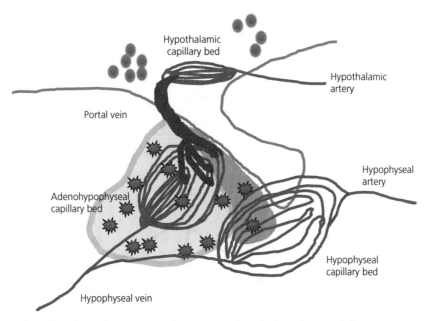

Figure 51.7 Hypothalamo-hypophyseal portal system. Neurohormones made in the hypothalamus diffuse into the hypothalamic capillary bed and the portal vein carries them to the adenohypophyseal capillary bed where they diffuse into the adenohypophysis to regulate secretion of hormones. The neurotransmitters produced in the neurohypophysis diffuse into a conventional hypophyseal capillary bed fed directly by the hypophyseal artery and drained by the hypophyseal vein.

the long bones of the body and it promotes protein accretion (builds muscle) while having a lipolytic effect that reduces adipose stores.

GH receptors can be found on many cells of the body, the most important being in the liver and adipose tissue. These receptors are linked to tyrosine kinases that mediate its biological functions in target tissues. When GH acts on the liver it will affect protein, lipid, and carbohydrate metabolism.

In many tissues (bone, mammary gland) the main action of GH on their activity is mediated by another hormone whose secretion is controlled by GH. A very important effect of GH on the liver is to cause the liver to secrete another hormone called **insulin-like growth factor (IGF)-1**. It is also known as **somatomedin C**. This 70-amino-acid hormone has a similar amino acid sequence to insulin. In fact, it is similar enough that IGF-1 can bind to insulin receptors and activate them, though not nearly as well as insulin itself does. The IGF-1 leaves the liver and is carried through the circulation to IGF-1 receptors on cartilage and bone cells, adipose tissue, mammary gland alveolar cells, and skeletal muscle. IGF-1 has a longer half-life in the blood than GH and blood levels are much more constant than GH levels. Production of IGF-1 following GH stimulation of the liver is not guaranteed. Undernutrition, particularly lack of protein in the diet, will cause the liver to fail to secrete IGF-1

In addition, a slightly different form of IGF called IGF-2, also known as **somatomedin A**, is produced in many tissues, such as cartilage and ovary, following stimulation by GH. In these tissues, IGF-2 acts as a paracrine hormone, binding to receptors on neighboring cells rather than entering the blood to act as an endocrine hormone. IGF-2 is made by the fetal liver in response

to GH and released into the fetal circulation. It is critical for normal embryonic development.

Growth hormone and IGF-1 are often considered to have anti-insulin effects. They enhance lipolysis by adipose tissues. GH reduces the uptake of glucose by adipose tissue and muscle by reducing sensitivity to insulin. It increases gluconeogenesis activity in the liver and kidney. The end result of these actions is an increase in blood glucose concentration. When IGF-1 binds to IGF-1 receptors on these tissues it generally increases protein synthesis within the tissue so that protein accretion occurs, and this is particularly important for muscle growth and hypertrophy. It also enhances proliferation of cells as part of the growth of a tissue. This is particularly important in growth of long bones.

Regulation of GH secretion

Secretion of GH is regulated primarily by two neurohormones produced by nuclei in the hypothalamus (Figure 51.8). One is **growth hormone-releasing hormone** (GH-RH) that stimulates secretion of GH by somatotropes. The other neurohormone inhibits GH release by somatotropes and is called **growth hormone release inhibitory hormone** (GH-IH), also known as **somatostatin**. The neurotransmitter dopamine released by nerve endings in the hypothalamus can also act directly on somatotropes and cause them to reduce GH secretion. The balance between these factors keeps GH secretion tightly regulated by the hypothalamus. GH secretion tends to be very episodic, so that blood concentrations will increase to very high levels from a baseline three to four times each day. GH levels might stay elevated for just a couple of hours following each surge in GH secretion. The plasma half-life of GH (time it takes

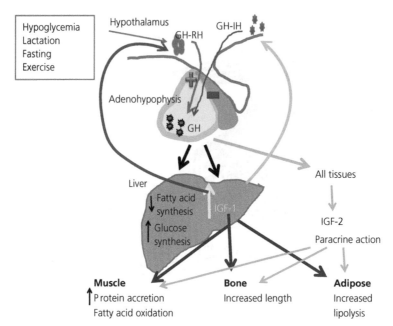

Figure 51.8 Growth hormone (GH) is secreted from the adenohypophysis and causes the liver to secrete a hormone called insulin-like growth factor (IGF)-1. IGF-1 acts on muscle, bone, and adipose tissues and modifies their metabolism. These tissues, as well as many other cells of the body, can also respond directly to GH by producing IGF-2. IGF-2 acts in a paracrine fashion to modulate metabolism in target cells. GH secretion is stimulated by growth hormone releasing hormone (GH-RH) produced in the hypothalamus in response to factors such as hypoglycemia, lactation, fasting, and exercise. IGF-1 feeds back on the hypothalamus causing hypothalamic neurons to secrete growth hormone inhibitory hormone (GH-IH), which reduces GH secretion from the adenohypophysis.

for blood concentration to fall by 50%) is about 20 min. In many species, the surge in blood GH concentration occurs at night, coinciding with lower secretion of GH-IH and dopamine into the hypothalamo-hypophyseal portal system, so essentially the "brakes" that normally suppress GH secretion are off.

Fasting, physical exercise, stress, high dietary protein, and low plasma glucose cause the hypothalamus to secrete more GH-RH. Thyroid hormones and the sex steroids can also impact the hypothalamus and also result in greater GH-RH stimulation of GH secretion, particularly around the time of puberty. GH is increased during lactation in most species and helps direct energy of the body toward the mammary gland and away from adipose tissue.

The following is a partial list of GH-RH secretagogues.

1 Hypoglycemia, fasting, aerobic exercise: these are all stimuli arising from a need to use fat rather than glucose for energy.
2 Melatonin: produced by the pineal gland during periods of darkness, it inhibits somatostatin release.
3 Xylazine and clonidine: α_2-adrenergic agonists useful in clinical assessment testing of adenohypophysis function.
4 Medroxyprogesterone acetate: synthetic progesterone used to prevent estrus in the bitch (see section on iatrogenic acromegaly).
5 Arginine: amino acid used in high amounts for growth of tissues.

The interplay between these factors determines GH secretion rate. In reality GH secretion is very episodic, and several spikes occur each day. How target tissues, such as bone, are able to signal or feedback on the pituitary to cease release of GH is unknown, though it seems likely that IGF-1 and IGF-2 are involved.

GH effects on specific tissues
Bone and cartilage

GH is necessary for elongation of the cartilage within the physis; specifically, it causes increased cell division in the physeal zone of proliferating cartilage. It also stimulates production of chondroitin sulfate by cartilage cells. This effect of GH is not mediated by its action on cartilage cell GH receptors. Instead GH causes cells in the liver to secrete IGF-1, which binds to IGF-1 receptors and directly stimulates cells in the zone of proliferating cartilage. It also stimulates the cartilage cells to produce IGF-2 locally, which has similar actions to IGF-1.

Deficiency of GH will lead to dwarfism. Interestingly, this is observed mostly in the larger breeds, such as German Shepherds and Great Danes. However, the majority of dogs (and people) with dwarfism produce adequate amounts of GH. In the majority of cases, dogs with short legs (Corgis, Dachshunds, etc.) have a genetic mutation in their fibroblast growth factor receptor gene that causes the reduced growth in length of the bones.

Excessive secretion of GH can cause **gigantism** in young growing animals. In adults, with closed physes, excess GH causes **acromegaly**. Usually this is due to a somatotrope tumor of the adenohypophysis secreting GH in an uncontrolled fashion. Flat bones of the face and the spacing between teeth can be affected.

Internal organs

GH deficiency leads to soft thin skin. Excess GH, as seen in acromegaly, can lead to hepatomegaly and cardiomegaly. The cardiomegaly can lead to congestive heart failure.

Protein metabolism

GH administration increases the uptake of amino acids from the blood and increases the rate of synthesis of new proteins. GH (usually through IGF-1) causes target cells to increase expression of protein-coding mRNA and it increases ribosomal activity.

Carbohydrate metabolism

GH is often described as diabetogenic, since administration of GH results in increases in blood glucose concentration.

1 GH decreases the sensitivity of cells to insulin: it reduces insulin receptor number on cells of muscle and adipose tissue.
2 Glycostatic effect: GH can spare glycogen in muscle, most likely by causing the cells to shift from using glucose to generate ATP to using more lipids for ATP generation.

Lipid metabolism

GH decreases synthesis of fatty acids from glucose by adipose tissue and liver. GH also increases lipolysis and mobilization of fats from body stores.

Syndromes of special concern to veterinary medicine

Cats

In aged cats, a **somatotrope pituitary tumor** sometimes develops and excessive secretion of GH occurs. These cats often have excessively high blood glucose, reminiscent of diabetes, but maintain lean body mass. They will have dramatically elevated blood insulin levels (as opposed to diabetic cats). They often develop cardiomegaly and congestive heart failure later in the disease.

Dogs

Endogenous progesterone can feed back on the hypothalamus and incite increased production of GH. This may be beneficial for initiation of lactation. However, when dogs are placed on high doses of synthetic progestins, usually to suppress estrus, it can induce **iatrogenic acromegaly**. In this very weird situation, the synthetic progestins cause cells within the mammary gland to abnormally produce and secrete GH.

Dairy cows

A recombinant form of bovine GH is administered to dairy cows to increase milk production. This is likely mediated by GH stimulation of IGF-1 production, which then has two effects.

1 It causes energy generated by absorption of nutrients from the diet to be repartitioned away from formation of triglyceride in adipose tissue and toward mammary gland production of proteins, lactose, and fats that will be incorporated into milk. This reduces adipose deposition and prevents dairy cows from becoming excessively fat in late lactation.
2 It inhibits apoptosis of alveolar cells. Normally, milk production declines over time due to the loss of alveolar cells by apoptosis. Growth hormone promotes a longer and higher level of milk production.

Prolactin

> **1** What is the main action of prolactin?

Prolactin is produced by cells in the pars distalis of the adenohypophysis called lactotropes. Prolactin maintains milk production in female mammals. It may also play a role in initiation of milk secretion in some species. In all species, the secretion of prolactin by the adenohypophysis occurs at a baseline level most of the time. However, when conditions are right (pregnancy or parturition) the hypothalamus secretes **prolactin-releasing hormone**, which increases secretion of prolactin by the pituitary. Estrogen levels in blood rise during each estrus cycle, causing increased release of prolactin and increased development of the mammary gland with each cycle during puberty. Estrogen also rises to high levels, particularly in ruminants, at the end of gestation to further development of mammary tissue to begin the process of lactation. The act of suckling by neonates also serves as a stimulus for prolactin secretion in some species, especially those giving birth to litters. When blood prolactin levels are excessively high, prolactin feeds back on the hypothalamus which secretes **prolactin release-inhibiting hormone** into the hypothalamo-hypophyseal portal system to inhibit prolactin secretion by lactotropes of the pituitary.

In rabbits, administration of prolactin alone to a lactating female that has been hypophysectomized (pituitary gland removed) can cause the animal to return to full milk production.

In ruminants, prolactin is just one of several hormones needed to initiate and sustain milk production. It works with estrogen and progesterone, along with placental lactogen produced by the fetal placenta in late gestation, to accelerate growth of the mammary gland. At parturition, prolactin secretion is greatly increased. Prolactin triggers increased production of casein within the Golgi apparatus of alveolar cells of the mammary gland.

Its role in males is not well defined, but low blood levels have been linked with reduced sexual behavior in males and very high levels may cause low testosterone levels by inhibiting secretion of LH from the adenohypophysis .

Thyroid function

> 1 How do the thyroid follicular cells use dietary iodine to form thyroid hormones?
>
> 2 How is thyroid hormone activated or inactivated inside target cells?
>
> 3 What is the most important factor affecting TRH secretion?
>
> 4 What is goiter and why does it occur in animals that are iodine deficient or fed plants containing goitrogens?
>
> 5 What are the clinical symptoms expected in a hyperthyroid cat and what are the cause of the symptoms?
>
> 6 What are the clinical symptoms expected in a hypothyroid dog?

Two lobes of the thyroid gland lie on each side of the trachea just below the larynx. In some species a bridge of thyroid tissue joins the two lobes. Thyroid tissue consists of numerous sac-like structures called **thyroid follicles** that vary in size. A single layer of epithelium lines each follicle and these cells synthesize the thyroid hormones (Figure 51.9). The lumen of each follicle is filled with a viscous protein-rich liquid called **colloid**. Within the connective tissue between thyroid follicles lies another collection of endocrine cells called the **C-cells** or **parafollicular** or **medullary** cells. These cells produce a hormone called **thyrocalcitonin**. Within the lobes of the thyroid gland or just outside the lobes of the thyroid gland of many species lie two to four (depending on species) parathyroid glands that produce PTH.

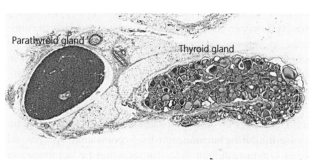

(A)

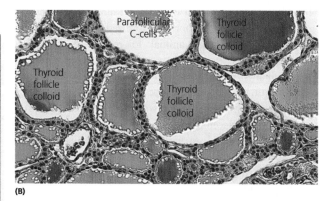

(B)

Figure 51.9 (A) Histomicrograph (2.5×) of the thyroid and parathyroid glands. (B) Photomicrograph (20×) of thyroid follicles and parafollicular C-cells. Iodinated thyroglobulin is stored within the colloid until secretion of thyroid hormones is required.

Thyrocalcitonin and PTH are discussed further in the section Parathyroid gland, thyroid C-cells, and calcium homeostasis.

Formation and release of thyroid hormones

The follicular cells of the thyroid produce two hormones that are derivatives of iodinated tyrosine, thyroxine and triiodothyronine. Ingested iodide is absorbed into the blood. Serum iodide is actively and very efficiently taken up by thyroid follicular cells using a Na^+/I^- cotransporter, with a Na^+ ion providing the driving force to bring the I^- into the cell across the basolateral membrane (Figure 51.10). The follicular cells produce a very large protein called thyroglobulin that contains a high number of tyrosine molecules. The thyroglobulin is exocytosed into the lumen of the thyroid follicle across the apical membrane. An enzyme system within the thyroid follicular cells generates hydrogen peroxide near the apical membrane. Another enzyme called thyroid peroxidase is also found in the apical membrane of the follicular cells. As the iodide is being pumped out into the lumen, thyroid peroxidase uses hydrogen peroxide to oxidize the iodide to elemental iodine. The iodine form is very reactive and will nonspecifically iodinate position 3 and/or position 5 on the tyrosine residues of thyroglobulin. If the tyrosine residue is iodinated at position 3 only, it is known as monoiodotyrosine. Under conditions providing normal dietary iodine, the majority of tyrosine residues are iodinated at both positions 3 and 5 to form diiodotyrosine (Figure 51.11). Thyroid peroxidase then catalyzes the fusion of two of these iodinated tyrosines end to end. If two diiodotyrosines are joined together by thyroid peroxidase, the resulting molecule (with four iodine atoms) is called thyroxine or T_4. If a monoiodotyrosine is joined with a diiodotyrosine, the result is a molecule with three iodine atoms and it is called triiodotyrosine or T_3. T_4 is preferentially produced by the thyroid follicle cells when there is sufficient iodine. Normally, thyroid hormone is synthesized at a ratio of 4 : 1 (T_4/T_3). During iodine deficiency the ratio may be just 1 : 3 (T_4/T_3). At this point, the thyroid hormone molecules are still attached to the large thyroglobulin molecule. They are stored in the colloid of the thyroid follicle until they need to be secreted.

When thyroid follicle cells are stimulated to secrete thyroid hormone by **thyroid-stimulating hormone (TSH)** produced by the adenohypophysis, iodinated thyroglobulin is endocytosed back into the cell and undergoes proteolysis, liberating both T_4 and T_3. The iodine atoms on the iodinated tyrosine residues of thyroglobulin that were not successfully united to form T_4 or T_3 molecules are very efficiently recycled within the follicle cell to iodinate new thyroglobulin molecules.

T_3 has a shorter half-life in blood than T_4 so circulating levels of T_4 are typically ninefold to tenfold greater than circulating T_3 concentrations. Because thyroid hormones are lipophilic they must be carried through the blood bound to a special protein called **thyroxine-binding globulin** (made by the liver). Albumin can also carry T_4 and T_3, though it has a lower affinity for the thyroid hormones. A small amount of the thyroid hormone is free in the circulation: it is in equilibrium with the much larger

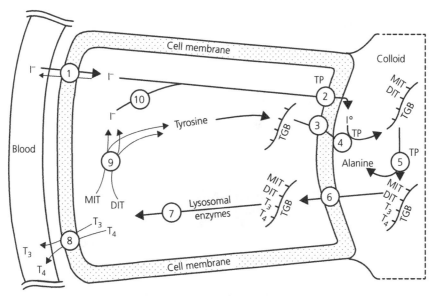

Figure 51.10 Follicular cell showing steps in the synthesis and release of triiodothyronine (T$_3$) and thyroxine (T$_4$). The numbers identify the major steps: 1, trapping of iodide; 2, oxidation of iodide; 3, exocytosis of thyroglobulin (TGB); 4, iodination of TGB; 5, coupling of iodotyrosines; 6, endocytosis of TGB; 7, hydrolysis of TGB; 8, release of T$_3$ and T$_4$; 9, deiodination and formation of monoiodotyrosine (MIT) and diiodotyrosine (DIT); 10, recycling of iodide. TP, thyroperoxidase. From Hedge, G.A., Colby, H.D. and Goodman, R.L. (1987) *Clinical Endocrine Physiology*. W.B. Saunders, Philadelphia. With permission from Elsevier.

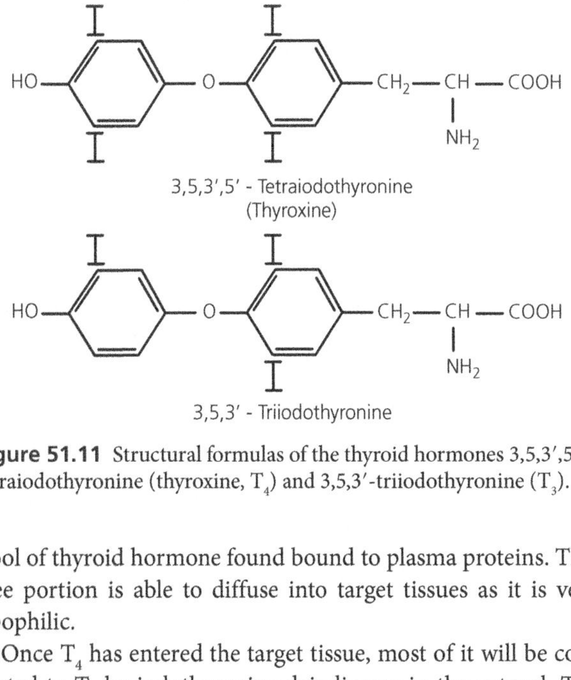

3,5,3',5' - Tetraiodothyronine
(Thyroxine)

3,5,3' - Triiodothyronine

Figure 51.11 Structural formulas of the thyroid hormones 3,5,3',5'-tetraiodothyronine (thyroxine, T$_4$) and 3,5,3'-triiodothyronine (T$_3$).

pool of thyroid hormone found bound to plasma proteins. This free portion is able to diffuse into target tissues as it is very lipophilic.

Once T$_4$ has entered the target tissue, most of it will be converted to T$_3$ by iodothyronine deiodinases in the cytosol. The iodothyronine deiodinase enzyme is unusual in that it contains selenium in the form of selenocysteine and its activity is diminished by selenium deficiency.

T$_3$ binds the nuclear thyroid hormone receptor with greater affinity than T$_4$ and so has about four times greater biological action than T$_4$; thus conversion of T$_4$ to T$_3$ is considered an activation step that occurs inside target cells. The thyroid hormone receptor–thyroid hormone complex then binds to thyroid response elements of the genome and causes transcription and translation of various genes.

Three isoforms of iodothyronine deiodinase are known. One type of iodothyronine deiodinase removes an alternative iodine from the T$_4$ molecule. The resulting compound is called reverse T$_3$. It has no biological activity. In this case the iodothyronine deiodinase has performed inactivation of T$_4$. How the different iodothyronine deiodinases are regulated to control inactivation or activation of T$_4$ remains unknown.

Control of thyroid hormone secretion

Neurons within the hypothalamus produce a tripeptide neurohormone called **thyrotropin releasing hormone (TRH)**, which enters the hypothalamo-hypophyseal portal system to stimulate thyrotrope cells in the adenohypophysis to release TSH (Figure 51.12). TSH enters the blood and stimulates secretion of thyroid hormones by the follicular cells of the thyroid gland.

The cortical brain responds to various external environmental cues such as colder weather to increase TRH secretion. In addition, internal environmental cues control TRH secretion. For example, leptin is a hormone made by adipose tissue when it is gaining triglyceride. It reacts with the hypothalamic neurons and stimulates TRH secretion. Lactation also increases TRH secretion. However, the most important regulator of TRH secretion is thyroid hormone itself. The brain has a certain requirement for thyroid hormones – they influence many aspects of the nervous system related to brain maturation and function, including neural cell migration, neuron differentiation, and the rate of conduction of action potentials down axons. When thyroid hormone levels decrease, the brain senses this and signals the hypothalamus to

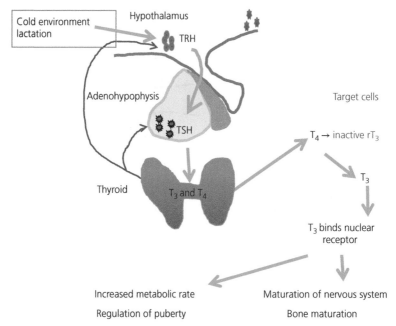

Figure 51.12 Regulation of thyroid hormones. The hypothalamus produces thyrotropin releasing hormone (TRH) in response to cold weather, lactation, and other factors. TRH reaches the adenohypophysis via the hypothalamo-hypophyseal portal system and stimulates adenohypophyseal production of thyroid-stimulating hormone (TSH). TSH then initiates mobilization of triiodothyronine (T_3) and thyroxine (T_4) from thyroglobulin stored in the colloid of the thyroid follicles. Nearly all cells have thyroid hormone receptors and are therefore targets for thyroid hormones. Secreted T_4 and T_3 are lipophilic and diffuse into their target tissues. T_4 can be converted to T_3 by cytosolic deiodinases. In some instances, when T_4 is plentiful, it can also be converted to reverse T_3 (rT_3), a biologically inactive compound. T_3 binds to the thyroid hormone receptor and stimulates transcription and translation of proteins and enzymes to increase metabolic rate and carry out other functions of thyroid hormones. The primary regulator of TRH secretion is negative feedback provided by T_3 and T_4 on the hypothalamus.

secrete TRH. When T_4 and T_3 in the blood are sufficiently high to fulfill thyroid hormone functions in the brain, the hypothalamus ceases secretion of TRH. Thyroid hormones (T_4 and T_3) also provide negative feedback directly on the adenohypophysis and cause reduced secretion of TSH.

Actions of thyroid hormones

Thyroid hormones increase the metabolic rate of cells. Little is known of the actual physiology involved in this action. Circulating thyroid hormone levels are increased during cold weather and during lactation. Most of the information on the actions of thyroid hormones has been gleaned from abnormally secreting thyroid glands, i.e., clinical cases of hypothyroidism or hyperthyroidism.

1 Thyroid hormones increase the basal metabolic rate. They determine how many calories are produced by the body at rest. Thyroid hormones increase the rate of lipolysis and glycolysis in cells. They also increase the conversion of cholesterol to bile salts, which has an unknown significance to energy status but can prove useful clinically as hypothyroid animals often suffer from elevated blood cholesterol levels.

2 Growth and development. Thyroid hormones permit maturation of the nervous system. When thyroid hormones are not produced or are insufficient in young animals and humans, this will result in reduced mental abilities. The long

bones do not grow or mature properly. Thyroid hormone affects the secretion of GH, which may explain why dwarfism is seen in chronic hypothyroidism of young animals.

3 Thyroid hormones impact release of sex hormones. Puberty is delayed and ovulation is impeded in hypothyroid females. Sperm production is greatly reduced in hypothyroid males.

4 Thyroid hormones are necessary for normal nerve conduction velocity. Hypothyroidism leads to slower reflexes and reduced mental abilities.

5 Thyroid hormones maintain the number of receptors for epinephrine and norepinephrine on tissues and so impact the effects of the sympathetic nervous system.

6 Skin integrity is maintained by thyroid hormones. Hypothyroid animals often exhibit hair loss, changes in skin and hair color, and seem predisposed to develop skin infections.

7 In amphibians, thyroid hormones control metamorphosis from one life form to another, an example being the metamorphosis of a tadpole into a frog.

Hypothyroidism

Hypothyroidism causes a general reduction in metabolic rate, characterized by slow heart rate, decreased body temperature, infertility, weight gain, and slower mental ability. Hypothyroidism can occur due to problems with thyroid hormone production (iodine deficiency, tumor, or atrophy of thyroid follicular cells), failure of the hypothalamus to secrete TRH, or failure of the adenohypophysis to secrete TSH.

Iodine-deficiency goiter: inability to iodinate tyrosine residues

Forage iodine concentrations are extremely variable and depend on soil iodine content. Soil near the oceans tends to provide adequate iodine to plants. However, in the Great Lakes region and in northwestern USA iodine concentrations in forages are generally low enough to result in iodine deficiency unless animal diets are supplemented. Iodine deficiency reduces thyroid hormone production, slowing the rate of oxidation of all cells. Iodine deficiency can cause enlarged thyroid glands, a condition called **goiter**. Since T_4 and T_3 are not produced, there is no negative feedback on hypothalamic production of TRH. TSH continues to be secreted in high amounts. This stimulates increased thyroglobulin production, which accumulates and distends the thyroid follicles. Under severe iodine deficiency conditions, the hyperplastic thyroid gland cannot compensate for the reduced availability of iodine. Animals become inappetant, have a slow heart rate, and often develop dermatological disorders. Iodine deficiency causes reduced fertility (males and females) and increased morbidity. Under conditions of marginal or deficient dietary iodine, the maternal thyroid gland becomes extremely efficient in uptake of iodine from the circulation and recycling of thyroid hormone iodine. Unfortunately, this leaves little iodine for the fetal thyroid gland and the fetus becomes hypothyroid. Often the first indication of iodine deficiency in a herd is enlargement of the thyroid (goiter) of newborn animals. Calves and lambs may be born hairless, weak, or dead. Fetal death can occur at any stage of gestation. Often the mothers will appear normal.

Autoimmune thyroiditis

This disorder is the most common cause of hypothyroidism in dogs. This is an autoimmune condition where the dog's immune system attacks the normal follicular tissue. It is akin to Hashimoto's syndrome in humans. The lack of thyroid hormone production causes weight gain and thinning of the hair coat with alopecia commonly observed in a bilaterally symmetrical pattern over the lower lumbar region. The tail may lose all its hair. Hypothyroid dogs can also develop acanthosis nigricans, or black pigmented skin, especially in the groin region.

Goitrogens

Goitrogens are compounds that interfere with the synthesis or secretion of thyroid hormones and cause hypothyroidism. Goitrogens fall into two main categories.

1 **Cyanogenic goitrogens** interfere with iodide uptake by the thyroid gland. Cyanogenic glucosides can be found in many feeds, including raw soybeans, beet pulp, corn, sweet potato, white clover, and millet and once ingested are metabolized to thiocyanate and isothiocyanate. These compounds alter iodide transport across the basolateral thyroid follicular cell membrane, reducing iodide retention. This effect is easily overcome by increasing supplemental iodine.

2 Thiouracil goitrins inhibit thyroid peroxidase. **Thiouracils** are found in cruciferous plants (rape, kale, cabbage, turnips, mustard), and **aliphatic disulfides** found in onions directly inhibit thyroid peroxidase preventing formation of monoiodotyrosine and diiodotyrosine. With goitrins, especially those of the thiouracil type, hormone synthesis is not restored to normal by increasing dietary iodine supplementation. The offending feedstuff needs to be reduced or removed from the diet.

Idiopathic thyroid atrophy

This can occur in some animals as they age.

Secondary to pituitary adenoma

Hypothyroidism occurs because the tumor reduces TSH production (uncommon in animals).

Hyperthyroidism

Hyperthyroidism is associated with increased heart rate, polyphagia, and weight loss.

Thyroid tumors that secrete excessive amounts of thyroid hormones

This is being increasingly diagnosed in cats. Since the symptoms often diminish when the cat is placed on a low-iodine diet, there is concern that this is occurring because diets are too high in iodine. It is an occasional finding in dogs due to development of a benign adenoma or, more rarely, a malignant carcinoma of the thyroid follicular tissue.

Cats are the animal most commonly affected by hyperthyroidism. They exhibit weight loss despite an insatiable appetite. They are often restless, continually walking and crying. They generally have tachycardia and in some cases the thyroid gland is palpably enlarged. Dogs and other species can also develop carcinoma of the thyroid resulting in excessive thyroid hormone production.

Graves' disease

This disorder is very rare in animals (unlike humans, where up to 2% of females will develop the condition). It has been diagnosed in dogs. In this case a very strange antibody is formed by the lymphocytes and secreted into the bloodstream. This antibody has the ability to mimic TSH – it will bind to TSH receptors on the thyroid follicular cells and initiate thyroid hormone secretion.

Parathyroid gland, thyroid C-cells, and calcium homeostasis

1 What are the main actions of parathyroid hormone and how this helps to increase blood calcium concentration?

2 How is vitamin D metabolized and what is the role of parathyroid hormone?

Most species have two pairs of **parathyroid glands**. One pair is located in the cranial portion of each thyroid lobe and one pair is often found near or within the cranial part of the thymus. Carotid arterioles supply them with blood. The parathyroid cells are very sensitive to a decline in blood calcium concentration. They have a **calcium-sensing receptor** on their surface that is actually a G protein-coupled receptor. As long as ionized blood calcium is normal (about 5 mg/dL in most mammals), the receptor is inactive. But if ionized calcium concentration falls, the receptor is activated. It initiates fusion of the PTH storage vesicle with the cell membrane and PTH is delivered into the bloodstream.

Parathyroid hormone has four major actions

1 PTH stimulates the kidney to reabsorb calcium from the glomerular filtrate. If the perturbation in blood calcium is small, this is often enough to correct the hypocalcemia. It also causes the kidney to excrete more phosphorus, though this is only a small effect in most animals (compared with humans).
2 PTH binds to its receptors on osteocytes and stimulates these cells to pump calcium from the fluids within bone canaliculi into the extracellular fluid and blood. This is sometimes referred to as **osteocytic osteolysis**.
3 PTH binds to its receptors on bone osteoblast cells. The osteoblasts respond by secreting a substance called **osteoclast-activating factor**, which causes nearby osteoclasts to become active. The osteoclasts then move toward the bone and begin to secrete acid and proteolytic enzymes to digest the organic matrix of the bone. Osteoclasts liberate calcium and phosphorus from the bone, which can then enter the blood to help restore blood calcium concentration.
4 PTH binds to its receptors on proximal renal tubule cells and stimulates the enzyme that converts 25-hydroxyvitamin D to a hormone called 1,25-dihydroxyvitamin D. Vitamin D can be made in the skin of many animals if they are receiving ultraviolet (UV)B irradiation from the sun (this does not occur in cats and dogs). The vitamin D can also be fed in the diet. Vitamin D is biologically inert. It is carried in the blood to the liver where it is hydroxylated at the C-25 position to form 25-hydroxyvitamin D, which is also biologically inert. Only after it has been hydroxylated at C-1 by the renal 1α-hydroxylase enzyme, which is active only when PTH has acted on the cell, does the vitamin become a hormone. The hormone 1,25-dihydroxyvitamin D stimulates the active transport of dietary calcium across the intestinal epithelium. Without 1,25-dihydroxyvitamin D most animals are unable to acquire enough calcium from the diet to support normal bone structure. By regulating blood 1,25-dihydroxyvitamin D concentrations, the animal can regulate the amount of calcium entering the blood from the diet. An exception is the horse and the rabbit, both hindgut fermenters. These animals have the intestinal mechanisms to absorb calcium activated all the time. They regulate blood calcium by increasing or decreasing urinary calcium loss. Thus they excrete any dietary calcium that is not needed. This is why these species often have chalky white-colored urine.

Thyroid calcitonin

> 1 How does calcitonin decrease blood calcium concentration?

The parafollicular cells or C-cells of the thyroid secrete a hormone called **calcitonin** (thyrocalcitonin). This hormone is secreted in response to elevated blood calcium levels. As a rule, animals only rarely experience hypercalcemia of sufficient magnitude to cause calcitonin secretion. However, in young animals suckling milk, a source of very available calcium, there is a short period following a meal when the blood calcium is slightly elevated. This causes calcitonin to be released for a short period after each meal.

Calcitonin has two major effects

5 Calcitonin binds receptors on renal tubules and inhibits renal tubular reabsorption of calcium. This allows more calcium to be excreted in the urine, lowering blood calcium levels.
6 Calcitonin binds to receptors on osteoclast cells and inhibits bone resorption activity by the osteoclasts, reducing liberation of calcium and phosphorus from bone.

Chapter 49 provides more details on calcium homeostasis as it relates to common bone and metabolic disorders observed in individual species.

Pituitary–adrenal axis

> 1 What are the three zones of the adrenal cortex and which hormones do they produce?
> 2 Aldosterone production is stimulated by changes in blood pressure and perfusion of the kidney. Describe how this is mediated.
> 3 What are the actions of aldosterone that cause sodium to be reabsorbed from renal tubular fluid?
> 4 Describe how stress causes cortisol to be secreted.
> 5 How does the hypothalamus control cortisol secretion?
> 6 Where are the receptors for the adrenal corticosteroids located? Do mineralocorticoids only act on mineralocorticoid receptors and do glucocorticoids only act on glucocorticoid receptors?
> 7 What are the major actions of cortisol on tissues, including the immune system?
> 8 Androgens are also made in the adrenal cortex. Where and what function could they serve in females?
> 9 Describe the symptoms expected in an animal with Addison's disease and explain why they occur.
> 10 Describe the symptoms expected in an animal with Cushing's syndrome and explain why they occur.

Two adrenal glands are located beneath the peritoneum cranial to each kidney. Each gland has two distinct layers, the adrenal cortex and the adrenal medulla.

Adrenocortical hormones

The adrenal cortex originates from the embryologic mesoderm. The cortex can be divided into three zones, with each zone secreting a different hormone (Figure 51.13). The outermost zone is called the **zona glomerulosa**. It produces hormones called **mineralocorticoids** that help regulate electrolyte balance in the animal. The middle zone is known as the **zona fasciculata** and it produces **glucocorticoid**s, important in glucose metabolism and stress responses. The innermost zone of the adrenal cortex is called the **zona reticularis** and it produces some glucocorticoids but is unique in that it also secretes **androgens** (Figure 51.14).

All the hormones produced by the adrenal cortex are produced from cholesterol. In the first step, common to all adrenocortical hormones, the side chain of the cholesterol molecule is cleaved off to form pregnenolone. This step is regulated by adrenocorticotropic hormone (ACTH) produced in the adenohypophysis. This step limits the rate of synthesis of all adrenocortical hormones. Hydroxylation reactions of various sites on pregnenolone can follow to produce each of the different adrenocortical hormones (Figure 51.15). Each zone of the adrenal cortex carries out a particular set of hydroxylation reactions. Adrenocortical hormones are not stored inside the adrenal cells awaiting a signal for secretion. When they need to be secreted they must be synthesized *de novo* from cholesterol. Adrenocortical hormones are lipid-soluble and diffuse from the cortical cells into the extracellular fluid. They are carried in the blood bound to special transport proteins, such as corticosteroid-binding globulin.

Mineralocorticoids

Mineralocorticoids help regulate the metabolism of sodium, potassium, and chloride ions. The major mineralocorticoid hormone produced in the zona glomerulosa is **aldosterone**. Smaller

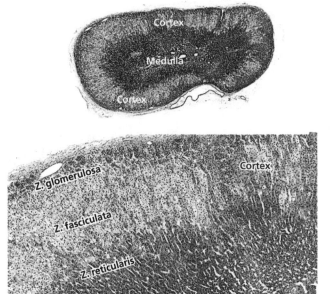

Figure 51.13 Histomicrograph of the adrenal gland and adrenal cortex.

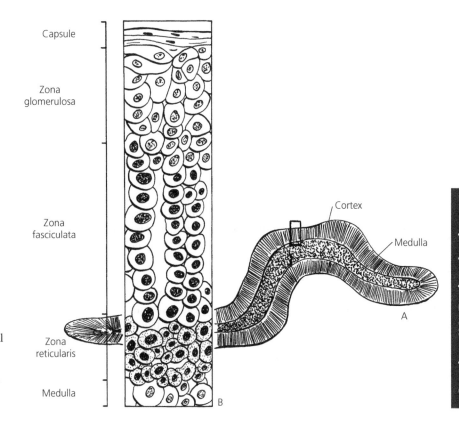

Figure 51.14 Schematic view of the adrenal cortex layers. From Reece, W.O. (2009) *Functional Anatomy and Physiology of Domestic Animals*, 4th edn. Wiley-Blackwell, Ames, IA. Reproduced with permission from Wiley.

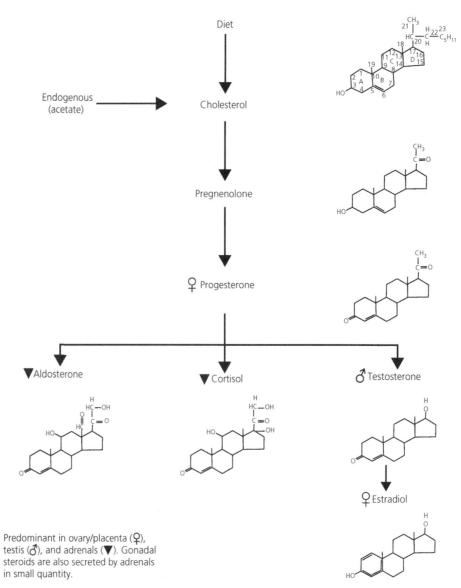

Figure 51.15 Structure of adrenal hormones. From Reece, W.O. (2004) *Dukes' Physiology of Domestic Animals*, 12th edn. Cornell University Press, Ithaca, NY. Reproduced with permission from Cornell University Press.

amounts of its precursor, deoxycorticosterone, are also secreted and it too has mineralocorticoid activity. Aldosterone is discussed here to illustrate the action of all mineralocorticoids. Synthesis and secretion of aldosterone is primarily regulated by the hormone angiotensin and the extracellular concentration of potassium.

Whenever arterial blood pressure decreases below normal or renal perfusion decreases, there is an increase in secretion of an enzyme called **renin** from the juxtaglomerular apparatus in the kidneys. The renin acts on **angiotensinogen,** a globular blood protein released into the blood by the liver. Renin converts this protein to **angiotensin I**. Angiotensin I is then converted to **angiotensin II** by enzymes found in the capillaries of the lungs. Angiotensin II circulates through the blood and when it reaches the adrenal glomerulosa it stimulates the cells to synthesize and

secrete aldosterone. Angiotensin II has effects independent of aldosterone, causing widespread vasoconstriction to raise blood pressure. It also causes constriction of efferent arterioles in the kidney to raise blood pressure while maintaining renal glomerular perfusion.

An increase in extracellular potassium concentration can also directly stimulate cells of the zona glomerulosa to begin producing aldosterone.

Aldosterone actions

Aldosterone stimulates renal tubular reabsorption of sodium in the ascending limb of the loop of Henle, in the collecting ducts, and in the distal renal tubules. Chloride follows the sodium passively to maintain electroneutrality. Aldosterone also increases renal secretion of potassium. Being a steroid hormone it diffuses into target tissue, binds to a nuclear receptor, and initiates transcription and translation of various proteins that comprise sodium ion channels in the apical membrane and sodium/potassium pumps in the basolateral membrane of the tubular epithelium. This allows sodium to be actively reabsorbed from renal tubular fluid and then pumped into the interstitial fluid. It also allows potassium to be secreted into the lumen of the renal tubules. Aldosterone stimulates renal conservation of sodium, and water follows sodium passively.

This helps determine total body sodium and water content. However, aldosterone does not directly respond to or control sodium concentration in the blood. Sodium concentration in blood is controlled more precisely by osmoreceptors in the hypothalamus that sense sodium concentration and control secretion of antidiuretic hormone to manipulate water loss or conservation to maintain normal blood sodium concentration.

Another hormone also plays a role in total body sodium and renal sodium excretion. **Atrial natriuretic peptide** is a hormone made by atrial cardiac muscle cells in response to high blood volume that stretches the atrial muscle beyond normal levels. Atrial natriuretic peptide has the opposite effects of aldosterone and the renin–angiotensin system. It increases renal loss of sodium and the presence of extra sodium in the urine causes an increase in water loss as well.

Glucocorticoids

Cortisol is the primary glucocorticoid produced within the zona fasciculata. **Corticosterone** is produced in smaller amounts in most mammals. However, in amphibians, reptiles, birds and rodents, corticosterone is the primary glucocorticoid produced.

Cortisol secretion is regulated by ACTH produced by corticotropes of the adenohypophysis (Figure 51.16). A smaller amount of corticotropin-like intermediate lobe peptide is made by cells in the pars intermedia. ACTH binds receptors on the surface of adrenal fasciculata cells and stimulates adenylyl cyclase activity. Increased intracellular cyclic AMP stimulates synthesis of cortisol. ACTH secretion is in turn controlled by neurons in the hypothalamus that secrete **adrenocorticotropic hormone-releasing hormone (ACTH-RH)** into the hypothalamo-hypophyseal portal system. Rising blood cortisol concentrations negatively feed back on ACTH secretion by the adenohypophysis and on ACTH-RH secretion by the hypothalamus. Despite its action to raise blood glucose concentration, low blood glucose does not directly stimulate cortisol secretion.

Many animals and humans normally exhibit a circadian rhythm of ACTH and cortisol secretion. In humans, cortisol secretion is highest early in the morning and lowest in the evening. Under stress conditions cortisol secretion can be more sustained, obliterating the ability to observe a circadian rhythm. Chronic stress can cause the zona fasciculata to hypertrophy. A small amount of cortisol is also secreted by zona reticularis cells.

Cortisol effects

Cortisol binds to nuclear receptors and stimulates or inhibits expression of specific genes. Cortisol is considered a "stress" hormone. Stress is a body's reaction to a challenge. That challenge can come from the environment being too hot or too cold. Many veterinary students find exams stressful! Stress can arise internally from factors such as pain or the need to fight an infection.

During stress, cortisol secretion causes blood glucose levels to increase by stimulating synthesis of enzymes involved in

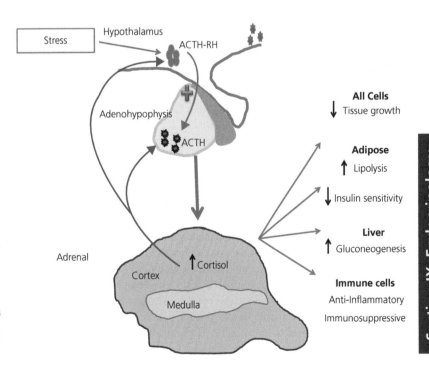

Figure 51.16 Adrenal glucocorticoid regulation. Stress and other factors cause the hypothalamus to secrete adrenocorticotropic-releasing hormone (ACTH-RH) which enters the hypothalamo-hypophyseal portal system and acts on the corticotrophs of the adenohypophysis, resulting in secretion of adrenocorticotropic hormone (ACTH). ACTH then stimulates the adrenal zona fasciculata cells to produce and secrete cortisol. Cortisol then interacts with glucocorticoid receptors in the nucleus of target cells and affects metabolism of a wide variety of cells. High cortisol concentrations in the blood feed back on the adenohypophysis and the hypothalamus to inhibit secretion of ACTH and ACTH-RH, respectively.

gluconeogenesis. The main substrates used for gluconeogenesis are amino acids derived from muscle. Cortisol also decreases sensitivity of adipose and lymphoid tissues to insulin, so less glucose is removed from the blood by these tissues. This leaves more glucose in the blood for use by the brain and muscle. Cortisol acts on adipose tissue to stimulate lipolysis so fatty acid levels in blood increase. It acts on muscle and other tissues to stimulate degradation of proteins so blood amino acid levels increase. Cortisol inhibits DNA synthesis and slows growth. Cortisol also potentiates the action of glucagon and epinephrine on glucose metabolism. This may be an adaptation to divert energy and amino acids away from growth activities to insure there are resources available to maintain the body during the stressful period.

At high concentrations, cortisol is **immunosuppressive**. It inhibits prostaglandin production produced by damaged tissues and reduces secretion of histamine by mast cells. Cortisol decreases phagocytosis and suppresses antibody formation. Cortisol also stabilizes granulocyte lysosomal membranes, preventing proteolytic enzymes from leaking out of these immune cells and damaging tissues. It causes loss of L-selectin on neutrophils and lymphocytes, preventing egress of these cells through postcapillary venules to a site of infection.

These **anti-inflammatory** actions reduce damage to tissue that might occur from a prolonged inflammatory response. Synthetic glucocorticoids are often administered to halt inflammatory responses that have gone beyond the useful stage of killing invading microbes and are now causing excessive tissue damage. Prolonged secretion of cortisol will cause atrophy of the thymus gland and cause lymphopenia. Excessively high secretion of cortisol is commonly observed in periparturient dairy cows. Often this is secondary to dystocia or some metabolic disease, such as hypocalcemia or ketosis. Unfortunately, this may immunosuppress the cow to the point that she is more susceptible to opportunistic infectious diseases such as mastitis or metritis.

Cortisol has psychoneural effects as well. Initially it causes euphoria and increased appetite, but this is followed later by depression. Cortisol also inhibits antidiuretic hormone (vasopressin) release and more water is excreted in the urine. This causes **polydipsia** (excessive thirst) and **polyuria** (excessive urine volume) in the animal due to the net loss of water from the body.

Adrenal androgens

Androgens are hormones that interact with male sex hormone receptors. Testosterone is the most important androgen and it is produced in the testes. The adrenal zona reticularis cells produce dehydroepiandrosterone and androstenedione. These androgens are not very active compared with testosterone in stimulating male sexual attributes. However, the androgens arising from the adrenals can circulate to various tissues such as adipose and be converted to testosterone. They can also be converted to estrogens, the female sex steroids. Females require

small amounts of testosterone to maintain bone density, muscle mass, and expression of estrous behaviors.

Adrenal androgen production can be stimulated by ACTH, but it appears that the adenohypophysis secretes a different hormone tentatively called adrenal androgen-stimulating hormone that stimulates the zona reticularis cells to produce adrenal androgens. Adrenal androgen production is not as great or as significant in most animals as it is in humans and other primates.

Redundancy in action of corticosteroids

Glucocorticoids such as cortisol have some mineralocorticoid activity, i.e., they can interact with mineralocorticoid receptors and have the same effects as aldosterone. They do not have the same affinity for the receptors as aldosterone, but they can exert some mineralocorticoid actions. Similarly, aldosterone has slight glucocorticoid activity. Synthetic corticosteroids used in veterinary medicine are usually more specific and will stimulate only glucocorticoid actions or only mineralocorticoid actions.

Addison's disease: hypoadrenocorticism

Addison's disease occurs when the adrenal glands fail to produce enough hormones for normal function. These animals have little or no cortisol in their blood. It occurs more frequently in dogs than it does in humans. In dogs, the cause is often an autoimmune disorder, where the body attacks the adrenal cortex and the ensuing damage reduces hormone production by all three layers of the adrenal cortex. Certain breeds of dog, such as Standard Poodles, seem more prone to develop Addison's disease. The lack of mineralocorticoids will often cause an upset in blood electrolytes, with sodium slightly below normal and potassium slightly above normal. The ratio of sodium to potassium in blood should be greater than 27 : 1. In dogs with Addison's disease the ratio is often below 24 : 1.

Often the animal will have elevated levels of ACTH in its blood, as there are no glucocorticoids being produced to inhibit ACTH-RH and ACTH production. When given exogenous ACTH, the animal produces little or no cortisol. Prolonged exposure to high levels of ACTH can induce darkening of the skin, as high ACTH concentrations can activate melanocyte-stimulating hormone receptors. Dogs with Addison's disease display a wide variety of symptoms that range from vomiting and diarrhea to lethargy and tremors. Hypoglycemia is often present due to the lack of glucocorticoids. The lack of mineralocorticoids can result in an Addisonian crisis, where potassium levels increase acutely and interfere with normal function of the cardiac muscle. Aldosterone deficiency causes sodium reabsorption to fail and leads to rapid loss of extracellular fluid volume.

Iatrogenic Addison's disease can also occur following chronic administration of glucocorticoids. During glucocorticoid treatment, the adrenal glands have essentially been dormant since the exogenous glucocorticoids acted on the hypothalamus and adenohypophysis to halt ACTH production. In most cases mineralocorticoid secretion is nearly normal, although prolonged lack of ACTH stimulation prevents conversion of cholesterol to pregnenolone. If glucocorticoid treatment is ended abruptly, the adrenal glands may not be able to reactivate and the animal will be without adrenal hormones. The animal will require glucocorticoid replacement therapy to survive. Tapering off the dose of glucocorticoid administered over a period of weeks usually allows the dormant cells to become active and this avoids iatrogenic Addison's disease. Rarely, a tumor in the adenohypophysis can cause cessation of ACTH secretion, resulting in Addison's disease.

Cushing's disease: hyperadrenocorticism

In Cushing's disease the adrenal gland produces excessive amounts of glucocorticoids. Rarely are the mineralocorticoids involved. Cortisol causes lipolysis and gluconeogenesis. It disrupts normal replacement of body muscle since it slows protein formation and accelerates protein degradation. The abdominal muscles are among the first affected and when they atrophy it gives the dog a pot-bellied appearance. In horses, swayback is common due to lumbar muscle deterioration. Affected animals often have elevated blood glucose concentration. Antidiuretic hormone secretion is reduced by high cortisol acting on the hypothalamus. As a result, the dog exhibits polydipsia and polyuria. Thin skin, hyperpigmented skin (because many of the adenohypophysis tumors also secrete melanocyte-stimulating hormone), and skin infections are common. The high cortisol levels have an immunosuppressive effect on the animal. Dystrophic calcification of the skin (calcinosis cutis) is a classical lesion of Cushing's disease in dogs. **Hirsutism** (long hair that does not shed) is a clinical symptom commonly observed in horses.

There are three causes of Cushing's disease.

1 *Pituitary tumors*: the most common cause of hyperadrenocorticism is a tumor that secretes ACTH in an uncontrolled fashion, i.e., the tumor cells do not require ACTH-RH stimulation to cause ACTH secretion and the cells do not respond to negative feedback from blood cortisol to cease ACTH secretion. These tumors are most common in dogs and older horses. In the horse, tumors commonly develop in the middle pituitary or pars intermedia of the adenohypophysis. They produce excessive amounts of corticotropin-like intermediate lobe peptide, which has essentially the same effects as ACTH.

2 *Tumor of the adrenal gland*: cells of the zona fasciculata may become benign tumors and secrete cortisol in an uncontrolled fashion. They do not require ACTH stimulation to produce the cortisol. More rarely, adrenal tumors secrete mineralocorticoids or androgens in excess.

3 *Iatrogenic Cushing's disease*: this occurs when animals are treated with excessive amounts of glucocorticoids for prolonged periods. They exhibit all the symptoms of a true Cushing's case when they are on the glucocorticoid. Then, when the glucocorticoid treatment is ended abruptly, many will go on to develop Addison's disease.

Diagnosis of Cushing's disease: dexamethasone suppression test

When normal animals receive a dose of the synthetic glucocorticoid dexamethasone, it causes endogenous cortisol levels to decline rapidly and dramatically. In animals with tumors of the pituitary or adrenals, blood cortisol levels do not change. Both the adrenal tumor and the pituitary tumor have lost the ability to respond to the negative feedback control provided by a rise in blood glucocorticoids.

Adenohypophysis gonadotropin–sex steroid axis

> 1 How is production of GnRH controlled?
>
> 2 FSH stimulates granulosa cells of the ovary to produce which hormones?
>
> 3 Which hormone do luteinized granulosa cells produce?

Gonadotropes within the pars distalis of the adenohypophysis produce two hormones, **follicle-stimulating hormone** (FSH) and **luteinizing hormone** (LH) (Figure 51.17). In females, FSH stimulates ovarian follicular development. It also causes the cells of the wall of the developing follicle to secrete estrogens. Estrogens induce changes in the reproductive tract and mammary gland necessary for successful reproduction. LH is responsible for inducing ovulation in many species. It also causes the cells comprising the ovulated follicle to change their phenotype to become progesterone-secreting cells and form a structure called the corpus luteum. Progesterone is necessary for preparing the uterus for implantation of a fertilized egg. In males, FSH stimulates the production of sperm within the **seminiferous tubules** of the testes. LH stimulates production of testosterone by the **interstitial cells (Leydig cells)**. Testosterone is required for further sperm production and maturation. Testosterone has secondary actions in the body to promote muscle growth, skin thickness, secondary male sexual characteristics such as a rooster's spurs, and sex drive.

Secretion of LH and FSH is stimulated by GnRH. This neurohormone is made in the hypothalamus and secreted into the hypothalamo-hypophyseal portal system. Many factors determine when and how much GnRH is to be secreted. These factors include daylength for many species that are seasonal breeders and signals from the pregnant uterus and fetal placenta. Age and plane of nutrition also impact the secretion of GnRH. High blood levels of testosterone negatively feed back on the hypothalamus to decrease GnRH and FSH and LH secretion in the male. In the female the situation is more complicated. Estrogen can have a stimulatory effect on GnRH secretion, when the objective is to induce ovulation of the developing follicle. At other times estrogen can decrease GnRH secretion. Progesterone can often feed back on the hypothalamus

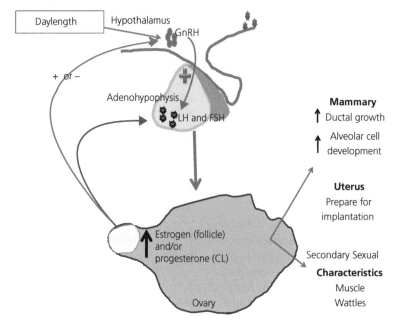

Figure 51.17 Regulation of sex steroid production in the female. Daylength, age, plane of nutrition, and other factors stimulate hypothalamic neurons to produce gonadotropin-releasing hormone (GnRH). GnRH reaches the adenohypophysis via the hypothalamo-hypophyseal portal system and stimulates release of luteinizing hormone (LH) and follicle-stimulating hormone (FSH) from the adenohypophysis. FSH circulates to the ovary and causes one or more follicles to begin to mature. FSH stimulates the granulosa cells in the wall of the developing follicle to secrete estrogen. Estrogens can influence the growth of the uterus and the mammary gland. Estrogen has a stimulatory effect on hypothalamic secretion of GnRH. This positive feedback eventually reaches an end point where sufficient GnRH secretion has been stimulated to cause a spike in LH secretion resulting in ovulation of the mature follicle. At other times in an animal's reproductive life, estrogen inhibits LH and FSH secretion by the adenohypophysis. LH stimulates the ovulated follicle to become a corpus luteum (CL). The luteinized granulosa cells now produce progesterone. Progesterone is vital for preparation of the uterus for implantation of the conceptus. It also plays a role in alveolar cell development in the mammary gland. Progesterone feeds back on the hypothalamus and adenohypophysis to inhibit GnRH and FSH and LH secretion, respectively.

to reduce GnRH secretion. Control of GnRH, LH, and FSH secretion varies considerably among species (see Chapters 52 and 53).

Function of the pars intermedia of the adenohypophysis

> 1 How does melanocyte-stimulating hormone allow a fish to alter its coloration?

The **pars intermedia** of the adenohypophysis is also known as the middle pituitary. These cells produce several hormones, the most important being **melanocyte-stimulating hormone (MSH)**, β-**endorphins** and **enkephalins**. MSH is particularly critical in lower vertebrates such as fish, reptiles, and amphibians. These animals have melanophore cells in their skin that can disperse or take up melanin granules. When the retina detects that the animal is in a dark background, MSH is released from the pars intermedia and the MSH binds receptors on the melanophores. This causes dispersion of the melanin granules and the animal's skin becomes a darker color. However, when the retina detects a light-colored or white background, the secretion of MSH ceases and the melanin granules are taken up in tight

aggregates in the cells, causing the skin color to lighten. In mammals there are no melanophores in the skin. In some mammals exposure of skin cells to UVA and UVB sunlight can cause increased MSH secretion and increased production of melanin in those skin cells. MSH and ACTH share similar amino acid sequences. Very high levels of ACTH in the blood can sometimes cause skin to darken (see section Addison's disease).

The cells of the pars intermedia also produce β-endorphin and enkephalin. These are **opioids** that provide analgesia: β-endorphin provides 80 times more pain relief than morphine. They are released following a traumatic injury and allow the animal to function, at least for a short while, without regard to the pain that would be expected to be debilitating. This allows animals with severe wounds to continue running to escape a predator or continue fighting to survive or bear the pain involved in completing the act of parturition.

Adrenal medulla

> 1 What role do the adrenal medullary cells play in the sympathetic nervous system?
>
> 2 What are the effects of epinephrine on blood flow and tissue metabolism to prepare the animal for fight or flight?

The adrenal medulla is ectodermal in origin. It is essentially a postsynaptic ganglia of the sympathetic nervous system that secretes neurotransmitter into the blood. The primary catecholamine produced by these postsynaptic neurons is epinephrine. An equal or smaller amount of norepinephrine is also produced, the amount depending on the species. Both of these catecholamines are produced by hydroxylation of the amino acid tyrosine.

Secretion of adrenal medulla hormones is part of the reaction of the sympathetic nervous system to stress. Secretion is stimulated by preganglionic sympathetic nerve fibers in the adrenal medulla that secrete acetylcholine onto nicotinic receptors of the adrenal medulla sympathetic postganglionic cells. The sympathetic postganglionic fibers have no axons and secrete their neurotransmitter into the blood. Adrenal medulla stimulation occurs when the animal is placed under stress, which may be pain, physical injury, or psychological fear.

Circulating epinephrine and norepinephrine bind to adrenergic receptors on target tissues. These include α- and β-adrenergic receptors and their subgroups α_1, α_2, β_1, and β_2. Most of these target tissues are also innervated by sympathetic postganglionic fibers that are also capable of releasing norepinephrine onto adrenergic receptors of these tissues. Stimulation of α receptors in the arterioles of most visceral organs causes contraction of arteriolar smooth muscle. This helps raise blood pressure and also restricts blood flow through the tissue, sparing blood for use by muscles. Epinephrine causes vasodilatation of skeletal muscle and liver arterioles so they can respond to the stressor. The catecholamines also increase heart rate, and force of contraction of each heartbeat. Circulating epinephrine, and to a lesser extent norepinephrine, have effects on metabolism as well. They increase the breakdown of glycogen in liver and muscle, causing a rapid increase in glucose availability. The glucose liberated from the liver enters the blood but the glucose liberated from glycogen in muscle is used by that muscle cell. Catecholamines also stimulate lipolysis of adipose tissue. They also increase basal metabolic rate. All these actions prepare the animal for a **flight or fight** response.

Neurohypophysis or posterior pituitary

> **1** Describe the path of axons from the paraventricular nucleus and supraoptic nucleus of the hypothalamus to the neurohypophysis.
>
> **2** What are the main effects of oxytocin and what controls its secretion?
>
> **3** Describe the main effects of antidiuretic hormone and how its secretion is controlled.

The neurohypophysis is essentially just the site where axons of nerves that reside in special nuclei within the hypothalamus terminate. The axons leave the hypothalamic nuclei and travel down the infundibulum or stalk of the pituitary to terminate in the area called the neurohypophysis. These nerve endings secrete two important neurotransmitters, **oxytocin** and **antidiuretic hormone**, into the blood. Both neurohormones are 9 amino acids in length. Both are produced in the nerve cell bodies and transported down the length of the axons in transport vesicles for storage at nerve endings until secreted (Figure 51.18).

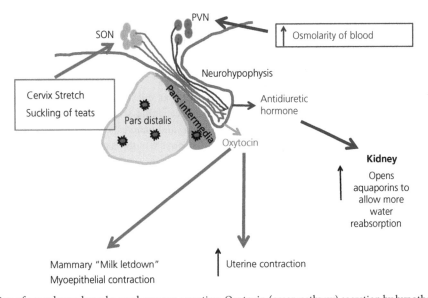

Figure 51.18 Regulation of neurohypophyseal neurohormone secretion. Oxytocin (green pathway) secretion by hypothalamic neurons is stimulated by suckling of the teat or stretch of the cervix during parturition. Oxytocin is secreted from the nerve terminals of the neurohypophysis and carried by the hypophyseal vein to the uterus where it stimulates increased contractions, or to the mammary gland to stimulate milk letdown. Hypothalamic osmoreceptor neurons initiate secretion of antidiuretic hormone (ADH) whenever the osmolarity rises above the normal set point (blue pathway). ADH causes aquaporins in the renal collecting ducts to open and allow water to flow to the renal interstitium from the tubular fluid. This adds water to the extracellular fluid, reducing the osmolarity.

Oxytocin

The neurons secreting oxytocin originate in the paraventricular nucleus. Oxytocin acts on smooth muscle of the uterus, increasing the strength of contractions of the uterus during the birthing process. Stretch of the cervix acts as a major stimulus for oxytocin release. Sensory afferent neurons carry the sensation of cervical stretch to the hypothalamus to initiate secretion of oxytocin. The oxytocin causes the uterus to contract and the fetus moves further into the cervix, stretching it further and causing the hypothalamus to secrete even more oxytocin. This positive feedback loop increases oxytocin concentrations and strength of uterine contractions until finally the fetus is expelled from the uterus. The cervix is no longer being stretched, and oxytocin secretion diminishes.

Oxytocin also acts on the smooth muscle cells surrounding individual alveoli within the mammary gland. These **myoepithelial cells** contract to cause milk to flow from the alveoli through the duct system to the teat end. In this case suckling or manual stimulation of the teat will be detected and transmitted by sensory afferents to the hypothalamus, which then initiates oxytocin release from the neurophypophysis.

Antidiuretic hormone (vasopressin)

Antidiuretic hormone (ADH), also known as vasopressin, is produced within neurons residing in the supraoptic nucleus of the hypothalamus. ADH regulates the water permeability of the renal distal tubules and collecting ducts. It regulates the number of aquaporins in the luminal membrane of the epithelium lining these sections of the renal tubule. Aquaporins are special channels that allow water, but not charged particles, to cross the lipid barrier of cell membranes. This allows water to move down its osmotic gradient from the renal tubular fluid to the extracellular fluid. When the concentration of ADH is low, water is not resorbed from the tubular fluid and dilute urine is produced. When ADH is high, water is resorbed from the tubular fluid to reduce water lost to urine. The main function of ADH is to help regulate extracellular fluid osmolarity. Osmolarity sensors in the hypothalamus increase neurohypophyseal secretion of ADH if the osmolarity increases and reduces ADH secretion if the osmolarity decreases. Hemorrhage or diarrhea can cause extracellular volume to decrease. Stretch and pressure receptors in blood vessels detect the decline in blood volume and this information is relayed to the hypothalamus and ADH is secreted.

THE ENDOCRINE PANCREAS

The bulk of the pancreas is an **exocrine gland** consisting of acini that secrete digestive enzymes into the lumen of the duodenum via the pancreatic duct. Endocrine pancreatic cells exist in small collections between the acini called the **islets of Langerhans** (Figure 51.19). The islets of Langerhans are highly vascularized and richly innervated by both vagal parasympathetic and splanchnic sympathetic fibers. At least four cell types are recognized. The great

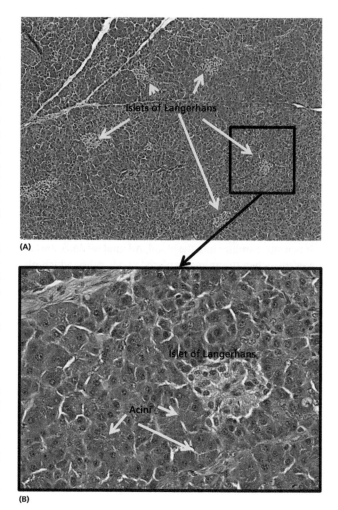

(A)

(B)

Figure 51.19 Histomicrograph of the pancreas showing (A) endocrine pancreatic islets of Langerhans and (B) exocrine pancreatic acini that produce digestive enzymes.

majority of cells, around 70%, are β cells that secrete insulin; 20% are α cells that secrete glucagon. The δ cells comprise somatostatin- and pancreatic polypeptide-secreting cells and each make up about 5% of the islet of Langerhans.

Insulin

1 How is insulin secretion is controlled?

2 What is GLUT-4 and what role does insulin have in controlling GLUT-4 expression in adipose and muscle cells?

3 Does glucagon affect GLUT-4 expression?

4 Do brain, mammary gland, and intestinal epithelium require insulin in order to take glucose from the blood?

5 What are the effects of insulin on liver, muscle, and adipose tissue?

6 Describe the symptoms expected in an animal with diabetes.

Insulin is a polypeptide hormone secreted by the β **cells** in response to hyperglycemia. In most mammals blood glucose is maintained at 80–90 mg/dL serum. In ruminants the normal blood glucose concentration is 55–65 mg/dL. Like all large protein hormones, insulin is synthesized in the Golgi apparatus and packaged into secretory granules awaiting secretion. The β cells have an insulin-independent facilitated glucose transporter (GLUT-2) that allows glucose to diffuse freely into the cell so that extracellular fluid glucose concentration directly affects glucose concentration inside the β cells. When the intracellular concentration of glucose rises above a certain level, it causes β-cell membrane depolarization, followed by an influx of calcium ions. The rise in intracellular calcium ions causes exocytosis of the secretory granules from the cell, raising blood insulin concentration.

Other factors can affect the amount of insulin secreted by β cells. Gastrin and secretin, hormones produced when a meal has entered the duodenum, can also stimulate insulin release, presumably in preparation for a rise in blood glucose that will be derived from the meal. Epinephrine, secreted by the adrenal medulla, shuts off insulin release. This promotes higher blood glucose as part of the fight or flight response. Somatostatin (pancreatic or intestinal origin) can also inhibit insulin secretion.

Insulin is required for glucose transport into adipose tissue and muscle

Insulin promotes the uptake of glucose from blood by insulin-dependent tissues, primarily muscle and adipose tissue. Adipose tissue and muscle cells have special **glucose transporter GLUT-4 molecules** packaged and stored within vesicles inside the cells. In this storage state they cannot be used to transport glucose. These insulin-dependent glucose transporter molecules are the primary means of bringing glucose into these tissues. Insulin is secreted in response to hyperglycemia and binds to insulin receptors, which are tyrosine kinases. In adipose tissue and muscle this triggers phosphorylation events that cause the transport vesicles to fuse with the cell membranes and GLUT-4 molecules translocate to the cell membrane. Now they can be used to transport glucose into the cell. When blood glucose levels return to normal, insulin secretion decreases and the GLUT-4 molecules are recycled back into the cytoplasm. Another cell type that requires insulin in order to allow entry of glucose is the pancreatic α cell that secretes glucagon. The implications of this are discussed further in the section on glucagon.

Most other tissues of the body can also respond to insulin, but have alternative glucose transporters that are not controlled by insulin to allow them to take up glucose from the blood. GLUT-1 transporters can be found on all cells, including adipose tissue and muscle. But they are present in only very small numbers on most tissues and allow just enough glucose into cells to sustain life. An exception is the red blood cell, where they are present in high numbers to accommodate the fact that erythrocytes can only use glucose as a fuel. GLUT-2 transporters are found in liver, intestinal epithelium, and pancreatic islet β cells. They are constitutively expressed in the cell membranes and allow glucose to diffuse across the cell membrane down its concentration gradient. This allows glucose to flow in or out of the cell, depending only on the glucose gradient. In the intestine these allow dietary glucose to be transported into the blood. In liver, it serves to let glucose into the cell and allows glucose produced by gluconeogenesis to leave the cell and enter the blood. GLUT-3 transporters are found in nervous tissue. They have threefold to fivefold the transport capacity of other GLUT molecules, which likely reflects the reliance of brain and nervous tissue on glucose to fuel their metabolic processes.

Effects of insulin

Nearly all cells have insulin receptors. Insulin's role is to promote storage of potential fuel to be used by the body when food is plentiful (Figure 51.20). Insulin also helps promote growth of many tissues. Insulin promotes the build-up of triglyceride in adipose tissue, glycogen in muscle and liver, and protein reserves in muscle. Insulin promotes amino acid uptake needed for growth. It also increases the activity of Na^+/K^+-ATPase pumps; this can cause extracellular potassium to move into cells at an accelerated rate. This is important to veterinarians treating diabetics with insulin: an overdose can cause extracellular potassium to decrease to levels that interfere with cardiac function, killing the patient.

Adipose tissue

The glucose provided to adipose tissue promotes glycerol formation. Glycerol combines with fatty acids delivered to adipose tissue to form triglycerides. Adipose tissue receives fatty acids from very low density lipoproteins (VLDL) produced in the liver. **Chylomicrons** synthesized by intestinal villous epithelium can deliver dietary triglycerides directly to adipose tissue for storage. Insulin inhibits lipolysis. The net effect is to promote adipose deposition.

Muscle

In smooth, striated, and cardiac muscle, insulin stimulates glycogen synthesis enzymes, promoting storage of glucose molecules in the form of glycogen. Insulin promotes the use of glucose as a fuel source. Insulin reduces fatty acid oxidation, further promoting use of glucose as a fuel. In the absence of insulin, muscles rely more on fatty acids as a fuel source. Insulin enhances amino acid uptake by muscle, which promotes muscle growth.

Liver

The liver does not require insulin to permit glucose uptake from blood. Insulin promotes fatty acid synthesis in hepatocytes and stimulates incorporation of those fatty acids and triglycerides into lipoprotein-bound vesicles such as VLDL for transport to adipocytes. Insulin stimulates glycogen synthesis.

Mammary gland

The mammary gland does not require insulin in order to remove glucose from the blood for milk production. This is important to the veterinarian because ketosis, a hypoglycemic disorder of

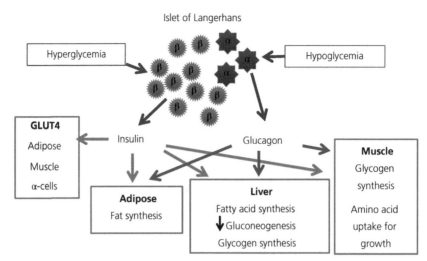

Figure 51.20 Regulation of insulin and glucagon secretion. Insulin-secreting β cells are very sensitive to changes in extracellular fluid glucose concentration. Whenever it rises above the normal set point, the β cells secrete insulin. Insulin has a variety of effects aimed at utilizing the surplus glucose for growth and fat synthesis as well as uptake of glucose from blood by muscle and adipose tissue. The green arrows point to the actions of insulin on various tissues. The actions of insulin reduce blood glucose concentration to the normal concentration. Glucagon is secreted by α cells of the pancreatic islets. These cells sense a decline in blood glucose concentration (which is dependent on presence of insulin since α-cell GLUT-4 requires insulin). Glucagon has the opposite effects on tissues that insulin has (red arrows). Glucagon inhibits fatty acid synthesis and glycogen synthesis and reduces uptake of amino acids for growth. It also stimulates gluconeogenesis, actions aimed at increasing blood glucose concentration back to normal concentrations.

dairy cows and goats, occurs partly because the mammary gland continues to remove glucose from the blood of the cow even when blood glucose is below normal. Insulin also has some effect on growth of the developing mammary gland alveolar cells.

Satiety centers
Insulin has the effect of inducing satiety and suppresses the appetite.

Diabetes mellitus
Diabetes mellitus occurs whenever there is failure of the β cells to produce insulin or there is failure of tissues to respond to insulin. Diabetes mellitus is discussed in detail in Chapter 47.

Glucagon

> 1 How is glucagon secretion controlled? How would insulin deficiency affect this?
>
> 2 What are the effects of glucagon on liver, muscle, and adipose tissue?

Glucagon is a 29-amino-acid peptide secreted by the α **cells** of the pancreas and in much smaller amounts by certain enteroendocrine cells of the small intestine. The α cells respond to a decline in blood glucose by secreting glucagon. Just as with insulin, a change in extracellular glucose is reflected by a similar change in intracellular glucose concentration. Low intracellular glucose causes glucagon secretory granules to be exocytosed,

raising blood glucagon concentration. Glucose diffusion into the α cell is dependent on GLUT-4 transporters, which are only present in the cell membrane when the cell is stimulated by insulin. Therefore, during diabetes mellitus the α cells will have low intracellular glucose levels and will be secreting great amounts of glucagon, even though extracellular glucose is already very elevated.

Glucagon actions
Glucagon's main effect is to try to return low blood glucose levels to normal levels. Its effects are opposite to the action of insulin. In the liver, glucagon stimulates **glycogenolysis**, causing release of glucose into the blood. It also stimulates the gluconeogenic enzymes needed to synthesize glucose from propionate and glycerol as well as amino acids. It stimulates release of amino acids from muscle cells and also stimulates glycogenolysis in muscle. At very high concentrations it can stimulate some lipolytic activity in adipose tissue.

Somatostatin

Somatostatin is a peptide hormone made by the δ **cells** of the pancreas. It is also made by enteroendocrine cells scattered throughout the intestinal tract. Somatostatin is also produced by hypothalamic neurons, where it often also called GH-IH. It is best known for its inhibition of GH secretion by the adenohypophysis. Somatostatin produced by the δ cells works in a paracrine fashion to inhibit secretion of both insulin and glucagon. In the intestine, somatostatin reduces cholecystokinin secretion, which has the effect of reducing pancreatic exocrine secretion of digestive enzymes. How somatostatin production is controlled remains unknown.

The Pineal Gland and Melatonin

> **1** How does exposure to sunlight affect melatonin secretion and how might this determine when a female of a species that is a seasonal breeder may begin to cycle sexually?

The **pineal gland** is a small collection of cells residing in the center of the brain in a groove where the two halves of the thalamus come together. It is often referred to as the **third eye** because its activity is influenced by the amount of light the animal is exposed to.

The pineal gland secretes a hormone derived from serotonin called **melatonin**. High levels of serotonin increase wakefulness; high levels of melatonin seem to induce a sleep state. In mammals and birds, light and dark information is transmitted from the retina of the eye to the pineal gland via various nerves (Figure 51.21). In reptiles and amphibians, the pineal gland is located in the forehead and seems to receive light cues directly through the skull. Secretion of melatonin is stimulated by darkness and inhibited by light. The pineal is responsible for regulating circadian rhythms that affect sleep patterns and determine the periodicity of estrous cycles in females. As daylength decreases more melatonin is secreted. This allows the animal to

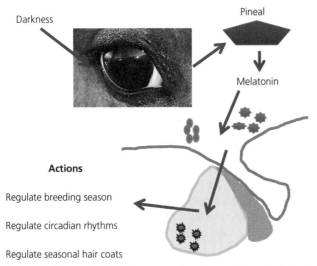

Figure 51.21 Pineal gland function and regulation. The pineal gland is located in the center of the brain and receives input from the retina (in mammals) or through the skull (birds and lower vertebrates). Light inhibits the pineal gland from producing melatonin, while darkness promotes melatonin secretion. Melatonin then diffuses to the hypothalamus and regulates secretion of hormones involved in seasonal breeding, circadian rhythms, and other functions that require the animal to know what season of the year it is and the number of hours of daylight.

anticipate seasonal changes and prepare for each season by influencing such activities as reproduction in seasonal breeders, adaptation to cold or warm weather, or preparation for migration. In seasonal breeders, melatonin can increase or decrease gonad size and development in the male, depending on the season where the animal is expected to be most fertile. In some arctic animals, such as snowshoe hares and arctic foxes, melatonin secretion can influence the color of the hair coat.

In domestic animals, light exposure is often utilized to manipulate melatonin secretion. As an example, in the wild, chickens would only lay eggs in the late spring and early summer. By keeping them exposed to 14–15 hours of light and 9–10 hours of darkness each day, the bird is induced to lay eggs year around.

Adipose tissue and leptin

Leptin is a peptide hormone secreted by adipose tissue that is full or filling with fat. It enters the blood and is carried to the hypothalamus where it signals satiety and depresses the appetite.

Overview of energy metabolism

Living organisms require a source of energy to sustain life. The bulk of the energy required by each cell is for maintenance of electrolyte composition inside and outside each cell. For instance, the electrogenic pump that moves three sodium ions out of the cell in exchange for two potassium ions coming into the cell requires energy in the form of ATP to power this pump. Other ion pumps keep cytosolic calcium low and maintain potassium, sodium, and chloride levels in blood relatively constant. Taken together, about 60% of all the energy utilized by mammals is dedicated to keeping the ion pumps operating. In mammals, another 10–15% of required energy is utilized for maintenance of body temperature; this is not a large expenditure in cold-blooded reptiles, amphibians, and fish, which gives them a distinct energetic advantage in warm climates. Mammals have the advantage in cooler climates where they can keep enzymes operating at their optimal temperatures. The remainder of the energy required for maintaining a body goes toward essential operations that include heart and respiratory muscle contraction, and energy for intermediary metabolism of processes such as replacement of tissue protein and replacement of senescent cells. If the animal is in a cold or hot environment, the energy required for maintenance increases and every function added to resting maintenance will incrementally increase energy needed by the body. Reproduction, lactation, exercise, and growth all require increased energy expenditure.

Energy is ultimately derived from dietary ingredients. The energy derived from food is generally described in terms of the amount of heat energy, or calories, it supplies. In the USA, use of the term "calorie" can be confusing. Physicists and animal scientists describe 1 calorie as the amount of heat required to increase the temperature of 1 g of water from 14.5 to 15.5°C. This is such a small amount of energy that animal nutritionists find it easier to describe energy needs in terms of 1000 calories, or kilocalories (kcal). In human nutrition, the kilocalorie is referred to as a Calorie (with a capital C). In many countries nutritionists describe energy used by the body in terms of how much work can be done by the heat utilized and therefore use the term joules (J) of energy. There are 4.18 J in a calorie. When a diet is fed to an animal, not all the heat contained within the foodstuff is available to the animal. A portion of the diet is likely to be indigestible and the potential calories within that material end up in the feces. Some calories that could be used by the body are also lost within the urine excreted each day and some potential calories are lost in respiration and eructation of substances such as methane. This loss can be substantial in herbivores. Some heat is also lost from the body during the digestive process due to inefficiencies of conversion of foodstuffs to absorbable nutrients and energy utilized in absorptive processes. The energy in a feedstuff that is retained by the body and which can be utilized by the body for maintenance, reproduction, etc. is referred to as the **net energy** of the feed. The net energy (calories) that would come from complete oxidation of the foodstuff outside the body is defined as the amount of energy in the food (as determined in a calorimeter) minus the energy contained in the feces, urine, and expelled gases collected after ingestion of the foodstuff. It is also necessary to subtract the heat lost during the digestive process. Since it is very difficult to measure the heat lost during the digestive process, the term **metabolizable energy** is often used to describe the energy an animal can derive from a foodstuff. In monogastric animals, each gram of sugar or starch can supply the animal with 4 kcal metabolizable energy. Herbivores often rely on fermentation of plant structural carbohydrates (cell wall components) for the bulk of their energy needs. This is somewhat less efficient in that only about 2 kcal metabolizable energy is derived from each gram of plant structural carbohydrate consumed. However, herbivores tend to consume large amounts of this material as it is generally abundant.

Proteins are best known as the building blocks for enzymes and cell proteins. However, their amino acids are also an important energy source for cells. Each gram of protein can supply about 4 kcal of metabolizable energy. Fats are much more energy dense and each gram can supply about 9 kcal metabolizable energy.

It is also possible to bring this back to a biochemical basis. The body transfers energy from nutrients to the cells by capturing the energy in the feedstuff in the form of chemical bonds. Phosphate and thioester bonds can capture energy during catabolism of nutrients and store that energy in a form that can be used by cells. The high-energy phosphate bond contained in 1 mol of ATP releases about 7.4 kcal of energy on hydrolysis to ADP. Creatine phosphate is found in muscle and some other cells and can capture and store energy. Creatine phosphate can convert ADP back into ATP when energy may be needed for muscle contraction. Phosphoenolpyruvate, produced during glycolysis, routinely provides phosphate bond energy to convert ADP to ATP. Thioesters are another type of high-energy bond. A thioester is a bond formed between a carboxylic acid and a thiol (SH) group. The most familiar thioester bonds may be those of coenzyme A. The thiol of coenzyme A can react with a carboxyl group of acetic acid (yielding acetyl-CoA) or a fatty acid (yielding fatty acyl-CoA). This imparts a high-energy potential to the acetate moiety, making it highly reactive and ready to take part in many types of reactions.

How does the animal derive energy from dietary components?

Carbohydrates

Glucose is the end product of digestion of starches, and dietary sugars contain glucose along with galactose and fructose. Glucose is used by virtually all cells of the body and is the sole, or at least the major, energy source for red blood cells and nervous tissue. Galactose and fructose are metabolized slightly differently but provide nearly the same energy to cells as glucose. All cells can carry out glycolysis, changing the 6-carbon sugars into two 3-carbon pyruvate or lactate molecules. These steps are performed in the cytosol of the cell and glycolysis yields a net gain of 2 ATP per molecule of glucose. It also yields two molecules of reduced nicotinamide adenine dinucleotide (NADH). Glycolysis can occur in the absence of oxygen.

In the presence of oxygen (aerobic metabolism) the pyruvate diffuses into the mitochondria and is oxidized to acetic acid and, with the energy provided by the thioester of coenzyme A, pyruvate is converted to acetyl-CoA for catabolism in the tricarboxylic acid (TCA) cycle. This step yields two more NADH molecules.

In the absence of oxygen (anaerobic), the pyruvate is used to accept electrons from NADH, converting the pyruvate to lactic acid. It is important to convert NADH back to NAD$^+$ so that glycolysis can continue. Failure to regenerate NAD$^+$ would leave the cell with no electron acceptor for the oxidation of glyceraldehyde 3-phosphate, and the energy-yielding reactions of glycolysis would stop (Figure 51.22).

The TCA cycle takes all the carbons, hydrogens, and oxygens of the pyruvate molecule and converts them to CO_2 and H_2O. Each acetyl-CoA entering the TCA cycle yields 1 ATP, releases 2 CO_2 molecules, and yields 3 NADH and 1 FADH$_2$ (flavin adenine dinucleotide). Therefore, for each glucose molecule that enters the TCA cycle (including the conversion of pyruvate to acetyl-CoA), the net yield is 8 NADH, 2 FADH$_2$, 2 ATP, and 6 CO_2 (Figure 51.23). The electrons of NADH and FADH$_2$ enter the mitochondrial electron chain and are used to reduce molecular oxygen (O_2) to H_2O. In this process, a large number of H$^+$ ions are placed on the outside of the outer mitochondrial membrane. This creates a H$^+$ gradient across the outer mitochondrial membrane and the potential energy of H$^+$ moving back into the

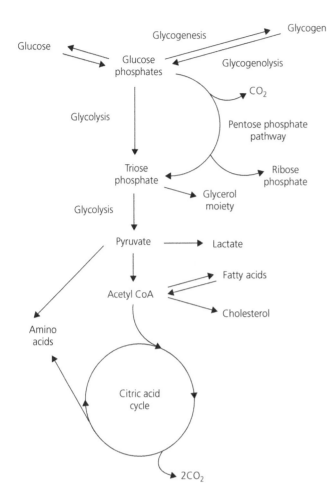

Figure 51.22 Overview of carbohydrate metabolism in animal cells. Most arrows represent sequences of reactions. From Reece, W.O. (2004) *Dukes' Physiology of Domestic Animals*, 12th edn. Cornell University Press, Ithaca, NY. Reproduced with permission from Cornell University Press.

mitochondria down its concentration gradient is utilized by an enzyme called ATP synthase to convert ADP to ATP. Each NADH and $FADH_2$ molecule sent through the electron transport chain can yield about 3 ATP. This process also regenerates NAD^+ and FADH for the glycolysis and TCA cycles to utilize (Figure 51.24).

For each glucose molecule undergoing complete oxidation via the TCA cycle and electron transport chain, a full accounting gives a yield of 36 ATP. Compare this with the 2 ATP net yield from anaerobic metabolism of glucose.

Fat metabolism

Fat can be a major energy source for the body. It can also be utilized to produce various phospholipids, eicosanoids, and steroids the body needs (Figure 51.25). Fat comes from three sources: (i) dietary triglycerides and free fatty acids in meals, and triglycerides made in the liver following meals and exported to other tissues; (ii) fat made in the liver can be packaged within VLDL and high-density lipoproteins; and (iii)

release of nonesterified fatty acids from triglycerides that were formed or stored in adipose tissue.

Triglycerides are taken into cells and broken down to free fatty acids and glycerol. The glycerol can be converted to pyruvate and be metabolized to yield similar energy to that derived from a single pyruvate molecule. The addition of ATP to glycerol yields dihydroxyacetone phosphate, which is used in gluconeogenesis. The fatty acids in the cytosol are combined with coenzyme A and ATP to form fatty acyl-CoA. This crosses the outer mitochondrial membrane and in the space between the inner and outer mitochondrial membranes the fatty acyl-CoA combines with carnitine, which ferries the fatty acyl-CoA across the inner mitochondrial membrane. The fatty acid can now undergo β-oxidation. In this process two carbon units are cleaved off the fatty acid molecules to react with coenzyme A to form acetyl-CoA molecules. The acetyl-CoA then enters the TCA cycle followed by the electron transport chain, as already described for the metabolism of glucose. Palmitate, a 16-carbon fatty acid, produces 34 ATP when it is oxidized. It is important to remember that β-oxidation of fats only occurs under aerobic conditions.

Protein amino acids as a source of energy

Proteins can also serve as an energy source. Proteins used for energy can come from the diet or they can come from catabolism of tissue and plasma proteins. Proteins are constantly being synthesized and degraded within the body. Some proteins, such as those of the liver and plasma, have half-lives of up to 6 months. However, many enzymes and receptor proteins have half-lives that can be measured in minutes or hours before they are catabolized and their amino acids recycled.

Proteins are broken down within cells (particularly hepatocytes) by a variety of proteolytic enzymes and the amino acids used to provide energy during the period between meals. A key step in this process is **transamination**. The amine group of the amino acid is transferred to the ketone group on another molecule. The original amino acid now becomes a **ketoacid**. These reactions are important for conversion of certain amino acids into nonessential amino acids that might be needed. However, the resulting ketoacids can also be used as sources of energy (Figure 51.26). The end result of these reactions is the conversion of some amino acids to pyruvate, which then can be converted to acetyl-CoA and enters the TCA cycle. Other amino acids can be converted to acetoacetyl-CoA and subsequently to acetyl-CoA, while some can be converted directly to acetyl-CoA. Still other amino acids can be converted to intermediates of the TCA cycle to generate ATP and the reducing equivalents (NADH and $FADH_2$) needed to drive mitochondrial electron transport and production of ATP.

Immediately after a meal, when the body is in the **absorptive phase** of digestion, there is a large influx of amino acids from the diet into the blood. It is not possible to store amino acids for later use, so they must be incorporated into proteins within cells when available or be lost. Muscle will typically accumulate proteins following a meal. The hormone controlling much of this

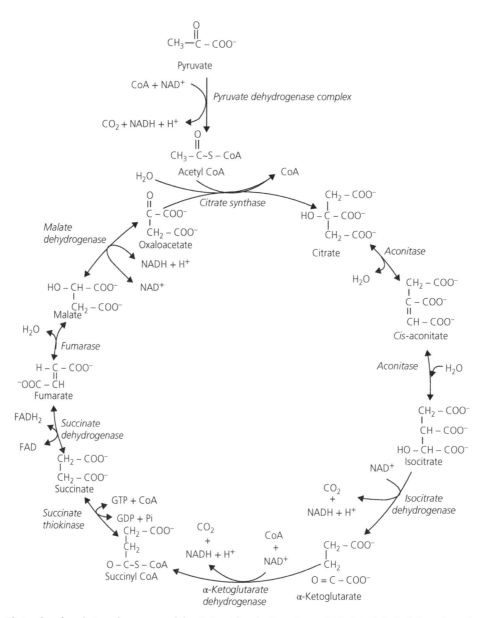

Figure 51.23 Oxidative decarboxylation of pyruvate and the citric acid cycle. From Reece, W.O. (2004) *Dukes' Physiology of Domestic Animals*, 12th edn. Cornell University Press, Ithaca, NY. Reproduced with permission from Cornell University Press.

action is insulin, secreted by pancreatic β cells in response to rising blood glucose levels following the typical meal. During this phase insulin stimulates the uptake of amino acids by various tissues to enable repair and growth (anabolism). GH (and associated IGFs) also promote protein accretion, but only if insulin levels are elevated. In muscle, the amino acids are used to replace depleted muscle proteins, and in a growing animal new muscle proteins can accumulate.

During the postabsorptive phase, these proteins are broken down when energy is required before the next meal (e.g., 6–10 hours after the last meal). Muscle protein is 7–10% alanine; however, about 30% of the amino acids leaving the muscle are alanine. As the muscle proteins break down they undergo

various transamination reactions and many of these reactions produce alanine. The alanine leaving the muscle is absorbed by the liver (along with other amino acids) and utilized to produce glucose, which is delivered into the circulation and used as an energy source for other tissues including muscle (Figure 51.27). The muscle protein-derived glucose is particularly important as a source of glucose for nervous tissue and red blood cells during periods between meals.

Gluconeogenesis

Immediately following most meals the diet provides a large influx of glucose and amino acids. The glucose is shunted into glycogen or fats (triglycerides) for storage. The amino acids are utilized for

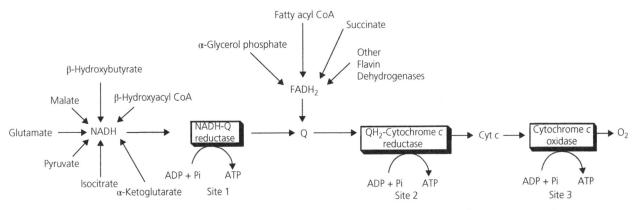

Figure 51.24 Electron transfer and oxidative phosphorylation in the respiratory assembly. Electron transfer from NADH and FADH$_2$ to O$_2$ occurs by enzyme-catalyzed oxidation–reduction reactions. The NADH-Q reductase complex catalyzes the transfer of electrons from NADH to Q (coenzyme Q or ubiquinone). The QH$_2$–cytochrome c reductase catalyzes electron transfer from Q to cytochrome c. Cytochrome c oxidase catalyzes electron transfer from cytochrome c to O$_2$. Proton gradients are generated by the three complexes that are enclosed by the rectangles and represent sites of ATP generation. The sequence of reactions for the transfer of electrons from NADH or FADH$_2$ results in a "pumping" of protons (H$^+$) out of the mitochondria, generating a proton gradient. ATP is synthesized when protons reenter the mitochondria. Pi, inorganic orthophosphate. From Reece, W.O. (2004) *Dukes' Physiology of Domestic Animals*, 12th edn. Cornell University Press, Ithaca, NY. Reproduced with permission from Cornell University Press.

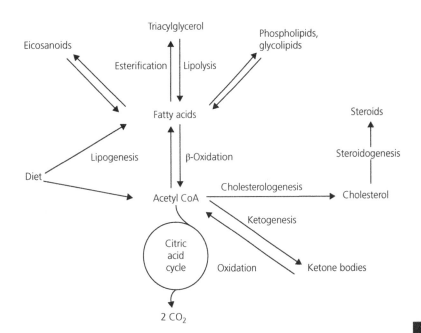

Figure 51.25 Overview of lipid metabolism. From Reece, W.O. (2004) *Dukes' Physiology of Domestic Animals*, 12th edn. Cornell University Press, Ithaca, NY. Reproduced with permission from Cornell University Press.

protein accretion in many tissues and as an energy source in the liver. The liver uses very little glucose for its own energy needs. Some 6–10 hours later (in a dog or cat), blood glucose levels will have fallen and it will be necessary for the animal to produce the glucose needed for nervous tissue and red blood cell function. The animal begins to draw down the energy stored in glycogen and triglycerides. The stored glycogen is sufficient to supply the body for only a short time, at most a few hours. Liver, muscle, and many other tissues of the body utilize fatty acids as energy sources during this time, **sparing glucose** for the nervous tissues and red blood cells. The liver and kidney (and to a much lesser extent the intestinal epithelium) begin to activate gluconeogenic

pathways to produce glucose. Gluconeogenesis is not simply the reverse of glycolysis, though many of the enzymes and reactions involved are the same (Figure 51.28). Three of the steps used in glycolysis can only be "reversed" to form glucose by induction of unique pathways that are under hormonal control.

1 Conversion of fructose 1,6-bisphosphate to fructose 6-phosphate is carried out by fructose 1,6-bisphosphatase. The activity of this enzyme is controlled by **glucagon** and the rate of gluconeogenesis correlates highly with the activity of this enzyme.

2 Glucose 6-phosphate can be converted to glucose only by glucose 6-phosphatase.

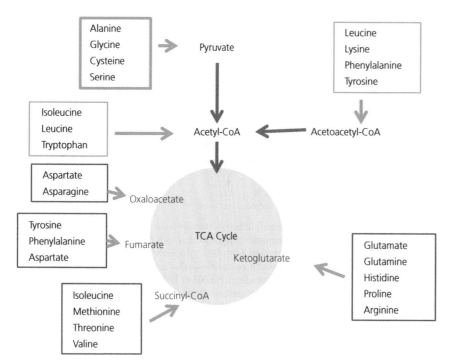

Figure 51.26 Conversion of amino acids to various intermediates of glycolysis and the TCA cycle for oxidation to produce energy.

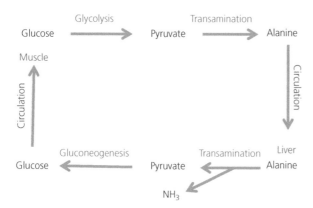

Figure 51.27 Glucose–alanine cycle. Muscle protein is catabolized and transamination reactions cause production of large amounts of alanine. The alanine enters the circulation and is taken up by the liver. Here it is used to transaminate ketoacids, forming pyruvate in the process. The pyruvate serves as a gluconeogenic precursor and the hepatocytes release the glucose back into the circulation where it can be used by muscle cells or other cells requiring glucose.

3 During glycolysis, phosphoenolpyruvate is converted to pyruvate. It is not possible to convert pyruvate back to phosphoenolpyruvate directly. To form glucose from pyruvate it is necessary to send pyruvate through the TCA cycle and then draw off the oxaloacetate produced and convert it to phosphoenolpyruvate using the enzyme phosphoenolpyruvate carboxykinase. To convert two pyruvate molecules to one glucose molecule requires expenditure of 6 ATP or GTP molecules and the use of 2 NADH molecules. The ATP required for gluconeogenesis are supplied primarily from fatty acid oxidation.

The main hormone stimulating gluconeogenic enzymes is glucagon, though glucocorticoids can also stimulate gluconeogenesis. Substrate availability (high acetyl-CoA and high citrate concentrations) also stimulates gluconeogenesis. Gluconeogenesis requires the presence of certain gluconeogenic precursors, including the following.

1 **Lactate**, from the anaerobic glycolysis of glucose in muscle, is converted to pyruvate.
2 **Propionate**, from the fermentation of carbohydrates, enters the TCA cycle as succinyl-CoA and is eventually converted to oxaloacetate. This is extremely important in ruminants and hindgut fermenters. Even carnivores exhibit a small amount of fermentation in the hindgut and produce some propionate.
3 **Glucogenic amino acids**, which are converted to pyruvate or various TCA cycle intermediates.
4 **Glycerol**, from adipose tissue as a result of lipolysis of triglycerides. Glycerol enters the gluconeogenic pathway as 3-phosphoglyceraldehyde. Note that all gluconeogenic precursors are at least three carbons in length. Carbons liberated from fatty acids as two-carbon acetyl-CoA units *do not* provide gluconeogenic precursors.

Synthesis of fats

Triglycerides are often supplied by the diet and can be incorporated directly into adipose tissue or be taken up by the mammary epithelium for secretion into milk. *De novo* synthesis of fatty acids takes place primarily in the liver, adipose tissue, and mammary gland. The starting material is acetyl-CoA, derived from carbohydrates (glucose) or amino acid catabolism. In ruminants, acetate produced during bacterial fermentation of carbohydrates, serves as the major source of acetyl-CoA. Fatty

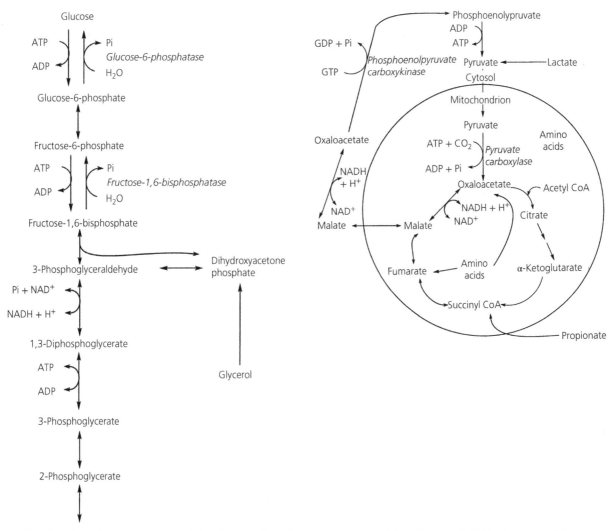

Figure 51.28 Pathway for gluconeogenesis (the column on the right is a continuation of the column on the left). The names of the enzymes of gluconeogenesis that are unique to the reversal of glycolysis are indicated. All reactants of every reaction are not indicated. The pathways for the conversion of major gluconeogenic compounds (glycerol, lactate, propionate, and amino acids) are indicated. Because pyruvate conversion to phosphoenolpyruvate is irreversible, pyruvate must be converted to oxaloacetate as a necessary intermediate for pyruvate synthesis and ultimate conversion to glucose. Because the reactions of glucose conversion to glucose 6-phosphate and of fructose 6-phosphate to fructose 1,6-bisphosphate are irreversible, alternate enzyme-catalyzed dephosphorylation reactions are necessary for the reverse of these two reactions for glucose synthesis. From Reece, W.O. (2004) *Dukes' Physiology of Domestic Animals*, 12th edn. Cornell University Press, Ithaca, NY. Reproduced with permission from Cornell University Press.

acid synthase combines acetyl-CoA with malonyl-CoA derived from the TCA cycle using the reducing power of NADPH. Two-carbon units continue to be added to form a long-chain fatty acid. Three fatty acids are combined with glycerol derived from glucose to form a triglyceride. Fats produced in the liver are ordinarily transported to other tissues, such as muscle, for catabolism or to adipose tissue for longer-term storage.

Summary of cell responses during the absorptive phase of metabolism

Shortly after a meal, when amino acids, glucose, and fats are present in high concentrations in the blood, the tissues respond by activating mechanisms to store these nutrients

for later use. The response of each tissue is outlined in the following sections.

Liver

Absorbed glucose

Glucose is converted to glycogen under the influence of insulin. Glucose can also be converted to fatty acids for incorporation into triglycerides. While some triglyceride is stored within hepatocytes, the bulk of the triglycerides synthesized are packaged with lipoproteins for export to other tissues of the body (primarily adipose tissue for storage and muscle for oxidation). Insulin stimulates fatty acid synthesis. Glucagon sharply inhibits fatty acid synthesis.

Absorbed amino acids

Amino acids taken up by the liver serve as the major fuel source for the liver during this time (hepatocytes use very little glucose). Amino acids can be converted to ketoacids during the various transamination reactions carried out in the liver. Some of these ketoacids are used for production of energy. Some of the ketoacids generated from amino acids are used for production of malonyl-CoA for fatty acid synthesis. Insulin stimulates the latter pathway.

Some amino acids are used for synthesis of plasma proteins and replacement of hepatocyte enzymes. This process is controlled by GH. GH effectively stimulates protein synthesis only if insulin levels are also elevated.

Absorbed fats

Chylomicrons produced within enterocytes transport diet-derived fats. The liver hepatocytes can take up chylomicron fats, but generally the majority of the absorbed dietary fat within chylomicrons is removed by muscle and adipose tissue.

Muscle
Absorbed glucose

Glucose is converted to glycogen under the influence of insulin. Remember that insulin is also required to allow the muscle cell to express the GLUT-4 proteins required to allow the muscle cell to remove glucose from the blood.

Absorbed amino acids

Amino acids are used for synthesis and replacement of muscle proteins. This process is controlled by GH. GH effectively stimulates protein synthesis only if insulin levels are also elevated.

Absorbed fats

Chylomicrons deliver fatty acids to the muscle for oxidation. This spares glucose so that it can be used by nervous tissue and red blood cells.

Adipose tissue
Absorbed glucose

Glucose will be utilized to produce glycerol, and can also be used to form fatty acids. Glycerol and the fatty acids can be combined to form triglycerides for storage within adipocytes. Insulin stimulates these processes; glucagon inhibits them. Remember that insulin is also required to allow the adipocyte to express the GLUT-4 proteins required to allow the adipocytes to remove glucose from the blood.

Absorbed amino acids

Only a small amount of protein is synthesized within adipocytes, largely to replace enzymes. Amino acids are used for synthesis and replacement of adipocyte proteins. This process is controlled by GH. GH effectively stimulates protein synthesis only if insulin levels are also elevated.

Absorbed fats

Chylomicrons deliver the bulk of their fatty acids to the adipocytes for storage. In ruminants the bulk of the acetate and butyrate produced during fermentation of carbohydrate is taken up by adipose tissue to produce fatty acids. This process is stimulated by insulin.

Mammary gland

The production of lactose, milk protein, and milk fat is largely under the control of GH, prolactin, placental lactogen, thyroid hormone, adrenal glucocorticoids, and insulin-like growth factors, with great variability between species in the relative importance of each hormone. The role of each hormone in controlling milk synthesis can also change depending on the stage of lactation.

Absorbed glucose

Glucose can be converted to the milk disaccharide lactose. The uptake of glucose from the blood is insulin independent. Glucose can also be used for *de novo* synthesis of milk fats in many monogastric mammals. Glucose is not as important for milk fat synthesis in ruminants – they use acetate.

Absorbed amino acids

A large amount of casein and whey protein is synthesized within mammary gland epithelial cells from dietary amino acids.

Absorbed fats

Chylomicrons deliver fatty acids to the mammary gland for secretion into the milk. In ruminants, acetate and butyrate produced during fermentation of carbohydrate are taken up by mammary epithelium to produce fatty acid.

Brain, nervous tissue, and red blood cells
Absorbed glucose

Glucose is taken up by these tissues independent of insulin. Glucose provides almost all of the energy for these tissues. Glucose undergoes glycolysis and is metabolized to lactate within red blood cells as they lack the mitochondria needed for complete oxidation of glucose.

Absorbed amino acids

Amino acids are used to replace enzymes in nervous tissue. Amino acids are not taken up by erythrocytes because these cells have no machinery to produce proteins. Neither erythrocytes nor nervous tissue can catabolize amino acids for energy purposes.

Absorbed fats

The lack of mitochondria prevents erythrocytes from using fats. Brain and nervous tissue also lack the enzymes needed to produce energy from fat. Certain fatty acids, especially the unsaturated essential fatty acids, are used for synthesis of glycerophospholipids and sphingolipids comprising myelin and nerve cell membranes. The blood–brain barrier prevents albumin-bound fatty acids from crossing into the brain. The brain does not utilize triglyceride within chylomicrons directly. Instead, brain and nervous tissue take up dietary essential fatty acids that have been packaged into VLDL by the liver.

Summary of cell responses during the postabsorptive phase of metabolism

Once the influx of nutrients from the diet ceases, the body must rely on stored energy to keep metabolic processes operating. Each tissue responds to hormonal stimuli to meet these needs. As a rule insulin is not elevated during the postabsorptive phase of metabolism because blood glucose levels are on the low end of normal range. Glucagon, glucocorticoids, and epinephrine may all be elevated during this phase of metabolism. A major driving force is to keep blood glucose levels within normal ranges so that the brain, nervous tissues, and erythrocytes, which rely on glucose for nearly all their energy needs, are able to function properly.

Liver

In order to help maintain normal blood glucose, the liver releases glucose that was incorporated as glycogen into the circulation. Both glucagon and epinephrine stimulate glycogenolysis. Gluconeogenic pathways are activated to allow production and release of glucose into the blood. Glucagon is the primary stimulus for gluconeogenesis. Glucocorticoids can also stimulate gluconeogenesis. The lack of insulin also allows gluconeogenesis as insulin is inhibitory to gluconeogenesis.

During the postabsorptive state the main source of energy for hepatocytes becomes free fatty acids liberated from adipose tissue or internal stores of triglyceride. Some of the fatty acids escape β-oxidation and are instead converted to ketone bodies (β-hydroxybutyrate and acetoacetate) for export to tissues that can use ketones as an energy source.

Protein synthesis is inhibited within the liver as a result of the lack of insulin. Glucagon stimulates the use of amino acids for gluconeogenesis. Fatty acid synthesis is also inhibited by the lack of insulin.

Muscle

Glycogen stores are converted back to glucose 6-phosphate (which cannot be transported out of the muscle cell) and metabolized by glycolysis to lactate. The lactate is released into the blood and taken up by the liver to support gluconeogenesis.

At rest muscle cells use fatty acid oxidation for most of their energy needs. During anaerobic high-intensity exercise the muscle cells rely on glycolysis of glucose stored in glycogen. Lactate is the end product of anaerobic muscle glycolysis. Glycogen stores are rather small and rapidly depleted, which is why sprinting is not a long-distance sport. During low-intensity sustained exercise the main fuels of the muscle cells are fatty acids and blood glucose. In this case, in a properly trained athlete that can exercise aerobically, the glucose is converted to pyruvate by glycolysis and enters the TCA cycle and mitochondrial electron transport for complete oxidation. Muscle cells are also capable of oxidizing ketones, released into the blood by the liver, as an energy source. Muscle protein formation is inhibited by the lack of insulin.

Adipose tissue

Triglycerides undergo lipolysis and free fatty acids and glycerol are released into the bloodstream. The free fatty acids are transported bound to albumin and taken up by various tissues (especially muscle and liver) by diffusion across cell membranes. The glycerol is taken up by liver hepatocytes and used for gluconeogenesis. In humans, epinephrine is the most potent stimulus of lipolysis in adipocytes. In other species, glucagon and glucocorticoids may be more important. In all species, the lack of insulin removes the inhibitory effect of insulin on lipolysis and allows lipolysis to proceed.

Mammary gland

During the postabsorptive phase the mammary gland does not normally alter its metabolism to any appreciable degree. It does not require insulin for uptake of glucose from the blood, so it will remove glucose from the blood to make lactose even if blood glucose concentrations are below normal. Lipolysis can actually increase the availability of free fatty acids available for milk fat synthesis, so it is possible to see milk fat concentrations increase in hypoglycemic animals. Normally, if amino acids are available, milk protein synthesis will continue unabated. However, if negative energy balance has caused a large increase in glucocorticoid secretion, protein synthesis will be reduced. Milk volume will also be reduced by high glucocorticoid levels.

Brain, nervous tissue, and red blood cells

These tissues are almost exclusively dependent on uptake of blood glucose for their energy. They continue to rely on the liver and other tissues to produce glucose and use alternative fuels (glucose sparing actions) so that they can utilize glucose all the time. However, during prolonged starvation, as blood glucose levels fall below normal, the brain and nervous tissue can produce the enzymes needed for oxidation of ketones. This adaptation to using ketones, in addition to glucose as an energy source, may take several days.

Self-evaluation

Answers can be found at the end of the chapter.

1 Cholesterol and arachidonic acid are the respective precursors of:
   A Tyrosine and peptide hormones
   B Steroid and prostaglandin hormones
   C Melatonin and prostaglandins
   D Epinephrine and steroid hormones

2 The hypothalamo-hypophyseal portal system is best described as:
  A A portal vein carries blood from capillary beds in the hypophysis to capillary beds in the hypothalamus
  B A portal vein carries blood from capillary beds in the juxtaglomerular apparatus to capillary beds in the hypothalamus
  C A portal vein carries blood from capillary beds in the hypothalamus to capillary beds in the adenohypophysis
  D A portal vein carries blood from capillary beds in the juxtaglomerular apparatus to capillary beds in the adrenal cortex

3 Growth hormone secretion is stimulated by all but one of these choices. Which one?
  A Growth hormone releasing hormone made in the adenohypophysis
  B Fasting
  C Lactation
  D Exercise

4 Which signal transduction pathway is incorrectly described?
  A Insulin receptors form a dimer on binding insulin, which activates the dimer to become an active tyrosine kinase enzyme
  B G protein-coupled receptors undergo a conformational change on bonding hormone that causes the Gα subunit of the G protein to activate adenylyl cyclase in the cell membrane
  C G protein-coupled receptor activation can cause intracellular magnesium ion concentrations to increase, stimulating protein kinase C activity
  D G protein-coupled receptor activation causes an increase in phopholipase C activity, which causes production of inositol trisphosphate and diacylglycerol

5 What is the stimulus for secretion of antidiuretic hormone?
  A Rise in blood calcium
  B Decreased sodium content of blood
  C Increase in osmolarity of the blood
  D Excessive glucose in the urine

6 Which factor stimulates secretion of oxytocin?
  A Milk letdown
  B Stretch of the cervix during parturition
  C Melatonin
  D Cortisol

7 The pineal gland secretes melatonin during:
  A Daylight
  B Darkness

8 Insulin-like growth factor 1 would be expected to:
  A Increase glycogen synthesis in muscle
  B Decrease liver gluconeogenesis
  C Increase lipolysis in adipose tissue
  D Decrease protein accretion in muscle

9 The most important factor inhibiting thyrotropin- releasing hormone production is:
  A Cold weather
  B Lactation
  C High TSH concentrations
  D High T_3 and T_4 concentrations

10 Glucagon secretion occurs when blood glucose is too low. Why would blood glucagon be increased in a diabetic dog?
  A Muscle cells cannot take up glucose, so glucagon needs to stimulate gluconeogenesis
  B Adipose cells are not able to form fatty acids well, so glucagon is needed to stimulate liver to form them
  C Glucagon is needed to stimulate amino acid uptake into muscle
  D Pancreatic α cells require insulin to activate the GLUT-4 transporter, so that during insulin deficiency the cells cannot sense the extracellular glucose concentration

11 Gonadotropin-releasing hormone secretion can be inhibited by all but one of these hormones. Which one?
  A Progesterone
  B Adrenocorticotropic hormone
  C Estrogen
  D Testosterone

12 The cells in the adrenal medulla are:
  A Preganglionic parasympathetic nerve cell bodies
  B Postganglionic parasympathetic nerve cell bodies
  C Preganglionic sympathetic nerve cell bodies
  D Postganglionic sympathetic nerve cell bodies

13 Cortisol has which one of the following physiologic effects?
  A Stimulates tissue growth
  B Decreases lipolysis by adipose tissue
  C Increases gluconeogenesis in the liver and kidney
  D Stimulates mast cells to release histamine

14 Decreased thyroid hormone secretion can:
  A Increase heart rate
  B Increase the appetite
  C Decrease ability to adapt to the cold
  D Increase milk production

15 A lamb is born hairless and dead. It has an enlargement of the throat just below the larynx. What could be the problem?
  A Calcium deficiency in the ewe
  B Iodine deficiency
  C Tumor in the adenohypophysis
  D Tumor in the neurohypophysis

Suggested reading

Etherton, T.D. and Bauman, D.E. (1998) Biology of somatotropin in growth and lactation of domestic animals. *Physiological Reviews* **78**:745–761.

Feldman, E.C. and Nelson, R.W. (1994) Comparative aspects of Cushing's syndrome in dogs and cats. *Endocrinology and Metabolism Clinics of North America* **23**:671–691.

Greco, D.S. (2007) Hypoadrenocorticism in small animals. *Clinical Techniques in Small Animal Practice* **22**:32–35.

McFarlane, D. (2011) Equine pituitary pars intermedia dysfunction. Veterinary Clinics of North America. *Equine Practice* **27**:93–113.

Scott-Moncrieff, J.C. (2012) Thyroid disorders in the geriatric veterinary patient. Veterinary Clinics of North America. *Small Animal Practice* **42**:707–725.

Answers

1 B
2 C
3 A
4 C
5 C
6 B
7 B
8 C
9 D
10 D
11 B
12 D
13 C
14 C
15 B

Male Reproduction in Mammals

William O. Reece

Iowa State University, Ames, IA, USA

The reproductive functions of the male involve the formation of sperm and the deposition of the sperm into the female. Sperm are produced in the seminiferous tubules of the testes and are then transported through the rete testes to the epididymides, where they are stored and matured. The production of sperm is a continuous process once it has been initiated. However, it can change in rate at times in some species, depending on the amount of daylight (photoperiod). The introduction of semen into the female is preceded by erection of the penis so that it can enter the tubular genitalia of the female. Entrance is followed by emission of sperm into the penile urethra, along with stored secretions of the accessory glands. Actual transport of semen through the penile urethra to the region of the cervix or into the uterus of the female is accomplished by ejaculation. The process of male reproduction is assisted by hormones and the autonomic nervous system.

Testes and associated structures

1 What are the seminiferous tubules?

2 Know the relative location of the Sertoli cells. Are they within the seminiferous tubules?

3 Know the relative location of the Leydig cells. Are they within the seminiferous tubules?

4 Which compartment of the seminiferous tubule provides a home for the spermatogonium? What must it move through to get into the other compartment? What is the name of the compartment where spermatozoa are finally formed?

5 What are the parts of the epididymis?

6 What is accomplished by storage of spermatozoa in the epididymis?

The two testes produce spermatozoa. Although they vary somewhat in size, shape, and location among species, they share a similar structure. The bull testicle and its associated genitalia are shown in Figures 52.1 and 52.2. The **seminiferous tubules** are convoluted and occupy the greatest portion of each testicle. The spermatozoa are produced within them. The testicle is surrounded by a connective tissue capsule called the **tunica albuginea**. Support of the seminiferous tubules is provided by connective tissue extensions (**septa** or **trabeculae**) into the testis from the tunica albuginea. A cross-section of the testicle (Figure 52.3) shows the relationship of the seminiferous tubules to each other and to their connective tissue support (interstitial tissue).

In addition to spermatozoa in various stages of development, two other important cell types are the **Sertoli cell** (sustentacular cell) and the **Leydig cell** (interstitial cell). The Sertoli cell provides a "nurse" function for developing spermatozoa. Processes from Sertoli cells surround spermatids and spermatocytes and provide intimate contact with all stages of spermatozoa production; in this respect they are known as sustentacular (supporting) cells. The arrangement of Sertoli cells and the details of seminiferous tubule compartments are shown in Figure 52.4. The Sertoli cells have their base at the periphery of the seminiferous tubules and extend toward the center. The basal

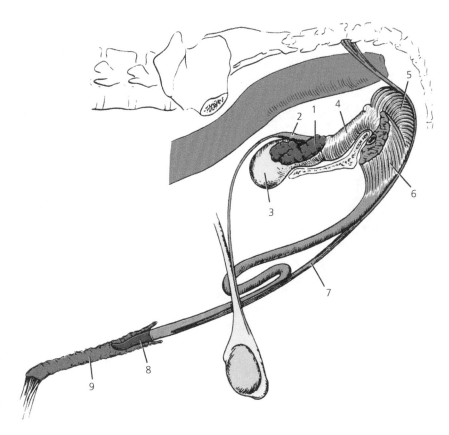

Figure 52.1 Genital organs of the bull. 1, Seminal vesicle; 2, ampulla of vas deferens; 3, bladder; 4, urethral muscle surrounding pelvic urethra; 5, bulbospongiosus muscle; 6, ischiocavernosus muscle; 7, retractor penis muscle; 8, glans penis; 9, preputial membrane and cavity. Adapted from Roberts, S.J. (1986) *Veterinary Obstetrics and Genital Diseases [Theriogenology]*, 3rd edn. Stephen J. Roberts, Woodstock, VT.

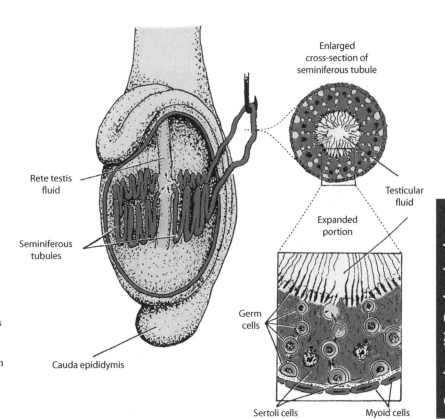

Figure 52.2 Detailed structure of the testicle. Only two of the many seminiferous tubule loops are shown. Testicular fluid is secreted by Sertoli cells into the lumen of the seminiferous tubules. Myoid cells are contractile cells contained within the basement membrane. Adapted from Hafez, E.S.E. and Hafez, B. (2000) *Reproduction in Farm Animals*, 7th edn. Lippincott Williams & Wilkins, Baltimore.

Section IX: Endocrinology, Reproduction, and Lactation

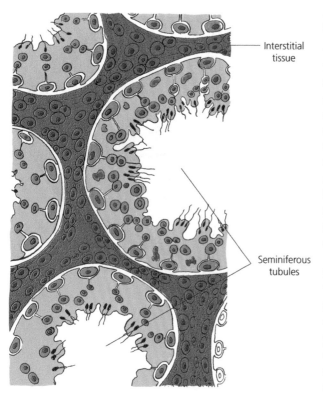

Figure 52.3 Relationship of the seminiferous tubules to each other and to the interstitial tissue. The interstitial tissue is occupied not only by the usual blood vascular network but also by Leydig cells (interstitial cells) and by connective tissue septa (provide support for seminiferous tubules) from the connective tissue capsule (tunica albuginea) of the testis. From Reece, W.O. (2009) *Functional Anatomy and Physiology of Domestic Animals*, 4th edn. Wiley-Blackwell, Ames, IA. Reproduced with permission from Wiley.

junction (tight junction) with adjacent Sertoli cells forms a blood–testis barrier that permits control of the environment within the tubule and also prevents spermatozoa from entering the interstitium. The Sertoli cells divide the seminiferous tubules into two compartments: (i) the **basal compartment**, which communicates with interstitial fluid and provides space for germinal epithelial cells; and (ii) the **adluminal compartment**, which is the space between Sertoli cells that communicates centrally with the lumen of the tubule. Division of a germinal epithelial cell (spermatogonium) in the basal compartment provides a replacement cell and another cell, which must move through the Sertoli cell junction to enter the adluminal compartment. Here, further divisions occur and spermatozoa are finally formed. The Sertoli cells secrete a fluid into the adluminal compartment; its composition favors the developing spermatozoa.

Epididymis

The **epididymis** is a collection and storage tubule for the testis (Figure 52.5). It begins at the pole of the testis in which blood vessels and nerves enter; this is known as the **head of the epididymis**. The head continues along one side of the testis as the **body of the epididymis**, which terminates before making a turn upward as the **tail of the epididymis**. The head of the epididymis receives sperm and adluminal fluid through efferent ducts from the rete testis (the intratesticular network of straight tubules that receives content from the convoluted seminiferous tubules). Spermatozoa move to the epididymis by the flow of fluid into the lumen of the seminiferous tubules from the adluminal spaces. Storage in the epididymis allows the spermatozoa to reach maturity and become motile. Reabsorption of much of the seminiferous tubular fluid occurs in the head of the epididymis.

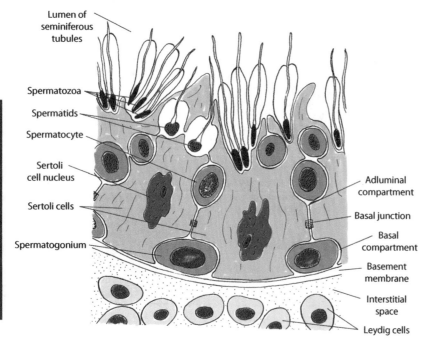

Figure 52.4 Schematic representation of the periphery of a seminiferous tubule. The Sertoli cells divide the seminiferous tubule into adluminal and basal compartments at their basal junction (tight junction). Leydig cells are in the interstitial space. The basal junction forms a blood–testis barrier whereby the tubule environment is controlled and spermatozoa are prevented from entering the interstitium. From Reece, W.O. (2009) *Functional Anatomy and Physiology of Domestic Animals*, 4th edn. Wiley-Blackwell, Ames, IA. Reproduced with permission from Wiley.

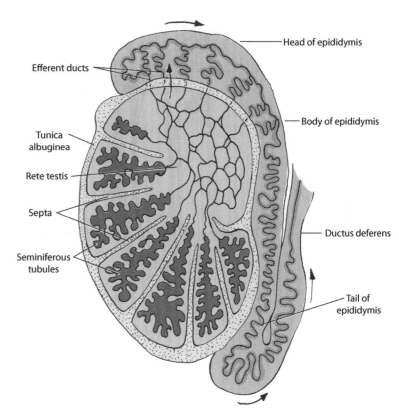

Figure 52.5 Relationship of the seminiferous tubules to the rete testis, efferent ducts, epididymis, and ductus deferens. The rete testis is a network of straight tubules connecting convoluted seminiferous tubules with the highly convoluted epididymal tubule via efferent ducts (extratesticular). The flow of spermatozoa with their fluids is shown by the arrows. From Reece, W.O. (2009) *Functional Anatomy and Physiology of Domestic Animals*, 4th edn. Wiley-Blackwell, Ames, IA. Reproduced with permission from Wiley.

Ductus deferens

The **ductus deferens** (see Figure 52.1), sometimes called the **vas deferens**, is the continuation of the duct system from the tail of the epididymis to the pelvic urethra. As the ductus deferens leaves the testis, toward the abdomen, it is enclosed along with the testicular artery, vein, and nerve, and lymphatic vessels within the **visceral layer** of the **vaginal tunic**. This combination of structures is known as the **spermatic cord** (Figure 52.6). The visceral layer of the vaginal tunic also envelops the testis and epididymis. It is derived from abdominal peritoneum of embryonic origin when the testes descended to the scrotum via the inguinal canal. The **inguinal canal** is an oblique passage from the abdominal cavity to the exterior of the body that extends from the **deep (interior) inguinal ring** to the **superficial (exterior) inguinal ring**. The inguinal rings are slits in the tendinous attachments of the two flat abdominal muscles to the pelvis. After the spermatic cord passes through the inguinal rings, the ductus deferens separates from the spermatic cord to proceed to the pelvic urethra (see Figure 52.1). The ductus deferens terminates in an enlarged glandular area (variable size among species) known as the **ampulla of the ductus deferens** (absent in the boar). The relationship of the terminal ductus deferens to the urinary bladder, accessory glands, and pelvic urethra is also shown in Figure 52.1.

Scrotum

The **scrotum** is a cutaneous sac containing the testes. The scrotum contains a subcutaneous layer of smooth muscle fibers, the **tunica dartos**, which contracts in cold weather and holds the testes closer to the abdominal wall. The scrotum is lined with the **parietal layer** of the vaginal tunic, which is a continuation of parietal peritoneum into the scrotum.

Descent of the testes

1 What structures compose the spermatic cord?

2 Read and understand the relationship of scrotal hernias to the visceral and parietal vaginal tunics.

3 What are cryptorchid testes?

It is helpful to describe the lining of the scrotum and covering of the testis in more detail because it explains the origin of scrotal or inguinal hernias frequently encountered in pigs. During embryonic development the testes are within the abdomen but outside the peritoneum. They have not yet entered the scrotum, but each has a fibrous connection to the scrotum known as the **gubernaculum testis**. As development and growth progress, the gubernaculum testis pulls the testes through the inguinal canal into the scrotum, creating a double-walled tube of peritoneum. The testis, epididymis, ductus deferens, and testicular vessels, nerves, and lymphatics are enveloped by the inner tube of peritoneum known as the visceral vaginal tunic. The vessels, nerves, lymphatics, and ductus deferens are the components of the spermatic cord (see Figure 52.6). The **cremaster muscle** (an extension of the external abdominal oblique muscle) lies on the spermatic cord and assists with drawing the testes closer to the

Section IX: Endocrinology, Reproduction, and Lactation

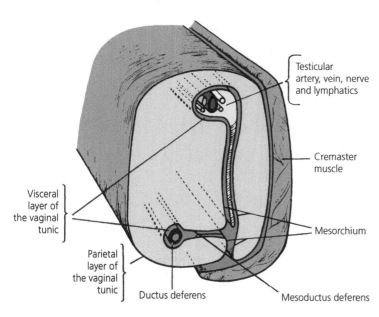

Testicular artery, vein, nerve and lymphatics

Cremaster muscle

Visceral layer of the vaginal tunic

Mesorchium

Parietal layer of the vaginal tunic

Ductus deferens

Mesoductus deferens

Figure 52.6 Cross-section of spermatic cord of mammals. Adapted from Frandson, R.D., Wilke, W.L. and Fails, A.D. (2009) *Anatomy and Physiology of Farm Animals*, 7th edn. Wiley-Blackwell, Ames, IA. Reproduced with permission from Wiley.

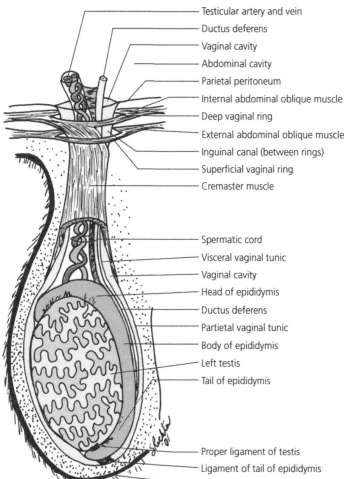

Testicular artery and vein
Ductus deferens
Vaginal cavity
Abdominal cavity
Parietal peritoneum
Internal abdominal oblique muscle
Deep vaginal ring
External abdominal oblique muscle
Inguinal canal (between rings)
Superficial vaginal ring
Cremaster muscle

Spermatic cord
Visceral vaginal tunic
Vaginal cavity
Head of epididymis
Ductus deferens
Partietal vaginal tunic
Body of epididymis
Left testis
Tail of epididymis

Proper ligament of testis
Ligament of tail of epididymis
Skin and "dartos" of testis

Figure 52.7 The descended adult bull testis featuring its relationship to the enveloping visceral vaginal tunic, spermatic cord, the inguinal canal, deep and superficial vaginal rings, vaginal cavity, and abdominal cavity. The deep vaginal ring is the location where the parietal vaginal tunic of the scrotum is continuous with the parietal peritoneum of the abdominal cavity. The proper ligament of testis and ligament of tail of epididymis are remnants of gubernaculum testis. Adapted from Reece, W.O. (2009) *Functional Anatomy and Physiology of Domestic Animals*, 4th edn. Wiley-Blackwell, Ames, IA. Reproduced with permission from Wiley.

abdominal wall. The outer tube of peritoneum is known as the parietal vaginal tunic, and it lines the scrotum (Figure 52.7). The testis and epididymis that are enveloped within the visceral vaginal tunic completely fill the scrotal cavity lined by the parietal vaginal tunic so that only a narrow space remains between the two tunics (the **vaginal cavity**). The vaginal cavity is continuous with the abdominal cavity at the deep vaginal ring (location where the parietal vaginal tunic of the scrotum is continuous with the parietal peritoneum of the abdominal cavity). The spermatic cord passes through the superficial and deep vaginal rings into the abdominal cavity. If the vaginal rings are too large, loops of intestine may enter the vaginal cavity to constitute what is known as an **inguinal hernia**. An inguinal hernia that has passed into the scrotum is known as a **scrotal hernia**. The herniated intestinal loops have the potential for strangulation (cut off blood supply) or for evisceration (removal from the abdominal cavity) at the time of castration.

Cryptorchid testes are those that fail to descend. This condition seems to be most prevalent in pigs and horses. When the testis is in the inguinal canal but not in the scrotum, the horse is referred to as a high flanker. Often the testis or testes are retained entirely within the abdominal cavity.

Accessory sex glands and semen

1 What composes the accessory sex glands? Which one is present in all the domestic animals? What is the relationship of the accessory sex glands to the pelvic urethra?

2 What is the collective name of the accessory gland secretions? What is the difference between seminal plasma and semen?

3 What function is served by seminal plasma?

4 What function may be served by the prostaglandins present in seminal plasma?

5 How large a number of sperm are present for each artificial insemination? Give an example.

The **accessory sex glands** provide secretions that empty into the pelvic urethra near their origin (Figure 52.8). They vary in size and shape among species and can be absent in some. The accessory sex glands are composed of the **ampullae of the ductus deferentes**, the **vesicular glands** (sometimes called seminal vesicles), the **prostate gland**, and the **bulbourethral glands** (sometimes called the Cowper glands). The ampullae (absent in the boar and dog) are enlargements of the terminal part of the ductus deferentes, and their secretion empties into the lumens of the ductus deferentes. The vesicular glands (absent in the dog) are paired glands that empty into the pelvic urethra along with the ductus deferentes. The prostate gland is present in all domestic animals. It is prominent in the dog, encircling the urethra. Enlargement can be a cause for obstruction of urine flow through the urethra; this condition is more common in older dogs. Multiple ducts from this gland empty directly into the urethra. The paired bulbourethral glands (absent in the dog) are the most caudal of the accessory glands. At the time of ejaculation, the accessory sex gland secretions (collectively known as **seminal plasma**) are mixed with sperm and fluid from the epididymides to form **semen**.

The seminal plasma provides an environment conducive to the survival of sperm within the female reproductive tract. It is rich in electrolytes, fructose, ascorbic acid, and other vitamins. Whereas fertilization can occur with sperm unaided by seminal plasma, the greatest fertilization potential is achieved with it. Species differ in the composition of seminal plasma, but it seems that each species has solved the same fundamental problems in a different way. However, one unvarying component among all species is fructose. The advantage of fructose as an energy

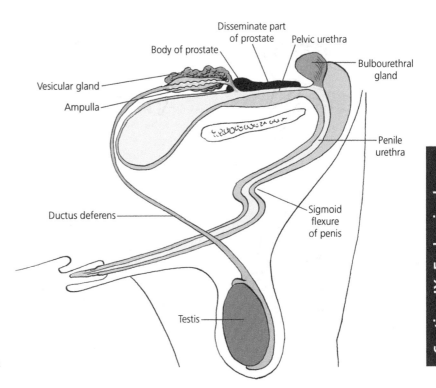

Figure 52.8 Disposition of the accessory glands that discharge into the pelvic urethra of the bull. Adapted from Reece, W.O. (2009) *Functional Anatomy and Physiology of Domestic Animals*, 4th edn. Wiley-Blackwell, Ames, IA. Reproduced with permission from Wiley.

source might be that it does not require metabolic energy for entrance into the spermatozoa.

Several **prostaglandins** (see Chapter 51) are present in seminal plasma. It is thought that they aid in fertilization in two ways: (i) prostaglandins react with cervical mucus and make it more receptive to sperm; and (ii) some of the prostaglandins present cause smooth muscle contraction, so it is believed that reverse peristalsis is initiated in the uterus and oviducts to facilitate transport of sperm toward the ovaries.

Most of the sperm in an ejaculate never reach the oviduct. In fact, only a few dozen might reach the vicinity of the oocyte, where only one is required for fertilization. Semen collected for artificial insemination is often diluted and mixed with extenders to obtain the greatest number of insemination units. The number of sperm intended for each artificial insemination varies among species, but approximates 10 and 125 million, respectively, for cattle and sheep, and 2 billion each for pigs and horses.

Penis and prepuce

1 Why is greater enlargement of the penis possible in the stallion than in the bull?

2 What is the urethral process of the ram penis?

3 How does the bulbus glandis of the dog penis participate in the "tie" associated with canine coitus?

4 Which domestic species have a sigmoid flexure of their penis?

5 Note the preputial diverticulum (pouch) in the boar and the double-folded prepuce in the stallion (Figure 52.9).

The **penis** is the male organ of copulation through which urine and semen pass by way of the penile urethra. The appearance of the penis of several farm animals and its association with other structures is shown in Figure 52.9. The **roots (crura)** of the penis begin at the caudal border of the pelvic ischial arch. The forward extension from the roots is known as the **body**, and the free extremity is known as the **glans**. The internal structure (Figure 52.10) is occupied mostly by **cavernous tissue** (commonly known as **erectile tissue**). Cavernous tissue is a collection of blood sinusoids separated by sheets of connective tissue. The stallion has a large amount of erectile tissue relative to connective tissue (Figure 52.10B), and greater enlargement is possible during erection than in the bull (Figure 52.10A), in which the ratio of erectile tissue to connective tissue is lower. The urethra is on the ventral aspect of the body of the penis (Figure 52.10).

The ram has a highly visible urethral process (see Figure 52.9B), and sometimes urethral calculi become lodged in its narrowed extremity. This can be corrected by amputation of the process. It is speculated that the function of the urethral process in the ram is to spray the cervical area with semen during ejaculation. The free end of such an extension would move in a circular pattern with the emission of fluid under pressure.

The dog has a **bulbus glandis** at the caudal part of the glans. The enlargement of the bulbus glandis is responsible for prolonged retention of the penis during coitus. Contraction of muscles in the vestibule of the female vagina caudal to the bulbus glandis assists this retention, commonly known as the **tie** (Figure 52.11).

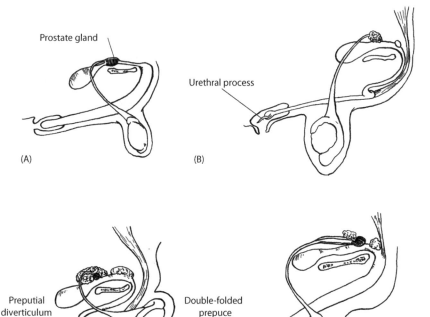

Figure 52.9 Comparative anatomy of the male reproductive organs of various domestic animals: (A) dog; (B) ram; (C) boar; (D) stallion. Note the encirclement of the pelvic urethra by the prostate in the dog, urethral process in the ram, preputial diverticulum in the boar, and double-folded prepuce in the stallion. Adapted from Reece, W.O. (2009) *Functional Anatomy and Physiology of Domestic Animals*, 4th edn. Wiley-Blackwell, Ames, IA. Reproduced with permission from Wiley.

The bull, ram, and boar have a **sigmoid flexure** of their penis, resulting in an S shape when not erect (see Figures 52.8 and 52.9). Erection causes extension of the flexure as shown for the bull in Figure 52.12.

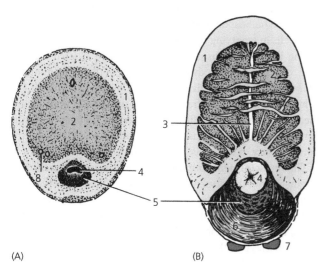

(A)   (B)

Figure 52.10 Transverse sections of the fibroelastic penis of a bull (A) and the musculocavernous penis of a stallion (B). 1, Tunica albuginea; 2, corpus cavernosum; 3, septum; 4, urethra; 5, corpus spongiosum; 6, bulbospongiosus; 7, retractor penis; 8, large thick-walled veins. Adapted from Dyce, K.M., Sack, W.O. and Wensing, C.J.G. (2002) *Textbook of Veterinary Anatomy*, 3rd edn. W.B. Saunders, Philadelphia. With permission from Elsevier.

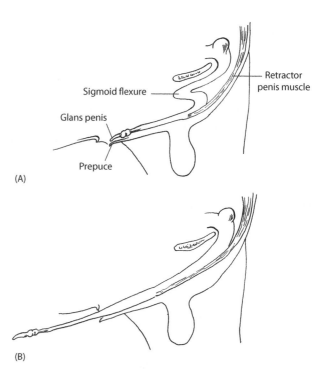

(A)

(B)

Figure 52.12 Penis of the bull. (A) Nonerect position with its characteristic sigmoid flexure. (B) Erect position with elimination of the sigmoid flexure and extension beyond the prepuce. The retractor penis muscle assists return of the penis to its nonerect position. Adapted from Reece, W.O. (2009) *Functional Anatomy and Physiology of Domestic Animals*, 4th edn. Wiley-Blackwell, Ames, IA. Reproduced with permission from Wiley.

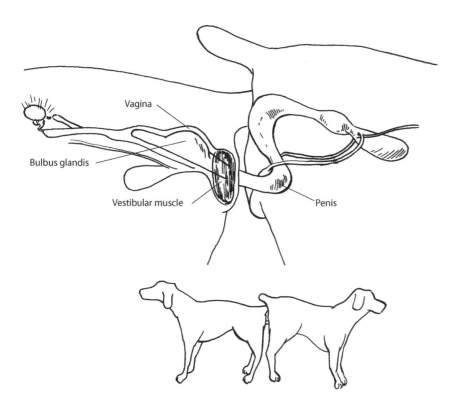

Figure 52.11 "Locking" phase or "tie" of canine coitus (lateral view). In the dog, erection involves primarily the glans penis. Enlargement of the bulbus glandis and contraction of vestibular muscles during intromission "lock" the dog's penis in the bitch's vagina. Adapted from Reece, W.O. (2009) *Functional Anatomy and Physiology of Domestic Animals*, 4th edn. Wiley-Blackwell, Ames, IA. Reproduced with permission from Wiley.

The **prepuce** is an invaginated fold of skin that surrounds the free extremity of the penis (see Figure 52.9). The stallion has a double-folded prepuce. Waxy accumulations known as **beans** sometimes form in the outer fold and must be removed manually. The boar has a **preputial diverticulum** (pouch) on the dorsal wall, which often contains decomposing urine and macerated epithelium. The fluid in the diverticulum also contains a **pheromone** (see Chapter 51) that induces sows to assume the immobile mating stance.

Muscles of male genitalia

> 1 Note the functions for the external cremaster muscle, the internal cremaster muscle, the urethralis and bulbospongiosus muscle, the ischiocavernosus muscles, and the retractor penis muscles.

The cremaster muscle is formed from the caudal fibers of the internal abdominal oblique muscle. It passes through the inguinal canal and attaches to the outer aspect of the parietal vaginal tunic (see Figures 52.6 and 52.7). This muscle pulls the testis up against the superficial vaginal ring, particularly in cold weather. The cremaster muscles are responsible for the testes being drawn into the abdominal cavity of the elephant, deer, and rabbit during times other than the breeding season.

A skeletal muscle, the **urethralis** (see Figure 52.1), is the pelvic continuation from the smooth muscle wall of the urinary bladder. Peristaltic action of this muscle assists in the transport of urine or semen through the pelvic urethra.

The **bulbospongiosus muscle** (Figures 52.1 and 52.13) is a striated muscle continuation of the urethralis. It continues throughout the length of the penis in the horse, but only proceeds for a short distance along the penile urethra in other animals. The bulbospongiosus muscle continues the action of the urethralis in emptying the urethra.

The **ischiocavernosus muscles** are paired striated muscles that converge on the body of the penis from their origins on the lateral sides of the ischial arch (see Figures 52.1 and 52.13). When these muscles contract, they pull the penis upward against the floor of the pelvis. Much of the venous drainage from the penis is obstructed because of the location of the veins on the dorsal surface of the penis, and erection is thereby assisted.

The **retractor penis muscles** are paired striated muscles that originate from the suspensory ligaments of the anus. They continue forward and converge caudal to the body of the penis (see Figures 52.12 and 52.13). After they join on the underside of the penis, they continue forward to the glans penis. The retractor penis muscles pull the flaccid penis back into the prepuce.

Blood and nerve supply

> 1 What is the function of the pampiniform plexus?
> 2 Where does stimulation occur to provide for the afferent side of the reflexes associated with erection and ejaculation?

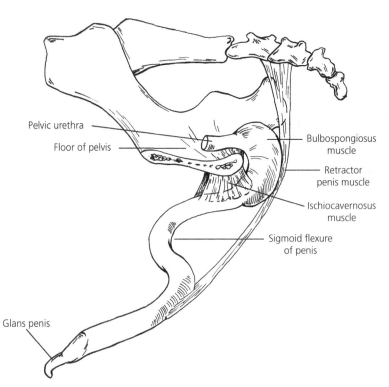

Pelvic urethra

Floor of pelvis

Bulbospongiosus muscle

Retractor penis muscle

Ischiocavernosus muscle

Sigmoid flexure of penis

Glans penis

Figure 52.13 Penis of the bull and some of its associated muscles. The bulbospongiosus muscle assists in emptying the urethra. The ischiocavernosus muscle assists in the erection process, and the retractor penis muscle assists in the return of the penis to the prepuce after intromission. Adapted from Reece, W.O. (2009) *Functional Anatomy and Physiology of Domestic Animals*, 4th edn. Wiley-Blackwell, Ames, IA. Reproduced with permission from Wiley.

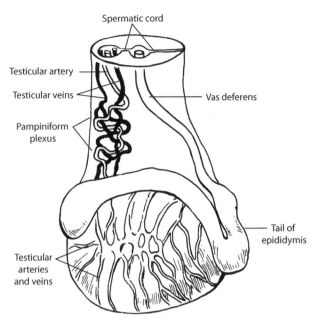

Figure 52.14 Lateral view of the stallion testis with emphasis on the pampiniform plexus. The pampiniform plexus is illustrated by the intertwining of the testicular artery and vein. This allows the cooler venous blood to cool the warmer arterial blood directed to the testis. Adapted from Reece, W.O. (2009) *Functional Anatomy and Physiology of Domestic Animals*, 4th edn. Wiley-Blackwell, Ames, IA. Reproduced with permission from Wiley.

Blood to the testicles is supplied by the testicular arteries. The testicular veins parallel the testicular arteries. Both artery and vein are enclosed within the spermatic cord (see Figure 52.6). A short distance above the testicle, the testicular vein is convoluted (the **pampiniform plexus**) and is in close association with the convoluted part of the testicular artery (Figure 52.14). Their closeness, and because they are convoluted and therefore longer, is the means whereby blood entering the testis is cooled by the venous blood leaving the testis. The arteries and veins are also close to the surface of the testes, and so direct loss of heat from the testes is favored. Spermatogenesis requires a cooler temperature than normal body temperature. Arterial blood to the penis provides for filling of the cavernous tissue and provides nutrition to the tissues. The exclusive supply is the artery of the penis, a terminal branch of the internal pudendal arteries. The blood supply to the penis of the horse is slightly different than that of other species and is more extensive.

In addition to autonomic nerve fibers to the testes, penis, and accessory sex glands, the penis is supplied by a spinal nerve, the pudendal nerve. Terminations of the pudendal nerve are located in the glans penis. Sensory stimulation of the glans provides the afferent side of reflexes associated with erection and ejaculation. Reflex centers for erection and ejaculation are located in the lumbar region of the spinal cord.

Spermatogenesis

> 1 Define spermatogenesis.
>
> 2 Spermatids undergo nuclear and cytoplasmic changes and develop a tail. What is this maturation phase called?
>
> 3 What is spermiation?
>
> 4 Where is the fertilizing ability of spermatozoa attained? Where are they stored? What happens to spermatozoa that are not ejaculated?
>
> 5 What function is served by the spermatogenic wave?
>
> 6 Describe the negative feedback system that relates to the production of testosterone by Leydig cells. Why is luteinizing hormone called interstitial cell stimulating hormone (ICSH)?
>
> 7 What is the role of testosterone in spermatogenesis?
>
> 8 What are the assumed roles of FSH in the male?
>
> 9 Aside from spermatogenesis, what are other functions of testosterone in the male?
>
> 10 What embryonic structures stimulated by testosterone become tubular portions of the male reproductive system?
>
> 11 What metabolic function is served by testosterone?
>
> 12 What are C-16 unsaturated androgens that are secreted by boar testes?

The term **spermatogenesis** refers to the entire process involved in the transformation of germinal epithelial cells (stem cells) to spermatozoa and can be divided into two phases: spermatocytogenesis and spermiogenesis. **Spermatocytogenesis** is the proliferative phase whereby spermatogonial cells multiply by a series of mitotic divisions followed by the meiotic divisions which produce the haploid (*n*) number of chromosomes (Figure 52.15).

The **stem cells (spermatogonia)** are located in the basal compartment of the seminiferous tubules (see Figure 52.4). The mitotic division of a spermatogonium results in one cell being a replacement for the cell that has just divided (it stays in the basal compartment). The other cell becomes a **type A spermatogonium**, which migrates through the Sertoli cell barrier to the adluminal compartment. Type A spermatogonia undergo mitotic division (sometimes involving several generations) until large numbers (variable among species) of **type B spermatogonia** have been produced. Type B spermatogonia undergo the last of the mitotic divisions, resulting in the formation of primary spermatocytes with 2*n* chromosome numbers. Primary spermatocytes undergo meiotic division (described previously) to form secondary spermatocytes, which in turn undergo meiotic division to form spermatids (*n* chromosome numbers). In the bull, 64 spermatids are formed from one type A spermatogonium.

The second phase of spermatogenesis, **spermiogenesis**, involves maturation of the spermatids while they are still in the adluminal compartment. Spermiogenesis comprises a series of nuclear and cytoplasmic changes and transformation from a nonmotile cell (not able to move) to a potentially motile cell in which a flagellum (tail) has formed. The mature spermatids

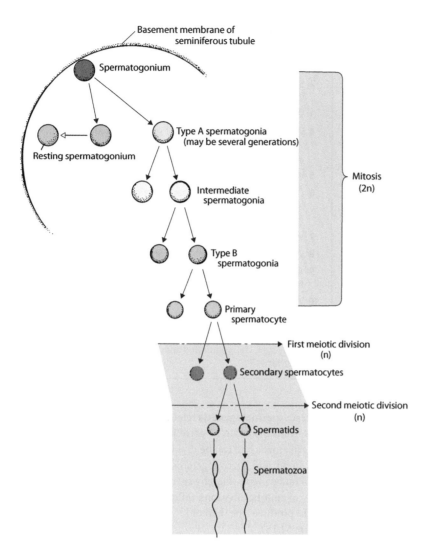

Figure 52.15 Diagrammatic representation of the stages of spermatogenesis in mammals. The chromosome number ($2n$, diploid; n, haploid) is also shown for each stage. Adapted from Pineda, M.H. (2003) The biology of sex. In: *Veterinary Endocrinology and Reproduction*, 5th edn (eds M.H. Pineda and M.P. Dooley). Iowa State Press, Ames, IA. Reproduced with permission from Wiley.

produced during the final phase of spermiogenesis are released into the lumen of the seminiferous tubules as **spermatozoa**.

The release of matured spermatids into the lumen of the seminiferous tubules is known as **spermiation**. Spermatozoa from several animal species are compared in Figure 52.16.

Epididymal transport

The newly formed spermatozoa are essentially immotile. They are transported to the epididymis by fluid secretions into the seminiferous tubules and rete testis and by activity of contractile elements in the testis that direct fluid flow to the head of the epididymis.

The fertilizing ability of an animal is attained progressively during the transit of spermatozoa through the epididymis. Changes include development of unidirectional (as opposed to circular) motility, changes in nuclear chromatin (DNA–protein complex), and changes in the nature of the surface of the plasma membrane.

The major site of sperm storage within the male reproductive tract is the tail (last portion) of the epididymis. About 70% of

the total number of spermatozoa in the ducts outside the rete testis (**excurrent duct system**) are found in the tail of the epididymis. Many of the spermatozoa formed in the testes are either phagocytized in the excurrent duct system or lost into the urine. About 85% of the daily sperm production in sexually inactive rams are voided in the urine.

Spermatogenic wave

If all segments of the seminiferous tubules were involved in the same activity at the same time, a continuous supply of spermatozoa would not be produced because for spermatocytogenesis (development from spermatogonia to spermatozoa) to proceed requires about 64 days (in the bull) in the adluminal compartment. While this development is continuing, a new type A spermatogonium migrates through the Sertoli cell barrier into the adluminal compartment to begin its development behind the developing type A spermatogonium that preceded it. In the bull, this occurs every 14 days. Since 64 days are required for development to spermatozoa, there will be 4.6 cycles (64/14)

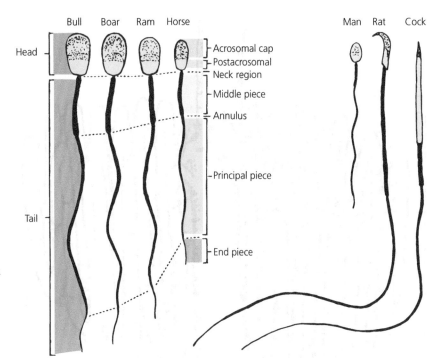

Figure 52.16 Comparison of the spermatozoa of farm animals and other vertebrates. The major structural features are given. Note the differences in the relative size and shape. Adapted from Hafez, E.S.E. and Hafez, B. (2000) *Reproduction in Farm Animals*, 7th edn. Lippincott Williams & Wilkins, Baltimore.

of development before the first cycle from a given area of seminiferous epithelium begins to arrive at the rete testis. A cycle is defined as a series of changes in a given area of seminiferous epithelium between two appearances of developmental stages. A portion of tubule at one stage is usually adjacent to portions of tubule in stages just preceding it or following it in time. This sequential change in stage of cycle along the length of the tubule is known as the **spermatogenic wave**. A spermatogenic wave that involves a 12-day cycle is illustrated in Figure 52.17. The wave involves a sequence of stages beginning with the less advanced stages in the middle of the loop to progressively more advanced stages nearer the rete testis. The stages proceed in opposite directions from the **site of reversal** at the middle of the loop toward the rete testis.

A large number of spermatozoa are produced daily in the normal male animal, about 6.0×10^9 spermatozoa in the bull and about 16.5×10^9 in the boar. In the bull, daily sperm production increases with age, reaching a maximum at about 7 years.

Hormonal control

Leydig and Sertoli cells are responsible for hormone production within the testes. The production of **testosterone** by Leydig cells is controlled by the gonadotropin known as **luteinizing hormone (LH)** (sometimes called **interstitial cell stimulating hormone**, or **ICSH**). Low levels of testosterone cause an increase in LH secretion by the anterior pituitary. The increase in LH secretion causes the Leydig cells in the testes to secrete testosterone; when increased, testosterone inhibits the further secretion of LH and testosterone levels are thus stabilized. A subsequent decline in testosterone again stimulates LH secretion, and the cycle is repeated; this is known as a negative feedback system.

The influence of testosterone on spermatogenesis requires that it diffuse from the interstitial tissues into the seminiferous tubules. Within the seminiferous tubules, it seems that testosterone maintains spermatogenesis by supporting the meiotic process.

Another gonadotropic hormone, **follicle-stimulating hormone (FSH)** from the anterior pituitary, stimulates production of an **androgen-binding protein** by the Sertoli cells. Androgen-binding protein is secreted into the lumen of the seminiferous tubules and binds with testosterone and other androgens to stabilize their concentrations and ensure appropriate amounts for spermatogenesis. It is also believed that FSH stimulates the secretion of estrogens by the Sertoli cells. The actual secretion of estrogen might arise from the intracellular conversion of testosterone (originating from Leydig cells) by the Sertoli cells. The Sertoli cells are also the source of a hormone known as **inhibin**, which inhibits secretion of FSH by the anterior pituitary.

Whereas LH is required continuously for spermatogenesis (testosterone-supported meiosis), FSH is not essential for the maintenance of spermatogenesis once it has been initiated. Initiation of spermatogenesis at puberty and after physiologic or pathologic interruptions requires FSH.

Other functions of testosterone

In addition to its spermatogenic activity, testosterone fulfills other functions in the peripheral circulation. After secretion of testosterone by Leydig cells into the interstitial space of the testes, a greater amount diffuses into the blood and lymphatic capillaries than that which diffuses into the seminiferous tubules. After entrance into the blood, testosterone is bound loosely with a plasma protein for its transport. Within 15–30 min, the

Section IX: Endocrinology, Reproduction, and Lactation

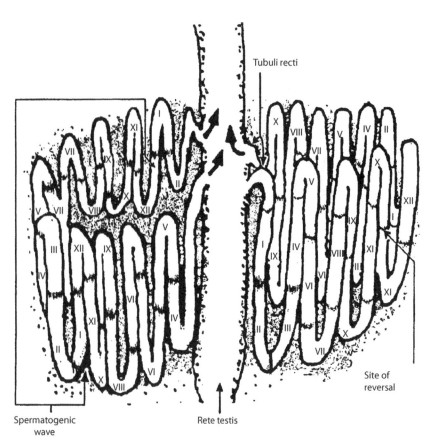

Tubuli recti

Site of reversal

Rete testis

Spermatogenic wave

Figure 52.17 A seminiferous tubule in which the wave of the seminiferous epithelium is schematically represented along the length of the tubule. The succession of stages I–XII (12-day cycle), the site of reversal in the middle of the tubule, and the relationship of the wave to the rete testis are shown. The more advanced stages of each wave are located nearer the rete testis. Any one tubule may have as many as 15 spermatogenic waves. Adapted from Hafez, E.S.E. and Hafez, B. (2000) *Reproduction in Farm Animals*, 7th edn. Lippincott Williams & Wilkins, Baltimore.

testosterone is released from the protein to be fixed to target tissues or to be degraded, mainly by the liver, into inactive products that are subsequently excreted.

Other functions of testosterone include the development and maintenance of **libido**, secretory activity of the accessory sex glands, and general body features associated with the male. Libido refers to sexual drive. It can be effectively eliminated by **castration** (removal of the testes). Castrated animals usually, but not invariably, lack libido. Small amounts of testosterone from other sources, such as the adrenal gland (interconversion potential), might be sufficient to provide libido in some animals.

The structural development and physiologic functioning (production of secretions) of the accessory sex glands are influenced by testosterone. In this regard, hyperactive prostate glands (enlargement) can be treated effectively by estrogen administration. The estrogen inhibits the secretion of LH, and testosterone production by the Leydig cells is suppressed. A reduced concentration of testosterone causes the hyperactive prostate gland to reduce its activity, and its size decreases.

General body features associated with the male (**secondary sexual characteristics**) are influenced by testosterone. These features include increased bone growth (heavier bones), greater muscling, thicker skin, and deeper voice (in the bull). During fetal growth, testosterone directs the descent of the testes. The presence or absence of testosterone determines the respective development of a penis and scrotum or a clitoris and vagina.

Before sexual differentiation in the embryo, the structures needed for the development of either sex are present. With normal male hormonal stimulation, the **Wolffian ducts** become tubular portions of the male reproductive system, and the **Müllerian ducts** regress. In the female the Müllerian ducts become tubular portions of the reproductive system, and the Wolffian ducts regress.

Metabolically, testosterone has protein anabolic functions that affect the greater muscling potential of males. It is probable that the thicker skin and laryngeal changes of the male are also related to this function of testosterone. Because of the desirability for more muscle and less fat in meat-producing animals, the current trend is to use noncastrated males for meat production. The protein anabolic effect obtained from testicular testosterone is thereby retained.

Other androgens

Testosterone is one of several steroid hormones classified as androgens. In addition to testosterone, the boar testes secrete large amounts of compounds known as **C-16 unsaturated androgens**. These androgens act as pheromones when they are excreted in boar saliva, and they cause the sow in heat to adopt the mating posture. When the C-16 unsaturated androgens are excreted in urine, they contribute to the characteristic odor of boar urine. These compounds are also responsible for the undesirable flavor of boar meat, which is known as **boar taint**.

Erection

> **1** How is erection of the penis accomplished?
>
> **2** Does erection accomplish straightening of the sigmoid flexure?
>
> **3** What is an approximate blood pressure within the corpus cavernosum penis of the bull during coitus? What is hematoma of the penis?

An increase in the turgidity of the penis is known as **erection**. It is caused by an increase in blood pressure within the cavernous sinuses of the penis as a result of greater blood inflow than outflow. The inflow of blood increases through vasodilation of the arteries caused by parasympathetic stimulation. The outflow of blood decreases through compression of the dorsal veins of the penis against the pelvis when the ischiocavernosus muscles contract. Contraction of the ischiocavernosus muscles also compresses the blood in the cavernous sinuses (now a closed system), which also assists erection by increasing blood pressure in the cavernous sinuses (see Figure 52.13).

Complete erection of the glans penis of the horse is delayed until after introduction of the penis into the vagina of the mare. Mounting of the mare compresses the prepuce against the vulva, and venous drainage from the prepuce is impaired. Complete erection of the glans is then possible because venous drainage from the glans is directed to the prepuce, which is blocked.

In animals with a sigmoid flexure, the filling of the cavernous sinuses, coupled with relaxation of the retractor penis muscles, causes the flexure to be eliminated and the penis to be straightened. Although animals with a sigmoid flexure have a higher ratio of connective tissue to cavernous tissue (see Figure 52.10), the length and diameter of the penis increase somewhat as a result of erection, in addition to penis straightening. Compared with the bull, ram, and boar, the penis of the horse has a lower ratio of connective tissue to cavernous tissue, and a relatively greater increase in the length and diameter of its penis occurs during erection.

Blood pressure within the corpus cavernosum penis of the bull has been measured during coitus. A pressure of approximately 14,000 mmHg was associated with peak activity, and peak activity was correlated with an increased intensity of ischiocavernosus muscle contraction that furthered compression of blood in the cavernous tissue. Higher pressures have been recorded. It is believed that these high pressures, coupled with cavernous tissue capsule weakness, might be the cause of rupture of the corpus cavernosum penis (hematoma of the penis) in some bulls. The usual rupture site is on the dorsal surface of the distal curve of the sigmoid flexure (see Figure 52.12).

Mounting and intromission

> **1** What are some causes for mounting failures?
>
> **2** Define intromission. Which domestic species has the longest and which has the shortest duration of intromission? What are causes for intromission failures?

Mounting is the stance assumed by the male by which the penis is brought into apposition with the vulva of the female. Successful mounting must be preceded by a receptive stance on the part of the female. Failures in mounting are encountered when there are injuries, weakness, or soreness in the hindlimbs of the male.

Introduction of the penis into the vagina and its maintenance within the vagina during coitus is known as **intromission**. Pelvic thrusts assisted by the abdominal muscles assist penetration of the penis into the vagina. The duration of intromission varies among species: it is shortest for the bull and ram and longest for the boar. Failures of intromission occur in some animals; causes include phimosis (constriction of the preputial orifice), hematoma of the penis (as in the bull), and congenital deformities. Final distension of the penis does not occur in the dog until after intromission. It is presumed that intromission is facilitated in the dog by the presence of the **os penis** (penis bone).

Emission and ejaculation

> **1** Differentiate between emission and ejaculation.

As sexual stimulation increases, a point is reached at which reflex centers in the spinal cord bring about **emission** and **ejaculation**. Emission precedes ejaculation. It results from sympathetic innervation whereby sperm and fluids in the vasa deferentia and ampullae are emptied into the urethra along with fluids from the other accessory glands (**seminal plasma**). The sympathetic innervation provides peristaltic movement for transport to the urethra and constricts the neck of the bladder to minimize reflux (backward flow) of sperm and fluids into the urinary bladder. Once emission has been accomplished, reflex peristalsis of the urethral muscles propels the urethral contents toward the external urethral orifice. The latter phase, peristalsis of the urethra, is assisted by contraction of the bulbospongiosus muscle, which in turn compresses the urethra. The combination of pressure and peristalsis forces the semen (mixture of seminal plasma and sperm and fluid from the epididymides) from the urethra to the exterior, the process of ejaculation. Stimulation for emission and ejaculation is derived from sensory nerves located in the glans penis.

Sperm and fluids are ejaculated near the opening of the cervix in cattle and sheep, directly into the uterus in swine, and partially into the uterus in the horse.

Factors affecting testicular function

> **1** When does testicular function become manifest?
>
> **2** How does puberty begin in the male?
>
> **3** What is the purpose for the influence of photoperiod on testicular function?
>
> **4** How does increasing photoperiod affect sheep and goats? Is this different in the stallion? Are cattle and swine influenced by photoperiod?
>
> **5** What gland mediates the photoperiod response?

Testicular function becomes manifest at the onset of **puberty**. It is believed that puberty is correlated with decreased sensitivity of the hypothalamus to testosterone, so that LH is secreted in greater amounts. An increased LH concentration stimulates the Leydig cells to secrete testosterone in greater quantities, and all aspects of testosterone function begin to appear. FSH is essential for the initiation of spermatogenesis at puberty.

In some species, changes in **photoperiod (length of daylight)** have a marked influence on testicular function. Photoperiod is also related to ovarian activity in the female of these same species. The purpose of this sensitivity to photoperiod is the coordination of birth with favorable weather conditions. Sheep and goats have major periods of testicular regression during increasing photoperiod, which is restored by decreasing photoperiod. In the stallion, decreasing photoperiod reduces testicular function. The pineal gland (also known as the pineal body) is an endocrine gland attached by a stalk to the dorsal wall of the third ventricle of the cerebrum. The pineal gland is inhibitory to the gonads and is the principal mechanism involved in the effect of photoperiod on testicular and ovarian function. The pineal gland mediates the photoperiod response in the ram and ewe and is probably involved in the response of the other species. Testicular function and photoperiod in cattle and swine are related only to a minor degree. When spermatogenesis is stopped during photoperiod inhibition, FSH is again required for its initiation.

Self-evaluation

Answers can be found at the end of the chapter.

1 Which one of the following cells lines the periphery of the seminiferous tubules, and provides a "nurse" function for developing spermatozoa?
   A Leydig cells
   B Spermatid
   C Sertoli cells
   D MPS cells

2 A scrotal hernia exists when a loop of intestine:
   A Descends to the scrotum within the spermatic cord
   B Descends to the scrotum in the vaginal cavity
   C Is in the peritoneal cavity
   D Occupies the pleural cavity

3 Seminal plasma is:
   A The same as semen
   B A component of blood
   C A collective name for accessory sex gland secretions
   D The fluid from the epididymides

4 Which one of the following accessory sex glands would obstruct urine flow when it becomes enlarged?
   A Bulbourethral glands
   B Ampullae of the ducti deferentes
   C Vesicular glands
   D Prostate gland

5 The pampiniform plexus:
   A Pampers the testicles
   B Assists warming of the testicles
   C Assists cooling of the testicles
   D Is a nerve network to the testicles

6 The maturation phase, whereby spermatids undergo nuclear and cytoplasmic changes and develop a tail, is known as:
   A Spermatidosis
   B Spermiation
   C Spermatogenesis
   D Spermiogenesis

7 Testosterone is produced by:
   A Leydig cells in response to stimulation by LH
   B Sertoli cells in response to stimulation by FSH
   C Leydig cells in response to stimulation by FSH
   D Sertoli cells in response to stimulation by LH

8 The spermatogenic wave:
   A Is a spectator performance at athletic events
   B Ensures a continuous supply of spermatozoa
   C Is an activity of the epididymis
   D Is a friendly acknowledgement

9 The function of luteinizing hormone in the male animal is to:
   A Stimulate the production of estrogen by Sertoli cells
   B Stimulate spermatogenesis
   C Stimulate the production of testosterone by the interstitial cells (Leydig cells)
   D Cool the testicle

10 Contraction of the ischiocavernosus muscle in the bull:
   A Pulls the testis up against the external inguinal ring
   B Assists in emptying the urethra
   C Pulls the penis upward against the floor of the pelvis, which obstructs venous outflow, thereby assisting erection
   D Pulls the flaccid penis back into the prepuce

Suggested reading

Brackett, B.G. (2004) Male reproduction in mammals. In: *Dukes' Physiology of Domestic Animals*, 12th edn (ed. W.O. Reece). Cornell University Press, Ithaca, NY.

Dyce, K.M., Sack, W.O. and Wensing, C.J.G. (1996) *Textbook of Veterinary Anatomy*, 2nd edn. W.B. Saunders, Philadelphia.

Frandson, R.D., Wilke, W.L. and Fails, A.D. (2009) *Anatomy and Physiology of Farm Animals*, 7th edn. Wiley-Blackwell, Ames, IA.

Hafez, E.S.E. and Hafez, B. (2000) *Reproduction in Farm Animals*, 7th edn. Lippincott Williams & Wilkins, Baltimore.

Pineda, M.H. (2003) Male reproductive system. In: *McDonald's Veterinary Endocrinology and Reproduction*, 5th edn (eds M.H. Pineda and M.P. Dooley). Iowa State Press, Ames, IA.

Answers

1 C

2 B

3 C

4 D

5 C

6 D

7 A

8 B

9 C

10 C

William O. Reece
Iowa State University, Ames, IA, USA

The reproductive functions of the female involve production of oocytes, provision of an environment for growth and nutrition of the fetus that develops after fertilization of a mature oocyte by a spermatozoon, to give birth at an appropriate time, and to continue the nutritional function through lactation. The complex relationships of hormones and tissue changes are coordinated in order to ensure successful perpetuation of the species.

Functional anatomy of the female reproductive system

1 When conducting a rectal palpation on a cow for the components of the female reproductive system, would one search dorsally (above) or ventrally (below)? What is the relative location of the urinary bladder?

2 Do all domestic animals (intact females) ovulate over the entire surface of the ovary?

3 Compare numbers of spermatozoa and oocytes that develop from one primary spermatocyte and one primary oocyte, respectively.

4 What is the process of oocyte formation known as?

5 What are primordial follicles? Does their number at birth, aside from those destined to become mature oocytes, continue throughout the reproductive life of the female?

6 What function is served by the uterine tubes?

7 What are fimbria?

8 What is the serous covering of the uterine tubes known as?

9 What function is served by the uterus?

10 Is the endometrium glandular throughout in all domestic animals (intact females)?

11 What function is served by the glandular secretion of the endometrium?

12 Is the cervix open at all times?

13 What composes the myometrium, and what is its function?

14 What is the major support for the gravid uterus?

15 What is the landmark junction between vagina and vulva? What is the vestibule of the vagina?

16 What is the fornix?

17 What is the major blood supply to the uterus? What is fremitus?

18 What function is served by the intertwining of the uterine artery and vein?

Dukes' Physiology of Domestic Animals, Thirteenth Edition. Edited by William O. Reece, Howard H. Erickson, Jesse P. Goff and Etsuro E. Uemura.
© 2015 John Wiley & Sons, Inc. Published 2015 by John Wiley & Sons, Inc.
Companion website: www.wiley.com/go/reece/physiology

Section IX: Endocrinology, Reproduction, and Lactation

The female reproductive system consists of two ovaries and the tubular genital tract composed of two uterine tubes, uterus, vagina, and the external genitalia (Figure 53.1). The mammary glands are an important part of the reproductive system as well, and they are described separately. The location of the reproductive system relative to the rectum and bladder is shown in Figure 53.2.

Ovaries

The **ovaries** are paired glands that provide for the development of oocytes and for the production of hormones. Each ovary is located caudal to its respective right or left kidney and is suspended from the dorsal wall of the abdomen by a reflection of the peritoneum, the **mesovarium**. The mesovarium is part of the **broad ligament** (Figure 53.3), an inclusive term that also refers to the suspensions of the uterine tubes (**mesosalpinx**) and uterus (**mesometrium**). The rather pendulous suspension of the ovaries provides for easy manipulation by rectal palpation in the cow and horse. The ovaries are described as almond-shaped in most species and as bean-shaped (kidney-shaped) in the

mare (Figure 53.4). In the sow the ovary resembles a cluster of grapes (berry-shaped) because of the larger number of protruding follicles. Ovulation (release of mature oocytes) occurs throughout the entire surface of the ovary in most species but is confined to an **ovulation fossa** (an indentation) in the mare; this gives the latter its bean shape.

The ovary has a surface or superficial layer of epithelium that is underlain by the **tunica albuginea**, a connective tissue covering of the entire ovary. Beneath the tunica albuginea is the **cortex**, which contains a large mass of follicles in various stages of development. The **medulla** is centrally located and contains loose connective tissue, blood vessels, lymphatics, and nerves.

Ovarian follicles

The follicles within the cortex are classified as (i) primordial (sometimes called primary) follicles, (ii) growing follicles, and (ii) Graafian follicles (Figure 53.5). The **primordial follicles** contain a single oocyte that is surrounded by a single layer of granulosa cells. The granulosa cells are derived from the superficial epithelium, and the oocytes are derived from mitosis of oogonia in the

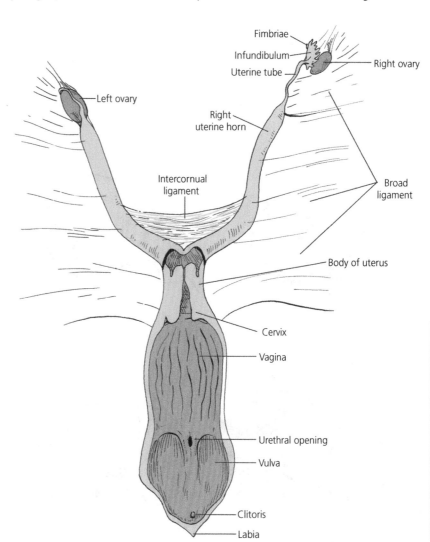

Figure 53.1 Reproductive tract of the cow (dorsal aspect). The body of the uterus, vagina, and vulva (vestibule of the vagina) have been laid open and the right ovary withdrawn from the infundibulum. The broad ligament (a downward reflection of the peritoneum) suspends the reproductive tract from the dorsolateral abdominal wall. Adapted from Reece, W.O. (2009) *Functional Anatomy and Physiology of Domestic Animals*, 4th edn. Wiley-Blackwell, Ames, IA. Reproduced with permission from Wiley.

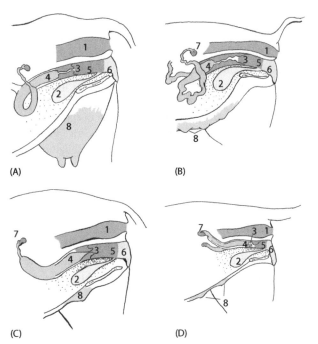

(A)

(B)

(C)

(D)

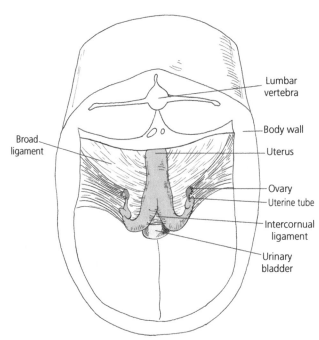

Lumbar vertebra

Body wall

Uterus

Ovary

Uterine tube

Intercornual ligament

Urinary bladder

Broad ligament

Figure 53.2 Location of reproductive organs relative to the rectum and urinary bladder: (A) cow; (B) sow; (C) mare; (D) bitch. Note species differences in anatomy of the cervix and mammary gland(s). 1, rectum; 2, urinary bladder; 3, cervix; 4, uterus; 5, vagina; 6, vulva; 7, ovary; 8, mammary gland(s). Adapted from Reece, W.O. (2009) *Functional Anatomy and Physiology of Domestic Animals*, 4th edn. Wiley-Blackwell, Ames, IA. Reproduced with permission from Wiley.

Figure 53.3 Dorso-cranial view of bovine female reproductive organs. The broad ligament is the inclusive term for the mesovarium, mesosalpinx, and mesometrium, which suspend the ovary, uterine tubes, and uterus, respectively, from the dorsolateral wall of the sublumbar region. The broad ligament is a reflection from the peritoneum. Adapted from Reece, W.O. (2009) *Functional Anatomy and Physiology of Domestic Animals*, 4th edn. Wiley-Blackwell, Ames, IA. Reproduced with permission from Wiley.

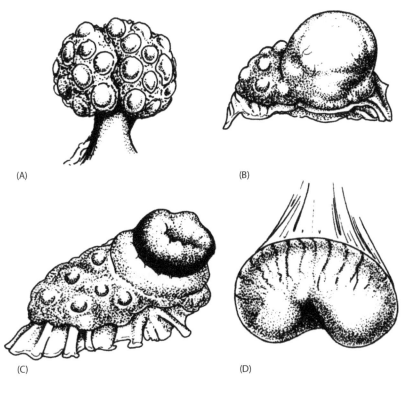

(A)

(B)

(C)

(D)

Figure 53.4 Ovarian differences resulting from species morphology and functional changes. (A) Sow ovary (berry-shaped). (B) Cow ovary (almond-shaped) with ripening follicle. (C) Cow ovary with fully developed corpus luteum. (D) Mare ovary (kidney-shaped) with ovulation fossa (indentation on the lesser curvature). From Dyce, K.M., Sack, W.O. and Wensing, C.J.G. (1996) *Textbook of Veterinary Anatomy*, 2nd edn. W.B. Saunders, Philadelphia. With permission from Elsevier.

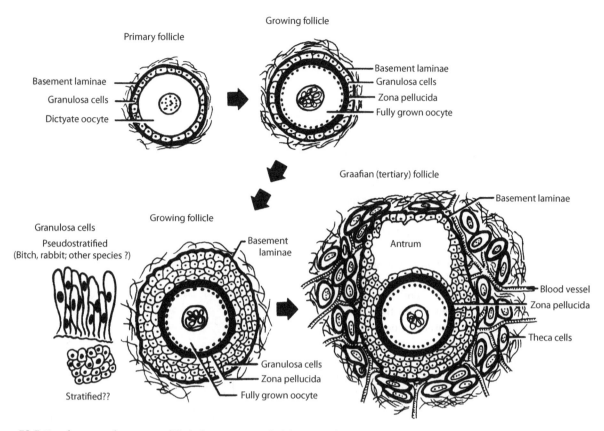

Figure 53.5 Development of an ovarian follicle from its primordial (primary) form to a Graafian follicle. Growing follicles are those that have begun growth from the resting stage as primordial follicles but have not developed thecal layers or an antrum. From Pineda, M.H. (2003) Female reproductive system. In: *McDonald's Veterinary Endocrinology and Reproduction*, 5th edn (eds M.H. Pineda and M.P. Dooley). Iowa State Press, Ames, IA. Reproduced with permission from Wiley.

embryonic genital ridge that then migrate to the ovary. **Growing follicles** are follicles that have begun growth from the resting stage as primordial follicles but have not developed a thecal layer or antrum (fluid-filled cavity; see Figure 53.5). They have two or more layers of granulosa cells surrounding the oocyte. Additional layers are added with continued growth. A zona pellucida that surrounds the oocyte may also be present. The zona pellucida provides pores through which processes of granulosa cells can interact with the oocyte surface. Also, sperm must first recognize and then contact and traverse the zona pellucida to reach the oocyte plasma membrane. **Graafian follicles** are those in which an antrum is clearly visible. Two layers of thecal cells, theca interna and theca externa, are also present (see Figure 53.5).

Follicle regression

Considerable **atresia (regression)** of the many primordial follicles occurs by birth and throughout the reproductive life of the female. At the end of the female's reproductive life, only a few primordial follicles remain, and even these undergo atresia soon thereafter. Growth of some number of primordial follicles does occur after birth and before puberty, but these never reach the Graafian follicle stage and regress. The growth that occurs before puberty is not hormone related and is probably controlled by an unknown intraovarian factor. The formation of Graafian follicles is hormone dependent and begins at puberty when tonic levels of luteinizing hormone (LH) and follicle-stimulating hormone (FSH) begin to rise and fall with each estrous cycle. Many of the follicles that undergo growth and maturation with each cycle never ovulate. Therefore, the number of primordial follicles that reach the Graafian follicle stage and proceed to ovulation is a very small fraction of the birth number.

Oogenesis

The process by which oocytes are formed is known as **oogenesis**. The oocyte of the primordial follicle is a primary oocyte that is in a quiescent (arrested) stage of meiosis. Meiosis resumes at the time of ovulation. Whereas four spermatozoa arise from one primary spermatocyte, only one oocyte develops from the reduction division of a primary oocyte. A polar body, which lacks sufficient cytoplasmic material for viability, develops when a primary oocyte divides to form a secondary oocyte. Another polar body is formed by the division of the secondary oocyte at the time of ovulation. The surviving oocyte has a haploid (n) number of chromosomes (similar to a spermatozoon) so that the union of a spermatozoon with an oocyte produces a cell with the diploid ($2n$) number of chromosomes.

Section IX: Endocrinology, Reproduction, and Lactation

Tubular genital tract

The tubular genital tract is the location for transport of spermatozoa to the oocyte. If fertilization occurs, the tract becomes the site for development of the fetus.

Uterine tubes

The **uterine tubes** are also called the oviducts and, less frequently, fallopian tubes. They are paired convoluted tubes that conduct oocytes from the ovaries to the respective horn of the uterus. The uterine tubes serve as the site for fertilization of released oocytes by spermatozoa in domestic species. The portion of each tube adjacent to its respective ovary expands to form the **infundibulum** (see Figure 53.1), and **fimbria** project from its free edge. The fimbria assist in directing the oocyte into the infundibulum at the time of ovulation.

The lumen of the uterine tubes are lined with secretory cells and ciliated cells. These cells provide an environment for the oocytes and transport the spermatozoa. Both longitudinal and circular smooth muscles are located within the walls of the uterine tubes, which assist in the transport of oocytes and spermatozoa by their contractions. The serous covering of the uterine tubes (see Figure 53.3) is known as the mesosalpinx, which is a continuation of the mesovarium and a part of the broad ligament (providing the serous support system for the internal genitalia).

Uterus

The uterus provides a place for development of the fetus if fertilization has occurred. The **uterus** consists of a **corpus (body)**, a **cervix (neck)**, and two **cornua (horns)**. The relative proportions of corpus, cornua, and cervix vary among species. The corpus is largest in the mare, less extensive in the cow and sheep, and small in the sow and bitch (Figure 53.6).

The mucous membrane lining the interior of the uterus (**endometrium**) is highly glandular. The glands are scattered throughout the entire endometrium of the uterus except in ruminants, in which the **caruncles** (mushroom-like projections from the inner surface that provide attachment for the fetal membranes) are nonglandular (Figure 53.7). The endometrium varies in thickness and vascularity with hormonal changes in the ovary and with pregnancy. The glandular secretion of the endometrium provides nutrients for the embryo before **placentation** (development of placental membranes), after which nutrition is provided by the mother's blood.

The **cervix** projects caudally into the vagina (see Figure 53.2). This heavy smooth muscle sphincter is tightly closed, except during estrus and at parturition (birth of young). The mucus seen at estrus is the secretion of cervical goblet cells. Goblet cell secretion of mucus during pregnancy and its outward flow prevents infective material from entering from the vagina.

The **myometrium** is the muscular portion of the uterus, composed of smooth muscle cells. The myometrium hypertrophies during pregnancy, increasing both in cell number and cell size. The principal function of the myometrium is aiding the expulsion of the fetus at parturition.

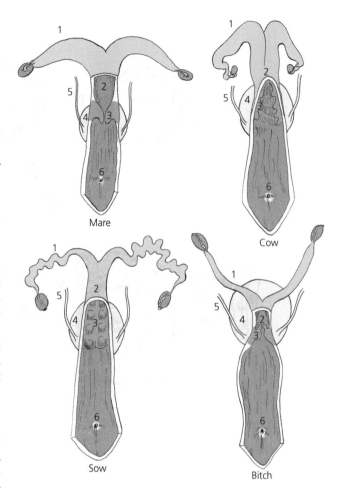

Figure 53.6 Genital tract comparisons among some domestic animals. 1, Uterine horn; 2, uterine body; 3, cervix; 4, urinary bladder; 5, ureter; 6, urethral opening. The genital tracts are opened dorsally near the body of the uterus, and the opening is extended caudally to the labia to show the cervix and urethral opening. Note that the relative proportions of uterine horns, uterine body, and cervix vary among species. The illustrations are not drawn to scale and do not compare size. Adapted from Reece, W.O. (2009) *Functional Anatomy and Physiology of Domestic Animals*, 4th edn. Wiley-Blackwell, Ames, IA. Reproduced with permission from Wiley.

The serous covering of the uterus is continuous with the mesosalpinx; in the uterus it is known as the mesometrium. The mesometrium provides a suspensory support, particularly for the nongravid uterus. It should be noted (see Figure 53.3) that there are two broad ligaments, each extending from the right or left sublumbar region and lateral pelvic wall to their respective ovary, uterine tube, uterine horn, and extending caudally onto the body of the uterus. The **gravid (pregnant) uterus** enlarges, and major support is provided by the abdominal wall (Figure 53.8).

Vagina

The **vagina** is the portion of the birth canal located within the pelvis, between the uterus cranially and the vulva caudally (see Figures 53.1 and 53.2). The vagina serves as a sheath for the male

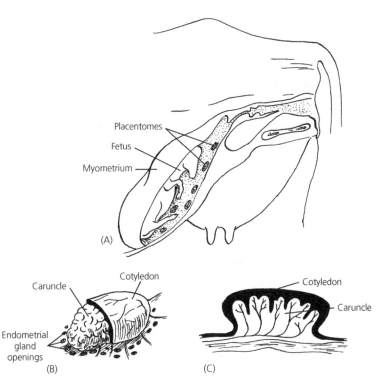

Figure 53.7 Relationship of the bovine fetal placenta to the maternal endometrium. (A) View of fetus within the uterus showing multiple placentomes. (B) Magnification of a placentome that is surrounded by a number of endometrial gland openings. Only a part of the fetal cotyledon is shown so that the underlying maternal caruncle and endometrial gland openings can be visualized. (C) Cross-section of a placentome. The contribution by the fetal placenta is known as the cotyledon, and the maternal contribution is known as the caruncle. Adapted from Reece, W.O. (2009) *Functional Anatomy and Physiology of Domestic Animals*, 4th edn. Wiley-Blackwell, Ames, IA. Reproduced with permission from Wiley.

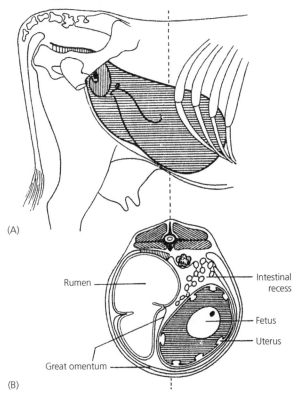

Figure 53.8 Position of the cow's uterus. (A) The nongravid uterus (vertical striping) compared with the 6-month gravid uterus (horizontal striping). (B) Location of the 6-month gravid uterus in transverse section (rumen on left and uterus on right side of abdomen). From Dyce, K.M. and Wensing, C.J.G. (1971) *Essentials of Bovine Anatomy*. Lea & Febiger, Philadelphia. Reproduced with permission from Wolter Kluwer.

penis during copulation. It is lined with stratified squamous epithelium, which is glandless. The **fornix** is the space formed cranial to the projection of the cervix into the vagina. In some animals the fornix is only visible dorsally, whereas in others it can completely encircle the cervix or be entirely absent (as in the pig).

External genitalia

The **external genitalia** consists of the **vulva**, **labia**, and **clitoris**. The vulva is the caudal portion of the female genitalia that extends from the vagina to the exterior. The external urethral orifice (opening) is the landmark junction of vagina and vulva. The **vestibule of the vagina** (Figure 53.9) is another name for the vulva. It is that part of the external genitalia between the vagina and the labia (lips of the vulva). The clitoris (female vestigial counterpart of the penis) is concealed by the lowest part of the vulva. The clitoris is supplied with erectile tissue and sensory nerve endings. The external part of the vulva is its vertical opening, the labia (see Figure 53.1).

Blood supply of female genitalia

The ovary and oviduct receive their blood supply from the **ovarian artery**, while the vagina receives its blood supply from the **vaginal artery** (Figure 53.10). The major blood supply to the uterus comes from the **uterine artery** (formerly called the middle uterine artery). The cranial part of the uterus is also supplied with blood from the ovarian artery, and the caudal part of the uterus receives blood from the vaginal artery. During pregnancy, the blood supply to the uterus increases dramatically. When the uterine artery is palpated, vibration of the blood within it can be felt. This is called **fremitus**, and is considered to

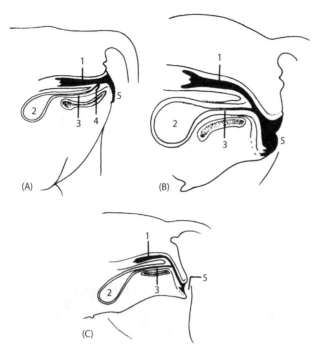

Figure 53.9 Species variations in position of the vestibule of the vagina: (A) cow; (B) mare; (C) bitch. The vulva, and hence the vestibule of the vagina, extends caudally from the external urethral orifice. 1, vagina; 2, bladder; 3, urethra; 4, suburethral diverticulum; 5, vulva. From Dyce, K.M., Sack, W.O. and Wensing, C.J.G. (2010) *Textbook of Veterinary Anatomy*, 4th edn. W.B. Saunders, Philadelphia. With permission from Elsevier.

be a good indicator of pregnancy. The ovarian artery is coiled and adheres closely to the uterine vein (Figure 53.11). Such an arrangement is important for diffusion of the hormone **prostaglandin (PG)F$_{2\alpha}$** (see Chapter 51) from the uterine vein to the ovarian artery in some species (e.g., cow and ewe, perhaps others). Early transport by this arrangement avoids the general circulation, where much of it would be inactivated by vascular endothelial cells in the lungs. Production requirements are lower because most of the PGF$_{2\alpha}$ produced goes only to the target organ (ovary) and avoids general circulation (and subsequent inactivation) to all body parts. PGF$_{2\alpha}$ at the ovarian site initiates **luteolysis** (termination of the corpus luteum).

Hormones of female reproduction

1 Are diethylstilbestrol and estradiol-17β both estrogens? Are they both steroids?

2 Which female steroid hormone has activities that are performed in concert with estrogens and usually requires previous estrogen priming?

3 Which female steroid hormone prevents contractility of the uterus during pregnancy?

4 What are the main functions of the gonadotropins in the female?

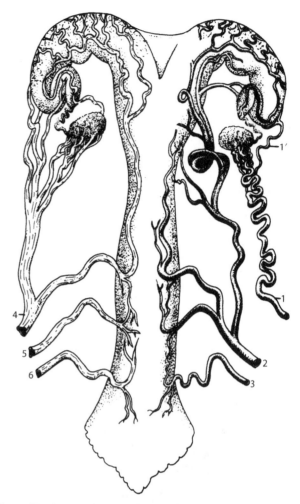

Figure 53.10 Ventral view of blood supply to the reproductive tract of the cow. The arteries are shown on the right side and the veins on the left. 1, ovarian artery; 1′, uterine branch; 2, uterine artery; 3, vaginal artery; 4, ovarian vein; 5, uterine vein; 6, vaginal vein. From Dyce, K.M., Sack, W.O. and Wensing, C.J.G. (2010) *Textbook of Veterinary Anatomy*, 4th edn. W.B. Saunders, Philadelphia. With permission from Elsevier.

5 Are tonic levels of the gonadotropins in the female increased or decreased by estrogens?

6 What is the role of the hypophysioportal system in the release of FSH and LH?

7 What is the significance of gradually increasing concentrations of estrogen over a period of time on LH release?

The principal hormones associated with ovarian cycling, pregnancy, and parturition are estrogens, progesterone, and gonadotropins.

Estrogens

Estrogens occur naturally and synthetically. The important estrogens in mammals are steroids, produced by the ovary (granulosa cells of follicles), placenta, and adrenal cortex. A common synthetic estrogen is **diethylstilbestrol**, which is not a steroid but a complex alcohol with estrogenic properties. The chemical structures of diethylstilbestrol and estradiol-17β (a steroid) are compared in Figure 53.12. Regardless of production site, steroids share a common biosynthetic pathway (Figure 53.13).

Estradiol-17β and estrone are estrogens that predominate in domestic nonpregnant and pregnant animals, respectively. Generally, the principal function of the estrogens is to cause cellular proliferation and growth of the tissues related to reproduction. Tissue responses caused by estrogens include:

1 stimulation of endometrial gland growth;
2 stimulation of duct growth in the mammary gland;
3 increase in secretory activity of uterine ducts;
4 initiation of sexual receptivity;
5 regulation of secretion of LH by the anterior pituitary gland;
6 possible regulation of $PGF_{2\alpha}$ release from the nongravid and gravid uterus;
7 early union of the epiphysis with the shafts of long bones, whereby growth of long bones ceases;
8 protein anabolism; and
9 epitheliotropic activity.

The protein anabolic effect of estrogens is less pronounced than that associated with testosterone. Its effect is probably associated more specifically with the sex organs rather than with a generalized effect. The epitheliotropic function manifests at estrus when the epithelium in the vagina proliferates and cornification is more prevalent.

Progesterone

Progesterone, like the estrogens, is a steroid sex hormone produced by the corpus luteum (CL) of the ovary, placenta, and adrenal cortex. Its place in the common biosynthetic pathway is shown in Figure 53.13. It is the principal progestational hormone. Certain synthetic and natural progestational agents are called **progestins**.

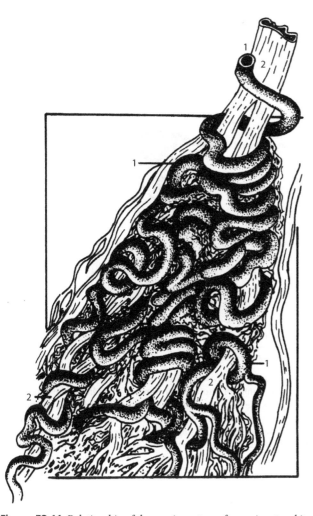

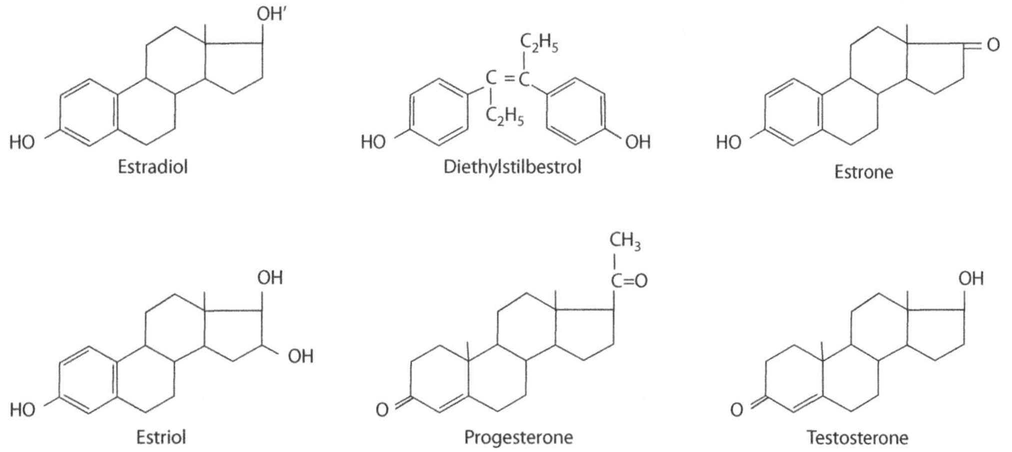

Figure 53.11 Relationship of the ovarian artery of a ruminant and its branches (1) with those of the uterine vein (2). The intertwining ensures a large area of contact. From Dyce, K.M., Sack, W.O. and Wensing, C.J.G. (2002) *Textbook of Veterinary Anatomy*, 3rd edn. W.B. Saunders, Philadelphia. With permission from Elsevier.

Figure 53.12 Chemical structure of some steroid hormones, and diethylstilbestrol. From Pineda, M.H. (2003) Female reproduction system. In: *McDonald's Veterinary Endocrinology and Reproduction*, 5th edn (eds M.H. Pineda and M.P. Dooley). Iowa State Press, Ames, IA. Reproduced with permission from Wiley.

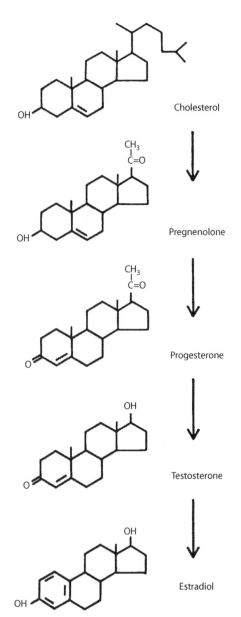

Figure 53.13 Biosynthesis of steroid hormones from cholesterol. From Hafez, E.S.E. and Hafez, B. (2000) *Reproduction in Farm Animals*, 7th edn. Lippincott Williams & Wilkins, Baltimore.

The activities associated with progesterone are often performed in concert with estrogens, and usually require previous estrogen priming. The functions of progesterone include (i) promotion of endometrial gland growth, (ii) stimulation of secretory activity of the oviduct and endometrial glands to provide nutrients for the developing embryo before implantation, (iii) promotion of lobuloalveolar growth in the mammary gland, (iv) prevention of contractility of the uterus during pregnancy, and (v) regulation of secretion of gonadotropins.

The interrelationships of the estrogens, progesterone, and gonadotropins are described later in the discussions of the estrous cycle and pregnancy.

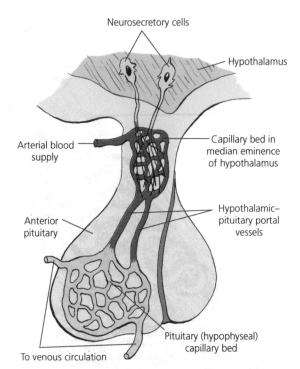

Figure 53.14 The hypophysioportal circulation involved with the secretion of anterior pituitary hormones. Cell bodies in the hypothalamus sense the need for a hormone and secrete a releasing hormone into the hypothalamic capillary bed. The releasing hormone enters the hypophyseal capillary bed and diffuses to specific cells, causing them to secrete their specific hormone. Adapted from Reece, W.O. (2009) *Functional Anatomy and Physiology of Domestic Animals*, 4th edn. Wiley-Blackwell, Ames, IA. Reproduced with permission from Wiley.

Gonadotropins

Follicle-stimulating hormone and **luteinizing hormone** are collectively referred to as the gonadotropins because of their role in stimulating cells within the ovary and testis (the gonads). FSH and LH are hormones secreted by cells within the anterior pituitary. Both are classified chemically as **glycoproteins**. A glycoprotein is a conjugated protein in which the nonprotein group is a carbohydrate.

The main function of FSH in the female is promotion of the growth of follicles. LH is important for the ovulatory process and the luteinization of the granulosa, an essential aspect of CL formation. Apparently, FSH and LH concentrations exist in the plasma at a tonic or basal level. These levels are controlled by negative feedback from the gonads. Tonic levels are increased by estrogen and decreased by progesterone.

The release of FSH and LH from the anterior pituitary is controlled by a releasing hormone from the hypothalamus. The circulatory system involved is known as the **hypophysioportal system** (Figure 53.14). A portal system begins with capillaries and terminates with capillaries. The hypothalamic capillaries receive a secretion from sensing cells in the hypothalamus known as **gonadotropin-releasing hormone (GnRH)**. GnRH is secreted in response to low levels of LH or FSH and is then followed by secretion of LH or FSH.

The concentrations of estrogens and progesterone also influence the amount of LH or FSH secretion. Generally, an increasing concentration of estrogen causes an increase in sensitivity of the anterior pituitary to GnRH, and results in increased release of gonadotropins. Progesterone decreases sensitivity of the anterior pituitary to GnRH, and LH and FSH concentrations decrease. These influences, particularly that of estrogen, depend on gradually increasing concentrations of estrogen over a period of time, which results in the preovulatory surge of LH release. Conversely, when estrogen concentration is basal and of short duration, LH and FSH secretions are suppressed.

Ovarian follicle activity

1 How do growing follicles become Graafian follicles?

2 What part of the Graafian follicle secretes androgens? Do androgens persist as androgens?

3 What hormones cause the formation of a fluid-filled space called an antrum?

4 What functions are served by the preovulatory (24 hours) surge of LH?

5 Do all animals ovulate before the end of estrus? What is the difference between spontaneous and reflex ovulation?

6 Does ovulation occur in all developing follicles? Do follicles continue to grow and develop during all phases of the ovarian cycle? What must be a characteristic of follicles for them to ovulate?

7 What changes are involved in the formation of the corpus luteum? How is the corpus luteum maintained?

8 What is the natural luteolytic substance that causes regression of the corpus luteum? Does acute regression of the corpus luteum occur in the bitch and queen?

9 Note the unique delivery system of the natural luteolytic substance.

10 What is a persistent corpus luteum, and what is its most probable cause?

When reproductive cycling begins, select follicles within the ovary are influenced by hormones and proceed through growth and maturity, followed by ovulation, and development and regression of the corpus luteum. These changes recur for other follicles at intervals characteristic for a species.

Follicular growth

Puberty is defined as the beginning of reproductive life, which in the female is usually marked by the beginning of ovarian activity. The formation of Graafian follicles from growing follicles is hormone dependent and begins at puberty when tonic levels of LH and FSH begin to rise and fall with each estrous cycle. Interstitial cells begin to surround the basement membrane of the granulosa cells to form the **theca**, which differentiates into a **theca interna** and **externa**. As the thecal cells are formed around the follicle, a capillary bed develops among them.

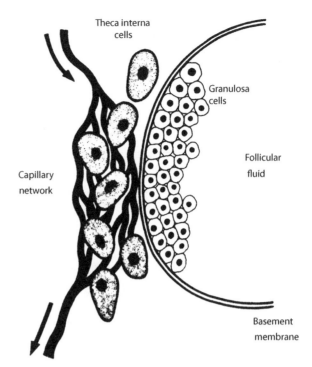

Figure 53.15 Formation of a Graafian follicle from a growing follicle. Wall structure. The theca interna cells are well supplied with blood. The basement membrane deprives granulosa cells of blood supply. From Baird, D.T. (1972) Reproductive hormones. In: *Reproduction in Mammals, Book 3* (eds C.R. Austin and R.V. Short). Cambridge University Press, Cambridge, UK. Reproduced with permission of Cambridge University Press.

These **thecal capillaries** increase in size and are concentrated in the theca interna close to the basement membrane that separates the theca interna cells from the granulosa cells (Figure 53.15). LH receptors form on the cells of the theca interna, and receptors for FSH and estrogen form on the granulosa cells.

During the hormone-dependent stage, under the influence of LH, **androgens** are produced by cells of the theca interna. The androgens diffuse from the theca interna to the granulosa cells. Under the influence of FSH, the granulosa cells convert the androgens to estrogens. The estrogens produced cause growth and division of the granulosa cells and, together with FSH, cause the granulosa cells to produce secretions that effect separation of the granulosa cells and formation of a space filled with **fluid (liquor folliculi)**, called an **antrum** (Figure 53.15). Also, FSH stimulates the formation of LH receptors on the granulosa cells. A surge of LH output (**preovulatory surge**) occurs about 24 hours before ovulation. In addition to its role in ovulation and formation of a corpus luteum, the LH surge causes a reduction in the number of FSH receptors on granulosa cells, so that the output of estrogen by the granulosa cells decreases.

Ovulation

When the oocyte is released into the abdomen from its protruding follicle, it is covered by those granulosa cells that immediately surrounded it just before ovulation; these are known as

Table 53.1 Factors related to female reproduction.

Animal	Onset of puberty (months)	Age first service (average)	Length of estrous cycle (days)	Length of estrus	Gestation period (days)
Mare	18 (10–24)	2–3 years	21 (19–21)	5 (4.5–7.5) days	336 (323–341)
Cow	4–24	14–22 months	21 (18–24)	18 (12–28) hours	282 (274–291)
Ewe	4–12 (first fall)	12–18 months	16.5 (14–20)	24–48 hours	150 (140–160)
Sow	3–7	8–10 months	21 (18–24)	2 (1–5) days	114 (110–116)
Bitch	6–24	12–18 months	6–12 months	9 (5–19) days	63 (60–65)

	Time of ovulation	Optimum time for service	Advisable time to breed after parturition
Mare	1–2 days before end of estrus	3–4 days before end of estrus; or second or third day of estrus	About 25–35 days or second estrus; about 9 days or first estrus only if normal in every way
Cow	10–15 hours after end of estrus	Just before middle of estrus to end of estrus	60–90 days
Ewe	12–24 hours before end of estrus	18–24 hours after onset of estrus	Usually the next fall
Sow	30–36 hours after onset of estrus	12–30 hours after onset of estrus	First estrus 3–9 days after weaning pigs
Bitch	1–2 days after onset of true estrus	2–3 days after onset of estrus; or 10–14 days after onset of proestrous bleeding	Usually first estrus or 2–3 months after weaning pups

Source: Frandson, R.D. and Spurgeon, T.L. (1992) *Anatomy and Physiology of Farm Animals*, 5th edn. Lea & Febiger, Philadelphia. Reproduced with permission from Wiley.

the **corona radiata**. The oocyte and granulosa cells are evacuated with an enveloping viscous (gelatinous) follicular fluid. At ovulation, the oocyte, together with its surrounding cells and gelatinous mass, is swept into the uterine tubes by motility of the fimbriae. The relationship of ovulation to estrus for domestic animals, and other factors involved in female reproduction, is given in Table 53.1.

Ovulation is spontaneous (no stimulation needed) in all the domestic species except the cat. The cat and other nonspontaneous ovulators (e.g., mink, rabbit, ferret) are **reflex ovulators**, in that coitus is required for ovulation to occur. Coital contact apparently brings forth an LH surge.

The selection of follicles for ovulation seems to occur primarily by chance. It is usually associated with the largest actively growing follicles present when the previous CL regressed (i.e., when progesterone decreased and FSH and LH output began to increase). Follicles continue to grow and develop during all phases of the ovarian cycle, with some impairment during the luteal phase, and the LH surge is necessary for ovulation to occur. Follicles close to full development, but without adequate LH receptors, do not ovulate in response to the LH surge and become atretic.

Corpus luteum formation and regression

Formation of the CL involves **luteinization of the granulosa**, by which the granulosa is converted from estrogen secretion to progesterone secretion (LH receptors on the granulosa cells were previously induced by FSH). The process is initiated by the preovulatory LH surge. The cavity of the ruptured follicle and the fibrin clot within serve as the framework on which the granulosa cells develop. Blood vessels from the theca externa invade

the developing CL, and it becomes vascularized. Maintenance of the CL is provided by LH derived from the LH surge and by the basal circulating levels of LH. In the sheep, prolactin, a gonadotropic hormone for some species, is required to maintain the CL, in addition to LH.

The uterus (endometrium) plays a major role in controlling the lifespan of the CL in nonpregnant mares, cows, sows, ewes, and does (goats), but is not active in CL regression in the bitch (dog) and queen (cat). $PGF_{2\alpha}$ is released by the nonpregnant uterus about 14 days after ovulation and is considered to be the natural luteolytic substance (causes regression of the CL). The venous return of uterine blood to the right heart and from there to the lung before transport of arterial blood to the ovary results in inactivation by the vascular endothelium of about 90% of $PGF_{2\alpha}$. To ensure that enough $PGF_{2\alpha}$ is delivered directly to the ovary for luteolysis, the anatomic arrangement of the uterine vein and ovarian artery is such that $PGF_{2\alpha}$ can diffuse from the vein to the artery and ovarian perfusion of $PGF_{2\alpha}$ can occur before circulation through the lungs (Figure 53.16). For $PGF_{2\alpha}$ to be effective when it enters the general circulation, it must either be secreted by the uterus in larger amounts, or be more resistant to degradation in the lungs, or both. Survival of $PGF_{2\alpha}$ in the general circulation is more important in the sow and mare.

The reason for final regression of the CL in the bitch and queen (bitch, 75 days; queen, 35 days) is not known. An acute lytic process does not occur.

Persistent corpus luteum

Prolongation of the luteal phase beyond 14 days to perhaps 1–5 months is known as **persistent corpus luteum**. The presence of a persistent CL prevents a return to the follicular phase and its next ovulation. The immediate reason for persistent CL is the failure of the endometrium to synthesize $PGF_{2\alpha}$. Often the failure is caused by an acute or chronic endometrial inflammation.

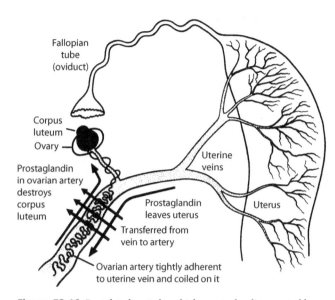

Figure 53.16 Postulated route by which prostaglandin secreted by the progesterone-primed uterus can enter the ovarian artery and destroy the corpus luteum in the ewe, and possibly other species. From Short, R.V. (1972) Role of hormones in sex cycles. In: *Reproduction in Mammals, Book 3* (eds C.R. Austin and R.V. Short). Cambridge University Press, Cambridge, UK. Reproduced with permission of Cambridge University Press.

Summary of ovarian cycle events

Events in the ovary associated with the cycle of hormone changes can be summarized as follows.

1 After regression of the CL (luteolysis caused by $PGF_{2\alpha}$), FSH and LH secretion increase (because of a decrease in the concentration of progesterone).

2 LH stimulates secretion of androgens by the theca interna cells, which diffuse into the granulosa cells.

3 FSH stimulates conversion of androgen to estrogen by the granulosa cells, and the estrogen concentration gradually increases.

4 FSH stimulates the formation of LH receptors on the granulosa cells.

5 Estrogen-rich fluid formed by the granulosa cells separates the granulosa cells and forms a pocket known as an antrum.

6 The gradually increasing estrogen concentration causes a preovulatory surge of LH release.

7 The LH surge promotes the maturation of oocytes by resuming meiosis through the first polar body stage.

8 The LH surge promotes the intrafollicular production of PGA and PGE, associated with rupture of the follicle.

9 Concomitant with PGA and PGE production is the formation of multivesicular bodies (MVB), which form as out-pockets of the exposed theca externa.

10 MVBs seem to secrete proteolytic enzymes that digest ground substance cementing the theca externa fibroblasts, allowing escape of the oocyte (ovulation).

11 The LH surge causes reduction in the number of FSH receptors on the granulosa cells, so the rate of conversion of androgen to estrogen diminishes.

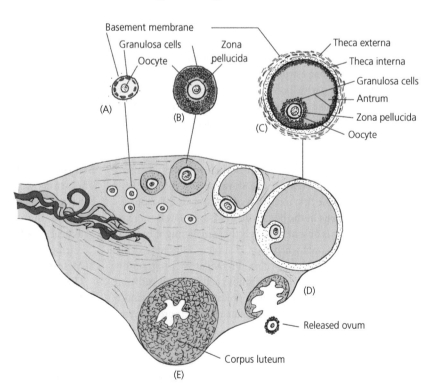

Figure 53.17 Sagittal section of an ovary. (A) Primary follicle. (B) Growing follicle. (C) Graafian follicle. (D) Ruptured follicle. (E) Corpus luteum. This schematic representation shows in sequence the origin, growth, and rupture of a Graafian follicle and a corpus luteum that develops from the remains of the ruptured follicle. Adapted from Reece, W.O. (2009) *Functional Anatomy and Physiology of Domestic Animals*, 4th edn. Wiley-Blackwell, Ames, IA. Reproduced with permission from Wiley.

Section IX: Endocrinology, Reproduction, and Lactation

12 LH attaches to granulosa cell LH receptors and begins the conversion of the granulosa from estrogen secretion in the follicular phase to progesterone secretion in the luteal phase.

13 At some point in the latter stages of these events, ovulation occurs, and the cavity previously occupied by the mature follicle becomes a CL.

14 The CL secretes progesterone, which causes a decrease in the output of FSH and LH by the anterior pituitary.

15 The CL regresses, and the output of progesterone begins to decrease.

16 A decrease in the level of progesterone causes FSH and LH secretion to increase, and the cycle is repeated.

The ovarian events are illustrated in Figure 53.17.

Sexual receptivity

> 1 What hormone is required for the initiation of sexual receptivity in all animals?
>
> 2 How does progesterone enhance receptivity in some domestic animal species?
>
> 3 What domestic animal species require estrogen synergism with progesterone?

If copulation is to occur near ovulation, the female must be receptive to the male. Initiation of sexual receptivity in all animals requires estrogen derived from the antral follicles. Also, in some species (e.g., bitch, ewe, sow, cow), progesterone acts synergistically with estrogen for manifestation of receptivity. Neurons associated with a "**sex center**" are located diffusely in the hypothalamus and are critical in initiating the mechanisms of sexual behavior as a response to hormones. It seems that progesterone (tonic levels) acts as a primer for the hypothalamic sexual centers so that estrogen becomes effective. During the postpartum (after parturition) period in some cows and sows, the low progesterone concentration fails to prime the sexual centers of the hypothalamus, and the animals are not sexually receptive at the time of the first postpartum ovulation. In sheep, the priming of the hypothalamus with progesterone is essential, after their seasonal anestrus, before sexual receptivity is manifested. Accordingly, ewes do not show sexual receptivity in conjunction with the first ovulation of the breeding season.

During **proestrus** in the bitch, when estrogen levels increase, sexual receptivity is absent although the female might be sexually attractive. It is only when the LH surge occurs near ovulation that sexual receptivity occurs. Preovulatory progesterone from the LH surge (luteinized granulosa cells) can be sufficient to prime the hypothalamus. Before proestrus, a long period of sexual inactivity (**anestrus**) occurs, during which progesterone levels are either low or nonexistent.

Some evidence has shown that GnRH has a role in the manifestation of sexual receptivity. Injection of GnRH without estrogen has been found to cause sexual posturing in some animals.

Also, the onset of sexual receptivity is correlated closely with the preovulatory LH surge as caused by GnRH release.

Progesterone is not synergistic with estrogen in manifesting sexual receptivity in the doe, queen, and mare.

Estrous cycle and related factors

> 1 How is an estrous cycle interval defined?
>
> 2 Know the stages of the estrous cycle and their relationships to ovarian activity.
>
> 3 Which steroid hormone predominates during the follicular periods?
>
> 4 Which stage of the estrous cycle is characterized by sexual receptivity?
>
> 5 Review photoperiod influence on the cat, horse, sheep, and goat. What does "turn-on" and "turn-off" time relate to?
>
> 6 How is nutrition related to puberty and postparturient resumption of ovarian activity?
>
> 7 Note species characteristics associated with their estrous cycles: cow – post-estrus ovulation; ewe – short estrous cycle interval; bitch – vaginal cytologic changes and classical pseudopregnancy; queen – reflex ovulation, signs of estrus, coital behavior.

The term **estrous cycle** refers to the rhythmic phenomenon observed in all mammals involving regular but limited periods of sexual receptivity (estrus) that occur at intervals characteristic of a species. **One cycle interval** is defined as the time from the onset of one period of sexual receptivity to the next (the ovulatory interval).

Animals are usually classified as **monestrous** or **polyestrous**. Monestrous animals are characterized by experiencing estrus once each year. Most wild carnivorous mammals are monestrous and, with some variation, the bitch is usually considered to be monestrous. Polyestrous animals, including most domestic species, have more than one period of estrus in a year. A seasonally polyestrous animal is one that has repeated estrous cycles within a physiologic breeding season (some part of a year), followed by a period of anestrus until the next breeding season.

Stages of estrous cycle

The estrous cycle can be divided into several stages according to behavioral or ovarian changes.

1 **Estrus**: the time of sexual receptivity, sometimes referred to as heat. Ovulation usually, but not always, occurs at the end of estrus.

2 **Metestrus**: the early postovulatory period, during which the CL begins development.

3 **Diestrus**: the period of mature luteal activity, which begins about 4 days after ovulation and ends with regression of the CL.

4 **Proestrus**: the period beginning after CL regression and ending at the onset of estrus. During proestrus, rapid follicle development leads to ovulation and to the onset of sexual receptivity.

The **follicular periods (proestrus and estrus)** are characterized by estrogen dominance. From the behavioral standpoint, the estrus/sexually receptive period encompasses estrus, and the diestrus/sexually nonreceptive period includes metestrus, diestrus, and proestrus.

Photoperiod

Among the domestic animals the seasonal breeders are considered to be the queen, doe, ewe, and mare. These animals are sexually inactive during certain times of the year. The resumption of sexual activity is correlated with conception, so that birth occurs when environmental conditions are more conducive to survival of the young.

The most important factor associated with seasonal breeding is **photoperiod** (relative lengths of alternating periods of light and dark). Both the queen and mare become **anestrous** (without estrous cycles) late in the fall ("turn-off" time) because of decreasing light, and ovarian cycles are resumed in late winter or early spring ("turn-on" time) by increasing light. The phenomenon in the ewe and doe is opposite to that of the queen and mare, in that the ovarian cycle has a turn-on time associated with a decrease in daylight and a turn-off time associated with an increase in daylight. Not only do differences in photoperiod response among species exist, but so do those within species as a result of genetic (breed) differences. Intraspecies difference is most apparent among sheep breeds and probably relates to their origin and related environmental differences. A representation of photoperiod influence on ovarian activity is shown for the queen, mare, ewe, and doe in Figure 53.18. Approximate dates of turn-on and turn-off vary according to distance from the equator and associated differences in photoperiods.

Nutrition

The influence of nutrition on the estrous cycle is most apparent at puberty and on reestablishment of the estrous cycle after parturition. Animals ingesting sound nutritional regimens reach puberty at an earlier age than nutritionally deprived animals. Consequently, breeding seasons can be delayed if calves are deprived of adequate nutrition. After parturition and during early lactation, cows can have a negative metabolic balance, which can result in an increased interval between parturition and resumption of ovarian activity.

Species characteristics

Whereas the general pattern of the estrous cycle is similar among the domestic species, differences are noted in duration, not only for the cycle but also for stages within the cycle. Duration of the cycle and for estrus is shown in Table 53.1 for domestic animals. The age of puberty onset also varies, and for some species it is affected by the breeding season for that species.

Cow

Smaller breeds of cows usually reach puberty at an earlier age than larger breeds (Jersey, 8 months; Holstein, 11 months). Behavioral changes associated with estrus include restlessness,

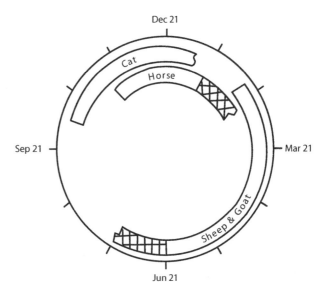

Figure 53.18 Effects of photoperiod on ovarian activity in the cat, horse, sheep, and goat at a latitude of 38.5° N (California). The open bars represent periods of ovarian inactivity (anestrus). The transition from anestrus to estrus (often erratic) is shown by the cross-hatched portion of the bars for the horse, sheep, and goat. From Stabenfeldt, G.H. and Edqvist, L. (1993) Female reproductive processes. In: *Dukes' Physiology of Domestic Animals*, 11th edn (eds M.J. Swenson and W.O. Reece). Cornell University Press, Ithaca, NY. With permission from Cornell University Press.

mounting activity, standing to be mounted, being more alert to other animals, and decreased appetite. At the same time, decreased milk production, mucus discharge from the vulva, and redness and relaxation of the vulva are noted. It is important to detect estrus so that the correct time for artificial insemination can be determined.

Most domestic animals ovulate toward the end of estrus, but the cow ovulates 12–14 hours after estrus. The most successful artificial insemination occurs when it is performed about 12 hours after the beginning of estrus. In the cow, therefore, insemination precedes ovulation, and optimum fertilization is coupled with expected spermatozoon and oocyte life and with capacitation. Capacitation refers to the modification of ejaculated or inseminated spermatozoa within the female reproductive tract, enabling the spermatozoa to fertilize oocytes. The fertile life for bovine spermatozoa (time in female genitalia) is 30–48 hours and for bovine oocytes (after ovulation) is 20–24 hours. The effect of time of insemination on conception rate in cattle is shown in Figure 53.19.

Mare

The onset of puberty in the mare occurs during the breeding season after birth. If the interval between birth and the next breeding season is short (e.g., summer birth), puberty can be delayed for 12 months. A wide range of age for puberty is seen in the mare, from 12 to 18 months.

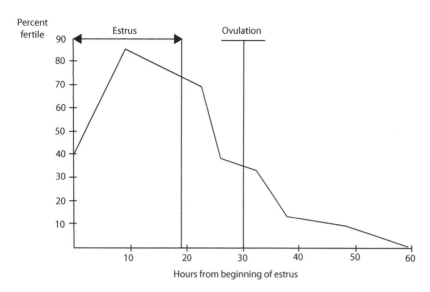

Figure 53.19 The effect of time of insemination on conception rate in cattle. Conception rate is best when inseminated about 10 hours from beginning of estrus. From Stabenfeldt, G.H. and Edqvist, L. (1993) Female reproductive processes. In: *Dukes' Physiology of Domestic Animals*, 11th edn (eds M.J. Swenson and W.O. Reece). Cornell University Press, Ithaca, NY. With permission from Cornell University Press.

The transition from winter anestrus to estrus in late winter or early spring is often erratic, in that follicles might be grown but not ovulated. This results in prolonged estrous periods. After the first ovulation, the length of the estrous cycle stabilizes, and the duration of estrus is 5–6 days.

Ovulation occurs about 24 hours before the end of estrus and causes the end of estrus, which is a good indication that ovulation has occurred. Signs of estrus in the mare are elevation of the tail, standing with the hindlegs apart, squatting and urinating, and rhythmically erecting the clitoris.

Ewe

Where lambs are normally born between December and March (in the northern hemisphere), puberty onset occurs the next fall, at about 8–9 months of age.

The estrous cycle in sheep is shorter than in the other domestic species because the antral phase of follicle growth is 3–4 days shorter. The physiologic breeding season lasts 6–7 months, during which repeated estrous cycles are observed in the absence of pregnancy.

A prominent sign of estrus is fluttering of the tail. Also, females separated from males by a barrier often assume a close proximity to the barrier.

Sow

Pigs born at any time of the year reach puberty at 6–7 months of age. Ovulation rates are more pronounced at the third estrus after puberty.

Signs of estrus include swelling of the vulva, restlessness, and decreased appetite. Application of pressure on the sow's back during estrus elicits the rigidity reflex that occurs during natural mating with a boar.

Ovulation occurs from both ovaries, and 14–16 oocytes can be released. Because of the large number of follicles or corpora lutea at any one time, the sow ovaries often appear to be lobulated (see Figure 53.4).

Doe

The breeding season and gestation periods are similar for goats and sheep, and puberty is reached at about the same age (8–9 months). Breeding is often delayed, however, until the next breeding season.

Signs of estrus in the doe are similar to those in the ewe. When mating occurs, intromission and ejaculation are accomplished rapidly, usually within several seconds.

Pseudopregnancy is a condition in which a female displays most of the signs of pregnancy but is not pregnant. Enlargement of the uterus occurs as a result of fluid accumulation. This phenomenon occurs in the goat and is believed to be caused by prolongation of the CL (see section Persistent corpus luteum). The injection of $PGF_{2\alpha}$ results in CL regression and discharge of the accumulated uterine fluid.

Bitch

The onset of puberty in the bitch occurs 2–3 months after she reaches adult size. Among breeds it ranges from 6 to 12 months of age.

The bitch has an unusually long period of ovarian inactivity (anestrus) that is unrelated to photoperiod or nutrition. Because of this she is sometimes considered to be monestrous. Estrous cycles are common at all times of the year. The stages of the estrous cycle are different from those of the other species in that each is longer. Proestrus and estrus are each 7–10 days long, and diestrus is prolonged, lasting 70–80 days.

The LH surge occurs at the end of proestrus, followed by ovulation in 24–48 hours. The bitch might be sexually attractive during proestrus but is not sexually receptive until after the LH surge. Progesterone secretion thereafter is essential for receptivity and although the estrogen level declines, sexual receptivity is maintained for 7–10 days.

Vaginal cytologic changes seem to be more pronounced in bitches than in other domestic species and have been correlated with each estrous cycle stage. Vaginal smears are useful for assessing the stage of estrus and for predicting the most suitable time for breeding. The principal cytologic changes are (i) thickening and cornification of the vaginal epithelium; (ii) loss of leukocytes because of the thickened epithelium; and (iii) appearance of erythrocytes from the developing vascular system of the endometrium.

Among those animals that show pseudopregnancy, it is most often seen in the bitch. In the absence of pregnancy the CL persists, and during the exaggerated diestrus progesterone continues to be produced for 50–80 days. This is a normal phenomenon in bitches because the uterus is not active in CL regression (production of $PGF_{2\alpha}$). The endometrium hypertrophies and endometrial glands develop, although no fetus is present. Some bitches have no other signs of the prolonged elevation of progesterone concentration, but others have mammary gland enlargement and relaxation of the pelvis. Occasionally, a maternal attitude develops that leads to nest building. Rarely, lactation begins and the bitch shows signs of labor.

The long period of progesterone dominance (long diestrus), coupled with the relatively long period of regression of the endometrium after luteolysis of the CL, predisposes the endometrium to pyometra (pus in the uterus). Pyometra is common in older bitches.

Queen

Cats born in the spring and summer months reach puberty in the next breeding season, at about 6–8 months of age. Cats born in the fall and early winter have their puberty delayed for 1 year, until the next breeding season. The breeding season is considered to be January to October in the northern hemisphere.

If the queen does not have coitus, ovulation does not occur and no luteal phase intervenes until the next cycle. However, the 8-day follicular phase is followed by an 8-day period of ovarian inactivity. If queens have coital contact but fail to conceive, a luteal phase prolongs the onset of the next proestrus, with a minimum time of 42 days between estrus. Pseudopregnancy occurs in queens if a luteal phase occurs without pregnancy. Development of the uterus, mammary glands, and abdomen is not as marked as in the bitch, and nest building and lactation seldom occur.

Signs of estrus in queens include an increase in affection, which can be shown to almost any object – humans, table legs, or other pieces of furniture. They also crawl with their thorax against the floor, roll about, and vocalize for prolonged periods.

Several coital contacts might be made, with intromission and ejaculation occupying only 10–15 s each time. A refractory period or lack of sexual receptivity occurs for 10–15 min after each intromission. During the first hour of contact, four or five intromissions and ejaculations might occur.

Pregnancy

> **1** Know the length of gestation for each of the domestic species (see Table 53.1).
>
> **2** What is a sperm reservoir? Where are important ones located?
>
> **3** What is capacitation? Name one capacitation change.
>
> **4** What is the zona reaction associated with fertilization? Where does fertilization normally occur?
>
> **5** What is uterine milk?
>
> **6** What is implied by implantation?
>
> **7** What is placentation? What membranes compose the fetal placenta?
>
> **8** Know the relationship of the placental membranes to each other and to the fetus and mother. Where are the branches of the umbilical arteries and veins located?
>
> **9** What is a persistent urachus?
>
> **10** Which animals have a cotyledonary placenta? What composes a placentome?
>
> **11** Which steroid hormone predominates during pregnancy? Where is it produced? Do the sources and duration of its production vary among species? When is the corpus luteum source needed by all species?
>
> **12** What function is served by pregnant mare serum gonadotropin (PMSG)?
>
> **13** What are some signs of pregnancy in the cow as observed by rectal palpation?

Pregnancy is the condition of the female in which unborn young are contained within the body. Pregnancy is also called **gestation**, and its length is frequently known as the **gestation period**, extending from fertilization through birth. Its length for various domestic animals is shown in Table 53.1. Pregnancy begins with fertilization, ends with parturition, and includes the essential aspects of implantation and placentation. Before fertilization, the oocyte and sperm are transported to appropriate sites in the uterine tubes.

Transport of oocyte and spermatozoa

At ovulation, the fimbriae of the uterine tubes (see Figure 53.1) are in close contact with the ovaries. The contractile activity of the fimbriae direct the shed oocyte into the funnel-shaped opening of the uterine tube. Within the uterine tube the oocyte is directed toward the uterus by cilia and by uterine tube motility.

The ejaculated spermatozoa are transported to the uterine tubes by increased motility within the uterus caused by the release of oxytocin at the time of coitus and by the presence of prostaglandins in semen. The oxytocin is effective because of the uterus being primed by estrogen. Another factor that assists in transport is thought to be the presence of a negative pressure (vacuum) in the uterus. Many spermatozoa are rapidly transported to the uterine tubes after ejaculation, but it is believed that these are not the ones destined for fertilization. Their presence might be coincidental with the spread of accessory fluids throughout the tubular genitalia. The spermatozoa destined

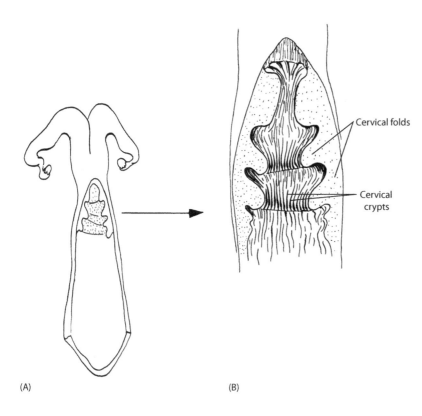

(A)   (B)

Figure 53.20 Dorsal view of the ruminant cervix. (A) The cervix has been cut open and its lateral walls reflected to show the folds and crypts. (B) Magnified view of the cervix. A mucous covering assists physical entrapment of spermatozoa destined for fertilization. The folds and crypts serve as sperm reservoirs and allow for capacitation of spermatozoa. Adapted from Reece, W.O. (2009) *Functional Anatomy and Physiology of Domestic Animals*, 4th edn. Wiley-Blackwell, Ames, IA. Reproduced with permission from Wiley.

for fertilization are transported more slowly from their sites of deposition (cervical canal, uterus, vagina) to **spermatozoa reservoirs**. The cervix of ruminants has prominent ridges and mucosal crypts that provide an extensive secretory surface (Figure 53.20). The cervical crypts and their mucous covering aid in the physical entrapment of spermatozoa and serve as spermatozoa reservoirs. Another important spermatozoa reservoir is located at the junction of the uterine horns with the uterine tubes.

Within the spermatozoa reservoirs, the spermatozoa undergo changes necessary for later penetration of the zona pellucida and fertilization of the oocyte. These changes, known as **capacitation**, require several hours. One important change involves the **acrosome**, in which channels are established for the escape of hyaluronidase and a proteolytic enzyme; these substances are essential for penetration of the ovum. Capacitated spermatozoa are released slowly from the spermatozoa reservoirs and proceed to the ampulla of the oviduct (dilated portion near the infundibulum) for fertilization. Ovulation occurs after the onset of estrus, so that insemination is accomplished before ovulation. This allows sufficient capacitation time and because the fertilizing lifespan is twice as long in spermatozoa as in oocytes, large numbers of spermatozoa are usually ready for fertilization at the time of ovulation. Oocytes retain viability for about 12–18 hours after ovulation in most domestic animals, while spermatozoa retain their fertilizing ability for 24–48 hours in the cow, ewe, and sow, for up to 90 hours in the bitch, and for 120 hours (5 days) in the mare.

Fertilization

Fertilization is the fusion of male and female gametes to form one single cell, the zygote. The first step in fertilization is penetration of the zona pellucida by the spermatozoon. This involves not only the enzymes **hyaluronidase** and **acrosin** (proteolytic enzyme from acrosome), but also spermatozoon motility. Motility ceases once contact with the oocyte has been made. In most domestic species, the second maturation division (meiosis) occurs when a spermatozoon penetrates the zona pellucida, whereas the first meiosis occurred a few hours before ovulation. The zona reaction occurs after penetration of the zona pellucida and protects the oocyte from further penetration by other spermatozoa. Penetration by more than one spermatozoon (**polyspermy**) is deleterious to normal development of the zygote.

Pronuclei develop from the nuclei of the spermatozoon and oocyte, which is followed by fusion of respective pronuclei to form a zygote with the diploid number of chromosomes. Fertilization is complete after the fused pronuclei have disappeared and are replaced by chromosome groups united in prophase of the first mitotic division.

Zygotes usually remain in the uterine tube for 3–4 days before being transferred to the uterus. Uterine motility is unfavorable for zygote survival, and estrogen dominance at estrus must be changed to progesterone dominance, which occurs with the formation of the CL. Progesterone has a quieting influence on the uterus and promotes development of a glandular endometrium that can secrete **uterine milk**, a nutrient medium for the embryo preceding its implantation. Cell division produces a

16- to 32-cell structure known as the morula. A cavity forms within the morula by 6–8 days of age, and the cell mass is called a blastocyst.

The period of the oocyte ends when the blastocyst attaches to the endometrium. This is the beginning of the embryonic period. The **embryonic period** is characterized by rapid growth; major tissues, organs, and systems develop and the major features of external body form become recognizable. The **fetal period** extends from this time until birth, and begins at about day 45 of gestation in the cow.

Implantation and placentation

The nutritive requirements of the developing blastocyst are satisfied by diffusion from yolk in the oocyte and by secretions of the uterine tube and uterus (uterine milk), until it becomes fixed in position in the uterus. **Implantation** of the embryo occurs when it becomes fixed in position and forms a physical and functional contact with the uterus. It occurs 2–5 weeks after

fertilization. The interval is shortest for the cat (2 weeks) and longest for cattle and horses (5 weeks).

Because the embryo continues to grow, the central mass of cells becomes further removed from the surface. Diffusion of nutrients is no longer adequate, and membranes develop concurrent with a circulatory system that provide for receiving nutrients from the dam. The development of extraembryonic membranes is known as **placentation**, and the collective name for the membranes is the **fetal placenta**, which consists of the **chorion**, **allantois**, and **amnion**. The relationship of the fetal membranes to the fetus is shown in Figure 53.21. The chorion is the outermost membrane and is the one most intimately associated with the endometrium. The amnion envelops the fetus and contains **amniotic fluid** in the amniotic cavity. The amniotic fluid is derived from fetal urine via the urethra, from secretions of the respiratory tract and oral cavity, and from the maternal circulation. The amniotic fluid protects the fetus from external shock, prevents adhesion of fetal skin with amniotic membrane,

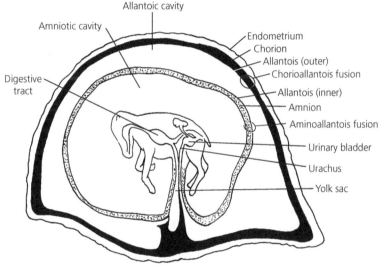

Figure 53.21 Fetus of horse within the placenta. The chorioallantois is the combination of the outer allantois with the chorion. Umbilical arteries and veins (not shown) occupy the space (blackened) between the outer allantois and chorion. The chorion is intimately associated with the endometrium. Attachment to endometrium not shown, and its extent varies with placental type. The inner allantois is fused with the amnion (stippled for contrast). From Reece, W.O. (2009) *Functional Anatomy and Physiology of Domestic Animals*, 4th edn. Wiley-Blackwell, Ames, IA. Reproduced with permission from Wiley.

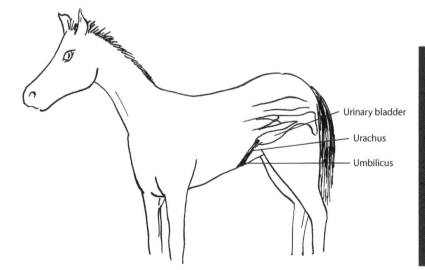

Figure 53.22 Diagrammatic view of persistent urachus in a foal. Failure of urachus closure at birth results in a continuous drip of urine at its umbilical exit. From Reece, W.O. (2009) *Functional Anatomy and Physiology of Domestic Animals*, 4th edn. Wiley-Blackwell, Ames, IA. Reproduced with permission from Wiley.

and assists in dilating the cervix and lubricating the birth passage at parturition. The allantois outer layer is fused to the chorion, and the inner layer of allantois is fused to the amnion. The space between the two layers of allantois is called the allantoic cavity. It is continuous with the cranial extremity of the urinary bladder by way of the urachus, which passes through the umbilical cord. When the urachus fails to close at birth, a continuous drip of urine is observed from the navel, a condition known as **persistent urachus** (Figure 53.22). Allantoic fluid originates from fetal urine and from secretory activity of the allantoic membrane. The fluid brings the chorioallantoic membrane into close apposition with the endometrium during early attachment and stores fetal excretory products. Branches of umbilical arteries and veins are distributed between the outer layer of allantois and the chorion. The yolk sac is connected to the fetal intestine (the remnant after birth is known as Meckel's diverticulum) and serves as a nutrition source early in development.

When the attachment (extension of chorionic villi) of fetal membranes to the endometrium is continuous throughout the entire surface of the fetal membranes, it is known as a **diffuse placenta**. A diffuse type of placenta is found in the horse and pig (Figure 53.23A). Ruminants have a **cotyledonary placenta**, in which attachment occurs only at the many mushroom-like projections from the endometrium (Figure 53.23B). The fetal cotyledons are attached to the maternal caruncles, a combination known as a **placentome**. The fetal placentas of the dog and cat are attached by a girdle-like band that encircles the placenta, called a **zonary placenta** (Figure 53.23C). The human placenta attachment is confined to a disk-shaped area and is called a **discoidal placenta** (Figure 53.23D).

A heifer calf born twin to a normal bull calf is sterile and is called a **freemartin**. This occurs when the female calf develops in the uterus with a normal male twin and they share the same blood supply (anastomosis of the placental blood vessels). When this occurs, the sex hormones from the earlier developing male twin pass across to the female twin, causing sexual differentiation of both male and female to proceed under control of male hormones. About 90% of heifer calves born twin to a bull calf are freemartins and can usually be detected clinically because of the shortened vagina (short advancement of a blunt instrument) and an enlarged clitoris.

Hormones

Pregnancy is maintained as a result of the predominance of progesterone. During gestation, progesterone is produced by the placenta and CL. The contribution from placental and luteal sources and the duration of their contribution varies among species. The CL source is needed by all species during early pregnancy, but is not needed by the mare and ewe after about 100 and 60 days, respectively. A CL is needed for most of pregnancy in the cow, bitch, and queen and for the entire pregnancy in the sow and doe. Although progesterone from the CL is not needed by the ewe, regression of the CL does not occur and luteal production continues, but placental production is dominant. Regression of the CL occurs in the mare about

midway, and the placenta is the sole source of progesterone for the maintenance of pregnancy.

In the mare, **endometrial cups** begin to be formed at about day 35 of gestation within the endometrium from cells migrating from the placenta. The cups begin to secrete a hormone known as **pregnant mare serum gonadotropin (PMSG)** at about 35 days, which

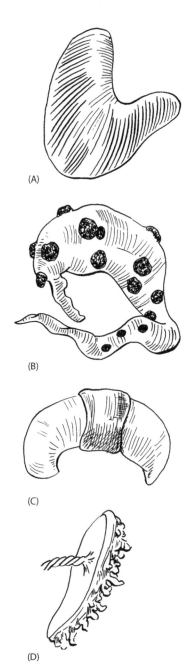

Figure 53.23 Placental types according to the distribution of chorionic projections (villi) on the endometrium. (A) Diffuse placenta of the horse and pig. (B) Cotyledonary placenta of ruminants. (C) Zonary placenta of the dog and cat. (D) Discoid placenta of the human and monkey. From Reece, W.O. (2009) *Functional Anatomy and Physiology of Domestic Animals*, 4th edn. Wiley-Blackwell, Ames, IA. Reproduced with permission from Wiley.

continues until about 130 days of gestation. PMSG helps to form new follicles, which ovulate and provide for additional corpora lutea. A greater supply of luteal progesterone is thereby ensured until the endometrial supply of progesterone is adequate for maintenance. All corpora lutea regress by about 150 days. Early pregnancy in the mare can be diagnosed by analyzing for the presence of PMSG.

Diagnosis

It is often of economic importance to determine whether an animal is actually pregnant. Pregnancy is obvious during the late stages when the size of the fetus, uterus, and fetal fluids have increased to the point at which the abdomen has enlarged and definite dropping of the abdominal wall has occurred (known as **bellying down**). Rectal palpation is a useful procedure for detecting earlier signs of pregnancy, particularly in the cow. The hand is inserted into the rectum and structures located outside of the rectal wall can be felt.

Using rectal palpation in the cow, early pregnancy is suggested if a corpus luteum is present and if one horn of the uterus is larger than the other. This condition can be apparent at 30–45 days. At about 3 months, the fetal membranes can be felt to slip away from the grasp when the uterus is lifted, and small caruncles in the uterine wall are palpable. Also at 3 months, a vibration or "buzzing" of blood in the uterine artery is palpable, known as fremitus. At 5–7 months the weight of the fetus causes the uterus to slip over the brim of the pelvis, and the cervix becomes taut. The ovaries and fetus are difficult to palpate when this occurs because of their distance from the palpator, but definite caruncles are palpable.

After the fetus has descended over the brim of the pelvis in the cow, it may be possible to detect pregnancy by an external technique known as **ballottement**. Pressure is exerted on the lower right abdominal wall (see Figure 53.8) with the fist or knee in an inward and upward direction and then is released, causing the fetus to rise and fall in its suspending fluids. The fall should be felt by the manipulator.

The use of radiography for the diagnosis of pregnancy has had limited application in veterinary medicine. Penetration of the rays is restricted in large animals, and exposure of the film is difficult. In small animals, such as the dog, exposure is adequate, but differentiation of a fetus is not possible until calcification of bones is adequate for contrast. This does not occur until about 45 days in the dog, and other means, such as palpation and observation, are often more useful for earlier diagnosis of pregnancy.

A biological test for the detection of pregnancy can be performed in the mare based on the production of PMSG by the endometrial cups (see previous section). Injection of serum taken from a mare at 40–130 days of pregnancy into a female rabbit that has been isolated from male rabbits for at least 30 days elicits ovarian follicles that rupture and form reddened corpora hemorrhagica about 48 hours after injection. The corpora hemorrhagica can be seen when the rabbit is butchered or observed by other procedures when placed under anesthesia. Because the rabbit does not ovulate and form corpora hemorrhagica unless coitus occurs, only the injected PMSG could have caused the ovulation.

Ultrasonography is currently the most used method for pregnancy diagnosis in small and large animals. The use of ultrasound for this purpose is being carried out by veterinary practitioners and theriogenologists. Transabdominal ultrasonography in the bitch is best used beyond 24 days of pregnancy where the amniotic vesicles are visible as black balls with a comma shaped tissue mass within them. Beyond 24–30 days, beating hearts can be seen. In the queen, it is best used beyond 16 days of pregnancy and the amniotic vesicles are seen similar to their appearance in the bitch. Beyond 16-25 days, beating hearts can be seen.

Transrectal ultrasonography is used for large animals. An example for the cow indicates that the embryo is well demarcated by approximately day 18, with a highly accentuated curve in it's anterior-posterior axis. Heartbeats are also visible at this time.

---

1 What are some signs of approaching parturition?

2 How is respiratory rate in the sow associated with closeness of farrowing? What happens to body temperature in the bitch just before parturition?

3 What functions are served by estrogen increase just before parturition?

4 What functions are served by $PGF_{2\alpha}$ at the time of parturition?

5 How do oxytocin and the presence of feet in the pelvic canal assist parturition?

6 What are the stages of labor?

7 What is meant by presentation of the fetus? How is it initiated?

8 What is the difference between an anterior and a posterior presentation? What is an example of an abnormal presentation?

9 What term is applied to difficulty encountered in expulsion of the fetus?

Parturition

Parturition, sometimes called labor, is the physiologic process by which the pregnant uterus delivers the fetus and fetal membranes from the mother.

Signs of approaching parturition

Throughout pregnancy the abdomen continues to enlarge, and its maximum size is reached just before parturition. The mammary glands also continue to enlarge and, within a few days of parturition, begin to secrete a milky material. Other signs include swelling of the vulva and a discharge of mucus from the vulva. The abdominal muscles relax, which causes the belly to drop and the rump to sink on both sides of the tailhead. It is believed that the hormone relaxin, in association with the increasing level of estrogen in late pregnancy, causes the relaxation of ligaments to enable the birth canal to enlarge. Also, it is thought that $PGF_{2\alpha}$ helps to relax the cervix. In addition to these physical signs, certain behavioral signs are characteristic, such as restlessness, frequent lying down and getting up, and frequent urination. The bitch and sow often attempt to build elaborate nests.

Respiratory rates are better indicators than milk letdown that sows are close to farrowing. Respiratory rates increase steadily and peak 6 hours before farrowing in almost all sows. In contrast, some sows produce colostrum as much as 3–4 days before farrowing. An example of the respiratory rate index can be obtained from the following data.

1 Respiratory rates average 54 breaths/min during the 24- to 12-hour period before farrowing.
2 From 12 to 4 hours before farrowing, respiratory rates are the highest, averaging 91 breaths/min.
3 The lowest respiratory rates are recorded between 6 and 18 hours after birth of the last piglet, averaging 25 breaths/min.

Rectal temperature changes have also been studied as indicators of impending parturition under the assumption that certain hormones influence body temperature. For example, progesterone increases the basal body temperature because it causes an increase in basal metabolic rate. However, with regression of the corpus luteum immediately preceding parturition (see further on), there is cessation of progesterone production, that is followed by a decrease in body temperature. Body temperature decrease is most dramatic and reliable in the bitch, in which a body temperature decrease of 2–3°C (4–5 °F) might be observed 6 or 8 hours before parturition. Body temperature has not been found to be a reliable indicator in other species..

Hormone changes

An important hormone change that occurs just before parturition is an increase in the production of estrogen. Estrone is produced by the fetoplacental unit as maturity of the fetus increases (approximately 3–4 weeks prepartum in the cow). The increase in production of cortisol by fetal adrenal cortices, concurrent with maturity of the fetus, initiates the prepartum increase in estrogen production. The secretion of estrogen assists in the production of uterine muscle contractile proteins before parturition. Estrogen might also be the signal for the secretion of $PGF_{2\alpha}$ that occurs in the immediate prepartum period (24–36 hours prepartum in the cow). $PGF_{2\alpha}$ initiates regression of the CL (if present) and subsequent lowering of progesterone levels. The increase in estrogen and decrease in progesterone levels convert the uterus from a state of quiescence to a state of potential contractility. The increase in estrogen level varies among domestic animals regarding time of occurrence before parturition (Figure 53.24). The length of increase is longest for the cow and shortest for the ewe.

Changes in maternal hormonal levels do not seem to play a major role in parturition in the mare. At parturition the mare has relatively high levels of progestogens and low levels of estrogens. However, $PGF_{2\alpha}$ level increases during foaling. The progesterone concentration does not decrease in the mare after $PGF_{2\alpha}$ secretion because no CL is present after about 150 days of pregnancy.

$PGF_{2\alpha}$ is also believed to increase the contractility of the uterus by permitting greater mobility of sarcoplasmic calcium. These early contraction increases might be important in positioning the fetus for delivery (presentation) through the pelvic canal. The presence of the fetus in the pelvic canal causes oxytocin to be

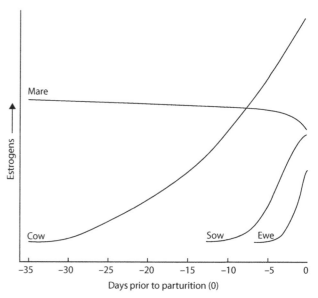

Figure 53.24 Estrogen patterns in the mare, cow, sow, and ewe before parturition. Negative numbers refer to days before parturition (0). From Edqvist, L.E. and Stabenfeldt, G.A. (1980) Reproductive hormones. In: *Clinical Biochemistry of Domestic Animals*, 3rd edn (ed. J.J. Kaneko). Academic Press, New York.

released from the posterior pituitary. In the presence of an estrogen-primed uterus, the muscle contractions increase in intensity to assist in expelling the fetus. $PGF_{2\alpha}$ also increases the sensitivity of the uterus to oxytocin, which enhances the rhythmic contractions of the uterine musculature during delivery. The uterus can only assist in the expulsion of the fetus and must have the coordinated contraction of the abdominal muscles. The presence of the feet in the pelvic canal and the consequent stimulation of the vagina provides for reflex contraction of the abdominal muscles, similar to the straining that occurs when one attempts to replace a prolapsed uterus. The abdominal and uterine muscle contraction, coupled with relaxed pelvic ligaments, separation of the pelvic symphysis, and dilatation of the cervix, provide for expulsion of the fetus. A summary of the events associated with parturition, beginning with the prepartum secretion of fetal cortisol and ending with expulsion of the fetus, is shown in Figure 53.25.

Stages

The three stages of parturition are as follows:
1 uterine contractions (contribute to dilatation of cervix and presentation of fetus);
2 contractions associated with expulsion of fetus (involve abdominal muscle contraction);
3 expulsion of fetal membranes.

The stages of labor and related events are summarized in Table 53.2.

In monotocous (single birth) species, the fetus lies on its back during gestation. Just before birth, a position is assumed in the uterus that is characteristic for the species (presentation). Presentation can be initiated by early contractions of the uterus.

A proper presentation for the bovine fetus is shown in Figure 53.26. The front feet are pointed toward the cervix, the head is extended and tucked between the feet, and the back of the calf is directed toward the sacral vertebrae. This is known as **an anterior or cranial presentation**. A **posterior or caudal presentation** with the hind feet extended into the pelvic canal is considered normal, but is less common. An example of an

abnormal presentation is one in which there might be an anterior presentation, but with a deviation of the head and neck. Abnormal presentations usually require correction before the fetus can be expelled successfully.

Difficulties are often encountered during parturition, and delays are observed in what are considered normal durations of each stage. Undue delay in providing assistance often aggravates the condition and can injure the mother and cause death to the fetus. Rules of thumb for the average duration of the three stages of labor in the mare, cow, buffalo, ewe, and sow are given in

↑Fetal cortisol (4 to 3 weeks prepartum)

↑Estrogen (fetoplacental unit)

↑Myometrial contractile proteins

↑PGF$_{2\alpha}$ (36 to 24 hours prepartum)

↑Relaxin

CL regression

↑Mobility of sarcoplasmic Ca^{2+}

↑Sensitivity to oxytocin

↓Progesterone

Myometrial contractile potential

Fetal feet in pelvis

Relaxation of pelvic ligaments; separation of pelvic symphysis

↑Oxytocin

↑Reglex contraction of abdominal muscles

Expulsion of fetus

Figure 53.25 Events of parturition beginning with the prepartum secretion of fetal cortisol and ending with expulsion of the fetus. PGF$_{2\alpha}$, prostaglandin F$_{2\alpha}$; CL, corpus luteum. From Reece, W.O. (2009) *Functional Anatomy and Physiology of Domestic Animals*, 4th edn. Wiley-Blackwell, Ames, IA. Reproduced with permission from Wiley.

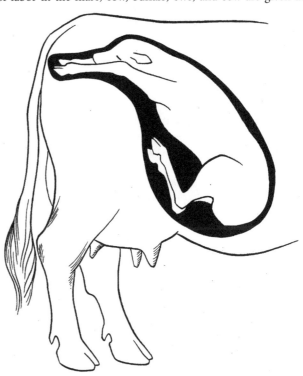

Figure 53.26 Normal presentation for the bovine fetus, known as a cranial or anterior presentation. From Frandson, R.D., Wilke, W.L. and Fails, A.D. (2009) *Anatomy and Physiology of Farm Animals*, 7th edn. Wiley-Blackwell, Ames, IA.

Table 53.2 Stages of labor and related events in farm animals.

Stage of labor	Mechanical forces	Period	Related events
I Dilation of cervix	Regular uterine contractions	Beginning of uterine contractions until cervix is fully dilated and continuous with vagina	Maternal restlessness, elevated pulse and respiratory rates Changes in fetal position and posture
II Expulsion of fetus*	Strong uterine and abdominal contractions	From complete cervical dilation to end of delivery of fetus	Maternal recumbency and straining Rupture of allantochorion and escape of fluid from vulva Appearance of amnion (water bag) at vulva Rupture of amnion and delivery of fetus
III Expulsion of fetal membranes	Uterine contractions decrease in amplitude	After delivery of fetus to expulsion of fetal membranes	Maternal straining ceases Loosening of chorionic villi from maternal crypts Inversion of chorioallantois Straining and expulsion of fetal membranes

*In polytocous species (sow) and twin-bearing species (sheep and goat), this stage cannot be separated from the next stage (III).
Source: Hafez, E.S.E. and Hafez, B. (2000) *Reproduction in Farm Animals*, 7th edn. Lippincott Williams & Wilkins, Baltimore.

Table 53.3 Average duration of the three stages of labor in farm animals (hours).

Animal	Stage I. Dilation of cervix	Stage II. Expulsion of fetus(es)	Stage III. Expulsion of fetal membranes
Mare	1–4	0.2–0.5	1
Cow, buffalo	2–6	0.5–1.0	6–12
Ewe	2–6	0.5–2.0	0.5–8
Sow	2–12	2.5–3.0	1–4

Source: Hafez, E.S.E. and Hafez, B. (2000) *Reproduction in Farm Animals*, 7th edn. Lippincott Williams & Wilkins, Baltimore.

Table 53.3. A difficulty encountered in expulsion of the fetus is referred to as a **dystocia**.

Involution of the uterus

> 1 What is meant by involution? What events characterize involution?
>
> 2 What is "foal heat" in the mare?
>
> 3 Is post-farrowing estrus (3–5 days after farrowing) in the sow fertile or nonfertile?

The process by which the uterus returns to its nonpregnant size after parturition is known as **involution**. The points of attachment of the fetal placenta to the endometrium slough, and the exposed endometrium heals by forming new epithelium. In addition to new epithelial growth, the myometrium contracts and the cells shorten.

Cow
Within 6–7 days postpartum, the upper two-thirds of the maternal caruncle sloughs into the uterus, becoming part of the fluids discharged. The epithelial cells of the caruncle must be shed for the placenta to be expelled. Within 21–35 days, all cellular repair has occurred and endometrial gland function is restored. The caruncles have retracted and cannot be palpated. Normally, estrus is observed at 45–60 days postpartum. Suckling by the calf, low energy intake, infections, and heavy lactation delay estrus.

Mare, ewe, and sow
Involution in the mare is rapid, but not complete, by the time of **foal heat**, which occurs within 6–13 days postpartum. Foal heat is usually accompanied by ovulation, and mares bred at this time can become pregnant. However, conception rates are lower when breeding occurs during the foal heat.

In the ewe and sow, about 24–28 days are needed for complete involution. In the sow, a nonfertile (no ovulation) estrus occurs 3–5 days after farrowing. Estrus combined with ovulation is usually inhibited throughout lactation. Sows not nursing their litters during the first week after farrowing have estrus with ovulation within 2 weeks. Weaning of pigs at any time induces estrus with ovulation in 3–5 days.

Resumption of estrus in the ewe and mare is consistent with the photoperiod of estrous activity characteristic for these species.

Bitch
The interplacental areas return to normal within a few weeks, but the placental sites require about 12 weeks to involute and heal. Estrus usually does not occur until after the young are weaned.

Self-evaluation

Answers can be found at the end of the chapter.

1 Intertwining of the ovarian artery with the uterine vein serves to:
  A Cool the ovary
  B Suspend the ovary
  C Transport $PGF_{2\alpha}$ from the uterus to the ovary
  D Transport spermatozoa from the uterus to the ovary

2 Fertilization of oocytes released by the ovary occurs in the:
  A Abdominal cavity
  B Uterine tubes
  C Uterus
  D Vagina

3 Which one of the following best describes the action of progesterone?
  A Increases libido
  B Increases blood supply and motility of the uterus
  C Increases endometrial development and glandular secretion of the endometrium, and decreases motility of the uterus
  D Assists follicular rupture and subsequent development of the corpus luteum

4 Tonic levels of LH and FSH in the female are increased by increases in:
  A Estrogen
  B Progesterone
  C Androgen

5 Which one of the following best describes the action of LH (luteinizing hormone) in the female?
  A Causes lysis or reduction in size of the corpus luteum
  B Increases the blood supply and motility of the uterus
  C Assists in the maturing of an ovarian follicle, its rupture, and subsequent development and maintenance of a corpus luteum
  D Stimulates the interstitial cells (Leydig cells) to secrete testosterone

6 What hormone has its concentration increased greatly just before ovulation (preovulatory surge), which assists ovulation and conversion of a ruptured follicle to a corpus luteum?
  A FSH
  B Estrogen
  C LH
  D Progesterone

7 Which one of the following best describes the action of FSH (follicle-stimulating hormone) in the female?

  A Causes lysis or reduction in size of the corpus luteum
  B Causes granulosa cells to convert androgen to estrogens
  C Assists in the maturing of an ovarian follicle, its rupture, and subsequent development and maintenance of a corpus luteum
  D Stimulates the interstitial cells (Leydig cells) to secrete testosterone

8 An estrous cycle interval is:

  A Diestrus to proestrus
  B One period of sexual receptivity to the next
  C The same in all animals
  D Puberty to the end of reproductive life

9 Pseudopregnancy is most commonly observed in the:

  A Bitch
  B Mare
  C Doe
  D Queen

10 A freemartin of the bovine species is:

  A A sterile female calf that develops in same uterus with a normal male twin and shares a common blood supply with the male while in the uterus
  B Same as answer A, except refers to the male as being sterile
  C Infrequently sterile (reproductively)
  D A calf with a free spirit

Suggested reading

Des Coteaux, L., Gnemmi, G., and Colloton, J. (2010) *Practical Atlas of Ruminant and Camelid Reproductive Ultrasonography.* Wiley Blackwell, Ames, IA.

Dyce, K.M., Sack, W.O. and Wensing, C.J.G. (2002) *Textbook of Veterinary Anatomy*, 3rd edn. W.B. Saunders, Philadelphia.

Frandson, R.D., Wilke, W.L. and Fails, A.D. (2009) *Anatomy and Physiology of Farm Animals*, 7th edn. Wiley-Blackwell, Ames, IA.

Hafez, E.S.E. and Hafez, B. (2000) *Reproduction in Farm Animals*, 7th edn. Lippincott Williams & Wilkins, Baltimore.

Pineda, M.H. and Dooley, M.P. (eds) (2003) *McDonald's Veterinary Endocrinology and Reproduction*, 5th edn. Iowa State Press, Ames, IA.

Root Krustritz, M.V. (2010) *Clinical Canine and Feline Reproduction.* Wiley Blackwell, Ames, IA.

Thompson, F.N. (2004) Female reproduction in mammals. In: *Dukes' Physiology of Domestic Animals*, 12th edn (ed. W.O. Reece). Cornell University Press, Ithaca, NY.

Answers

1	C	6	C
2	B	7	B
3	C	8	B
4	A	9	A
5	C	10	A

Section IX: Endocrinology, Reproduction, and Lactation

54 Lactation

Patrick J. Gorden and Leo L. Timms
Iowa State University, Ames, IA, USA

Milk, nature's most perfect food and an essential nutrient for neonatal development, is a unique liquid composed of emulsified lipid globules encased in a distinctive and essential protein membrane, colloidal suspended protein particles that also chelate and deliver many minerals, in an aqueous solution of other special proteins and carbohydrates, minerals and vitamins, and water which provides proper viscosity for nursing removal as well as sole hydration and nutrition for neonates. Milk is secreted from a specialized cutaneous gland. The tubuloalveolar structure of the mature mammary gland originates from the ectoderm during fetal development and differentiates throughout an animal's growth and gestation. **Lactation** is defined as the combined process of **milk secretion** and **milk removal** and is the final stage of the reproductive cycle. Lactation requires synchronous physiological processes to maintain homeorhesis of the dam and nutrient acquisition essential for milk formation.

While the anatomical structures and physiological processes that result in lactation are similar across species, and the milk product itself contains common nutrients in different proportions across a class of animals called **Mammalia**, the evolution of how young are born and some of the structures are uniquely different. The most primitive nonextinct mammals are found in the subclass **Prototheria** and are called **monotremes** (i.e., they possess a cloaca) and include the duck-billed platypus and two types of echidna. These are egg-laying mammals that hatch very immature young. They have no teat or nipple and milk is secreted through over 100–150 glands and ducts directly on to the abdominal fur. Echidna developed a brood pouch to carry their egg and young, and an areola region. Next in evolution came the subclass **Theria**. **Methatheria**, which today includes only **marsupials**, exhibit live birth, though the young are still very immature, through use of a **chorio-vitelline placenta**. These animals possess inguinal mammary glands covered by a pouch, and some (like kangaroos) have separate mammary glands that can independently differentiate as their young mature and thus can feed age-specific milk to two joeys of different ages. **Eutheria**, the class that comprises more than 95% of the 4500 mammalian species, have a **true placenta**, longer gestation, and give birth to more advanced and developed young. Probably the most notable mammal is the dairy cow, which has the ability to produce over 15 gallons (57 L) of milk daily. This equates to more than 10% of her body weight on a daily basis, although other species, metabolically and energetically, produce similar amounts of energy per unit of metabolic body weight.

While there are numerous mammalian species for which much is known about the mammary gland, the vast amount of material that has been chronicled about the cow makes it an excellent model for this chapter, with important species variations noted where appropriate.

Dukes' Physiology of Domestic Animals, Thirteenth Edition. Edited by William O. Reece, Howard H. Erickson, Jesse P. Goff and Etsuro E. Uemura.
© 2015 John Wiley & Sons, Inc. Published 2015 by John Wiley & Sons, Inc.
Companion website: www.wiley.com/go/reece/physiology

Section IX: Endocrinology, Reproduction, and Lactation

Functional anatomy of the mammary gland

1 What are the primary areas where mammary glands are found and do they have different numbers of openings/teat or glands?

2 How do the medial and lateral suspensory ligaments of the bovine mammary gland differ?

3 What is the basic functional unit responsible for milk secretion of the mammary gland?

4 Where are myoepithelial cells located and what is their function?

5 Why is the streak canal different and very important?

6 What is the primary structure responsible for retention of milk within the udder of cattle?

7 How many liters of blood circulate through bovine mammary gland to produce 1 L of milk?

8 What is the purpose of a collateral venous blood supply in the lactating ruminant?

9 What is principal lymph node associated with lymphatic outflow from the bovine udder?

10 Are the sensory nerve fibers required for secretion or ejection of milk?

External anatomy

The entire exterior surface of the mammary gland is covered by skin with varying degrees of coverage by hair, another characteristic of mammals. The skin helps protect the glandular tissue but provides very little mechanical support. The mammary glands and external teats of various species are located in different areas of the body. Each species has not only distinct locations (thoracic, abdominal, and/or inguinal) and numbers of mammary glands, but also varying numbers of ducts or openings/teats (Table 54.1).

Internal anatomy

In dairy cattle, the mammary gland can weigh up to 60 kg; however, it should be noted that the size of the udder has little correlation with the productivity of the cow. Each udder of cattle is divided into four mammary glands, with each gland having separate glandular tissue, milk collection system, and teat. The individual glands are separated by connective tissue, which is usually defined externally by the contours of the udder. Each half of the udder, containing two mammary glands, is supplied by independent blood, nervous, and lymphatic systems.

Supportive structures

In cattle, the mammary gland is suspended by medial and lateral suspensory ligaments made of fascial sheets that essentially surround and support the gland. The **elastic medial suspensory ligament** originates from the linea alba cranially and prepubic tendon caudally. It is divided into right and left lamellae by loose connective tissue, allowing each half of the ligament to support its corresponding udder half. **Fibrous lateral suspensory ligaments** are composed of dense connective tissue originating from the subpubic and prepubic tendons and function to support and enclose the lateral aspects of the udder. The lateral suspensory ligament helps protect the superficial mammary blood vessels and lymph structures as well. Both the medial and lateral suspensory ligaments are thicker dorsally and become thinner as they approach the udder. As the ligaments extend ventrally, they intertwine with the connective tissue network surrounding the glandular parenchyma. Eventually, the medial and lateral suspensory ligaments anastomose on the ventral aspect of each half of the gland to form a sling-like support structure.

Table 54.1 Variation in mammary gland locations, numbers, and openings per teat.

Order	Common name	Gland position			Total glands	Openings per teat
		Thoracic	Abdominal	Inguinal		
Marsupialia	Red kangaroo		4		4	15
Marsupialia	Opossum		13		13	8
Carnivora	House cat	2	6		8	3–7
Carnivora	Domestic dog	2	6	2	10	8–14
Rodentia	House mouse	4	2	4	10	1
Lagomorpha	Rabbit	4	4	2	10	8–10
Cetacea	Whale			2	2	1
Proboscidea	Elephant	2			2	10–11
Perissodactyla	Horse			2	4	2
Artiodactyla	Cattle			4	2	1
Artiodactyla	Sheep			2	2	1
Artiodactyla	Goat			2	2	1
Artiodactyla	Pig	4	6	2	12	2
Primate	Human	2			2	15–25

Source: adapted from Akers, R.M. (2002) *Lactation and the Mammary Gland*. Iowa State University Press, Ames, IA.

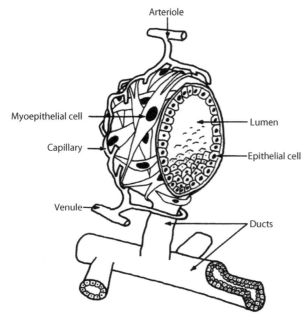

Figure 54.1 An alveolus surrounded by blood vessels and myoepithelial cells in the mammary gland. Drawn by C.B. Choi. From Reece, W.O. (2004) *Dukes' Physiology of Domestic Animals*, 12th edn. Cornell University Press, Ithaca, NY. Reproduced with permission from Cornell University Press.

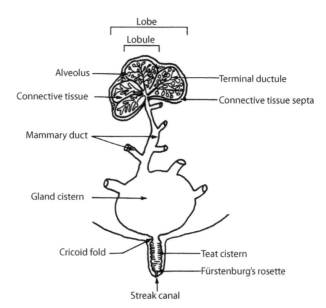

Figure 54.2 Duct and lobuloalveolar systems of the bovine mammary gland. From Reece, W.O. (2004) *Dukes' Physiology of Domestic Animals*, 12th edn. Cornell University Press, Ithaca, NY. Reproduced with permission from Cornell University Press.

Milk production, collection, and transport systems

Milk synthesis and secretion is achieved by the mammary gland through **specialized sebaceous glands**, each with a fluid volume capacity of approximately 1 mm³, called **alveoli**. A single layer of secretory epithelium bound together by tight junctions, the zona occludens, is arranged in a cylindrical fashion to form the alveoli. Multiple alveoli are grouped together between connective tissue septa into units known as lobules. Further bundling of the lobules occurs to form lobes (Figures 54.1 and 54.2).

Bands of **smooth muscle**, known as **myoepithelial cells**, surround each individual alveolus and milk ducts. The myoepithelial cells are responsible for contracting in response to oxytocin resulting in milk release and movement from the alveoli down the ducts, also known as **milk letdown**. The myoepithelial cell bodies sit in close association with capillary beds responsible for supplying nutrients to the alveolar cells and oxytocin for contraction.

Secretory ducts drain each individual alveolus and lead to larger ducts called **lactiferous ducts**. These combine into larger duct systems and eventually dump into the gland cistern. From the gland cistern, milk flows through the teat cistern and streak canal to exit the teat. Two layers of cuboidal epithelium line the entire duct system, gland cistern, and teat cistern.

The transition from the teat cistern to the **streak canal** is an area known as **Fürstenberg's rosette**, which is composed of loose folds of double-layered columnar epithelium, each containing multiple secondary folds. Starting at Fürstenberg's rosette, the epithelium becomes stratified squamous and this epithelial type remains continuous with the skin of the teat. The major difference between the epithelium of the streak canal and the external skin is that the teat canal epithelium contains **keratin** that functions to trap bacteria that may invade the teat. As milk flows through the streak canal, the keratin peels off along with any trapped bacteria, thus removing bacteria from the teat. In cattle, there is a small ring of smooth muscle called the **teat sphincter muscle** that functions as a sphincter to retain milk within the teat.

Between subsequent milkings or periods of suckling, milk is stored in the alveoli and the gland and teat cisterns. There are tremendous species differences in storage capacity of the different structures, with cows storing only 20–30% of their milk as cisternal milk after a 10- to 12-hour inter-milking interval. In comparison, goats store up to 80% of their milk in the cisterns while sows store no milk in cisterns between periods of suckling.

Blood networks

The grid of arteries and veins that supply the mammary gland is vast in order to account for the large amount of blood flow through the udder daily and the nutrients required to synthesize copious amounts of milk. It is estimated that at least 500 L of blood flow through the udder for every liter of milk produced by a moderate-producing dairy cow. During lactation, this equates to approximately 10% of cardiac output. Blood supply for the udder of the cow originates from the caudal aorta, divides into right and left iliac arteries, and continues to flow bilaterally to supply the right and left halves of the udder. Each of the iliac arteries divides into external and internal iliac arteries, with the only significant vessel to the mammary gland from the internal

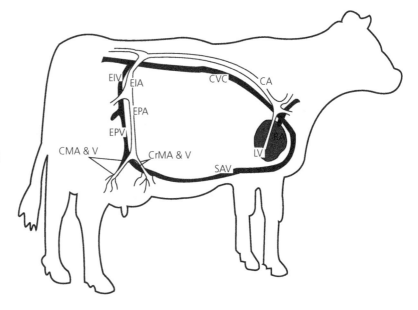

Figure 54.3 Blood circulation to and from the udder. RA, right atrium; LV, left ventricle; CA, caudal artery; CVC, caudal vena cava; EIV, external iliac vein; EIA, external iliac artery; EPA, external pudic artery; EPV, external pudic vein; CMA&V, caudal mammary artery and vein; CrMA&V, cranial mammary artery and vein; SAV, subcutaneous abdominal vein. Drawn by W.L. Keller. From Reece, W.O. (2004) *Dukes' Physiology of Domestic Animals*, 12th edn. Cornell University Press, Ithaca, NY. Reproduced with permission from Cornell University Press.

iliac artery being the perineal artery, which supplies a small amount of blood to the caudal udder. The external iliac artery provides the majority of the blood by branching into the prepubic artery until it courses through the internal inguinal ring, after which it courses as the external pudendal artery until the blood enters the mammary gland and then this main supply is known as the mammary artery. Before the artery enters the mammary gland, it has a sigmoid flexure to protect the artery against stretching. The mammary artery branches into cranial and caudal mammary arteries to supply the respective areas of the udder. The right and left mammary arteries interconnect behind the medial suspensory ligament. There is also a potential for collateral circulation via the perineal artery connecting with the caudal mammary artery. The mammary arteries continue to branch and supply the various areas of the udder, with multiple small branches coming together above the teat to form a plexus through which the walls of the teats are supplied (Figure 54.3).

Blood returns to the heart in similarly named veins to the caudal vena cava. However, a system is in place for blood return via a **collateral route** when blood flow becomes obstructed during recumbency. One such mechanism is through the perineal vein via connections with the caudal mammary vein. The most prominent collateral route found in the cow, sheep, and goat comprises the tortuous subcutaneous abdominal veins commonly called milk veins, which direct blood to the heart by way of the cranial vena cava. The subcutaneous abdominal veins develop in late pregnancy when the cranial and caudal superficial epigastric vessels unite. This union occurs as valves present in the cranial and caudal epigastric veins of the young animal become incompetent as pregnancy progresses and blood flow through the mammary gland increases. Although very large, these subcutaneous abdominal veins are not essential for milk production.

Animals that have mammary glands in different locations have a different path for blood supply. In the sow, the caudal glands receive blood via the route supplied by the caudal aorta as described here. However, the cranial glands are supplied from the external and internal thoracic arteries.

Lymph network

Blood flow through the udder during lactation results in a large amount of **lymph** (1.6 times the volume of milk). Lymph flows through an extensive network of vessels to the **supramammary lymph nodes** located in the mammary fat pad above the caudal glands, although there may be some mammary lymph passing through the prefemoral lymph nodes. There is great variation in the number and size of the supramammary lymph nodes. Efferent vessels leave the supramammary lymph node and traverse the inguinal ring into the abdomen and then possibly through the deep inguinal, external iliac, or prefemoral lymph nodes en route to the systemic circulation (Figure 54.4).

In prepartum cattle or cattle with mastitis, udder edema can occur as a result of loosening of the tight junctions between the epithelial cells of the alveoli or from increased pressure within the parenchyma from milk secretions, thus occluding the lymph vessels. This allows milk components, with osmotic potential, to leak into the interstitial space and results in reduced clearance of lymph. In cases where excessive lymph accumulation occurs, the deep inguinal node may be palpated per rectum in the cow.

Nerve supply

The mammary gland possesses both **sensory and motor nerves**. Mammary nerves do not make any direct connection with alveolar cells and have no direct effect on milk secretion; however, sensory nerves are important in the milk ejection process. Ventral branches of the first through fourth lumbar nerves

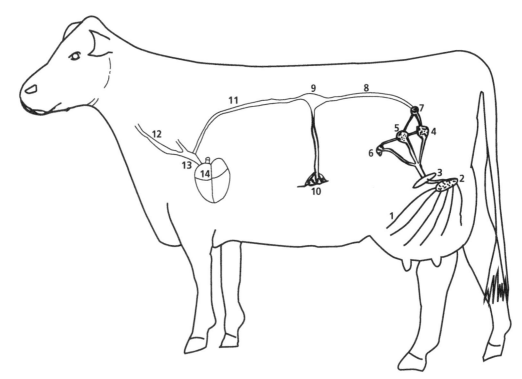

Figure 54.4 Lymphatic system of the cow showing lymph flow from the udder to the anterior vena cava. 1, Lymphatic vessels of udder; 2, supramammary lymph gland; 3, inguinal ring; 4, deep inguinal lymph gland; 5, external iliac lymph gland; 6, prefemoral lymph gland; 7, internal iliac lymph gland; 8, lumbar lymph trunk; 9, cisterna chyli; 10, intestinal lacteals; 11, thoracic lymph duct; 12, jugular vein; 13, anterior vena cava; 14, right atrium. From Anderson, R. (1985) Mammary gland. In: *Lactation* (ed. B.L. Larson). Iowa State University Press, Ames, Iowa.

supply the sensory nerve supply to the udder. The first and second nerve ventral branches unite, providing innervation to a small part of the cranial udder, primarily the skin. Ventral branches of the second, third, and fourth lumbar nerves come together to form the inguinal nerve. The inguinal nerve passes through the inguinal canal with the blood vessels that supply the mammary gland and then divides into cranial and caudal inguinal nerves. The cranial inguinal nerve innervates the cranial part of the front quarter, including the teat. The caudal inguinal nerve branches again into cranial and caudal branches, with the cranial branch (or branches) innervating the lateral skin of the front quarter and the caudal portion of the front quarter, although there is very little impact on the glandular tissue of the front quarter. The caudal branch of the caudal inguinal nerve innervates the glandular tissue, the caudal portion of the front quarter, and the entire rear quarter. Additionally, it supplies the area around the supramammary lymph node and the skin of the rear quarter, with the exception of the caudal portion above the base of the rear teat, which is supplied by the superficial perineal nerve. The complexity of sensory nerve innervation complicates local anesthesia of the udder but the intricacy of teat surgery is reduced, as the nerves of the teat essentially run vertically within the teat wall (Figure 54.5).

The skin of the teat has an abundant number of sensory receptors, especially near the teat sphincter. Stimulation of the sensory nerves is essential for milk letdown from the alveoli via the neurohormonal reflex responsible for oxytocin release.

The motor nerve supply contains nerve fibers from the sympathetic system but there appears to be no parasympathetic nerve innervation, despite the cutaneous origin of the mammary gland. The motor nerves originate from the lumbar sympathetic plexus and its primary activity is to induce vasoconstriction and muscular constriction of the teat sphincter.

Primary immune system defenses

Secretions of the mammary gland provide an opportunistic environment for bacterial growth if bacteria gain entrance to the gland. Immune function is unique in comparison to other parts of the body and it is compromised in various stages of lactation. The majority of new infections that develop in the mammary gland enter through the streak canal, so anatomical and physiological barriers provide the primary lines of immune system mammary defense. The smooth muscle of the teat sphincter closes the entrance to the streak canal, which prevents entrance of bacteria, but there are periods when the muscular activity of the sphincter is decreased, namely immediately after machine milking or during decreased muscular activity associated with periparturient paresis, which allows for easier access by microorganisms.

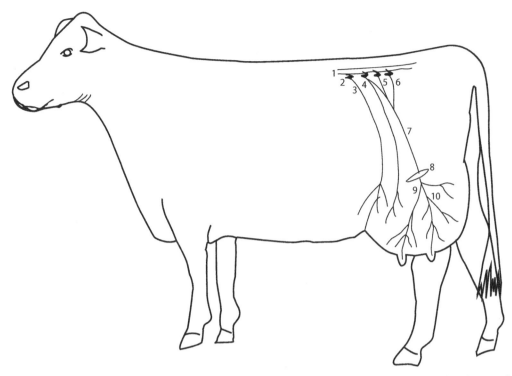

Figure 54.5 Nerves of the udder having afferent and efferent components that connect to the spinal cord. 1, Spinal cord; 2, ganglia of sympathetic nerve trunk; 3, first lumbar nerve; 4, second lumbar nerve; 5, third lumbar nerve; 6, fourth lumbar nerve; 7, inguinal nerve; 8, inguinal ring; 9, anterior inguinal nerve; 10, posterior inguinal nerve. From Anderson, R. (1985) Mammary gland. In: *Lactation* (ed. B.L. Larson). Iowa State University Press, Ames, Iowa.

Like other parts of the body, the skin that lines the teats and the udder, as well as the streak canal, provides a physical and chemical barrier to bacterial invasion. The skin and the lining of the streak canal have a normal flora of bacteria present that inhibit colonization by bacterial pathogens. In addition, keratin lines the surface of the streak canal. Keratin contains lipid and protein compounds that are antibacterial in nature. Keratin functions to prevent invasion by bacteria by first binding bacteria to its surface and then bacterial-laden keratin is expelled through controlled desquamation during the process of milk secretion. In addition, keratin desiccation can help form a keratin plug in the streak canal, thus blocking the streak canal during nonlactating periods.

Many of these primary anatomical and physiological mechanisms are highly heritable, including udder and teat size and shape, teat length and teat end shape, teat placement, udder depth, teat sphincter, and keratin.

Mammogenesis, lactogenesis, galactopoiesis, and involution

1 What mammary parenchymal structural development takes place between birth until pregnancy, including through puberty?

2 What is isometric and allometric growth and when does this occur during mammogenesis? Why is proper feeding important during these times?

3 When does the most structural development of the mammary gland take place?

4 What is the cause of accelerated mammary growth during pregnancy?

5 What are the two stages of lactogenesis and what blocks these through late pregnancy?

6 What changes in mammary secretory cells occur after exposure to hormones of the lactogenic complex? What are the hormones of the lactogenic complex?

7 What are the characteristics of mammary involution and what brings about involution?

Successful lactation is required to complete the reproductive process in most mammalian species, with the physiology of reproduction and lactation being intimately interdependent. It requires coordinated growth processes that start *in utero* and continue through delivery of the first young, and to some extent into early lactation, by a process called **mammogenesis**, or mammary growth and development. **Lactogenesis** is defined as the initiation of lactation, where alveolar cells differentiate into milk-producing and -secreting cells and tissue, while **galactopoiesis** is defined as maintenance and/or enhancement of an

Table 54.2 Major hormones affecting mammary gland development or function.

Endocrine gland	Hormone secreted	Major mammary effect
Anterior pituitary	Adrenocorticotropic hormone (ACTH)	Stimulates adrenal secretion of cortisol
	Follicle-stimulating hormone (FSH)	Estrogen secretion
	Growth hormone (GH)	Stimulates milk production
	Luteinizing hormne (LH)	Progesterone secretion
	Prolactin (PRL)	Lactogenesis, cell differentiation, milk protein gene expression
	Thyroid-stimulating hormone (TSH)	Stimulates thyroid gland to secrete thyroxine and triiodothyronine
Posterior pituitary	Oxytocin	Milk ejection reflex
Hypothalamus	Growth hormone-releasing hormone	Stimulates GH secretion
	Somatostatin	Inhibits GH secretion
	Thyrotropin-releasing hormone	Stmulates TSH secretion (as well as PRL and GH)
	Corticotropin-releasing hormone	Stimulates ACTH secretion
	Prolactin-inhibiting hormone (dopamine)	Inhibits PRL secretion
Thyroid	Thyroxine, triiodothyronine	Stimulate oxygen consumption, protein synthesis
	Thyrocalcitonin	Calcium and phosphorus metabolism
Parathyroid	Parathyroid hormone	Calcium and phosphorus metabolism
Pancreas	Insulin	Glucose metabolism (species variation)
Adrenal cortex	Glucocorticoids (cortisol, corticosterone)	Lactogenesis, cell differentiation milk protein gene expression
Adrenal medulla	Epinephrine	Inhibition of milk ejection reflex (peripheral)
Ovary	Estrogen	Mammary duct growth
	Progesterone	Mammary lobuloalveolar development, inhibition of lactogenesis
Placenta	Estrogen	*See* Ovary
	Progesterone (species dependent)	
	Placental lactogen	Mammary development

Source: Akers, R.M. (2002) Overview of mammary development. In: *Lactation and the Mammary Gland*. Iowa State Press, Ames, IA. Reproduced with permission from Wiley.

established lactation. **Involution** involves both anatomical and physiological changes (immediate, short and long term) associated with cessation of milking.

All processes associated with lactation, from mammogenesis to galactopoiesis through involution, are regulated by hormonal interactions with the mammary gland and exchanges with other tissues of the body. Endocrine glands most intimately associated with successful lactation include the hypothalamus, pituitary, adrenal, ovaries, and placenta but other endocrine glands have influence as well (Table 54.2).

Mammogenesis

Mammogenesis or growth and development of the mammary gland takes place during various reproductive epochs beginning in the fetal or prenatal period and continuing through parturition, and early lactation in some species. Mammogenesis is a unique interaction of ectodermally derived tissue or parenchyma (milk ductal and secretory epithelial cells) with mesoderm tissue or stroma (myoepithelial cells, adipocytes, fibroblasts, and cells associated with the vascular, neural, and immune systems). Mammary growth, particularly in terms of parenchymal tissue, is correlated with milk yield. While a large proportion of this growth occurs during pregnancy, especially late gestation, there is compelling evidence that alteration in growth in all periods prior to this can compromise future lactation and production. Also, the mammary gland is one of the few tissues in mammals which can repeatedly undergo cycles of growth, functional differentiation, and regression.

Fetal development

The first indicator of mammary development is slight thickening of the embryonic ventrolateral ectoderm, known as the mammary band, at about the time limb buds begin to lengthen (30 days in bovine). The sequence of developmental events is similar across species in relation to different gestation lengths. These ectodermal cells proliferate and condense into cell masses that define where mammary glands will form (mammary streak, lines, crest) around 35 days. The ectodermal mass will grow into the mesoderm (mammary hillock) and then form a dome-shaped hemispherical structure (mammary bud: 43 days in bovine; 49 days in human). These tissue layers are always separated by a distinct basement membrane. Up to this stage females and males develop identically. Following this, males and females grow slightly differently, with males growing slower in most species, but male rats, mice, and horses stop teat formation. The proliferating ectoderm moves deeper into the mesenchyme, forming the primary sprout (days 60–80). In species where there are multiple ducts exiting each teat, the inner layer of the primary bud proliferates and produces secondary buds for each future exiting duct (10–25 in humans) and each of these develops an epithelial cord or sprout that will ultimately form lactiferous ducts. Secondary sprouts grow and branch from the primary sprout around 100 days. At this time, the process of forming the lumen in this solid core of epithelial cells, called canalization, starts at the proximal end of the primary sprout and proceeds in both directions. The canalized primary sprout becomes the gland and teat cistern around 130 days and ultimately the streak canal, while the secondary sprouts become major lactiferous ducts. Expansion and canalization continue until canals are lined with only a couple of layers of epithelial cells. At the same time, rapid growth of the mesenchyme around the bud raises this area, resulting in early teat formation. Blood and lymph vessels start to develop in a dense mesenchyme with many fibroblasts in the area associated with the bud and sprout. Development of udder shape, including the fat pad, begins. The size and development of this pad and mesenchyme is critical, as it dictates future parenchymal growth. Hormones involved during this period include growth hormone and adrenocorticoids, as well as local factors such as insulin-like growth factors (IGF), all involved in cellular and nutrient metabolism. As the teat develops, the tip invaginates from the outside, resulting in the surface cells keratinizing and forming the streak canal and keratin layer.

Mammogenesis in growing animals: birth to parturition
Birth to puberty
At birth, teats are well developed with the gland canalized to the inner ectoderm growth, nonsecretory tissue known as stroma is well formed, while no secretory or glandular parts have yet developed. Prepubertal mammary growth in most species is **isometric** (same as body growth rate) and is mostly associated with ductal elongation and associated stromal tissue development. Hormones involved are similar to those of the fetal period. However, in cattle **allometric** growth (faster than body growth rate) starts at 3–4 months of age and continues after puberty for a few months.

Feeding and nutrition during this period are critical. Recent research evaluating accelerated feeding and growth of preweaned calves (i.e., during the isometric period where parenchymal tissue increases 20 fold) has shown effects on mammary tissue that result in increased future milk production. Overfeeding energy during the allometric phase, especially the prepubertal phase, can result in excess fat deposition and possible inhibition of parenchymal growth and future milk production.

Puberty to conception
Mammary growth is allometric through the first few estrous cycles and then resumes isometric growth until conception. Much of parenchymal growth is characterized by elongation and/or branching of the ductal system, with this enhanced growth as well as stromal growth (especially blood vessels) under the influence of **estrogen**, therefore resulting in greater growth in females. This enhancement of stromal tissue, especially vascularity, is the subject of much research related to estrogenic effects and mammary tumor development and cancer. In species like rodents, the elongating ducts can have terminal end buds (TEB), which are actively growing ectodermal tissue under estrogen stimulation with limited branching. In ruminants, humans, and other species, this ductile development is also associated with branching (possibly due to

both estrogen and progesterone associated with longer luteal phases and permissive prolactin effects) and results in terminal ductile lobular units (TDLUs). TDLUs are developmental and functional parenchymal units held together by loose intralobular connective tissue and surrounded by a denser interlobular connective tissue resulting in lobular and lobe development.

Conception to parturition
Factors associated with the maternal–conceptus axis enhance allometric growth, with 45–95% of total mammary growth during this period. This growth is exponential in relation to fetal and placental growth, with most growth during the last trimester of pregnancy. This parenchymal growth involves extensive lobuloalveolar growth. Early pregnancy is characterized by ductal elongation and branching, with mid to late pregnancy associated with alveolar development. Alveoli are formed by a single epithelial cell layer or ball that will differentiate into milk secretory cells that secrete into the hollow lumen and duct, while surrounded by myoepithelial cells, composed of smooth muscle, and blood vessel networks. Optimal mammary growth, especially in late gestation, requires both estrogen and progesterone and the simultaneously elevated levels of both steroid hormones that are associated with pregnancy and the placenta, in addition to the previously mentioned mammogenic hormones. This growth also requires concurrent secretion of prolactin (PRL) and growth hormone (GH), and is further enhanced by placental lactogen, a placenta-derived hormone in some species that possesses PRL and GH activity. This increase and permissiveness of prolactin is important in most species but essential in rodents to diminish TEB and allow rapid ductile branching and alveolar development. Insulin and IGFs are also involved in mammary cell mitosis during pregnancy, and thyroid hormones are involved in overall metabolic rate and oxygen consumption of the body. Alveolar cells proliferate through the prepartum period until differentiated into secretory cells via an orchestrated hormonal profile, which includes a decrease in progesterone due to luteolysis via ovarian prostaglandin release prior to parturition.

Although pregnancy is considered essential for mammary growth, development, and lactation, programs to induce lactation in many species, including humans, have been developed. These programs often include simultaneous steroid hormone (estrogen and progesterone) administration followed by properly timed administration of PRL agonists and then a corticosteroid. Programs focused on enhancement of PRL only, via teat stimulation and/or compounds that enhance PRL or mammary blood flow, have resulted in milk production, but this is often limited compared to when all hormones are synchronized. Any of these programs must be accompanied by appropriate medical supervision and are illegal in food-producing animals in the USA.

Lactogenesis
In order for a lactation to be successful, three distinct events must occur: (i) prepartum proliferation of alveolar epithelial cells, (ii) biochemical and structural differentiation of the

epithelial cells, and (iii) synthesis and secretion of milk components. Lactogenesis or initiation of lactation is this process of differentiation whereby mammary alveolar cell acquire the ability to secrete milk. It is defined by a two-stage mechanism. The first stage of lactogenesis consists of partial enzymatic and cytological differentiation of alveolar cells with limited secretion. The second stage begins with copious secretion of all milk components shortly before parturition and extends several days postpartum in most species. High progesterone in late pregnancy blocks lactogenesis. A drop in progesterone near parturition allows the **lactogenic complex** to initiate cell differentiation and lactation. Estrogen has a stimulatory effect on PRL secretion. Glucocorticoids become less bound to globulin proteins and the PRL– glucocorticoid complex initiates differentiation and early enzymatic activities to produce and secrete milk. Other hormones involved include GH, IGF, insulin, and thyroid hormones. At the onset of the lactation, alveolar cells have undergone dramatic maturation of rough endoplasmic reticulum, smooth endoplasmic reticulum, and Golgi apparatus under the influences of PRL and glucocorticoids, resulting in cellular ability to synthesize and secrete protein, fat, and lactose.

Galactopoiesis

Galactopoiesis or maintenance of lactation requires preservation of alveolar cell numbers, synthetic activity per cell, and efficacy of the milk ejection reflex. Hormones involved are similar to those of the lactogenic complex, with the PRL–glucocorticoid complex involved in milk synthesis and secretion with other supportive hormones. Although all hormones are important, PRL is the dominant regulator in rodents, plus GH in many other species.

Lactation performance

After parturition, milk production increases at a high rate to peak yield and then daily milk yield decreases gradually until the end of lactation. This lactation curve is similar in all species, with the major differences being the height of the peak and the persistency and length of the lactation. In dairy cattle, peak production normally occurs 8–12 weeks after parturition and can easily exceed 45 kg per day in an older Holstein cow.

Once peak production has occurred, loss of daily milk production occurs due to decreased efficiency and some loss of secretory cells, most likely through apoptosis. The rate of decrease in daily milk yield after peak production throughout the remainder of the lactation is defined as **persistency**, with animals that have a smaller decline in production being more persistent. Age of the animal and pregnancy status affect persistency's contribution to the lactation curve most significantly, assuming that nutritional support is adequate. Production in primiparous animals usually declines by approximately 6% per month while older cows typically decline by 9% per month. Cattle that do not become pregnant can lactate indefinitely but the economics of milking those animals usually limits their productive lactation length 1–2 years if they do not become pregnant. As dairy

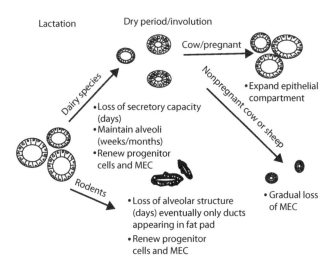

Figure 54.6 Comparison of structural changes during mammary involution in dairy animals and rodents. MEC, mammary epithelial cells. From Akers, R.M. (2002) Overview of mammary development. In: *Lactation and the Mammary Gland.* Iowa State Press, Ames, IA. Reproduced with permission from Wiley.

animals age, milk production per lactation increases, suggesting that mammary growth continues with successive lactations.

A hormonal complex controls lactation but unless milk is removed frequently, synthesis of milk will not persist. Conversely, intense suckling or milking to provide adequate milk removal will not sustain lactation indefinitely. Oxytocin is required for milk removal or ejection. Both milk synthesis and secretion and milk removal are integral processes for lactation persistency.

Involution

Involution is the process following cessation of milking that results in structural and physiological changes in the mammary gland. Secretory activity is decreased due to increased pressure and levels of the hormone feedback inhibitor of lactation (FIL). Rodents lose alveolar structure quickly (days) and only have ducts appearing in the fat pad due to decreased PRL. Dairy cows lose secretory activity over a longer period and can maintain their alveolar structures for weeks to months (Figure 54.6).

Milk secretion and synthesis

1 What are the five methods of transport of milk constituents into the alveolar lumen?

2 What is the major milk carbohydrate, what sugars comprise it, what enzymes make it, and where is it synthesized?

3 What are the two major classes of milk proteins, what are they synthesized from and where, and where are they packaged?

4 Do different species have different ratios of the two major protein classes? Why?

5 What are the unique features of α, β, and κ casein? What do these features accomplish?

6 What is the major form of lipids in milk and what are the major precursors of milk fatty acids and milk fat? What enzymes are essential to fatty acid synthesis and where does fatty acid synthesis take place? Where are triglycerides assembled?

7 What enzyme is present on the cell membrane that increases tissue uptake as well as disassembly of triglycerides during uptake?

8 How are calcium, phosphorus, magnesium, sodium, chloride, and potassium found in milk? Why are they different? What is usually the mineral with the highest content in milk?

9 Why should caution be exerted (from a mineral standpoint) when feeding milk components and formulas from one species to another?

10 Why are there interests in iodine and selenium in milk?

The alveolar cell undergoes extensive differentiation to enable the synthesis and secretion of milk (Figure 54.7). Other metabolic changes, including increase in appetite (food and water), gastrointestinal tract size and function, nutrient metabolism,

and weight loss, must also be coordinated to support lactation demands.

Mammary gland metabolism

The onset of lactation places a tremendous nutritional drain on the body. In the dairy cow, energy requirements for lactation can reach 80% of net energy from intake and lactose production can utilize 85% of circulating glucose. In order to meet these nutrient demands, there is a tremendous increase in nutrient and water intake and associated hypertrophy of the gastrointestinal tract, liver, and heart in addition to the mammary gland. In an attempt to meet the unmet nutrient demands from intake, body nutrient stores are employed through lipolysis and some, but limited, muscle catabolism. It is estimated that a dairy cow will lose 50 kg or more of body weight during the first 1–2 months of a new lactation in an attempt to establish nutrient homeorhesis. To conserve glucose for the synthesis of lactose, ruminants have developed glucose-sparing mechanisms in the mammary gland and other tissues of the body (i.e., myocytes) to preferentially use other metabolites, such as nonesterified fatty

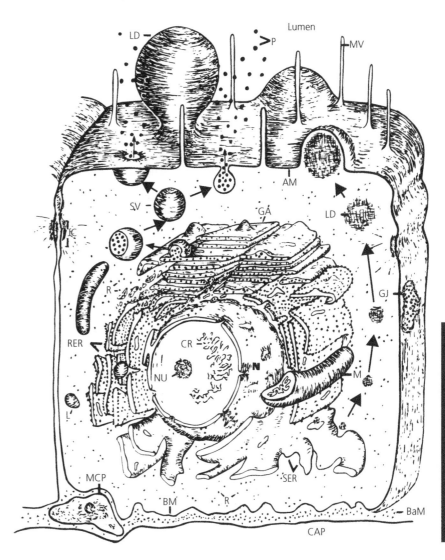

Figure 54.7 Diagrammatic representation of a secretory cell in the alveolar epithelium of the lactating mammary gland. AM, apical plasma membrane; BM, basal plasma membrane; BaM, basement membrane; CAP, capillary; CR, chromosomes; GA, Golgi apparatus; GJ, gap junction; JC, junctional complex; L, lysosome; LD, lipid droplet (globule); M, mitochondrion; MCP, myoepithelial cell process; MV, microvilli; N, nucleus; NU, nucleolus; P, protein (casein) micelle; R, ribosomes (free and bound); RER, rough endoplasmic reticulum; SER, smooth endoplasmic reticulum; SV, secretory vesicle. Precursors from the blood capillary (CAP) enter the cell and exit into the lumen as milk constituents. From Reece, W.O. (2004) *Dukes' Physiology of Domestic Animals*, 12th edn. Cornell University Press, Ithaca, NY. Reproduced with permission from Cornell University Press.

Table 54.3 Changes in serum concentrations of presumptive homeorhetic and homeostatic hormones, tissue sensitivity, and tissue responsiveness in selected tissues during pregnancy and lactation.

	Mid pregnancy	Late pregnancy	Early lactation
Homeorhetic hormones			
Progesterone	↑	↓	↓
Placental lactogen		↑	↓
Estrogens		↑	↓
Prolactin	—	—	↑
Growth hormone			↑
Leptin	?	?	?
Homeostatic hormones			
Insulin		↑	↓
Glucagon	—	—	—
CCK and somatostatin	?	?	?
Tissue sensitivity			
Insulin	↑	↓	↓
Catecholamines		↑	↑
Tissue responsiveness			
Insulin		↓	↓
Catecholamines	↓	↑	↑
Liver			
Gluconeogenesis			↑
Ketogenesis			↑
Adipose tissue			
Lipogenesis	↑	↓	↓
Fatty acid esterification	↑	↓	↓
Lipolysis		↑	↑
Glucose utilization		↓	↓
Skeletal muscle			
Protein synthesis		↓	↓
Protein degradation		↑	↑
Glucose utilization		↓	↓

CCK, cholecystokinin; ↑, increase; ↓, decrease; —, no change; ?, unknown for ruminants. It should also be understood that not all ruminants are necessarily equivalent (e.g., there are differences in placental lactogen in cows vs. sheep). *Source*: Akers, R.M. (2002) Overview of mammary development. In: *Lactation and the Mammary Gland*. Iowa State Press, Ames, IA. Reproduced with permission from Wiley.

acids (NEFAs) and ketone bodies, as energy sources for metabolic activities. Metabolic and hormonal changes that take place during mid to late pregnancy and into lactation are shown in Table 54.3.

Secretion of milk components

During lactation, the components of milk are secreted across the mammary epithelium and/or into the lumen by one of five routes: (i) membrane route, (ii) Golgi route, (iii) milk fat route, (iv) transcytosis, and (v) paracellular route.

Membrane route

Interstitial fluid-derived substances like water, urea, glucose, and some ions utilize the **membrane route**. After these compounds cross the basolateral membrane of the alveolar epithelial cell, they traverse the cytoplasm and then diffuse across the apical membrane of the cell into the alveolar lumen.

Golgi route

Products that utilize the **Golgi route** must first by synthesized within the cell and then packaged into secretory vesicles within the Golgi apparatus. Once these materials are packaged, vesicles bud from the stacks of Golgi membranes, travel to the apical membrane where they fuse with the membrane and release their contents, leaving their membrane behind. Substances that are secreted via the Golgi route include lactose, casein, whey proteins, citrate and calcium.

Milk fat route

When milk fat droplets are secreted into milk via the **milk fat route**, a portion of apical membrane surrounds the droplets. During the process of milk fat droplet budding through the apical membrane, portions of the cytoplasm and other cellular substances from the epithelial cell can be trapped in the milk fat droplet. Examples of substances that are typically secreted in this manner include any lipid-soluble material found in the cell, including drugs and hormones. However, due to the random nature in which cytoplasm is incorporated into the fat droplet, any cellular components or cytoplasmic substances could be secreted in this manner.

Transcytosis

Transcytosis involves the transport of vesicles derived from the basolateral membrane via endocytosis or pinocytosis, which then migrate across the cellular cytoplasm and are secreted into milk via exocytosis. Examples of products transported via transcytosis include immunoglobulin during lactation and albumin.

Paracellular route

Paracellular transport involves the passage of materials from the interstitial fluid, between adjacent cells, and into the milk. During colostrogenesis, much of the immunoglobulin and other serum-derived proteins move into the mammary secretions via the paracellular route prior to the formation of tight junctions. However, after parturition, maturation of the tight junctions prevents paracellular transport of most materials, like immunoglobulins, unless the tight junctions are disrupted. Disruption of tight junctions can occur through diapedesis of leukocytes, bouts of mastitis, administration of supraphysiologic doses of oxytocin, or prolonged intervals between milk removal. Higher levels of serum proteins like bovine serum albumin (BSA) and higher levels of sodium and chloride result due to leakage, and lactose synthesis will decrease via downregulation of α-lactalbumin to maintain osmotic balance.

Biosynthesis of milk components

Milk carbohydrates (lactose)

Lactose is the primary carbohydrate in milk of most species and relies on the supply of glucose from direct digestion of sugars and starches by nonruminants, indirect digestion to propionate in ruminants, and conversion of propionate and/or gluconeogenic amino acids in the liver. An initial glucose molecule enters the cell and is phosphorylated, which fixes glucose inside the cell. Some glucose molecules are then converted to galactose via an epimerase enzyme and uridine triphosphate (UTP). Lactose is formed in the Golgi apparatus by combining glucose and galactose under the control of **lactose synthase** (a two-enzyme complex of **galactosyltransferase**, which is common in tissues, and mammary-specific **α-lactalbumin**). Lactose is packaged in secretory vesicles along with specific proteins to be exported from the cell. As the vesicle awaits secretion from the cell, substantial water is incorporated into the vesicle due to the osmotic effect of lactose. Lactose is the major contributor to milk osmolarity.

Milk proteins

Most milk proteins are synthesized in the rough endoplasmic reticulum from blood amino acids that result from digestion of feed protein, ruminally derived bacterial protein, or limited body protein catabolism. The cellular process for assembly of these proteins is similar to that of other protein-synthesizing cells. The two major classes of protein made are **casein** and **whey**, with a small amount of nonprotein nitrogen, mainly urea, which can be used diagnostically to evaluate protein and energy feeding interactions in ruminants. Different species contain different proportions of protein classes (cow, 79% and 21%; sow, 58% and 42%; human, 35% and 65% casein and whey proteins, respectively) due to the neonate's ability to handle and differentially digest each protein class. Whey proteins are packaged in the Golgi secretory vesicles and include β-lactoglobulin and α-lactalbumin, immune proteins such as lactoferrin and lysosomal enzymes, and protein hormones. Casein is phosphorylated in the Golgi and this allows other minerals such as Ca, Mg, Zn, Fe, Cu, and Mn to bind, forming natural organic chelation products. **α and β Casein** contain high amounts of calcium phosphate and link together to form protein colloids called casein micelles. **κ Casein** is situated on the outside of the micelle. It has less calcium phosphate but has a carbohydrate chain that restricts micelles from coagulating. The micelle is packaged in the Golgi secretory vesicle. During digestion, low pH (<4.6) and/or the presence of rennin enzyme hydrolyzes the carbohydrate and the micelles coagulate to form clots or curds, which aid in slowing down passage and enhancing digestion. Milk proteins have an excellent amino acid profile and are highly digestible.

Milk fat or lipids

Milk fat is primarily composed of **triglycerides** that are composed of variable mixtures of fatty acids, depending on dietary availability of free fatty acids, with the balance of the fat globule composed of diglycerides, monoglycerides, free fatty acids, phospholipids, cholesterol, and cholesterol esters.

In bovines, milk fat is approximately 98% triglyceride with high amounts of saturated fatty acids due to partial or full hydrogenation in the rumen. Circulating chylomicrons and lipoproteins containing triglycerides interact with **lipoprotein lipase**, an enzyme on the cell that helps tissues sequester lipids and breaks down triglycerides on entry into the cell. Three pathways exist for the synthesis of milk fat in the mammary gland. However, glucose-sparing mechanisms and the availability of precursors limit the application of all three pathways in most species. A significant portion of milk fat is derived directly from the diet, with much of this being C_{16} or larger fatty acids, including the essential fatty acids linoleic and linolenic. In cattle, this accounts for approximately half of the milk fat, including most of the C_{18} fatty acids and approximately 30% of the C_{16} fatty acids. In an attempt to spare glucose for synthesis of lactose, ruminants acquire the other half of their fatty acids through *de novo* synthesis in the mammary epithelial cells, using acetate and β-hydroxybutyrate as the precursors. In nonruminant species, metabolism of glucose by the epithelial cell provides acetyl-CoA, which can be used as the carbon primer for fatty acid synthesis. Fatty acid synthesis occurs in the mammary cell cytoplasm and requires **acetyl-CoA carboxylase** as well as a four-enzyme system called **fatty acid synthetase** to link two carbon chains together.

Synthesis and transfer of triglycerides within the epithelial cell begins near the smooth endoplasmic reticulum, although the exact transport mechanism is not well understood. Accumulation of triglycerides and other lipid products within the cytoplasm results in the formation of microdroplets, which coalesce into larger droplets as they translocate to the apical membrane where they are secreted.

Other components

Milk provides all the essential vitamins and minerals in appropriate quantities for specific neonatal growth. Milk is a rich source of calcium and phosphorus but also contains magnesium, potassium, chloride, and sodium. These minerals are derived from the blood and the balance between milk and blood is maintained via active transport mechanisms. Calcium, phosphorus, and magnesium are chelated to casein, while sodium, chloride, and potassium are secreted as highly available free ions and controlled through sophisticated pumping and feedback mechanisms. Potassium provides the highest concentration of mineral in most species but calcium is highest in the pig. Differences in ion concentrations in relationship to neonatal kidney function is critical when considering feeding artificial milk to other species as it is often these ion differences that lead to renal issues. Iodine is highly sequestered in milk, outcompeting the thyroid, so concerns about iodine in milk due to chelated iodine-containing feed products led to establishment of a legal limit in milk. Also, during the Japan typhoon in 2011 that damaged nuclear plants and released radioactive materials (including iodine), milk from animals around the world was specifically monitored because of the mammary gland's ability to sequester iodine. Organic selenium, usually fed as selenium-rich yeast, can increase selenium levels in milk and milk products; this has stimulated interest with regard to human consumption but concerns have been expressed about the potential for selenium toxicity at the animal level. Vitamins in milk are also absorbed from the blood. Increasing concentrations of vitamins in the blood of cows will generally result in an increase in milk concentrations.

Concentrations of lactose, sodium, and potassium are usually constant in milk. These components, along with chloride, dictate the osmotic balance between milk and blood. Maintaining osmotic balance in milk dictates the volume of milk produced. Paracellular leakage of sodium and chloride during mastitis leads to decreased lactose via downregulation of α-lactalbumin to maintain osmotic balance.

Physiological control of milk secretion and milk removal

> 1 Is mammary gland milk secretion always at a constant rate? If not, what factors affect the rate of milk secretion into the alveolar lumen?
>
> 2 What is the major factor affecting milk secretion rate and sustained lactation?

> 3 What are the major physical and chemical factors that affect milk secretion rate?
>
> 4 What hormone is essential in the milk letdown or ejection process? Where is the hormone made, how does it get to the mammary gland, and what target tissue does it affect?
>
> 5 What factors cause the release of oxytocin? Which factor results in the highest oxytocin release?
>
> 6 Why should the lag time between teat stimulation and milking machine attachment be 90–120 s?

Control of milk secretion

Once initiated, secretion of milk by alveolar epithelial cells is a continuous process but secretion does not occur at a constant rate over time. Maintenance of secretion throughout an individual lactation cycle requires regular removal of milk from the gland. Rate of milk secretion depends on available storage capacity within the gland. Rate of milk secretion is fastest immediately after milk removal via suckling or milking and slows dramatically by 10–12 hours. Implementing a shorter interval between subsequent bouts of milk removal can increase milk production capacity. Approximately 35 hours after the most recent milk removal, milk secretion essentially stops.

Control of milk secretion is achieved through both physical and chemical interactions. **Physical limitations** are achieved through the build-up of pressure within the alveoli, resulting in an inverse relationship between intramammary (IMM) pressure and milk secretion rate. As milk pressure builds up, supporting structures, such as blood vessels, will be displaced, which in turn will limit the delivery of nutrients to alveolar cells. Pressure within the gland is highest at milking or suckling time, when teat stimulation causes oxytocin release and contraction of myoepithelial cells, resulting in milk letdown. During this time, IMM pressure is approximately 35–55 mmHg. As the milk removal process continues, pressure will drop to near zero independently of the amount of milk removed. Within 1 hour of milking, pressure will increase to a level of approximately 8 mmHg and continues to increase steadily until the next milking. In dairy cattle, high- and low-yielding cows experience the same change in absolute pressure but the pressure per unit of newly secreted milk is lower in high-yielding cows.

Chemical control of milk secretion appears to occur at the local level through a protein fraction called **feedback inhibitor of lactation (FIL)**, which is secreted by mammary epithelial cells. Milk secretion rate is inversely proportional to FIL concentration in the alveoli. FIL's mode of action is not fully understood, but it apparently works to slow milk secretion rate by suppressing key enzymes in epithelial cells, thus slowing secretion of key milk components. Over time, increasing concentrations of FIL stimulate intracellular breakdown of casein, reduces the number of PRL receptors on mammary epithelial cells, and inhibits differentiation of mammary epithelial cells.

Milk removal

Removal of milk from the mammary gland is accomplished when milk is released from the alveolar areas of the gland into the ducts and gland and teat cisterns, and subsequently expelled from the teat during the process of suckling or machine milking. Milk letdown is achieved when oxytocin is released from the posterior pituitary into the bloodstream and interacts with oxytocin receptors on the myoepithelial cells surrounding the alveoli. This hormone–receptor interaction causes contraction of the myoepithelial cells, which essentially squeezes the milk from the alveolar lumen and releases it into the ducts leading to the gland cistern.

Release of oxytocin from the posterior pituitary is accomplished through either tactile stimulation of the sensory receptors on the teat or conditioned responses from higher brain centers in response to external stimuli (i.e., the cry of a dam's offspring, visual sight of the neonate, or approaching the milking parlor by dairy cattle). Tactile stimulation of the teat end occurs either through suckling by the neonate or by mechanical stimulation of the teat end during udder preparation practices associated with machine milking.

After mechanical stimulation, elevations in oxytocin concentrations can be detected in the jugular vein within 30 s independent of level of milk production, stage of lactation, season, or other potential influencing factors. In machine-milked dairy cattle, basal levels of oxytocin in the blood range from 1 to 5 pg/mL between milkings and reach 10–100 pg/mL following oxytocin release, depending on the effectiveness of stimulation. More efficient stimulation and suckling of a calf produce higher levels of oxytocin, but it has been shown that a level of 10 pg/mL is sufficient to produce adequate alveolar milk release via myoepithelial cell contraction. The appearance of alveolar milk in the teat cistern varies widely depending on the degree of udder fill, with alveolar milk reaching the teat in 40–50 s in cows with full udders whereas it may take up to 3 min in cows with a low udder fill. Therefore, it is recommended that the lag time from teat stimulation to milking unit attachment should be 90–120 s in an attempt to achieve uniform milk letdown across the entire herd during machine milking.

Once milk letdown is initiated, the entire volume of milk stored within the alveoli is not immediately released. Oxytocin has a half-life of 2–3 min once it interacts with the receptor, which is shorter than the average milking time, so that maximum removal of the alveolar fraction of milk requires continuous stimulation of the teat throughout the milk removal process. This is only accomplished during machine milking by the movement of the liner wall of the milking unit around the teat end. Therefore, continued stimulation of the teat end via liner wall movement will cause pulsatile release of oxytocin throughout the milking process, insuring complete milk-out of the udder minus a residual volume of 5–20% of the total milk (alveolar and cisternal) volume, which cannot be removed unless exogenous oxytocin is administered.

Evacuation of milk from the teat occurs because a pressure difference is established between the milk in the teat cistern and the area outside the teat. This pressure difference must be sufficient to overcome the resistance to milk flow created by the teat sphincter and duct resistance. The udder assists with milk evacuation via the increased hydrostatic pressure that is achieved by milk letdown. The young calf initiates a vacuum inside its mouth during the suckling process that allows milk to flow from the teat, while the goat kid clamps the teat with the mouth and uses the tongue to squeeze the teat and mechanically express milk from the teat. Therefore, the calf mimics the process utilized by machine milking while the goat kid mimics the process of hand milking.

It has long been thought that catecholamines (epinephrine and norepinephrine) interfere with the milk removal process by causing severe contraction of smooth muscle. However, recent research indicates that these hormones only affect milk removal at supraphysiologic levels, unless oxytocin levels are insufficient. It appears that interference with milk letdown by certain animals (i.e., immediate postpartum first-lactation cows) may be the result of reduced or nonexistent release of oxytocin. Administration of exogenous sources of oxytocin to such animals is the most common therapy for overcoming this lack of oxytocin. However, extreme care must be exercised when deciding to utilize this therapy, for multiple reasons. First, exogenous administration of oxytocin causes elevated levels for several hours afterwards, which results in early accumulation of cisternal milk that leads to increased risk for development of mastitis. Secondly, chronic exogenous administration can lead to addiction to the hormone within 1 week of use, with a constant requirement for exogenous administration that will need to be implemented throughout the entire lactation. Efforts to break the addiction through withholding the exogenous source of oxytocin will require 48 hours or longer to take effect, resulting in an irreversible reduction in lactational performance and an increased risk for the development of new IMM bacterial infections.

Factors affecting lactation

1 Are milk production and components influenced by parents? If so, what percentage of the variation in milk production and milk components (lactose, fat, and protein) are explained or accounted for by genetic inheritance?

2 What is the most limiting nutrient in early lactation? Why?

3 What is the most variable milk component? What are some causes for this wide variation?

4 What factors affect or result in milk fat depression?

5 Does milking more frequently impact milk production?

6 What is rBST? How does it enhance milk production?

7 At what temperature in dairy cows does heat stress start to alter physiology? What changes take place during heat stress?

8 What is mastitis and what is the primary cause for mastitis?

9 What milk compositional changes take place when mastitis occurs?

10 What is the normal range of pH in milk?

Genetics or heritability

Milk yield and milk components or composition are highly heritable traits. **Heritability (h^2)** is defined as the amount of variation that can be explained by genetics or inheritance. In dairy cattle, h^2 of milk production is 0.25–0.27 (or 25–27% of variation due to genetics), while h^2 of lactose, protein, and fat is 0.55, 0.49, and 0.58, respectively. Genetic correlations between fat and protein percentage are 0.5 (there is a positive effect on one when selecting for the other), while genetic correlations between milk production and fat and protein percentage are –0.2 and –0.1, respectively.

Nutrition and physiological and environmental factors

Milk production in the dairy cow follows a typical pattern throughout the stages of lactation. At the onset of lactation following parturition, milk production starts at a high rate and increases steadily throughout the first 8–12 weeks of lactation. During much of this period, the cow cannot consume sufficient amounts of energy and protein from her diet to match the nutrient outputs of milk production. Cows will mobilize stored energy reserves through lipolysis of body fat and stored protein reserves through muscle catabolism to meet nutrient demands. In addition, she must mobilize vast amounts of minerals, like calcium, in early lactation from bone storage. **Energy** is the most limiting nutrient in early lactation and has a direct relationship to the amount of milk produced because the content of lactose in milk is tightly regulated and the osmotic tie that lactose creates for the movement of water into milk.

Protein requirements in dairy cattle are very specific and require proper proportions of ruminally degradable and ruminally undegradable protein in order to maximize milk production. Underfeeding of specific protein requirements can cause a dramatic reduction in milk production. However, feeding protein in excess of requirements or of energy availability within the rumen will require the cow to expend energy to eliminate excess protein from the body by means of urea nitrogen. Dairy cattle nutritionists often use milk urea nitrogen content as a means of monitoring protein and energy nutrition balance of lactating cows.

The most variable component in milk is fat content. Hereditary and nutritional interventions have a strong influence on milk fat content. Feeding adequate amounts of fiber to ruminant animals results in sufficient supplies of ruminally derived acetate which, along with β-hydroxybutyrate, is essential for *de novo* fat synthesis within the mammary secretory cells.

Biohydrogenation of dietary fats in the bovine rumen produces an important source of **conjugated linoleic acids (CLAs)** that provide many health benefits to humans. Milk and dairy products are the primary source of CLAs in the diets of most humans. However, alterations in rumen fermentation can create particular geometric isomers of CLA, specifically *cis*-10, *trans*-12 CLA, which can dramatically reduce milk fat production in dairy cattle by blocking fatty acid uptake at the mammary

gland level. Specific situations that may alter rumen metabolism and create milk fat depression include induction of rumen acidosis through overfeeding of concentrates and/or underfeeding of fiber, inclusion of excessive levels of dietary vegetable fats, and inclusion of the ionophore monensin in the diet. Monensin selects for the bacteria in the rumen that produce the volatile fatty acid propionate at the expense of acetate production.

As has been discussed, milk secretion depends on the continued release of PRL and removal of the negative feedback associated with build-up of milk components and the hormone FIL. Extensive research has manipulated milk removal intervals in an attempt to increase milk production. Milking cows twice daily has been shown to increase milk production by approximately 20–40% per day compared with once-daily milking depending on stage of lactation. Milking thrice daily has been shown to produce an additional 5–20% over milking twice daily. More recent research has demonstrated that milking cows four to six times daily for a defined period during the first 14–21 days of lactation will result in higher production per day throughout the remainder of the lactation, despite reducing the number of milkings after the defined period. This physiological phenomenon appears to occur through proliferation of additional secretory cells or enhanced functional differentiation in a population of preexisting nonsecretory cells.

By far the most common galactopoietic treatment utilized by today's dairy industry is the treatment of cows with **recombinant bovine somatotropin (rBST)**. rBST increases milk production by stimulating the mammary secretory epithelium to increase its metabolic rate, decrease cell aging, and improve nutrient utilization and partitioning, rather than through differentiation of new epithelial cells. Currently, the only rBST product marketed increases milk production during the period of treatment and calls for cows to be redosed every 14 days or milk production will return to pretreatment levels.

All animal species are exposed to outdoor weather conditions and will be exposed to temperature conditions outside their thermoneutral zone, which will increase the animal's maintenance nutrient requirements. In the US dairy industry, **heat stress** begins to occur around 20°C with breeds typical for the industry and costs millions of dollars in lost income each year. Heat stress increases the maintenance requirement in Holstein cattle by 25–30% but there is also a concurrent decrease in dry matter intake, resulting in negative energy balance and decreased daily milk production. However, the resulting decreased dry matter intake only accounts for approximately 50% of the reduction in milk production, indicating that other adaptations in metabolism are taking place to reduce heat increment. Normally, cows in negative energy balance would shift homeorhetic mechanisms to alter metabolism, such as decreasing insulin levels and increasing lipolysis from stored reserves. However, recent research has shown that many animal species implement an impaired lipolysis regulated by increased circulating levels of insulin, which results in increased utilization of glucose by hepatocytes and myocytes. Utilization of stored lipids as energy sources will increase the heat increment, so it appears that dairy animals preferentially utilize glucose as the predominant energy source in an attempt to maintain thermoneutrality, at the expense of milk production. In contrast, during periods of cold stress cattle increase dry matter intake to account for increased maintenance nutrient requirements. Increased dry matter intake prevents daily milk production loss until the temperature drops below −20°C.

There are typically variations in milk composition during seasonal changes, with levels of milk fat, protein, total solids, and nonfat solids generally higher during winter months and lowered fat and protein contents during summer months.

Metabolic disturbances and mastitis
Metabolic disturbances

The onset of lactation creates a tremendous demand for energy, protein, and minerals to support high levels of milk production. In an attempt to maintain energy homeorhesis, species undergo extensive lipolysis to provide NEFAs for the liver to metabolize and produce energy sources for other tissues, along with ketone bodies, in an attempt to spare glucose for galactopoiesis. Incomplete oxidation of NEFAs results in the development of ketone bodies, which are released into the blood and can be used by other body tissues as an energy source. Ketone bodies can accumulate in tissues, including milk, and excessive ketone presence will cause **ketosis** to develop. Assessment of milk ketone levels is often used by veterinarians to detect and monitor ketosis levels in dairy herds.

In the biosynthesis of milk fat, the mammary gland incorporates circulating NEFAs into milk fat. It is common for postpartum dairy cows to have high concentrations of blood NEFAs, which are incorporated into milk fat and can result in milk fat concentrations in excess of 6% in the first month of lactation. Elevated milk fat levels in the postparturient period are often used as a metric to monitor NEFA mobilization and ketosis in dairy cattle, with a milk fat/protein ratio of 1.4 or 1.5 or more used as a signal or indicator of potential problems.

At parturition, there is a tremendous need for calcium in order to support colostrum and milk synthesis. Colostrum has a calcium concentration of approximately 2.1 g/L while milk has a calcium concentration of 1.22 g/L. The postparturient animal must supply this calcium from her circulating pool and from extravascular sources such as bone and the diet. If these sources are insufficient to meet the demand, subclinical or clinical **hypocalcemia** will develop that will limit metabolic functions of the animal, alter muscular activity, may result in the animal becoming nonambulatory and, if not corrected, could lead to death. Calcium homeostasis is essential for proper function of the immune system and therefore important in limiting postpartum diseases.

Mastitis

Mastitis is defined as an inflammation of the mammary gland but in most situations the changes in milk are subclinical, with no change in the visible appearance of the milk. Subclinical mastitis results in the greatest economic losses associated with mastitis in dairy cattle. Estimates indicate that only 25% of all mastitis losses are associated with cases where the milk is visually abnormal, known as **clinical mastitis**. Most cow dairy farms experience a 25–40% incidence of clinical mastitis on an annual basis. The majority of the IMM infections are bacterial in origin but there are also instances where yeasts and algae are the causative agents.

The highest percentage of new IMM infections occurs during the nonlactating period, known as the **dry period**. More specifically, the majority of new IMM infections occur during the first 2 weeks after initiation of the dry period and the last 2 weeks of the dry period. The reason for these periods of increased susceptibility to new infections is suppression of mammary defense mechanisms, including loosening of the teat sphincter due to increased IMM pressure, preferential consumption of milk components by phagocytic cells, and suppression of the functionality of the immune cells associated with parturition. Also, milk is not being flushed from the mammary gland at these times, which is an important mechanism for bacterial clearance.

Prevalence of mastitis on dairy farms is often monitored by the degree of elevation of the **somatic cell count (SCC)** within the milk. Uninfected cows typically have a SCC below 200,000 cells/mL, with most of the cells being epithelial cells and macrophages. When a new IMM infection occurs, the SCC rapidly increases with a swift influx of neutrophils to control the infection. Depending on clinical severity of the infection, the mammary gland may exhibit either very little long-term damage or, in cases of severe mastitis, the individual glands of the udder may cease lactating because of secretory cell apoptosis or PRL dysfunction. In very severe cases, the cow may die from endotoxemia as a result of toxins produced by the pathogen. IMM infections alter the consistency of milk as a result of altered secretory cell metabolism and the increased presence of serum products, such as serum albumin, in the milk due to disruption of the tight junctions between secretory cells. In comparison with low-SCC milk, elevated SCC causes a drop in lactose content to maintain osmotic balance due to increased leakage of sodium and chloride. During bouts of mastitis, there are (i) minimal changes in milk fat percentage but increased lipolysis and rancidity due to milk fat globule membrane disruption and host and bacterial lipases present in milk; (ii) minimal change in total protein content but casein concentration drops significantly due to enhanced degradation in alveolar lumen and milk; and (iii) there is a dramatic increase in serum proteins and soluble inflammatory polypeptides. These changes can result in decreased utility of the milk for processors due to decreased cheese yields and increased potential for rancidity due to alterations in fatty acid composition.

Mastitis therapy

Therapy for IMM infections is the principal reason antimicrobial products are used on dairy farms and results in substantial consumption of other products, like anti-inflammatory drugs.

Antimicrobial products can be administered directly into the milk via the IMM route or indirectly via systemic administration. Both routes result in effective therapeutic levels in the milk if the proper pharmacologic principles are considered. In general, the IMM route results in high concentrations of drug at the site of infection provided local inflammation does not prevent diffusion of the product. Systemic drugs that are weak bases, hydrophobic, nonionized, and not highly protein bound can successfully pass across the cellular membrane of the secretory epithelium and achieve therapeutic concentrations in milk.

Normal milk has a pH range of 6.5–6.8, while mastitic milk typically has a pH range of 6.9–7.2, which may alter the effectiveness of antimicrobials. In addition, disruption of the tight junctions between secretory cells may allow compounds that normally do not diffuse across intact epithelial membranes to more easily move into milk.

Milk residues

No matter what type of drug is systemically administered, the molecule and/or its metabolite will end up in milk at some concentration. Clearance of drugs from milk occurs primarily through removal of milk from the gland during the milking or suckling process and through diffusion of drugs into the blood. In the drug approval process, pharmaceutical companies have to present pharmacokinetic data in order for proper withdrawal times to be established for milk and meat products before human consumption. However, it must be remembered that these withdrawal periods are established on healthy animals and some drugs exhibit different pharmacodynamics in ill animals. Neonates consuming milk products from treated animals may ingest sufficient quantities of pharmaceutical residues to develop residues that violate regulations.

Residues in milk can also result from a variety of products that are intentionally or accidentally ingested or administered topically or systemically. Examples of compounds or metabolites that could result in a milk residue include mycotoxins, parasiticides, pesticides, hormones, detergents, and disinfectants. Veterinarians must be aware of residue prevention strategies for both milk and meat when treating food animal species.

Biological function of milk

1 Does milk composition vary in different species? Why?

2 What is colostrum and what is its function?

3 What are somatic cells? What is a normal SCC and cell types in uninfected mammary glands? What about SCC and cell types in infected glands?

4 What is lactoferrin? When is lactoferrin high in cows, humans, and horses?

Milk provided through lactation assures that reproduction is successful via delivery of essential components for growth and health of the neonate. Bovine milk has become a staple in the diets of humans, including its inclusion as the major ingredient in infant formulas. Milk provides energy via lactose, fat, and protein as well as proteins for amino acid requirements, through both casein and whey proteins. Milk also contains essential minerals and vitamins such as calcium, phosphorus, thiamine, and riboflavin, in addition to a source of metabolic water.

Nutritive value and species differences

Milk composition for 30 mammalian species is shown in Table 54.4. As can be seen from the table, there is tremendous variation between species depending on the distinct evolutionary requirements of the neonate. Milk from the Holstein dairy cow contains approximately 3.5% fat, 3.2% protein, and 4.6% lactose. Marine species, for example the hooded seal, produce milk that is 50% fat, 6% protein with almost no lactose. Newborn seal pups only nurse for approximately 4 days but gain tremendous strength and insulation during this period, and in fact double their birth weight while nursing. Rapidly growing species, like the rabbit and rat, tend to have milk with high protein content to support precipitous muscular development. In contrast, milk from the guinea pig contributes minimally to total growth of the neonate. It should also be noted that factors like breed, environmental stressors, nutrition, and nursing habits of the young can contribute substantially to composition variation within a species.

Colostrum

Colostrum, the first secretion of the mammary gland prior to parturition, provides important, and in some cases essential, components for health and survival of the neonate. Compared with milk, the composition of colostrum is considerably higher in solids, protein, and ash components (specifically zinc, iron, folic acid, choline, riboflavin, and vitamins A, E, and B_{12}) (Table 54.5). It has been estimated that at birth a newborn calf only has enough energy stores, in the form of fat and glycogen, to last for approximately 18 hours without colostrum consumption.

Farm animal species, such as cattle, sheep, and pigs, have epitheliochorial placentas containing six layers, thus preventing transfer of immunoglobulins from the dam to the fetus. In these species, adequate colostrum consumption is essential for survival of the neonate. The predominant immunoglobulin in these species is IgG but IgM and IgA are also present and provide the neonate with the systemic and gut-associated immunity essential in early life. Dogs and cats have an endotheliochorial placenta that allows moderate transfer of immunoglobulins; they thus acquire immunoglobulins *in utero*, as well as through colostrum consumption. Immunoglobulin transfer occurs across the hemochorial placenta of species like human, monkeys, and rabbits. In rabbits, the immunoglobulin concentration in colostrum is much lower and composed mostly of IgA and IgM

Table 54.4 Composition of milks of various animals.

| | Percentage by weight | | | | | | | |
| | Water | Fat | Protein | | | Lactose | Ash | Energy (kcal/100 g) |
			Casein	Whey	Total			
Aardvark (*Orycteropus afer*)	68.5	12.1	9.5	4.8	14.3	4.6	1.4	184
Bat, fringed (*Myotis thysanodes*)	59.5	17.9	ND	ND	12.1	3.4	1.6	223
Bear, black (*Ursus americanus*)	55.5	24.5	8.8	5.7	14.5	0.4	1.8	280
Buffalo, water (*Bubalus bubalis*)	82.8	7.4	3.2	0.6	3.8	4.8	0.8	101
Camel (*Camelus dromedarius*)	86.5	4.0	2.7	0.9	3.6	5.0	0.8	70
Cow (*Bos taurus*)	87.3	3.9	2.6	0.6	3.2	4.6	0.7	66
Dog (*Canis familiaris*)	76.4	10.7	5.1	2.3	7.4	3.3	1.2	139
Dolphin (*Tursiops truncatus*)	58.3	33.0	3.9	2.9	6.8	1.1	0.7	329
Donkey (*Equus asinus*)	88.3	1.4	1.0	1.0	2.0	7.4	0.5	44
Echidna (*Tachyglossus aculeatus*)	63.2	19.6	8.4	2.9	11.3	2.8	0.8	233
Elephant, Indian (*Elephas maximus*)	78.1	11.6	1.9	3.0	4.9	4.7	0.7	143
Goat (*Capra hircus*)	86.7	4.5	2.6	0.6	3.2	4.3	0.8	70
Guinea pig (*Cavia porcellus*)	83.6	3.9	6.6	1.5	8.1	3.0	0.8	80
Hedgehog (*Erinaceus europaeus*)	79.4	10.1	ND	ND	7.2	2.0	2.3	100
Horse (*Equus caballus*)	88.8	1.9	1.3	1.2	2.5	6.2	0.5	52
Human (*Homo sapiens*)	87.1	4.5	0.4	0.5	0.9	7.1	0.2	72
Kangaroo, red (*Macropus rufus*)	80.0	3.4	2.3	2.3	4.6	6.7	1.4	76
Manatee (*Trichechus manatus*)	87.0	6.9	ND	ND	6.3	0.3	1.0	88
Opossum (*Didelphis virginiana*)	76.8	11.3	ND	ND	8.4	1.6	1.7	142
Pig (*Sus scrofa*)	81.2	6.8	2.8	2.0	4.8	5.5	1.0	102
Rabbit (*Oryctolagus cuniculus*)	67.2	15.3	9.3	4.6	13.9	2.1	1.8	202
Rat (*Rattus norvegicus*)	79.0	10.3	6.4	2.0	8.4	2.6	1.3	137
Reindeer (*Rangifer tarandus*)	66.7	18.0	8.6	1.5	10.1	2.8	1.5	214
Seal, fur (*Callorhinus ursinus*)	34.6	53.3	4.6	4.3	8.9	0.1	0.5	516
Sheep (*Ovis aries*)	82.0	7.2	3.9	0.7	4.6	4.8	0.9	102
Shrew, tree (*Tupaia belangeri*)	59.6	25.6	ND	ND	10.4	1.5	ND	278
Sloth (*Bradypus variegatus*)	83.1	2.7	ND	ND	6.5	2.8	0.9	62
Squirrel, gray (*Sciurus carolinensis*)	60.4	24.7	5.0	2.4	7.4	3.7	1.0	267
Yak (*Bos grunniens*)	82.7	6.5	ND	ND	5.8	4.6	0.9	100
Zebu (*Bos indicus*)	86.5	4.7	2.6	0.6	3.2	4.7	0.7	74

ND, not determined.
Source: Park, S. and Lindberg, G.L. (2004) The mammary gland and lactation. In: *Dukes' Physiology of Domestic Animals*, 12th edn (ed. W.O. Reece). Cornell University Press, Ithaca, NY. Reproduced with permission from Cornell University Press.

Table 54.5 Composition of bovine colostrum and normal whole milk.

Constituent	Colostrum (%)	Whole milk (%)
Total solids	23.9	12.9
Lactose	2.7	5.0
Fat	6.7	4.0
Protein	14.3	3.2
Casein	5.2	2.6
Albumin	1.5	0.47
Immunoglobulin	6.0	0.09
Ash	1.1	0.7
Vitamin A (ng/dL)	295.0	34.0
Specific gravity (g/mL)	1.056	1.032

Source: Park, S. and Lindberg, G.L. (2004) The mammary gland and lactation. In: *Dukes' Physiology of Domestic Animals*, 12th edn (ed. W.O. Reece). Cornell University Press, Ithaca, NY. Reproduced with permission from Cornell University Press.

(Figure 54.8). Differences in the amounts and isotypes of immunoglobulin can be seen across species and serum and mammary secretions (Table 54.6). In addition to immunoglobulins and other growth and development nutrients, colostrum possesses a multitude of immune proteins and cells for early immunological protection, as well as factors that enhance digestion.

Internal secondary immune defense systems

Deeper within the mammary gland, white blood cells and soluble defense mechanisms, such as lactoferrin, immunoglobulins, and complement, coordinate in an attempt to control IMM infections. White blood cells provide the primary defense mechanism in the mammary gland. The milk from an uninfected mammary gland can have a SCC ranging from 20,000 to 200,000 cells/mL, with the predominant white blood cell being macrophages. When bacterial invasion occurs, neutrophils

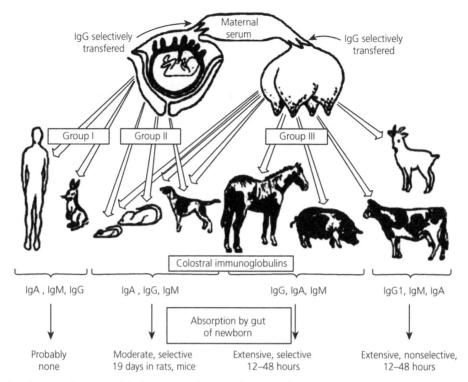

Figure 54.8 Transfer of maternal immunoglobulin (universal carrier of passive immunity in all species) to offspring in representative species. Transfer in group I is *in utero*, via colostrum in group III, and mixed in group II. The relative concentration of immunoglobulin in colostrum is depicted by the size of the immunoglobulin designation. Relative absorption and timing of absorption by the newborn gut are also shown. From Guidry, A.J. (1985) Mastitis and the immune system of the mammary gland. In: *Lactation* (ed. B.L. Larson). Iowa State University Press, Ames, IA.

Table 54.6 Concentration (mg/mL) of immunoglobulins in serum and mammary secretions of three representative species.

	Serum	Colostrum	Milk
Human			
IgG	12.10	0.43	0.04
IgA	2.50	17.40	1.00
IgM	0.93	1.60	0.10
Bovine			
IgG	18.90	50.50	0.80
IgA	0.50	3.90	0.20
IgM	2.60	4.20	0.05
Porcine			
IgG	21.50	58.70	3.00
IgA	1.80	10.70	7.70
IgM	1.10	3.20	0.30

Source: Akers, R.M. (2002) Overview of mammary development. In: *Lactation and the Mammary Gland*. Iowa State Press, Ames, IA. Reproduced with permission from Wiley.

quickly invade the area of infection in response to proinflammatory cytokines. It is common for a cow with an IMM infection to have 500,000 or more somatic cells present in the milk, comprising predominantly neutrophils.

Cows that develop a new IMM infection, in a previously uninfected gland, have been shown to have a delayed cellular immune response due to difficulties in cellular migration and an inherent reduction in phagocytic capacity in milk. However, recent discoveries have shown that IMM neutrophils have an additional bacterial control mechanism called **neutrophil extracellular traps (NETs)** that, unlike phagocytic activity, function very efficiently in milk. NETs are antibacterial webs of extracellular DNA and histones along with other granular and nuclear proteins that are produced very rapidly to trap new bacterial infections.

Bacterial phagocytosis is enhanced via opsonization with antibody, with or without the participation of complement. IgG1 is the predominant immunoglobulin in the uninfected gland and is thought to be an important contributor to the early mammary defense mechanism through recognition of new infections. IgG2 opsonization of bacteria increases phagocytosis by neutrophils, whereas opsonization by IgG1 and IgG2 increases bacterial phagocytosis by macrophages. IgA in milk functions to agglutinate bacteria, prevent multiplication of bacteria, prevent adherence to mucosal linings, and to bind and neutralize toxins. In normal milk, immunoglobulin levels are below 0.1% but during colostrogenesis immunoglobulin levels reach approximately 6%.

Fürstenberg's rosette is significant within the mammary gland in antigen recognition. While this structure has enjoyed much notoriety in veterinary textbooks throughout the years, its clinical significance has only recently been defined. Recent observations have determined that there are lymphoid-associated germinal centers in this area, called **Fürstenberg's rosette associated lymphoid tissue (FALT)**, much like those found in the gut or the bronchus, that play an important role in antigen processing within the mammary gland. Several types of lymphocytes are present in milk, much like in blood. Natural killer lymphocyte subsets participate in antibody-dependent cell-mediated cytotoxicity; B lymphocytes are responsible for antigenic memory and antibody production, while T lymphocytes are responsible for producing cytokines to help regulate immune function. In milk, the ratio of CD4$^+$ (T helper cells) to CD8$^+$ (T suppressor cells) is lower than in blood. In addition, the functionality of the immune system of the mammary gland can be affected by the stage of lactation of the animal. For example, in the postpartum dairy cow, increased phenotypic expression of CD8$^+$ suppressor lymphocytes may reduce phagocytic activity in the mammary gland. Additionally, different bacteria have been shown to alter cytokine expression and thus gain a competitive advantage in milk.

Lactoferrin is found in mammary secretory cells and neutrophils. It is an iron-binding glycoprotein that is typically found in the iron-deficient form, apolactoferrin. The iron-binding properties of apolactoferrin make the mineral unavailable to iron-dependent bacteria. Lactoferrin is extremely important during mammary involution and is 100-fold higher during this period in dairy cows. Lactoferrin is present in high concentrations in milk of humans and mares throughout lactation.

Immune function within the mammary gland is a complex arrangement with varying degrees of immunosuppression throughout lactation. Despite this, and the vast exposure to microorganisms, the mammary gland does a remarkable job in controlling IMM infections.

Self-evaluation

Answers can be found at the end of the chapter.

1 Concerning the functional anatomy of the mammary gland (choose all correct answers):
   A The capacity of the lactating bovine udder is closely related with empty udder weight because the ratio of parenchyma to stroma is relatively constant
   B The functional unit of the lactating mammary gland is the alveolus, which comprises a single layer of secretory epithelial cells that synthesize and secrete milk into the lumen
   C To produce 1 L of milk, approximately 1200 L of blood needs to circulate through the mammary gland
   D In the bovine udder, both afferent and efferent nerves are required for the processes of secretion and ejection of milk

2 For mammary growth, differentiation, and lactation, which of the following are correct (choose all correct answers)?
   A Growth of the mammary gland (mammogenesis) is the major determinant of bovine milk yield since the number of secretory cells directly influence milk yield
   B Mammary involution is characterized by a decrease in secretory cell numbers. If a cow enters the dry period in advanced stages of pregnancy, the decrease in cell number is much less than if the animal enters the dry period in the early stages of pregnancy
   C Accelerated mammary growth during pregnancy is the result of increased and synchronous secretion of estrogen and growth hormone
   D While most mammary secretory cell proliferation occurs by the end of pregnancy, an additional increase in cell number continues throughout the entire lactation

3 During milk synthesis and secretion (choose all correct answers):
   A Glucose is the primary energy substrate in the nonruminant, whereas glucose (propionate) and acetate are the main energy sources in ruminants
   B The major milk proteins synthesized for export in bovine mammary tissues are the casein and whey proteins
   C Fats in bovine milk are characterized as mixed triglycerides with a large proportion of short-chain fatty acids (C$_4$ to C$_{16}$)
   D Minerals in milk are derived from the blood, whereas vitamins are absorbed from the diet or are synthesized in the rumen

4 Regarding the physiology of milking (choose all correct answers):
   A The milk secretion rate depends on the pressure that accumulates within the mammary gland and on feedback regulation by specific milk components
   B While a pressure differential is needed to overcome sphincter resistance to milk flow, suckling by calves does not generate sufficient vacuum to counteract teat sphincter resistance
   C The milking machine uses vacuum for milk removal. A sustained vacuum will causes milk to flow quickly without damaging the teat
   D Residual milk is milk that is left in the udder after a normal milking or suckling (about 10–20% of total milk). A cow with a high percentage of residual milk has a high persistency of lactation

5 Concerning the biological function of milk (choose all correct answers):
   A A newborn calf acquires passive immunity through the colostrum, which is its only source of immunoglobulins
   B The milk of cows may serve as the sole or major component of the diet of human infants, and it is a valuable source of protein and calcium for the elderly
   C While there is a wide difference in milk composition among species and even within species, the composition of bovine milk is consistent among and within breeds of cattle
   D Residues found in milk enter only through the secretion process or through infusion via the streak canal and can result in residues that may be harmful to human health

6 Which factors affect lactation (choose all correct answers)?
   A Although nutrients (carbohydrates, lipids, protein, minerals, vitamins, and water) are of immense importance for growth and

lactation, protein is considered the most limiting nutrient because it is necessary for the proper metabolism of all the remaining nutrients

B Increasing the dietary protein (e.g. above 19%) has little effect on milk yield and milk protein content. However, increasing fat content in the diet of the lactating cow significantly increases fat content in milk

C Increasing the frequency of milking increases milk yield, for example milking twice daily yields at least 40% more milk than milking once daily. However, the milk yield response to more frequent milking diminishes with increasing frequency

D Heat stress reduces feed intake and alters glucose utilization by tissues other than the mammary gland, causing a rapid decline in milk yield. The decrease in milk yield during cold stress is primarily due to increased requirements to maintain body core temperature.

7 Concerning the immune system of the mammary gland (choose all correct answers):

A Macrophages are the primary white blood cell found in the noninfected gland of the bovine

B Neutrophils invade rapidly in response to new intramammary infections and are very effective at phagocytosis in milk

C IgG and IgA play important roles in milk during an intramammary infection

D Cytokines play an important role in regulating the inflammatory response within the mammary gland during infection and show similar properties as those found in serum

Suggested reading

Akers, R.M. (2002) *Lactation and the Mammary Gland.* Iowa State Press, Ames, IA.

Anderson, R.R., Collier, R.J., Guidry, A.J. *et al.* (1985) In: *Lactation* (ed. B.L. Larson). Iowa State University Press. Ames, IA.

Lippolis, J.D., Peterson-Burch, B.D. and Reinhardt, T.A. (2006) Differential expression analysis of proteins from neutrophils in the peri-parturient period and neutrophils from dexamethasone treated dairy cows. *Veterinary Immunology and Immunopathology* **111**:149–164.

Rhoads, M.L., Rhoads, R.P., VanBaale, M.J. *et al.* (2009) Effects of heat stress and plane of nutrition on lactating Holstein cows: I. Production, metabolism, and aspects of circulating somatotropin. *Journal of Dairy Science* **92**:1986–1997.

Answers

1 B	**5** A, B, D
2 A, B	**6** C, D
3 A, B, C, D	**7** A, C
4 A	

55 Avian Reproduction

Patricia A. Johnson
Cornell University, Ithaca, NY, USA

One of the obvious differences between birds and mammals is that there is no well-defined estrous cycle or pregnancy. Birds are oviparous and the embryo must have everything it needs when the egg is laid. As a result there are significant modifications in the reproductive physiology as well as anatomy between birds and mammals. For example, the production and accumulation of yolk is necessary for birds as is the formation of a protective shell. These adaptations require specific endocrine underpinnings.

Chickens (*Gallus domesticus*) are the most numerous domesticated birds and have been extensively studied. In addition, turkeys (*Meleagris gallopavo*), ducks (*Anas platyrhynchos*), and Japanese quail (*Coturnix coturnix japonica*) are other domesticated species which have also been heavily studied. The commercial importance of these types of birds has stimulated investigation of their basic physiology, while commercial pressures have also promoted genetic selection that has made them differ from many free-living avian species. For example, selection for increased numbers of eggs laid has resulted in strains of chickens that lay 250–270 eggs per hen annually, while the tendency for these strains to cease laying and incubate their eggs has been nearly eliminated. These traits are of obvious commercial advantage for egg production but would be maladaptive in a natural environment. Likewise, the selection for large breast size in turkeys has made natural mating impossible and necessitated artificial insemination in turkey production. Information in this chapter is primarily derived from domestic species since that is the topic of this book and intensive work with these species, because of their commercial interest, has provided much information about their basic reproductive physiology.

Photoperiodism

> 1 How is photoperiodic information received by birds?
>
> 2 How is relative refractoriness different from absolute refractoriness?
>
> 3 What is the photosensitive phase?
>
> 4 How is photorefractoriness terminated?
>
> 5 What is the endocrine mediator of photoperiodic information?

Photoreceptors

The most significant environmental cue for reproductive activity in birds is the photoperiod. Although nutritional cues, rainfall, and social interactions are involved in stimulating reproductive activity in some species, the vast majority of temperate-zone birds, including the common domesticated species, use photoperiod as a cue. Light that affects reproductive stimulation and timing is perceived by **photoreceptors** that are located in the hypothalamus. Many experiments has shown that light must pass through the avian skull and that the pineal gland and eyes are not critical for perception of daylength. When light

Dukes' Physiology of Domestic Animals, Thirteenth Edition. Edited by William O. Reece, Howard H. Erickson, Jesse P. Goff and Etsuro E. Uemura.
© 2015 John Wiley & Sons, Inc. Published 2015 by John Wiley & Sons, Inc.
Companion website: www.wiley.com/go/reece/physiology

Section IX: Endocrinology, Reproduction, and Lactation

was prevented from penetrating through the skull by fitting ducks with light-impermeable hats or by injection of dye under the skull, the birds were not able to respond to photostimulation. Similarly, photoperiodic information was found to be equally well received by blind and sighted birds. Several studies have indicated that these photoreceptors are located in the hypothalamus and near the ventricles. Some neurons in these areas contain protein material (opsin-like) similar to that contained in retinal photoreceptors. Light perception in the brain results in the release of **gonadotropin-releasing hormone (GnRH)** with subsequent release of gonadotropins and stimulation of the gonads (Figure 55.1).

Photostimulation

In considering the effect of light on avian species, it is important to realize that light is photostimulatory by causing birds to become reproductively competent and active when the duration of light is sufficient. In addition, light also acts to time events in the reproductive cycle (as described more fully in section

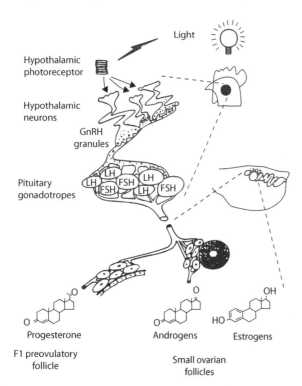

Figure 55.1 Diagrammatic representation of the effect of light on the stimulation of the hypothalamic–pituitary–gonadal axis. Hypothalamic photoreceptors activate neurons containing gonadotropin-releasing hormone (GnRH). GnRH-I is released into the pituitary portal vessels and transported to the pituitary gland. In response, luteinizing hormone (LH) and follicle-stimulating hormone (FSH) are released from the pituitary gland. These hormones stimulate the ovary (as shown) or testis. In response to the gonadotropins, follicle development and steroid secretion are stimulated in the female and sperm production and androgen production in the male. From Etches, R.J. (1996) *Reproduction in Poultry*. CAB International, Cambridge, UK. Reproduced with permission from CAB International.

Ovulatory cycle). A long day for most domesticated species is a period of light longer than 12 hours, although the bird does not have to experience this as continuous light. For stimulatory effects on the reproductive system, light must occur during the **photosensitive phase**, which is set by the time of dawn and usually occurs at least 12 hours after dawn. As long as light falls during the photosensitive phase, photostimulation will occur, even if a period of darkness occurs between the hours of dawn and the onset of the photosensitive phase. In addition, this period of sensitivity will occur on each day.

Photorefractoriness

In general, the response to the lighting schedule is profoundly influenced by the previous photoperiod that a bird experienced. That is, a light/dark schedule of 13/11 hours can be either stimulatory or inhibitory depending on the previous exposure of the bird. If the bird perceives that daylength is increasing, it is stimulatory. In contrast, perception of a decreasing photoperiod leads to photo-induced regression. Additionally, prolonged exposure to a long daylength eventually leads to an inability to be stimulated by that daylength, a phenomenon known as **absolute photorefractoriness**. In quail, a phenomenon termed **relative photorefractoriness** occurs, whereby although gonadal regression does not occur on prolonged long days, if the length of daylight decreases, regression immediately ensues. This occurs even if the decrease in photoperiod makes the daylength longer than that which originally stimulated the bird. Exposure to a period of short daylengths is necessary to break both absolute and relative photorefractoriness and to cause the bird to regain photosensitivity.

Thyroid gland

Interestingly, the thyroid gland has been found to be of great importance for the photoperiodic response in birds (also true in mammals). In the absence of the thyroid gland, birds do not develop photorefractoriness but maintain gonadal stimulation during a prolonged period of long days. Recent studies have shown hypothalamic photoreception affects thyroid-stimulating hormone (TSH) production in the pars tuberalis of the pituitary gland. On long days, there is an increase in the hypothalamic concentration of thyroid deiodinase type 2, which increases local production of bioactive thyroid hormone (T_3). Elevated bioactive thyroid hormone appears to cause morphological changes in the GnRH nerve terminals and glial cells, facilitating GnRH secretion (Figure 55.2).

Gonadotropin-releasing hormone

The stimulatory effect of light on birds is mediated through changes in the hypothalamic decapeptide, GnRH. Interestingly, avian GnRH has been found to exist in two forms, **GnRH-I** (which differs from the mammalian form in one amino acid) and **GnRH-II**. These forms differ from each other in three amino acids at positions 5, 7 and 8. Although both GnRH-I and GnRH-II stimulate luteinizing hormone

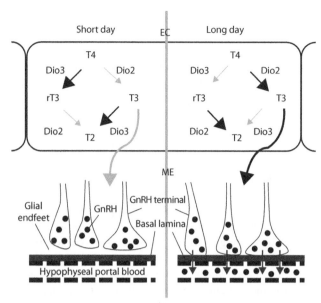

Figure 55.2 Type 2 deiodinase (Dio2) converts the prohormone thyroxine (T_4) to bioactive triiodothyronine (T_3) under long day (LD) conditions, while type 3 deiodinase (Dio3) metabolizes thyroid hormones under short day (SD) conditions in birds and mammals. In quail, LD-induced T_3 appears to induce morphological changes in the gonadotropin-releasing hormone (GnRH) nerve terminals and glial processes, thereby causing GnRH secretion into the hypophyseal portal blood. T_2, diiodothyronine; rT_3, reverse triiodothyronine; EC, ependymal cells; ME, median eminence. Reproduced with permission of the Society for Reproduction and Development from Ikegami K, et al.: Seasonal time measurement during reproduction. *J Reprod Dev* 2013; 59: 327–333.

release *in vivo*, GnRH-II is more potent than GnRH-I in stimulating LH release from chicken pituitary cells *in vitro*. Despite these findings, GnRH-I is believed to be the physiologically relevant form for stimulating gonadotropin release from the pituitary gland. GnRH-I containing neurons have been localized to the median eminence area of the hypothalamus in contrast to GnRH-II containing neurons and GnRH-II release has not been detected in the median eminence area. This evidence is supported by results indicating that immunization against GnRH-I causes involution of the reproductive system, with no effect on reproductive function after immunization against GnRH-II.

Chicken **luteinizing hormone (LH)** and **follicle-stimulating hormone (FSH)** have been isolated and purified and the hormones used to develop specific antibodies. This has permitted the validation of specific radioimmunoassays, which have contributed to the knowledge about avian reproductive physiology. The avian gonadotropins are dimeric glycoprotein hormones, similar to their mammalian counterparts. Specific LH and FSH binding sites on ovarian follicles, which vary with respect to follicle development, have been characterized. Additionally, the patterns of expression of the mRNAs for the LH and FSH receptors during stages of follicle development have been characterized.

Male reproductive function

1 What are the main cell types in the avian testis?
2 What is the function of the excurrent duct system in the male?
3 How is semen deposited in the female?
4 What is the effect of avian body temperature on spermatogenesis?
5 How do the gonadotropins regulate testis function in birds?
6 What determines testis size?
7 What is a primary impediment to use of cryopreserved avian semen?

Testes

Similar to mammals, the testes of birds have the dual functions of hormone (androgen) and gamete production. The testes in birds are paired and internal. They are located near the cephalic end of the kidneys and ventral to them. In general, the testes of a male that is reproductively competent are very large. There is a small epididymis and a ductus deferens that conducts sperm to the cloacal opening (Figure 55.3). In some species of birds, most notably the songbirds, the ductus deferens elongates at the distal end and is called the **seminal glomus**. When the glomus is filled with sperm, it protrudes on either side of the cloaca and, although not a scrotum, indicates breeding condition. Another secondary sex characteristic that is associated with testis growth and function is the **cloacal gland** of Japanese quail (*Coturnix coturnix japonica*). The cloacal gland is located within the cloaca and is androgen dependent. Production of a foam-like substance is highly correlated with testosterone secretion and the foam is deposited into the cloaca of the female at the time of mating, although the function of this adaptation is not known. Androgens are required to induce the growth of the comb and wattles in roosters.

The testes are composed of **seminiferous tubules** with **interstitial cells** dispersed among the tubules. The seminiferous tubules contain spermatogonia and developing germ cells in close association with Sertoli cells. There are tight junctions between adjacent Sertoli cells which contribute to a carefully regulated environment within the seminiferous tubule. The Sertoli cells are responsive to, and regulated by, FSH and testosterone. The interstitial or Leydig cells secrete several androgens including testosterone and androstenedione, although the major androgen in the blood is testosterone. In response to stimulatory photoperiods or as sexual maturity approaches, increasing amounts of circulating LH stimulate the differentiation of the Leydig cells. The mature Leydig cells are then capable of LH-stimulated androgen production.

Accessory sex organs

The seminiferous tubules connect to the excurrent duct system of the testis at the **rete testis**. This duct system consists of efferent ducts, connecting ducts, and epididymal ducts. The epididymal ducts connect to the distal deferent duct and this

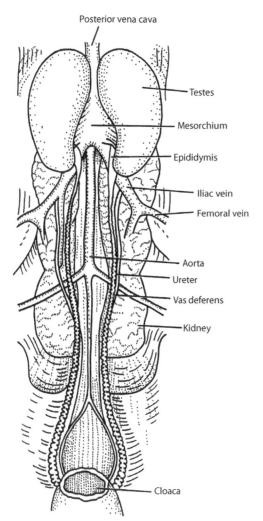

Figure 55.3 Reproductive organs of a rooster. From Sturkie, P.D. (1976) *Avian Physiology*, 3rd edn. Harcourt, Inc. Orlando, FL. Reproduced with permission from Springer-Verlag GmbH & Co.

because sperm does not flow through it but rather along the spiral groove. Chickens and turkeys have a small erectile phallus on the ventral part of the cloaca that becomes erect prior to mating. It becomes engorged with lymph-like fluid during sexual arousal. Each ductus deferens opens into a small papilla on the dorsal wall of the cloaca. Semen from the ductus deferens flows out along the longitudinal groove of the phallus. Insemination is by **cloacal contact**; the male and female cloacas are placed in close apposition, rather than a true intromission.

Spermatogenesis

There are approximately eight to twelve different morphological changes that occur during **spermiogenesis** (transformation of spermatids to sperm cells) in most domestic avian species. Spermatogenesis in birds takes place within the seminiferous tubules and there are distinct cellular associations along the tubules, which contain germ cells in different stages of development. Maturation proceeds from the periphery to the lumen as in mammals and the cellular associations change with time at any position as maturation progresses. The series of stages is referred to as the cycle of the seminiferous epithelium, while the complete series of stages within the seminiferous tubule is called a spermatogenic wave.

Although avian testes are internal, this does not mean that spermatogenesis is insensitive to temperature. A variety of experiments have demonstrated that spermatogenesis is well adapted for the warm body temperature of birds (~41°C). Spermatogenesis was disrupted both when avian testes were exposed to lower body temperature by creation of an artificial scrotum and when the testes were warmed by incubation in warm saline.

Endocrine regulation of the testis

In male chickens, sexual maturity is not defined as the production of first gametes, as in the hen, because the first sperm have poor fertilizing ability. By the end of the pubertal phase in chickens (18–19 weeks), testicular size is maximal and fertility is optimal. The Leydig cells produce androgens, principally testosterone and androstenedione. Male levels of the pituitary hormone FSH rise during development. In chickens maintained on long days, levels of FSH begin to rise at 11 weeks and plateau at 19 weeks. In these same birds, LH is elevated at 7–15 weeks, suggesting that LH rises earlier than FSH. In general, male chickens have significantly higher plasma LH levels compared with females throughout development. Measurable levels of immunoreactive **inhibin** are detected in the plasma of males, although there is no apparent inverse relationship during development between inhibin and FSH in male chickens as has been observed in female chickens.

The testes of birds are regulated by conventional negative feedback mechanisms between the gonads and the pituitary hormones LH and FSH. That is, removal of one or both testes results in elevation of the gonadotropins. Furthermore, removal of just one testis leads to compensatory hypertrophy of the remaining testis. The time of unilateral testis removal determines

conducts semen to the cloaca. Through the absorption of **seminiferous tubule fluid**, sperm concentration is markedly increased with transport through the system. In addition, sperm acquire the capacity for motility as they pass through the excurrent duct system, although sperm within the deferent duct do not appear motile. Interestingly, sperm motility does not appear to be essential for fertility since testicular sperm have the potential to fertilize oocytes if they are placed into the oviduct above the vagina. It has been shown that testicular and epididymal germ cells of the rooster contain aromatase activity and estrogen receptors are present in the **efferent ducts** and **epididymis**. Similar to mammals, estrogen action in the avian efferent ducts is critical for reabsorption of seminiferous tubule fluid. Neither prostate gland nor seminal vesicles are present in birds.

The anatomy of the **phallus** differs somewhat among birds. Birds lack the true penis present in mammals. Ducks and geese have a well-developed phallus (pseudopenis) which is spirally twisted and serves as an intromittent organ. It is not a true penis the extent of compensation. It appears that full compensation, both with respect to size and sperm output, occurs when the testis is removed early in life at less than 4 weeks of age. Some level of compensation is observed, however, when removal occurs up to 8 weeks of age. This extent of functional compensation appears to be related to overlap with the time of Sertoli cell mitosis. While the absolute period for Sertoli cell mitosis is not known in birds, this does seem to limit the capacity for compensatory hypertrophy.

As has been observed in mammals, there is a linear relationship in birds between testis size and sperm production. That is, increased size is associated with increased sperm output. Although a variety of factors such as photoperiod, genetics, and age influence sperm production, size of the gonads is very important. As mentioned already, thyroid hormones are involved in seasonal reproductive activity in birds and mammals. Interestingly, it has been shown that treatment with drugs that cause hypothyroidism during a critical phase of development (apparently associated with Sertoli cell mitosis) is associated with a dramatic increase in testis size. Treatment with a goitrogen in chickens aged between 6 and 12 weeks resulted in a doubling of testis weight (and increased sperm production) at maturity. This finding may have implications for increasing sperm output in male birds of commercial interest or for conservation purposes.

Cryopreservation of semen

Cryopreservation of spermatozoa and **artificial insemination (AI)** have been investigated for their application to domesticated as well as nondomesticated avian species. Work has been done in a variety of species but most research has been on the chicken. Chickens were the first animals to be bred using cryopreservation of spermatozoa and AI, although wide utilization of the technology in birds has been hampered by technical problems. Sperm storage in the female (described more fully in section Sperm storage) implies that the function of frozen/thawed semen must be evaluated both for fertility as well as for the duration of fertility. Protocols have been developed for freezing and thawing spermatozoa from chickens and turkeys, with relatively good fertility after AI. The procedures are somewhat laborious, however, because of the need to dilute or remove the cryoprotectant glycerol, which has been found to have a contraceptive effect when inseminated into the hen's vagina. Other cryoprotectants such as dimethylacetamide and methylacetamide have been examined that do not require removal prior to insemination in chickens. Some of these other compounds have shown good promise of effectiveness. While progress has been made in cryopreservation and AI in avian species, the technology has not advanced to the level utilized in mammals. Furthermore, it has become very clear that there are significant species differences in spermatozoa susceptibility to damage from freezing and thawing. This has made the utilization of this technology for preservation of germplasm from other avian species not yet broadly applicable. Other

procedures, such as creation of germline chimeras and interspecies germ cell transfer, are currently being developed to assist in the conservation of avian genetic resources.

Female reproductive function

> 1 What regulates the asymmetric pattern of ovary and oviduct development in birds?
> 2 Where is yolk made and how is it accumulated?
> 3 What cell types are present in the avian follicle?
> 4 How is the oviduct specialized for formation of the egg?
> 5 How is sperm stored in the hen?
> 6 What are the steroidogenic cell types in the ovary?
> 7 What hormone induces the preovulatory LH surge in birds?
> 8 How are the growing follicles arranged on the avian ovary and which follicles are susceptible to atresia?
> 9 What is the length of an ovulatory cycle in the chicken?
> 10 What hormones are involved in oviposition?

Anatomy of the reproductive tract

In most female birds including the domestic species, only the left ovary and oviduct develop. As in mammals, both male and female avian embryos possess undifferentiated **Müllerian** and **Wolffian** ducts early in embryonic development. About halfway through the incubation period in the male chick, the Müllerian ducts have involuted and disappeared. The right Müllerian duct of the female disappears soon after while the left Müllerian duct continues to develop into the left oviduct. When **anti-Müllerian hormone (AMH)** was implicated in the regression of Müllerian ducts in male mammals, it was hypothesized and later established that AMH had a role in regression of the Müllerian ducts in male birds and of the right Müllerian duct in female birds. In birds, both embryonic gonads express AMH, although estrogen secretion from the left ovary is greater than that from the right ovary. Estrogen inhibits the action of AMH on the left side and so the tract on that side is preserved. Occasionally, a remnant of the right oviduct can be observed at the distal end where it would join the cloaca. There is some plasticity in the development of the reproductive system, because removal of the left ovary results in formation of a right testis if done early in life. In contrast, if the ovariectomy is done on an older hen, a right ovotestis develops. Some species of birds such as hawks and falcons have two ovaries and oviducts. The excellent flight ability of these species seems to detract from the argument that a unilateral reproductive tract increases efficiency of flight in other birds. This pattern of reproductive tract development seems to be determined very early in the embryo. In chickens, the primordial germ cells migrate to the presumptive gonad in a ratio of 5 : 1 with respect to the left and right side. In contrast, this ratio is 1 : 1 in falcons, which generally have two ovaries.

Follicle growth

As shown in Figure 55.4, the ovary of a bird consists of follicles in various stages of development. During the breeding season or during photostimulation of domestic birds, the yolk-filled follicles are arranged in a **hierarchy**. The largest follicle is the one that will ovulate next, the second largest after that, and so on. It is not known what regulates the hierarchy but the follicles in the hierarchy have been characterized with respect to steroid secretion and other parameters as described in subsequent sections. The **yolk** that accumulates in the follicles is made in the liver under the influence of estradiol. Lipoproteins, specifically **very low density lipoproteins (VLDL)**, and the protein **vitellogenin** are produced in the liver in response to estrogen. After synthesis in the liver, the lipoproteins are transported in the blood to the ovary where they are incorporated into the growing follicles by a receptor-mediated process as depicted in Figure 55.5. The hierarchical follicles are very well vascularized, which is likely important for the transfer of large amounts of yolk. The yolk that is accumulated by the growing follicle is deposited in concentric layers. This can be demonstrated by administration of a different color of lipid-soluble dye on sequential days. After a number of days, the yolk exhibits concentric rings of colored yolk, a result of the pattern of yolk accumulation. The effect of estradiol on the avian liver can also be replicated in the male by administration of estradiol. This will result in the synthesis and secretion of yolk components into the blood.

The cell types of an avian follicle are similar to those of a mammal (Figure 55.6). The **oocyte** is large and yolk-filled (unlike mammals). The oocyte is surrounded by a vitelline membrane. The **germinal disk region**, which contains the

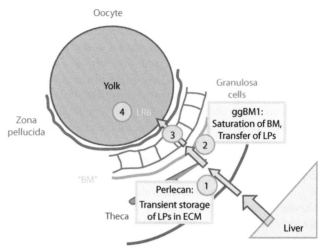

Figure 55.5 Proposed multistep scheme for yolk precursor transport from the liver to the oocyte. Four steps have been identified by biochemical and cell biological approaches. Following transport from the liver to follicles via the circulation, macromolecules enter follicles and traverse the thecal cell layers, where they intermittently associate with perlecan (1), followed by further passage to and through the so-called basement membrane ("BM") via interaction with *Gallus gallus* basement membrane protein 1 (ggBM1). (2) Subsequently yolk precursors diffuse through gaps between the granulosa cells and through the zona pellucida (3) in order to reach the major yolk precursor receptor on the oocyte surface (lipoprotein receptor with 8 ligand-binding repeats, LR8) (4), which mediates their uptake to form yolk. From Schneider, W.J. (2009) Receptor-mediated mechanisms in ovarian follicle and oocyte development. *General and Comparative Endocrinology* 163: 18-23). Reproduced with permission from Elsevier.

nuclear material, is an opaque structure on the surface of the oocyte under the vitelline membrane. In birds, the heterogametic sex is the female with a ZW sex chromosome complement (the male is ZZ). As a result of this, embryo sex in birds is determined at ovulation with extrusion of the first polar body. The **granulosa cell layer** is an avascular layer surrounding the vitelline membrane. This is surrounded by a basement membrane and outside this is the vascularized **theca layer**, which consists of a **theca interna** and **theca externa** and connective tissue. Each follicle is suspended on a stalk.

Anatomy of the oviduct

The avian **oviduct** is basically a conduit from the ovary to the cloaca, with individual regions specialized for particular functions (Figure 55.7). The oocyte spends varying amounts of time in each section (specific times indicated here refer to the chicken). The fimbriated end of the **infundibulum** becomes active at the time of ovulation and engulfs the ovum. There are some sperm storage glands in the infundibulum, which is the location of fertilization. The egg spends approximately 15–30 min here. The next section of the oviduct is the **magnum** which, as the name suggests, is the longest part of the oviduct. Albumen (produced in response to estrogen) is deposited here over the course of 2–3 hours. The egg remains in the **isthmus** for 1–1.5 hours and this where the inner

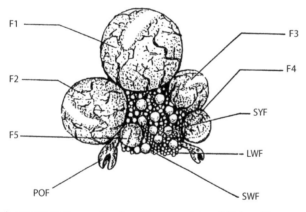

Figure 55.4 Ovary of the hen. The preovulatory follicles of the hierarchy are identified according to size, with the F1 follicle being the largest follicle and the next follicle to ovulate, followed by the F2 follicle, the second largest follicle, etc. The postovulatory follicle (POF) is the structure remaining after ovulation of the oocyte. Small follicles are classified according to size: small yellow follicle (SYF; 6–12 mm in diameter), large white follicle (LWF; 2–5 mm in diameter), and small white follicle (SWF; <2 mm in diameter). From Cupps, P.T. (1991) *Reproduction in Domestic Animals*, 4th edn. Harcourt, Inc., Orlando, FL. Reproduced with permission from Elsevier.

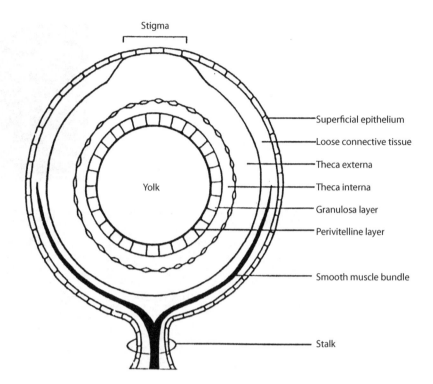

Figure 55.6 Anatomical structure of the preovulatory follicle. From Cupps, P.T. (1991) *Reproduction in Domestic Animals*, 4th edn. Harcourt, Inc., Orlando, FL. Reproduced with permission from Elsevier.

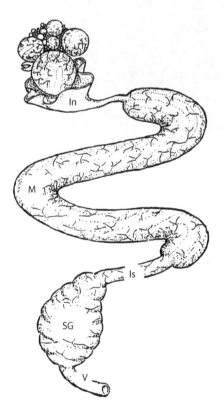

Figure 55.7 Oviduct of the chicken. In, infundibulum; M, magnum; Is, isthmus; SG, shell gland; V, vagina. From Cupps, P.T. (1991) *Reproduction in Domestic Animals*, 4th edn. Harcourt, Inc., Orlando, FL. Reproduced with permission from Elsevier.

and outer shell membranes are deposited. The egg spends the greatest amount of time (approximately 20 hours) in the **shell gland** (or uterus) where the shell is added. Water and salts as well as pigmentation are also added to the egg in the shell gland. The **uterovaginal junction** is the main site of sperm storage tubules. The **vagina** is the part of the oviduct leading from the shell gland to the cloaca and has no role in egg formation.

Sperm storage

Inseminated sperm are stored in the **sperm storage tubules** of the uterovaginal junction and are released and transported to the infundibulum for fertilization. Only motile and morphologically normal sperm enter the sperm storage tubules and inseminated sperm remain fertile for 7–14 days in chickens and 40–50 days in turkeys. Sperm storage also occurs in feral species of birds (for varying lengths of time) where the advantage of sperm storage is quite apparent. If a female loses a clutch of eggs, another fertile clutch of eggs can be laid and incubated without the need for a male. Sperm initially populate the sperm storage tubules in the caudal end and progressively fill the more cranial tubules, thus filling the sperm storage tubules in a stratified manner. Interestingly, sperm from the last male has precedence in fertilization, so a majority of progeny would be sired by the most recent insemination.

Ovarian endocrinology

The ovary of a reproductively active hen contains a mixture of cell types and growing follicles in different stages of development. Hormone production from the ovary of many

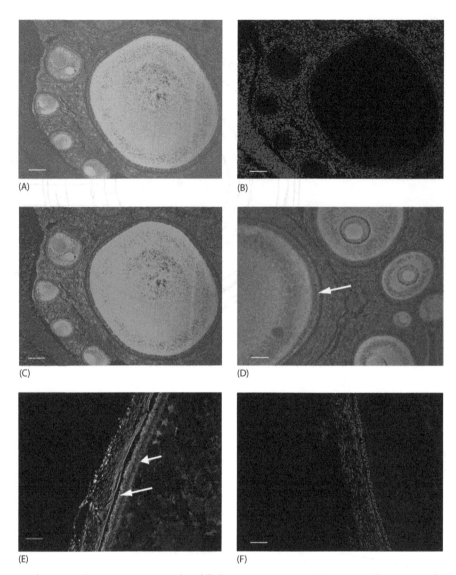

Figure 55.8 Immunocytochemistry of GDF-9 expression in hen follicles. Primary antiserum was against the C-terminal region of mouse GDF-9 (JH131) and secondary antiserum was goat anti-rabbit IgG (Alexa Fluor 488). Propidium iodide was used to identify nuclei. (A) Section through the ovary containing various sized follicles. Strong fluorescence is seen in all oocytes pictured, the largest of which is approximately 300 μm in size. (B) Propidium iodide staining of the same section viewed in (A), showing the nuclei of cells surrounding the oocytes. (C) Overlay of (A) and (B). (D) Similar section as viewed in (C) but in this panel the arrow indicates GDF-9 staining in the granulosa layer. (E) GDF-9 staining of pedunculated oocyte (6 mm). GDF-9 staining is most intense at the periphery of the oocyte (indicated by short arrow), just under the vitelline membrane and adjacent to the granulosa layer (arrow). Scattered positive staining can also be observed within the oocyte in areas of cytoplasm among the yolk platelets. Propidium iodide staining indicates the nuclei of cells in the granulosa and theca layers. (F) Negative control with normal rabbit serum used in place of the primary antiserum. Scale bar = 50 μm. From Johnson, P.A., Dickens, M.J., Kent, T.R. and Giles, J.R. (2005) Expression and function of growth differentiation factor-9 in an oviparous species, *Gallus domesticus*. *Biology of Reproduction* 72: 1095–1100. Reproduced with permission from the Society for the Study of Reproduction.

domestic species has been well characterized with respect to follicle size and hormone secreted during development. The steroidogenic cell types in the avian ovary are the granulosa and theca layers. The theca layer can be distinguished as a theca interna and externa layer. Theca externa cells are characterized by the presence of **aromatase**. The theca interna produces primarily **androgens**, while **estrogens** are derived from the theca externa. **Progesterone** is produced in greatest

quantities by the granulosa layer from the large follicles. LH stimulates steroidogenesis in both the theca and granulosa layer and LH receptor mRNA and receptor number increase dramatically in the granulosa layer with follicle development. In contrast, there is little change in LH receptor mRNA throughout follicle development in the theca layer, although a considerable amount is expressed at all stages. FSH receptors exist on the theca cells throughout follicle development but

FSH receptors are most abundant on the granulosa cells from small pre-hierarchical follicles.

Similar to mammals, it appears that the oocyte interacts with the surrounding somatic cells in a manner that facilitates follicle development. The oocyte hormones **growth differentiation factor (GDF)-9** and **bone morphogenetic factor (BMP)-15** have been demonstrated in chicken oocytes. Expression of GDF9 mRNA is localized in the oocyte and depicted in Figure 55.8.

The relative quantities of the primary steroidogenic hormones secreted by the large follicles in the ovarian hierarchy of the chicken are illustrated in Figure 55.9. The granulosa layer of the largest follicle is the main source of progesterone, while the small growing follicles produce most of the estrogen in the hen. In the chicken, a preovulatory surge of progesterone (in contrast to estrogen in most mammals) from the largest follicle induces LH release which causes ovulation. The protein hormone inhibin is produced in the granulosa cells of the hen. A distinct pattern of expression of inhibin subunits has been noted during follicle development and the hormone seems to act in a conventional negative feedback manner with FSH. AMH is also expressed in the granulosa cells of the hen, with the most abundant level of expression occurring in small growing follicles (<5 mm in size) as well as in follicles not yet accumulating yolk (Figure 55.10). There is evidence that the chicken oocyte has a role in the regulation of AMH expression and AMH increases granulosa cell proliferation. The postovulatory follicle remains after ovulation and although it has a role in the timing of oviposition, it does not continue to produce progesterone. Surgical removal of the postovulatory follicle after ovulation delays oviposition of the egg.

Follicle selection

The ovarian follicles are arranged in a hierarchy, with the follicle that will ovulate next called F1, the follicle that will ovulate on the subsequent day termed F2, and so on. These follicles are very well vascularized, likely important for the transfer of large quantities of yolk from the blood. The hierarchical follicles are selected from a pool of small growing follicles. The nonhierarchical follicles in the chicken are usually described as white follicles (small and large, ranging in size from 1 to 5 mm; SWF and LWF, respectively) and small yellow follicles (SYF; 5–12 mm). These follicles are so named because of their accumulation of white or yellow yolk. The mechanism responsible for the maintenance of the follicular hierarchy is not known nor is it known what factor(s) is involved in the selection of the next growing follicle to join the hierarchy.

The follicles which make up the hierarchy of domestic birds almost always ovulate. **Atresia** or apoptosis (programmed cell death) of the large hierarchical follicles can occur under certain circumstances, such as during the transition to broody behavior or at the end of the breeding season. In general, however, it appears that most follicular atresia occurs in the population of small growing follicles which have not yet been selected into the

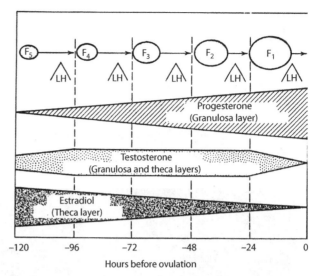

Figure 55.9 A schematic representation of changes in steroid concentrations of granulosa and theca layers during follicular maturation. The "capped" LH represents the preovulatory LH surge which occurs 4–6 hours before ovulation. From Bahr, J.M., Wang, S.C., Huang, M.Y. and Calvo, F.O. (1983) Steroid concentrations in isolated theca and granulosa layers of preovulatory follicles during the ovulatory cycle of the domestic hen. *Biology of Reproduction* 29:326–334. Reproduced with permission from the Society for the Study of Reproduction.

hierarchy. It is logical that atresia is a rare occurrence in the large follicles since yolk formation and deposition is energetically demanding.

Many birds produce a **clutch** or **sequence** of eggs that are laid over consecutive days. The number of eggs laid depends on whether the species is classified as determinant or indeterminant. In **determinant** species, a specific number of eggs are matured and ovulated. If the eggs are removed or lost, the female does not replace them immediately. It may be the next season before another group of eggs is matured and ovulated. In contrast, most domestic species such as the domestic hen are classified as **indeterminant** layers. In these species, if eggs are sequentially removed from the nest as they are laid, the hen will continue to ovulate and lay eggs to attain a theoretical clutch. Obviously, this trait is exploited in commercial laying operations where eggs are removed immediately after lay.

Ovulatory cycle

In domestic species, a distinct pattern of **ovulation** time, and hence time of **oviposition**, occurs. In the chicken, ovulations occur at approximately 26-hour intervals. Each ovulation is followed in approximately 26 hours by an oviposition. In chickens, the first egg of the sequence is usually laid early in the morning of a conventional photoperiod (14L/10D or 15L/9D, where L is hours of daylight and D is hours of darkness), with sequential eggs being laid at progressively later times on succeeding days.

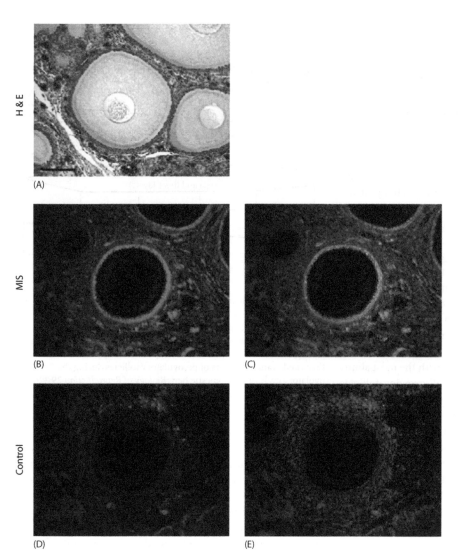

H&E

(A)

MIS

(B)

(C)

Control

(D)

(E)

Figure 55.10 Immunohistochemistry of anti-Müllerian hormone (AMH) expression in the hen ovary. (A) H&E-stained section through the ovary containing various-sized follicles. (B) Section stained with AMH antiserum, showing predominant cytoplasmic staining in the granulosa layer. (C) Section stained with AMH antiserum as well as propidium iodide (PI) to indicate nuclei. (D) Negative control with rabbit IgG used in place of the primary antiserum. Some autofluorescence due to red blood cells is seen in this panel. (E) Negative control stained with PI. Scale bar on (A) = 50 μm. From Johnson, P.A., Kent, T.R., Urick, M.E. and Giles, J.R. (2008) Expression and regulation of anti-Mullerian hormone in an oviparous species, the hen. *Biology of Reproduction* 78:13–19. Reproduced with permission from the Society for the Study of Reproduction.

When the final egg of the sequence has been laid (usually late in the afternoon), no ovulation occurs on that day and as a result no oviposition occurs on the next day (skip day). On the skip day an oocyte is ovulated, and on the subsequent day that egg is laid early in the morning and the sequence repeats (usually with a similar number of eggs). The number of eggs in the sequence of domestic species is dependent on the strain, phase of the laying cycle, and age of the hen.

The unusual pattern of ovulation in domestic species is dictated by the time when LH surges are initiated as well as by the rate of follicle development. The so-called **open period** for initiation of LH surges appears to be restricted to a particular time of the day. In chickens, the open period for LH release occurs during the dark phase. Each ovulation is preceded by a preovulatory surge of plasma LH. In birds, the LH surge is induced by progesterone and preovulatory surges of progesterone and LH occur approximately 4–6 hours before ovulation. Elevation in the plasma concentration of testosterone (and, less usually, estrogen) also precedes ovulation.

Oviposition

Each ovulation is followed by an oviposition. Most typically, the oviposition occurs approximately 24–26 hours after ovulation. For all ovipositions except the last of the sequence, ovulation occurs soon after the egg is laid. Various hormonal influences have been implicated in the oviposition of the egg. **Prostaglandin** secretion from the preovulatory follicle as well as from the postovulatory follicle is involved in oviposition. The contribution of the postovulatory follicle is thought to be the most significant since removal of the postovulatory follicle delays oviposition for several days, whereas delay after removal of the preovulatory follicle is less. In addition, the concentration of the posterior pituitary hormone **arginine vasotocin** rises at the time of oviposition.

Broodiness

---

1 How common is broodiness in birds? Does it vary among species?

2 Is the ovary active during broodiness?

3 What is the pituitary hormone most often associated with broodiness?

4 How is prolactin regulated in birds?

5 Can broodiness be controlled in turkeys?

Broodiness is observed when egg production declines and the hen begins to incubate her eggs. This is associated with a decrease in food consumption. Among domestic birds, broodiness is rare in laying strains of hens, is observed in broiler strains of hens, and is common and troublesome in turkeys. During broodiness when the hen is incubating, plasma concentrations of gonadotropins are very low and regression of the ovary occurs. Plasma concentration of **prolactin** is high. Broodiness has been very well studied in turkeys because it is a commercial problem when turkey hens become broody with consequent reduction in egg production. Interestingly, in birds, pituitary prolactin secretion is regulated primarily by stimulatory hypothalamic effects, unlike in mammals. The primary prolactin-releasing factor has been identified as vasoactive intestinal polypeptide (VIP). Experiments in turkeys have shown that immunization against VIP is very effective in reducing broodiness. Treated hens show a dramatic reduction in incubation behavior compared to uninjected control or carrier-immunized turkeys.

Self-evaluation

Answers can be found at the end of the chapter.

1 What is the neuroendocrine factor that mediates the effects of light on the reproductive system of a hen?

2 Where is sperm produced in the avian testis?

3 What is the primary site of the sperm storage tubules?

4 What hormone causes the regression of the right oviduct in many birds?

5 What hormone stimulates the preovulatory LH surge in birds?

Suggested reading

Bakst, M.R. (1998) Structure of the avian oviduct with emphasis on sperm storage in poultry. *Journal of Experimental Zoology* **282**:618–626.

Dunn, I.C. and Millam, J.R. (1998) Gonadotropin releasing hormone: forms and functions in birds. *Poultry and Avian Biology Reviews* **9**:61–85.

El Halawani, M.E., Silsby, J.L., Rozenboim, I. *et al.* (1995) Increased egg production by active immunization against vasoactive intestinal peptide in the turkey (*Meleagris gallopavo*). *Biology of Reproduction* **52**:179–183.

Etches, R.J. (1996) *Reproduction in Poultry.* CAB International, Cambridge, UK.

Ikegami, K. and Yoshimura, T. (2013) Seasonal time measurement during reproduction. *Journal of Reproduction and Development* **59**:327–333.

Johnson, A.L. and Woods, D.C. (2009) Dynamics of avian ovarian follicle development: cellular mechanisms of granulosa cell differentiation. *General and Comparative Endocrinology* **163**:12–17.

Tajima, A. (2013) Conservation of avian genetic resources. *Journal of Poultry Science* **50**:1–8.

Whittow, G.C. (ed.) (2000) *Sturkie's Avian Physiology, 5th edn.* Academic Press, San Diego, CA.

Answers

1 Hypothalamic photoreceptors detect light and increase the secretion of GnRH-I into the pituitary portal system. GnRH-I acts at the level of the pituitary gland to stimulate the release of the gonadotropins LH and FSH. The gonadotropins stimulate steroid synthesis and ovarian follicular development. In response to steroid secretion, the oviduct grows and becomes functionally developed. Estrogen acts on the liver to stimulate synthesis of yolk, which is secreted into the blood and accumulated by the growing follicles through a receptor-mediated process. Follicle growth eventually results in ovulation of the largest follicle. The stimulatory effects of long daylengths on the gonads are exerted when photosensitive birds are exposed to light during a restricted time of day, termed the photosensitive phase.

2 Sperm is produced in the seminiferous tubules. These tubules contain spermatogonia and developing germ cells in association with Sertoli cells. Sertoli cells are regulated by FSH and testosterone. The interstitial cells lie outside the tubules, are sensitive to LH, and produce androgens.

3 The primary site of sperm storage tubules is at the uterovaginal junction. In addition to this site, there are also some sperm storage tubules in the infundibulum. As the name suggests, sperm are stored in these tubules between matings. Sperm fill the tubules, with the most recent at the proximal opening and therefore first to be released for fertilization. During the ovulatory cycle, sperm are released at periodic intervals and make their way to the infundibulum, the site of fertilization. Recent evidence indicates that progesterone stimulates the release of sperm from the sperm storage tubules. Sperm can be stored for varying intervals in different species, permitting prolonged fertility in the absence of the male.

4 Anti-Müllerian hormone (AMH) has been implicated in the regression of the right oviduct. In birds, both male and female embryonic gonads produce AMH. The Müllerian ducts in the male are also regressed during embryonic development. Estrogen secretion from the left ovary is believed to inhibit the action of AMH on the left oviduct.

5 This surge is stimulated by progesterone, secreted primarily by the largest follicle. In the hen, a preovulatory LH surge precedes ovulation by about 4–6 hours. The granulosa layer of the largest follicle is the primary source of progesterone and the capacity of this layer to secrete progesterone increases with follicle development. The initiation of the LH surge seems to be restricted to the dark phase in chickens and, as a result, LH surges, ovulation and hence oviposition are generally restricted to a particular part of the day.

Index

Page numbers in *italics* denote figures, those in **bold** denote tables.

Dukes' Physiology of Domestic Animals, Thirteenth Edition. Edited by William O. Reece, Howard H. Erickson, Jesse P. Goff and Etsuro E. Uemura.
© 2015 John Wiley & Sons, Inc. Published 2015 by John Wiley & Sons, Inc.
Companion website: www.wiley.com/go/reece/physiology